SYSTEMIC PATHOLOGY / THIRD EDITION

Volume 8 The Kidneys
The Urinary Tract

SYSTEMIC PATHOLOGY / THIRD EDITION

General Editor W. St C. Symmers

Volume Editors

M. C. Anderson **Female Reproductive System**
I. D. Ansell **Male Reproductive System**
M. E. Catto and A. J. Malcolm **Bone, Joints and Soft Tissues**
B. Corrin **The Lungs**
C. W. Elston and I. O. Ellis **Breasts**
I. Friedmann **Nose, Throat and Ears**
K. Henry and W. St C. Symmers **Thymus, Lymph Nodes, Spleen and Lymphatics**
P. D. Lewis **Endocrine System**
B. C. Morson **Alimentary Tract**
K. A. Porter, R. C. B. Pugh and I. D. Ansell **The Kidneys / The Urinary Tract**
W. B. Robertson **Cardiovascular System**
D. Weedon **The Skin**
R. O. Weller **Nervous System, Muscle and Eyes**
S. N. Wickramasinghe **Blood and Bone Marrow**
D. G. D. Wight **Liver, Biliary Tract and Pancreas**

For Churchill Livingstone
Publisher: Timothy Horne
Editorial Co-ordination: Editorial Resources Unit
Copy Editor: Patricia Croucher
Production Controller: Mrs Lesley W Small
Design: Design Resources Unit
Sales Production Executive: Hilary Brown

SYSTEMIC PATHOLOGY / THIRD EDITION

General Editor W. St C. Symmers

Volume 8

The Kidneys

EDITED BY

K. A. Porter

MD(Lond) DSc(Lond) FRCPath

Emeritus Professor of Pathology, University of London, UK;
Honorary Consultant Histopathologist, St Mary's Hospital, London, UK;
Formerly Chairman of the Department of Pathology, St Mary's Hospital Medical School, London, UK

The Urinary Tract

EDITED BY

R. C. B. Pugh

MB BChir MD FRCS FRCPath

Formerly Consultant Pathologist, St Peter's and St Paul's Hospitals and Institute of Urology, London, UK

REVISED BY

I. D. Ansell

MA FRCPath

Consultant Histopathologist, City Hospital, Nottingham, UK;
Clinical Teacher, Nottingham University Medical School, Nottingham, UK

CHURCHILL LIVINGSTONE
EDINBURGH LONDON MADRID MELBOURNE NEW YORK AND TOKYO 1992

CHURCHILL LIVINGSTONE
Medical Division of Longman Group UK Limited

Distributed in the United States of America by Churchill Livingstone Inc., 650 Avenue of the Americas, New York, N.Y. 10011, and by associated companies, branches and representatives throughout the world.

First published 1992

ISBN 0-443-03171-1

British Library Cataloguing in Publication Data

CIP catalogue record for this book is available from the British Library.

Library of Congress Cataloging in Publication Data

Porter, K. A.
The Kidneys / K. A. Porter. The urinary tract / R. C. B. Pugh; revised by I. D. Ansell. — 3rd ed.
p. cm. — (Systemic pathology; v. 9)
Includes index.
1. Urinary organs—Disease. 2. Kidneys—Diseases. I. Pugh, R. C. B. Urinary tract. II. Ansell, I. D. (Ian David). 1938– III. Title. IV. Series.
[DNLM: 1. Kidney Diseases—pathology. 2. Urologic Diseases––pathology. QZ 4 S995 1986 v. 9]
RB111.S97 1987 vol. 9
[RC873.9]
616.07 s—dc20
[616.6'1]
DNLM/DLC
for Library of Congress 91-23093
CIP

Printed and bound in Great Britain by
Butler & Tanner Ltd, Frome and London

Preface

Major advances have occurred in the fields of nephrology and urology since publication of the second edition of *Systemic Pathology* in 1978. In that edition diseases of the kidneys, ureters, bladder and urethra were considered in two chapters, one written by Professor A. C. Thackray of the Department of Pathology at the Middlesex Hospital Medical School, London and the other by me. For the 1992 edition this entire volume has had to be devoted to the two subjects, reflecting the enormous growth in our knowledge; the description of the diseases of the kidneys now appears in Part 1 and an account of the disorders of the urinary tract in Part 2.

I have again written Part 1, but Part 2 has been written by Dr R. C. B. Pugh who kindly agreed to take over this task from Professor Thackray. The great experience and international reputation of Roger Pugh, who until a few years ago was Consultant Pathologist at St Peter's Hospitals and the Institute of Urology, London, is evident in the quality of his contribution. Because I was slow completing Part 1 it became necessary to update Dr Pugh's three chapters and Dr I. D. Ansell, another expert uropathologist and Consultant Histopathologist at the City Hospital, Nottingham, did this very competently and at short notice. I am most grateful for his help.

The account of the diseases of the kidneys and urinary tract in this volume differs greatly from that in the two chapters in the second edition. The text has been completely rewritten and expanded to incorporate information derived from recent molecular, immunological, histochemical, electron microscopical and genetic techniques. Many new sections have been added. The pathological changes that occur in uraemia and in patients maintained by dialysis are now considered, including the increasingly important problems of beta$_2$-microglobulin amyloidosis, acquired renal cystic disease, malignancy and aluminium toxicity. An account of the development of the kidneys is included. Renal involvement in various hereditary metabolic disorders and other hereditary diseases, such as neurofibromatosis type 1 and cystic fibrosis, are considered. The renal changes in Waldenström's macroglobulinaemia, light chain deposition disease, immunotactoid glomerulopathy and fibrillary glomerulopathy are discussed. There are sections on the renal complications of infections with HIV, Hantavirus and various fungi, protozoa and metazoa. Chapters have been added that discuss renal disease caused by poisoning, occupational hazards, drug and alcohol dependence, and by therapeutic and diagnostic agents. Descriptions of oncocytoma, rhabdoid tumour of the kidney, clear cell sarcoma of the kidney, and the renal complications of extrarenal cancer have been added. The chapter on renal transplantation discusses the transmission of disease from host to graft, disease arising de novo in the graft, and changes caused by immunosuppressive treatment, including lymphomas and cyclosporin nephrotoxicity. In addition to this new material, much fuller, up-to-date accounts have been provided for the many disorders that were poorly understood at the time of the previous edition.

We have also tried to present some of the nephrological and urological complications of diseases that are major problems in the developing and hotter countries of the world. Examples are schistosomiasis, filariasis, malaria and infections by the Hantaan and hepatitis viruses. Throughout the volume space has been devoted to subjects in proportion to their clinical importance, the light they shed on fundamental biological processes, and their significance as current growing areas of interest.

A number of people have been crucial in the preparation of this volume. Miss Sarah Chantler, my secretary, prepared the manuscript and sought out and checked all the references. Her unfailing energy, enthusiasm and good humour were an enormous support which ensured that the project was completed. I cannot thank her enough. Mr Adrian Roberts, who for many years has run the electron microscopy unit in the Department of Pathology at St Mary's Hospital Medical School, prepared the majority of the illustrations for Part 1 of the text. He did this at great inconvenience on evenings and weekends when he would undoubtedly have far rather been with his family. I am most grateful. Two of my sons, Tom and David, with unruffled patience helped with the final word processing; they also collaborated with my wife, Jane, to produce the index. I would like to thank all three very much; they must be relieved that at last it is all over.

But the whole undertaking ultimately depended upon the skills of the scientific staff who produced the sections and electron micrographs for analysis. Over the years Miss Jill Collar, working with Mr Adrian Roberts, has consistently taken the most beautiful electron micrographs; Miss Karen Hennessy, Miss Lynn McMullen, Mr William Russell and Mr Niall MacHugh have prepared excellent sections and some of the electron micrographs; and Dr Marian Ruszkiewicz has made the most elegant and reliable immunoperoxidase preparations. I am deeply indebted to them all.

Supplementary illustrations and other material have been generously provided by my close colleagues Dr Victoria Cattell and Dr H. Terry Cook, and by friends and other individuals whose names appear in the appropriate legends.

Dr Pugh wishes to acknowledge the valued help of his many colleagues, clinical and pathological, medical and secretarial, during his time at St Paul's Hospital when he established his special interest in urological pathology. In particular he wishes to thank Dr Katherine Cameron for the many years when she shared the workload of the pathology department at St Paul's and her many contributions to the teaching and research which emanated from that centre.

Dr Ansell would like to express his gratitude to Roger Pugh for kindling his interest in uropathology and for his help and support over the last 20 years. He would also like to thank Mrs Dorothy Clayton for secretarial help, the department of photography at the City Hospital Nottingham for the preparation of the photographs and Mr Keith Gordon for the photomicrographs.

I shall also like to thank the staff of Churchill Livingstone, particularly Mrs Janice Urquhart and Mr Timothy Horne, for their patience and their help.

Finally I am especially grateful to Professor W. St C. Symmers for reading through the whole manuscript and suggesting numerous improvements, and for his continual encouragement and assistance.

Newbury, Berks, UK, 1991 K.A.P.

Contents

PART 1

The Kidneys

K. A. Porter

1

K. A. Porter

Structure and effects of ageing and reduction in mass

ANATOMY AND HISTOLOGY OF THE KIDNEYS

GROSS APPEARANCES

Each kidney weighs about 150 g in the adult male and about 135 g in the adult female and is enclosed by a thin, translucent, fibrous *capsule*. Small blood vessels pass through the capsule into the underlying parenchyma. The surface of normal kidneys of adults is usually smooth; grooves divide the surface of the kidneys of the newborn into many small lobes. This fetal lobation usually disappears in infancy or early childhood but quite commonly traces of the fissures persist into adult life and these must not be confused with scars. Small stellate veins are usually clearly visible on the renal surface, deep to the capsule.

When longitudinally sectioned the surface of the kidney shows a peripheral *cortex* and an inner *medulla* (Fig. 1.1). The cortex forms a layer about 4–6 mm in thickness; it covers the medulla and dips between the pyramids as the *septa* or *columns of Bertin*.[1] The cortex is composed of glomeruli and renal tubules. Groups of faint striations in the cortex are visible to the unaided eye as the *medullary rays*; they are formed by the limbs of Henle, the collecting tubules and the straight parts of the proximal convoluted tubules.

The medulla is composed of several wedge-shaped renal *pyramids*, each of which tapers to the hilum. Most of the length of the collecting tubules is in the medulla. The apex of each pyramid is the *papilla* and it is from numerous small openings on its surface that urine enters the renal pelvis. At the poles of the kidney the papillae may be compound

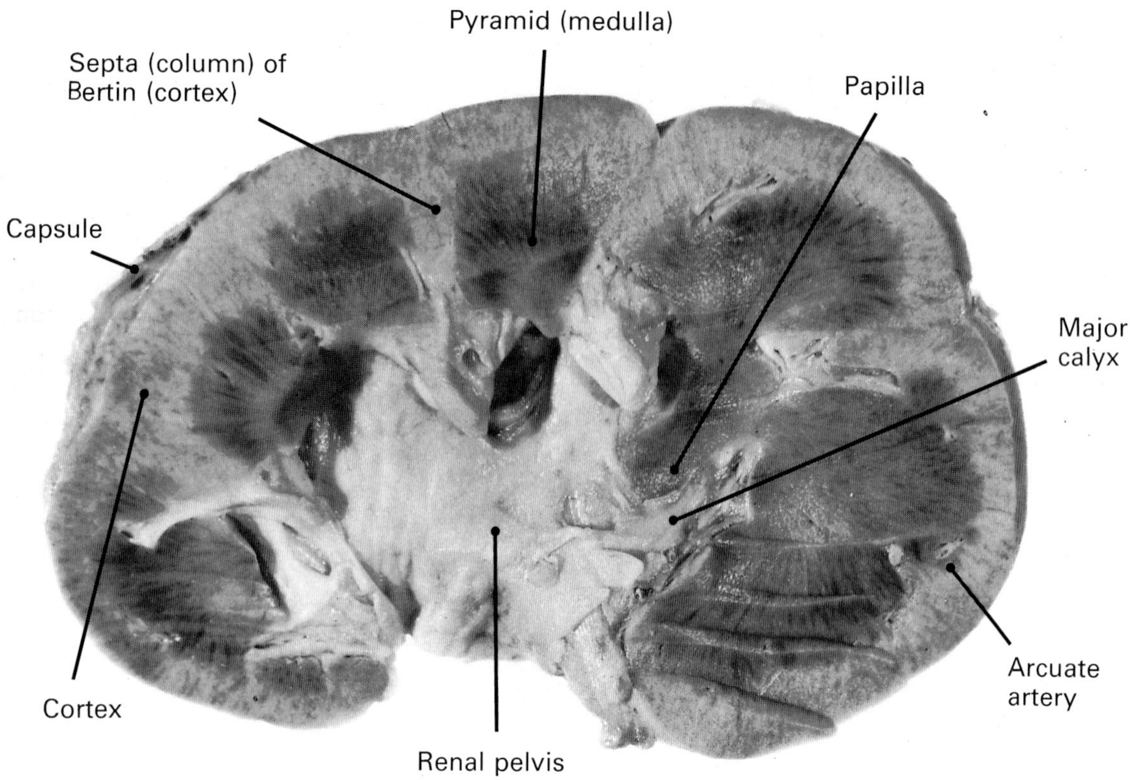

Fig. 1.1 Longitudinally sectioned human kidney

and may drain as many as three fused pyramids. It is the compound papillae that allow reflux of urine up the ducts of Bellini in certain patients with vesicoureteric reflux (see p. 436). At the junction of cortex and medulla the arcuate arteries are visible.

Although all obvious external division of the kidney into lobes has usually disappeared in the adult, the 14 or so lobes still exist within the kidney, each consisting of a central pyramid covered at base and sides by cortex.

The hilum of the kidney contains the *pelvis*, formed by the union of three or four *major calyces* and about 12 *minor calyces*. The minor calyces are cup shaped and closely invest the papillae. The pelvis forms the funnel-shaped upper end of the ureter.

THE BLOOD SUPPLY

The main *renal artery* of each kidney comes from the abdominal aorta. At the hilum it usually divides into *anterior and posterior divisions* that pass respectively in front of and behind the pelvis. These divisions then subdivide into vessels that supply the apical, upper, middle, lower and posterior segments of the kidney.[1,2] There are no collateral connexions between the segments: the five *segmental arteries* are virtually end-arteries.[3] The segmental arteries give rise to the *arcuate* branches at the corticomedullary junction. From the arcuate arteries a series of perpendicular branches, the *interlobular arteries*, radiates into the cortex (Fig. 1.2); it has recently been proposed that the term cortical radial artery should be used to describe these vessels. Smaller branches, the *afferent arterioles*, arise from the interlobular arteries and supply the individual glomeruli. From the glomerulus emerges the *efferent arteriole*. In most of the cortex the efferent arterioles are about half the diameter of the afferent arterioles and, after a short course, they break up into the abundant network of *peritubular or intertubular capillaries* that

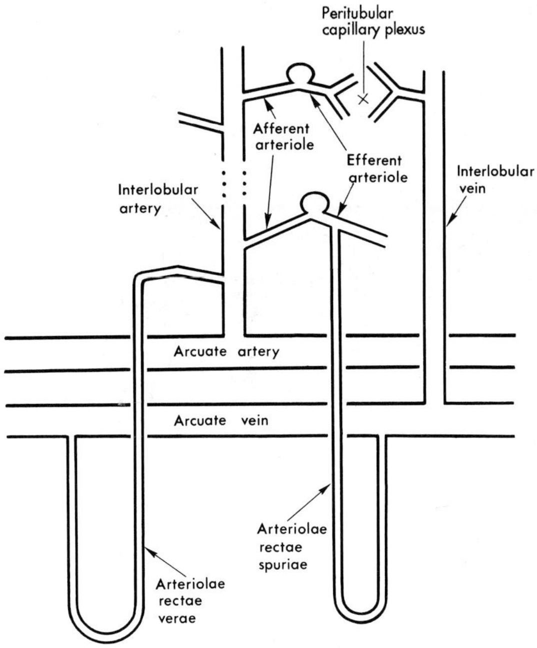

Fig. 1.2 Diagram to show the blood supply of the cortex and medulla of the kidney.
Reproduced by permission of Professor R.H. Heptinstall from: Systemic pathology, 1st edn. London: Longman, 1966

ramify round the tubule. The efferent arterioles emerging from the juxtamedullary glomeruli are much larger: it is their continuation as the *arteriolae rectae spuriae* that provides the main blood supply of the papillae. The medulla is also supplied by the *arteriolae rectae verae* which originate directly from the interlobular arteries in the juxtamedullary zone; they are formed when glomeruli become sclerosed (see p. 25). The arteriolae rectae verae and the arteriolae rectae spuriae are collectively known as the *vasa recta.* The peritubular capillaries drain into the *interlobular veins* and thence into the *arcuate veins.* The vasa recta loop back as the *venulae rectae* to empty directly into the arcuate veins. The arcuate veins return the blood through the *segmental veins* into the main *renal vein.*

The endothelial cells lining the interlobular and larger arteries synthesize von Willebrand factor,[4] store it in rod-shaped Weibel–Palade[5] bodies (Fig. 1.3) and release it by exocytosis. Von Willebrand factor is a large complex glycoprotein that causes platelets to adhere to the subendothelial collagen fibrils after vascular injury. It is a component of factor VIII and essential for the normal clotting of blood. The concentration of von Willebrand factor is raised in patients with renal allografts who are receiving high doses of the immunosuppressive but nephrotoxic drug cyclosporin A (see p. 661).

In the mouse erythropoietin messenger RNA has been detected in the endothelial cells of the peritubular capillaries suggesting that this is the site in the kidney where erythropoietin is produced.[6] Lack of the hormone in chronic renal failure causes a debilitating anaemia which is corrected by giving recombinant human erythropoietin (see p. 36).

LYMPHATIC DRAINAGE

Lymph capillaries are found round the afferent arterioles and drain into deep lymphatics that accompany the interlobular, arcuate and segmental vessels at the hilum. The walls of the lymph capillaries are formed by unfenestrate endothelium that lacks a basement membrane. There are no pericytes.

THE GLOMERULI

Each glomerulus or renal corpuscle has a diameter of about 250 μm and consists of a lobulate *tuft* of capillaries formed by division of the afferent arteriole and surrounded by Bowman's capsule. The point where the afferent arteriole enters the glomerulus and the efferent arteriole leaves is called the *vascular pole* of the glomerulus.

Bowman's capsule

The capsule is composed of a parietal layer and of a visceral layer that results from invagination of the original epithelial vesicle by the capillary tuft. The *parietal epithelium* is usually flattened, shows scattered, short microvilli and rests on a thick basement membrane. Both the basement membrane and the lining epithelium are continuous with the corresponding structures of the associated proximal convoluted tubule. Between the parietal and visceral layers of Bowman's capsule is *Bowman's space.* In paraffin sections this is nor-

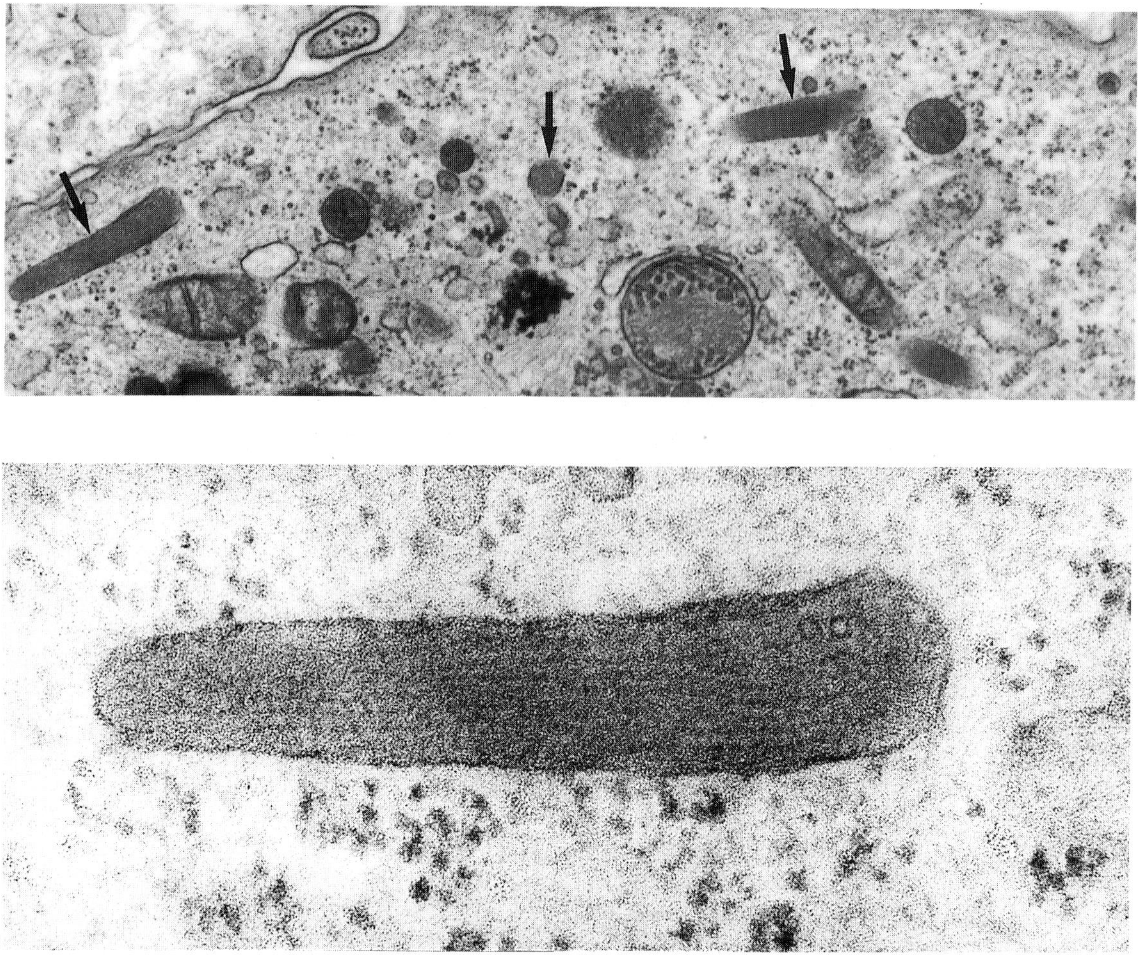

a

b

Fig. 1.3 Electron micrograph of part of an endothelial cell lining an interlobular artery. In the cytoplasm there are three Weibel–Palade bodies (**a**, arrows), each containing parallel fine tubules (**b**). These bodies contain von Willebrand factor. (**a**) × 51 250; (**b**) × 128 125

mally from 7 to 14 μm wide. The *visceral epithelium* is described below.

Glomerular tuft

The glomerular tuft consists of about eight convoluted *capillaries* that arise from the afferent arteriole and unite again at the hilum of the glomerulus to emerge as the efferent arteriole. They are covered by the invaginated visceral layer of Bowman's capsule. Injection studies suggest that anastomoses exist between the glomerular capillary loops.[7] The capillaries are supported by a central branching tree-shaped core, the mesangium, which extends from the hilum.

Endothelial cells

The walls of the glomerular capillaries are lined by large, flattened endothelial cells that fit closely together by tight cell junctions (Figs 1.4, 1.5).[8] Over most of the capillary wall the endothelial layer is very thin and studded with many circular *pores* measuring up to 100 nm (1000 Å) in diameter (Fig. 1.6). These pores are known as *fenestrations*; they account for about 29% of the surface area of the capillary lining and in man they are only rarely closed by a membrane (except in the developing glomerulus).[9] The capillary endothelium therefore allows the passage each day of about 170 litres of fluid and solute and offers no anatomical barrier to the passage of even the largest molecules. The endothelial cells have a

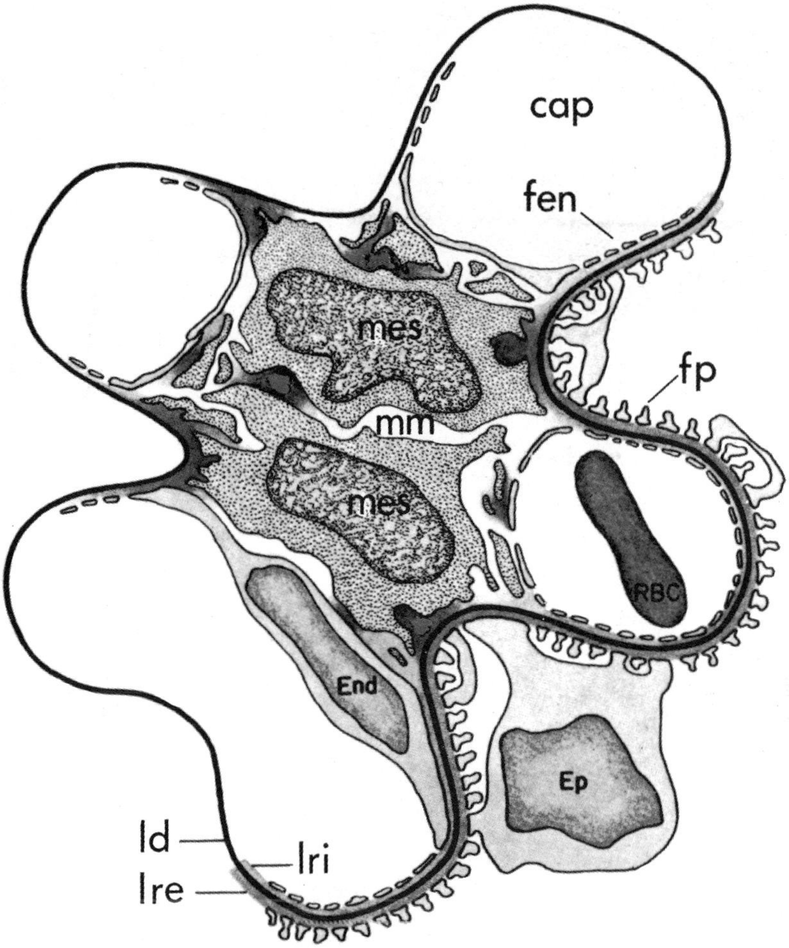

Fig. 1.4 Diagram of part of a glomerulus. cap, lumen of capillary loop; End, main body of endothelial cell, with nucleus; Ep, visceral epithelial cell; fen, fenestrated endothelial lining of capillary; fp, epithelial foot processes; ld, lamina densa of capillary basement membrane; lre, lamina rara externa of capillary membrane; lri, lamina rara interna of capillary basement membrane; mes, mesangial cell; mm, mesangial matrix.
Reproduced with modifications, by permission from: Latta H, Maunsbach AB, Madden SC. J Ultrastruct Res 1960; 4: 455 (Fig. 10)

negatively charged cell coat which is up to 12 nm in thickness.[10] The nucleus and main cytoplasmic mass of the endothelial cells are usually situated on the mesangial side of the capillary and bulge into the lumen (Fig. 1.5a). The glomerular endothelial cells, in common with those lining the peritubular capillaries and larger blood vessels, express many alloantigens, including those of both classes I and II of the major histocompatibility complex (Fig. 1.7),[11] the A and B blood group antigens and the erythrocyte antigens Pr and Gd. They also express antigens unique to vascular endothelial cells.[12]

Capillary basement membrane

The endothelial cells rest on a capillary basement membrane that is relatively thick, measuring about 315 nm, but the range is wide – 250–350 nm. The capillary basement membrane, which is thinner in infants and children,[13] is a compound membrane, being formed by the basement membranes of both the endothelium and the epithelium which fuse during development of the glomerulus. The membrane consists of a central *lamina densa* with less dense zones on each side, the *lamina rara externa* and *lamina rara interna* (Figs 1.4, 1.5). The relative prominence of the three zones varies according to the age of

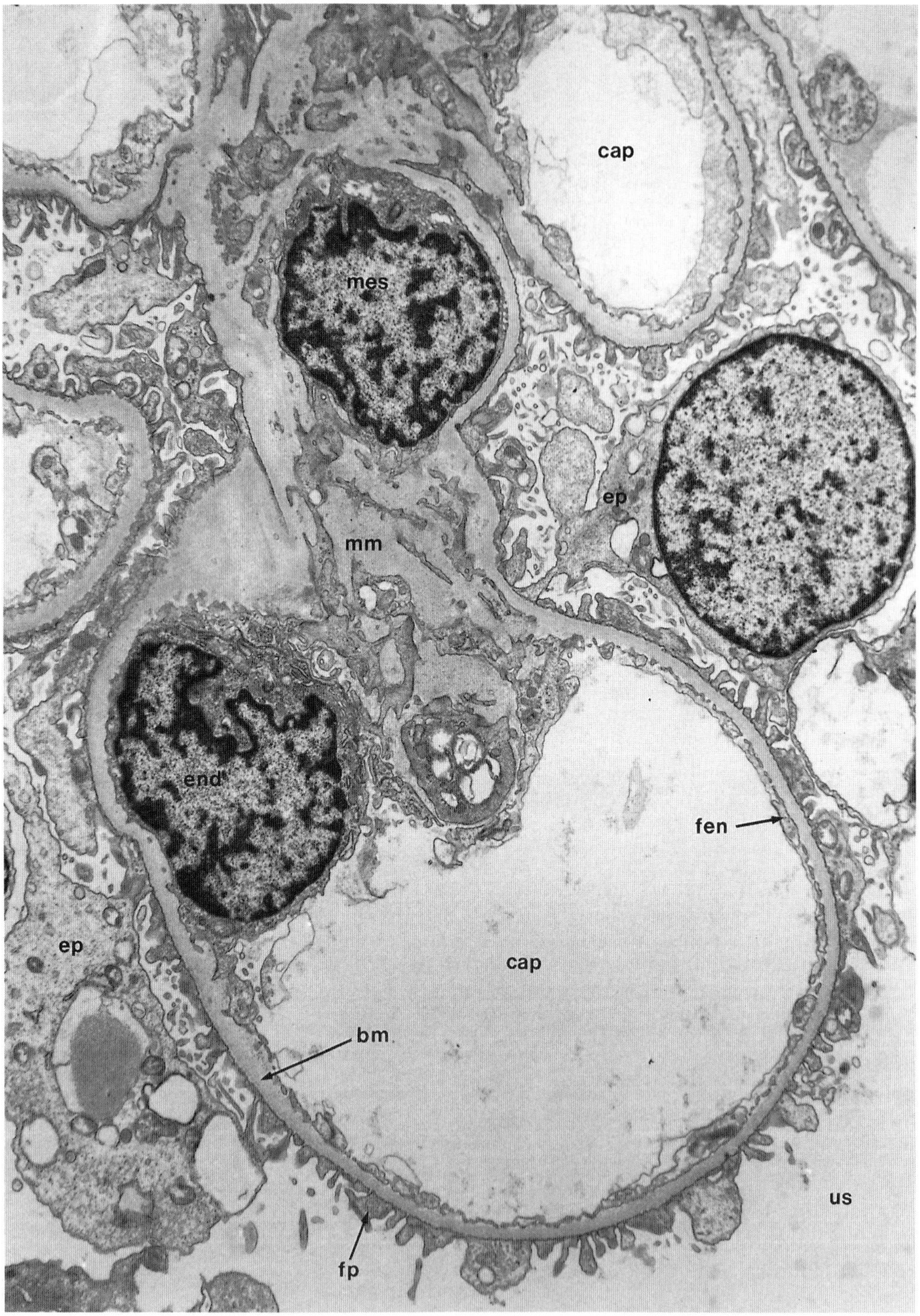

a

Fig. 1.5 Electron micrographs of part of a normal glomerulus. (**a**) A relatively low power view of the whole cross-section of a capillary. (**b**) The wrinkling and thickening of the glomerular basement membrane where it covers the mesangium, in contrast to the smoothness and relative thinness of the membrane where it surrounds capillaries. (**c**) Part of a capillary wall in greater detail. bm, capillary basement membrane; cap, capillary lumen; end, main body of endothelial cell, with nucleus; fen, fenestrated endothelium; ep, visceral epithelial cell; fp, visceral epithelial cell foot processes; ld, lamina densa of capillary basement membrane; lre, lamina rara externa of capillary basement membrane; lri, lamina rara interna of capillary basement membrane; mes, mesangial cell; mm, mesangial matrix; us, urinary space; arrow heads, mesangial angles; fs, filtration slit. (**a, b**) × 7200; (**c**) × 28 240

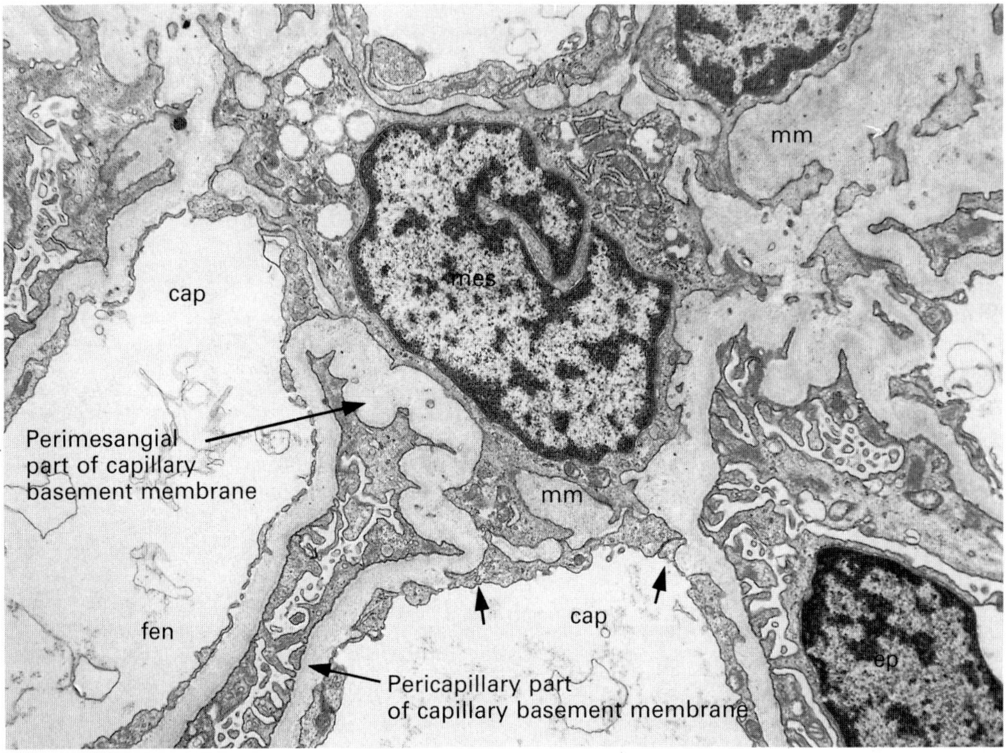
mm
cap
mes
Perimesangial part of capillary basement membrane
mm
cap
fen
ep
Pericapillary part of capillary basement membrane

b

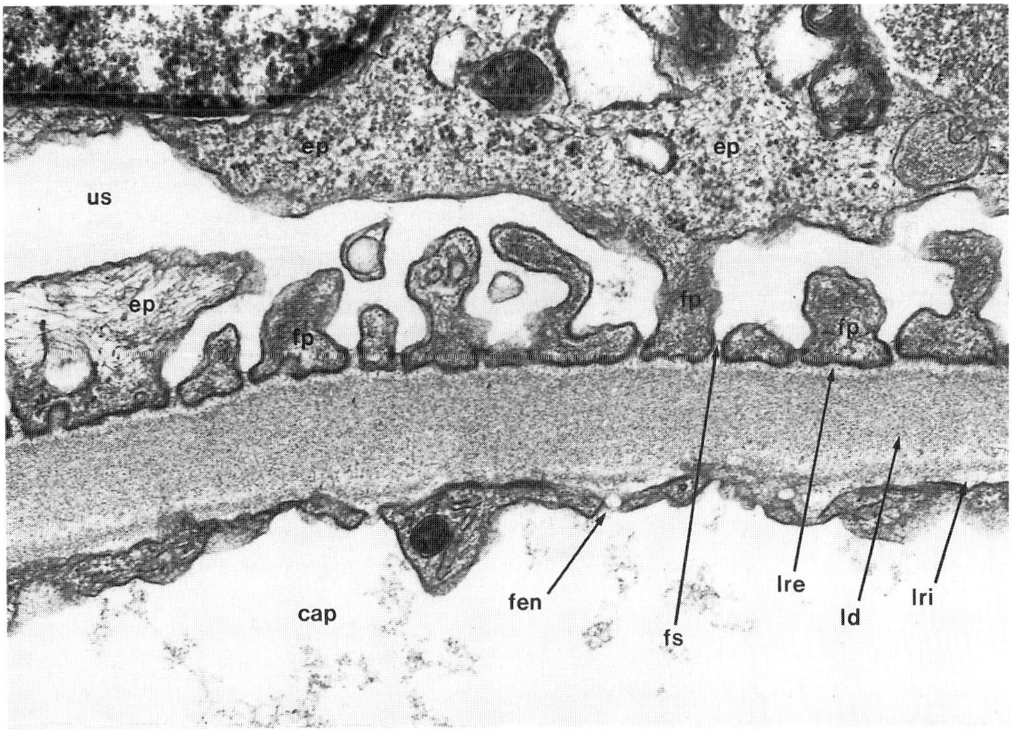
ep
ep
us
ep
fp
fp
fp
cap
fen
fs
lre
ld
lri

c

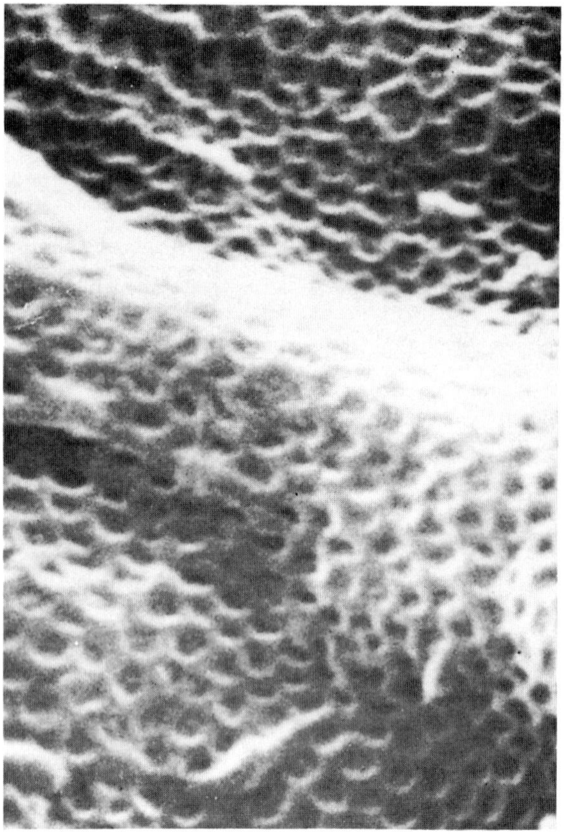

Fig. 1.6 Inner surface of normal glomerular capillary, as seen by scanning electron microscopy. The very thin endothelial lining has many circular depressions: these are the fenestrations.
× 45 000
Reproduced by permission from: Fujita T, Tokunaga J, Miyoshi M. Arch Histol Jap 1970; 32: 99 (Fig. 11)

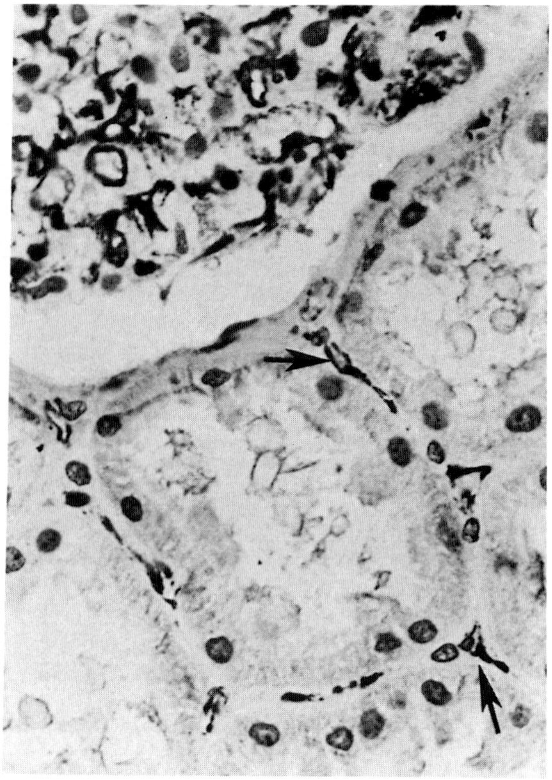

Fig. 1.7 Normal kidney stained for HLA-DR, a class II major histocompatibility antigen, by the avidin-biotin-peroxidase method. There is prominent staining of glomerular and peritubular capillary endothelium. Tangentially sectioned endothelial cells (arrows) could be misinterpreted as interstitial dendritic cells.
× 490
Reproduced by permission from: Alpers CE, Beckstead JH. Clin Immunol Immunopathol 1985; 36: 129 (Fig. 1)

the individual and the way in which the tissue is processed. The lamina rara interna of the glomerular capillary basement membrane is in direct contact with the blood stream through the endothelial fenestrae. It is made up of a network of approximately 3-nm fibrils that are tightly packed in the lamina densa and loosely arranged in the lamina rara interna and externa. Type IV procollagens, various proteoglycans, laminin and entactin are integral components of this network.[14] Type IV collagen is largely concentrated in the lamina densa while heparin sulphate proteoglycan is found mainly in the lamina rara interna and externa.

The sulphated glycosaminoglycans form gels with specific sieving properties and electrically are highly negatively charged. The collections of heparin sulphate proteoglycan, regularly distributed at 60-nm intervals, are referred to as the *anionic sites* of the basement membrane (Fig. 1.8). They enable the glomerular basement membrane to act as a selective charge and size barrier to the filtration of circulating macromolecules.[15] Cationic (i.e. positively charged) particles pass through the glomerular capillary basement membrane more easily and anionic (i.e. negatively charged) particles less easily than neutral particles of comparable size.[16] This phenomenon is be-

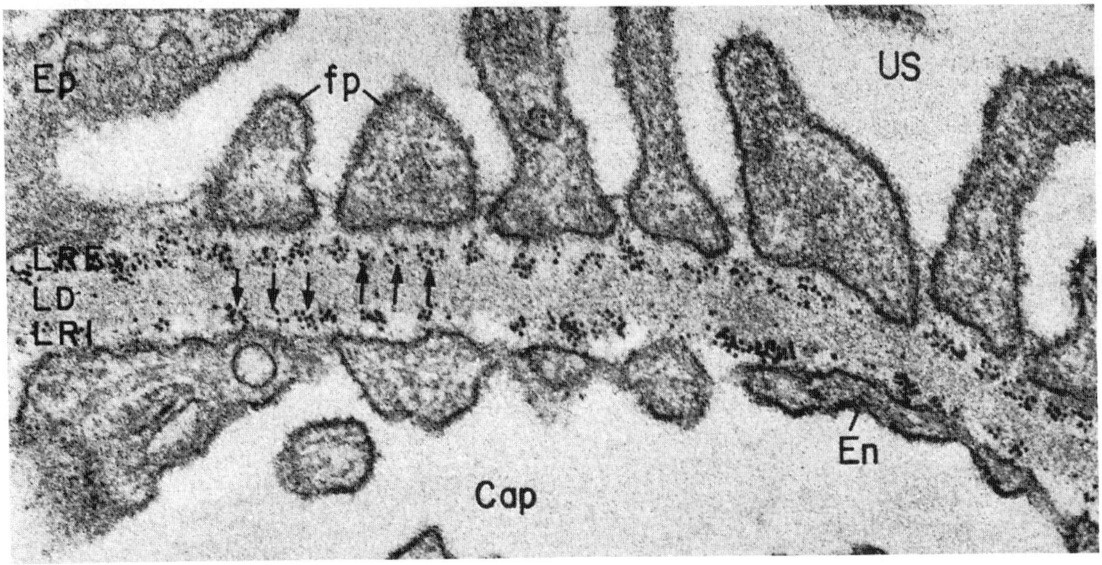

Fig. 1.8 Demonstration of collections of particles of negatively charged heparin sulphate-proteoglycan in the lamina rara interna (LRI) and lamina rara externa (LRE) in the glomerular capillary basement membrane of a rat. The rat had been injected intravenously with cationized ferritin which has bound to the strongly anionic heparin sulphate-proteoglycan (arrows). US, urinary space; Ep, part of visceral epithelial cell; fp, foot processes of epithelial cells; Cap, glomerular capillary lumen; En, fenestrated endothelium.
× 85 600
Reproduced by permission from: Kanwar YS, Farquhar MG. J Cell Biol 1979; 81: 137 (Fig. 1)

lieved to be due to electrostatic interaction between the charges on the particles and the fixed negative charges in the basement membrane.

Two antigens important in renal disease are present in the glomerular capillary basement membrane. One is called Goodpasture antigen because autoantibodies are formed against it in some cases of Goodpasture's syndrome (see p. 218). This antigen is located in the lamina densa in a globular non-collagenous domain of type IV procollagen.[17,18] The glomerular capillary basement membrane lacks Goodpasture antigen in some cases of Alport's syndrome (see p. 77). The second antigen is amyloid P component which is a non-fibrillar glycoprotein of the pentraxin family that is identical to a normal circulating plasma protein, serum amyloid P component, and structurally very similar to C-reactive protein, an acute phase reactant. Amyloid P component is a normal constituent of other vascular basement membranes and elastic microfibrils throughout the body.[19] In the glomerular capillary basement membrane it is confined to the lamina rara interna.[20] It is absent in patients with Alport's syndrome whose glomerular capillary basement membrane lacks Goodpasture antigen (see p. 77).[21]

The glomerular capillary basement membrane is stained well by the periodic acid-Schiff and periodic acid-methenamine silver (hexamine silver) methods. The membrane does not completely surround any of the capillaries, being absent over the region of the capillary wall that is adjacent to the mesangium (Fig. 1.5a). This gap provides a direct path into the mesangium for the disposal of macromolecular substances barred from filtration by the basement membrane.

Visceral epithelial cells (podocytes) On their outer surface the glomerular capillaries are covered by the epithelial cells of the visceral layer of Bowman's capsule (Figs 1.4, 1.5, 1.9). This visceral epithelium consists of large cells with a complex structure. The thickest part of each, which contains the nucleus, tends to be located inside the curve of a capillary loop. Extending in various directions from this central mass are cytoplasmic processes that vary greatly in width. From these arise secondary and tertiary processes that encircle the

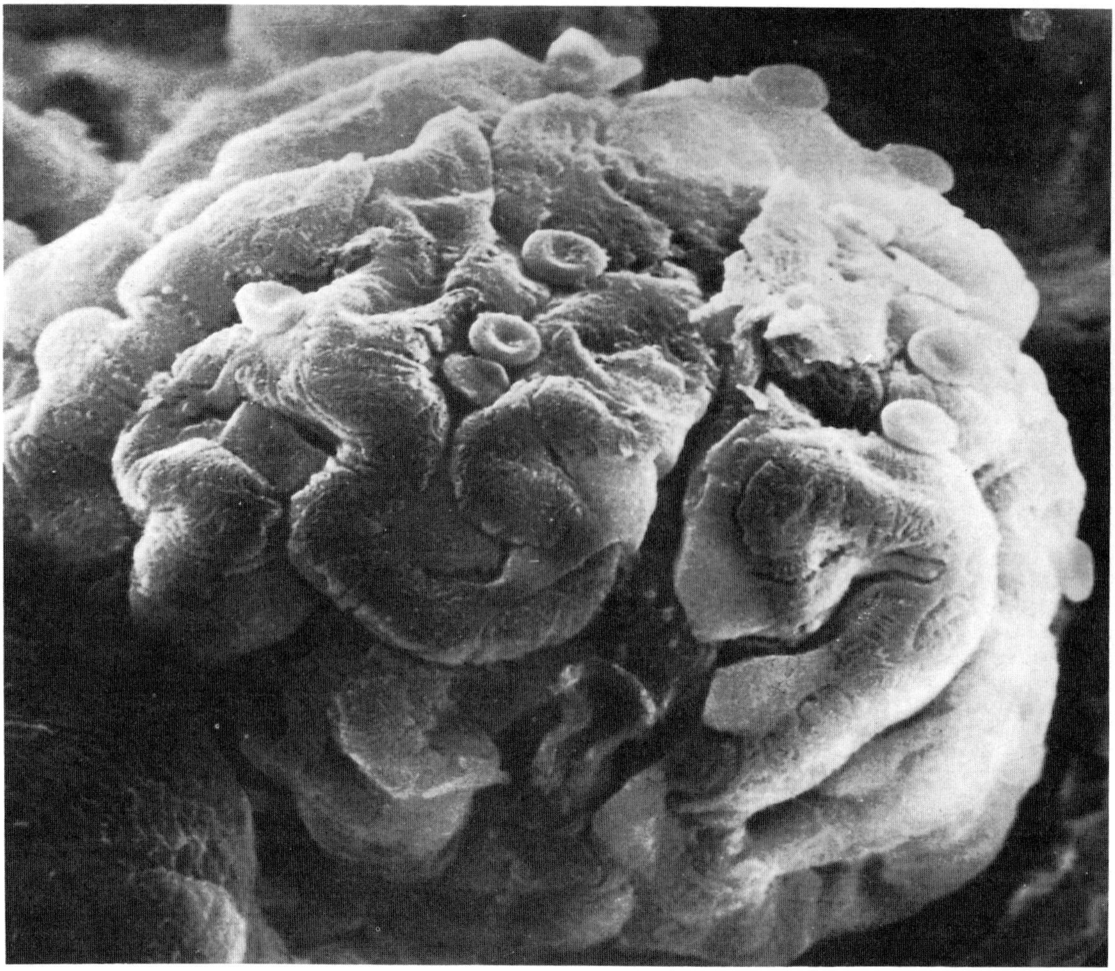

Fig. 1.9 Scanning electron micrograph of normal glomerulus. The capillary loops are encircled by branching visceral epithelial cells (see also Fig.1.10). The presence of the red cells on the surface of the glomerulus is an artefact accompanying the preparation of the specimen.
× 7060
Reproduced by permission from: Arakawa M. Lab Invest 1970; 23: 489 (Fig. 3)

capillaries (Fig. 1.10). All the branches are covered with many short, thin *foot processes*, which are attached to the outside of the capillary basement membrane. Each epithelial cell sends foot processes to several capillary loops, where they alternate with similar processes from other epithelial cells. On the capillary basement membrane the epithelial foot processes are separated from one another by about 20–50 nm. This space, called the *filtration slit* or slit pore, is closed by a fine membrane, the *slit diaphragm* (Fig. 1.5c), which consists of a central bar that is connected by many parallel bridging subunits to the outer aspect of the foot processes (Fig. 1.11). Between the cross-bridges there are a series of rectangular pores.[22,23] The outer surface of the foot processes is covered by a strongly anionic (i.e. negatively charged) cell coat, 15–80 nm thick, which fills the filtration slit and covers the outer surface of the slit diaphragm. The presence of the polyanionic cell coat is probably responsible for maintaining the shape and interrelationship of the foot processes by their mutual repulsion. All along the surface of the visceral epithelial cells, including the sides of the foot processes, there are small pits. The pits possess a bristle coat on their cytoplasmic aspect and are identical to the clathrin-coated vesicles that occur in other organs. The coated pits at the

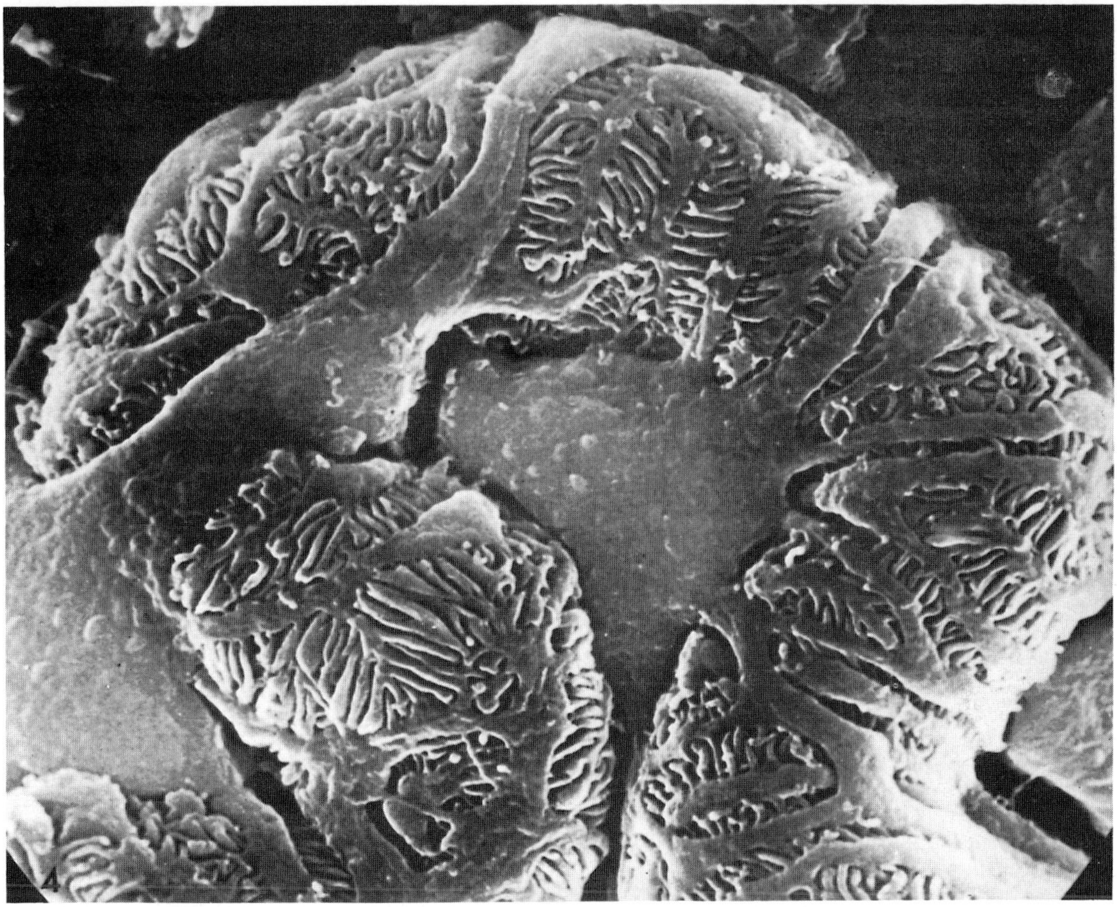

Fig. 1.10 Higher magnification of one of the capillary loops of the normal glomerulus illustrated in Fig.1.9. The branching processes from the two visceral epithelial cells (epl, ep2) encircle the capillary and interdigitate with one another. × 17 300
Reproduced by permission from: Arakawa M. Lab Invest 1970; 23: 489 (Fig. 4)

base of the foot processes are the sites where in the rat an epithelial antigen (gp 330) and circulating antibody to that antigen meet to form the initial immune complexes in Heymann's nephritis, a disease that resembles human membranous glomerulonephritis (see p. 202). The cytoplasm of the foot processes contains fine filaments of actin and heavy meromysin and may therefore be contractile;[24,25] there are also many microtubules and other organelles. The visceral epithelial cells are a major source of basement membrane renewal;[26,27] they synthesize collagen type IV, laminin and heparin sulphate. Receptors for the third component of complement (C3b)[28] and the easily crystallizing fragment (Fc) of immunoglobulin G (IgG)[29], obtained by splitting the IgG molecule by papain, have been demonstrated on the membrane of human visceral epithelial cells. The possible role of these receptors in glomerulonephritis remains speculative. The epithelial cells, although probably not phagocytic, do have the capacity to endocytose and pinocytose; they take up macromolecules which have crossed the major filtration barrier in the capillary basement membrane and prevent them reaching the urinary space.

The mesangium

This ramifying structure fills the centrilobular region of the glomerular tuft and supports the capillaries (Figs 1.4, 1.5).[30] It contains at least

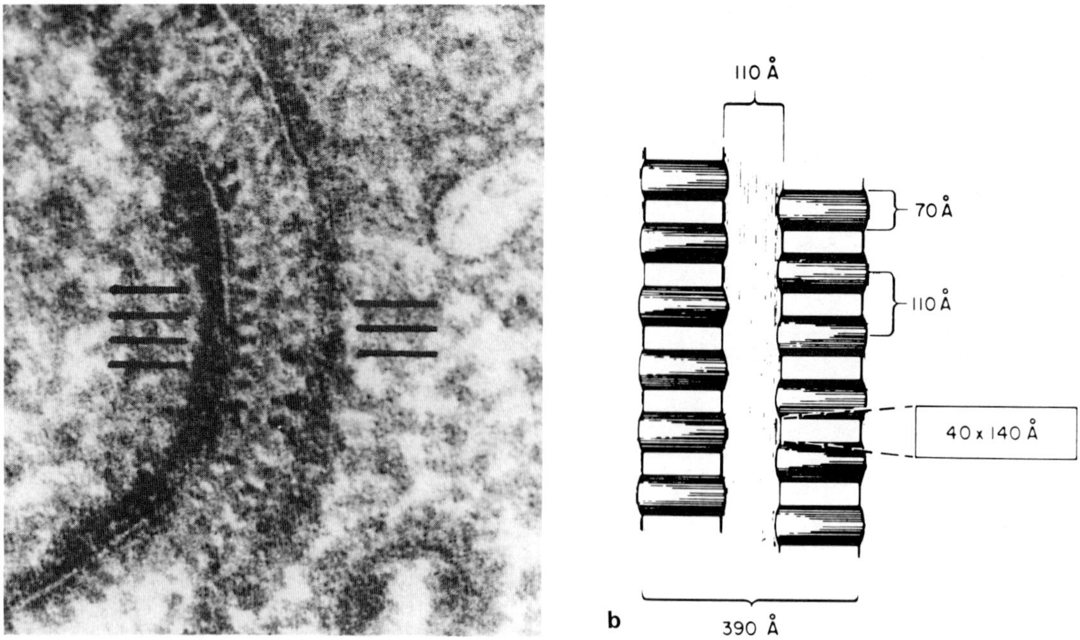

Fig. 1.11 (**a**) Slit diaphragm that closes the space between the foot processes of the glomerular visceral epithelial cells. In the region marked by lines the central bar is flanked by many cross bridges. There are rectangular pores between the cross bridges. (**b**) Diagram of glomerular slit diaphragm showing central bar, cross bridges and pores.
(**a**) × 195 000
Reproduced by permission from: Rodewald R, Karnovsky MJ. J Cell Biol 1974; 60; 423 (Figs 3, 4)

two, and perhaps more, functionally distinct cell populations, surrounded by matrix.

In paraffin wax sections 2 μm thick or resin sections 1 μm thick a maximum of two mesangial cells is seen in each mesangial area at the periphery of the glomerulus. A greater number of mesangial cells is present in the central ('stalk') area of the mesangium. The number of mesangial cells is increased in several diseases of the kidney, in particular in some forms of glomerulonephritis (see p. 153).

The predominant cell population in the mesangium is composed of *intrinsic mesangial cells*. These cells originate in the kidney and have an irregular nucleus and many fine branching cytoplasmic processes (Figs 1.12, 1.13). They bear receptors for angiotensin II (see p. 19) and atrial natriuretic peptide (ANP) on their surfaces (ANP augments sodium and water excretion and is formed in electron-dense secretory granules within atrial myocytes). In the cytoplasm of the intrinsic mesangial cells there are a number of organelles, including microfilaments which contain actomysin, indicating that these cells are modifed smooth muscle cells or myofibroblasts.[31] They are continuous with the lacis cells of the juxtaglomerular apparatus (see p. 17; Fig. 1.15b) with a graded transition of cell types from one to the other.[32] Contractile activity of the intrinsic mesangial cells could be involved in regulation of glomerular blood flow. The intrinsic mesangial cells produce interleukin I during the 'gap' (G1) in the cell cycle which precedes the synthetic (S) phase during which the DNA is replicated.[33] Interleukin 1 is a polypeptide mediator involved in the regulation of the immune and inflammatory systems.[34] It acts as a growth factor for mesangial cells, stimulating their proliferation. The local production of interleukin 1 by intrinsic mesangial cells may be an important determinant controlling the extent of cellular proliferation and extracellular matrix production during the course of chronic forms of glomerulonephritis. The intrinsic mesangial cells do not phagocytose and they do not express HLA-DR antigens (class II molecules encoded by the D region of the human major histocompatibility

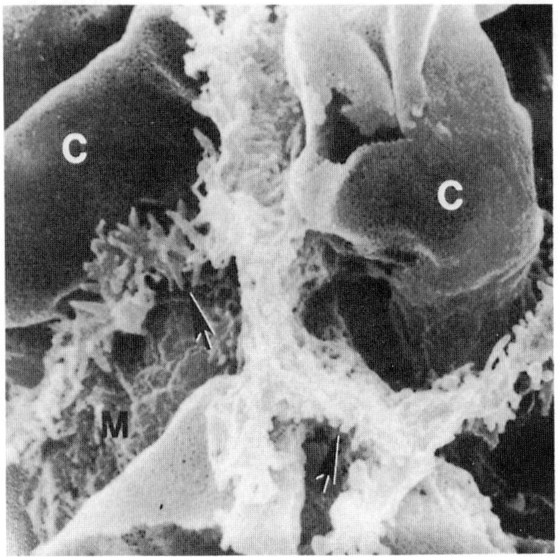

Fig. 1.12 Scanning electron micrograph of mesangial cell (M) and its processes extending along the centrilobular aspect of the glomerular capillaries (C) to contact adjacent mesangial cells. Anchoring processes (arrows) protrude into the mesangial matrix. The glomerular capillary basement membranes and the mesangial matrix have been removed by digestion with enzymes.
× 6000
Reproduced by permission from: Jones DB. Lab Invest 1985; 52: 453 (Fig. 7)

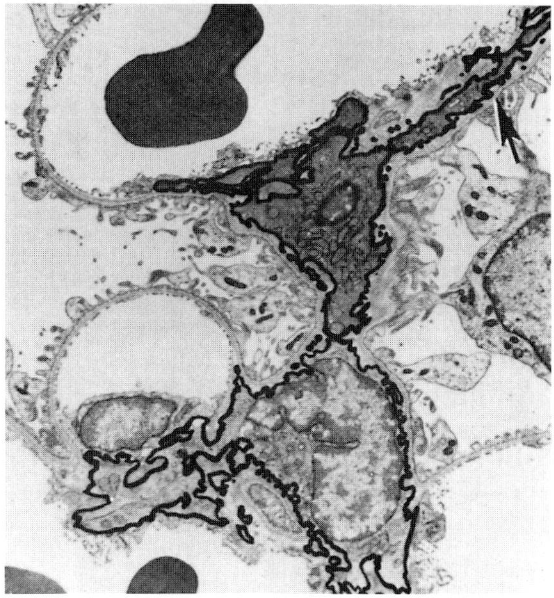

Fig. 1.13 Transmission electron micrograph of a rat glomerulus on which the complex contours of the mesangial cell plasma membranes have been traced with Indian ink. An anchoring process (arrow) is inserted into the mesangial matrix.
× 5250
Reproduced by permission from: Jones DB. Lab Invest 1985; 52: 453 (Fig. 8)

complex or MHC; they are equivalent to mouse immune associated, Ia, antigen. These antigens are discussed on p. 618).[34–37]

A second cell population in the mesangium is composed of *mononuclear phagocytes* (Fig. 1.14) that have the morphology and functional characteristics of monocytes and macrophages.[35] They express surface receptors for the Fc fragment of immunoglobulins and the third component of complement (C3b). In the rat, these cells originate from the bone marrow,[36,37] circulate in the blood stream as monocytes, migrate into the mesangium and stay there for a few days.[38] They seem to be analogous to the fixed tissue phagocytes such as Kupffer cells. Most mononuclear phagocytes in the glomeruli of normal human kidneys lie within capillary lumens: only 1% are in the mesangium, i.e. about one cell in each whole glomerulus.[39] The numbers of mononuclear phagocytes in the mesangium are greater in rats (9.14 ± 0.2 per glomerulus in normal Lewis rats)[38] and in both experimental animals and man they increase in some forms of immune mediated glomerulonephritis.[40]

In rats, a substantial subset (between 35 and 70%) of the mesangial mononuclear phagocytes express class II MHC antigens.[36–38] Expression of these antigens occurs in mononuclear phagocytes derived from the circulating monocytes after they have resided in the mesangium for 3–4 days.[38] The factors responsible for inducing the expression of class II MHC antigens in these cells are unknown. No mesangial mononuclear phagocytes expressing class II MHC antigens have yet been clearly identified in man. Suggestive staining using the immunoperoxidase method to identify HLA-DR antigens has been found by some workers,[41] but the fact that the endothelial cells are strongly positive makes exact cell localization difficult.[42]

The *matrix* that surrounds the mesangial cells, and is synthesized by them, is amorphous and contains closely packed negatively charged (anionic) filaments 1.2–2.5 nm wide composed of various collagen types, fibronectin, laminin and entactin.[43]

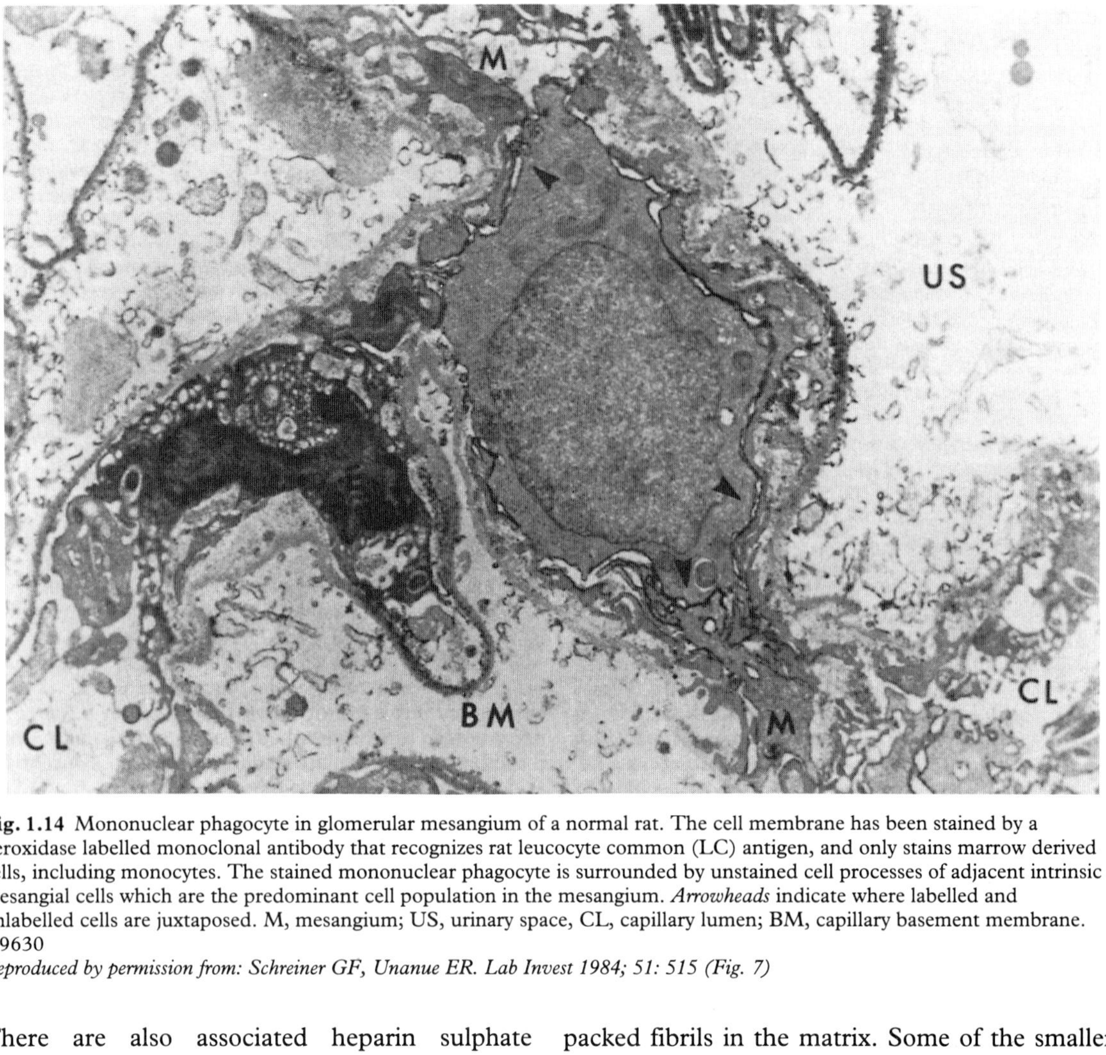

Fig. 1.14 Mononuclear phagocyte in glomerular mesangium of a normal rat. The cell membrane has been stained by a peroxidase labelled monoclonal antibody that recognizes rat leucocyte common (LC) antigen, and only stains marrow derived cells, including monocytes. The stained mononuclear phagocyte is surrounded by unstained cell processes of adjacent intrinsic mesangial cells which are the predominant cell population in the mesangium. *Arrowheads* indicate where labelled and unlabelled cells are juxtaposed. M, mesangium; US, urinary space, CL, capillary lumen; BM, capillary basement membrane. × 9630
Reproduced by permission from: Schreiner GF, Unanue ER. Lab Invest 1984; 51: 515 (Fig. 7)

There are also associated heparin sulphate proteoglycans. It has the same staining properties and electron density as the lamina densa of the glomerular capillary basement membrane, but its complete biochemical structure is unknown and there is some evidence that it differs antigenically from the glomerular basement membrane. Also the anionic fibrils are closely packed and more extensive than the lattice of negatively charged heparin sulphate proteoglycan in the glomerular capillary basement membrane.

Plasma flows continuously into the mesangium from the glomerular capillaries through fenestrae in the lining endothelium. As there is no capillary basement membrane over this part of the mesangium, even macromolecules enter unimpeded but they are trapped and filtered out by the closely packed fibrils in the matrix. Some of the smaller particles are then endocytosed by the intrinsic mesangial cells and any aggregated proteins or immune complexes are taken up by monocytes which migrate into the mesangium. The use of particles that can be easily followed in the glomerulus, such as colloidal carbon, thorium dioxide, ferritin protein conjugates and polyvinyl alcohol, suggests that the plasma leaves the mesangium by three routes: through the overlying visceral epithelium into the urinary space, through endothelial fenestrations into the efferent glomerular capillaries, and through channels in the mesangial matrix into the matrix between the lacis cells of the juxtaglomerular apparatus.[43] One consequence of the first route is that any macromolecules in the plasma accumulate against the capillary basement membrane. Electron-dense deposits are frequently found here in human glomerulonephritis: it has been called the *para-mesangial region*. Only a small part of the plasma flowing through the mesangium leaves by the second and third routes.

Factor VIII is found in the mesangium; it is not known whether the mesangium stores or manufactures this substance.

THE JUXTAGLOMERULAR APPARATUS AND GRANULAR PERIPOLAR CELLS

The juxtaglomerular apparatus[44,45]

The juxtaglomerular apparatus (Fig. 1.15) is situated at the hilum of the glomerulus and is normally inconspicuous. It consists of granular cells, lacis cells and the macula densa. Unmyelinated sympathetic nerve endings are associated with these structures.

Granular cells

The granular cells of the juxtaglomerular apparatus are modifed smooth muscle cells (myoepithelial cells) found in the wall of the terminal part of the afferent arteriole on the outer aspect of the muscular layer. They are more numerous in the glomeruli in the superfical cortex. In the rat the granules stain intensely with Bowie's method[46] but in man they are difficult to demonstrate. Ultrastructurally there are two main types of granule: a crystalline, often rhomboidal, form called a protogranule, and a round, membrane-bound storage granule (Fig. 1.16). The rhomboidal granules are commonest near the Golgi apparatus and are precursors of the round granules that are found mainly in the peripheral cytoplasm. The use of peroxidase-labelled, highly specific, monoclonal antibodies and ultrastructural immunochemistry shows that the granules contain both active renin (an aspartyl peptidase) and angiotensin II (an octapeptide).[47,48] The contents of the granules are secreted from the surface of the cells by exocytosis.

Lacis cells

The lacis cells, which are so named because of their supposedly lace-like arrangement, lack renin granules, although they may contain lipofuscin. The lacis cells lie in the arch formed by the afferent and efferent arterioles and are in intimate

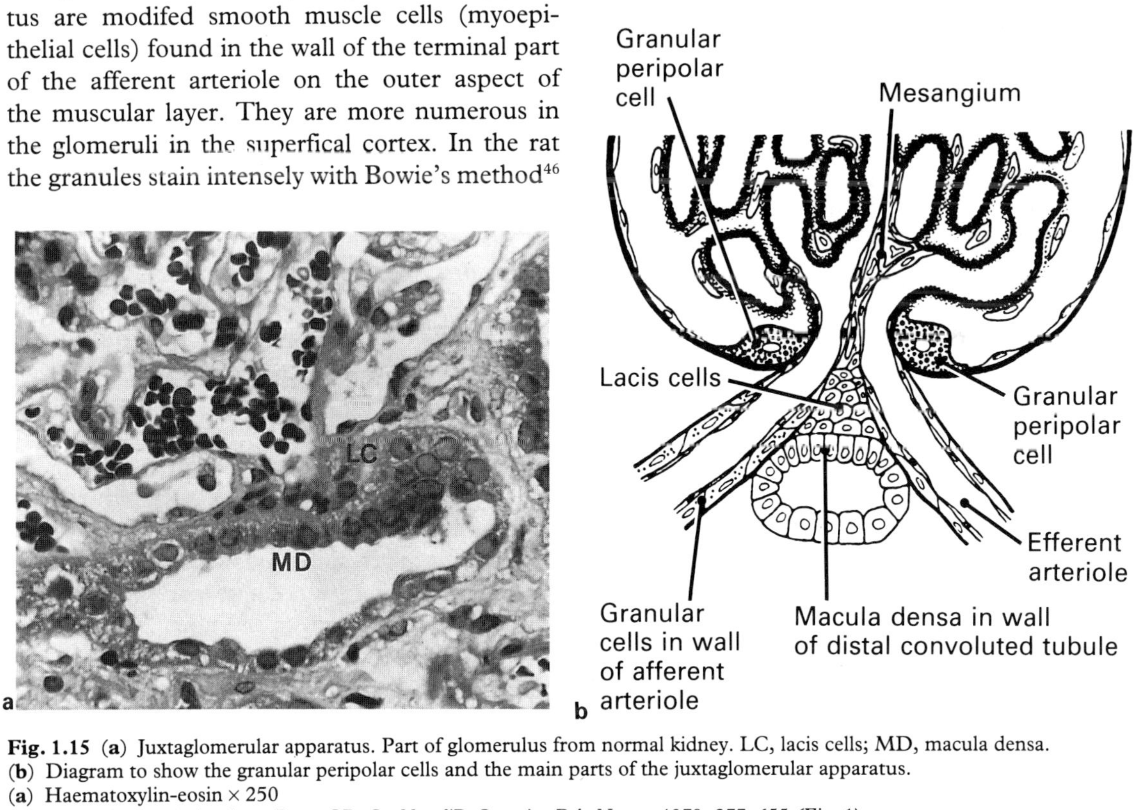

Fig. 1.15 **(a)** Juxtaglomerular apparatus. Part of glomerulus from normal kidney. LC, lacis cells; MD, macula densa. **(b)** Diagram to show the granular peripolar cells and the main parts of the juxtaglomerular apparatus.
(a) Haematoxylin-eosin × 250
Reproduced by permission from: Ryan GB, Coghlan JP, Scoggins BA. Nature 1979; 277: 655 (Fig. 1)

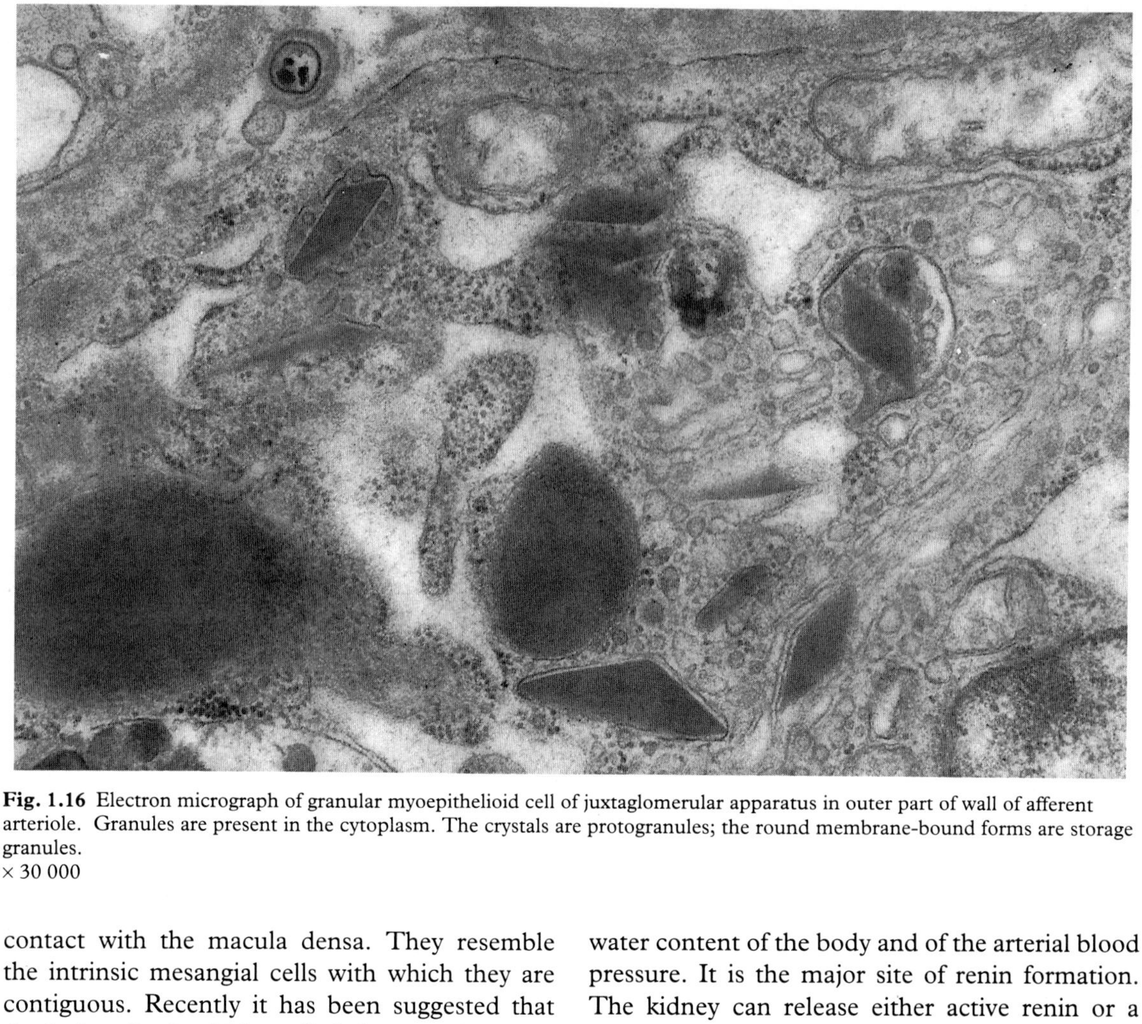

Fig. 1.16 Electron micrograph of granular myoepithelioid cell of juxtaglomerular apparatus in outer part of wall of afferent arteriole. Granules are present in the cytoplasm. The crystals are protogranules; the round membrane-bound forms are storage granules.
× 30 000

contact with the macula densa. They resemble the intrinsic mesangial cells with which they are contiguous. Recently it has been suggested that the lacis cells should be called the *extraglomerular mesangial cells*.

Macula densa

The macula densa is the part of the circumference of the distal convoluted tubule that lies nearest the hilum of the glomerulus. The cells are narrower and often taller than other cells of the distal convoluted tubule. The nuclei of the macula densa lie close together. The tubular basement membrane is deficient in this sector and the macula densa lacks the Tamm–Horsfall glycoprotein which is present in the rest of the ascending thick limb of the loop of Henle.

The juxtaglomerular apparatus is concerned mainly with the regulation of the sodium and water content of the body and of the arterial blood pressure. It is the major site of renin formation. The kidney can release either active renin or a mixture of active and inactive (proenzyme) renin, depending on the stimulus.[49] Up to 60% of the renin in the blood is inactive.[50] Renin is secreted predominantly into the renal interstitium and subsequently enters the circulation via the peritubular capillaries and, to a lesser extent, the lymphatics. Several stimuli can cause the juxtaglomerular cells to release their renin,[51] but the most important are a fall in the pressure in the afferent arteriole, which is sensed by stretch receptors within the vessel wall, a decrease in the amount of sodium or chloride arriving at the macula densa, and direct stimulation of the sympathetic nerves. The released active renin cleaves a plasma alpha$_2$-globulin, called angiotensinogen, and releases an inactive decapeptide known as angiotensin I. An enzyme, angiotensin-converting enzyme (ACE), which is identical to kinase II and is ubiquitously distributed in vascular endothelium, converts angiotensin I to a potent vasoconstrictor octapeptide, angiotensin II. Angiotensin II also causes the release of aldosterone from the adrenal cortex; this stimulates the distal nephron to reabsorb sodium ions, causing extracellular fluid retention. The renin–angiotensin–aldosterone system therefore maintains blood pressure by vasoconstriction and by increased blood volume. Under normal circumstances, the increased renin secretion is quickly countered by a negative feedback mechanism. Increased renin secretion plays a role in certain forms of hypertension (see pp. 310, 318).

Granular peripolar cells

The granular peripolar cells are modified epithelial cells encircling the vascular pole of the glomerulus within Bowman's space.[52,53] They lie on the basement membrane of Bowman's capsule at the junction between the parietal and visceral epithelial cells (Figs 1.15, 1.17). Their cytoplasm contains large numbers of closely packed granules which react positively with Bowie's stain (see p. 17). The granules are mostly round, 100 nm to 1 μm in diameter, have a membrane and contain fine fibrillar and granular electron-dense material. Granular peripolar cells are found in all kidneys but their incidence varies widely, with 3–28% of glomeruli showing these structures. They are found predominantly in the glomeruli in the superficial cortex. The granules in the peripolar cells do not contain renin (Fig. 1.18); preliminary findings suggest that they contain a kallikrein-like protease. The function of the granular peripolar cells is unknown but as their secretion enters directly into the glomerular filtrate, they may control some aspect of tubular reabsorption.

THE TUBULES

The capsular space of the glomerulus (Bowman's space) continues directly into the *proximal convoluted tubule* which meanders around the parent glomerulus (Fig. 1.19). It is lined by cubical epithelial cells that show intense enzyme activity, and have finely granular eosinophile cytoplasm, a round basal nucleus, a brush border on their luminal aspect and indistinct cell boundaries. The brush border is composed of microvilli that increase

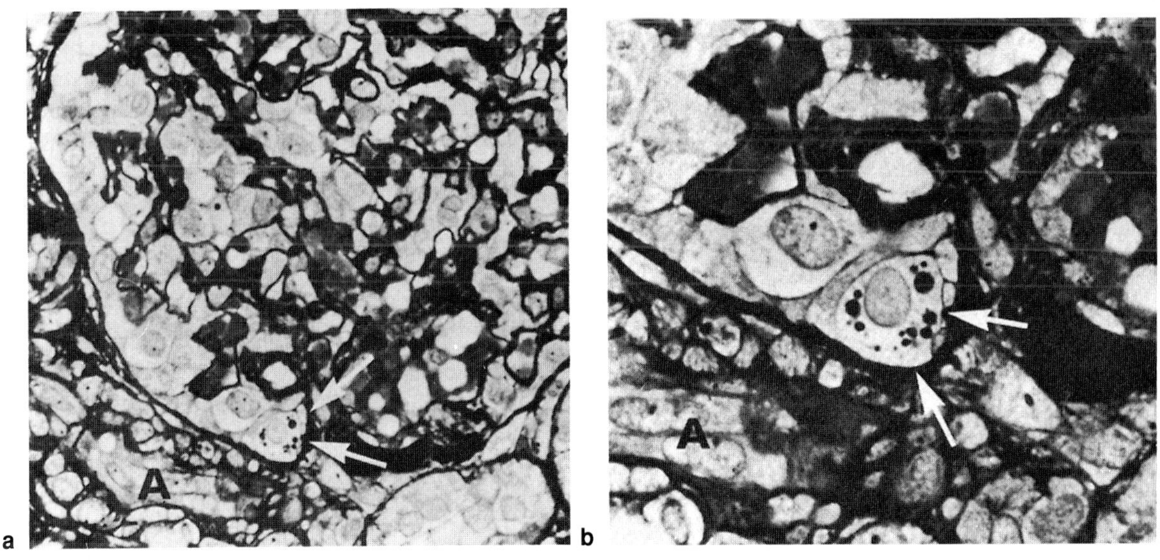

Fig. 1.17 (**a, b**) A peripolar cell with large cytoplasmic granules (arrows) lying on the basement membrane of Bowman's capsule and at the junction between the parietal and visceral epithelial cells. A, afferent arteriole.
Toluidine blue: (**a**) × 360; (**b**) × 800
Reproduced by permission from: Gardiner DS, Lindop GBM. Histopathology 1985; 9: 675 (Fig. 2)

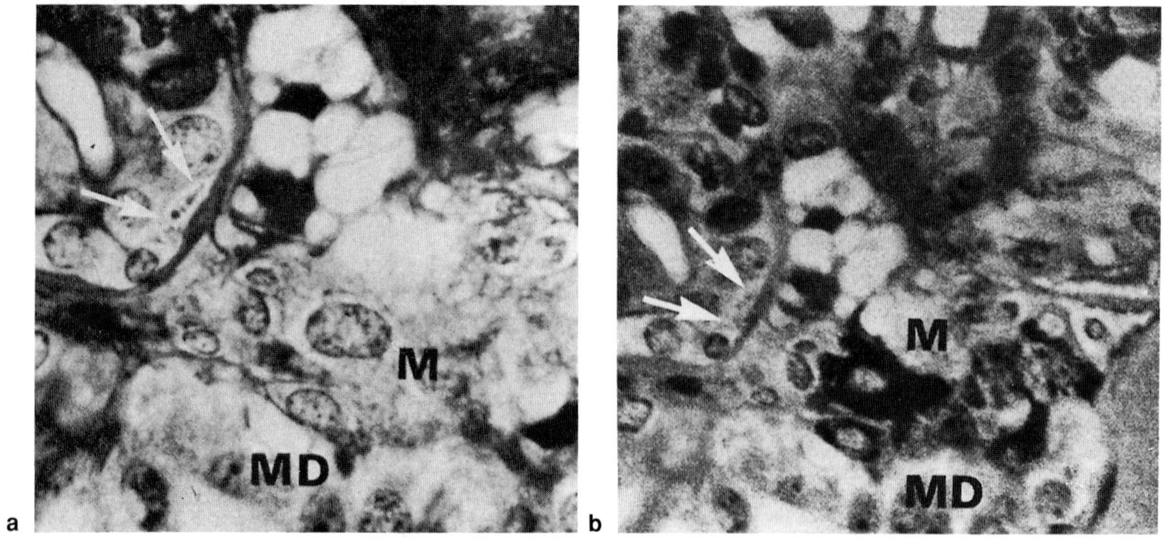

Fig. 1.18 (**a**) A granular peripolar cell (arrows) rests on the basement membrane of Bowman's capsule. Granular cells of juxtaglomerular apparatus (M) lie in the wall of the afferent arteriole. MD, macula densa.
(**b**) Same section stained with peroxidase-antiperoxidase (PAP) technique for renin. The granular cells of the juxtaglomerular apparatus stain strongly positive but the granules of the peripolar cells are negative.
(**a**) Dawes and Hilliers trichrome × 800;
(**b**) peroxidase-antiperoxidase × 500
Reproduced by permission from: Gardiner DS, Lindop GBM. Histopathology 1985;9:675 (Fig. 4)

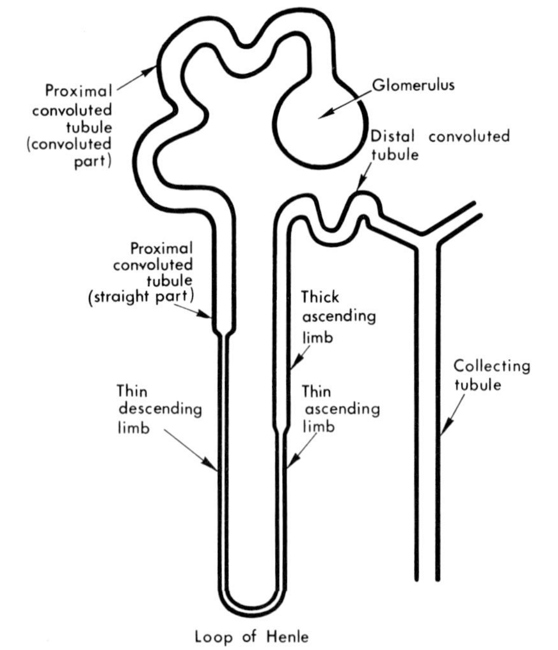

Fig. 1.19 Diagram to show the main parts of the nephron. The limbs of Henle extend variable distances into the medulla.
Reproduced by permission of Professor R. H. Heptinstall from Systemic pathology, 1st edn. London: Longman, 1966

the tubular surface area about 40-fold (Figs 1.20, 1.21). The granularity of the cytoplasm is caused by the presence of large numbers of mitochondria. The cell boundaries are indistinct because adjacent cells have irregular interlocking surfaces; in addition, at the base of the epithelial cells there are large numbers of infoldings of the basal plasma membrane (Fig. 1.20).The basal and lateral infoldings further increase the surface area of the cells. Reabsorbed droplets of IgG, IgA and albumin that have escaped through the glomerular filter are common in the cytoplasm (Fig. 1.22).

The proximal convoluted tubule assumes a relatively straight course in the medullary ray and then becomes narrowed to form the *thin descending limb of Henle's loop*, which extends into the medulla for a variable distance before looping back as the *thin ascending limb*. This thin segment of the tubule is much smaller in diameter than the proximal convoluted tubule and is lined by flatter epithelium with a few mitochondria and only small numbers of short microvilli. In the papilla the thin segment is in very close proximity to the

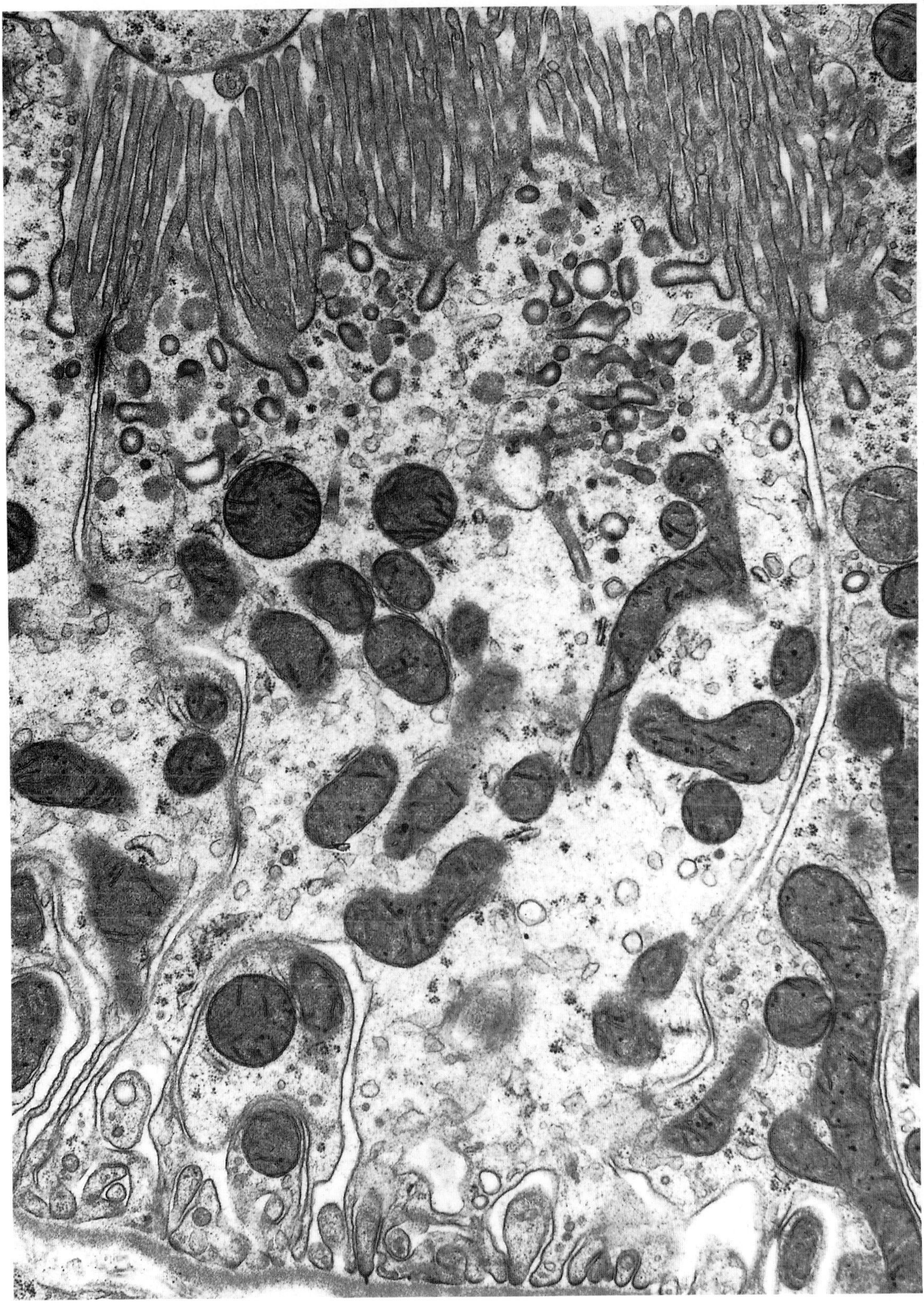

Fig. 1.20 Electron micrograph of part of a normal human proximal convoluted tubule. The microvilli comprising the brush border can be seen in the upper part of the photograph. The cytoplasm contains numerous elongated mitochondria. At the base of the epithelial cells there are large numbers of infoldings of the basal plasma membrane.
× 9500

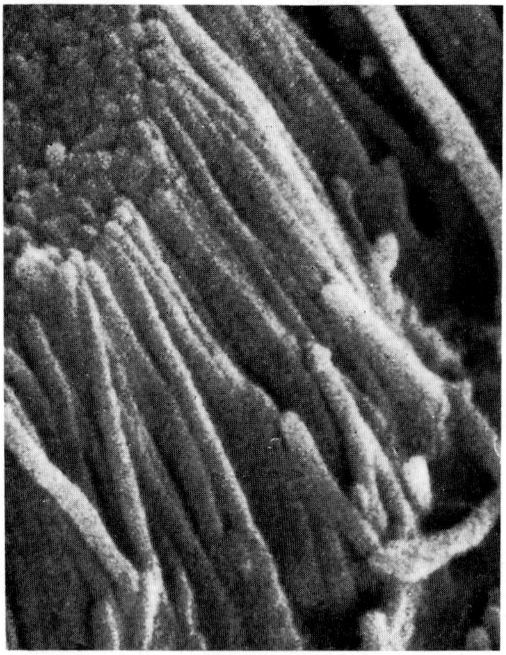

Fig. 1.21 Scanning electron micrograph of the microvilli of a normal proximal convoluted tubule.
× 20 000
Reproduced by permission from: Bulger RE, Siegal FL, Pendergrass R. Am J Anat 1974; 139: 483 (Fig. 8)

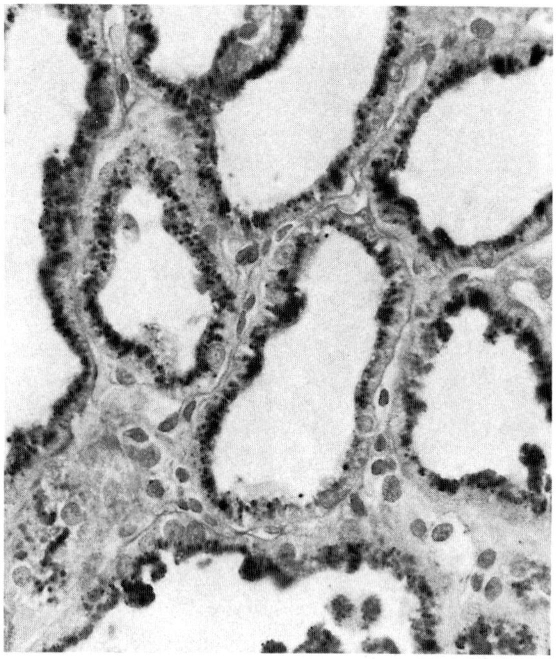

Fig. 1.22 Human renal tubules. There are globules of IgG in the cytoplasm of the epithelial cells lining the proximal convoluted tubules.
Peroxidase labelled anti-IgG × 350

vasa recta (Fig. 1.23). In the outer part of the medulla the thin ascending limb of Henle's loop gives way to the *thick ascending limb*, which runs in the medullary ray of the cortex back to the vicinity of the parent glomerulus. The epithelium of the ascending limb is taller than that of the descending limb, but it is still less tall than that of the proximal convoluted tubule. There is no brush border because the microvilli are both small and few in number. The cells of the thick ascending limb contain many large basal mitochondria and show intense enzyme activity.

When the ascending limb reaches the vicinity of the glomerulus it becomes the *distal convoluted tubule* and is closely associated with the afferent and efferent arterioles. In this part of its course the distal convoluted tubule forms the macula densa which is part of the juxtaglomerular apparatus (see p. 18). The distal convoluted tubule is relatively short and is much less convoluted than the proximal convoluted tubule. It is lined by cuboidal cells that lack both eosinophile granules and a brush border. Each day these cells, together with those of the thick ascending limb of Henle's loop, secrete 10–140 mg of an alpha$_1$-glycoprotein called Tamm–Horsfall protein (Fig. 1.24).[54] The cells of the macula densa do not produce the protein. In the presence of albumin Tamm–Horsfall protein comes out of solution as a gel and forms the matrix of casts (see p. 494). The distal convoluted tubule continues as the *connecting piece*. Several connecting pieces from adjacent nephrons join to form an early *collecting tubule*. By a series of unions of collecting tubules of different orders, the *ducts of Bellini* are formed: these discharge at the surface of a papilla. The epithelial cells lining the collecting tubules are cubical, stain palely with eosin, have clear outlines and a central nucleus, and lack a brush border.

THE INTERSTITIUM

In the renal cortex the interstitium is sparse be-

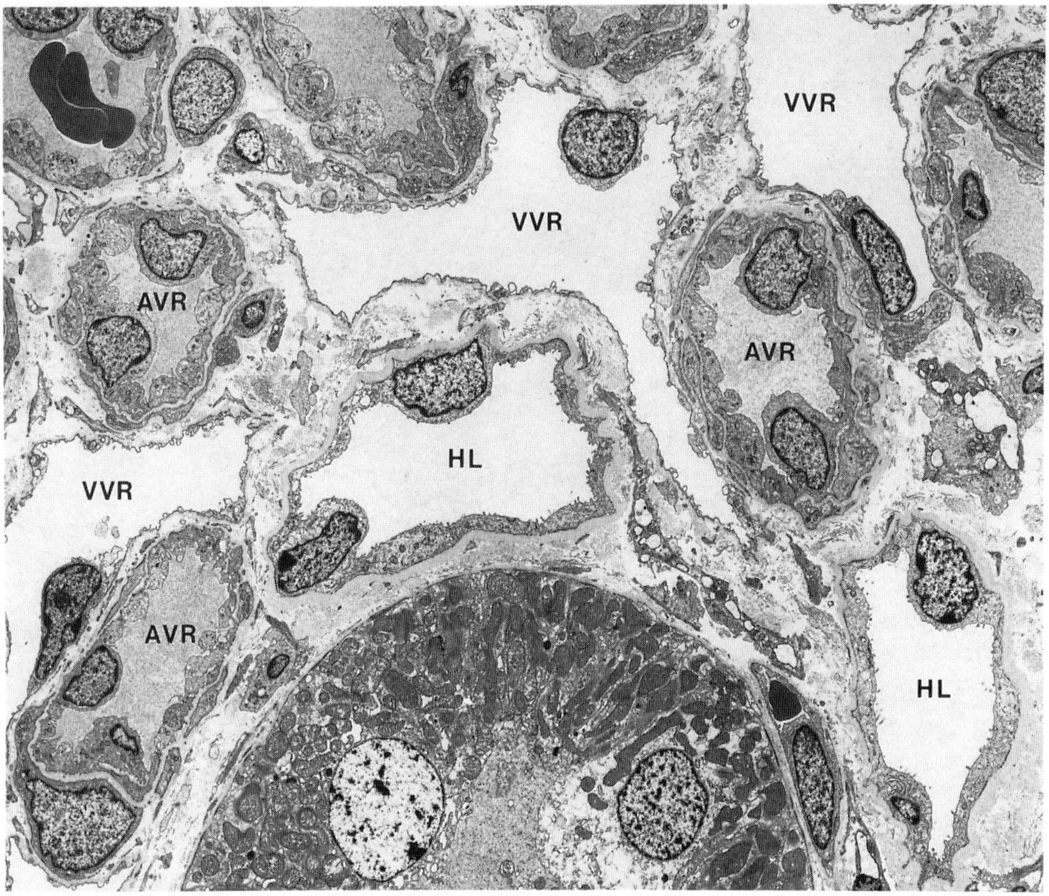

Fig. 1.23 Electron micrograph of normal renal papilla. The thin descending limb of Henle's loop (HL) is lined by flat epithelium with only short microvilli. It is in very close proximity to the arterial vas rectum (AVR) and the venous vas rectum (VVR).
× 2180

cause the tubules are packed very close. Fine fibrils and occasional cells are present, however. The interstitium is much more prominent in the medulla, where there are apparently specific *interstitial cells*, situated close to many of the small blood vessels and to be found particularly between Henle's loop and the vasa recta. They have elongated processes and their cytoplasm contains lipid droplets, cisternae and a prominent Golgi apparatus. There is some evidence that they are secreting cells, producing prostaglandins, in particular PGE_2 which probably controls salt and water secretion, and an antihypertensive lipid called neutral lipid factor.[55] In rats, some of the stellate interstitial cells bear major histocompatibility complex (MHC) class II antigens.[37] and are often referred to as *dendritic cells* because it is thought that they may function in a similar way to the antigen-presenting dendritic cells that are found in the skin. However, in humans careful analysis of the so-called interstitial cells which exhibit HLA-DR antigens has shown them to be endothelial cells lining the vasa recta, veins and peritubular capillaries.[42] No specific interstitial cell that contains class II histocompatibility antigens has yet been found in humans.

EFFECTS OF AGEING ON THE KIDNEYS

The gross and microscopic appearances of the kidneys in premature and full-term babies and in infancy and childhood are described on page 50.

By the age of 20 years the nephrons in the kid-

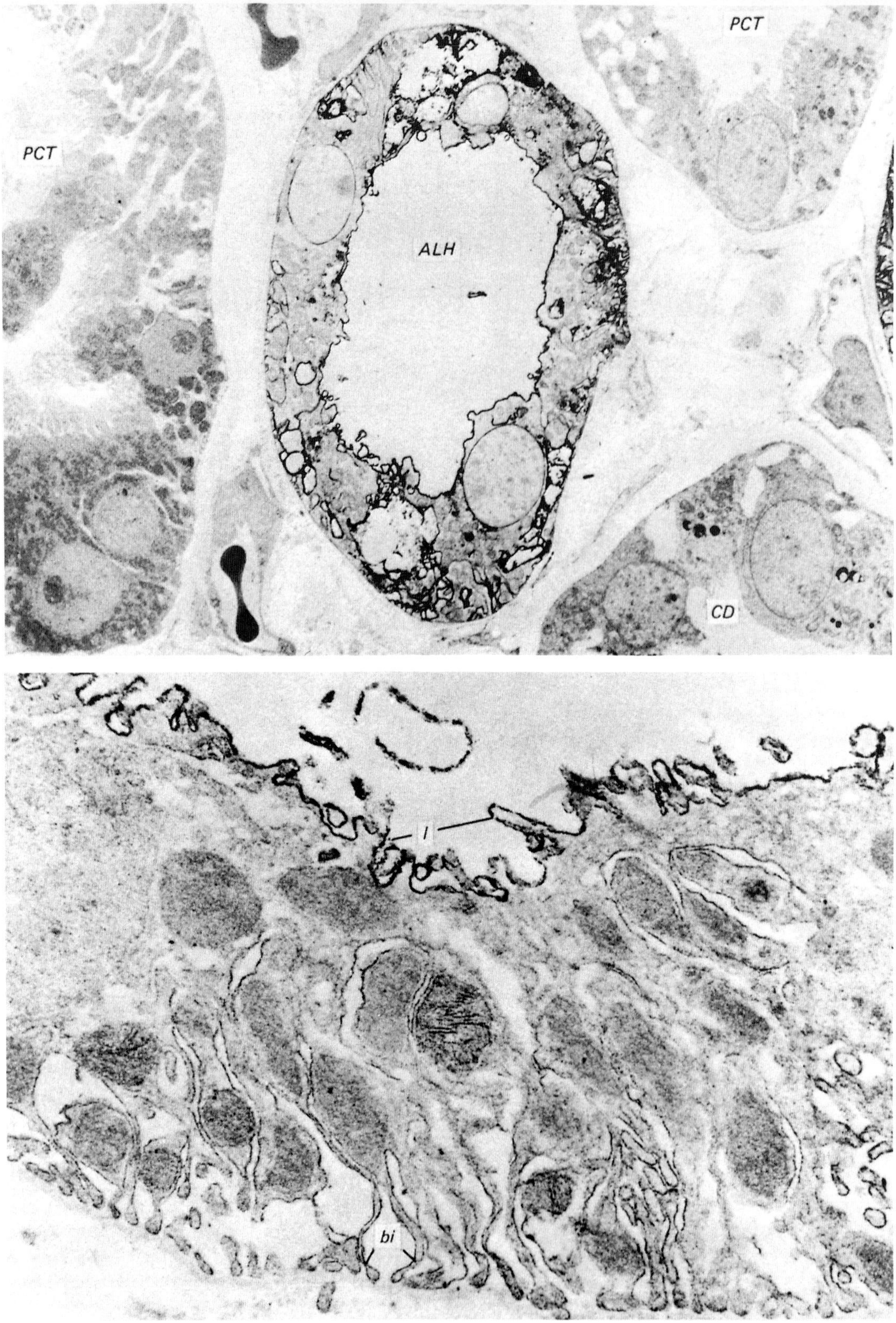

Fig. 1.24 Immuno-electron micrographs of a thick ascending limb of Henle's loop (ALH) (**a**) and part of distal tubule (**b**). Black granules demonstrate the presence of Tamm–Horsfall glycoprotein on the plasma membranes of the cells of both these parts of the tubule. It is absent from the proximal convoluted tubule (PCT). CD, collecting ducts; l, lumenal surface; bi, infoldings of basal membrane. Peroxidase labelled antibody to human Tamm–Horsfall protein: (**a**) × 21 800; (**b**) × 2180

Reproduced by permission from: Sikri KL, Foster CL, MacHugh N, Marshall RD. J Anat 1981; 132: 597 (Figs 6, 5) ney have reached maturity and they change little until the age of 30 years when they begin to shrink. The weight and volume of the kidney then decreases 20–30% in the next 60 years.[56] This loss is primarily cortical and seems to be related to atherosclerotic involvement of the intrarenal vasculature.[57,58] The reduction in the size of the kidney probably accounts for the dramatic changes that occur in renal function with ageing. For example, the glomerular filtration rate of healthy octagenarians is only half to two-thirds that found in young adults.[59] The number of functioning glomeruli declines roughly in accord with the changes in renal weight, while the size of the remaining glomeruli increases.[60]

The sequence of glomerular structural changes with ageing has been elucidated by combining microangiographic and histological techniques.[61–63] The glomerular capillary basement membrane progressively wrinkles and then thickens. This stage is accompanied by simplification of the glomerular tuft, progressive loss of cells and the formation of free anastomoses between a reduced number of glomerular capillary loops. Eventually the wrinkled and thickened glomerular capillary basement membrane collapses and condenses into a small, compact eosinophile mass that stains positively with periodic acid-Schiff reagent, a condition referred to as *global sclerosis*. Collagen is also often laid down on the inner side of Bowman's capsule (Figs 1.25–1.27). In most of the renal cortex the related afferent and efferent arterioles atrophy, but in the juxtamedullary zone a direct channel forms between the afferent and efferent arterioles producing arteriolae rectae verae.[62]

The number of globally sclerotic glomeruli rises with increasing age. Up to the age of 40 years fewer than 3% of the glomeruli have undergone sclerosis but after this the incidence slowly climbs so that by the age of 70 years very roughly 25–30% of the glomeruli are sclerotic; however there is a lot of variation between individuals.[64,65] One study indicates that the 90th percentile for the percentage of sclerotic glomeruli, in people without overt renal disease, can be calculated for any age by subtracting 10 from half the person's age.[66] No racial or sex related differences in the baseline incidence of global sclerosis of glomeruli have been recorded in any age group.[66]

Associated with the glomerular loss the renal tubules decrease in number, the proximal tubules shrink in length and diameter and the distal tubules develop diverticula.[67] The afferent arterioles show increased spiralling and small amounts of homogeneous PAS-positive material, usually referred to as *hyalin*, appears in their walls. The renal arteries develop fibrous intimal thickening and an increase in the number of layers of elastic in the internal elastic lamina (usually called reduplication of the lamina).

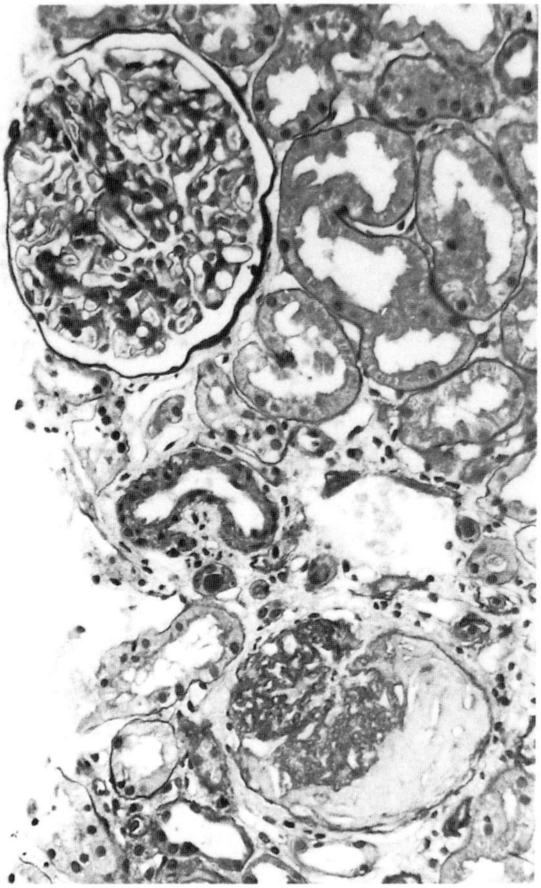

Fig. 1.25 Kidney from an 80-year-old man. A glomerulus (lower part of picture) has undergone global sclerosis and collagen has been laid down on the inner side of Bowman's capsule.
Periodic acid-Schiff × 250

DIET AND AGEING KIDNEYS

It has been suggested that the protein-rich diet characteristic of modern Western society may

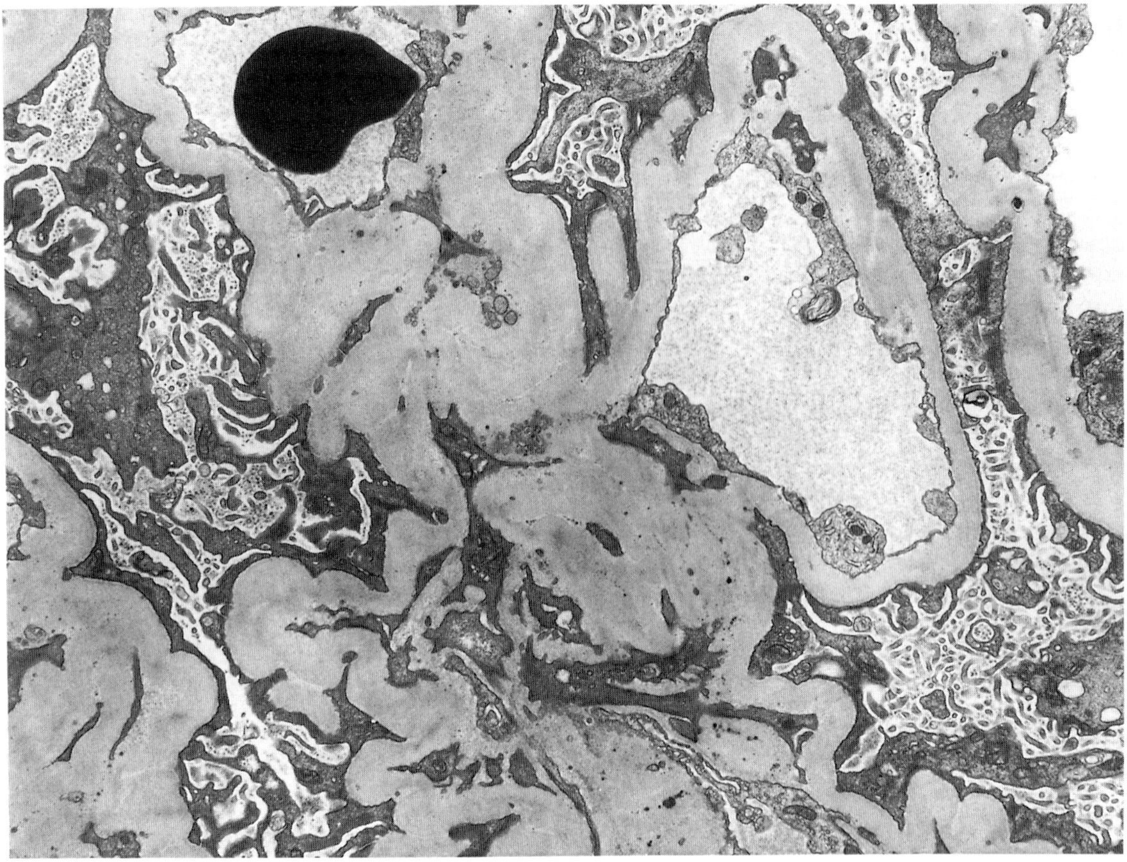

Fig. 1.26 Electron micrograph of part of a glomerulus from the kidney shown in Figure 1.25. The capillary basement membranes are irregularly thickened, wrinkled and collapsed and the cellularity of the glomerulus is reduced. × 8000

contribute to these changes in ageing kidneys by inducing chronic renal hyperfiltration and hyperperfusion (see below).[68,69]

Certainly, in rats, reducing the amount of protein in the diet markedly delays the onset of ageing changes in the kidneys and prolongs the animals' life. Simply restricting the amount of food eaten, without decreasing protein consumption (this is accomplished by increasing the casein content of the diet), also greatly slows down the ageing changes in the kidneys and the animals live longer.[70]

It seems likely that the reduction in calories is the major factor responsible for the beneficial effect of protein or general food restriction on the kidneys. The underlying mechanism is not known. Decreasing the amount of food consumed does not influence systemic blood pressure or retard the increase in serum lipids that occurs with age. Rats that eat less, however, remain more active than those on a normal diet, and this may be important; exercise has been shown to reduce the progression of glomerulosclerosis in rats that have had five-sixths of their total renal mass removed.[70]

EFFECTS OF REDUCING THE AMOUNT OF RENAL TISSUE: THE SOLITARY KIDNEY

When the amount of renal tissue is reduced the remaining nephrons hypertrophy and their function increases. The glomerular microcirculation adapts, resulting in a marked increase in the filtration rate within the individual surviving nephrons.

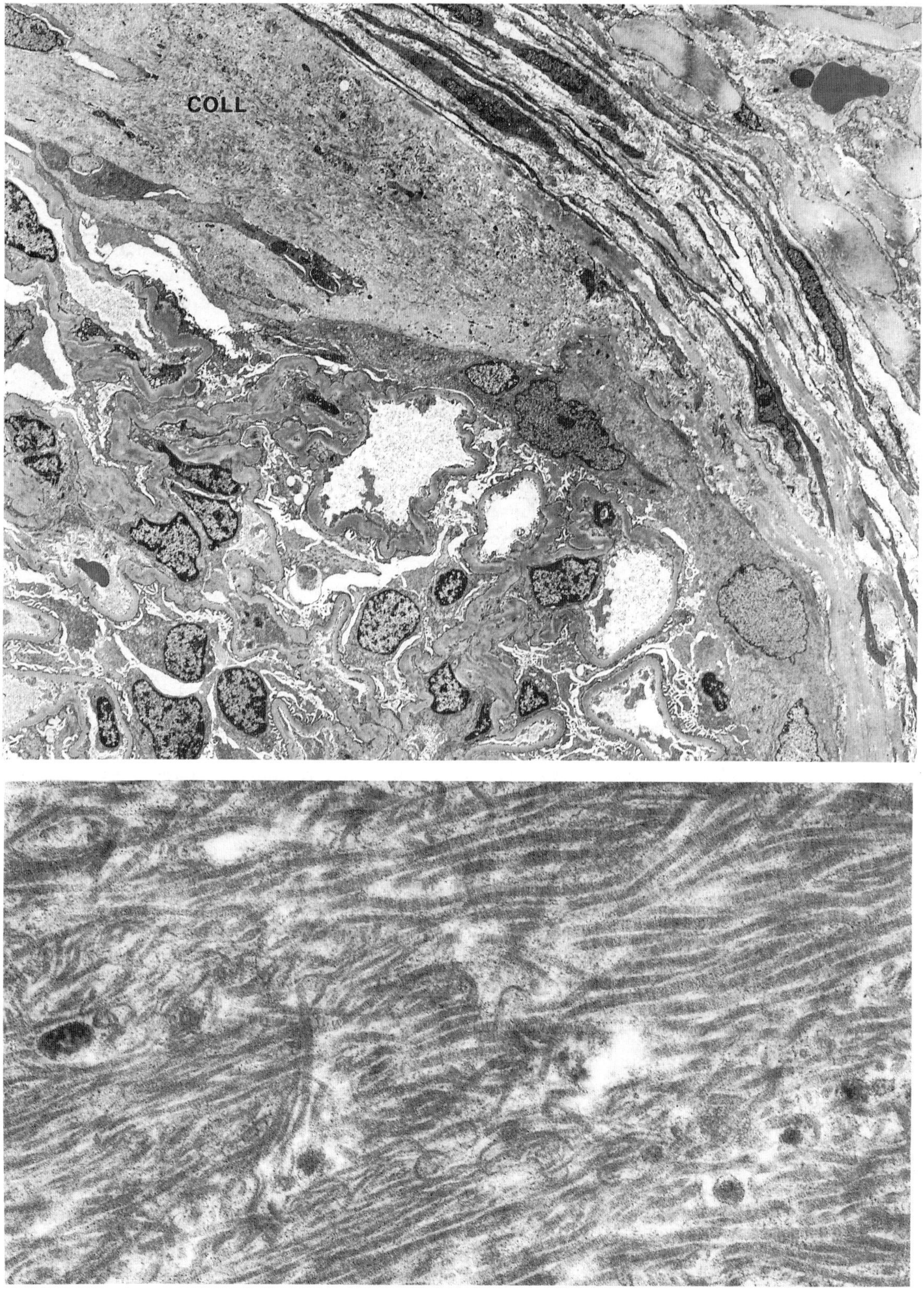

a

b

Fig. 1.27 Electron micrographs of part of another glomerulus from the kidney shown in Figure 1.25. In (**a**) collagen (COLL) can be seen on the inner side of Bowman's capsule beneath the parietal epithelium. (**b**) shows the characteristic periodicity of the collagen fibrils.
(**a**) × 2025; (**b**) × 40 000

The magnitude of this increase correlates closely with the amount of renal tissue that has been lost: in this way the reduction in glomerular filtration rate is minimized. However, a growing body of evidence suggests that single nephron hyperfiltration eventually injures the glomeruli.[69,71] It has long been known that removal of approximately five-sixths of the total renal mass in the rat leads within the next 3 weeks to a syndrome of progressive proteinuria, azotaemia and glomerular sclerosis. Following the reduction in renal mass the glomeruli enlarge, their visceral epithelial cells develop cytoplasmic vacuoles and the foot processes become obliterated. At the same time the glomerular capillary wall loses its ability to retain within the capillary lumen large molecules bearing negative electron charges and this accounts for the progressive proteinuria. Evidence of focal and segmental injury to endothelial and epithelial cells next appears and homogeneous PAS-positive material accumulates under endothelial cells near the hilum of some glomeruli. The term *hyalinosis* is given to this last lesion. As more of this material accumulates and encroaches on the capillary lumen foamy macrophages and extracellular lipid droplets appear. Over the following few weeks foci of hyalinosis develop in more and more of the glomeruli and by 11 weeks about 75% of glomeruli are affected. Coincidental with these changes the amount of mesangial matrix increases and progressive glomerular sclerosis occurs.[72]

The mechanisms involved in producing these injuries in rats are not known but the combined effects of intrarenal hypertension and hyperperfusion lead to an increased passage of ultrafiltrate and macromolecules across the glomerular capillary walls with overloading of the mesangium. This may stimulate both increased matrix deposition giving glomerular sclerosis and accumulation of hyaline material beneath the endothelium producing focal and segmental hyalinosis.

These changes following reduction of renal mass can be ameliorated by giving the rats a low protein diet which reduces the single nephron glomerular filtration rate.[73]

From these findings in the rat three hypotheses have been put forward. The first is that damage caused by hyperperfusion of individual surviving nephrons may account for the progressive glomerular sclerosis and fall in renal function that occurs in some renal diseases even when the initiating process has apparently either ceased spontaneously or been controlled by treatment. For example, patients with vesicoureteric reflux (see p. 444) often develop progressive glomerular sclerosis in the absence of active urinary tract infection or hypertension, and despite surgical correction of the reflux. Hyperperfusion damage may also account for the development of glomerular sclerosis in children born with reduced numbers of functioning nephrons (oligomeganephronia; – see p. 56) and in the only kidney of patients born with unilateral renal agenesis (see p. 55). The latter example implies that patients who have undergone unilateral nephrectomy may be at risk. The evidence for this is at present equivocal. Proteinuria and focal glomerulosclerosis in the remaining kidney has been found in some patients after unilateral nephrectomy for calculous disease;[74] nephrectomy in these patients usually does not result in increased morbidity or mortality for at least 15 years after the operation.[75] Kidney donors followed for over 20 years show an unimpaired glomerular filtration rate which is raised to 70–80% of the normal, two kidney, rate. Some donors develop mild proteinuria that does not progress; others become hypertensive but the incidence of hypertension does not differ from that in a control population. It would seem that hyperfiltration secondary to 50% reduction of renal mass in humans does not lead to loss of function if the remaining kidney is normal.[76,77]

The second hypothesis is that a high dietary protein intake in the presence of renal injury contributes to the increased perfusion of the surviving glomeruli and accelerates their destruction.[68] Some evidence in patients suggests that protein restriction may slow the deterioration of function in some renal diseases. As a result, controlled multicentre clinical trials of protein restriction in renal failure are now being attempted to test this hypothesis.

The third hypothesis is that the functional burden imposed on the nephrons by a lifetime of eating a high protein diet leads to the progressive sclerosis that occurs in ageing (see p. 25).[68]

SIMPLE RENAL CYSTS

Autopsies and routine abdominal computed tomography examinations reveal that about 50% of people over the age of 50 years have one or more unsuspected cysts in their kidneys.[78] These benign and usually asymptomatic cysts are rare in infants or children[79] but become progressively more common with increasing age.[78] Although little is known about their aetiology and pathogenesis simple cysts are discussed in this chapter because they are associated with ageing and are thought to be caused neither by a congenital malformation nor a non-developmental hereditary disease.

Clinical features

Simple cysts rarely cause symptoms. Occasionally large cysts present as a palpable abdominal mass and infrequently symptoms arise from rupture, haemorrhage, infection or ureteral obstruction. There have been isolated instances of simple cysts compressing adjacent blood vessels, causing renal ischaemia and hypertension reversible after surgical decompression.[80]

Gross and microscopic appearance

Simple cysts are usually unilocular, solitary and in the cortex; sometimes they are multiple and bilateral: rarely they occur in the medulla. They vary from a few millimetres to many centimetres in diameter and generally contain clear, pale yellow fluid. Larger cysts often project above the renal surface.[81] The cysts are lined by discontinuous flattened epithelium. The capsule consists of collagen and the adjacent renal parenchyma is compressed.

Differential diagnosis

When simple cysts are multiple and bilateral they must be distinguished from the milder examples of autosomal dominant polycystic kidney disease that are occasionally seen in older people. This is usually easily done by looking for the presence or absence of autosomal dominant transmission and for evidence that other organs are involved. In the very rare instance where, after doing this, uncertainty remains, chromosomal evidence of polycystic disease should be sought using a linked DNA probe derived from the alpha-globin region on the short arm of chromosome 16 (see page 62).

Pathogenesis

The pathogenesis of simple renal cysts is unknown. One theory is that they arise from the small diverticula that appear on the distal renal tubules with increasing frequency as people age (see page 25).[67,82] It is suggested that closure of the neck connecting one of these diverticula to the tubule from which it arose, leads to the formation of a simple cyst which then progressively enlarges; this process is facilitated if any intrarenal or urinary obstruction is present.[83] What causes a diverticulum to appear and then sequestrate to form a cyst is not known.

REFERENCES

Anatomy and histology of the kidneys

1. Hodson CJ. The renal parenchyma and its blood supply. Curr Probl Diagn Radiol 1978; 7:1–32
2. Sykes D. The arterial supply of the human kidney with special reference to accessory renal arteries. Br J Surg 1963; 50: 368–374.
3. Graves FT. The anatomy of the intrarenal arteries and its application to segmental resection of the kidney. Br J Surg 1954; 42: 132–139.
4. Warhol MJ, Sweet JM. The ultrastructural localisation of von Willebrand factor in endothelial cells. Am J Pathol 1984; 117: 310–315.
5. Weibel ER, Palade GE. New cytoplasmic components in arterial endothelia. J Cell Biol 1964; 23: 101–112.
6. Eschbach JW, Adamson JW. Recombinant human erythropoietin: implications for nephrology. Am J Kidney Dis 1988; 11: 203–209.
7. Fourman J, Moffat DB. The blood vessels of the kidney. Oxford: Blackwell, 1971.
8. Pease DC. Electron microscopy of the vascular bed of the kidney cortex. Anat Rec 1955; 121: 701–721.

9. Moffat DB. New ideas on the anatomy of the kidney. J Clin Pathol 1981; 34: 1197–1206.
10. Latta H, Johnston WK. The glycoprotein inner layer of glomerular capillary basement membrane as a filtration barrier. J Ultrastruct Res 1976; 57: 65–67.
11. Von Willebrand E, Lautenschlager I, Inkinen K, Lehto V-P, Virtanen I, Häyry P. Distribution of the major histocompatibility complex antigens in human and rat kidney. Kidney Int 1985; 27: 616–621.
12. Cerilli J, Brasile L, Galouzis T, Lempert N, Clarke J. The vascular endothelial cell antigen system. Transplantation 1985; 39: 286–289.
13. Jorgensen F, Bentzon MW. The ultrastructure of the normal human glomerulus. Thickness of glomerular basement membrane. Lab Invest 1968; 18: 42–48.
14. Kanwar YS. Biology of disease. Biophysiology of glomerular filtration and proteinuria. Lab Invest 1984; 51: 7–21.
15. Kanwar YS, Farquhar MG. Anionic sites in the glomerular basement membrane. In vivo and in vitro localisation to the laminae rarae by cationic probes. J Cell Biol 1979; 81: 137–153.
16. Brenner BM, Hostetter TH, Humes HD. Molecular basis of proteinuria of glomerular origin. N Engl J Med 1978; 298: 826–833.
17. Weislander J, Barr JF, Butkowski RJ, Edwards SJ, Bygren P, Heinegard D, Hudson BG. Goodpasture antigen of the glomerular basement membrane: localisation to non-collagenous region of type IV collagen. Proc Natl Acad Sci USA 1984; 81: 3838–3842.
18. Butkowski RJ, Weislander J, Wisdon BJ, Barr JF, Noelken ME, Hudson BG. Properties of the glomerular domain of type IV collagen and its relationship to the Goodpasture antigen. J Biol Chem 1985; 260: 3739–3747.
19. Pepys MB, Baltz ML. Acute phase proteins with special reference to C-reactive protein and related proteins and serum amyloid A protein. Adv Immunol 1983; 34: 141–212.
20. Dyck RF, Lockwood CM, Kershaw M, et al. Amyloid P component is a constituent of normal human glomerular basement membrane. J Exp Med 1980; 152: 1162–1174.
21. Melvin T, Kim Y, Michael AF. Amyloid P component is not present in the glomerular basement membrane in Alport-type hereditary nephritis. Am J Pathol 1986; 125: 460–464.
22. Rodewald R, Karnovsky MJ. Porous substructure of the glomerular slit diaphragm in the rat and mouse. J Cell Biol 1974; 60: 423–433.
23. Scheeberger EE, Levey RH, McCluskey RT, Karnovsky MJ. The isoporous substructure of the human glomerular slit diaphragm. Kidney Int 1975; 8: 48–52.
24. Trenchev P, Dorling J, Webb J, Holborow EJ. Localisation of smooth muscle-like contractile proteins in kidney by immunoelectron microscopy. J Anat 1976; 121: 85–95.
25. Andrews PM. Investigations of cytoplasmic contractile and cytoskeletal elements in the kidney glomerulus. Kidney Int 1981; 20: 549–562.
26. Kurtz SM, Feldman JD. Experimental studies on the formation of the glomerular basement membrane. J Ultrastruct Res 1962; 6: 19–27.
27. Striker GE, Savin V, Agodan L, Killen P. Glomerular cells *in vitro*. Contr Nephrol 1976; 2: 25–31.
28. Kazatchkine M, Fearon DT, Appay MD, Mandet Ch, Bariety J. Immunochemical study of the human glomerular C3b receptor in normal kidney and in seventy five cases of renal disease. J Clin Invest 1982; 69: 900–912.
29. Mancilla-Jimenez R, Appay M-D, Bellon B, Kuhn J, Bariety J Druet P. IgG Fc membrane receptor on normal human glomerular visceral epithelial cells. Virchows Arch [A] 1984; 404: 139–158.
30. Michael A, Keane WF, Raij L, Vernier RL, Mauer SM. The glomerular mesangium. Kidney Int 1980; 17: 141–154.
31. Latta H. The multipotential nature of mesangial cells. Biol Cell 1980; 39: 245–248.
32. Latta H, Maunsbach AB. Relations of the centrilobular region of the glomerulus to the juxtaglomerular apparatus. J Ultrastruct Res 1962; 6: 562–578.
33. Lovett DH, Szamel M, Ryan JL, Sterzel RB, Gemsa D, Resch K. Interleukin I and the glomerular mesangium 1. Purification and characterisation of a mesangial cell-derived autogrowth factor. J Immunol 1986; 136: 3700–3705.
34. Dinarello CA. Interleukin 1. Rev Infect Dis 1984; 6: 51–95.
35. Camazine SM, Ryan GB, Unanue ER, Karnovsky MJ. Isolation of phagocytic cells from the rat renal glomerulus. Lab Invest 1976; 35: 315–326.
36. Schreiner GF, Kiely JM, Cotran RS, Unanue ER. Characterisation of resident glomerular cells in the rat expressing Ia determinants and manifesting genetically restricted interactions with lymphocytes. J Clin Invest 1981; 68: 920–931.
37. Gurner A, Smith J, Cattell V. The origin of Ia antigen expressing cells in the rat kidney. Am J Pathol 1987; 127: 342–348.
38. Gurner A, Smith J, Cattell V. In vivo induction of Ia antigen in resident leucocytes in the normal rat renal glomerulus. Lab Invest 1986; 55: 546–550.
39. Marshall RJ, MacIver AG. The monocyte/macrophage population of the normal human kidney. J Pathol 1984; 143: 275–280.
40. Cook HT, Smith J, Salmon JA, Cattell V. Functional characteristics of macrophages in glomerulonephritis in the rat. O_2^- generation, MHC class II expression, and eicosanoid synthesis. Am J Pathol 1989; 134: 431–437.
41. Hart DNJ, Fuggle SV, Williams KA, Fabre JW, Ting A, Morris PJ. Localisation of HLA-ABC and DR antigens in human kidney. Transplantation 1981; 31: 428–433.
42. Alpers CE, Beckstead JH. Monocyte/macrophage derived cells in normal and transplanted human kidneys. Clin Immunol Immunopathol 1985; 36: 129–140.
43. Latta H, Fligiel S. Mesangial fenestrations, sieving, filtration and flow. Lab Invest 1985; 52: 591–598.
44. Lindop GBM, Lever AF. Anatomy of the renin–angiotensin system in the normal and pathological kidney. Histopathology 1986; 10: 335–362.
45. Barajas L, Salido E. Juxtaglomerular apparatus and the renin–angiotensin sytem. Lab Invest 1986; 54: 361–364.
46. Bowie DJ. A method for staining the pepsinogen granules in gastric glands. Anat Rev 1935; 64: 357–367.
47. Celio MR. Angiotensin II immuno-reactivity coexisting with renin in the human juxtaglomerular epithelioid cells. Kidney Int 1982; 22: suppl 12, S30–S32.
48. Cantin M, Gutkowska J, Lacasse J, et al. Ultrastructural

immunocytochemical localisation of renin and angiotensin II in the juxtaglomerular cells of the ischaemic kidney in experimental renal hypertension. Am J Pathol 1984; 115: 212–224.
49. Webb DJ, Cumming AMM, Adams FC et al. Renal secretion of inactive renin and extraction of angiotensin II in renal artery stenosis in man: factors determining renal vein renin ratio. J Hypertens 1985; 2: suppl 3, 255–258.
50. Leckie BJ, McIntyre GD. Binding of human renin to plasma proteins and comparison with plasma active and inactive renin. J Hypertens 1985; 3: 73–80.
51. Barajas L, Powers K. The structure of the juxtaglomerular apparatus (JGA) and the control of renin secretion: an update. J Hypertens 1984; 2: suppl 1, 3–12.
52. Ryan GB, Coghlan JP, Scoggins BA. The granulated peripolar cell: a potential secretory component of the renal juxtaglomerular complex. Nature 1979; 277: 655–656.
53. Gardiner DS, Lindop GBM. The granular peripolar cell of the human glomerulus: a new component of the juxtaglomerular apparatus. Histopathology 1985; 9: 675–685.
54. Sikri KL, Foster CL, McHugh N, Marshall RD. Localisation of Tamm–Horsfall glycoprotein in the human kidney using immunofluorescence and immunoelectron microscopical techniques. J Anat 1981; 132: 579–605.
55. Dunn MJ. Renal prostaglandins. In: Dunn MJ, ed. Renal endocrinology. Baltimore: Williams and Wilkins, 1983: 1–74.

Effects of ageing on the kidneys

56. Lindeman RD. Kidney and body fluids. In: Masoro EJ, ed. CRC handbook of physiology in ageing. Boca Raton: CRC, 1981: 75–191.
57. Hollenberg NK, Adams DF, Solomon HS et al. Senescence and the renal vasculature in normal man. Circ Res 1974; 34: 309–316.
58. Kasiske BL. Relationship between vascular disease and age-associated changes in the human kidney. Kidney Int 1987; 31: 1153–1159.
59. Rowe JW, Andres R, Tobin JD, Norris AK, Shock NW. The effect of age on creatinine clearance in men: a cross sectional and longitudinal study. J Gerontol 1976; 31: 155–163.
60. Goyal VK. Changes with age in the human kidney. Exp Gerontol 1982; 17: 321–333.
61. McManus JFA, Lupton CH. Ischaemic obsolescence of renal glomeruli. The natural history of the lesions and their relation to hypertension. Lab Invest 1960; 9: 413–434.
62. Ljungqvist A, Lagergren C. Normal intrarenal arterial pattern in adult and ageing human kidney. A micro-angiographical and histological study. J Anat 1962; 96: 285–300.
63. Takazakura E, Sawabu N, Handa A, Takada A, Shinoda A, Takeuchi J. Intrarenal vascular changes with age and disease. Kidney Int 1972; 2: 224–230.
64. Kaplan C, Pasternack B, Shah H, Gallo G. Age related incidence of sclerotic glomeruli in human kidneys. Am J Pathol 1975; 80: 227–234.
65. Kappel B, Olsen S. Cortical interstitial tissue and sclerosed glomeruli in the normal human kidney, related to age and sex. A quantitative study. Virchows Arch [A] 1980; 387: 271–277.
66. Smith SM, Hoy WE, Cobb L. Low incidence of glomerulosclerosis in normal kidneys. Arch Pathol Lab Med 1989; 113: 1253–1255.
67. Darmady EM, MacIver AG. Renal pathology. London: Butterworths, 1980: 57.
68. Brenner BM, Meyer TW, Hostetter TH. Dietary protein intake and the progressive nature of kidney disease. N Engl J Med 1982; 307: 652–659.
69. Shimamura T, Morrison AB. A progressive glomerulosclerosis occuring in partial five-sixths nephrectomized rats. Am J Pathol 1975; 79: 95–101.
70. Masoro EJ, Yu BP. Diet and nephropathy. Lab Invest 1989; 60: 165–167.

Effects of reducing the amount of renal tissue: the solitary kidney

71. Hostetter TH, Rennke HG, Brenner BM. Compensatory renal haemodynamic injury: a final common pathway of residual nephron destruction. Am J Kidney Dis 1982; 1: 310–314.
72. Olson JL, De Urdaneta AG, Heptinstall RH. Glomerular hyalinosis and its relation to hyperfiltration. Lab Invest 1985; 52: 387–398.
73. Hostetter TH, Olson JL, Rennke HG, Venkatachalam MA, Brenner BM. Hyperfiltration in remnant nephrons: a potentially adverse response to renal ablation. Am J Physiol 1981; 241: F85–93.
74. Zucchelli P, Cagnoli L, Casanova S, et al. Focal glomerulosclerosis in patients with unilateral nephrectomy. Kidney Int 1983; 24: 649–655.
75. Vincenti F, Amend WJC, Kaysen G, et al. Long-term renal function in kidney donors. Substantial compensatory hyperfiltration with no adverse effects. Transplantation 1983; 36: 626–629.
76. Fotino S. The solitary kidney: a model of chronic hyperfiltration in humans. Am J Kidney Dis 1989; 13: 88–98.
77. Schmitz A, Christensen CK, Christensen I, Solling K. No microalbuminuria or other adverse effects of long standing hyperfiltration in humans with one kidney. Am J Kidney Dis 1989; 13: 131–136.

Simple renal cysts

78. Tada S, Yamagishi J, Kobayashi H, Hata Y, Kobari T. The incidence of simple renal cysts by computed tomography. Clin Radiol 1983; 34. 437–439.
79. Siegel MJ, McAlister WH. Simple cysts of the kidney in children. J Urol 1980; 123: 75–78.
80. Rose HJ, Pruitt DW. Hypertension, hyperreninemia with a solitary renal cyst in an adolescent. Am J Med 1976; 61: 579–581.
81. Clarke BG, Hurwitz IS, Dubinsky E. Solitary serous cysts of the kidney: biochemical, cytologic and histologic studies. J. Urol 1956; 75: 772–778.
82. Fetterman GH. Microdissection in the study of normal and abnormal renal structure and function. Pathol Annu 1970; 5: 173–205.
83. Baert L, Steg A. Diverticula on distal tubules, simple renal cysts, and ureteral obstruction. Causal relationship. Urology 1978; 11:221–224.

2

K. A. Porter

Pathological changes in uraemia and dialysis

PATHOLOGY OF URAEMIA

When renal function becomes impaired, the plasma urea concentration rises (a condition called *azotaemia*). Initially this produces no symptoms, but when the glomerular filtration rate falls below about 10% of normal a clinical syndrome, termed *uraemia*, may be produced. Uraemia is always associated with an increase in plasma urea and plasma creatinine concentration; oliguria (a total daily urinary output of less than 400 ml) is frequent but not invariable. The patients have symptoms of gastrointestinal, neurological, mental, haematological and vascular disorders together with twitching of the muscles and a foetid or ammoniacal odour to the breath. If untreated they die in coma. The retention of phenols, guanidines, indoles, abnormal amino acids and undetermined substances, including 'middle molecules' of MW 500–3000 daltons, have all been blamed as the cause of the symptoms.[1,2] Hypertension, anaemia, circulatory failure and sodium depletion with dehydration, acidosis, hypercalcaemia and potassium retention, may all play a part in producing the syndrome. The raised plasma urea contributes to gastrointestinal irritation due to the conversion of urea to ammonia, but is otherwise probably relatively unimportant.

The renal insufficiency that results in uraemia may be due to three main categories of causes.[3]

The first of these is *prerenal* and is due to inadequate perfusion of the kidney by blood. Causes of prerenal uraemia are:

1. A fall in effective arterial blood volume due to:
   a. Decrease in intravascular blood volume because of either haemorrhage or plasma loss after burns.
   b. Decrease in extravascular fluid because of protracted vomiting or diarrhoea, diabetes insipidus or excessive sweating.
   c. Expansion of volume of vascular bed in sepsis, anaphylaxis and ganglionic blockage.
   d. A shift of fluid from within vessels to the surrounding tissues as with ascites, pancreatitis and peritonitis.
2. Cardiac failure, due to either congestive cardiac failure or massive pulmonary embolus.

Glomerular filtration falls and the plasma urea concentration rises rapidly as the reduced amount filtered is largely reabsorbed. Creatinine, not being reabsorbed, shows much less increase in plasma concentration. The mechanisms involved in prerenal failure have recently been reviewed.[4] The second category of causes of uraemia is *renal* and is the result of intrinsic renal disease, such as glomerulonephritis or interstitial nephritis, vascular disease such as malignant hypertension or microscopic polyarteritis, some other systemic disease involving the kidneys such as systemic lupus erythematosus or amyloidosis, renal injury due to some nephrotoxin such as one of the aminoglycosides, or acute tubular necrosis. The third category is *postrenal*, a synonym for urinary tract obstruction.

In uraemia histopathological changes may be encountered in the heart, arteries, lungs, gastrointestinal tract, pancreas, haemopoietic system, lymphoid system, nervous system or bones and joints.

HEART

Pericarditis[5]

A serofibrinous pericarditis of some degree is present in 30–50% of patients with uraemia, but in only about 6–17% does it produce signs or symptoms. Some patients who are on dialysis may later develop pericarditis which is often characterized by bleeding and in about 20% of cases is complicated by tamponade. They are referred to as having *dialysis-associated pericarditis* as opposed to *classic uraemic pericarditis*.

Many cases of uraemic pericarditis rapidly respond to dialysis and heal with the production of fibrous tissue. Occasionally this gives rise to constrictive pericarditis. Uraemic pericarditis is often thought to be caused by one or more of the biochemical alterations seen in uraemia, but how this may come about is far from clear. In some cases fluid overload appears to be an important contributory factor because, although the capacity to dilute urine in chronic renal failure becomes severely limited only at very low glomerular filtration rates, overhydration will lead to water retention.

In dialysis-associated pericarditis a number of studies indicate that the level of uraemia is not the most important factor and in some cases it would appear to be a viral pericarditis.

Oxalate deposits[6]

In uraemic patients extensive deposits of calcium oxalate are often found in the myocardial interstitium, and within the muscle fibres. The deposits are usually surrounded by chronic inflammatory cells and fibrosis.[6] Congestive cardiac failure may result and crystal deposits in the bundle branches can lead to conduction disturbances.[7] Oxalic acid is a metabolic end-product whose sole route of excretion is the kidney. In patients with uraemia the plasma concentration of oxalate is chronically elevated which results in tissue deposits and secondary oxalosis (see p. 545).[8]

Calcification of the myocardium

Myocardial calcification may occur as a consequence of secondary hyperparathyroidism. It may involve the atrioventricular node and conduction bundles.

Cardiac enlargement

Cardiac enlargement is common in uraemia mainly

because of the increased incidence of hypertension in these patients, but other factors such as anaemia, hypervolaemia and high cardiac output due to inappropriately large arteriovenous shunts used for haemodialysis also contribute. It has been suggested that there is a specific uraemic cardiomyopathy but this remains controversial.

ARTERIES

When secondary hyperparathyroidism is present *calcium deposits* are found in the media of many arteries. In secondary oxalosis *deposits of calcium oxalate* are common in arterial walls. Many patients with chronic renal failure show type IV hyperlipoproteinaemia[5] and *severe atherosclerosis* but there is no clear evidence that the progress of this lesion is accelerated by uraemia.

LUNGS[9]

Pleuritis (pleurisy)

A fibrinous pleuritis occurs in about 20% of patients with uraemia. There may also be pleural effusion, sometimes haemorrhagic.

Pulmonary oedema

Pulmonary oedema is a well-recognized complication of uraemia. Microscopically the pulmonary septa are widened and the alveoli and smaller bronchioles contain a fibrin-rich fluid. Organization may occur with the production of areas of fibrosis. The oedema is probably caused by a combination of high hydrostatic pressure in the central circulation, low intravascular protein pressure and increased permeability of the pulmonary capillaries.

Pulmonary infections

Pulmonary infections are a major cause of death in acute renal failure and an important cause of morbidity and mortality in chronic renal failure. Increased susceptibility to infection results from the deleterious effects of uraemia on the patient's defences. Delayed hypersensitivity and the ability of phagocytes to ingest bacteria are impaired. The incidence of tuberculosis among patients with chronic renal failure is higher than in the general population. In the USA the incidence is 3.6–6.1% in patients with uraemia compared with 0.015% in the general population; in India the incidence in one centre was 11.5% compared with 1.3% in the general population.[10]

Pulmonary calcification

Pulmonary calcification may occur in alveolar septa and is associated with fibrosis. The incidence does not correlate with the severity or duration of uraemia. Plasma calcium and parathyroid hormone levels are normal. Pulmonary calcification in uraemic patients may run a brief, fatal course. The aetiology is not known.

GASTROINTESTINAL TRACT[11]

Uraemic gastroenterocolitis

The commonest lesions are oedema and punctate haemorrhages in the mucosa and submucosa affecting mainly the oesophagus, stomach, ileum and proximal colon. Less frequently there are confluent and superficial ulcers which are most marked in the ileum and colon. Bleeding into the gut lumen may occur from any of these lesions and spontaneous perforation of the colon has been reported. The tendency to bleed that occurs in uraemia seems to be the factor that initiates these lesions. Mucosal and submucosal haemorrhage is followed by bacterial invasion, necrosis and ulceration. There is no correlation between the plasma urea concentration and the occurrence of uraemic gastroenterocolitis.

Other lesions

About 60% of patients with uraemia develop *duodenitis*, 22% *gastritis* and 13% *oesophagitis*. *Parotitis* and *stomatitis* may also occur.

PANCREAS[11]

Acinar dilatation, flattening of epithelial lining cells and inspissation of secretions are common in the pancreas in uraemia, whether treated with haemodialysis or not. Involvement is often unsuspected despite symptoms. In one series 56% of the uraemic patients had significant pancreatic dis ease. Although none had ever been diagnosed as having had pancreatic disease, 86% had complained of epigastric pain, nausea or vomiting at some time during their course and 81% had at least one record of a raised level of serum amylase.[12] Acute pancreatitis is relatively uncommon except after renal transplantation.[13]

HAEMOPOIETIC SYSTEM[14]

Anaemia

Anaemia is almost always present in uraemia; it is usually normochromic and normocytic, the reticulocyte index is low relative to the severity of the anaemia, and the serum iron is normal or high. The anaemia is caused primarily by a decrease in erythropoietin due to damage and loss of the sites of production in the kidney. Erythropoietin is very low or absent from the plasma of most uraemic patients who have anaemia. The anaemia is least severe in patients with adult polycystic disease (see p. 61);[15] patients whose non-functioning, previously shrunken kidneys develop acquired cystic disease (see p. 39) frequently show a striking rise in haemoglobin and serum erythropoietin levels despite an unchanged uraemic state.[16] Why the erythropoietin levels rise is unknown. Treatment of this anaemia is now possible. The gene coding for erythropoietin has been cloned[17] and recombinant human erythropoietin has been used to treat patients.[18] Iron deficiency is only common in those uraemic patients who are treated by chronic haemodialysis. The red cells adhere to the dialysis membrane and up to 11 ml may be lost in this manner at each dialysis. Some reduction in the life span of the red cells also occurs in all uraemic patients. This is caused by reversible damage to the Na-K-ATPase in the red cell membrane brought about by unidentified substances in the plasma. Many of these patients require regular blood transfusions with their attendant risks of hepatitis, acquired immunodeficiency syndrome and iron overload. About 75% of anaemic patients also have an acquired abnormality of pentose-phosphate shunt which results in decreased generation of phosphorylated nicotinamide-adenine dinucleotide (NADPH) and of reduced glutathione. This defect makes the haemoglobin vulnerable to oxidative damage and some patients develop haemolysis when exposed to oxidizing drugs such as primaquine, quinidine, sulphonamides and nitrofurantoin.

Tendency to haemorrhage[19]

Patients with uraemia often develop haemorrhagic complications. These have been attributed predominantly to platelet dysfunction which induces decreased platelet adhesiveness and aggregation in response to adenosine diphosphate (ADP), and decreased release of platelet factor III. The platelet dysfunction is caused by elevated plasma concentrations of toxic metabolites such as guanidinosuccinic acid, phenols and urea. The level in the plasma of the prostacyclin $PG1_2$ is also raised in uraemic patients and may contribute to decreased platelet function by inhibiting platelet aggregation. All these substances are readily removed by dialysis.

Granulocyte dysfunction

The number of granulocytes in uraemic patients is normal but their chemotactic function is abnormal; this may account for the increased incidence of bacterial infections in uraemia. Granulocyte dysfunction is only partly corrected by haemodialysis.

MONONUCLEAR PHAGOCYTE SYSTEM

Macrophages are important in the host's defence against infection, particularly systemic infection with *Streptococcus pneumoniae* and other encapsulated organisms, because these cells have Fc_γ receptors which recognize bacteria that are coated with antibody. The function of the receptors is impaired in uraemia.[20]

Monocytes express two Fc_γ-receptor proteins, $Fc_\gamma RI$ and $Fc_\gamma RII$. The defect in uraemia seems to lie in $Fc_\gamma RI$ function. The expression of this receptor is regulated by steroid hormones and other analogues; alterations in the metabolism of the hormones in patients with end-stage renal disease may be the cause of the depressed expression of the $Fc_{\gamma}RI$ receptor.[20]

LYMPHOID SYSTEM

A number of T (thymus dependent) lymphocyte functions, including delayed cutaneous hypersensitivity, skin allograft rejection and *in vitro* response to mitogens, are impaired in untreated uraemia.[21] Some of these defects are reversed by dialysis. Their practical significance in uraemic patients is in doubt because the most prevalent organisms responsible for infections in this group of patients are those which typically cause infections in individuals with granulocyte dysfunction or granulocytopenia rather than in those with abnormalities of T lymphocytes.

NERVOUS SYSTEM[22]

Encephalopathy

The major change is degeneration of neurones with relative preservation of glial components. Lesions are commonest in the sensory nuclei of the brain stem, the reticular formation and the cerebral cortex.

Myopathy

The onset is insidious and affects particularly the quadriceps and hip flexors and the shoulder abductors. There is atrophy of type II muscle fibres and variation in size of fibres.

Neuropathy

About 50% of uraemic patients have clinical or electromyographic evidence of *peripheral neuropathy*. In affected nerves there is loss of large myelinated fibres and swelling and fragmentation of the myelin sheath in many of the survivors. As a response to the axonal injury there is chromatolysis and dispersion of the Nissl substance in the anterior horn cells of the spinal cord. In addition to peripheral neuropathy, uraemia may injure the autonomic nervous system. It is not known which circulating toxins are responsible for these injuries.

REPRODUCTIVE SYSTEM[23]

In uraemia *testicular abnormalities* are common, ranging from impaired spermatogenesis to germinal cell aplasia and alterations in the morphology of the interstitial cells. *Cystic ovarian disease* is also more common. The pathogenesis is complex, involving both hypothalamic-pituitary dysfunction and direct uraemic intoxication of reproductive tissue.

BONES AND JOINTS[24]

Renal osteodystrophy[25]

Patients with uraemia develop a wide range of metabolic bone diseases, none of which is specific for chronic renal failure. These disorders are frequently, though not invariably, found in combination and are collectively described as renal osteodystrophy. Pathologically, there may be various combinations of osteitis fibrosa cystica, osteomalacia, osteosclerosis, generalized osteoporosis and subchondral resorption of bone. There are geographical differences with osteitis fibrosa cystica predominating in the USA and osteomalacia in the UK. Renal osteodystrophy is probably caused by a variety of metabolic derangements: these include impaired vitamin D metabolism, phosphate retention, skeletal resistance to parathormone and disordered calcium and phosphate metabolism.[26]

Arthritis[24]

Acute arthritis

Acute arthritis may occur in uraemic patients. It is most commonly caused by crystals of either sodium urate, which give *gout*, or calcium pyrophosphate dihydrate, which produce *pseudogout*. Acute gouty arthritis is commonest in patients with chronic renal disease due to lead intoxication. Calcium pyrophosphate dihydrate is deposited in cartilage, producing chondrocalcinosis affecting particularly the knees, wrists, symphysis pubis and shoulders. When crystals of calcium pyrophosphate dihydrate are shed into the joint space they induce an acute arthritis. Both gout and pseudogout are more frequent in patients with hyperparathyroidism.

Bone and joint infections

Uraemic patients are more likely to develop osteomyelitis and infective arthritis.

PATHOLOGICAL CHANGES IN URAEMIC PATIENTS UNDERGOING DIALYSIS

Long-term haemodialysis prolongs uraemia, modifies its symptoms and is associated with new disorders.

ALUMINIUM INTOXICATION

Aluminium intoxication causes three disorders: a neurological syndrome, called dialysis encephalopathy; a severe form of osteomalacia; and a worsening of the anaemia of uraemia. All three occur together in many patients undergoing dialysis with dialysate prepared from tapwater that contains large amounts of aluminium. The oral administration of aluminium-containing phosphate-binding gels to uraemic patients may also cause aluminium intoxication. These gels are used to trap phosphorus in the small intestine and reduce the amount that is absorbed, avoiding the risk of nephrocalcinosis and renal osteodystrophy; however, the aluminium in the gels is absorbed. The problem is avoided if calcium carbonate is used instead of aluminium hydroxide.

DIALYSIS ENCEPHALOPATHY[27]

Dialysis encephalopathy is a progressive neurological disease which usually causes death in 6–8 months. It is characterized by speech impediments (e.g. dysarthria and dyspraxia), myoclonus, grand mal seizures and dementia. Neuropathological changes are slight with loss of Purkinje cells from the cerebellum and non-specific gliosis, accumulation of lipofuscin and focal oedema.

Aluminium is toxic to the central nervous system partly because it inhibits a number of enzymes, including hexokinase (a magnesium-dependent phosphorylating enzyme) and synaptosomal Na-K-ATPase and Mg-ATPase. Aluminium also displaces magnesium from adenosine triphosphate (ATP), which prevents the transfer of phosphate, and aluminium inhibits calmodulin activity. Finally, aluminium displaces copper from some of its metalloenzymes; copper is essential for brain cytochrome oxidase activity.

Aluminium-associated osteomalacia[28,29]

This form of osteomalacia is associated with bone pain, fractures, severe skeletal deformity and a myopathy; serum alkaline phosphatase is usually normal or low and serum calcium normal or slightly raised. It is unresponsive to vitamin D and to calcitriol. Although there are radiological and biochemical clues to the diagnosis, undecalcified bone biopsy is the only certain way of making the diagnosis. Histochemical stains, using aluminon, the ammonium salt of aurine tricarboxylic acid,[30] reveal aluminium in the mineralizing layer of the osteoid (Fig. 2.1). In vitro, aluminium impairs hydroxyapatite maturation and collagen synthesis by osteoblasts.[31,32] Insulin-dependent diabetics and patients who have undergone parathyroidectomy are particularly at risk, probably because in both conditions there is a decrease in bone formation which allows more time for the deposition of aluminium on quiescent bone surfaces.

Aluminium-induced anaemia[33]

Aluminium causes a hypochromic microcytic non-iron-deficiency anaemia and is one factor responsible for a worsening anaemia in a patient who is being treated with haemodialysis.

Prophylaxis of aluminium intoxication

The incidence of all three conditions can be greatly reduced by ensuring that the dialysate contains less than 10 μg of aluminium per litre. A few cases also occur in small children with uraemia who have been given large doses of aluminium-containing phosphate-binding gels to control their serum phosphate levels and reduce their chances of developing metastatic calcification. However, many uraemic patients undergoing long-term dialysis receive moderate doses of aluminium compounds which they retain. Since such patients now survive for 20 years or more, the fear is that

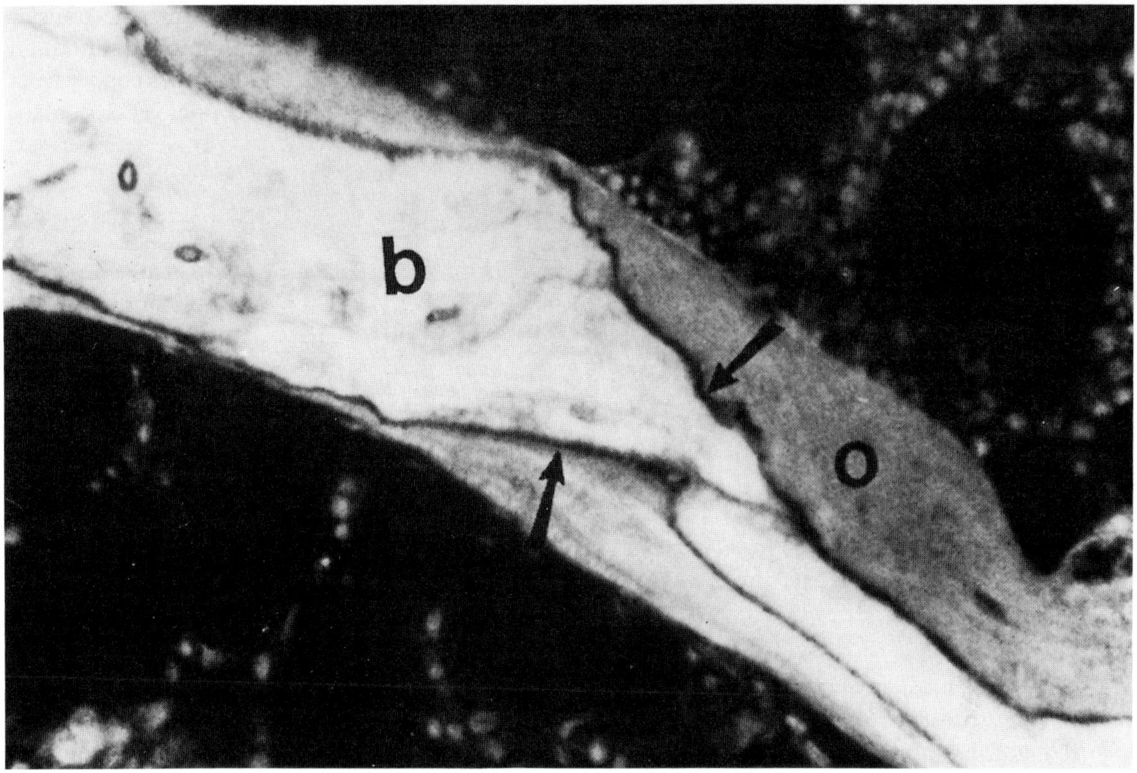

Fig. 2.1 Aluminium deposition in the mineralizing layer of the osteoid. The aluminium stains an intense red and is the dark linear deposit (arrows) at the interface between calcified bone (b) and osteoid (o). Aurine tricarboxylic stain × 36
Reproduced by permission from: Faugere M-C, Malluche HH. Kidney Int 1986; 30: 717 (Fig. 1).

this ever-increasing accumulation of aluminium in the body may eventually lead to aluminium toxicity. Patients with plasma aluminium levels higher than 100 µg/l are most at risk and may require modification of their aluminium therapy.

ACQUIRED RENAL CYSTIC DISEASE

About 44% of patients whose lives are prolonged by dialysis develop multiple small cysts in both kidneys.[34–37] The disorder is rare in patients who have been dialysed for less than 3 years but it becomes increasingly common and severe as the duration of dialysis increases. Usually no symptoms are produced but bleeding may occur into the renal collecting system causing blood clots and macroscopic haematuria. Haemorrhage within the kidney or extending retroperitoneally may cause pain in the loin or abdomen. The diagnosis of cystic disease is established by computed tomography (Fig. 2.2). Acquired cystic disease may stabilize or regress after renal transplantation.[38] The major importance of acquired cystic disease of the kidney is its association with tumours (see p. 40).

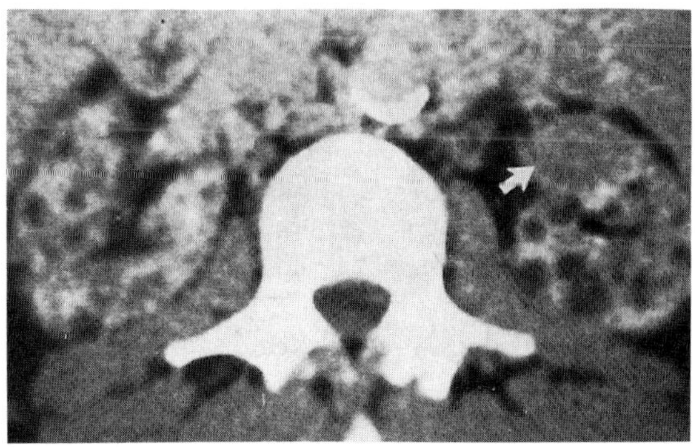

Fig. 2.2 Post-contrast computed tomography scan. There are multiple cysts in both kidneys and a small tumour (arrow) in the left kidney.
Reproduced by permission from: Levine E, Grantham JJ, Slusher SL, Greathouse JL, Krohn BP. Am J Roentgenol 1984; 142: 125 (Fig. 1B)

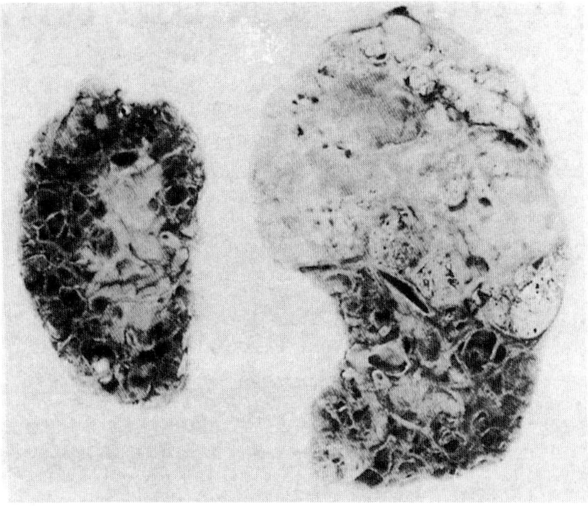

Fig. 2.3 Acquired cystic change in both kidneys with large tumour at upper pole of right kidney and small one at lower pole.
Reproduced by permission from: Ratcliffe PJ, Dunnill MS, Oliver DO. Br Med J 1983; 287: 1855 (Fig. 2)

The cortex is most affected but some cysts also occur in the medulla. Most of the cysts are less than 0.5 cm in diameter and contain either clear or blood-stained fluid (Fig. 2.3). Usually the affected kidneys remain small but occasionally they enlarge and come to resemble those of autosomal dominant polycystic disease. Microdissection suggests that the cysts begin as tubular dilatations or pouches. The majority of the cysts are lined by cuboidal or columnar epithelium with a large vesicular nucleus and granular eosinophile cytoplasm; some of the lining cells have a brush border. A few cysts are lined by a multilayer epithelium which has papillary projections and frequent mitoses. Calcium oxalate crystals are common in the cyst walls and lumens.

The pathogenesis of acquired renal cystic disease is not known, but there is evidence to suggest that when large numbers of nephrons are lost there is increased production of poorly defined chemicals, collectively referred to as renotropic factors, that cause hyperplasia and cystic change in the tubules.[39] The process may be aggravated by tubular obstruction from oxalate crystal deposition and interstitial fibrosis.

RENAL TUMOURS

About 10–20% of patients with acquired renal cystic disease also have renal tumours.[34,35,40] Most appear to be benign but 3–6% are malignant (Fig. 2.3). The benign tumours are adenomas and either arise in the cyst wall and are papillary, projecting into the cyst cavity, or they arise between the cysts and are composed of tubular structures. The malignant tumours are usually adenocarcinomas (Fig. 2.4); they sometimes extend into the renal veins or show systemic metastases. About 7% of the adenocarcinomas are bilateral. Renal cell carcinomas occurring in association with acquired renal cystic disease are discussed further on page 571. Transitional cell carcinomas also occur occasionally in the pelvis, calyces and ureter.

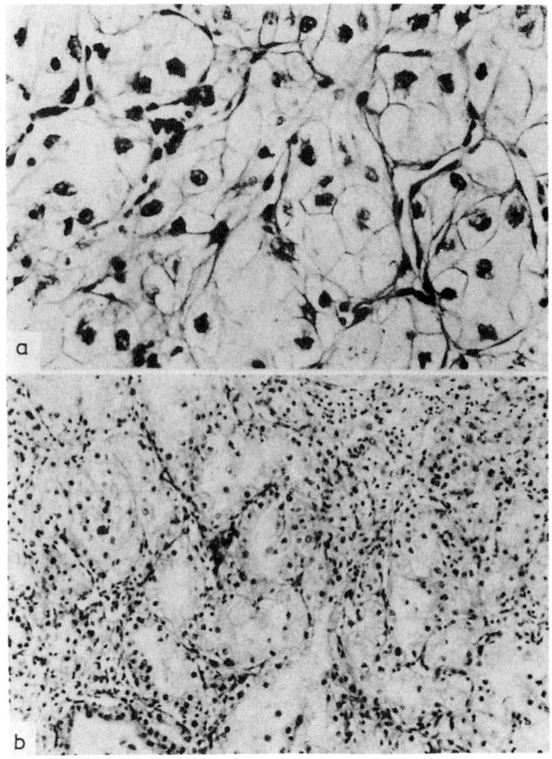

Fig. 2.4 Renal cell carcinoma arising in acquired polycystic kidney. Same case as shown in Figure 2.3.
(**a**) Typical clear cell adenocarcinoma in upper pole of right kidney.
(**b**) Metastatic tumour in lung.
Haematoxylin-eosin **a** × 204; **b** × 80
Reproduced by permission from: Ratcliffe PJ, Dunnill MS, Oliver DO. Br Med J 1983; 287: 1855 (Fig. 3)

AMYLOIDOSIS – β_2-MICROGLOBULIN IN TYPE

White nodules of amyloid, compressing the median

nerve, are sometimes found in the perineurium or on the synovium inside the carpal tunnel of patients on chronic haemodialysis who develop the carpal tunnel syndrome (see below).[41,42] Amyloid deposits are also found in bone in chronic haemodialysis patients who develop a severe arthropathy with shoulder and joint pain and stiffness,[43,44] or present with pathological hip fractures.[45] The bone deposits appear as lytic defects in skeletal radiographs (Fig. 2.5a). Deposits sometimes occur in the rectum,[46] stomach or colon[47] and there may be progression to systemic amyloidosis.[48,49]

Amyloidosis is a disorder characterized by extracellular deposits of an abnormal protein that is insoluble in physiological fluids (see p. 344). The deposits may be localized or systemic. They stain pinkish-orange with Congo red and display a pathognomonic green birefringence when viewed in polarized light. The ultrastructure of all types of amyloid is the same: a feltwork of unbranched fibrils 7.5–10 nm in diameter (Fig. 2.6). Associated with the protein fibrils there is a small quantity of a non-fibrillar glycoprotein of the pentraxin family known as amyloid P component (the letter P was used because of its pentagonal ultrastructure). The chemical composition of the fibrils is not constant; it differs with the underlying disorder that has caused the amyloid to form.[50] Amyloid P component is always the same. Amyloid is classified according to the chemical composition of the fibrils (see p. 344).

The subunits of the fibrils in the amyloid deposits encountered in uraemic patients who have been dialysed for long periods are composed of β_2-microglobulin (Fig. 2.5b).[46,51] This low molecular weight protein, which has been identified as the light chain of HLA-A, -B and -C antigens, is non-covalently attached to MHC class I heavy chains and is essential to their serological specificity and cell surface expression.[52] As a result of metabolism and degradation of HLA, β_2-microglobulin is dissociated from the heavy chain and appears in the extracellular fluid and plasma. About 95% of all free β_2-microglobulin is filtered by the normal glomerulus and subsequently almost completely reabsorbed and catabolized by the cells of the proximal tubules.[53] In patients with advanced renal insufficiency, filtration and catabolism are impaired or non-existent and greatly increased serum concentrations of β_2- microglobulin occur.

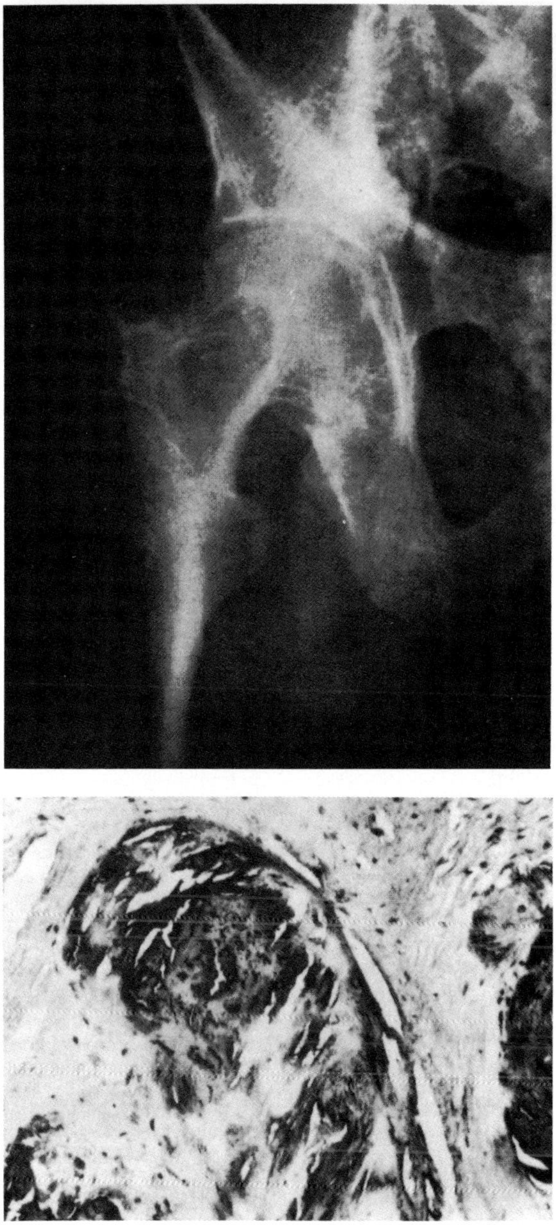

a

b

Fig. 2.5 (**a**) Radiograph showing amyloid, β_2 -microglobulin in type, producing osteolytic lesion in neck of femur. (**b**) Light microscopy of amyloid deposit seen in (**a**). The amyloid has been stained with human anti-β_2-microglobulin. (**b**) Immunoperoxidase with haematoxylin counterstain × 125

Reproduced by permission from: Bardin T, Zingraff T, Noël L-H, et al. Am J Med 1987; 83: 419 (Figs 1, 3)

There is little or no clearance of the protein by the commonly used dialysis membranes[54] and β_2-microglobulin accumulates in the tissues where it is transformed into insoluble amyloid fibrils.

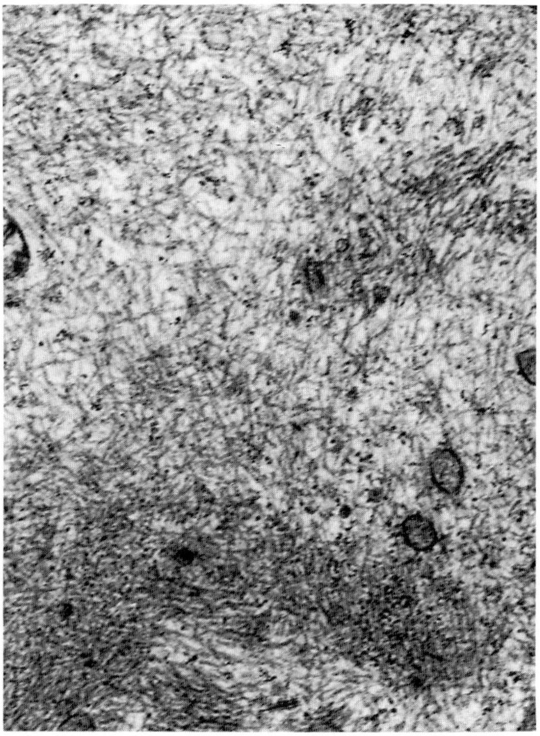

Fig. 2.6 Fibrillar structure of amyloid (β_2-microglobulin in type) from synovial nodule in chronically dialysed patient suffering from carpal tunnel syndrome.
Electron microscopy × 37 760

The incidence of β_2-microglobulin-related amyloidosis is increasing as the number of long-term haemodialysis patients rises. This could have important implications for the future of dialysis. There is evidence that the use of highly permeable polyacrylonitrile dialysis membranes rather than the standard cuprophane membranes allows clearing of β_2-microglobulin from the circulation.[55] This has prompted some dialysis units to abandon the use of cuprophane membranes in treating long-term patients.[56] It remains to be seen if haemodialysis which ensures β_2-microglobulin excretion close to the normal catabolic rate of the protein will prevent dialysis amyloidosis. β_2-microglobulin-associated amyloidosis has also been reported in patients on continuous ambulatory peritoneal dialysis (CAPD).[57]

CARPAL TUNNEL SYNDROME

About 12% of patients treated by chronic haemodialysis develop a carpal tunnel syndrome and the incidence rises with duration of dialysis.[58] In some the syndrome is caused by deposition of β_2-microglobulin-derived amyloid in the perineurium of the median nerve, the synovium of the flexor tendons and the transverse carpal ligament.[59] In others no appreciable changes are found in biopsies of these structures and the pathogenesis remains obscure.[58]

EOSINOPHILIA

Eosinophilia is often present in uraemia but is particularly frequent in patients being treated by haemodialysis.[60] The raised count is reflected in the composition of any cellular infiltrate that may occur in the kidneys of these patients. The cause of the eosinophilia is not known. It may be part of a reaction to the cellulose membranes that are commonly used in haemodialysis: the eosinophil count falls when the membranes are changed to ones composed of polyacrylonitrile.[61]

DIALYSIS-ASSOCIATED PERICARDITIS

This has been discussed earlier (see p. 34).

URINARY STONES

Urinary matrix calculi are common in patients on haemodialysis.[62] They are also occasionally seen in the kidneys of patients with chronic renal failure who are not on dialysis. The calculi are composed of protein, have a microfibrillar structure and seem in part to be derived from β_2-microglobulin. It has been suggested that calculi, by obstructing nephrons, may contribute to the progression of renal failure and the genesis of acquired renal cystic disease.[63]

OSTEONECROSIS (AVASCULAR NECROSIS)

Occasionally patients on maintenance haemodialysis, who have never received corticosteroid treatment, develop osteonecrosis. In a few of these patients β_2-microglobulin-associated amyloidosis is responsible. In others the pathogenesis is unknown.

INFECTIOUS HEPATITIS[64]

Infectious hepatitis is a major problem for patients with end-stage renal disease and for staff caring for these patients. In the early years of haemodialysis most cases were caused by the hepatitis B virus (HBV), but in recent years non-A, non-B hepatitis has emerged as the most frequent cause. Hepatitis A, which is rarely transmitted by blood, has never been a problem among dialysis patients. Dialysis patients when infected with HBV only occasionally develop symptoms of acute hepatitis but they are very likely to become chronic carriers of hepatitis B virus surface antigen (HB_sAg). This is because of changes in their immune responses induced by uraemia (see p. 37). About 60% of the patients who become carriers develop chronic active hepatitis, chronic persistent hepatitis or cirrhosis.[65] Healthy dialysis staff, on the other hand, when infected frequently develop acute symptomatic disease and rarely become carriers. However, these days screening blood products for HBV, avoiding pricks with contaminated needles, decontamination of equipment and other infection control measures have led to a great reduction in the occurrence of hepatitis B both in dialysis patients and in staff. With the development of hepatitis B vaccines the protection of patients and staff is now possible but the present vaccines, although highly efficient for dialysis staff, do not appear to be as immunogenic or as effective in dialysis patients.

Despite the successful control of hepatitis B infection, hepatitis in dialysis patients still occurs. Other forms of viral hepatitis have emerged, particularly that due to hepatitis C. The incidence of this form of hepatitis is low in Britain but has been as high as 20–27% in some hospital dialysis units in Spain[66] and the USA.[67] Some of these patients progress to chronic liver disease; in one series of 29 patients, eight still had elevated transaminase levels 5–7 years later and liver biopsy revealed chronic persistent hepatitis in two.[68]

INFECTION WITH HUMAN IMMUNODEFICIENCY VIRUS (HIV)

At present reports of the acquired immunodeficiency syndrome are rare in patients on dialysis but evidence of HIV infection is more frequent (5% in one series).[69] To prevent the spread of HIV among this susceptible population they should be regularly screened for markers of HIV and seropositive patients should be segregated from those who are seronegative during dialysis sessions.[70]

RUPTURE OF THE SPLEEN

Spontaneous rupture of the spleen has been reported in haemodialysis, one centre seeing four cases in as many years.[71] One patient was suffering from amyloidosis, but in the other three there was no obvious predisposing condition.

AORTIC AND MITRAL VALVE CALCIFICATION[72]

Calcification of the aortic and mitral valves is more frequent in patients maintained on dialysis than in age-matched controls; in a few cases it is severe and produces aortic stenosis or, less frequently, mitral stenosis. Premature calcification of the valves is associated with increased plasma levels of calcium and phosphate and metastatic calcification caused by hyperparathyroidism and failure to control blood phosphate levels by diet and drugs. Other factors are increased mechanical stress on the valve cusps, due to increased cardiac output (caused by anaemia and/or arteriovenous fistula) and hypertension, and hyperlipidaemia.

HAEMOSIDEROSIS

Severe overloading with iron, from repeated blood transfusions, intravenous iron dextran and oral iron with vitamin supplements, is a problem of increasing clinical significance in long-term haemodialysis patients. In one series of unselected haemodialysis patients 41% had ferritin levels higher than 2000 ng/ml, the normal being 10–36 ng/ml.[73] Autopsies on dialysis patients often show haemosiderosis.[73,74] Sometimes there are also bone changes similar to those seen in aluminium-induced osteomalacia but with striking linear staining for iron at the mineralization front of trabecular bone.[73] The availability of recombinant human erythropoietin to treat the anaemia of patients receiving dialysis should prevent the complications of iron overload in the future (see p. 36).

REFERENCES

The pathology of uraemia

1. Bergstrom J, Furst P. Uraemic toxins. Kidney Int 1978; suppl 13, 9–12.
2. Powell D, Bergstrom J, Dzurik R, Gulyassy P, Lockwood D, Philips L. Toxins and inhibitors in chronic renal failure. Am J Kidney Dis 1986; 7: 292–299.
3. Blachley JD, Henrich L. The diagnosis and management of acute renal failure. Semin Nephrol 1981; 1: 11–18.
4. Badr KF, Ichikawa I. Prerenal failure: a deleterious shift from renal compensation to decompensation. N Engl J Med 1988; 319: 623–629.
5. Ayus JC, Frommer JP, Young JB. Cardiac and circulatory abnormalites in chronic renal failure. Semin Nephrol 1981; 1: 112–123.
6. Salyer WR, Hutchins G. Cardiac lesions in secondary oxalosis. Arch Intern Med 1974; 134: 250–252.
7. Lewis RD, Lowenstam HA, Rossman GR. Oxalate nephrosis and crystalline myocarditis. Case report with postmortem and crystallographic studies. Arch Pathol 1974; 98: 149–155.
8. Thompson CS, Weinman EJ. The significance of oxalate in renal failure. Am J Kidney Dis 1984; 4: 97–100.
9. Brigham KL, Bernard G. Pulmonary complications of chronic renal failure. Semin Nephrol 1981; 1: 188–197.
10. Al-Sulaiman MH, Dhar JM, Al-Hasani MK. Tuberculous interstitial nephritis after kidney transplantation. Transplantation 1990; 50: 162–164.
11. Zelnick EB, Goyal RK. Gastrointestinal manifestations of chronic renal failure. Semin Nephrol 1981; 1: 124–136.
12. Avram MM. High prevalence of pancreatic disease in chronic renal failure. Nephron 1977; 18: 68–71.
13. Rutsky EA, Robards M, van Dyke JA, Rostand SG. Acute pancreatitis in patients with end-stage renal disease without transplantation. Arch Intern Med 1986; 146: 1741–1745.
14. Fried W. Hematologic abnormalities in chronic renal failure. Semin Nephrol 1981; 1: 176–187.
15. Chandra M, Miller ME, Garcia JF, Mossey RT, McVicar M. Serum immunoreactive erythropoietin levels in patients with polycystic kidney disease as compared with other haemodialysis patients. Nephron 1985; 39: 26–29.
16. Ratcliffe PJ, Dunnill MS, Oliver DO. Clinical importance of acquired cystic disease of the kidney in patients undergoing dialysis. Br Med J 1983; 287: 1855–1858.
17. Jacobs K, Shoemaker C, Rudersdorf R, et al. Isolation and characterisation of genomic and cDNA clones of human erythropoietin. Nature 1985; 313: 806–810.
18. Winearls CG, Oliver DO, Pippard MJ, Reid C, Downing MR, Cotes PM. Effects of human erythropoietin derived from recombinant DNA on the anaemia of patients maintained by chronic haemodialysis. Lancet 1986; 2: 1175–1177.
19. Di Minno G, Martinez J, McKean M-L, De La Rosa J, Burke JF,Murphy S. Platelet dysfunction in uraemia. Multifaceted defect partially corrected by dialysis. Am J Med 1985; 79: 552–559.
20. Ruiz P,Gomez F, Schreiber AD. Impaired function of macrophage Fc_γ receptors in end-stage renal disease. N Engl J Med 1990; 322: 717–722.
21. Kurz P, Kohler H, Meuer S, Hutteroth T, Meyer zum Buschenfelde K-H. Impaired cellular immune responses in chronic renal failure: evidence for a T cell defect. Kidney Int 1986; 29: 1209–1214.
22. Reese GN, Appel SH. Neurologic complications of renal failure. Semin Nephrol 1981; 1: 137–150.
23. Emmanouel DS, Lindheimer MD, Katz AI. Endocrine abnormalities in chronic renal failure: pathogenetic principles and clinical implications. Semin Nephrol 1981; 1: 151–175.
24. Kovarsky J. Rheumatologic complications of chronic renal failure. Semin Nephrol 1981; 1: 198–207.
25. Teitelbaum SL. Renal osteodystrophy. Hum Pathol 1984; 15: 306–323.
26. Lee DBN, Goodman WG, Coburn JW. Renal osteodystrophy: some new questions on an old disorder. Am J Kidney Dis 1988; 11: 365–376.

Pathological changes in uraemic patients undergoing dialysis

27. Alfrey AC. Dialysis encephalopathy. Clin Nephrol 1985; 24: suppl 1, S15–19.
28. Visser WJ, van de Vyver FL. Aluminium-induced osteomalacia in severe chronic renal failure (SCRF). Clin Nephrol 1985; 24: suppl 1, S30–S36.
29. O'Connor M, Garrett P, Dockery M, et al. Aluminium-related bone disease. Correlation between symptoms, osteoid volume, and aluminium staining. Am J Clin Pathol 1986; 86: 168–174.
30. Buchanan MRC, Ihle BU, Dunn C. Haemodialysis-related osteomalacia: a staining method to demonstrate aluminium. J Clin Pathol 1981; 34: 1352–1354.
31. Blumenthal NC, Posner AS. In vitro model of aluminium induced osteomalacia: inhibition of hydroxyapatite formation and growth.Calcif Tissue Int 1984; 46: 439–441.
32. Lieberker M, Grosse B, Cournot-Witmer G, Thic CL, Balsan S. In vitro effects of aluminium on bone phosphatases. A possible interaction with PTH and vitamin D_3 metabolites. Calcif Tissue Int 1982; 34: 280–284.
33. Kaiser L, Schwartz KA. Aluminium-induced anemia. Am J Kidney Dis 1985; 6: 348–352.
34. Dunnill MS, Millard PR, Oliver D. Acquired cystic disease of the kidneys: a hazard of long-term intermittent maintenance haemodialysis. J Clin Pathol 1977; 30: 868–877.
35. Grantham JJ, Levine E. Acquired cystic disease: replacing one kidney disease with another. Kidney Int 1985; 28: 99–105.
36. Hughson MD, Buchwald D, Fox M. Renal neoplasia and acquired cystic disease in patients receiving long-term dialysis. Arch Pathol Lab Med 1986; 110: 592–601.
37. Narasimhan N, Golper TA, Wolfson M, Rahatzad M, Bennett WM. Clinical characteristics and diagnostic considerations in acquired renal cystic disease. Kidney Int 1986; 30: 748–752.
38. Ishikawa I, Yuri T, Kitada H, Shinoda A. Regression of acquired cystic disease of the kidney after successful renal transplantation. Am J Nephrol 1983; 3: 310–314.
39. Yamamoto N, Kanetake H, Yamada J. In vitro evidence from tissue cultures to prove existence of rabbit and human renotropica growth factor. Kidney Int 1983; 23: 624–631.
40. Noronha IL, Ritz E, Waldherr R, Stein G, Fassbinder W. Renal cell carcinoma in dialysis patients with acquired renal cysts. Nephrol Dial Transplant 1989; 4: 763–769.

41. Clanet M, Mansat M, Durroux R, et al. Syndrome du canal carpien, ténosynovite amyloide et hémodialyse périodique. Rev Neurol (Paris) 1981; 137: 613–624.
42. Walts AE, Goodman MD, Matorin PA. Amyloid, carpal tunnel syndrome and chronic hemodialysis. Am J Nephrol 1985; 5: 225–226.
43. Bardin T, Zingraff J, Shirahama T, et al. Hemodialysis-associated amyloidosis and beta$_2$-microglobulin. Clinical and immunohistochemical study. Am J Med 1987; 83: 419–424.
44. Munoz-Gomez J, Bergad A, Barado E, et al. Amyloid arthropathy in patients undergoing periodic haemodialysis for chronic renal failure: a new complication. Ann Rheum Dis 1985; 44: 729–733.
45. Di Raimondo CR, Casey TT, Di Raimondo CV, Stone WJ. Pathologic fractures associated with idiopathic amyloidosis of bone in chronic hemodialysis patients. Nephron 1986; 43: 22–27.
46. Gejyo F, Odani S, Yamada T, et al. β_2-microglobulin: a new form of amyloid protein associated with chronic haemodialysis. Kidney Int 1986; 30: 385–390.
47. Takahashi S, Morita T, Koda Y, Murayama H, Hirasawa Y. Gastrointestinal involvement of dialysis-related amyloidosis. Clin Nephrol 1988; 30: 168–171.
48. Theaker JM, Raine AEG, Rainey AJ, Heryet A, Clark A, Oliver DO. Systemic amyloidosis of β_2-microglobulin type: a complication of long term dialysis. J Clin Pathol 1987; 40: 1247–1251.
49. Ogawa H, Saito A, Hirabayashi N, Hara K. Amyloid deposition in systemic organs in long-term hemodialysis patients. Clin Nephrol 1987; 28: 199–204.
50. Cohen AS, Shirahama T, Sipe JD, Skinner M. Amyloid proteins, precursors, mediator, and enhancer. Lab Invest 1983; 48: 1–4.
51. Gejyo F, Yamada T, Odani S, et al. A new form of amyloid protein associated with chronic hemodialysis was identified as β_2-microglobulin. Biochem Biophys Res Commun 1985; 129: 701–706.
52. Creswell P, Springer T, Strominger JL, Turner MJ, Grey HM, Kubo RT. Immunological identity of the small subunit of HLA antigens and β_2-microglobulin and its turnover on the cell membrane. Proc Nat Acad Sci 1974; 71: 2123–2207.
53. Karlsson FA, Wibell L, Evrin PE. β_2-microglobulin in clinical medicine. Scand J Clin Lab Invest 1980; 40: suppl 154, 27–37.
54. Vincent C, Revillard JP, Galland M, Traeger J. Serum β_2-microglobulin in haemodialysed patients. Nephron 1978; 21: 260–268
55. Kleinman KS, Coburn JW. Amyloid syndromes associated with hemodialysis. Kidney Int 1989; 35: 567–575.
56. Hauglustaine D, Waer M, Michielsen P, Goebels J, Vandeputte M. Haemodialysis membranes, serum β_2-microglobulin, and dialysis amyloidosis. Lancet 1986; 2: 1211–1212.
57. Benhamou CL, Bardin T, Noël LH, et al. Beta-2-microglobulin amyloidosis as a complication of peritoneal dialysis treatment. Clin Nephrol 1988; 30: 346 (letter).
58. Spertini F, Wauters JP, Poulenas I. Carpal tunnel syndrome: a frequent, invalidating, long-term complication of chronic hemodialysis. Clin Nephrol 1984; 21: 98–101.
59. Bardin T, Kuntz D, Zingraff J, Voisin M-C, Zelmar A, Lansaman J. Synovial amyloidosis in patients undergoing long-term haemodialysis. Arthritis Rheum 1985; 28: 1052–1058.
60. Baukenroth R, Spinowitz BS, Galler M, Goldin RA, Rascoff JH, Charytan C. Comparison of eosinophilia in patients undergoing peritoneal dialysis and hemodialysis. Am J Kidney Dis 1986; 8: 186–191.
61. Vanherweghem J-L, Leon M, Goldman M, Lietar N, Gamar N, Thayse C. Membrane-related eosinophilia in hemodialysis. Kidney Int 1988; 33: suppl 24, S73–74.
62. Bommer J, Ritz E, Tschope W, Waldherr R, Gebhart M. Urinary matrix calculi consisting of microfibrillar protein in patients. Kidney Int 1979; 16: 722–728.
63. Mickisch O, Bommer J, Bachmann S, Waldherr R, Mann JFE, Ritz E. Multicystic transformation of kidneys in chronic renal failure.Nephron 1984; 38: 93–99.
64. Shusterman N, Singer I. Infectious hepatitis in dialysis patients. Am J Kidney Dis 1987; 9: 447–455.
65. Galbraith R, El Sheikh N, Portmann B, et al. Immune response to HB_sAg and the spectrum of liver lesions in HB_sAg positive patients with chronic renal disease. Br Med J 1976; 1: 1495–1497.
66. Esteban JI, Esteban R, Viladomiu L, et al. Hepatitis C virus antibodies among risk groups in Spain. Lancet 1989; 2: 294–297.
67. Seaworth B, Garrett L, Stead W, et al. Non-A, non-B hepatitis and chronic dialysis – another dilemma. Am J Nephrol 1984; 4: 235–239.
68. Galbraith RM, Portmann B, Eddleston A, et al. Chronic liver disease developing after outbreak of HB_sAg-negative hepatitis in haemodialysis unit. Lancet 1975; 2: 886–890.
69. Goldman M, Vanherwieghem J-L, Liesnard C, et al. More on AIDS in patients on dialysis. N Engl J Med 1986; 314: 1386–1387 (letter).
70. Favero MS. Recommended precautions for patients undergoing haemodialysis who have AIDS or non-A, non-B hepatitis. Infect Control 1985; 6: 301–305.
71. Lloveras J-J, Prevost F, Goudable C, Durand D, Ton That H, Suc JM. Rupture of the spleen in hemodialysed patients. Clin Nephrol 1986; 26: 160–161 (letter).
72. Maher ER, Young G, Smyth-Walsh B, Pugh S, Curtis JR. Aortic and mitral valve calcification in patients with end-stage renal disease. Lancet 1987; 2: 875–877.
73. Hakim RM, Stivelman JC, Schulman G, et al. Iron overload and mobilization in long-term hemodialysis patients. Am J Kidney Dis 1987; 10: 293–299.
74. Ali M, Ayemi AO, Rigolosi R, et al. Hemosiderosis in hemodialysis patients. JAMA 1980; 224: 343–345.

3

K. A. Porter

Development and congenital malformations of the kidneys

DEVELOPMENT OF THE KIDNEYS[1,2]

A clear understanding of the embryology of the kidney and ureter is necessary because about 4% of babies are born with some developmental abnormality of these organs.

During evolution three different forms of excretory system have developed. In the human embryo this evolutionary process is repeated with the serial and overlapping production of the pronephros, the mesonephros and the metanephros. They develop from two longitudinal masses of mesoderm (the *nephrogenic cords*) that lie one on each side of the primitive aorta (Fig. 3.1). The pronephros and the mesonephros regress during early embryonic life.

PRONEPHROS (HEAD KIDNEY)

The pronephros functions as an adult organ only in amphioxus and in certain lampreys. In the human embryo it is rudimentary and non-functional. It begins to appear about 20 days after conception and consists of about seven pairs of tubules formed as dorsolateral sprouts from the nephrotomes of the 7th to 14th mesodermal segments. One end of each tubule, a ciliated *nephrostome*, drains the coelomic cavity; the other empties into the *pronephric duct* which opens into the cloaca. Adjacent to each nephrostome an offshoot from the dorsal aorta branches to form a cluster of capillaries which invaginates the coelomic mesothelium to produce a primitive *glomerulus*. The pronephros is soon replaced, its cephalic segments beginning to regress even before the most caudal units are formed.

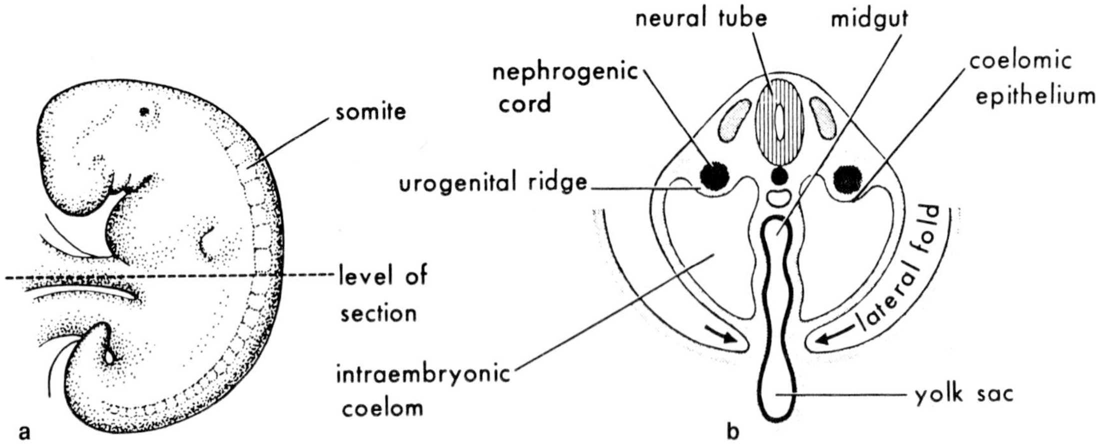

Fig. 3.1 (**a**) Lateral view of a 26-day-old human embryo. (**b**) Diagram of transverse section through the embryo at the level marked in (**a**) showing the nephrogenic cords of the intermediate mesoderm.
Reproduced by permission from: Moore KL. The developing human, 4th edn. Philadelphia: WB Saunders, 1988: 247 (Figs 13.1 C, D)

MESONEPHROS (MIDDLE KIDNEY, WOLFFIAN BODY)

The mesonephros replaces the pronephros and is the permanent kidney of fish and amphibians; in human embryos any function is brief. It begins to appear about 24 days after conception and by about 28 days the pronephros has almost disappeared. The mesonephros arises lower in the embryo in the region of about the 10th to the 28th mesodermal segments. The nephrogenic cord segments into solid masses which hollow out into S-shaped tubules. One end of each tubule communicates with the original pronephric duct, now the *mesonephric* or *Wolffian excretory duct*; the other end cups itself about a cluster of blood vessels arising from a branch of the dorsal aorta to form a glomerulus. About 40 pairs of primitive nephrons are present in each mesonephros at any one time (Fig. 3.2). Each tubule consists of a proximal, thick-walled secretory segment and a distal thinner excretory segment which empties into the Wolffian duct. The mesonephros starts to regress at about the 5th week and by the 11th week it has been replaced by the metanephros.

METANEPHROS[3–6]

The metanephros, or permanent kidney of humans (and all reptiles, birds and mammals) begins to develop early in the 5th week of intrauterine life and starts to function about 6 weeks later, excreting urine into the amniotic fluid. It arises from two different sources. The collecting tubules, renal pelvis and ureter develop from the lower end of the Wolffian duct, whereas the glomeruli and tubules differentiate from the caudal end of the nephrogenic cord.

Formation of collecting tubules, pelvis and calyces

During the 5th week of embryonic life a metanephric diverticulum or *ureteric bud* arises from the Wolffian duct near where it enters the cloaca. The ureteral bud elongates and grows dorsocranially into that part of the nephrogenic cord (the *metanephric mesoderm*) that is going to differentiate into the glomeruli and tubules. The expanded cranial end of the ureteric bud forms the pelvis. The ureteric bud also branches and as it grows and divides the major and minor calyces appear. The latter then give rise to straight and arched collecting tubules (Fig. 3.3). The metanephric mesoderm, or metanephric blastema, covers the branching ureteric bud as a cap of densely packed cells that segments to correspond to branches of the ureteric bud. It is generally thought that the branches of the ureteric bud induce the formation of nephrons in the metanephrogenic mesenchyme.

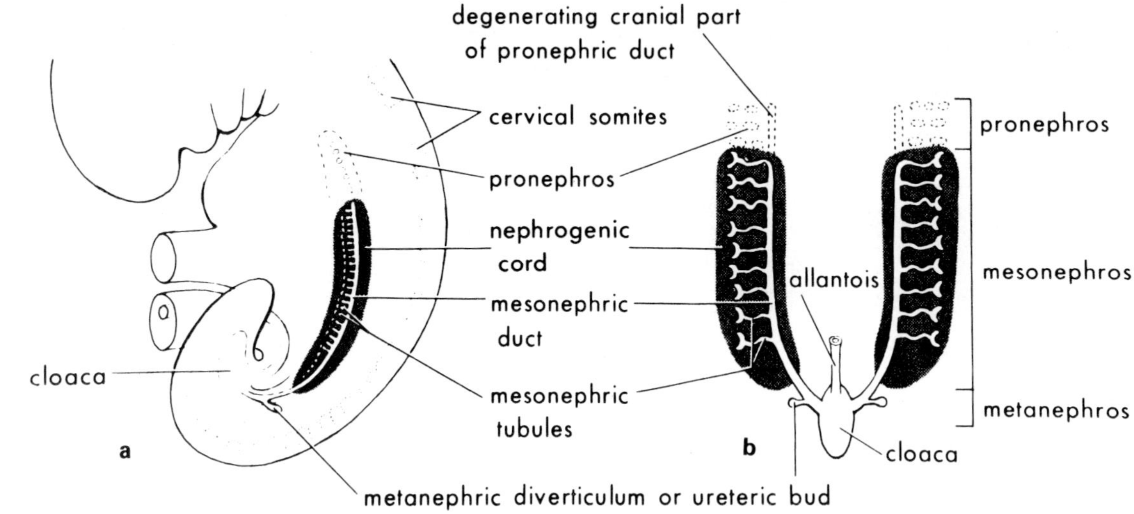

Fig. 3.2 (**a**) Diagrammatic lateral view of a 32-day-old human embryo showing the extent of the mesonephros. (**b**) Diagramatic ventral view of same embryo.
Reproduced by permission from: Moore KL. The developing human, 4th edn. Philadelphia: WB Saunders,1988: 247 (Fig. 13.2)

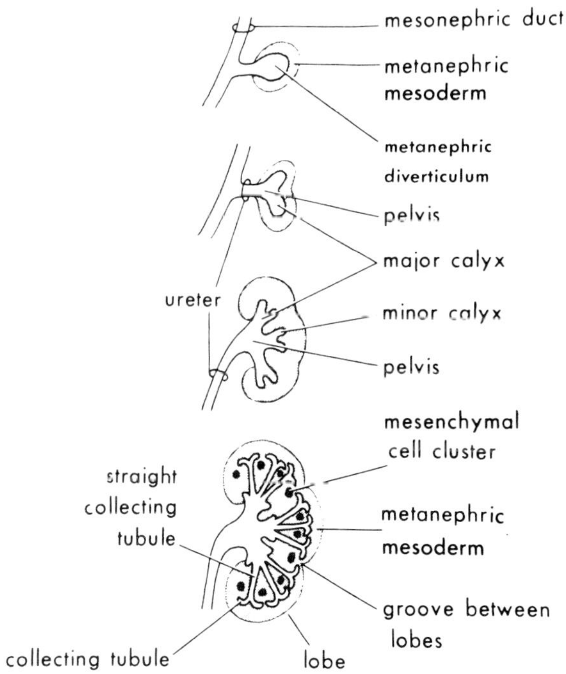

Fig. 3.3 Diagrams showing the development from the 5th to the 8th weeks of the ureteric bud (metanephric diverticulum) into the ureter, pelvis, calyces and collecting tubules.
Reproduced by permission from: Moore KL. The developing human, 4th edn. Philadelphia: WB Saunders,1988: 250 (Fig. 13.5)

By the time the minor calyces have developed the nephrogenic tissue exists as discrete lobes that will still be obvious at birth (fetal lobation).

Formation of glomeruli and secretory tubules

Adjacent to the blind end of each arched collecting tubule (Fig. 3.3) clusters or caps of mesenchymal cells in the metanephric mesoderm form *metanephric vesicles* (Fig. 3.4A) which elongate into S-shaped *metanephric tubules* (proglomeruli; Fig. 3.4B). Each metanephric tubule then makes contact with an arched collecting tubule and the two soon become confluent (Fig. 3.4C). The metanephric tubule continues to grow and differentiates into the distal convoluted tubule, the loop of Henle and the proximal convoluted tubule. The blind proximal tubular end becomes invaginated by a cluster of capillaries to form a glomerulus (Fig. 3.4C, D). Mesangial cells probably enter the glomerulus with these capillaries. As the kidney develops the most recently formed nephrons are located at the periphery of each renal lobe, while the older, progressively more differentiated nephrons, lie near the hilum (Figs 3.4D, 3.5). At about the 36th week, growth of the ureteric bud ceases, no more nephrons are formed and further growth

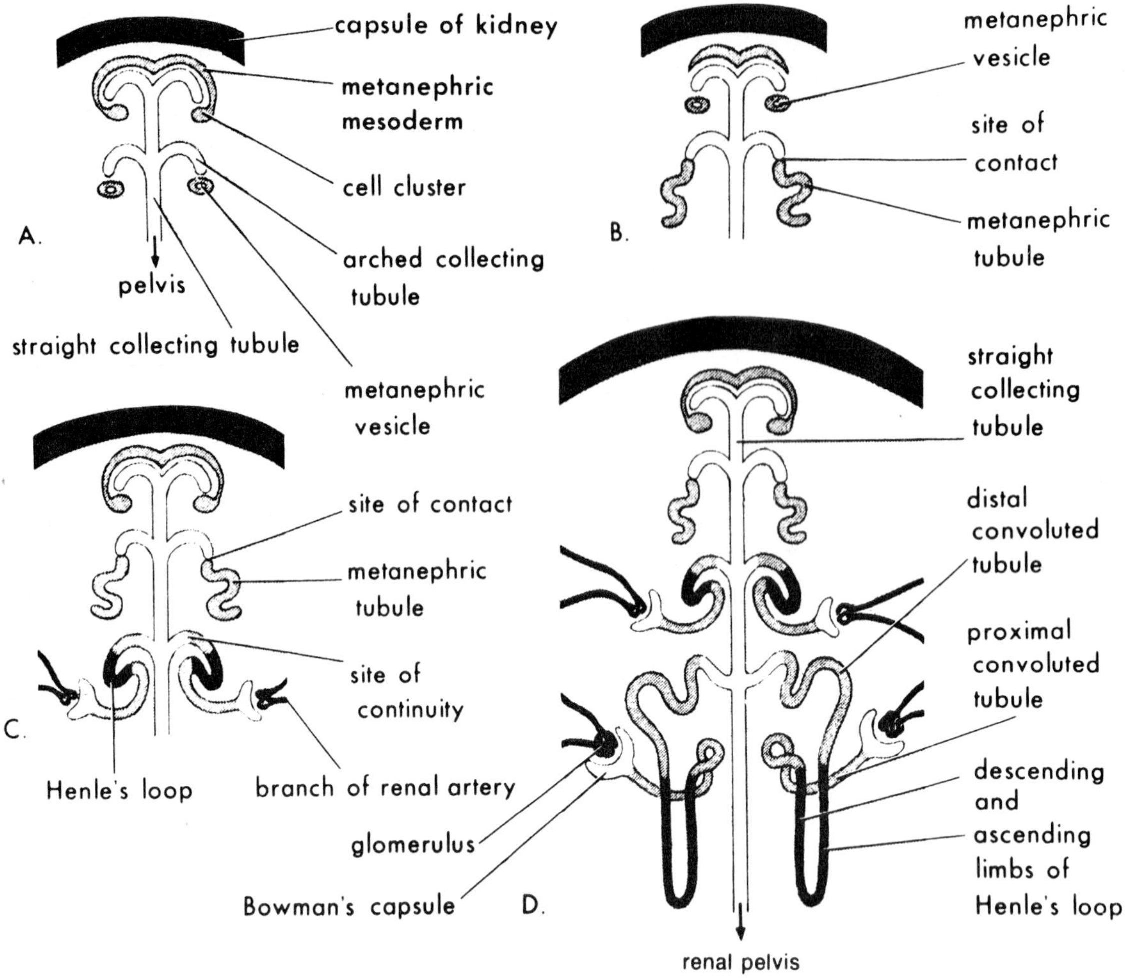

Fig. 3.4 Diagrams showing stages in development of secretory tubule and glomerulus.
Reproduced by permission from: Moore KL. The developing human, 4th edn. Philadelphia: WB Saunders, 1988: 251 (Fig: 13.6)

of the kidney results entirely from hypertrophy of existing nephrons. Each kidney contains 1–1.5 million nephrons.

Changes in position of kidneys and of their vascular supply

When the kidneys are first formed they are in the pelvis, but they gradually come to lie in the abdomen. This change in position occurs because the caudal part of the embryo grows away from the kidneys, eventually leaving them behind the peritoneum on the posterior abdominal wall (Fig. 3.6). As the kidneys occupy progressively higher levels they rotate so that the hilum of each comes to face anteromedially instead of ventrally. The arterial supply to the kidneys also alters. Initially the renal arteries are branches of the middle sacral and common iliac arteries. Later the kidney becomes vascularized by arteries that originate from the aorta at continuously higher levels. The original lower vessels usually degenerate. The final renal arteries do not appear until about the 9th intrauterine week.

MATURATION OF THE KIDNEYS[6,7].

At full term the capsular surface of the kidneys is

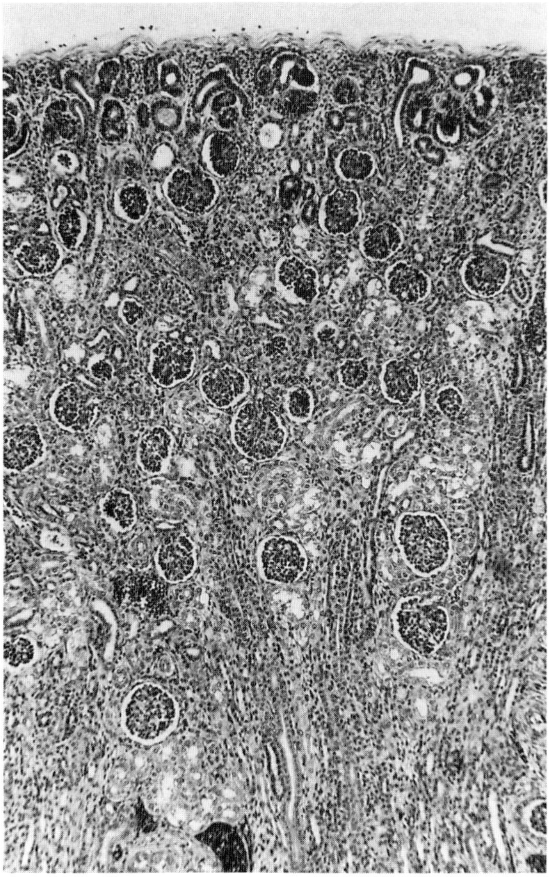

Fig. 3.5 Renal cortex of a 25-week fetus showing progressive maturation of nephrons from the capsular surface (top) to the depths of the renal lobe.
Haematoxylin-eosin × 80

still divided into lobes. Microscopically, many of the glomeruli and tubules are immature, the least differentiated being situated at the periphery of the lobes, i.e. beneath the renal capsule and adjacent to the interlobar grooves.

Glomeruli

These differ in size: the most immature ones at the lobar periphery are smaller than the more differentiated ones in the corticomedullary zone. The average size of the glomeruli present at birth is nearly half that of adult glomeruli (average diameter of glomeruli in full term infants 130 μm; in adults 250 μm). Moreover, the tubules are smaller and more closely arranged in the newborn. This means that when sections of kidneys of full-term infants are examined by light microscopy approximately five times as many glomeruli are seen in a given field as in an adult kidney.

The glomeruli of infants appear more cellular than adult glomeruli. This is because the capillary

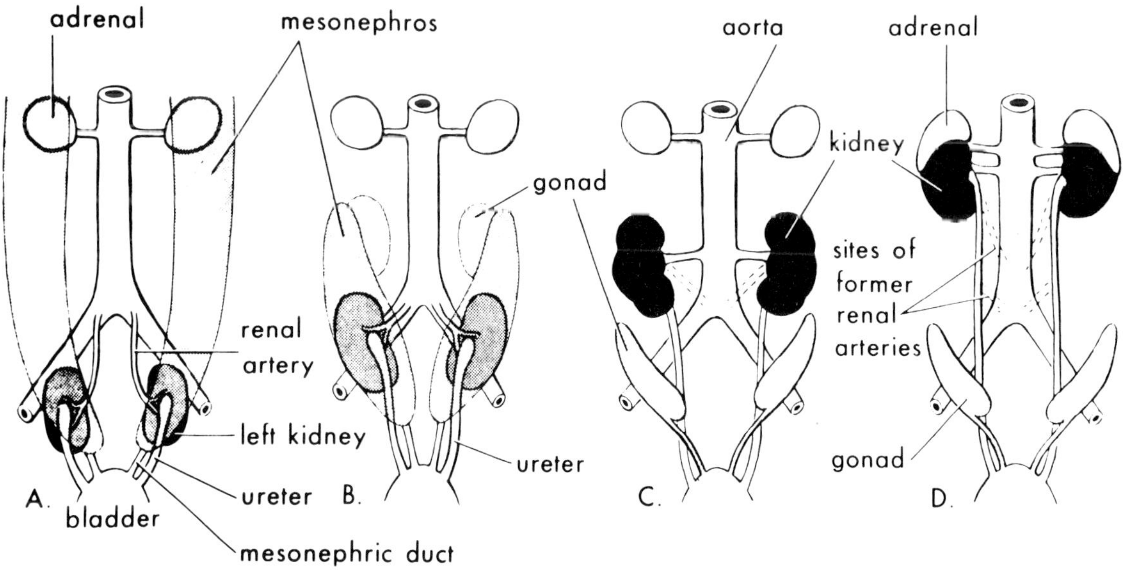

Fig. 3.6 Diagrams showing medial rotation and change in position of kidneys from pelvis to abdomen.
Reproduced by permission from: Moore KL. The developing human, 4th edn. Philadelphia: WB Saunders, 1988: 252 (Fig. 13.8)

a b

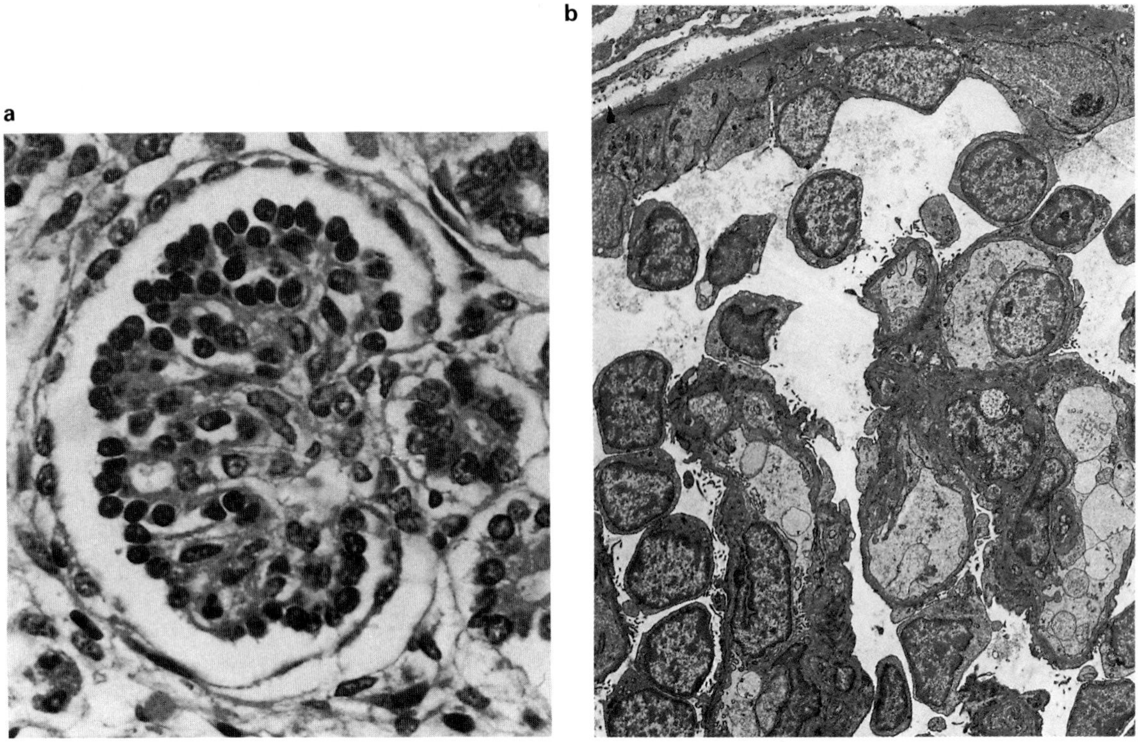

Fig. 3.7 a, b Glomerulus from the superficial cortex of a 6-month-old infant. (**a**) There is a corona of cuboidal visceral epithelial cells covering the glomerular tuft. (**b**) Part of a glomerulus. The visceral epithelial cells are cuboidal and the parietal epithelium lining Bowman's capsule is tall.
(**a**) Haematoxylin-eosin × 150; (**b**) electron micrograph × 1925

tufts are covered by a corona of large cuboidal, deeply staining, visceral epithelial cells and the parietal epithelial cells lining Bowman's capsule are tall resembling the epithelium of proximal convoluted tubules (Fig. 3.7). The more superficial and immature the glomeruli the more prominent the epithelial cells. As the glomeruli mature the epithelial cells become progressively flatter except for the epithelium close to the tubular neck which may remain high for a longer period. The superficial subcapsular immature glomeruli also appear to have few open capillary lumina. As the glomerulus matures the glomerular capillary loops expand and the number of visible capillary lumina increases.

By the age of 2 years all the glomeruli are the same size. Gradually more and more of the glomeruli assume a mature appearance, but cuboidal visceral epithelial cells are occasionally found in a few glomeruli in children up to the age of 12 years. The glomeruli continue to increase in size throughout childhood and adolescence and attain adult size at about the age of 20 years.[8]

Tubules

These are smaller in infants than in adults but their appearance on light microscopy is otherwise similar. The proximal convoluted tubules grow rapidly during the first few months of infancy but from 1 year onwards the growth rate slows. By the age of 15 years the mean length of the proximal convoluted tubule is about twice that of an infant of 1 year.[7,8] The length and volume vary according to the position of the nephron. Tubules of the outer cortical nephrons are usually shorter than those arising from the juxtamedullary zone. In the normal adult the mean length of tubule is approximately 19.5 mm. Little is known about the differentiation and maturation of the tubules in the human kidney.

Interstitium

This is usually inconspicuous in the full-term infant and haemopoiesis at this site has ceased.

Arteries and arterioles

Initially the interlobular arteries and arterioles have a thick concentric adventitia but these vessels assume their mature appearance after 3–4 years.

CONGENITAL GLOMERULOSCLEROSIS (NEONATAL GLOMERULOSCLEROSIS)

About 40% of kidneys in normal infants contain scarred glomeruli.[9] The number of glomeruli affected is small – usually about 1% (Fig. 3.8)[10] Their capillary walls become wrinkled, thickened and collapsed. The tuft shrinks, becomes acellular and ends up as a small compact eosinophilic mass that stains mauve with the periodic acid-Schiff method and brown with Van Gieson. Collagen is progressively laid down internal to Bowman's capsule, beginning in the hilar region, and eventually forming a fibrous mass that envelops the collapsed glomerular tufts. This process seems to be essentially the same as that which in adults produces glomerular obsolescence, often as a consequence of ischaemia. The first glomeruli to undergo sclerosis are in the juxtaglomerular zone at about 2 months of age; later, towards the end of the first year, it is the subcapsular glomeruli that are affected.

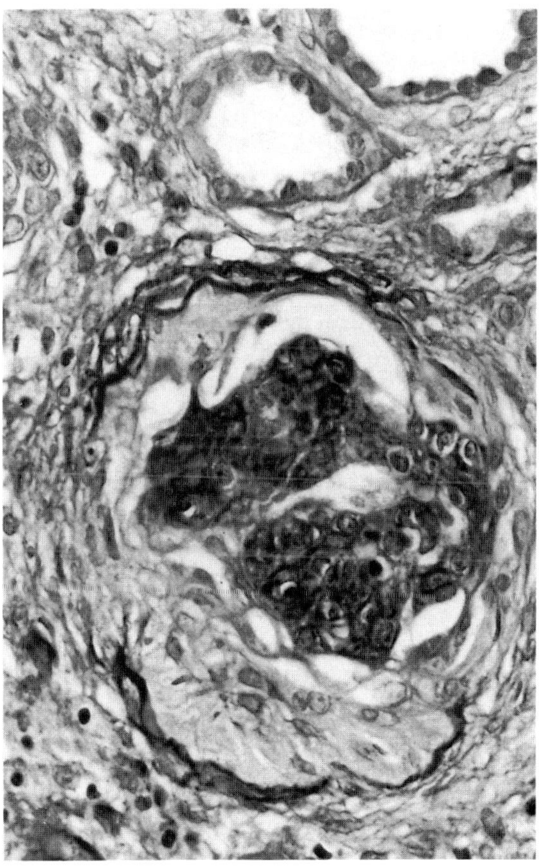

Fig. 3.8 Congenital glomerulosclerosis. Scarred glomerulus from the superficial cortex of a kidney from a 9-month-old infant.
Periodic acid-Schiff × 150

Congenital glomerulosclerosis is probably caused in the majority of instances by involution of glomeruli from nephrons that have in some way not completed their development. For example, as far as the subcapsular glomeruli are concerned, the glomeruli and secretory tubules may have failed to connect with the ampullae of the ureteral bud.[6] It is also possible that the arterial supply is inadequate to sustain more than the normal 15 generations of nephrons and any excess undergo ischaemic obsolescence.[7]

EXCESSIVE NEONATAL GLOMERULOSCLEROSIS (NEONATAL GLOMERULONEPHRITIS, NEONATAL PYELONEPHRITIS, GLOMERULAR DYSPLASIA)

Sclerosis of more than 30% of the glomeruli is occasionally found in the kidneys of infants who develop a nephrotic syndrome or renal failure. In some of these cases the infants have had a severe urinary infection[11] while in others the mother has suffered from rubella[12–14] or some other infection during pregnancy (Fig. 3.9).

CONGENITAL MALFORMATIONS OF THE KIDNEYS

RENAL AGENESIS

Bilateral agenesis (renal aplasia)

When both kidneys fail to develop the infant is ei-

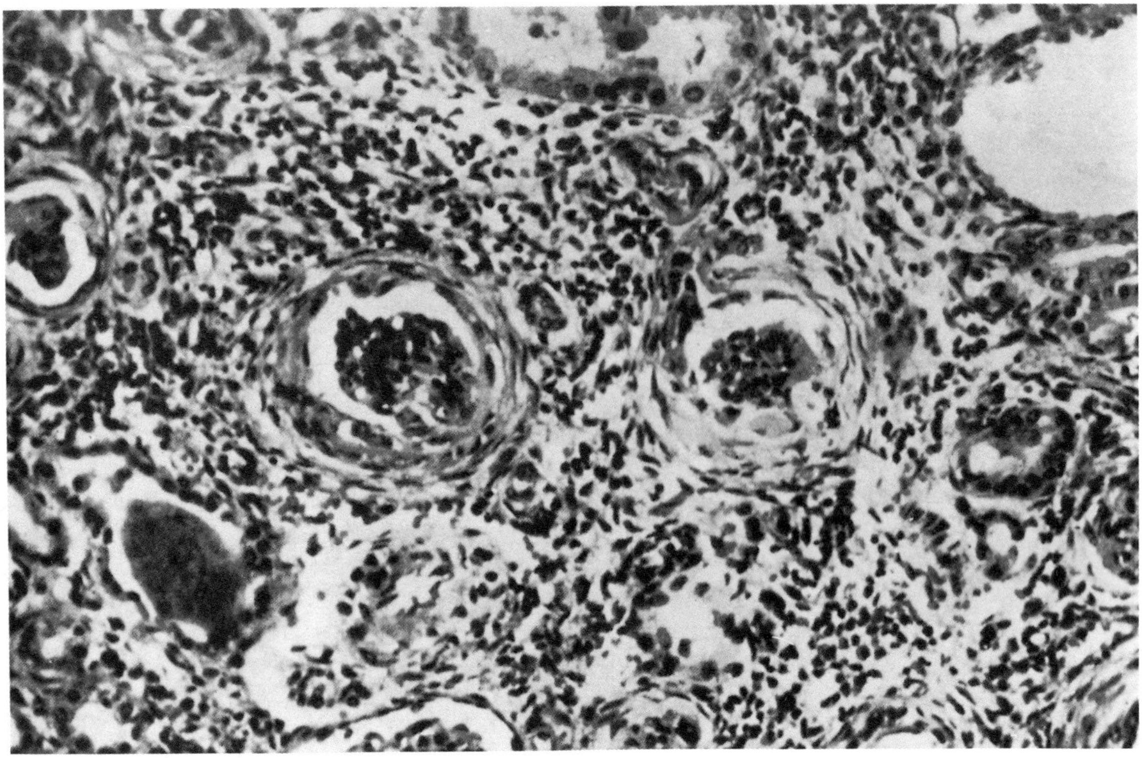

Fig. 3.9 Excessive neonatal glomerulosclerosis. Many of the glomeruli are undergoing sclerosis. This infant died of renal failure at the age of 20 weeks.
Haematoxylin-eosin × 165

ther stillborn or dies shortly after birth. This condition is rare, occurring about once in every 6400 births.[15] It is commoner in boys and monozygotic twins. In bilateral agenesis a deficiency of amniotic fluid (*oligohydramnios*) becomes marked after 14 weeks of gestation because urine is not being excreted; ultrasonography can usually detect the lack of kidneys from about the 24 week. The facial features of these infants are characteristic (*Potter's facies*):[16] the eyes are wide-set, the nose is broad and flattened, the chin is receding, the ears are large and low-set, and the inner canthus of each eye is usually prominent (Fig. 3.10).

There is almost always a bilateral pulmonary hypoplasia and other major malformations; in particular, deformities of the lower limbs, and anomalies or absence of the bladder, urethra and gonads, are present in about 75% of cases of bilateral renal agenesis.[17] Amnion nodosum (minute meconium granulomas studding the amniotic surface) is also frequent. None of these abnormalities is specific for bilateral renal agenesis. They also occur in infants with bilateral renal dysplasia or infantile polycystic disease. As they are probably caused by oligohydramnios, they are also found in infants with normal kidneys in whom there has been chronic leakage of amniotic fluid.[18]

The parents of infants with bilateral renal agenesis are more likely than other adults to have asymptomatic renal malformations, most often unilateral agenesis: the frequency of unilateral agenesis in these relatives is about 4.5% compared with 0.3% in other age- and sex-matched adults.[15] The parents also have an increased risk of having another severely affected child.

The underlying defect in bilateral renal agenesis is not known but in most cases it is probably more basic than simple failure of both ureteric buds to form. No environmental causal factor has so far been recognized, there are no characteristic chromosomal abnormalities and there is no agreement on the pattern of inheritance.

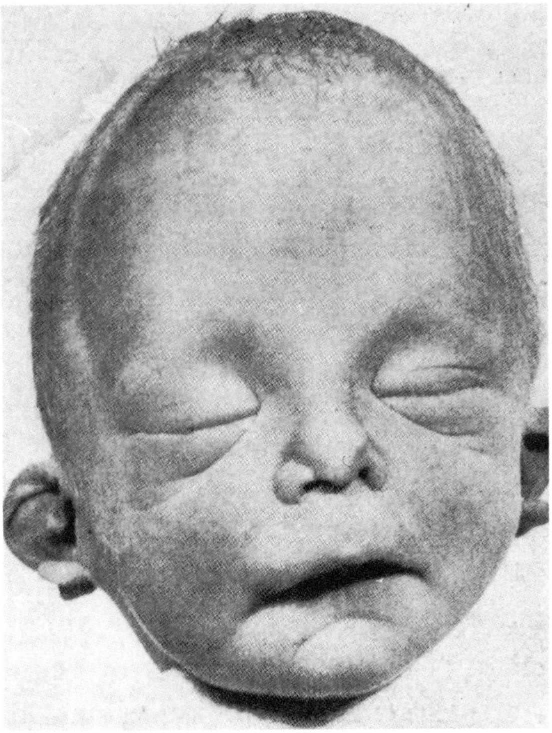

Fig. 3.10 Characteristic facial appearance associated with bilateral renal agenesis.
Reproduced by permission from: Potter EL. Am J Obstet Gynecol 1946;51:885 (Fig. 1)

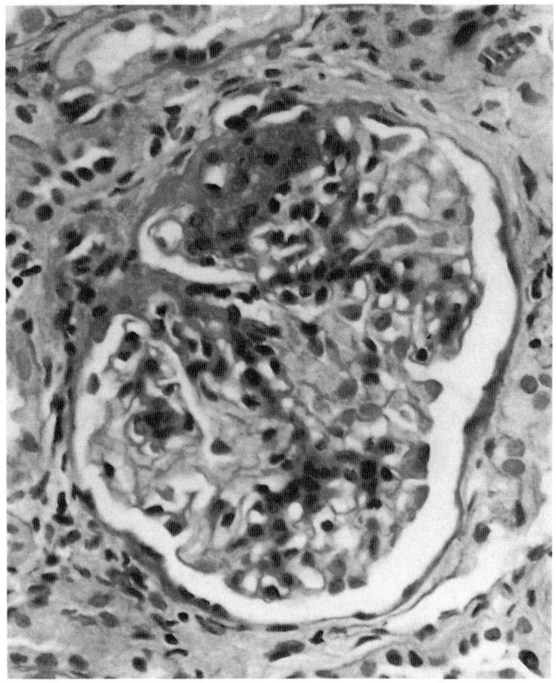

Fig. 3.11 Segmental sclerosis and hyalinosis in glomerulus from only kidney of an 18-year-old man with unilateral renal agenesis.
Periodic acid-Schiff × 150

Unilateral agenesis

The failure of one kidney to develop is compatible with a normal span of life because the single kidney that does form undergoes compensatory enlargement. However, it is most frequently encountered in stillborn infants because severe malformations in other organ systems, such as oesophageal atresia and various forms of congenital heart disease, are commonly present. It occurs in 1 in every 1000 infants and there is a familial tendency.[19] The ureter is absent on the affected side in more than half the cases. The left kidney is more frequently absent than the right. Boys are likelier than girls to have the defect. Most cases seem to be due to failure of the ureteric bud on one side to make contact with the mesenchyme of the nephrogenic cord.

Apart from being roughly twice the size of the normal organ the solitary kidney is usually normal. However, focal and segmental glomerulosclerosis (Fig. 3.11) (see p. 204) may develop, with proteinuria and progression to renal failure in early adult life.[20,21] The incidence of this complication is not known. In a review of 9200 autopsies, seven cases of unilateral renal agenesis were found; of these, two patients (29%) had died of chronic renal failure with focal and segmental sclerosis present in the solitary kidney. This is most certainly an overestimate of the incidence because the cases were selected in that they had been referred to a medical centre and then had died. Occasionally focal and segmental glomerulosclerosis in solitary kidneys is caused by vesicoureteric reflux and/or by pyelonephritis (see p. 443); in others it may be that the solitary kidney contains less than a critical number of nephrons, which causes the glomerular filtration rate per individual nephron to rise, leading to glomerular damage (see p. 26). The process is self-perpetuating, because with every glomerulus that becomes sclerotic, there is a further increase in perfusion of the remaining nephrons.

The possibility of unilateral agenesis in any case

makes confirmation of the presence of two kidneys obligatory before performing nephrectomy.

RENAL HYPOPLASIA

A truly hypoplastic kidney has five or fewer calyces and is small, but otherwise normal. The number of calyces is best determined by opening the renal pelvis and counting the papillae that protrude into it.[22] Many kidneys that are described as hypoplastic are in fact not hypoplastic but dysplastic (see p. 58). True hypoplasia is a very rare anomaly. It is most frequently bilateral.[23] The prognosis will depend upon the volume of functional renal parenchyma. If marginal, life is sustained until some minor degree of acquired disease precipitates progressive renal insufficiency and death. Bilateral renal hypoplasia accounts for about 20% of the cases of chronic renal failure below the age of 16 years.[24]

Oligomeganephronic renal hypoplasia (oligomeganephronia)

This rare form of hypoplasia is characterized by reduction in number and increase in size of the nephrons.[25,26] The kidneys are very small. Most patients present in infancy with fever, vomiting and dehydration. Hyperfiltration in the surviving nephrons initially maintains the glomerular filtration rate at an acceptable level, but by adolescence these children develop focal and segmental glomerulosclerosis (see p. 204) with progressive proteinuria and eventual renal failure.[27] The aetiology and pathogenesis of oligomeganephronic renal hypoplasia are not known. One possibility is that the ureteric bud prematurely ceases to induce the formation of nephrons in the metanephrogenic mesenchyme. Advanced maternal age, viral infections and, more rarely, genetic factors have been suggested as the cause of this arrest. In monozygotic twins non-concordant for oligomeganephronic renal hypoplasia, it has been suggested that passage of blood through arteriovenous shunts in the placenta may lead to decreased renal blood flow and decreased renal size in the donor twin.[28]

DUPLICATION OF THE RENAL PELVIS

Some degree of duplication of the renal pelvis is present in about 10% of the population.

SUPERNUMERARY KIDNEY[29]

An extra mass of renal tissue that has no parenchymatous connexion with the normally developed kidneys is one of the rarest of renal anomalies. Such a supernumerary kidney usually lies caudal to one of the normal kidneys, has only one or two calyces and drains into the normal ureter on the same side. The supernumerary kidney becomes infected in about two-thirds of cases and symptoms then develop.

RENAL ECTOPIA

One or both kidneys may be in an abnormal position. Most ectopic kidneys lie below the level of the second or third lumbar vertebra in the iliac fossa, or on the brim of the pelvis or in the pelvic cavity.

Simple ectopia[30,31]

Simple ectopia involves malposition of a kidney that lies on its (developmentally) proper side of the body (Fig. 3.12). It results from failure of the kidney to 'ascend' from the pelvis during early intrauterine life. The cause of this failure is not known. The ectopic kidney is disc shaped because it has not been subjected to compression during development. The pelvis and ureter arise from the anterior flat surface. The ureter is short and enters the bladder either normally or through an ectopic orifice.

Crossed ectopia[30,32]

In this condition both kidneys are on the same side of the abdomen. The crossed kidney usually lies caudal to the uncrossed organ and the two are often fused. Sometimes the lower pole of the uncrossed kidney joins the upper pole of the misplaced organ, producing an S-shaped structure.

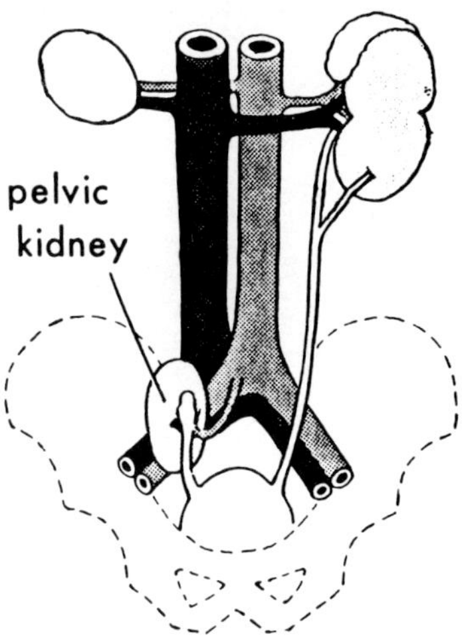

Fig. 3.12 Diagram showing simple renal ectopia. *Reproduced by permission from: Moore KL. The developing human, 4th edn. Philadelphia: WB Saunders, 1988: 254 (Fig. 13.10B)*

More extensive fusion will produce a 'cake' or 'pancake' kidney (Fig. 3.13). Crossed ectopia is the result of displacement of one ureteric bud across the midline into the nephrogenic ridge of the opposite side.

The arterial supply to ectopic kidneys is derived from branches of the aorta near its bifurcation or from the common iliac arteries. The urinary drainage of ectopic kidneys is often inefficient and this predisposes to pyelonephritis. However, in most cases the condition is asymptomatic throughout life.

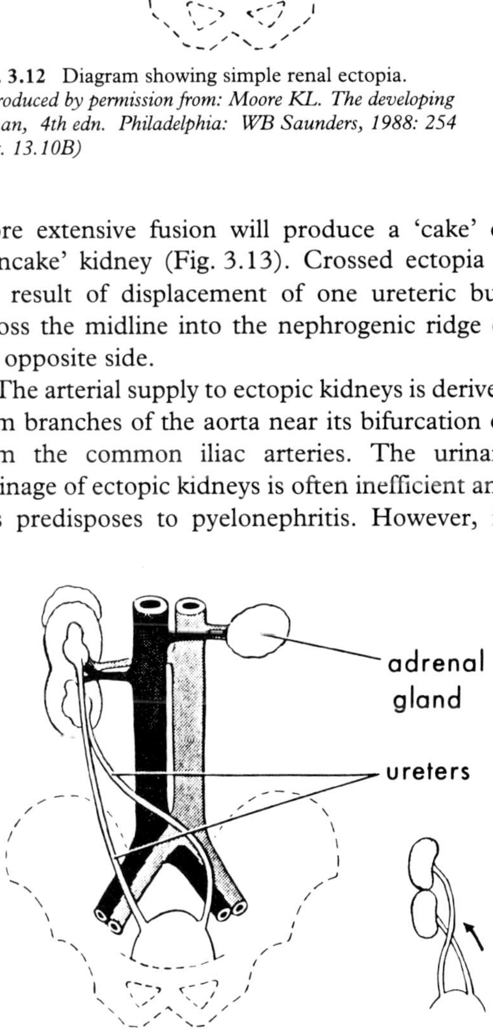

Fig. 3.13 Diagram showing crossed renal ectopia. *Reproduced by permission from: Moore KL. The developing human, 4th edn. Philadelphia: WB Saunders, 1988: 254 (Fig. 13.10D)*

FUSION OF THE KIDNEYS[33,34]

Some degree of renal fusion is found once in about 250 necropsies. Usually a broad isthmus of renal tissue connects the lower poles of the kidneys across the midline, forming a *'horseshoe' kidney* (Fig. 3.14). The pelves that drain the two halves of the horseshoe are directed more anteriorly than is normal and the two ureters are angulated anteriorly as they cross the isthmus. Fusion of the kidneys is thought to be due to the two ureteric buds becoming attached to each other. Their normal migration and medial rotation is then blocked by the inferior mesenteric artery. What causes the fusion of the ureteric buds is unknown.

This anomaly is twice as common in males as in females. it is often associated with other congenital abnormalites.[35] Patients with a horseshoe kidney may suffer episodes of nausea, vomiting and abdominal pain that can be relieved by bending the trunk forward (Rovsing's syndrome). Symptoms and changes in the urine that suggest infection occur in about 30% of cases. Stones are particularly likely to form in the isthmus and secondary hydronephrosis is responsible for most of the operations on horseshoe kidney. Nephroblastoma and adenocarcinoma have been encountered in patients with horseshoe kidney;[33] the incidence of nephroblastoma is approximately twice that expected in the populations studied (see p. 589).

PERSISTENT FETAL LOBATION

In the fetus the nephrogenic tissue exists as fairly discrete lobes that will still be demarcated at birth by interlobar grooves (see p. 50). These lobations may persist into adult life to a variable extent (Fig. 3.15); rarely this is extreme, giving a *cotyledonous kidney*.

Another rarity is *displacement or inversion of a renal lobe* which may disturb the excretory urogram and simulate a neoplasm.[36]

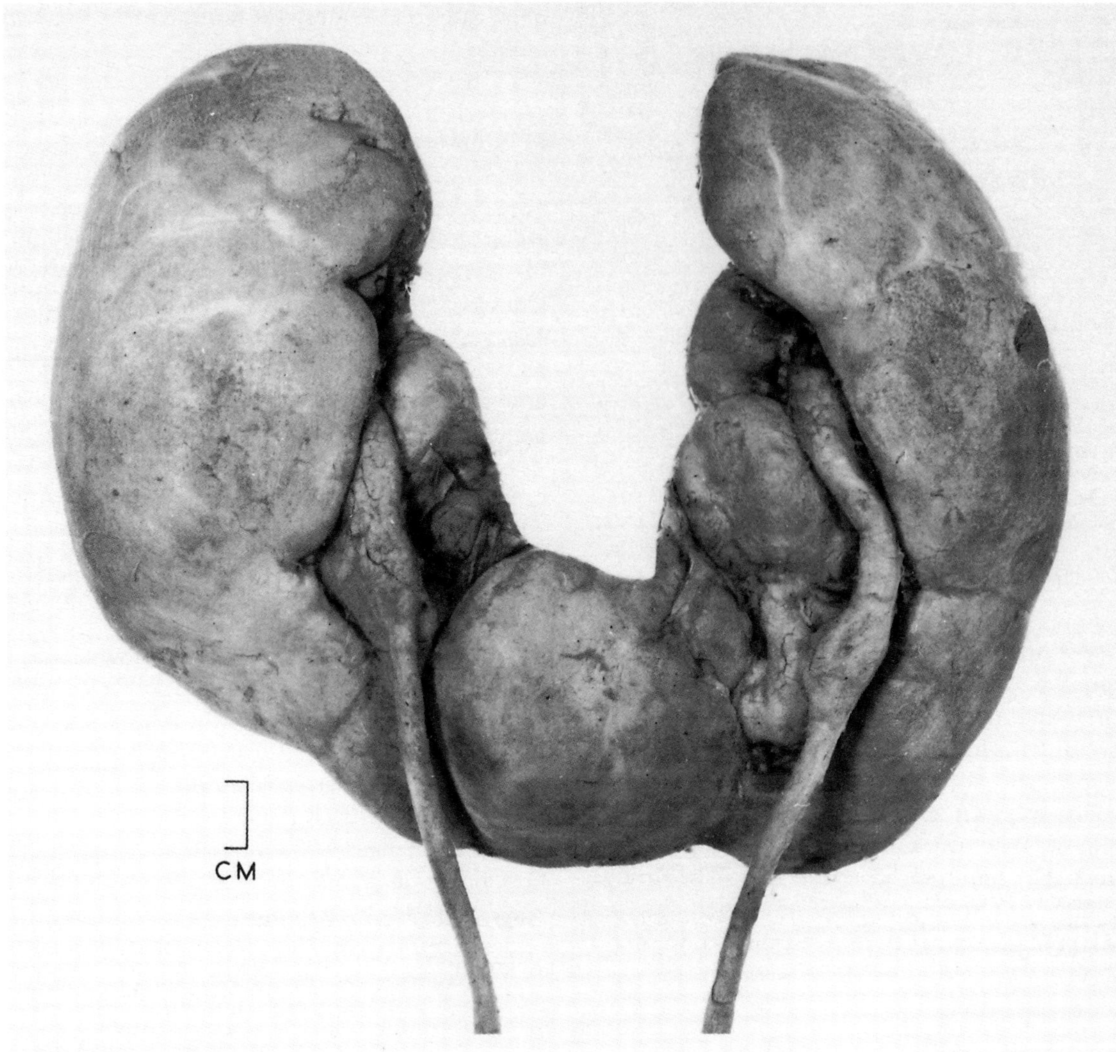

Fig. 3.14 'Horseshoe' kidney with fusion of the lower poles across the midline.
Specimen from the Pathology Museum, Charing Cross and Westminster Medical School, London, UK. Reproduced by permission of the Curator, Dr F. J. Paradinas.

ANOMALIES OF ROTATION[37]

Rotational abnormalities are rare in orthotopic kidneys, i.e. kidneys that are lying in their normal anatomical site. The commonest is that in which the kidney remains disc shaped and its pelvis and ureter arise from the anterior rather than the medial surface. Anomalies of rotation may produce partial obstruction at the ureteropelvic junction.

RENAL DYSPLASIA[6,38,39]

Renal dysplasia is brought about by disturbed differentiation of nephrogenic tissue, with production and persistence of structures not seen in normal development. It seems not to be hereditary. Other names that have been used for this condition are unilateral polycystic disease and multicystic disease and, inappropriately, aplasia. Many kidneys described as 'hypoplastic' are in fact dysplastic (see p. 56).

The two structures that characterize dysplasia are:[38,39]

1. Primitive ducts which are lined by columnar epithelium (often ciliated) and surrounded by concentric collars of cellular mesenchyme and

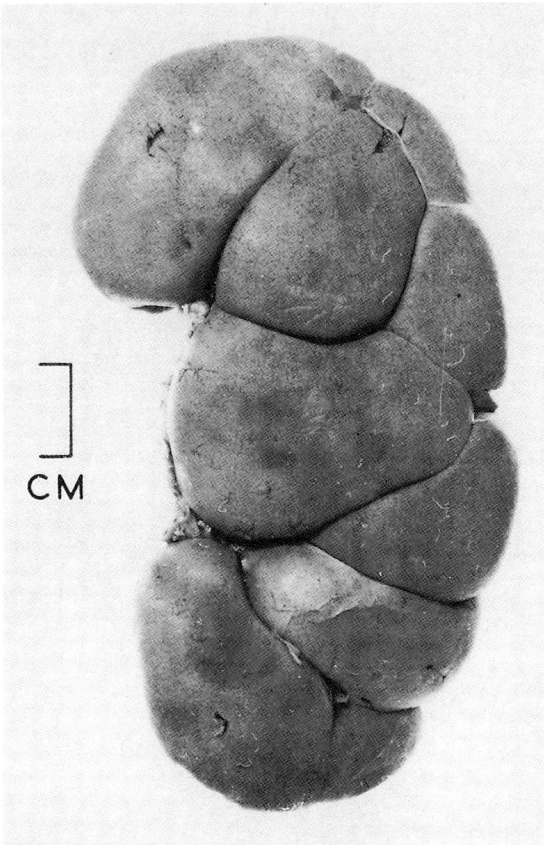

Fig. 3.15 Persistant fetal lobation in the kidney of a boy aged 8 years.
Specimen from the Pathology Museum, Charing Cross and Westminster Medical School, London, UK. Reproduced by permission of the Curator, Dr F. J. Paradinas.

smooth muscle (Fig. 3.16). These are the most common in the medulla and are thought to be derived from the branches of the ureteric bud.
2. Islands of cartilage (Fig. 3.16). These are usually cortical and are produced by the metanephrogenic tissue. They may later calcify or ossify. Cartilage is present in only a proportion of the kidneys that contain primitive ducts.

Other elements that are often present are immature ductules lined by hyperchromatic epithelium, abundant cellular mesenchymal stroma and primitive tubules and glomeruli. Renal dysplasia may be unilateral or bilateral and within a kidney may be complete, segmental or focal.

Complete renal dysplasia[6,40]

Complete renal dysplasia is usually unilateral.

Unilateral complete renal dysplasia

Unilateral complete renal dysplasia is the commonest cystic disease of the kidneys in the newborn. It affects both sexes equally. The left kidney is affected oftener than the right and malformations of other organ systems are frequent. The lesion is sporadic without a familial tendency. In infancy it usually presents as a palpable mass. Later in life calcium or bone in a dysplastic kidney may be detected radiologically.

The dysplastic kidney consists of a disorderly mass of cysts of various sizes (Fig. 3.17). The mass resembles a bunch of grapes. Calyces and pelvis are not present and the stem of the ureter is often absent or atretic. Unilateral renal dysplasia does not predispose to hypertension.

Bilateral total renal dysplasia

Bilateral total renal dysplasia is associated with Potter's facies (see p. 54). Death occurs in the first few days after birth.

Segmental renal dysplasia

Segmental renal dysplasia is a rare condition which usually involves the upper pole of the kidney and is almost always associated with duplication of the renal pelvis and ureter. The ureter that drains the dysplastic segment may obstruct the ureter that drains the normally differentiated part of the kidney, producing hydronephrosis and predisposing to chronic pyelonephritis.

Focal renal dysplasia

Occasionally, histological examination of grossly cystic kidneys of patients with various teratological syndromes may show the presence of numerous dysplastic foci. Such syndromes include the Meckel–Gruber syndrome[41] (dysencephalia splanchnocystica) and the Dandy–Walker syndrome.[42] In addition to polycystic disease affecting the kidneys predominantly, the Meckel–Gruber syndrome comprises dwarfism characterized by shortness of

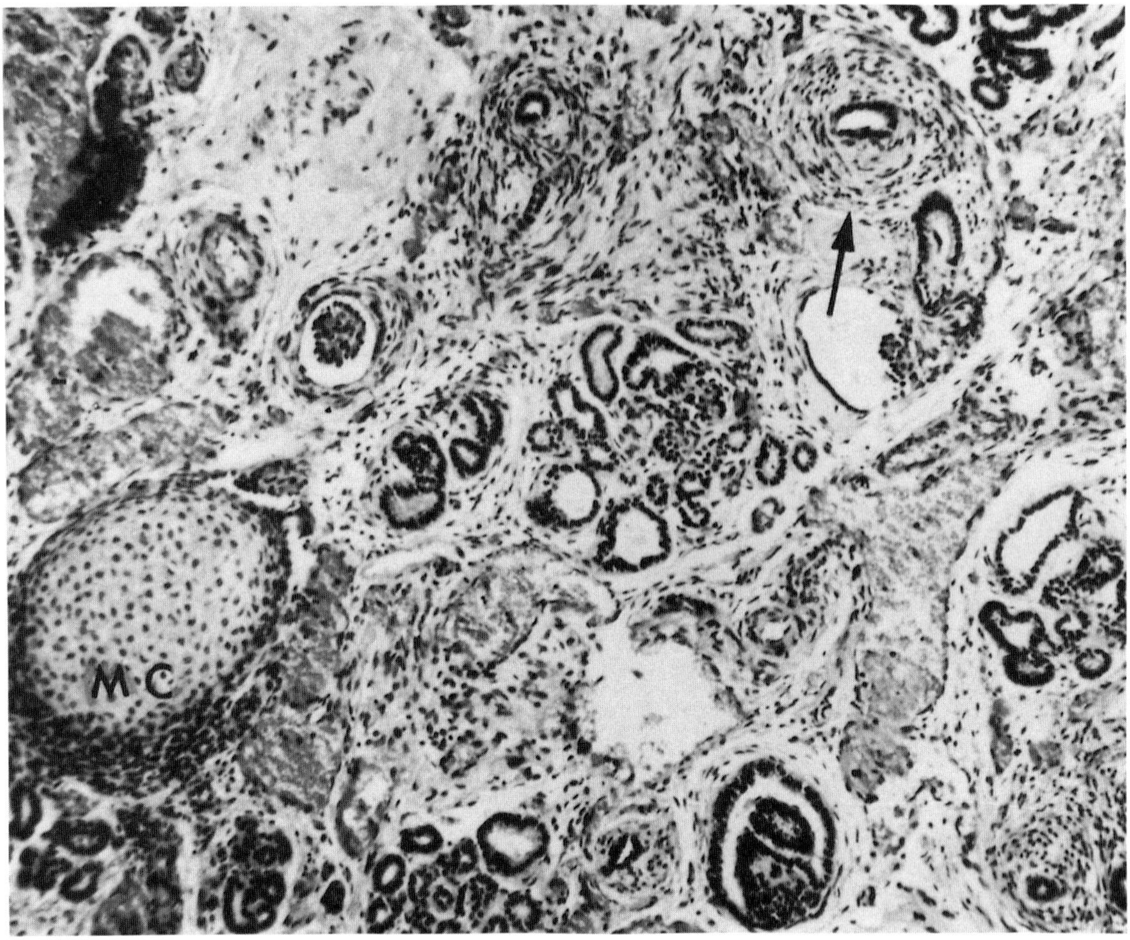

Fig. 3.16 Renal dysplasia. A primitive duct (arrow) and metaplastic cartilage (MC) are surrounded by cellular mesenchymatous stroma and clusters of primitive tubules and glomeruli.
Haematoxylin-eosin x 100
Reproduced by permission from: Bernstein J. Pediatr Clin North Am 1971; 18: 395 (Fig. 2)

the proximal part of the limbs, polydactyly, hare lip and cleft palate, malformation or absence of the eyeballs and malformation of the skull accompanying major abnormalities of the brain. The affected child is stillborn or dies in infancy. The Dandy–Walker syndrome comprises enlargement of the fourth ventricle of the brain with separation of the cerebellar hemispheres and consequent dolichocephaly; it is less frequently accompanied by polycystic disease.

Urinary tract obstruction in associaton with renal dysplasia

Many cases of renal dysplasia, particularly bilateral dysplasia, are associated with obstructive anomalies of the urinary tract. The obstruction is usually complete and sited in the lower urinary tract, where the anomaly may be urethral atresia or stenosis, valves in the urethra, contracture of the bladder neck, or hypertrophy of the verumontanum. In these cases marked cystic dilatation of Bowman's space in the subcapsular glomeruli is found in addition to the microscopical features of renal dysplasia.

Obstruction of the urinary tract may be an important factor in the pathogenesis of renal dysplasia. Microdissection studies have suggested that cystic dysplasia is due to premature cessation of branching of the ampullary portion of the col-

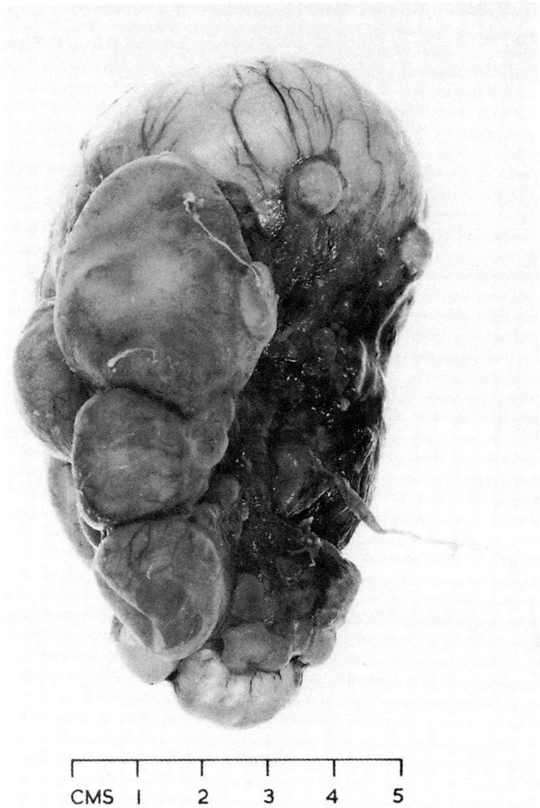

Fig. 3.17 Unilateral complete renal dysplasia. Kidney consists of a mass of various sized cysts. The ureter is atretic. *Reproduced by permission from: Risdon RA. J Clin Pathol 1971; 24: 65 (Fig. 6)*

lecting ducts, with resulting cyst formation and failure to induce normal nephron production in the metanephric blastema.[43] Urinary tract obstruction may be the cause of this inhibition of ampullary activity.

GLOMERULOCYSTIC DISEASE

Glomerulocystic disease is a rare type of congenital renal cystic disease characterized by dilatation of Bowman's space in almost all of the glomeruli. To be classified as glomerulocystic disease the cortical cysts must occur in a kidney without dysplastic changes or evidence of urinary tract obstruction. Also the tubules must be normal. It is associated with a high incidence of congenital abnormalities in other organs and renal failure that usually occurs in early childhood[44] but may be deferred until early adult life.[45] The mode of inheritance is not known but an autosomal dominant pattern has been suggested. A familial variant of glomerulocystic disease has been described[46] in which there were no major extrarenal malformations, the renal papillae were absent and there was stable chronic renal failure starting during the first few months of life.

POLYCYSTIC RENAL DISEASE

In this condition much of the renal parenchyma is converted into cysts of varying size. There are two distinct forms of the disease, one that is autosomal dominant and occurs predominantly in adults and the other that is autosomal recessive and is found almost exclusively in infants. The dominant variety is much more frequent than the recessive form.

Autosomal dominant polycystic kidney disease (adult polycystic kidney disease)

Autosomal dominant polycystic kidney disease is the most common inherited renal disorder. It is a systemic disease characterized by enlargement of both kidneys due to focal cystic dilatation of the tubules in various segments along the entire length of the nephron. There are often accompanying extrarenal manifestations, in particular hepatic cysts and mitral valve prolapse. This form of polycystic renal disease occurs approximately once in every 400–1000 live births[47] and accounts for about 12% of all end-stage renal disease.[18] Females are more frequently affected than males.

Most people older than 20 years who carry the gene for autosomal dominant polycystic renal disease have some manifestations of the condition; the way the disease presents and develops varies.[49] End-stage renal failure occurs in about half the patients with the gene. A few cases are detected in infancy, but most do not become clinically apparent until about the age of 25–40 years. Patients rarely develop end-stage renal failure before the age of 30 years.[49]

Inheritance

The condition is inherited as an autosomal dominant; genetic mapping, using highly polymorphic DNA probes, has shown that the polycystic kidney disease locus is closely linked to that for the alpha-chain of haemoglobin and also with phosphoglycolate phosphatase on the short arm of chromosome 16.[50,51] Attempts are now being made to isolate and clone the gene responsible for the disease. A complication is that two Italian families with the classical autosomal dominant polycystic kidney disease have been described in whom the abnormal DNA is not linked to the alpha-globin locus.[52,53] These findings suggest either that the gene causing the disease is translocated to another chromosome in some families, or that mutations in two separate genes may lead to indistinguishable phenotypes, i.e. may cause pathological changes that cannot at present be differentiated from one another.[52] Current evidence suggests that families whose mutant gene is not linked to chromosome 16 represent less than 10% of the patients with autosomal dominant polycystic kidney disease.[54]

Clinical features

The presenting symptom is most commonly flank pain which may be accompanied by renal colic. Hypertension, gross haematuria, symptoms of urinary tract infection and palpable abdominal masses are also common. Hypertension occurs in 50–75% of those carrying the mutant gene. Intermittent proteinuria is present in nearly 70% of patients with this disorder but it is rarely severe. Renal calculi are frequent and erythrocytosis occurs in some patients.[55] Erythrocytosis is caused by increased production of erythropoietin. The erythropoietin-producing cells are possibly stimulated by local hypoxia consequent either on spatial distortion by cysts or narrowing of arteries and arterioles secondary to infection or hypertension. The intravenous pyelogram usually shows that the pelvis of each kidney is elongated and the calyces characteristically distorted. Ultrasonography and computed tomography are more sensitive in detecting the disease[56] but, unfortunately, polycystic disease cannot be excluded by this means. Thirty-four per cent of patients at risk in the second decade and 14% in the third will go on to develop cysts after a negative ultrasonogram. The low sensitivity of diagnostic techniques in this critical age range imposes severe limitations on genetic counselling.[57] However, early prenatal diagnosis is now possible using a linked DNA probe derived from the alpha-globin region.[54,58]

Gross appearance of the kidneys

The kidneys maintain their general shape but become huge. They may weigh more than 1000 g each (Fig. 3.18). Almost always both kidneys are affected equally. Spherical cysts are present throughout the cortex and medulla and bulge from the capsular surface, producing an appearance referred to as bosselation. The contents of the cysts vary from clear yellow fluid to gelatinous red or brown material if there has been haemorrhage. Cholesterol crystals are sometimes present. The calyces and renal pelvis are structurally normal but greatly distorted.[6]

Light microscopy

Most of the cysts are lined by flat epithelium (Fig. 3.19). Some are lined by epithelium of the type normally found in the proximal parts of the tubules. In others the epithelium resembles that of the distal parts of the tubules or of the collecting ducts. Hyperplasia of the tubular epithelium with formation of polyps is common, particularly late in the disease and especially in those patients being treated by dialysis. Microscopic adenomas of limited clinical significance are occasionally present. Renal carcinomas are no more common than would be expected by chance association alone.[59] A few cysts contain a glomerular tuft. Scattered, small areas of normally differentiated renal parenchyma are present between the cysts. In these foci there may be hypertensive vascular changes and evidence of pyelonephritis. The juxtaglomerular renin-containing cells are often increased in number and extend into the walls of the interlobular arteries; a few cells with renin granules occur in the fibrous tissue apart from vessels.[60] The cysts may partially regress after chronic dialysis or successful renal transplantation.

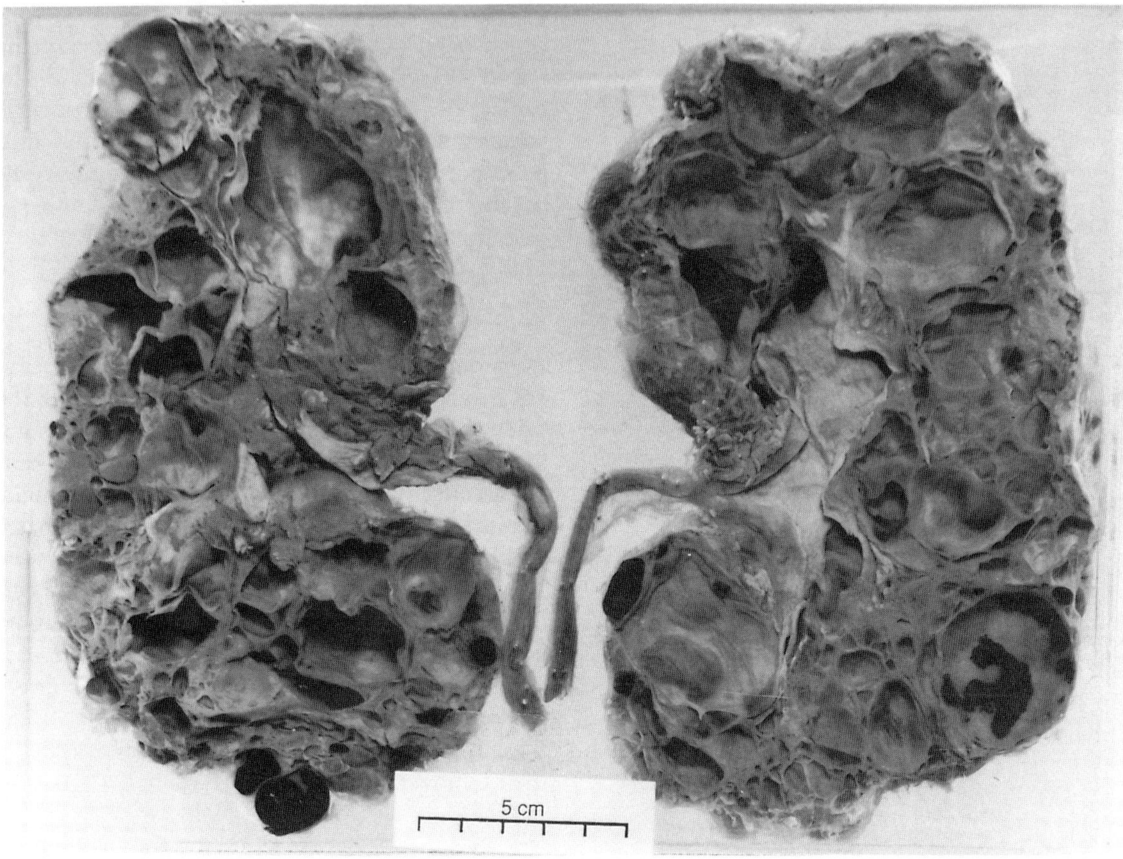

Fig. 3.18 Autosomal dominant polycystic kidney disease.

Numerous glomerular and tubular microcysts have been reported in the kidneys of fetuses as early as the 12th week of gestation in patients diagnosed as having autosomal dominant polycystic kidney disease by chorionic villus biopsy and genetic linkage analysis using an appropriate marker.[61]

Changes in other organs

About 40% of patients with autosomal dominant polycystic renal disease have *cysts of the liver*,[55,62,63] about 10% have one or more *cysts in the pancreas*[55,62] and a few have *cysts in the spleen, ovaries, testes or lungs. Berry aneurysms of the cerebral arteries* occur in about 15% of patients.[62,64,65] *Mitral valve prolapse* is found in 26% of patients with the disease and in 14% of unaffected family members, compared with 2% of controls.[66] Autosomal dominant polycystic kidney disease is also associated with an increased incidence of *other cardiac valvular abnormalities, diverticulosis, abdominal aortic aneurysms* and *annuloaortic ectasia*.

Differential diagnosis

The main distinction that has to be made is between autosomal dominant polycystic kidney disease and *acquired cystic disease*.[67] In autosomal dominant polycystic kidney disease the kidneys tend to be large, they are diffusely cystic and their surfaces are bosselated; in acquired cystic disease the kidneys are often normal sized, focally cystic and their surfaces are smoother. The cysts are usually larger and more variable in size in autosomal dominant polycystic kidney disease than in acquired cystic disease. Renal tumours, mostly

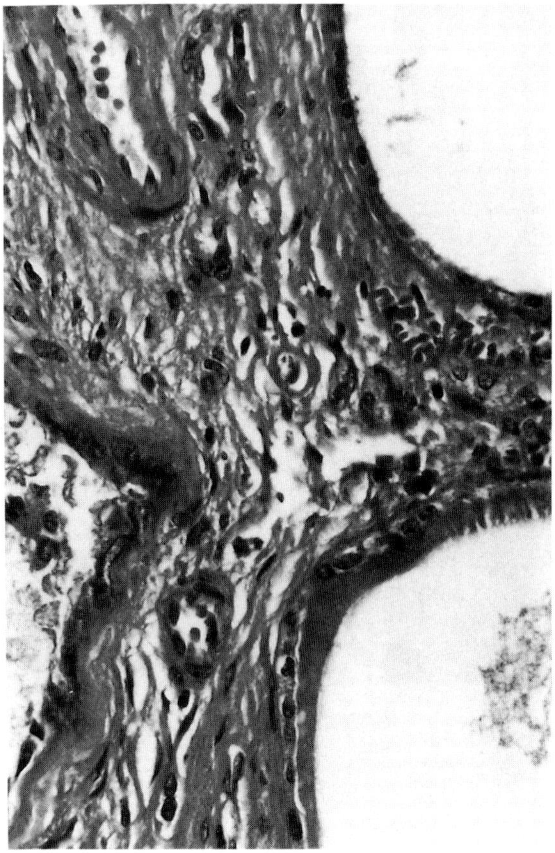

Fig. 3.19 Autosomal dominant polycystic kidney disease. Cyst on upper right of photograph is lined by flattened epithelium; those on lower right and lower left parts of picture by epithelium resembling that of proximal and distal tubules, respectively.
Haematoxylin-eosin × 100

adenomas, occur in about 20% of cases of acquired cystic disease; they are rare in autosomal dominant polycystic kidney disease.

The differentiation of autosomal dominant polycystic kidney disease from *autosomal recessive polycystic kidney disease* is much easier because the cysts in the autosomal recessive disease are radially arranged and fusiform, unlike the spherical cysts of the autosomal dominant condition.

Complications

Renal calculi. Stone formation is a fairly common complication, occurring in 20% of one series of 751 patients with autosomal dominant polycystic kidney disease.[68] Very little is known about the mechanism responsible for the frequency with which nephrolithiasis occurs. Obstruction of the collecting system is clearly one factor; the low urinary pH values and the frequency of hypocitric aciduria suggest that metabolic factors may also be important. Just over half the stones are composed of uric acid; the other half are mainly calcium oxalate, often with a uric acid core.[68]

Renal transplantation

Autosomal dominant polycystic kidney disease does not recur in transplanted kidneys, which is evidence against the hypothesis that a circulating factor is responsible for the disease. The survival of patients after renal transplantation and the survival of grafts over a period of 15 years are not significantly different from those in other diseases. There is a small risk of complications related to the disease, such as aortic dissection, rupture of an intracranial aneurysm and infection of cysts.[69] After renal transplantation the polycystic kidneys tend to decrease in size in most patients; occasionally they enlarge dramatically, necessitating their removal: the cause is uncertain.[70]

Prognosis

The chance of developing renal insufficiency increases with advancing age in people who carry the mutant gene; end-stage renal failure occurs in about 50% of patients older than 50 years. Those who survive to their sixtieth year without renal insufficiency are unlikely to require dialysis or renal transplantation.[55] Approximately 10% of patients with adult polycystic renal disease die from subarachnoid haemorrhage caused by rupture of an intracranial berry aneurysm.[6] Other causes of death are myocardial infarction and sepsis.

Pathogenesis

The cause of autosomal dominant polycystic kidney disease is unknown. Several hypotheses have been formed on the basis of various experimental and clinical observations. Three main theories currently prevail.[71]

The first proposes that increased distensibility or compliance of the tubular basement membrane is the primary defect. Supporting this notion is the increased incidence of hepatic and pancreatic cysts, cerebral aneurysms, colonic diverticulae and mitral valve prolapse in autosomal dominant polycystic kidney disease; all of these lesions suggest that basement membranes generally are defective. The notion is that in autosomal dominant polycystic kidney disease there is a disordered synthesis of extracellular matrix, analogous to Marfan's syndrome and Ehlers–Danlos syndrome. As a result of this postulated defect the tubular basement membranes are abnormally compliant and permit unrestrained distension of the tubules. Support for this hypothesis comes from studies of an autosomal recessive polycystic kidney disease that occurs in a particular strain of mice.[72] In these animals expression of kidney basement membrane genes for the alpha-1 chain of type IV collagen and the B1 and B2 chains of laminin are abnormal.

The second hypothesis is that hyperplasia of tubular cells, with or without the formation of tiny polyps, causes partial obstruction of tubular lumina and leads to cyst formation. Dilatation occurs as the consequence of the increased intraluminal pressure.[73]

A third hypothesis regards cysts as being formed because of abnormal outward growth of the tubular epithelial cells. Support for this suggestion comes from animal models of cystic disease in which the cells lining renal cysts sometimes appear to multiply in a manner reminiscent of those that form adenomas. In one mouse strain with autosomal polycystic kidney disease there is increased expression of the proto-oncogenes c-*fos*, c-*myc* and c-Ki-*ras*, which is consistent with abnormal regulation of the growth of the tubular cells.[74]

The three theories are not mutually exclusive. It is also probable that the basic underlying genetic defect, whatever it may be, is susceptible to environmental and other influences.

Autosomal recessive polycystic kidney disease (infantile polycystic kidney disease)

This rare disorder, occuring about once in every 16 000 live births, is due to an autosomal recessive gene. At present there are no markers linking it to a particular chromosome. The disease appears in siblings and is commoner in girls. The disease invariably affects both kidneys, which are massively enlarged at birth due to abnormal expansion and growth of the collecting ducts. Most patients die in infancy or early childhood but survival to reproductive age has been recorded.[75,76]

All patients with infantile polycystic renal disease have hepatic abnormalities. These take the form either of multiple epithelial cysts or of biliary dysgenesis, proliferation of the bile ductules and portal fibrosis. In one study, 38% of patients were found to have hepatic cysts by ultrasound.[63] Malformations of other parts of the body are infrequent.

Clinical features

The greatest danger to the few who live beyond the perinatal period is severe systemic hypertension. Portal hypertension secondary to the liver changes may also occur.

Renal changes

The kidneys may each weigh as much as 150–400 g (normal weight at birth is about 15 g). Their capsular surface is studded with miliary opalescent spots but there is no bosselation. On the cut surface the normal pattern of the cortex and medulla is replaced by the presence of innumerable, radially arranged, fusiform cysts (Fig. 3.20). The calyces, pelves and ureters are normal. Microscopically, the cysts are lined by cuboidal epithelium. Microdissection reveals that the cystic lesions are confined to the collecting ducts and tubules, i.e. that part of the nephron derived embryologically from the ureteric bud (see p. 48).

Pathogenesis

The pathogenesis of the infantile form of polycystic renal disease is unknown. Similar hypotheses to those suggested for the dominant form of the condition have been advanced. In the two mutant strains of mice that have autosomal recessive polycystic kidney disease, abnormal regulation of basement membrane gene expression is present in one[72] and altered replication of tubular epithelial cells in the other.[74]

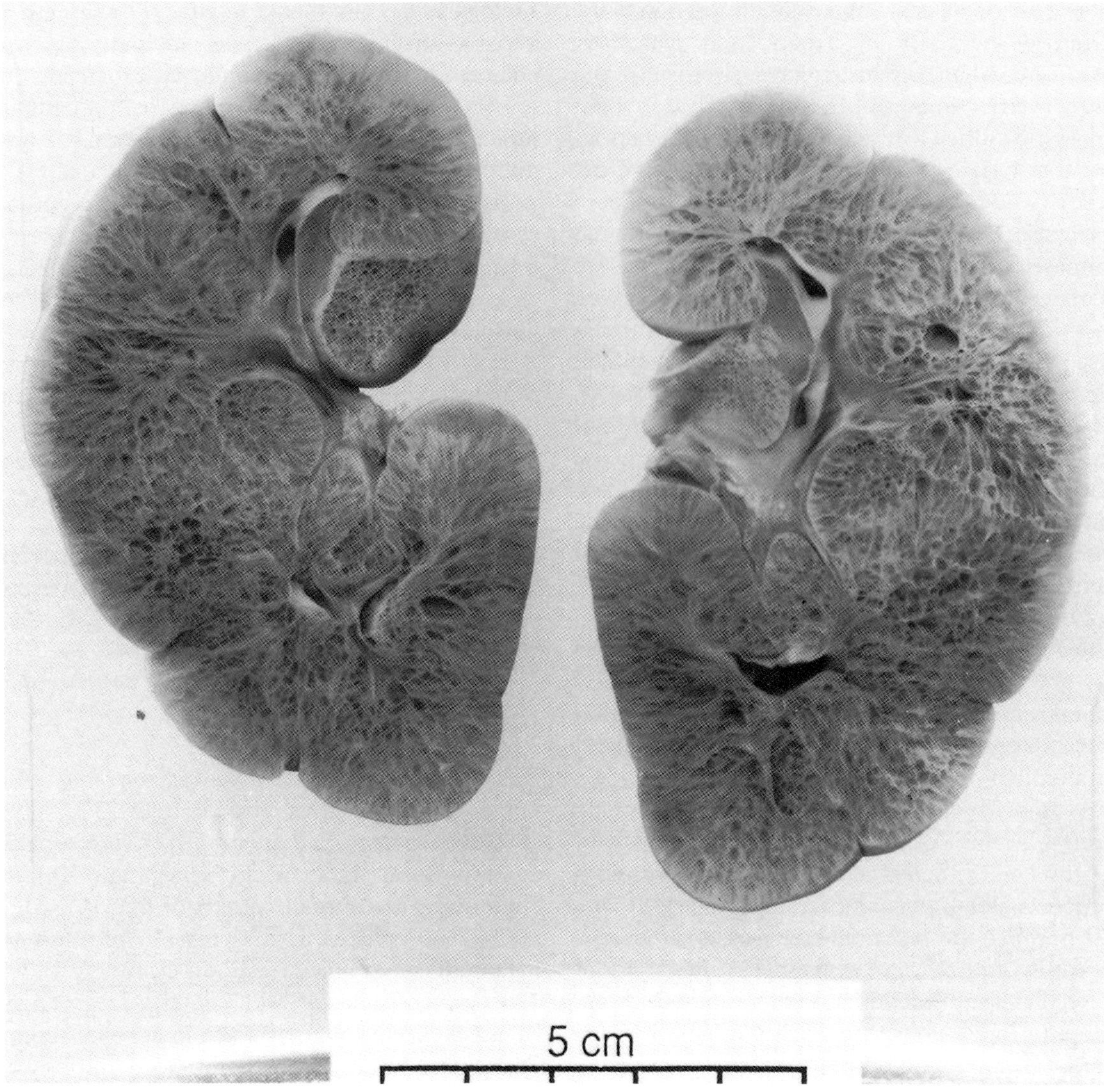

Fig. 3.20 Autosomal recessive polycystic kidney disease.

RENAL CYSTIC DISEASE ASSOCIATED WITH CONGENITAL HEPATIC FIBROSIS

Congenital hepatic fibrosis is the term that has been used to describe a condition affecting young patients who present with features of portal hypertension, including ascites, hepatosplenomegaly and bleeding oesophageal varices.[77] There is marked portal fibrosis in the liver of these patients, accompanied by bile duct proliferation but without gross cyst formation. The condition is thought to be due to an autosomal gene.

Although renal function is not significantly impaired in congenital hepatic fibrosis, about half the patients have many spherical cysts throughout the cortex and medulla of both kidneys. The cysts are separated by broad areas of normal parenchyma.

The pathogenesis of renal cystic disease associated with congenital hepatic fibrosis is not known.

MEDULLARY CYSTS

Medullary sponge kidney[78,79]

In this fairly common disorder dilated collecting

ducts are found in one or more renal papillae. Most of the patients are between 30 and 50 years old. It is commoner in women than in men. In the absence of complications there are usually no symptoms but occasionally there may be microscopic haematuria or attacks of gross haematuria. Serious illness can result from two common complications – urinary infection and stone formation (see p. 534)[80] – which may occur together or separately giving dysuria and renal colic. However, the infections can usually be controlled with antibacterial treatment and calculi prevented by thiazide diuretics and inorganic phosphates, so renal insufficiency is rare. Sandy material may be present in the urine. Somatic asymmetry, in the form of congenital hemihypertrophy, has been present in several cases.[81]

In 75% of cases both kidneys are affected. Tiny cysts, less than 0.5 cm in diameter, are present in one or more of the renal papillae (Fig. 3.21). The cysts are lined by columnar or cuboidal epithelium, communicate with collecting ducts and frequently contain spherical laminated PAS-positive calculi composed of apatite, a mixture of phosphates of calcium. The cortex may show evidence of pyelonephritis but is free of cysts.

a

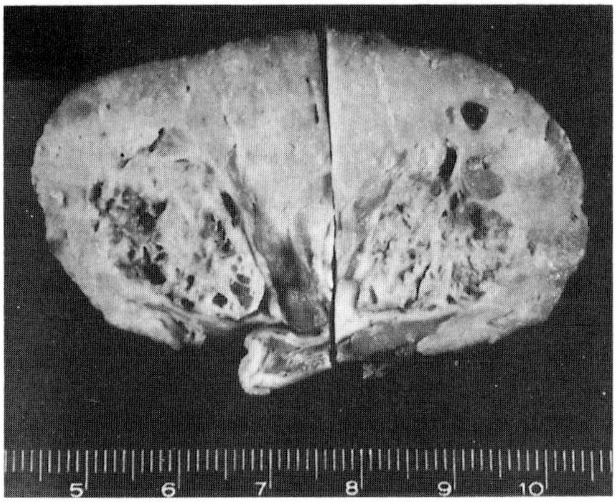

b

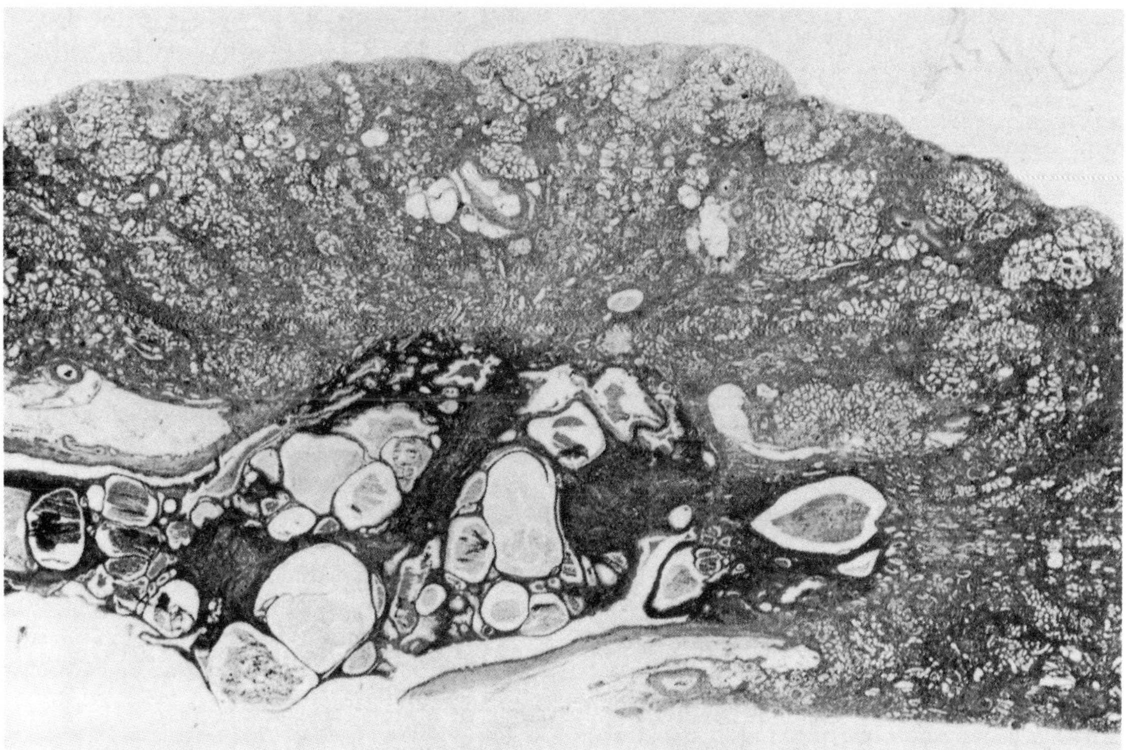

Fig. 3.21 a, b Medullary sponge kidney. (**a**) Gross appearance of cut surface showing medullary cysts. (**b**) Cysts and surrounding dense stroma confined to the medulla.
(**b**) Masson trichrome × 3
Reproduced by permission from: Levitt MH, McCoy RC, Fetter BF. J Urol 1974; 112: 710 (Figs 1, 2)

The diagnosis is usually made by intravenous urography, which demonstrates the characteristic cysts in the renal papillae. The calculi, although small, are often visible in plain radiographs. The prognosis of uncomplicated cases is good. In patients with extensive calculi or with persistent urinary infection progressive renal damage may occur. The pathogenesis of the medullary sponge kidney is unknown. A congenital malformation of collecting ducts has been suggested but the evidence for this is not strong.

Nephronophthisis–medullary cystic disease complex[6,82,83]

This term refers to a heterogeneous group of hereditary disorders characterized pathologically by progressive tubular atrophy, progressive interstitial fibrosis and variable numbers of tiny cysts, predominantly in the outer medulla at the junction with the cortex. These disorders account for 10–20% of cases of renal insufficiency in childhood and adolescence. The sexes are affected approximately equally. Among the inheritance patterns that have been recognized is an autosomal dominant form referred to as *medullary cystic disease,*[83] an autosomal recessive condition known as *familial juvenile nephronophthisis*[84] and a group of autosomal recessive conditions called *renal–retinal dysplasia* because of associated ocular abnormalities such as retinitis pigmentosa, tapetoretinal pigmentary degeneration, retinal dysplasia or cataracts.[85] The recessive forms are commoner and become apparent in the first 10 years of life; the dominant form often appears in early adulthood. Sporadic forms without a family history of renal disease also occur with an onset in adolescence.

Clinical features

Clinically there is polyuria, polydipsia, enuresis, normochromic normocytic anaemia, growth retardation and progression to renal failure. The only radiological finding is a reduction in the size of the kidneys. The cysts do not fill with contrast material.

Renal changes

Both kidneys are usually smaller than normal and the subcapsular surfaces are granular. The cortex is narrow and in the outer medulla there are cysts that are usually less than 0.5 cm in diameter (Fig. 3.22). They are lined by flattened or cuboidal epithelium. When renal failure has developed most of the glomeruli are sclerosed, tubular atrophy is widespread and there is interstitial fibrosis. At this stage minute cysts are often present in the cortex as well. Thickening of some of the tubular basement membranes is particularly pronounced, while others may be extremely thin.

Pathogenesis

The cause of the renal damage is unknown. The cysts are inadequate to explain the widespread destruction of glomeruli and tubules. An inherited metabolic abnormality, resulting in a nephrotoxic agent which causes localized thickening of the tubular basement membranes and consequent partial obstruction of the urine flow and cystic dilatation, has been considered as the initiating event but no agent has been identified. As staining with antitubular basement membrane antibody is often reduced the membrane may lack some normal antigenic component and it has been speculated that this may be the fundamental defect.[86] The disease does not recur in renal transplants.

MULTILOCULAR CYSTS[87,88]

Solitary or rarely bilateral multilocular cysts that do not communicate with the renal pelvis, in which there is no communication between locules, and which are lined by epithelium and contain no differentiated renal elements within the cysts, are rare. Some can be difficult to differentiate from renal carcinomas because of proliferation of the epithelium. About 50% occur in children but they are not familial. Multilocular cysts in both children and adults are benign.

The pathogenesis of multilocular cysts is unknown. Those occurring in children are generally thought to represent mature variants of nephro-

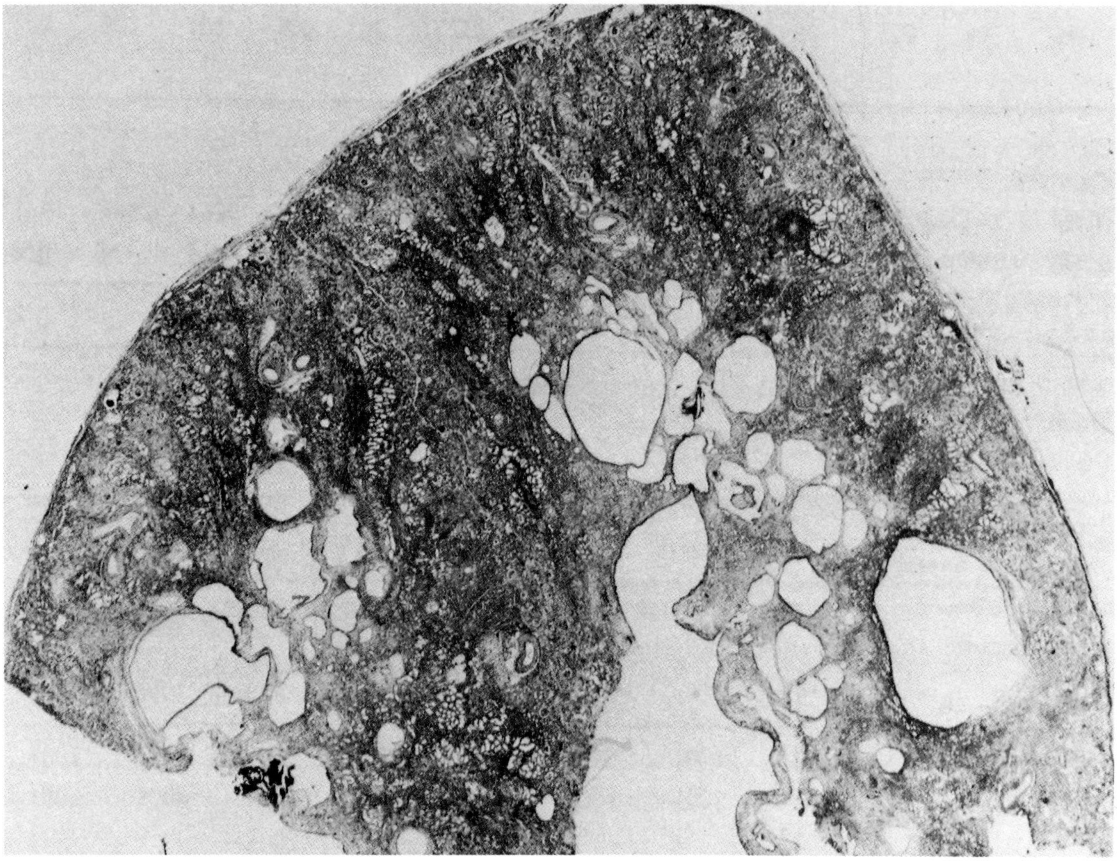

Fig. 3.22 Nephronophthisis. Section of part of kidney removed from a boy aged 14 years at the time of renal transplantation. The child had suffered from familial juvenile nephronophthisis for 6 years. Many small cysts are present in the medulla. Haematoxylin-eosin × 9
Reproduced by permission from: van Collenburg JJM, Thompson MW, Huber J. Clin Nephrol 1978; 9: 55–62 (Fig. 1)

blastoma; they are sometimes referred to as *cystic nephromas* (see p. 598).[89] Multilocular cysts in adults are considered by some to be hamartomatus masses of developmental origin.[90]

OTHER RARE DEVELOPMENTAL ANOMALIES

Many other rare developmental disorders have been described.[91,92] A few of the more important are given below.

Cystic kidneys

Examples of cystic kidneys are autosomal recessive syndromes such as Zellweger's cerebro-hepato-renal syndrome, Michel's syndrome and short rib polydactyly, and autosomal dominant syndromes such as von Hippel–Lindau's disease and Alpert's syndrome.

Von Hippel–Lindau disease

Von Hippel–Lindau disease (VHLD) is an uncommon condition characterized by angiomatous cysts of the cerebellum, tumours or cysts of abdominal organs (chiefly pancreas and kidneys), and angiomatosis of the retina. Renal cell carcinoma occurs commonly in these patients (see p. 571).[93] Early recognition of VHLD and prompt surgical intervention are essential if malignancy is to be avoided. Genetic counselling of young family members in their child-bearing years is also important because this autosomal dominant condition does not become clinically apparent until early or middle adult life.

Tuberous sclerosis

Tuberous sclerosis, in which there may be diffuse cystic change in the kidneys, is discussed on page 113.

Renal dysplasia

Examples of renal dysplasia are the branchio-oto-renal syndrome,[92] the VATER association[92] and Beckwith–Wiedemann's syndrome (see p. 589).

Tubulointerstitial nephritis

Progressive tubulointerstitial nephritis occurs in Jeune's syndrome, Laurence–Moon–Biedl–Bardet syndrome and Alström's syndrome. The first two disorders are also accompanied by renal cysts. All three conditions are discussed on page 476.

Renal agenesis

Unilateral renal agenesis occurs in the LEOPARD syndrome[92] and the Klippel–Feil syndrome.[92]

REFERENCES

Development of the kidneys

1. Moore KL. The developing human. Clinically orientated embryology, 4th edn. Philadelphia: WB Saunders, 1988.
2. Pansky B. Review of medical embryology. New York: MacMillan, 1982.
3. Osathanondh V, Potter EL. Development of human kidney as shown by microdissection: I. preparation of tissue with reasons for possible misinterpretation of observation. II. Renal pelvis, calyces and papillae. III. Formation and inter-relationship of collecting tubules and nephrons. Arch Pathol 1963; 76: 271–276.
4. Osathanondh V, Potter EL. Development of human kidney as shown by microdissection: V. Development of vascular patterns of glomerulus. Arch Pathol 1966; 82: 403–411.
5. Potter EL. Normal and abnormal development of the kidney. Chicago: Year Book Medical, 1972.
6. Kissane JM. Development of the kidney. In: Heptinstall RH, ed. Pathology of the kidney, Vol 1, 3rd edn. Boston: Little, Brown and Co, 1983: 61.
7. Darmady EM, MacIver AG. Renal pathology. London: Butterworth, 1980: 43.
8. Fetterman GH, Shuplock NA, Phillipp FF, Gregg HS. The growth and maturation of human glomeruli and proximal convolutions from term to adulthood. Studies by microdissection. Pediatrics 1965; 35: 601–619.
9. Emery JL, MacDonald MS. Involuted and scarred glomeruli in the kidneys of infants. Am J Pathol 1960; 36: 713–723.
10. Thomas MA. Congenital glomerulosclerosis. Pathology 1969; 1: 105–112.
11. Porter KA, Giles HMcC. A pathological study of five cases of pyelonephritis in the newborn. Arch Dis Child 1956; 31: 303–309.
12. Swan CA. A study of three infants dying from congenital defects following maternal rubella in the early stages of pregnancy. J Pathol Bacteriol 1944; 56: 289–295.
13. Tedeschi CG, Helpern MM, Ingalls TH. Pathological manifestations in an infant after maternal rubella in the sixteenth week of gestation: report of a case. N Engl J Med 1953; 249: 439–442.
14. Beale MG, Strayer DS, Kissane JM, Robson AM. Congenital glomerulosclerosis and nephrotic syndrome in two infants. Speculations and pathogenesis. Am J Dis Child 1979; 133: 842–845.

Congenital malformations of the kidneys

15. Roodhooft AM, Birnholz JC, Holmes LB. Familial nature of congenital absence and severe dysgenesis of both kidneys. N Engl J Med 1984; 310: 1341–1345.
16. Potter EL. Facial characteristics of infants with bilateral renal agenesis. Am J Obstet Gynecol 1946; 51: 885–888.
17. Fantel AG, Shepard TH. Potter's syndrome: non-renal features induced by oligoamnios. Am J Dis Child 1975; 129: 1346–1347.
18. Perlman M, Williams J, Hirsch M. Neonatal pulmonary hypoplasia after prolonged leakage of amniotic fluid. Arch Dis Child 1976; 51: 349–353.
19. Carter CO, Evans K, Pescia G. A family study of renal agenesis. J Med Genet 1979; 16: 176–188.
20. Kiprov DD, Colvin RB, McCluskey RT. Focal and segmental glomerulosclerosis and proteinuria associated with unilateral renal agenesis. Lab Invest 1982; 46: 275–281.
21. Thorner PS, Arbus GS, Celermajer DS, Baumal R. Focal segmental glomerulosclerosis and progressive renal failure associated with a unilateral kidney. Pediatrics 1984; 73: 806–810.
22. Boissonnat P. What to call hypoplastic kidney. Arch Dis Child 1962; 37: 142–148.
23. Kanasawa M, Moller J, Good RA, Vernier RL. Dwarfed kidneys in children. The classification, etiology and significance of bilateral small kidneys in 11 children. Am J Dis Child 1965; 109: 130–140.
24. Broyer M. Chronic renal failure. In: Royer P, Habib R,

Mathieu H et al, eds. Pediatric nephrology. Philadelphia: Saunders, 1974: 358.
25. Royer P, Habib R, Mathieu M, Courtecuisse V. L'hypoplasie rénal é bilatéral é congénitale avec reduction du nombre, et hypertrophie des nephrons chez l'énfant. Ann Pédiatr (Paris) 1962; 9: 133–146.
26. Wing LNg, Cheung MF, Chan CW, Yu CL. Oligomeganephronic renal hypoplasia. Pathology 1980; 12: 639–645.
27. McGraw M, Poucell S, Sweet J, Baumer R. The significance of focal segmental glomerulosclerosis in oligomeganephronia. Int J Pediatr Nephrol 1984; 5: 67–72.
28. Acker KJ van, Roodhooft AM, Melis K. Monozygotic twins non-concordant for oligomeganephronic renal hypoplasia: artery–vein placental shunting as a possible pathogenetic mechanism. Clin Nephrol 1986; 25: 165–168.
29. Carlson HE. Supernumerary kidney. A summary of fifty-one reported cases. J Urol 1950; 64: 224–229.
30. Thompson GJ, Pace JM. Ectopic kidney. A review of 97 cases. Surg Gynecol Obstet 1937; 64: 935–943.
31. Malek RS, Kelalis PP, Burke EC. Ectopic kidney in children and frequency of association with other malformations. Mayo Clin Proc 1971; 46: 461–467.
32. Abeshouse BS. Crossed ectopia with fusion. Review of the literature and a report of four cases. Am J Surg 1947; 73: 658–683.
33. Kolln CP, Boatman DL, Schmidt JD, Flocks RH. Horseshoe kidney: a review of 105 patients. J Urol 1972; 107: 203–204.
34. Pitts WR, Muecke EC. Horseshoe kidneys: a 40-year experience. J Urol 1975; 113: 743–746.
35. Boatman DL, Kolln CP, Flocks RH. Congenital anomalies associated with horseshoe kidney. J Urol 1972; 107: 205–207.
36. Jensen N-H, Mortensen NP. Displaced renal lobe simulating tumour. Acta Radiol (Diagn) 1978; 19: 458–459.
37. Weyrauch HM. Anomalies of renal rotation. Surg Gynecol Obstet 1939; 69: 183–199.
38. Bernstein J. The morphogenesis of renal parenchymal maldevelopment (renal dysplasia). Pediatr Clin North Am 1971; 18: 395–407.
39. Risdon RA. Renal dysplasia. Part 1. A clinico-pathological study of 76 cases. J Clin Pathol 1971; 24: 57–65.
40. Risdon RA. Renal dysplasia. Part II. A necropsy study of 41 cases. J Clin Pathol 1971; 24: 65–71.
41. Hsia YE, Bratu M, Herbordt A. Genetics of the Meckel–Gruber syndrome (dysencephalia splanchnocystica). Pediatrics 1971; 48: 237–247.
42. Kudo M, Tamura K, Fuse Y. Cystic dysplastic kidneys associated with Dandy–Walker malformation and congenital hepatic fibrosis. Report of two cases. Am J Clin Pathol 1985; 84: 459–463.
43. Osathanondh V, Potter EL. Pathogenesis of polycystic kidneys. I, II, III, IV, V. Arch Pathol 1964; 77: 459–465.
44. McAlister WH, Siegel HM, Shackleford G, Askin F, Kissane JM. Glomerulocystic kidney. Am J Radiol 1979; 133: 536–538.
45. Carson RW, Bedi D, Cavallo T, Du Bose TD. Familial adult glomerulocystic kidney disease. Am J Kidney Dis 1987; 9: 154–165.
46. Rizzoni G, Loirat C, Levy M, Milanesi C, Zachello G, Mathieu H. Familial hypoplastic glomerulocystic kidney. A new entity? Clin Nephrol 1982; 18: 263–268.
47. Wyngaarden JB. Human heredity. In: Wyngaarden JB, Smith LH eds. Cecil — textbook of medicine, 17th edn. Philadelphia: Saunders, 1982: 6.
48. Vollmer WM, Wahl PW, Blagg CR. Survival with dialysis and transplantation in patients with end-stage renal disease. N Engl J Med 1983; 309: 1553–1558.
49. Milutinovic J, Fialkow PJ, Agodoa LY, Phillips LA, Rudd TG, Sutherland S. Clinical manifestations of autosomal dominant polycystic kidney disease in patients older than 50 years. Am J Kidney Dis 1990; 15: 237–243.
50. Reeders ST, Breuning MH, Davies KE, et al. A highly polymorphic DNA marker linked to adult polycystic kidney disease on chromosome 16. Nature 1985; 317: 542–544.
51. Reeders ST, Breuning MH, Coriney G, et al. Two genetic markers closely linked to adult polycystic kidney disease on chromosome 16.Br Med J 1986; 292: 851–853.
52. Kimberling WJ, Fain PR, Kenyon JB, Goldgar D, Sujansky E, Gabow PA. Linkage heterogeneity of autosomal dominant polycystic kidney disease. N Engl J Med 1988; 319: 913–917.
53. Romeo G, Devoto M, Costa G, et al. A second genetic locus for autosomal dominant polycystic kidney disease. Lancet 1988; 2: 8–10.
54. Gabow PA, Grantham JJ, Bennett W, et al. Gene testing in autosomal dominant polycystic kidney disease: results of National Kidney Foundation Workshop. Am J Kidney Dis 1989; 85: 87.
55. Delaney VB, Adler S, Bruns FJ, Licinia M, Segel DP, Fraley DS. Autosomal dominant polycystic kidney disease: presentation, complications, and prognosis. Am J Kidney Dis 1985; 5: 104–111.
56. Gardner KD, Evan AP. Cystic kidneys: an enigma evolves. Am J Kidney Dis 1984; 3: 403–413.
57. Sahney S, Weiss L, Levine NW. Genetic counselling in adult polycystic kidney disease. Am J Med Genet 1982; 11: 461–468.
58. Reeders ST, Zerres K, Gal A, et al. Prenatal diagnosis of autosomal dominant polycystic kidney disease with a DNA probe. Lancet 1986; 2: 6–8.
59. Gregoire JR, Torres VE, Holley KE, Farrow GM. Renal epithelial hyperplastic and neoplastic proliferation in autosomal dominant polycystic kidney disease. Am J Kidney Dis 1987; 9: 27–38.
60. Graham PC, Lindop GBM. The anatomy of the renin-secreting cell in adult polycystic kidney disease. Kidney Int 1988; 33: 1084–1090.
61. Waldherr R, Zerres K, Gall S, Enders H. Polycystic kidney disease in the fetus. Lancet 1989; 2: 274–275 (letter).
62. Dalgaard OZ. Bilateral polycystic disase of the kidneys: a follow-up of two hundred and eighty four patients and their families. Acta Med Scand 1957; suppl 328, 10–15.
63. Gabow PA, Ikle DW, Holmes JH. Polycystic kidney disease: prospective analysis of nonazotemic patients and family members. Ann Intern Med 1984; 101: 238–247.
64. Kulla L, Deymeer F, Smith TW, Weiner M, Mullins TF. Intracranial dissecting and saccular aneurysms in polycystic kidney disease. Arch Neurol 1982; 39: 776–8.
65. Iglesias CG, Torres VE, Offord KP, Holley KE, Beard CM, Kurland LT. Epidemiology of adult polycystic kidney disease, Olmsted County, Minnesota: 1935–1980. Am J Kidney Dis 1983; 2: 630–639.

hood with persistent recurrent haematuria were described.[2] Subsequently they developed renal failure.[3] In 1927 Alport redescribed the same family, emphasizing the occurrence in successive generations of progressive nephritis and adding that nerve deafness was present in these patients as well as in some other members of the family, and that the nephropathy was more severe in the males than in the females.[4] The condition received little further attention until 1951 when a careful and detailed study of a very large affected family was published.[5] Since then many other families have been described from various parts of the world and it has become clear that expression of either the renal or hearing defects may be variable within families. Also the occurrence of spontaneous mutations means that sporadic cases will be met. Inherited ocular defects may accompany the renal disease.

Strictly the term Alport's syndrome should be confined to those cases that have sensorineural deafness; the term *hereditary nephritis without deafness* should be applied to the other patients. Many workers, however, use the label Alport's syndrome to embrace all families with inherited nephritis, with or without deafness.

It is probable that many cases go undetected; Alport's syndrome and hereditary nephritis without deafness must be considered in any child or young adult with unexplained persistent haematuria. Alport's syndrome and hereditary nephritis without deafness are uncommon causes of chronic renal failure. Only 0.6% of patients listed in the registry of the European Dialysis and Transplantation Association (EDTA) in 1982 had this diagnosis.[6]

Mode of inheritance

Hereditary nephritis, including Alport's syndrome, is genetically heterogeneous. The majority of cases appear to be transmitted as an X-linked dominant trait, but autosomal dominant, sex-linked dominant, and autosomal recessive forms occasionally occur.[7] The estimated frequency of the X-linked gene in the population is 1 in 5000.

Clinical features

The commonest presenting manifestation is haematuria, which usually occurs intermittently from the age of about 5 years. Occasionally it is noted even in infancy. The haematuria is usually microscopical and asymptomatic with episodes of gross haematuria; it is often accompanied by progressive proteinuria and sometimes by pyuria. Occasionally advice is not sought until the patient is in renal failure. Although male and female members of a family develop the renal disease with equal frequency, affected females rarely develop renal failure whereas affected males frequently die in uraemia before the age of 40 years unless treated by dialysis or renal transplantation.

Bilateral nerve deafness is the most frequently associated extrarenal defect and occurs in about 50% of the patients, producing Alport's syndrome. The hearing loss is usually in the high tone range and may be detected by audiometry before the patient is aware of any disability.

Ocular abnormalities are less common and include bilateral anterior lenticonus, cataracts and rupture of the lens capsule.[8] Symmetrical bilateral pale yellow granulations around the fovea also occur and appear to be characteristic of Alport's syndrome and hereditary nephritis without deafness.[9]

Serology

The levels of complement in the serum are consistently normal.

Renal changes

Gross appearance of the kidneys

At necropsy the kidneys are shrunken and their subcapsular surface is pale and finely granular, as in end-stage sclerosing glomerulonephritis. Linear yellow streaks may be present in the cortex.

Light microscopy

In the first few years of life the glomeruli either appear normal or show only slight diffuse thickening of the capillary basement membrane. Increased numbers of immature glomeruli may be seen. The tubules contain red cell casts; usually there are also some small foci of tubular atrophy, with surrounding interstitial fibrosis and infiltration by mononuclear cells.

Later the thickening of the glomerular capillary basement membrane becomes more pronounced, there is segmental mesangial proliferation and segmental areas of sclerosis and hyalinosis appear (Fig. 4.1). Epithelial crescents sometimes occur and adhesions form between the glomerular tufts and Bowman's capsule. The process is focal: some glomeruli progress to obsolescence while others long remain normal. The areas of tubular atrophy, marked interstitial fibrosis and cellular infiltration progressively increase in size. Groups of fat-laden foam cells may be found in the interstitium and cause the yellow streaks that are seen grossly. Arteriolar and arterial changes are usually slight.[10]

None of these features is diagnostic, but the unusual mixture of glomerulonephritic and interstitial nephritic changes should suggest the possibility. The accumulation of foam cells in the interstitium in the absence of raised blood lipid levels should also make one think of Alport's syndrome.

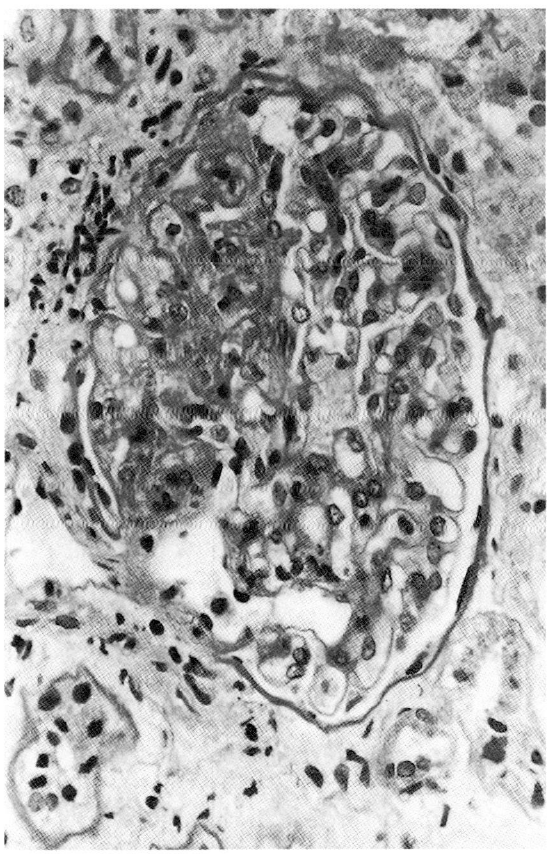

Fig. 4.1 Alport's syndrome. The glomerulus shows segmental sclerosis, capillary wall thickening and mesangial cell proliferation. Adjacent tubules are atrophic. Periodic acid-Schiff × 250

Electron microscopy

The most characteristic change is segmental thickening and splitting of the lamina densa of the glomerular capillary basement membrane into multiple, thin, irregular, interwoven layers, separated by clear spaces that sometimes contain small dark particles, measuring up to 90 nm in diameter, which may be lipid (Fig. 4.2). The term 'basket weave' is sometimes applied to the pattern formed by the interwoven layers of the lamina densa. The severity of the glomerular basement membrane splitting is directly proportional to the grade of proteinuria and the clinical course.

Elsewhere the glomerular capillary basement membrane may be exceptionally thin because of segmental reduction in the lamina densa to about a third of its normal thickness.[11] These basement membrane changes usually occur early, before the appearance of light microscopic changes; they are not specific. However, marked thickening and splitting of the basement membrane in the absence of other glomerular changes strongly suggest a diagnosis of Alport's syndrome. Minor degrees of splitting occur in a variety of glomerular diseases.

The foot processes of the visceral epithelial cells are usually obliterated. The mesangial matrix is increased in amount but appears structurally normal. Thickening and splitting of the tubular basement membrane is frequent but is also non-specific.

Immunofluorescence/immunoperoxidase microscopy

In most cases there is no localization of immunoglobulins or complement in the capillary walls. Occasionally focal deposits of IgM and/or complement are found.[12]

Changes in other organs: the hearing defect

Only non-specific changes have been found in the

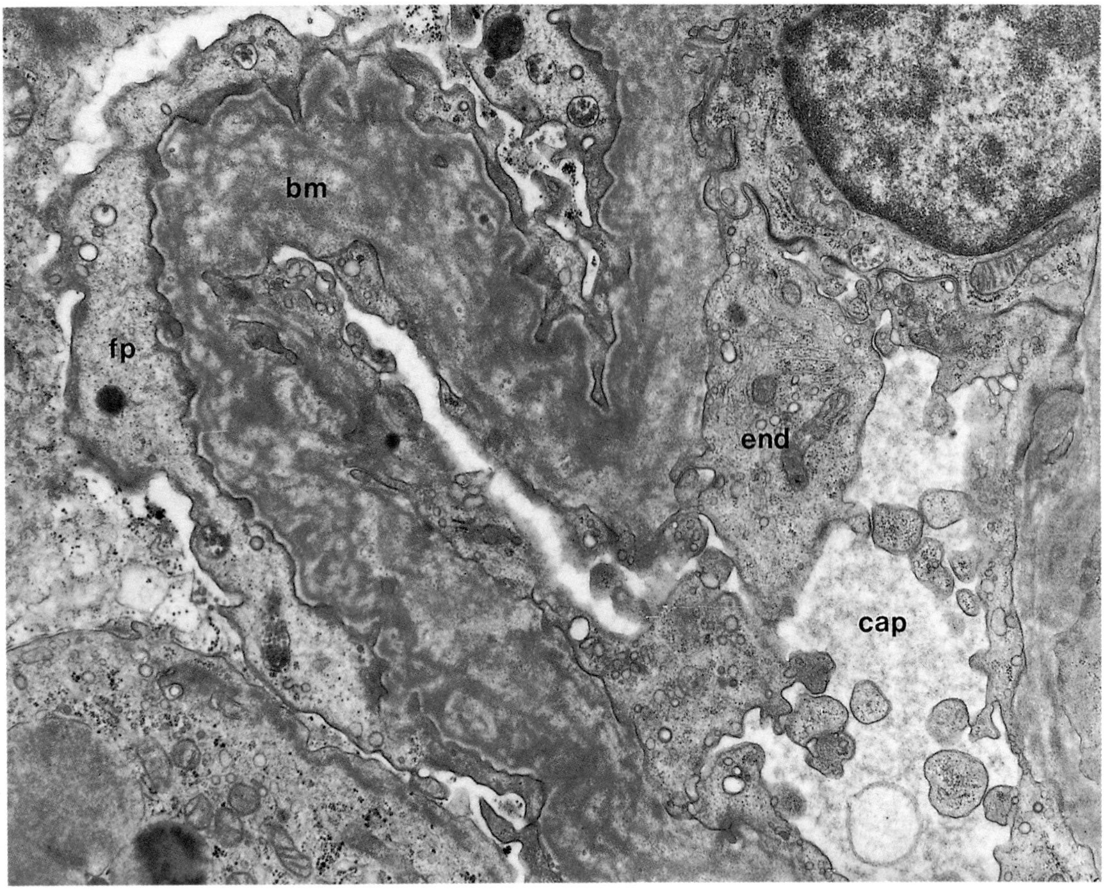

Fig. 4.2 Alport's syndrome. Electron micrograph of part of a glomerular loop. The thickened basement membrane (bm) consists of multiple irregular layers separated by clear spaces containing small particles. The epithelial foot processes (fp) are obliterated. cap, capillary lumen; end, endothelium.
× 11 000

cochleovestibular nerves and in the temporal bones.

Differential diagnosis of cause of haematuria in children

A monoclonal antibody which specifically recognizes the Goodpasture antigen has been used to identify patients with Alport's syndrome in whom the Goodpasture antigen is abnormal. In these patients there is no binding, or greatly reduced binding, of the antibody to the glomerular capillary basement membrane and distal tubular basement membrane compared with controls in whom there is strong linear binding of the antibody to these sites.[13]

Glomerular basement membrane antigens, including the Goodpasture antigen, are excreted in urine. It has been suggested[14] that Goodpasture antigen is absent or reduced in the urine of patients with Alport's syndrome – if this is confirmed then patients with mild disease could be identified by assaying the level of Goodpasture antigen in the urine using a monoclonal antibody to that antigen.

Renal transplantation

Patients with Alport's syndrome who receive a normal renal allograft sometimes develop anti-glomerular basement membrane antibodies (see p. 672), presumably because they react to the Goodpasture antigen which is present in the graft but was absent from their own kidneys.[15,16] The incidence of linear fixation of IgG along glomerular capillary basement membranes of renal allografts in patients whose original disease was Alport's syndrome is much higher than in graft recipients with other renal diseases. The linear fixation is usually transient and not accompanied by glomerular changes and deterioration of renal function. Occasionally it is associated with crescentic glomerulonephritis and rapid failure of the graft.[15,17] Awareness of this rare complication is important because early treatment by plasmapheresis may save the graft. The basement membrane and other changes associated with Alport's syndrome do not recur in renal transplants.

Prognosis

Major prognostic factors are the patient's sex and the mode of inheritance.[18] The presence of deafness does not appear to be a significant factor independent of the patient's sex (deafness is more common in males).

Sex

End-stage renal disease occurs approximately 20–25 years later in women than in men. In one series the median renal survival in males was 32 years in Alport's syndrome and 34 years in hereditary nephritis without deafness, compared with 61 years and 57 years respectively in females. It has been suggested that the renotrophic effect of androgens may hasten the course of the disease in men; in IgA, membranous and diabetic nephropathies, females also have a better prognosis.[18]

Mode of inheritance

The mode of inheritance strongly influences prognosis. Median survival is approximately 25 years longer among male patients with autosomal dominant than among those with X-linked disease. The same difference also applies to women with Alport's syndrome and hereditary nephritis without deafness.[18]

Pathogenesis

The mechanism of renal damage is unknown but it is probable that the glomerular basement membrane changes are all secondary to deficient synthesis and repair of a chemically abnormal basement membrane and are steps in the progression to glomerular collapse and sclerosis.[11] The abnormality may be in a structural gene at a locus governing the composition of basement membrane in glomerulus, lens capsule and inner ear.[19]

Immunological studies which have attempted to define the biochemical defects in the composition of the glomerular basement membrane indicate that Goodpasture antigen (a component of normal glomerular basement membrane against which antibodies are directed in some cases of Goodpasture's syndrome – see p. 11) may be reduced in quantity, or absent from the glomerular basement membrane of various subsets of patients with Alport's syndrome.[20] It has been suggested that the amount of Goodpasture antigen present is related to prognosis – absence of the antigen indicating a poor prognosis and slight reduction indicating a good prognosis.[21] Most patients lacking Goodpasture antigen are males.

In those patients whose glomerular capillary basement membrane is deficient in Goodpasture antigen, amyloid P component, a known constituent of normal glomerular basement membrane (see p. 11), is also absent.[22] The relationship between these two basement membrane substances is unknown. They may be bound to each other by electrostatic forces or they may be normally bound to another unknown antigen which is missing or modified in Alport's syndrome.

In X-linked Alport's syndrome evidence has been produced that a gene (COL 4A5) that codes for the $\alpha5$ chain of type IV collagen, located on the X chromosome at Xq22, is defective.[23] Three different mutations of this gene have been shown in three kindreds with Alport's syndrome. The degree of deafness seems to be directly correlated with the severity of the defect in the gene.

Type IV collagen is the major component of glomerular basement membranes; at the C terminus of the molecule is the NC1 domain composed of dimers and monomers of molecular weights 24 kDa, 26 kDa and 28 kDa. The non-collagenous NC1 domain cross links collagen type IV molecules in the formation of glomerular basement membrane and contains the Goodpasture antigen.

Indirect evidence suggests that, as a result of the genetic defect, the monomers and Goodpasture antigen are either absent from the glomerular basement membrane or present but structurally altered; the cross linking of the type IV molecules is incomplete resulting in splitting of the lamina densa.[24]

Variants on Alport's syndrome

Some cases of Alport's syndrome are accompanied by hyperprolinaemia.[25] The association is probably coincidental, the two conditions being inherited separately. Other less frequent associations include a haematological syndrome of thrombocytopenia with giant platelets.[26]

THIN GLOMERULAR BASEMENT MEMBRANE SYNDROME (BENIGN FAMILIAL HAEMATURIA; THIN MEMBRANE NEPHROPATHY)

In 1966 a benign form of familial haematuria was described.[27] The condition, which is inherited as an autosomal dominant trait, has no extrarenal manifestations and affects both sexes with equal frequency and intensity.[28] It is associated with glomerular basement membranes that appear unusually thin; it is not possible to be more definite than this because information about membrane width in appropriate controls is scanty.

More recently some sporadic cases of isolated haematuria, for which no cause could be found, have been shown to have glomerular capillary basement membranes that are thinner than normal when an arbitrary value for normality is used.[29,30] This value has been based on control groups with various diseases, or on published values for controls who were not matched for age or sex, both factors which affect glomerular basement membrane width.

As the familial and sporadic cases have in common isolated haematuria and glomerular capillary basement membranes thought to be thinner than normal, the terms 'thin glomerular basement membrane syndrome' and 'thin membrane nephropathy' have been coined to describe these conditions.

The incidence of thin glomerular basement membrane syndrome is not known. It is identified infrequently, probably because electron microscopy is necessary for the diagnosis and this examination is still not done in many renal units. The results of studies in Holland[31] and England[32] suggest that it is as common as IgA nephropathy in patients with persistent microscopic haematuria. Examination of renal transplant donor kidneys indicates that it may occur in as many as 5–9% of the general population.[33]

It is still uncertain whether the glomerular basement thinning is responsible for the haematuria.

Clinical features

The haematuria is asymptomatic, persistent and microscopic but there may also be recurrent episodes of gross haematuria. Mild proteinuria is sometimes present. In these familial cases both children and adults are affected but the diagnosis is usually made in childhood. A similar, possibly identical, condition occurs sporadically, particularly in adults.[29,30]

Renal changes

Light microscopy

Characteristically, in children the light microscope reveals no glomerular abnormality; in adults global sclerosis can occur in variable numbers of glomeruli. There may be red cell casts in the tubules.

Electron microscopy

There is widespread thinning of most of the glomerular capillary basement membranes caused by a reduction in the width of the lamina densa (Fig. 4.3);[28–30,34,35] the narrowed lamina densa is often prominent giving the membrane a trilaminar appearance such as is seen in the glomerulus of a mouse.[36] Thinning of the basement membrane is easy to recognize if it is extreme. However, the detection of lesser degrees of thinning depends very much on the accuracy of the method used in measuring the membrane width. Even if the measurements are accurate and representative their interpretation is difficult because there are no adequate data giving the range of variation in glomerular capillary basement membrane widths in normal males and females at different ages. Also comparison of measurements obtained by different groups of observers can be misleading unless it is known that identical methods were used in the preparation of the samples; in particular the embedding medium will affect the apparent width of the membrane. However, having said this it is generally agreed that capillary basement membranes with a harmonic mean measurement of 200 nm or less in children or 250 nm or less in adults are abnormally thin if the measurements are made using the method reported by Osawa et al.[37] or Steffes et al.[38] on sections cut from material embedded in Epon 812 resin.[30,39]

Rarely there are small gaps or breaks in the thin membrane. Lamination, segmental thickening and splitting of the glomerular capillary basement membrane are not found in children with thin basement membrane syndrome; in adults small segmental areas may show minor degrees of these changes.[29] Partial obliteration of epithelial foot processes is present in some cases. Scanty electron-dense deposits are found in the mesangium of a few of the adults.

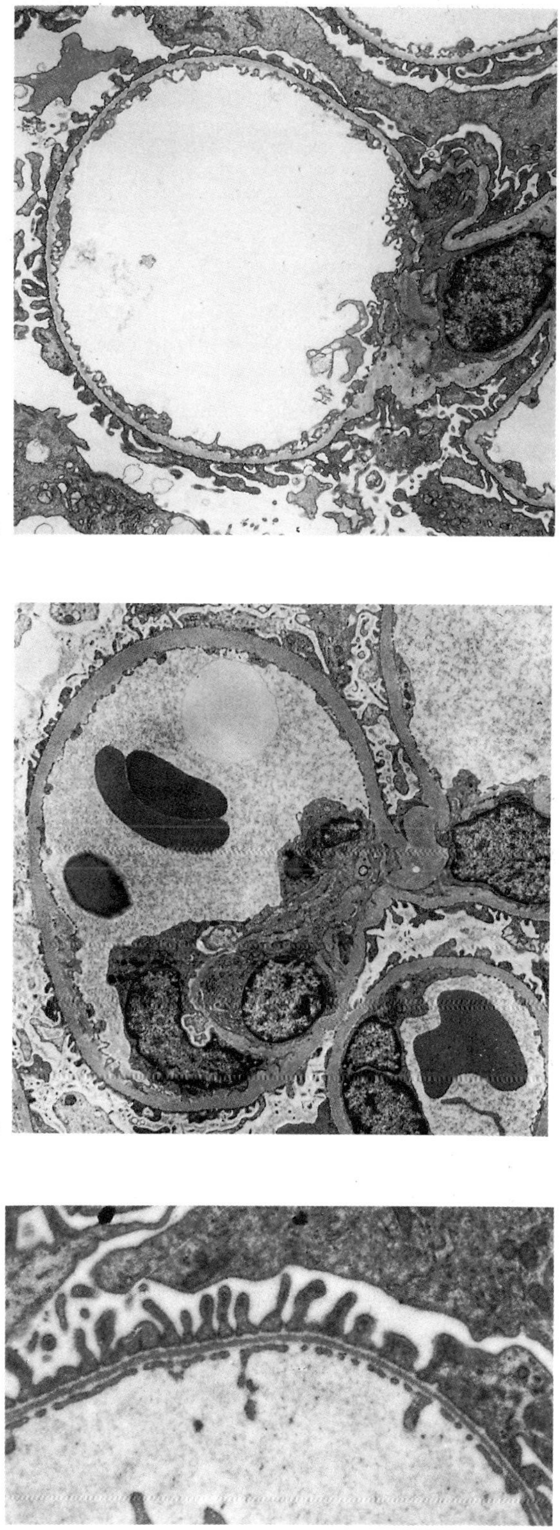

Fig. 4.3 Thin glomerular basement membrane syndrome. Markedly attenuated glomerular capillary basement membrane (**a**), compared with normal (**b**). (**c**) Glomerular capillary basement membrane with a trilaminar appearance such as is seen in the glomerulus of a mouse. Electron micrographs: (**a, b**) × 4800; (**c**) × 11 000

Immunofluorescence/immunoperoxidase microscopy

No deposits of immunoglobulin or complement have been found in the childhood cases but scanty deposits of C3 and IgM occur in a few of the adults.[29]

Differential diagnosis

Extensive thinning of the glomerular capillary basement membrane is seen in the early stages of *Alport's syndrome*. However, it is often accompanied by abnormalities of the Goodpasture antigen and sometimes by marked splitting and lamination of the basement membrane (see pp. 75–77). Neither of these features is found in the thin glomerular basement membrane syndrome.[40] Segmental, as distinct from widespread, thinning of the glomerular capillary basement membrane is seen in a variety of glomerulopathies. Capillary dilatation from any cause can lead to local attenuation of the membrane.

Prognosis

The long-term prognosis is excellent in those familial cases whose parents have haematuria but are otherwise normal. The outlook for the sporadic cases is less certain; in one series four of the 14 patients had impaired renal function.[29]

Pathogenesis

This is not known. It has been suggested that the glomerular capillary basement membrane does not mature properly and stays in its infantile state (see p. 7).[34] In some of the sporadic cases the basement membrane abnormality may be acquired. The cause of the haematuria also remains unknown. It seems likely that the thin glomerular basement membrane allows erythrocytes to escape into Bowman's space. Ruptures or defects in the membrane are observed only exceptionally in these cases,[28] but such gross lesions are probably unnecessary for the passage of cells across the glomerular basement membrane, which may have the properties of a thixotropic gel.[41] Systems exhibiting biological thixotropy have the ability to undergo localized reduction in viscosity under the influence of pressure alone, followed by a comparatively slow recovery to their original consistency.

NAIL–PATELLA SYNDROME (HEREDITARY ONYCHO-OSTEODYSPLASIA)

The nail–patella syndrome is a rare hereditary disorder in which hypoplasia or aplasia of the patellae, deformity of the elbows consequent on hypoplasia of the head of the radius, and the presence of bilaterally symmetrical, horn-like processes projecting from the centre of the gluteal surface of the ilium are associated with dysplasia of the nails, particularly the nail of the thumbs and of the big toes, and nephropathy.[42,43] It is transmitted as an autosomal dominant trait with a frequency of approximately twenty-two per million persons. The locus for the nail–patella syndrome and loci for adenylate kinase and the ABO blood groups are closely linked on chromosome 9.[44,45]

Clinical features

Renal involvement is evident in 30–40% of patients, usually in the form of asymptomatic proteinuria which is occasionally severe enough to cause the nephrotic syndrome.

Renal changes

Light microscopy

There is focal and segmental thickening of the basement membrane of the glomerular capillaries. This may be accompanied later by segmental increase in the number of mesangial cells and in the amount of mesangial matrix. Eventually, the condition progresses to glomerular hyalinization and sclerosis. In the later stages there is also focal interstitial infiltration of mononuclear cells, fibrosis, and atrophy of tubules.

Electron microscopy

In all patients, even those without proteinuria, segments of the basement membrane of the glomerular capillaries are irregularly widened by electronlucent areas, giving a 'moth-eaten' appearance to the membrane. Within the lucent areas are bundles of collagen fibrils (Fig. 4.4). Phosphotungstic acid may be needed to demonstrate the fibrils. Lucent foci containing fibrils are also present in the mesangium of some cases. Obliteration of the foot processes of the epithelial cells is common.[42,43]

Immunofluorescence/immunoperoxidase microscopy

Usually there are no deposits of immunoglobulin or complement. In rare cases small amounts of IgM and C3 have been found distributed focally and segmentally in the wall of the glomerular capillaries and afferent arterioles.[42]

Differential diagnosis

Collagen fibrils commonly appear in the capillary basement membrane involved in any area of scarring following healing of a segmental focus of glomerular inflammation. However, the fibrils are confined to the scar and are not found in bundles elsewhere as they are in the nail–patella syndrome.

Renal transplantation

There has been no recurrence of the disease in the

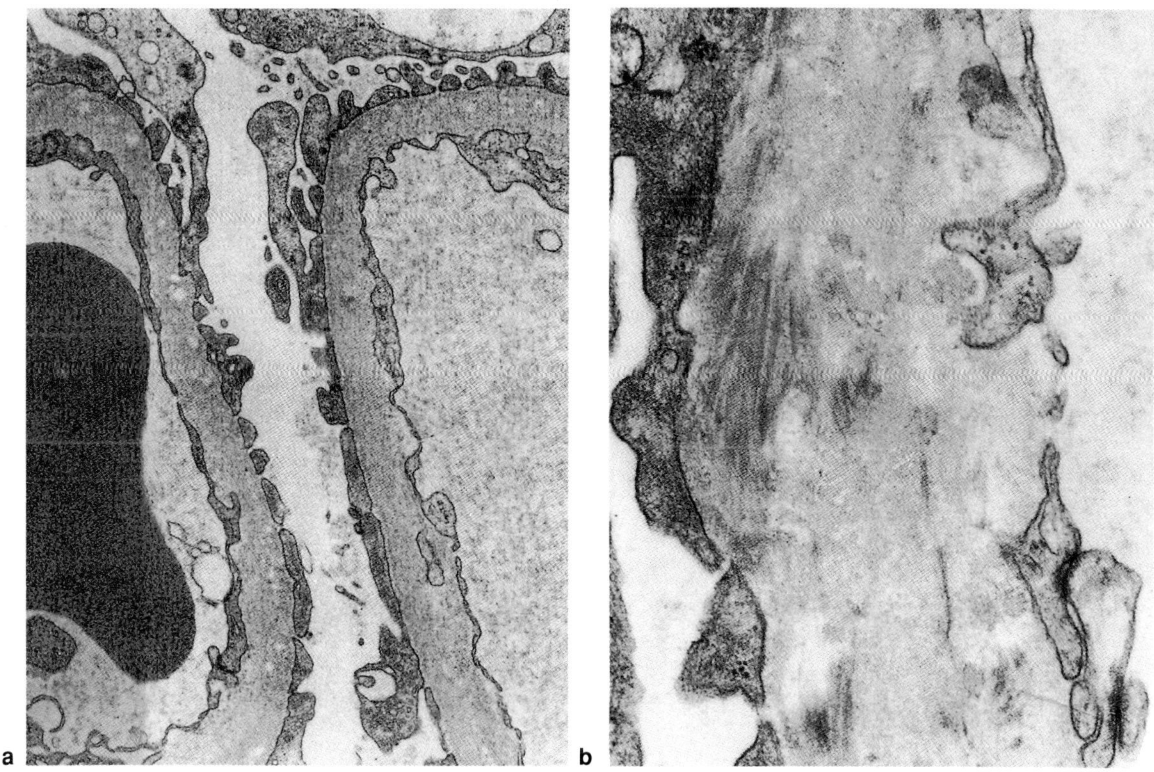

Fig. 4.4 Nail–patella syndrome. (**a**) Part of two glomerular capillary loops. The basement membrane is thickened and contains irregular lucent areas (moth-eaten appearance). (**b**) The basement membrane has been stained with phosphotungstic acid revealing bundles of collagen fibrils.
(**a**) Electron micrograph × 11 000; (**b**) electron micrograph, phosphotungstic acid × 44 000
Reproduced by permission from: Taguchi T, Takebayashi S, Nishimura M, Tsuru N. Ultrastruct Pathol 1988; 12: 175–183 (Figs 2, 4)

graft in the few cases that have been studied for periods of up to a year after transplantation.[46]

Prognosis

Renal failure develops in the second to fourth decades in about 25% of the patients with proteinuria.

Pathogenesis

The underlying cause of the nail–patella syndrome is not known. An enzymic defect in collagen metabolism has been postulated. It is unclear how the glomerular capillary basement membrane defects lead to progressive renal disease in some cases.

In two of three patients the glomerular capillary basement membranes failed to stain with the monoclonal antibody P1 which reacts with the Goodpasture antigen.[47] In the third patient and in two cases in another study the Goodpasture antigen stained normally. The reason for the lack of staining in some cases is not clear; it is possible that in nail–patella syndrome the primary biochemical abnormalities (whatever they are) secondarily affect the molecules bearing the Goodpasture antigen, leading to loss or alteration of the antigenic sites.

Variants of the nail–patella syndrome

Four patients with glomerular lesions typical of the nail–patella syndrome but lacking the bony and nail changes have been reported.[46,47] These may represent a partial or uneven gene penetrance or manifestations of only a portion of the gene complex involved in this syndrome.[48] The other possibility is that the presence of collagen-containing lucent areas in the glomerular basement membrane is not restricted to nail–patella syndrome but can occur in other forms of hereditary nephritis.[49]

CONGENITAL NEPHROTIC SYNDROME OF FINNISH TYPE

The congenital nephrotic syndrome of Finnish type is a rare condition that appears during the first 3 months of life and is inherited as an autosomal recessive trait.[50] It was first reported from England[51] but it is commonest in Finland where it affects one in every 8200 newborns;[52] this is probably because the autosomal recessive gene is most likely to be expressed in a relatively small and stable community where consanguineous marriage is more frequent.[53] In other countries and races the incidence of the syndrome is extremely low. Without treatment most of the infants with this condition die before the age of 1 year.

Clinical features

The baby is usually premature and the placenta is large, weighing more than a quarter of the birth weight of the child. The cranial sutures and fontanelles tend to be wide and the nose small and snub. There is often a calcaneovalgus deformity; this may involve one or both feet. Pyloric stenosis and oesophageal dysfunction occur in about 20% of the infants. Marked proteinuria is present from birth. The nephrotic syndrome occurs in half the cases during the first postnatal week and affects all the infants by 3 months.[53] Coagulation abnormalities are common and thrombosis of the renal and other large veins may occur. Serum immunoglobulin levels are extremely low despite normal maternal levels of IgG, IgM and IgA; the agammaglobulinaemia is probably due to a high renal clearance of immunoglobulin in utero.[54] The infant does not thrive and without treatment most die from intercurrent infections or electrolyte disorders within the first year.

The proteinuria in the congenital nephrotic syndrome of Finnish type commences in utero and the disease may be detected as early as the 15th week of gestation by demonstrating a markedly raised concentration of alpha-fetoprotein in the amniotic fluid.[55] There has been one report of a false normal result.[56]

Renal changes

Light microscopy

In about three-quarters of the cases there is

marked dilatation of the proximal convoluted tubules leading to the formation of small cysts, initially at the corticomedullary junction but later throughout the cortex (Fig. 4.5).[53] These changes are even present in utero and dilated tubules and microcysts have been recorded in the kidneys of affected fetuses aged 18–20 weeks.[57] The proportion of immature (fetal) glomeruli with dilatation of Bowman's space frequently appears increased but this is not confirmed by quantitative analysis.[58] In the mature glomeruli there is a segmental increase in the number of mesangial cells and there is more mesangial matrix than is normal. Arteriolar medial hypertophy is common. As the disease progresses, periglomerular fibrosis, glomerular sclerosis and interstitial fibrosis occur.[53]

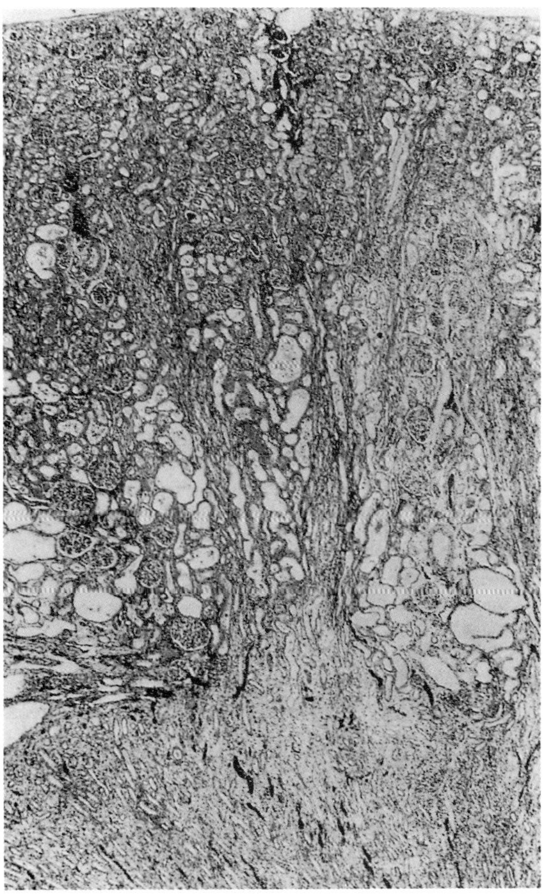

Fig. 4.5 Congenital nephrotic syndrome of Finnish type. Dilated tubules forming microcysts are present at the corticomedullary junction.
Haematoxylin-eosin × 60
Reproduced by permission from: Hallman N, Norio R, Rapola J. Nephron 1973; 11: 105 (Fig. 2)

Electron microscopy

The glomerular visceral epithelial cells are hypertrophied and there is widespread obliteration of their foot processes (Fig. 4.6). The capillary basement membrane is thin and the mesangium is expanded and hypercellular; neither shows electron-dense deposits.[59,60]

Immunofluorescence/immunoperoxidase microscopy

Deposits of immunoglobulin, complement and fibrinogen are not found.[59]

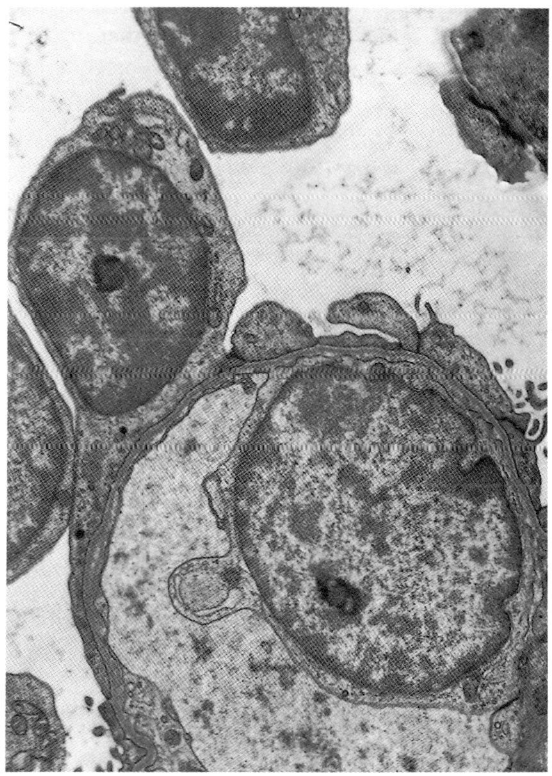

Fig. 4.6 Congenital nephrotic syndrome of Finnish type. Electron micrograph of part of a glomerular capillary. There is obliteration of the epithelial foot processes and the capillary basement membrane is thin.
× 6560

Changes in the placenta

In the enlarged placenta the villi and stroma are oedematous and there is patchy persistence of the cytotrophoblast.

Renal transplantation

In one series 70% of the patients survived long enough to receive a renal transplant and 80% of those transplanted were alive 2 years later.[61] There is no evidence that the disease affects the transplanted normal kidney. The heavy proteinuria ceases after successful transplantation and does not recur.[63]

Prognosis

Untreated patients usually die during the first year; all are dead by 4 years. The disease is completely resistant to corticosteroid therapy but careful nutritional management, prompt treatment of complications and early renal transplantation have greatly improved the outlook for these children.

Pathogenesis

This is unknown. However, the number of anionic sites in the lamina rara externa of the glomerular capillary basement membrane is decreased in affected infants.[62] This alteration in the electrostatic barrier to the filtration of macromolecules through the glomerulus can produce proteinuria in experimental animals (see p. 131) and could explain the heavy proteinuria in infants with congenital nephrotic syndrome of Finnish type. It has been postulated that the decrease in the anionic sites may be caused by an inherited failure of synthesis or altered turnover of either glomerular heparin sulphate or proteoglycan or both.[63]

DIFFUSE MESANGIAL SCLEROSIS
(congenital nephrotic syndrome of French type)

A few infants who develop the nephrotic syndrome during the first year of life have a characteristic lesion in their renal glomeruli consisting of mesangial sclerosis without cellular proliferation (Fig. 4.7). The condition was first recognized in France[64] but has since been described in other countries. It is familial and is probably inherited as an autosomal recessive trait.[64–67]

Clinical features

The onset of the nephrotic syndrome is at various times during the first year of life, but usually after 3 months. Renal failure develops and if renal transplantation cannot be performed, death occurs before the age of 3 years.

Renal changes

Light microscopy

The striking feature is a marked increase in the amount of mesangial matrix in the glomeruli (Fig. 4.7). This occurs without an increase in the number of mesangial cells. As the disease progresses all the glomeruli are converted into shrunken spheres of material staining positively with periodic acid-Schiff and there is widespread tubular atrophy and interstitial fibrosis.[64]

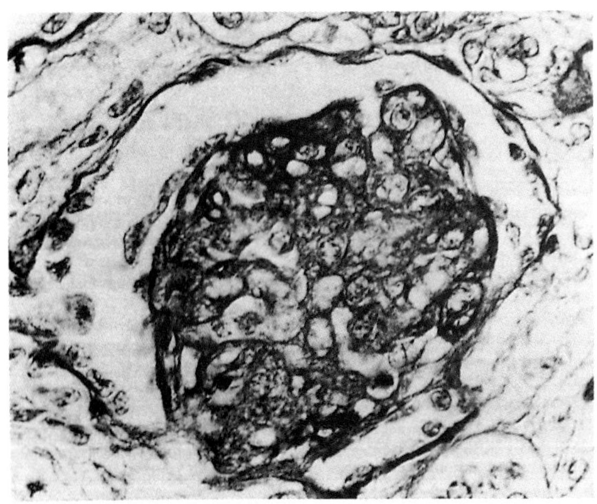

Fig. 4.7 Diffuse mesangial sclerosis. The glomeruli show global mesangial sclerosis.
Periodic acid-Schiff × 250
Reproduced by permission from: Hallman N, Noris R, Rapola J. Nephron 1973; 11: 105 (Fig. 5)

Electron microscopy

In addition to great expansion of the mesangial matrix, there may be irregular thickening of the glomerular capillary basement membrane.[67]

Immunofluorescence/immunoperoxidase microscopy

In most cases immunoglobulins and complement have not been found in the glomeruli.

Renal transplantation

The results of renal transplantation and information about whether there is recurrence of the disease are not available.

Pathogenesis

This is unknown. Even the pattern of inheritance is not certain because too few patients have been studied.

RENAL INVOLVEMENT IN HEREDITARY METABOLIC DISORDERS

DISORDERS OF LYSOSOMAL ENZYMES

Fabry's disease (Fabry–Anderson disease)

Fabry's disease, first described by Fabry[68] and Anderson[69] in 1898 as a dermatological curiosity, is a rare inborn error of glycosphingolipid catabolism occurring in about one in forty thousand births.[70] The condition is inherited as an incompletely recessive trait through a gene on the middle of the long arm of the X chromosome; the α-galactosidase gene has been isolated and characterized. Males, therefore, are usually affected but females may have biochemical and histopathological evidence of the disease and occasionally show clinical symptoms.[71] Deficient activity of an enzyme, α-galactosidase A (which catalyses the hydrolysis of various glycosphingolipids and glycoproteins), results in accumulation of globotriaosylceramide and, to a lesser extent, galabiosylceramide and blood group B substances in the plasma and their deposition and storage in the lysosomes of various cells. Globotriaosylceramide is the approved name for the substance previously known as α-galactosyl-lactosyl-ceramide, ceramide trihexoside or trihexosylceramide. Galabiosylceramide was formerly called digalactosylceramide. Deposits are common in the endothelial and smooth muscle cells of blood vessels and in the epithelial cells of the cornea, glomeruli and renal tubules; they also occur in macrophages, heart muscle and ganglion cells of the autonomic nervous system. Biochemical analysis of α-galactosidase activity in cells, urine or serum allows specific diagnosis of the disease and the detection of heterozygous females;[72] more precise carrier detection can be achieved by direct demonstration of the basic molecular defect. Prenatal diagnosis is based on analysis of amniocytes and samples of chorionic villi.

Clinical features

In hemizygous males the disease usually begins before puberty and runs a progressive course. It ends in chronic renal failure or death from coronary thrombosis or sequelae of high blood pressure, most commonly in the third or fourth decade, but sometimes later. The manifestations are protean but often include cutaneous and mucosal haemangiomas (angiokeratomas), painful paraesthesia made worse by hot weather, recurrent 'shooting' pains in the extremities and signs and symptoms of renal disease, coronary heart disease and sometimes vascular disease affecting the brain. Hypertension is common. Renal involvement is usually shown by proteinuria and microscopical haematuria. When women are affected it is usually later in life and less severely; extrarenal manifestations, particularly the skin lesions, are often absent.[71,72]

Renal changes[73]

Light microscopy In males there is marked vacuolation of the cytoplasm of the glomerular visceral epithelial cells and, to a lesser extent, of the mesangial cells and endothelium (Fig. 4.8). Vacuoles are also present in the distal convoluted

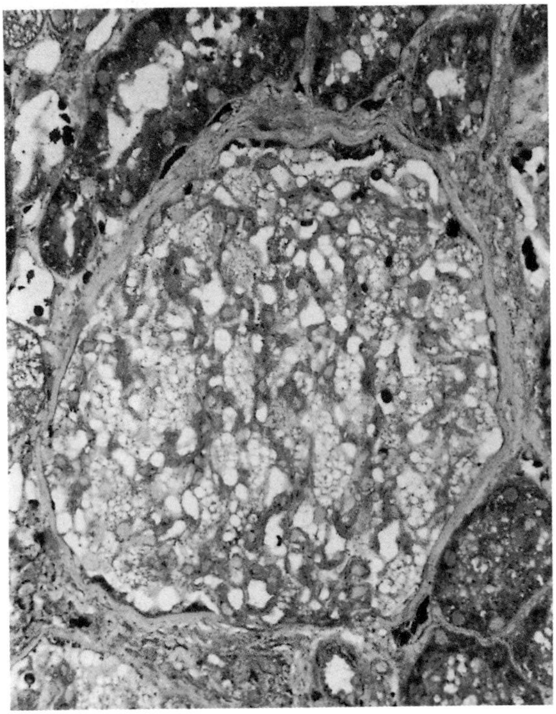

Fig. 4.8 Fabry's disease. A glomerulus showing marked vacuolation of epithelial cells. This appearance is common to several storage diseases and is not pathognomonic. The stored trihexosyl ceramide has been extracted during processing leaving empty cytoplasmic vacuoles. Methyl violet × 640

tubules and in the walls of arteries. These vacuoles contained globotriaosylceramide but this material is easily extracted by lipid solvents and is lost during processing in paraffin sections. In frozen sections globotriaosylceramide can be demonstrated as fine granules which are birefringent, stain with lipid stains and are strongly positive with the periodic acid-Schiff reaction. With increasing age the glomeruli undergo segmental and global sclerosis, there is tubular atrophy and interstitial scarring, and there is severe hyaline change in arteriolar walls. The renal changes in females are similar but less severe.

Electron microscopy The deposits are osmiophilic and appear as round or ovoid myelin-like bodies which are either membrane bound or free in the cytoplasm. Most are composed of closely packed electron-dense membranes arranged in parallel or concentric lamellae, sometimes giving the effect of a zebra's stripes (Fig. 4.9). Some are more homogeneous electron-dense structures (Fig. 4.10) The deposits are commonest in the cytoplasm of the visceral epithelial cells, but are also present in the cytoplasm of endothelial, mesangial, tubular and interstitial cells and in the endothelial and muscle cells of the arterial walls.

Immunofluorescence/immunoperoxidase microscopy Deposits of immunoglobulin or complement have not been reported.

Differential diagnosis

Vacuolation of the cytoplasm of glomerular epithelial cells is a feature of several metabolic disorders, including the mucopolysaccharidoses (see p. 93) and mucolipidoses (see p. 87).

The ultrastructural appearance of multiple myelin-like deposits is almost diagnostic, but for unequivocal identification of Fabry's disease biochemical analysis of tissue or blood must be performed. Deposits in tubular epithelial cells in the urine of patients with Fabry's disease can be identified by using a fluorescein-labelled antibody to globotriaosylceramide.[74]

Renal transplantation

A transplanted normal kidney will not provide the deficient enzyme but there is often a decrease in circulating ceramide hexoside substrate levels sufficient to ease neuropathic pain. The fall in substrate is probably caused partly by its increased clearance and partly by increased red cell survival with the abolition of uraemia; much of the circulating ceramide in uraemia comes from destroyed red cells.

Globotriaosylceramide may accumulate within a grafted kidney. In one case widespread recurrence of the disease occured within 6 months of transplantation.[74] However, at least five patients with Fabry's disease have survived more than 5 years after transplantation and one kidney retained normal function with only occasional small myelin-like bodies in the vascular endothelium 8 years after transplantation.[75]

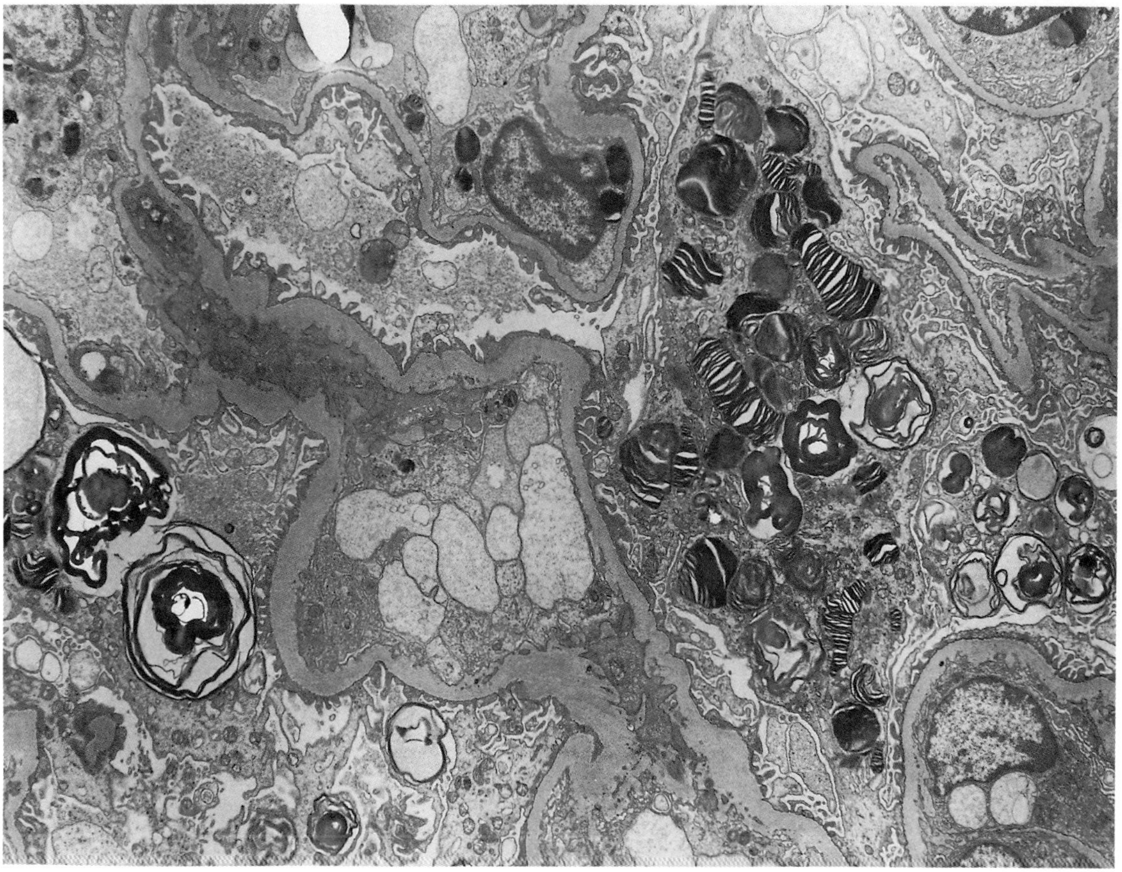

Fig. 4.9 Fabry's disease. Electron micrograph. Lamellar ('zebra') bodies are present in the visceral epithelial cells, endothelial cells and mesangial cells of a glomerulus.
× 8000

Prognosis

Without dialysis or renal transplantation most affected males will die from renal failure by the age of 50 years.

Mucolipidosis type II (I-cell disease)

Mucolipidosis type II is an autosomal recessive disorder. It is one of a heterogeneous group of inherited storage diseases which are characterized by the intracellular accumulation of both mucopolysaccharides and lipids.[76] In mucolipidosis type II various macromolecules, especially glycosaminoglycans and lipids, accumulate in the lysosomes of mesenchymal cells, histiocytes and renal epithelium. The macromolecules can be seen as coarse granules or inclusions in the cytoplasm of fibroblasts cultured from affected individuals; they stain positively with periodic acid-Schiff and Sudan black and sometimes with alcian blue. The inclusion-bearing fibroblasts have been called inclusion (I) cells and are the explanation for the alternative name for this condition, I-cell disease.[77] In this condition numerous hydrolases are either missing from the lysosomes or if present their activity is greatly reduced; serum levels of these enzymes, however, are elevated. The reason for this anomaly is that a primary defect in *N*-acetylglucosamine-1-phosphotransferase causes inadequate production of a recognition marker on

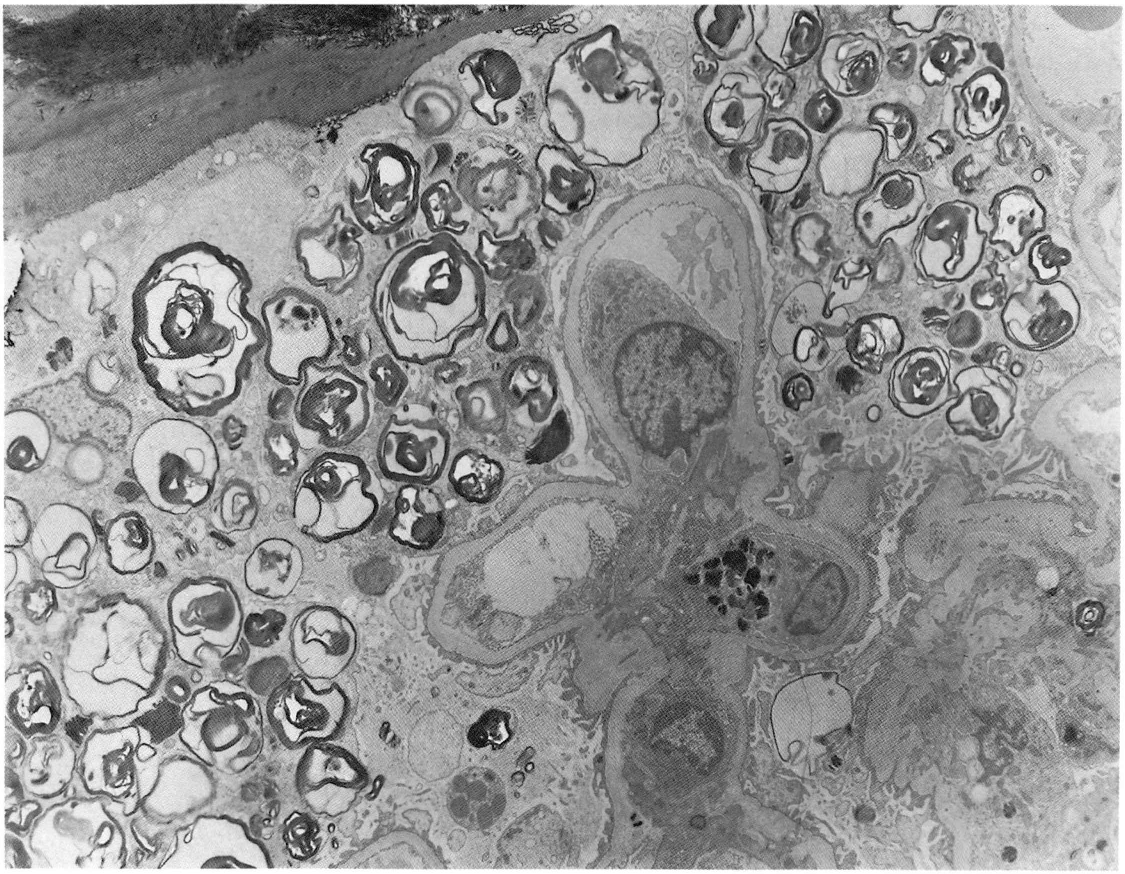

Fig. 4.10 Fabry's disease. Electron micrograph. Round and oval osmiophilic myelin-like bodies in cytoplasm of mostly visceral epithelial cells of a glomerulus.
× 8000

the molecules of the hydrolases which cannot then enter the lysosomes.[73,78]

Clinical features

Affected individuals have coarse facial features resembling those in Hurler's syndrome, hypertrophic gums, severe psychomotor retardation, skeletal abnormalities and cardiac insufficiency; they seldom survive childhood.[79] Renal manifestations are infrequent, but there may be slight proteinuria and haematuria. Renal failure is rare. The excretion of urinary mucopolysaccharides is not increased.

Renal changes

Light microscopy[73,80] The glomerular epithelial cells are swollen and their cytoplasm is vacuolated. The vacuoles contain glycosaminoglycans which stain strongly with cationic dyes such as colloidal iron or alcian blue at low pH (Fig. 4.11), and glycolipids which stain with periodic acid-Schiff and Sudan black. Similar vacuoles are present in the interstitial fibroblasts and sometimes in the epithelial cells of the collecting duct.

Electron microscopy[73] The cytoplasm of the visceral epithelial cells contains multiple membrane-bound vacuoles containing variously sized collections of lamellated lipid in a clear matrix (Fig. 4.12). The vacuoles are lysosomes grossly distended with glycosaminoglycans and lipids.

Niemann–Pick disease (sphingomyelinosis)[73]

Niemann–Pick disease is an autosomal recessive storage disorder in which sphingomyelin accumu-

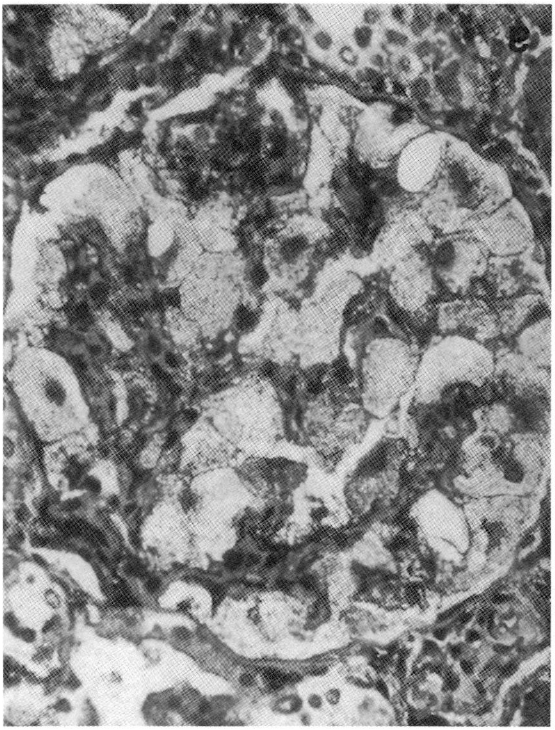

Fig. 4.11 Mucolipidosis type II (I-cell disease). Renal glomerulus showing marked swelling of the epithelial cells and vacuolation of their cytoplasm. The vacuoles contain glycosaminoglycans that have been stained light blue. Alcian blue × 400
Reproduced by permission from: Faraggiana T, Churg J. Hum Pathol 1987; 18: 661 (Fig. 6A)

lates, particularly in macrophages, neurones and hepatocytes. Clinical manifestations become evident by the age of 6 months. Typically the affected child has a protuberant abdomen because of hepatosplenomegaly. There are at least five variants. In types A and B the defect is a marked reduction in the amount of the lysosomal enzyme sphingomyelinase in many tissues. Sphingomyelinase breaks down sphingomyelin into ceramide and phosphorylcholine. The enzyme defect in other variants is not known.

Renal changes

The kidneys are involved in about 50% of cases but rarely causes this disturbance of function.

Light microscopy In paraffin sections there are large vacuolated cells in the interstitium and in the glomerular capillaries and mesangium; there is also vacuolation of the cytoplasm of glomerular visceral epithelial cells, tubular epithelial cells and endothelial cells lining arteries (Fig. 4.13a). In frozen sections the vacuoles contain sphingomyelin which can be demonstrated by the ferric haematoxylin method of Elleder, and cholesterol which stains by the Schultz method. These substances are extracted during the processing of paraffin sections.

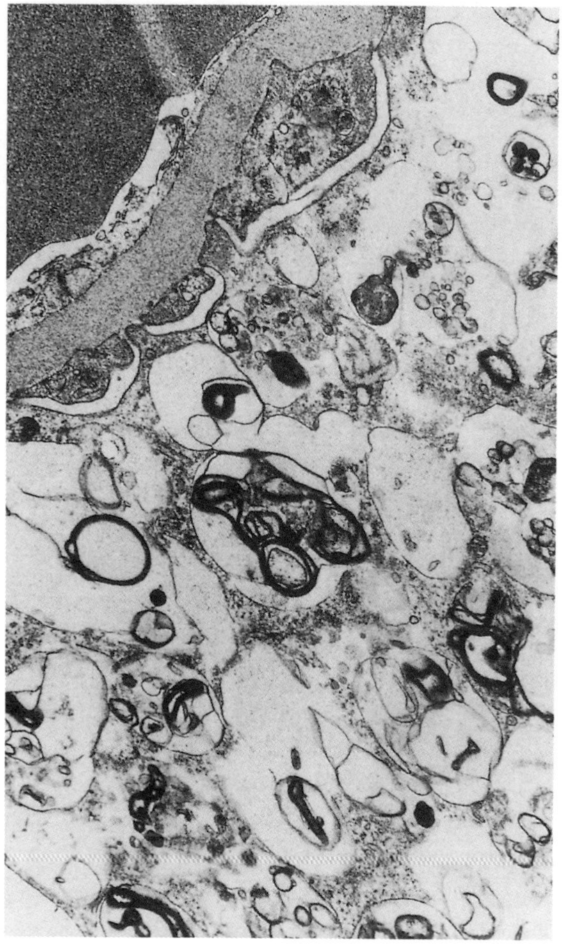

Fig. 4.12 Mucolipidosis type II (I-cell disease). Electron micrograph of part of a glomerulus showing a visceral epithelial cell. The cytoplasm contains many vacuoles which are distended lysosomes. These contain glycosaminoglycans which appear as a clear matrix and lipid which can be seen as black lamellar structures.
× 16 800
Reproduced by permission from: Faraggiana T, Churg J. Hum Pathol 1987; 18: 661 (Fig. 6B)

Electron microscopy Ultrastructurally the vacuoles are distended secondary lysosomes con-

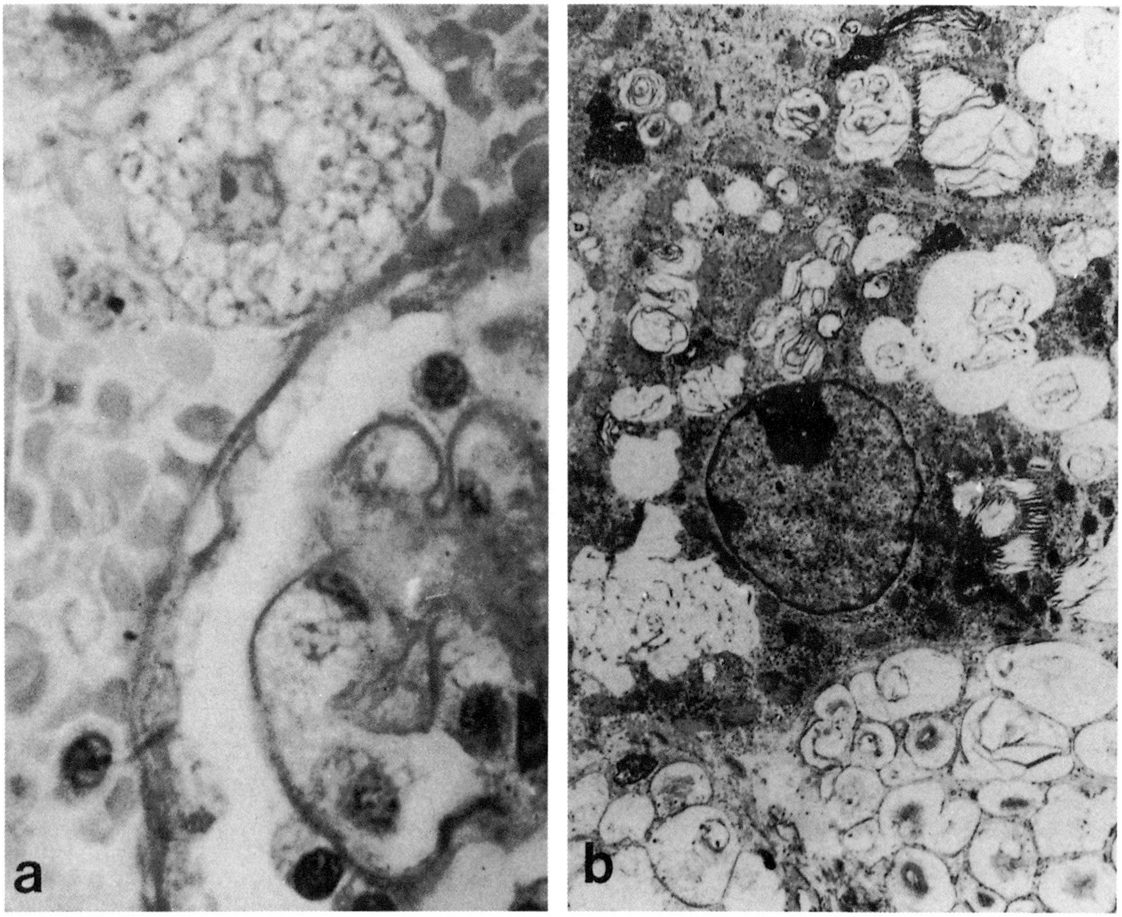

Fig. 4.13 Niemann–Pick disease. (**a**) In the interstitium there is a large cell with vacuolated cytoplasm; another is present within the glomerulus. (**b**) Electron micrograph of one of the swollen vacuolated cells. The vacuoles are distended lysosomes which contain lamellae of lipid.
(**a**) Haematoxylin-eosin × 1600; (**b**) electron micrograph × 10 700
Reproduced by permission from: Faraggiana T, Churg J. Hum Pathol 1987; 18: 661 (Fig. 2)

taining osmiophilic granules and myelin-like lamellae (Fig. 4.13b).

Diagnosis

Biochemical analysis of affected cells is necessary to establish the diagnosis unequivocally.

Gaucher's disease (cerebrosidosis)[73]

In this autosomal recessive disease glucosylceramide accumulates in the tissues because there is a reduction in the activity of the lysosomal enzyme glucosylceramidase, which catalyses the hydrolysis of glucosylceramide into ceramide and glucose. Glucosylceramide collects in massive amounts in the reticuloendothelial cells throughout the body. The spleen and liver are mostly affected, but rarely the kidney is involved, usually after splenectomy. There are generally no signs or symptoms of the renal involvement. The adult form of the disease (type I) is particularly frequent in Ashkenazi Jews; one in every 2500 newborns is affected.

Renal changes

Light microscopy Characteristic large Gaucher cells, with clear cytoplasm containing linear inclusions giving an appearance of crumpled tissue paper, are found in the lumens of the glomerular

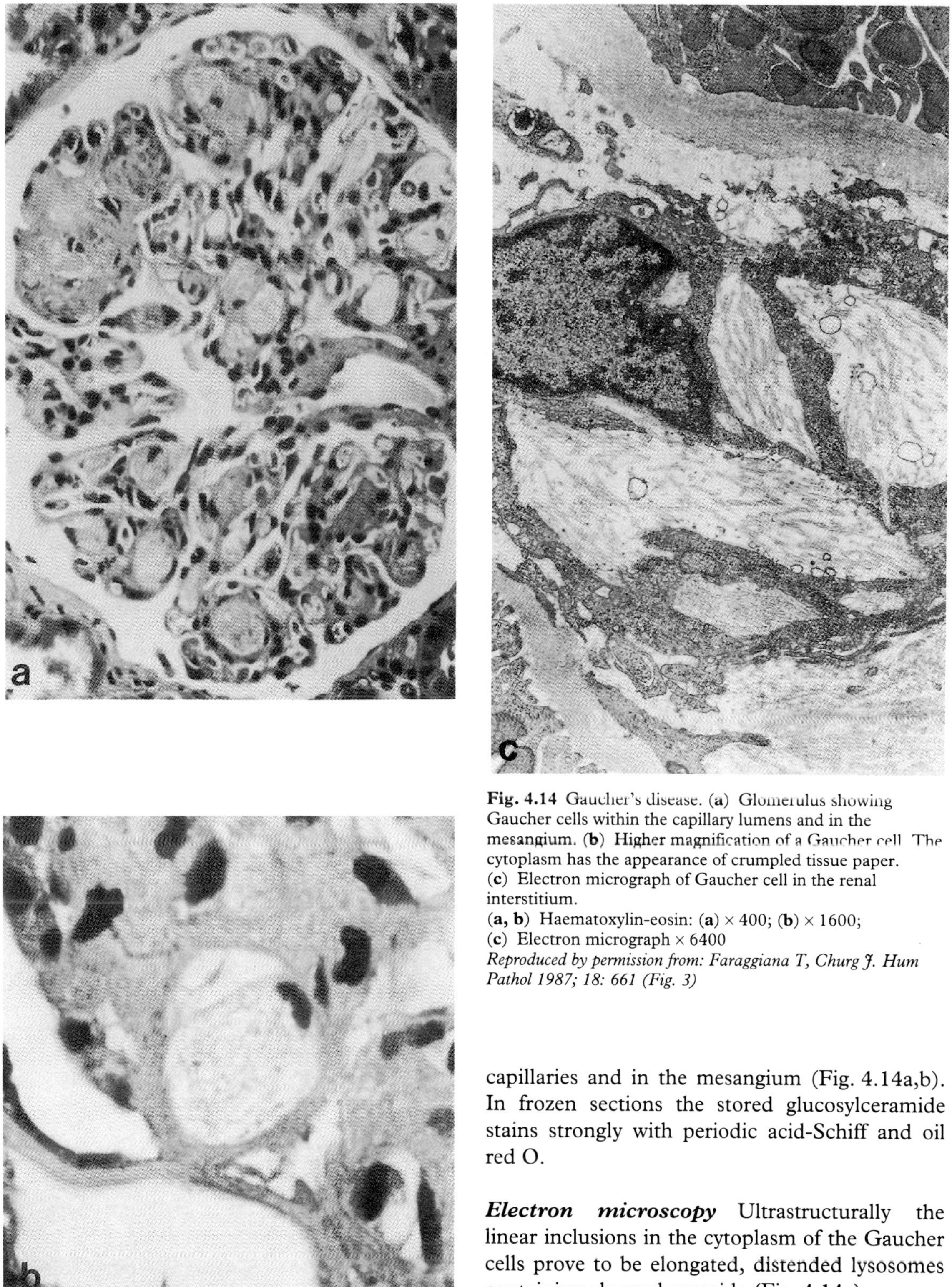

Fig. 4.14 Gaucher's disease. (**a**) Glomerulus showing Gaucher cells within the capillary lumens and in the mesangium. (**b**) Higher magnification of a Gaucher cell. The cytoplasm has the appearance of crumpled tissue paper. (**c**) Electron micrograph of Gaucher cell in the renal interstitium.
(**a, b**) Haematoxylin-eosin: (**a**) × 400; (**b**) × 1600;
(**c**) Electron micrograph × 6400
Reproduced by permission from: Faraggiana T, Churg J. Hum Pathol 1987; 18: 661 (Fig. 3)

capillaries and in the mesangium (Fig. 4.14a,b). In frozen sections the stored glucosylceramide stains strongly with periodic acid-Schiff and oil red O.

Electron microscopy Ultrastructurally the linear inclusions in the cytoplasm of the Gaucher cells prove to be elongated, distended lysosomes containing glucosylceramide (Fig. 4.14c).

Metachromatic leucodystrophy (sulphatidosis)[73]

Metachromatic leucodystrophy is an autosomal recessive storage disease in which cerebroside sulphate (galactosyl sulphatide) accumulates in the brain and other organs, particularly the kidney.[81,82] The stored material displays a reddish-brown metachromasia when stained with cresyl violet or toluidine blue. The incidence of metachromatic leucodystrophy is about one in 40 000 births. The cause is inadequate levels of arylsulphatase A, an enzyme that catalyses the hydrolysis of cerebroside sulphate to give galactocerebroside and sulphate. The locus determining the expression of arylsulphatase A activity is on chromosome 22.

Renal changes

In the kidney large deposits of cerebroside sulphate are found in the epithelial cells of the distal collecting duct, distal convoluted tubules and the thin loop of Henle. The same material may be present in the tubular lumen and in interstitial macrophages. Renal function is usually unaffected, but rarely when storage occurs in the proximal tubular cells there may be proximal tubular acidosis.[83] Renal tubular cells shed in the urine contain metachromatic cerebroside sulphate.

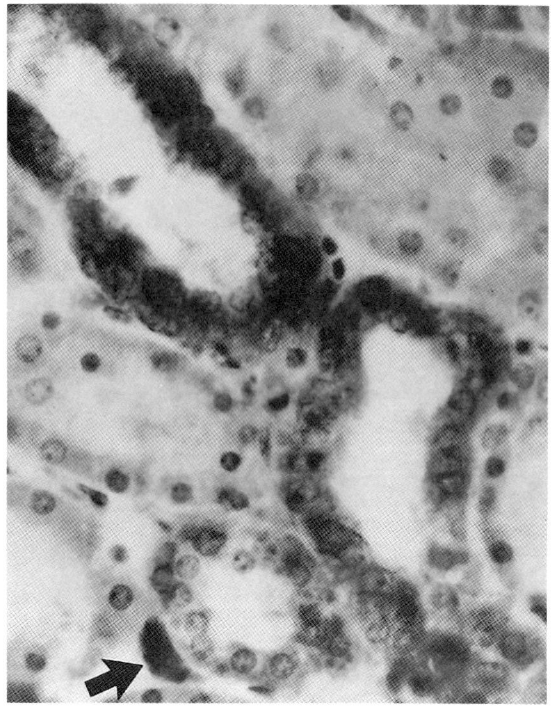

Fig. 4.15 Metachromatic leucodystrophy. Metachromatic material is present in the cells of the tubules and in an interstitial cell (arrow).
Cresyl violet Hirsch and Pfeiffer – technique × 540
Reproduced by permission from: Wolfe HJ, Pietra GG. Am J Pathol 1964; 44: 921 (Fig. 5)

Light microscopy The affected tubular cells are swollen and have vacuolated cytoplasm. In frozen sections the cerebroside sulphate stains with Sudan black and alcian blue. Reddish-brown metachromasia occurs after staining with cresyl violet using the technique described by Hirsch and Pfeiffer[84] (Fig. 4.15).

Electron microscopy The lysosomes are distended by cerebroside which appears as thin lamellae in a clear matrix.[73]

Diagnosis

The levels of arylsulphatase A should be measured in blood leucocytes or skin fibroblasts.

Gangliosidoses[85]

There are two main groups of autosomal recessive ganglioside storage diseases, both due to a deficiency or lack of a lysosomal enzyme. The first group, called G_{M1} gangliosidosis, is caused by lack of G_{M1} ganglioside beta-galactosidase. The second, called G_{M2} gangliosidosis, is due to deficiency of either hexosaminidase A (Tay–Sachs disease) or hexosaminidases A and B (Sandhoff's disease). The brain and peripheral nerves are mostly affected. The kidney is involved in G_{M1} gangliosidosis and very slightly in Sandhoff's disease; it is not affected in Tay–Sachs disease.[73]

Renal changes

G_{M1} gangliosidosis In G_{M1} gangliosidosis the kidneys are frequently affected in both the infantile form (type 1) and the juvenile form (type 2).

Light microscopy. In the glomeruli the visceral and parietal epithelial cells contain cytoplasmic vacuoles giving them a foamy appearance. Similar cells are present in the mesangium, endothelium, interstitium and tubules, particularly the loops of Henle.[85]

Electron microscopy. The vacuoles are bounded by a membrane and appear empty.

Sandhoff's disease In Sandhoff's disease, a G_{M2} gangliosidosis, clear vacuoles have been described in the loop of Henle. By electron microscopy they may be empty or contain lamellar lipid bodies.

Farber's lipogranulomatosis[73]

This rare autosomal recessive storage disease is caused by a deficiency of a lysosomal enzyme, acid ceramidase, that cleaves ceramide into sphingosine and fatty acid. Ceramide accumulates in various tissues and is associated with a granulomatous infiltration. A previously healthy infant between 2 and 4 months old develops painful swollen joints and pulmonary infiltrates. The kidneys are sometimes involved, usually with no functional changes. In early lesions the interstitium contains macrophages laden with clear cytoplasmic vacuoles; later, interstitial granulomas occur.[86] The stored ceramide stains well with periodic acid-Schiff but is only faintly stained by Sudan black.

Wolman's disease[73,87]

In this rare autosomal recessive disease, which usually leads to death before the age of 6 months, the lysosomes lack the enzyme acid lipase that hydrolyses cholesteryl esters in low density lipoproteins as they are removed from the plasma by the tissues. The structural gene for the acid lipase enzyme is on the long arm of chromosome 10. The result is accumulation of cholesteryl esters and triglycerides in the liver, spleen, adrenals and lymph nodes. The kidneys are only slightly affected. Cells with foamy cytoplasm occur in the interstitium and in the glomerular mesangium. In frozen sections the foamy cytoplasm stains positively with oil red O and Sudan black, and Schultz's technique for cholesterol is positive.

Mucopolysaccharide storage diseases

These diseases are caused by inherited lack of specific lysosomal enzymes that degrade dermatin sulphate, heparin sulphate or keratin sulphate, singly or in combination. Incompletely degraded mucopolysaccharides accumulate in the tissues and are excreted in the urine. There are 10 mucopolysaccharidoses. Nine are autosomal recessively inherited; the tenth, Hunter's syndrome, is an X-linked recessive disorder. They have a combined incidence of about one in 10 000 births.

In most of the types the patients are short and hirsute, their joints are stiff, they are deaf, arteriosclerosis develops early in the aorta and coronary arteries, the trachea and bronchi become narrowed, the liver and spleen enlarge and deposits in the brain lead to mental and neurological deterioration. Death occurs before age 10 in Hurler's syndrome but in some of the other forms patients may survive until old age.

Renal changes

The kidney is often involved in the mucopolysaccharidoses but function is rarely impaired.

Light microscopy The accumulation of acid mucopolysaccharides in the cytoplasm gives a foamy appearance to the visceral and parietal epithelial cells of the glomeruli. Prominent vacuolization is also present in the cytoplasm of the epithelial cells of Henle's loop, distal convoluted tubule and collecting ducts. The tubular lumen contains hyaline casts. In paraffin sections the stored material stains strongly with alcian blue and colloidal iron. There is no metachromasia with acid cresyl blue and toluidine blue. Sudan black is also negative.[88]

Electron microscopy The glomerular visceral and tubular epithelial cell cytoplasm is distended by huge lysosomes swollen by clear unstained mucopolysaccharides. A few laminated inclusions are also present.[88]

DISORDERS OF TRANSPORT

Cystinosis

Cystinosis, which is quite distinct from primary cystinuria (see p. 96), is a rare disorder of metabolism in which there is widespread deposition of cystine crystals in the lysosomes of cells that exhibit phagocytosis and pinocytosis. Characteristically, cystine deposits are therefore most obvious in the cells of the mononuclear phagocyte system (reticuloendothelial system) in the bone marrow, spleen, lymph nodes, liver, intestines and lungs, and in cells of the eyes and kidneys. The crystals are also found in circulating neutrophils and monocytes and in fibroblasts. Cystinosis is caused by defective transport of cystine across the lysosomal membrane because of a fault in the carrier protein; this prevents the egress of cystine which accumulates within the lysosomes to levels 50–100 times normal.[89] At these high concentrations crystals form within the lysosomes.

The disease is inherited as an autosomal recessive characteristic.

Clinical features

Although the abnormal intralysosomal storage of cystine affects most organs from birth, the clinical manifestations and prognosis are largely determined by whether cystine is deposited in the kidney. There are three distinct clinical forms – infantile, adolescent and adult. Cystine is deposited in the kidney in the first and second of these forms but not in adult cystinosis. The three types are genetically distinct but it is not known whether they result from different alleles at a single locus or mutations at multiple loci.

Infantile cystinosis (nephropathic cystinosis) This is the commonest form. It usually becomes evident about 6 months after birth[90]. Its manifestations include aminoaciduria, glycosuria, hyperphosphaturia, proteinuria, polyuria, hypophosphataemia, chronic acidosis and electrolyte disturbances. The level of cystine in the plasma is normal. Cystine is not lost in the urine to the extent that is characteristic of cystinuria (see p. 96) and cystine stones are very rarely formed. Photophobia is a frequent manifestation because of accumulation of cystine crystals in the cornea. Progressive renal failure develops and there is often a severe degree of dwarfism associated with rickets that is resistant to treatment with vitamin D.

The combination of rickets, aminoaciduria, glycosuria and hyperphosphaturia is frequently known as Fanconi's syndrome. As at least 11 distinct syndromes are currently attributed by name to Guido Fanconi,[91] an eponymous designation of the condition under discussion must necessarily include other names if confusion is to be reduced. Alternatives are de Toni–Debré–Fanconi syndrome and Abderhalden–Lignac syndrome. The syndrome is not unique to cystinosis; it is also a characteristic feature of type 1 tyrosinaemia, hereditary fructose intolerance, Wilson's disease, galactosaemia and one form of glycogen storage disease (see p. 103).

In the later stage of their disease many patients with cystinosis become hypothyroid and require thyroxine.

Adolescent cystinosis (juvenile or late-onset cystinosis) This milder, but nevertheless fatal, variant does not become evident until adolescence. Renal tubular defects are absent or mild, but there is proteinuria of glomerular origin.

Adult cystinosis This form is benign. It is usually not discovered before adult life. There is no renal involvement.

Diagnosis

In all three clinical forms of cystinosis it is possible to observe cystine crystals in the cornea on examination with the slit-lamp. This is the usual way in which the adult form is detected. Confirmation of the diagnosis can be obtained by microscopical examination of bone marrow aspirates.

The concentration of free cystine in cultured dermal fibroblasts, peripheral leucocytes amd amniotic cells is raised in all forms of cystinosis. The level is highest in the infantile form and lowest in the adult form. Measurement of the cystine content enables prenatal diagnosis and the detection of heterozygotes.

Heterozygotes

Those who are heterozygous for the abnormal gene are generally healthy and suffer no renal disturbance. They accumulate cystine to a much smaller degree.

Renal changes

Light microscopy The kidneys are involved in the infantile and adolescent forms of cystinosis. In the *infantile form*, atrophy of the epithelial cells of the beginning of the proximal part of the tubules is an early change and accounts for the distinctive 'swan-neck' lesion that is found on microdissection of the nephrons. Later, widespread atrophy of the tubules, interstitial fibrosis and focal infiltration by mononuclear cells tend to dominate the picture. The glomeruli show focal and segmental sclerosis, increased cellularity of the tufts and thickening of the wall of the capillaries; adhesions and occasional epithelial crescents may be found.[92] A striking and characteristic feature is the presence of numerous multinucleate visceral epithelial cells in the glomeruli (Fig. 4.16). The changes in the glomeruli eventually lead to their obliteration.

In tissue that has been fixed in alcohol, birefringent crystals of cystine can sometimes be demonstrated in the cells in the interstitium, in the epithelial cells of the tubules and, occasionally, in the cells of the glomeruli.

In the *adolescent form*, the changes in the glomeruli and interstitium are less severe. The 'swan-neck' lesion has been described only once.

Electron microscopy Cystine crystals, usually within lysosomes, are often seen in the epithelial and mesangial cells of the glomeruli (Fig. 4.17), in the epithelial cells of the tubules and in interstitial cells, even when they are scarce or apparently absent on light microscopy. The shape of the crystals varies; angular forms are particularly frequent. There is obliteration of the foot processes of the epithelial cells.[92,93]

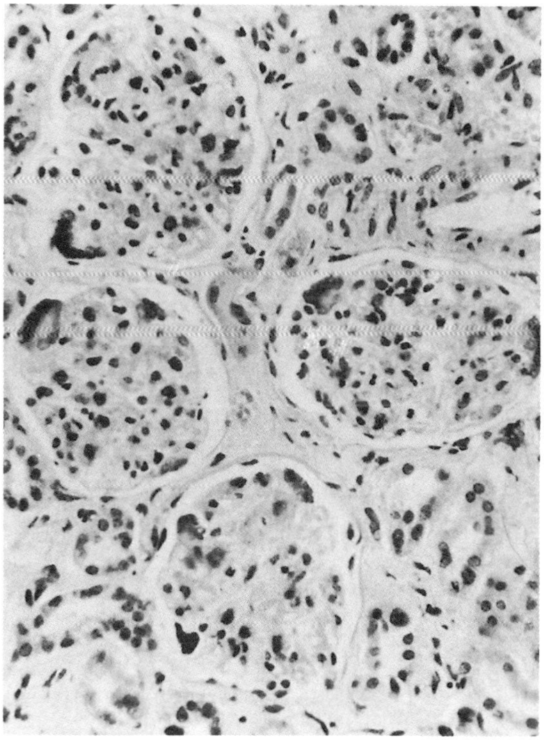

Fig. 4.16 Cystinosis. Some visceral epithelial cells in the glomeruli are multinucleate. There is also tubular atrophy. Haematoxylin-eosin × 300
Reproduced by permission from: Spear GS, Slusser RJ, Schulman JD, Alexander F. Johns Hopkins Med J 1971; 129: 83 (Fig. 10)

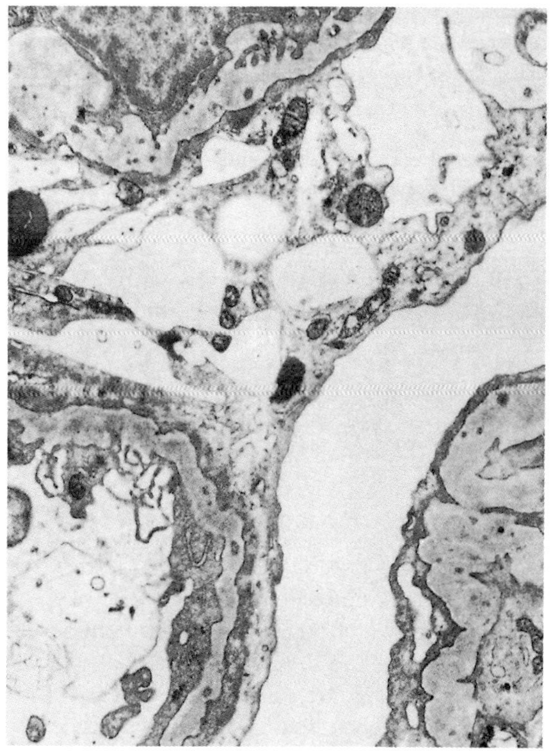

Fig. 4.17 Cystinosis. Electron micrograph of part of a glomerulus. The cytoplasm of a visceral epithelial cell in the upper left of the picture contains clear areas from which cystine has been dissolved out.
× 8880
Reproduced by permission from: Spear GS, Slusser RJ, Schulman JD, Alexander F. Johns Hopkins Med J 1971; 129: 83 (Fig. 5)

Renal transplantation

A series of 24 patients with cystinosis has been studied for periods of up to 4.5 years after receiving a renal allograft,[94] and in another group of 10 patients two have survived beyond 5 years.[95] Cystine accumulates in the interstitium and glomerular mesangium as a result of infiltration by cystine-laden host cells; it also accumulates occasionally in the tubular lumen although not in the tubular epithelium. Usually there are no deleterious effects. Since a functioning renal allograft does not correct the primary metabolic defect, non-renal manifestations of cystinosis, such as photophobia and hypothyroidism, persist.

Prognosis

Without dialysis or renal transplantation most children with infantile cystinosis die from chronic renal failure before puberty. Treatment with cysteamine may be beneficial but this is not yet clear. Cysteamine enters the lysosomes and reacts with cystine to form cysteine and a cysteine-cysteamine mixed disulphide, both of which traverse the lysosomal membrane in a normal fashion.[96] Patients with adolescent cystinosis, who are not treated by dialysis or renal transplantation, usually die between the ages of 15 and 20 years. Adult cystinosis does not shorten life.

Pathogenesis

The defects in glomerular and tubular functions are presumed to be secondary to the accumulation of cystine in the cells, but the mechanism involved is far from being understood.

Cystinuria

Cystinuria is an inherited disorder of amino acid transport in which there is impairment in the reabsorption of cystine and other dibasic amino acids from the glomerular filtrate by the cells of the proximal segment of the tubules; there is a similar functional defect in the mucous membrane of the small intestine.[97] The urine contains large amounts of cystine, together with ornithine, arginine and lysine. Cystinuria is transmitted as an autosomal recessive characteristic; the homozygous abnormality is present in about one in 20 000 people.

The only recognizable clinical disorder or pathological change in cystinuria is cystine urolithiasis (see p. 542).

Bartter's syndrome

Bartter's syndrome is an uncommon disorder characterized by hypokalaemia, hypochloraemic acidosis, raised levels of renin and aldosterone in the plasma, normal blood pressure and hyperplasia of the juxtaglomerular apparatus.[98] Other associated abnormalities, which are not always present, include a decreased sensitivity to angiotensin II and noradrenalin, impaired urinary concentrating ability that is unresponsive to vasopressin, increased excretion in the urine of prostaglandins, kinins and kallikrein, and growth retardation. The syndrome is commonest in females and blacks. Most cases are discovered in childhood, 50% before the age of 5 years. The disorder is probably inherited as an autosomal recessive trait. Very similar symptoms may be

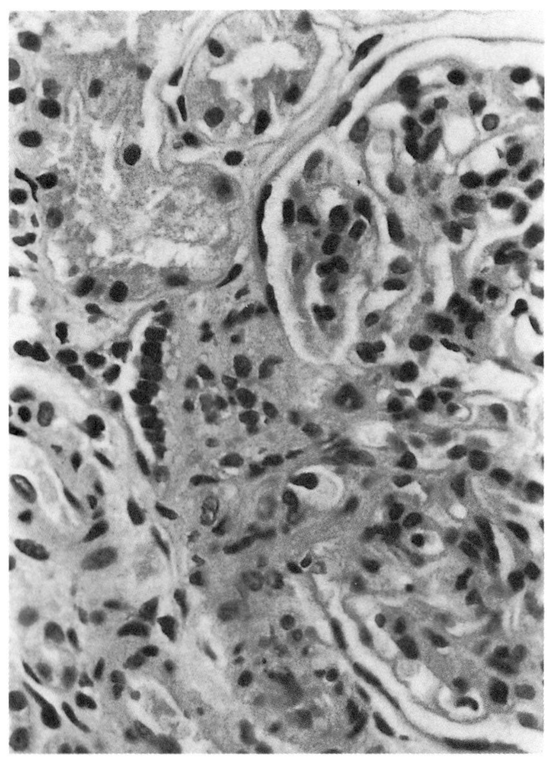

Fig. 4.18 Bartter's syndrome. Hyperplasia of the juxtaglomerular apparatus. The macula densa is prominent. Periodic acid-Schiff × 500

produced by conditions associated with long-term hypokalaemia; these conditions may have a renal origin or be caused by chronic laxative abuse, familial chloride diarrhoea and chronic surreptitious vomiting.

Renal changes

There is hyperplasia and hypergranularity of the cells of the juxtaglomerular apparatus (Fig. 4.18). The granules are mainly large and amorphous rather than protogranules (Fig. 4.19) and the macula densa is prominent. The interstitial cells in the medulla are also often hyperplastic and the proximal convoluted tubules are vacuolated; both these changes are related to the hypokalaemia.[99]

Pathogenesis

Bartter's syndrome probably has more than one underlying cause.[100] One group of patients appear to have an isolated defect in potassium transport which results in loss of protein in the urine. A second group have defects in the transport of sodium and chloride which leads to loss of salt; potassium loss is secondary to enhanced exchange of sodium and potassium in the distal tubules and increased urine flow. The third group includes patients with a defect in the transport of chloride in the thick ascending limb of Henle's loop; this results in potassium loss for the same reasons as in the second group of patients.

DISORDERS OF LIPOPROTEIN AND LIPID METABOLISM

Familial lecithin-cholesterol acyltransferase deficiency

Lecithin-cholesterol acyltransferase plays a major

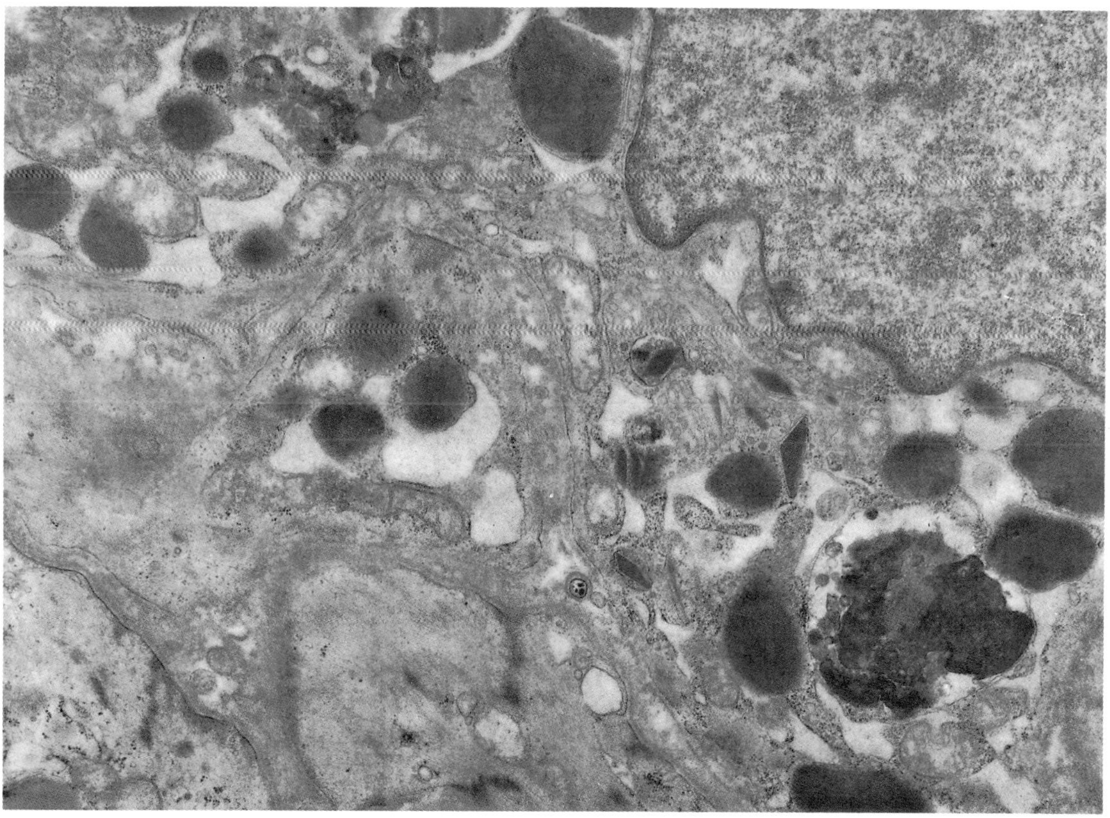

Fig. 4.19 Bartter's syndrome. Electron micrograph of granular cell in wall of afferent arteriole. Most of the granules are large and amorphous; there are only a few small angular protogranules.
× 30 000

role in converting free cholesterol into cholesterol esters in the plasma. Absence of this enzyme results in the accumulation of free cholesterol in the tissues. Familial deficiency of lecithin-cholesterol acyltransferase was first described in Norway in 1968;[101] subsequently other affected families have been reported from several parts of the world but it remains a rare disease. The deficiency is inherited as an autosomal recessive trait and the responsible gene is located on chromosome 16.[102] Several different enzymic phenotypes probably exist in this disease.

Clinical features

Both sexes are affected. Proteinuria, with or without mild microscopic haematuria, begins in childhood and persists. Diffuse corneal opacities and haemolytic anaemia are almost always present. The serum lipids and lipoproteins are abnormal with increased levels of free cholesterol, triglycerides and phospholipids and greatly reduced levels of cholesterol esters. Renal failure develops in the fourth or fifth decade.[103]

Renal changes

Light microscopy[104] The glomerular capillary basement membrane is diffusely thickened and contains multiple tiny holes giving a honeycomb appearance. This change is best seen when the sections are stained with periodic acid-silver methenamine (Fig. 4.20). Cells with foamy cytoplasm are also sometimes present in the glom-

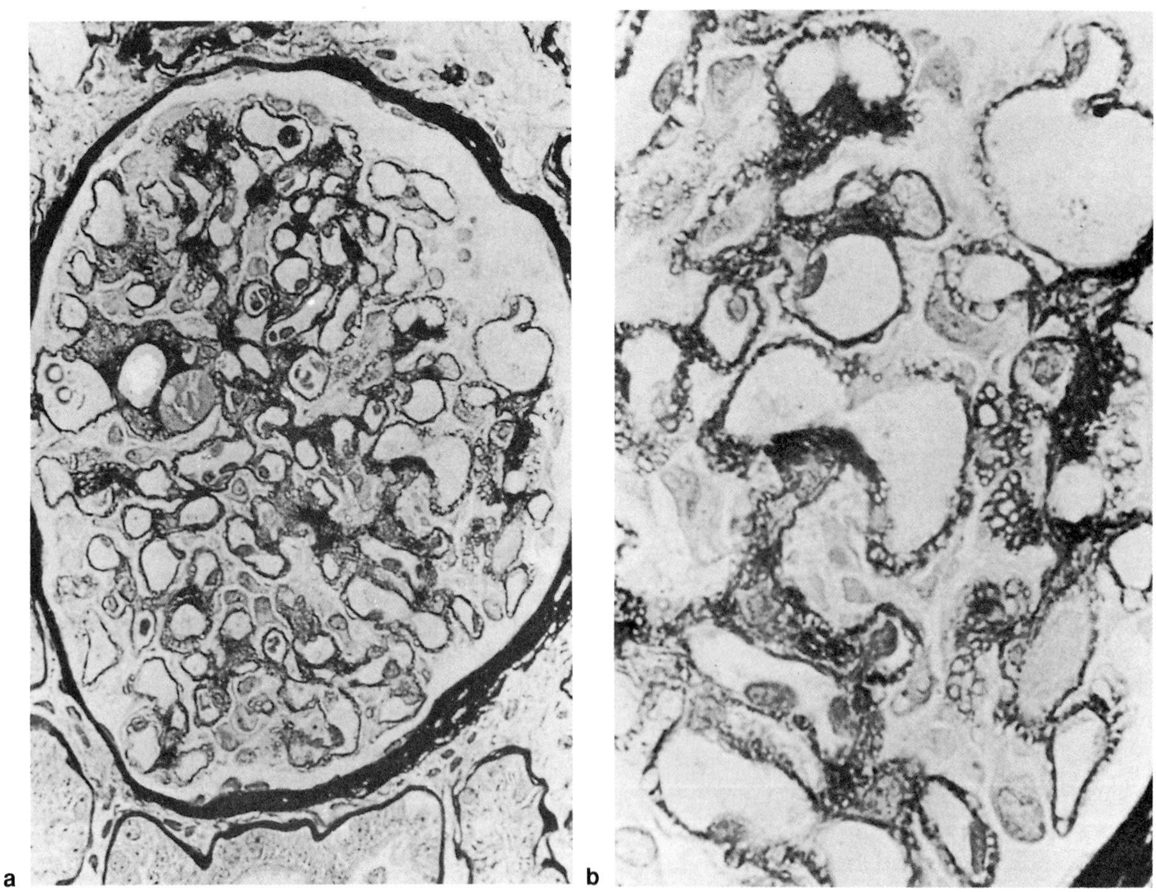

Fig. 4.20 Familial lecithin-cholesterol acyltransferase deficiency. (**a**) Glomerulus with diffusely thickened and mottled capillary basement membranes and thickened Bowman's capsule. (**b**) The capillary basement membrane and the mesangium have a marked honeycomb appearance.
Methenamine silver: (**a**) × 400; (**b**) × 1000
Reproduced by permission from: Ohta Y, Yamamoto S-I, Tsuchida H et al. Am J Kidney Dis 1986; 7: 41 (Figs 2, 3)

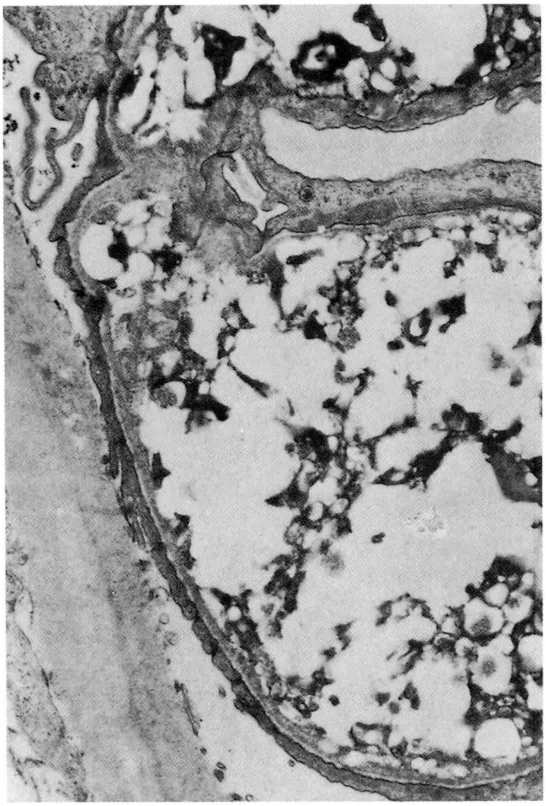

a

erulus. Frozen sections stained for fat show that some glomerular capillaries are filled with lipid, most of it extracellular. Bowman's capsule is thickened and contains lipid. Fat is also present in the interstitium and in the subendothelial region of the wall of small arteries. Progressive accumulation of fat in the mesangium eventually leads to sclerosis of the glomerulus.

Electron microscopy[73,104,105] Lipid deposits of various sizes and density are present on or within the glomerular capillary basement membrane and

Fig. 4.21 Familial lecithin-cholesterol acyltransferase deficiency. (**a**) Electron micrograph. The lumen of a glomerular capillary is filled with amorphous lipid. (**b**) Electron micrograph. Part of a glomerular capillary. There are large accumulations of small lipid vesicles and granular material in the mesangium and on the subendothelial aspect of the capillary basement membrane. (**a**) × 11 000; (**b**) × 7500
(**a**) *Reproduced by permission from: Ohta Y, Yamamoto S-I, Tsuchida H et al. Am J Kidney Dis 1986; 7: 41 (Fig. 6)*
(**b**) *Reproduced by permission from: Faraggiana T, Churg J. Hum Pathol 1987; 18: 661 (Fig. 9A)*

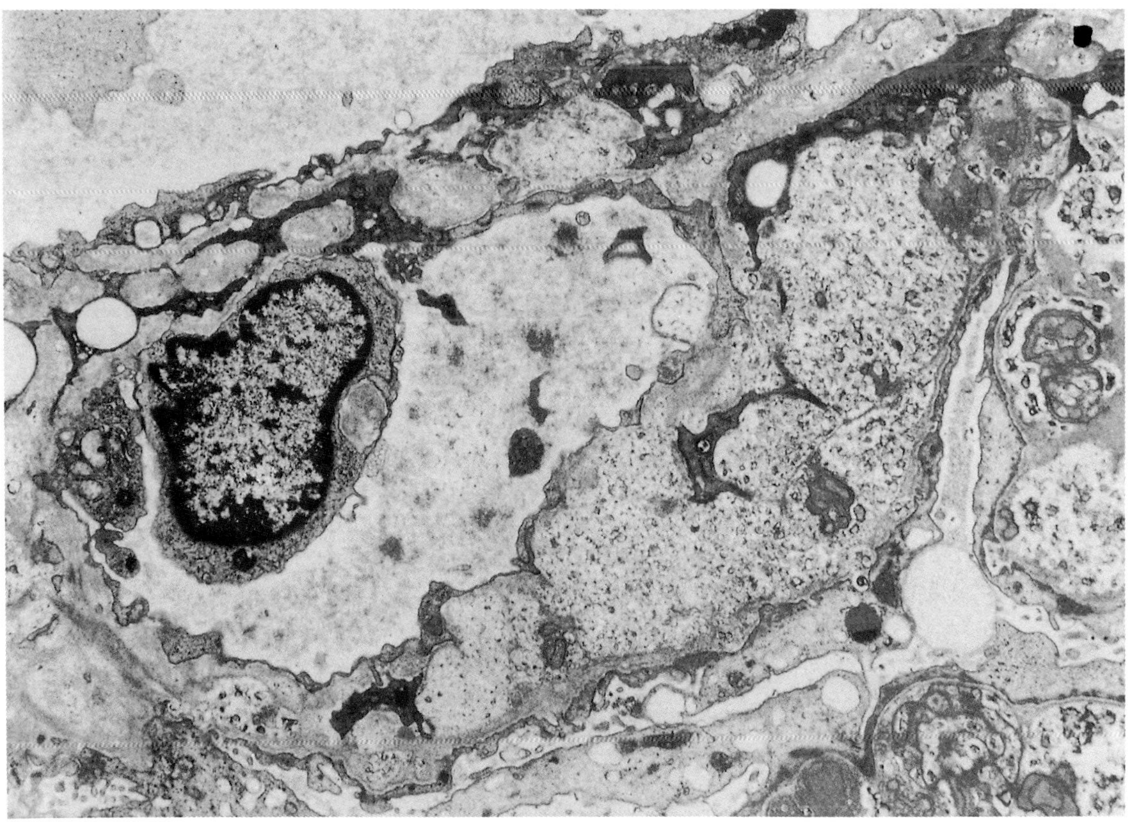

b

in the mesangium. They often appear as vacuoles or vesicles containing irregular profiles of very electron-dense material (Fig. 4.21). The basement membrane deposits are usually subendothelial but are sometimes subepithelial. In some glomeruli the capillary lumen becomes filled with lipid and the endothelial lining cells are destroyed (Fig. 4.21). Similar collections of lipid are found in the interstitium; most are extracellular.

Immunofluorescence/immunoperoxidase microscopy There is positive staining for apolipoprotein-B along the capillary walls and in mesangial regions.[105]

Differential diagnosis

The same light microscopic and electron microscopic changes can occur in the kidney in *Alagille's syndrome* (see p. 116) and in patients with *hyperlipidaemia due to cholestatic liver disease.*

Renal transplantation

Lipid deposits soon occur in the grafted kidney; they were obvious in a kidney examined 5 months after transplantation.[106]

Batten's disease (ceroid lipofuscinosis)[73,107]

The term Batten's disease is used to describe a group of autosomal recessive diseases that have in common mental retardation, neurological symptoms and the storage in neurones and various organs of a complex lipid resembling lipofuscin. The kidney may be involved in the infantile, late infantile and juvenile variants. The lipid is seen in the glomerular capillary endothelial cells, in the distal tubular epithelium and as tubular casts. It is autofluorescent, not extractable by common lipid solvents, and stains with periodic acid-Schiff and Sudan black even in paraffin sections. In the electron microscope the deposits appear as osmiophilic globules with a granular matrix in the infantile form and as curved lamellae in the late infantile form.

Familial hypercholesterolaemia (type IIa hyperlipoproteinaemia)

Familial hypercholesterolaemia is inherited as an autosomal dominant trait with a gene dosage effect, i.e. homozygotes are more severely affected than heterozygotes. It is a consequence of a mutation in the gene encoding the receptor for plasma low density lipoprotein. This receptor is located on the surface membrane of most body cells. It normally binds low density lipoprotein and aids the cell in taking up the lipoprotein and delivering it to lysosomes. In the lysosomes low density lipoprotein is broken down and its cholesterol released for use in the synthesis of cell membranes, steroid hormones and bile acids. Any inherited deficiency in the low density lipoprotein receptors leads to a reduction in the rate of removal of low density lipoprotein from the plasma. As a consequence the level of low density lipoprotein in the plasma rises and the excess is deposited in macrophages and other cells. The prevalence of heterozygotes is about one in five hundred persons and of homozygotes about one in one million persons.

Renal changes

The kidney is a frequent site of lipid storage in this disorder but only occasionally are there renal symptoms.

Light microscopy The lipid deposition is mostly in macrophages in the interstitium; there is only mild infiltration of the tubular epithelium and the glomerular mesangium.[108] In frozen sections the lipid is stained by Sudan black and the Schultz reaction is positive. In the occasional case with the nephrotic syndrome lipid masses (sometimes called 'thrombi') are found in the glomerular capillaries (Fig. 4.22).

Electron microscopy Most of the lipid lies free in the cytoplasm of affected cells; only a small proportion is within lysosomes.

Familial type III hyperlipoproteinaemia (remnant hyperlipoproteinaemia)

Patients with familial type III hyperlipopro-

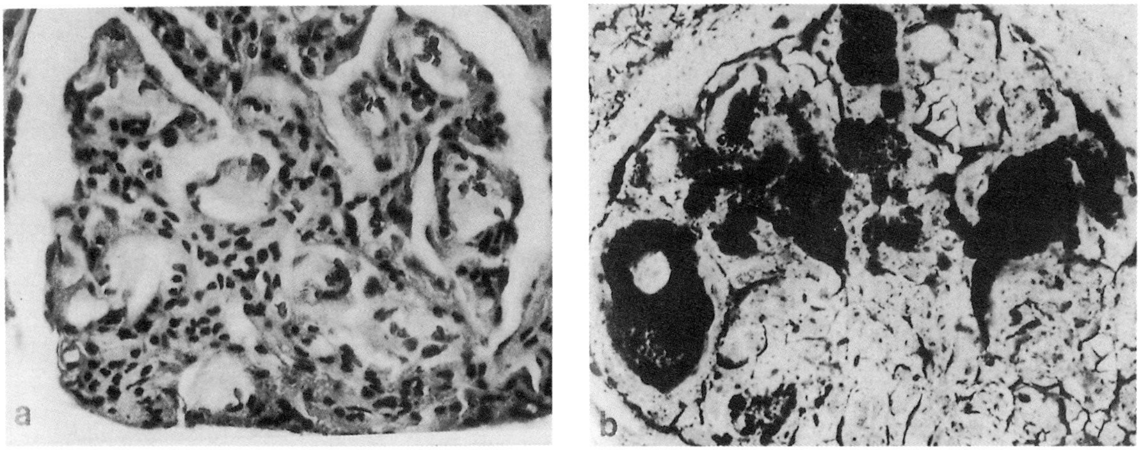

Fig. 4.22 Familial hypercholesterolemia. (**a**) The glomerular capillaries contain large lipid masses. (**b**) The intracapillary lipid stains positively with oil red O.
(**a**) Haematoxylin-eosin × 400; (b) oil red O × 400
Reproduced by permission from: Faraggiana T, Churg J. Hum Pathol 1987; 18: 661 (Fig. 8)

teinaemia have raised plasma concentrations of cholesterol and triglycerides. The cause is an inherited defect at the genetic locus that specifies the structure of apoprotein E, a substance that normally binds to hepatocyte surface receptors and promotes the uptake of remnant lipoproteins (particles derived from the partial catabolism of very low density lipoproteins and chylomicrons). The defective locus produces an abnormal apoprotein E (designated E^d); remnant lipoproteins are not cleared from the circulation and they accumulate in scavenger and other cells. After the age of 20 years affected individuals develop cutaneous xanthomas and severe atherosclerosis. The disease affects about one in 10 000 persons.

Renal changes

The kidney is frequently involved but renal symptoms are unusual.

Light microscopy Lipid deposition is normally seen as severe atherosclerosis in the renal artery. Sometimes many of the glomeruli contain collections of foamy cells (Fig. 4.23); most of these are in the mesangium but a few are swollen endothelial cells.[109] In frozen sections the lipid is stained by oil red O. There are also usually a few foam cells in the interstitium. Tubular epithelial cells contain only a little fat.

Phytanic acid storage disease (Refsum's disease)[73,110]

In this rare disease phytanic acid, a branched chain fatty acid, accumulates in the blood and various tissues, particularly the heart, liver, nerves and kidneys. This happens because these patients lack an enzyme, phytanic acid α-hydrolase, which is needed if phytanic acid, consumed in dairy products and ruminant fats, is to be oxidised and degraded.

Clinical features

The main clinical manifestations are retinitis pigmentosa, peripheral neuropathy and cerebellar ataxia. Renal involvement may be shown by lipiduria (the presence of oval fat bodies in the urine), mild glycosuria and impairment of tubular function and the glomerular filtration rate. In most patients signs and symptoms of the disease occur by the age of 20 years but in a few they commence much later. The diagnosis is made by demonstrating elevated levels of phytanic acid in the plasma and impaired phytanic acid oxidation in cultures of the patient's fibroblasts. Heterozygotes do not accumulate phytanic acid and remain asymptomatic. Plasmapheresis combined with a diet low in phytanic acid arrests progress of the disease and prevents relapses.

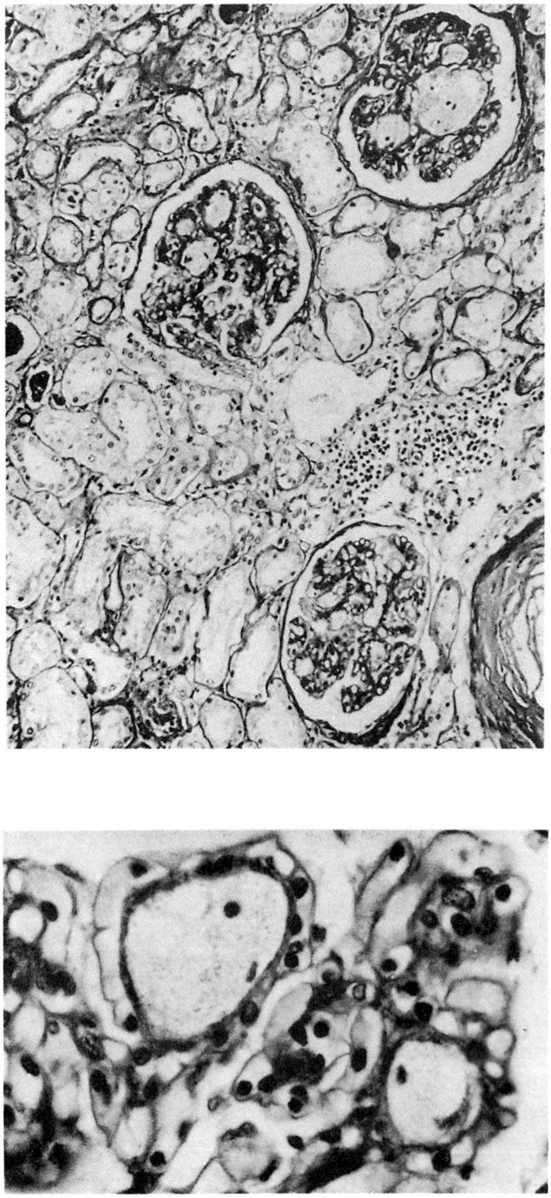

Fig. 4.23 Familial type III hyperlipoproteinemia. (**a**) The glomeruli contain clusters of foam cells. (**b**) Part of glomerulus showing mesangial location of foam cells. Periodic acid-Schiff: (**a**) × 120; (**b**) × 500
Reproduced by permission from: Amatruda JM, Margolis S, Hutchins GM. Arch Pathol 1974; 98: 51 (Figs 9, 11)

Renal changes

There is extensive vacuolation of the cytoplasm of the proximal and distal tubular epithelial cells and slight vacuolation of the glomerular visceral epithelial cells (Fig. 4.24). The vacuoles are positive for fat when frozen sections are stained with oil red O. In the electron microscope the tubular and glomerular epithelial cells contain lipid vacuoles of various sizes.[110]

DISORDERS OF CARBOHYDRATE METABOLISM

Glycogen storage diseases (glycogenoses)

Inherited defects may involve many of the enzymes concerned in the synthesis and degradation

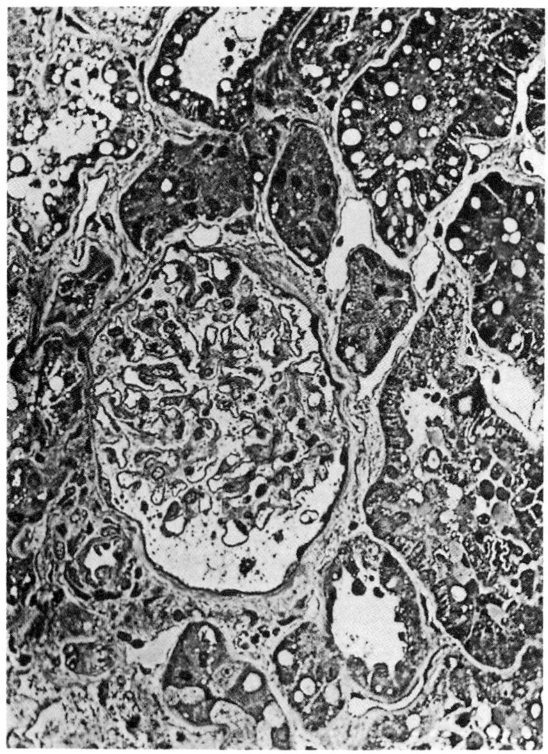

Fig. 4.24 Phytanic acid storage disease (Refsum's disease). The tubular epithelial cells and glomerular visceral epithelial cells contain large vacuoles from which lipid was removed in the processing of the tissue.
Haematoxylin-eosin x 450
Reproduced by permission from: Pabico RC, Gruebel BJ, McKenna BA et al. Am J Med 1981; 70: 1136 (Fig. 1)

of glycogen but it is only in von Gierke's and Pompe's glycogen storage diseases that the kidney is affected. Both diseases are inherited as an autosomal recessive trait. In young children renal function is usually unimpaired although there may be glycosuria and aminoaciduria. Later, in adolescence and adult life, chronic renal disease is a frequent and serious complication of von Gierke's disease. In one series 70% of patients aged 13 years or older had persistent proteinuria; hypertension and haematuria were also common. Progressive renal failure developed in 43% of the patients with proteinuria.[111]

Von Gierke's disease (glycogen storage disease type I)[111,112]

Glycogen storage disease type I is caused in most cases by a deficiency of the enzyme glucose-6-phosphatase; in a few patients the system for transporting glucose-6-phosphate across the microsomal membrane is defective. About one in every 100 000 newborns is affected. Children with the defect are stunted and have huge abdomens because of massive enlargement of the liver due to glycogen storage. Signs and symptoms appear in the first year of life. The glomerular filtration rate is increased by approximately 50%.[113] Hyperuricaemia is common and many patients develop gout in adolescence (see p. 106). As the children grow up microalbuminuria often appears and may progress to frank proteinuria. Hypertension may also occur. Hepatic adenomas that may undergo malignant transformation have also been described.

Pompe's disease (glycogen storage disease type II)[114]

Glycogen storage disease type II is caused by deficiency of the lysosomal enzyme α-1,4-glucosidase. The incidence of the disease is about the same as for von Gierke's. The heart is the main site of glycogen storage and is greatly enlarged; cardiac failure is common in the first year of life.

Renal changes

The kidneys are enlarged and pale.

Light microscopy There is severe vacuolation of the tubular cells affecting particularly the proximal convoluted tubules. After alcohol fixation masses of granular glycogen in the cytoplasm of the cells are stained red by Best's carmine. Glycogen is also present in interstitial cells. Focal segmental glomerulosclerosis (see p. 204) in various stages of progression is found in those patients with proteinuria; it is the cause of the renal failure that may develop.[111] This progressive renal damage may be due to the glomerular hyperfiltration (see p. 26).[113]

Electron microscopy[115] Particles of glycogen are scattered throughout the proximal tubular cytoplasm and also packed into greatly distended lysosomes. In von Gierke's disease there is often thickening, lamellation and segmental intramembranous and subepithelial glycogen deposition in the glomerular capillary basement membranes (Fig. 4.25). Glycogen is also present in the mesangium and in the glomerular epithelial, mesangial and endothelial cells.[116,117]

Primary hyperoxaluria

Primary hyperoxaluria is a general term for two autosomal recessive errors of metabolism which are characterized biochemically by the continuous excessive synthesis and urinary excretion of oxalic acid, and pathologically by the recurrent formation of bilateral calcium oxalate stones, and nephrocalcinosis. The pattern of urinary organic acid excretion is the basis for classification of the disease into two types. Type I is an uncommon but not rare metabolic disturbance and patients with this form of the disease excrete in the urine excessive amounts of glycolic and glyoxylic acids as well as oxalic acid. The cause is a deficiency of peroxisomal alanine : glyoxylate aminotransferase[118] which is only found in any quantity in the liver. The enzyme lack leads to excessive synthesis of oxalate and glycolate. Type II has only been found in a few patients and they excrete in the urine excessive amounts of L-glyceric acid as well as oxalic acid, but the amounts of glycolic and glyoxylic acids are normal. The cause is a deficiency of leucocyte D-glyceric dehydrogenase: this leads to faulty pyruvate metabolism which results in its excessive reduction to L-glyceric acid. Both types

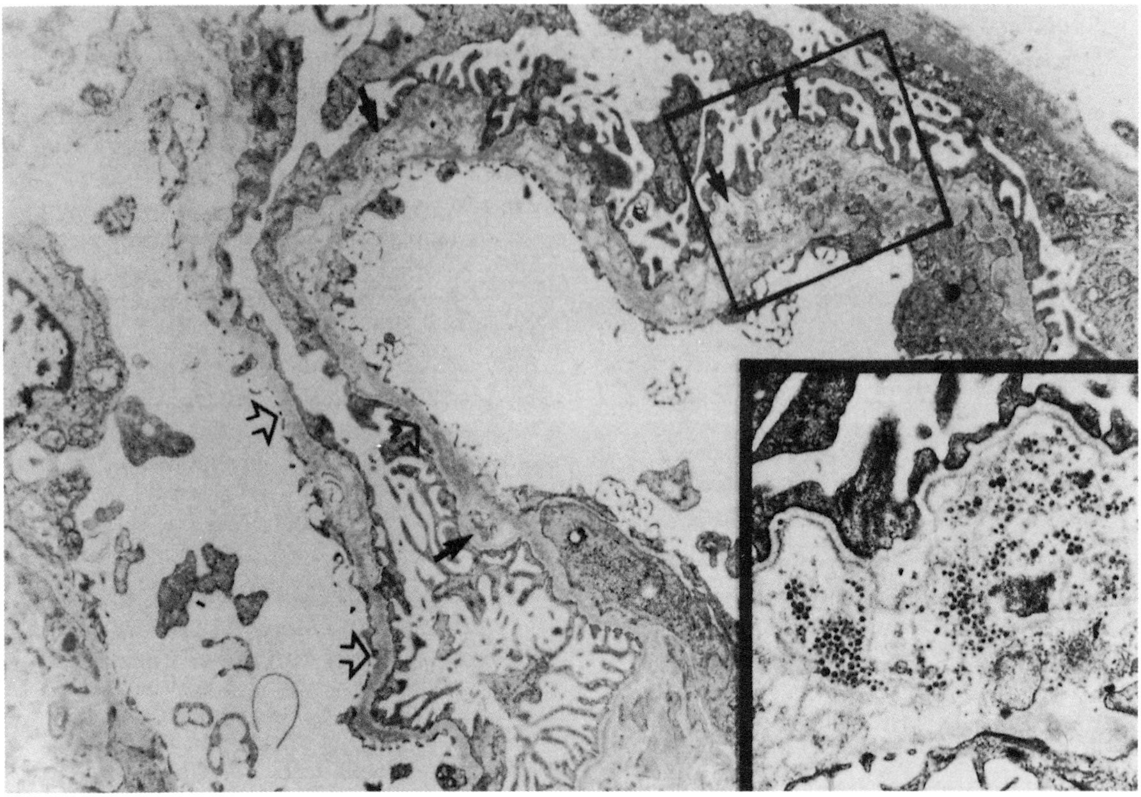

Fig. 4.25 Von Gierke's glycogen storage disease. Electron micrograph of part of a glomerulus. The capillary basement membranes are thickened and irregular, with lamellation and focal deposits of glycogen (solid arrows). There are a few remaining areas of normal basement membrane (open arrows). Inset: Glycogen deposits in the basement membrane. × 6400; inset, × 16 000
Reproduced by permission from: Jonas AJ, Verani RR, Howell RR, Conley SB. Am J Kidney Dis 1988; 11: 264 (Fig. 2)

of primary hyperoxaluria produce the same clinical features and pathological changes.

Clinical features[119]

Evidence of renal involvement commonly appears before the age of 10 years. It may include haematuria, urinary infection and symptoms of urinary stones. Occasionally the disease presents with proteinuria, renal insufficiency or retardation of growth. The disease usually leads to progressive renal failure and, if dialysis or renal transplantation is not available, death in uraemia before adolescence. However, primary hyperoxaluria is phenotypically heterogeneous and severe forms which lead to death in infancy, and mild forms which remain symptomless until early adult life, are encountered.

Primary hyperoxaluria type I can be detected prenatally by assaying alanine : glycoxylate aminotransferase in fetal hepatic tissue obtained by biopsy.

Renal changes[120]

Gross appearances The kidneys are granular and reduced in size; they may be coarsely scarred. They feel gritty when cut. The calyces and pelvis are often dilated and usually contain fine particles of calcific material and many small stones.

Light microscopy Large numbers of crystals are present in the dilated lumen of the proximal and distal convoluted tubules and in the collecting tubules (Fig. 4.26). They are also found between the epithelial cells and the basement membrane of the tubules. They are birefringent and arranged usually in the form of rosettes and sheaves. There

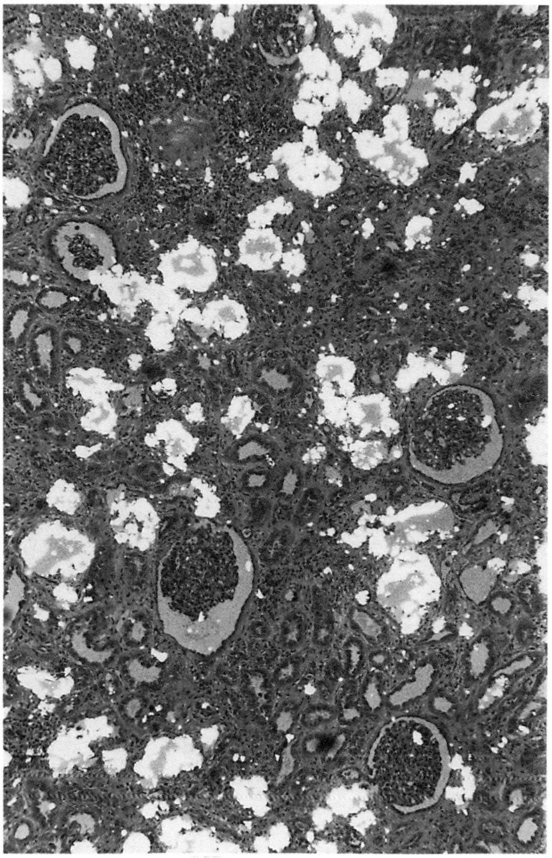

Fig. 4.26 Primary hyperoxaluria. There are numerous birefringent intratubular and interstitial calcium oxalate deposits.
Haematoxylin-eosin, partially polarized light × 155

is also focal atrophy of the tubules and widespread interstitial fibrosis. Interstitial deposits of crystals are often accompanied by the formation of multinucleate giant cells of foreign body type and by patchy infiltration of the adjoining tissue by mononuclear cells. The interlobular and arcuate arteries show various degrees of endarteritis obliterans. Crystals may be present in the wall of some of the larger arteries.

The crystalline material has been identified as calcium oxalate by chemical analysis and by X-ray crystallography.

Renal transplantation

Oxalate deposition readily occurs in renal allografts in patients with type I hyperoxaluria (see p. 670); there are no reports of renal transplantation in cases of type II hyperoxaluria. Treatment with pyridoxine, which reduces urinary excretion of oxalate in some patients, long-term diuresis and administration of neutral phosphate will keep oxalate deposition in the graft to a minimum for many years,[121] but good graft function will not prevent further extrarenal deposition which leads to severe oxalate-induced bone and vascular disease. Combined hepatic and renal transplantation has been successfully used to overcome these problems; the liver graft provides the patient with the missing peroxisomal alanine : glyoxylate aminotransferase and the underlying genetic defect is corrected.[122,123]

Pathogenesis

Calcium oxalate has a very low solubility and therefore tends to form urinary calculi and to be deposited in the tissues. The deposition of oxalate in the kidneys and the formation of stones lead to renal impairment, decreased excretion of oxalate, raised levels of oxalate in the blood, and deposition of oxalate crystals in many tissues. Once established, this vicious spiral may cause rapid deterioration in the patient's condition.

Diabetes mellitus

Primary diabetes mellitus is characterized by insulin deficiency and glucagon excess. There are two major forms of the primary disease: insulin-dependent diabetes (type 1) and non-insulin-dependent diabetes (type 2). Both types appear to be genetically distinct; neither follows simple patterns of Mendelian inheritance. That the disease has a genetic background in most cases is generally accepted, but the nature and mechanisms of that genetic contribution are unclear.

Renal changes

Renal disease is frequent in diabetes mellitus and is described on page 330.

DISORDERS OF PURINE METABOLISM

Hyperuricaemia and gout[124]

The biochemical hallmark of gout is hyperuricaemia, but this also occurs in the absence of gout. Gout is classified as primary when it is neither a consequence of an acquired disorder nor a late and subordinate manifestation of an inborn error of metabolism which leads initially to a clinical disorder unlike gout, e.g. patients with glycogen storage disease (see p. 103) have hyperuricaemia from infancy and may develop gout at about the age of 10 years.

Probably primary gout always has an hereditary basis but the precise metabolic defect and its genetic pattern have been identified in only a few subsets. In one such subset there is a complete deficiency of the enzyme hypoxanthine-guanine phosphoribosyltransferase, in another it is partial deficiency of the same enzyme and in a third subset it is overactivity of 5-phosphoribosyl-α-1-pyrophosphate synthetase. All three defects are inherited as X-linked disorders. The first defect is associated with the Lesch–Nyhan syndrome (gout, choreoathetosis, spasticity, mental retardation and self-mutilation). About 25% of the asymptomatic blood relatives of persons with primary gout have hyperuricaemia. Renal disease is common in patients with primary gout (see pp. 343, 541 and 542).

Renal changes

These are described under gout (see p. 340).

DISORDERS OF BLOOD

Sickle cell disease and trait

The predominant type of haemoglobin in human red cells is haemoglobin A; it is composed of four polypeptide chains – two alpha chains and two beta chains. An inherited error may lead to one of the amino acids in the polypeptide chains being replaced by another. The commonest example of this is where an uncharged valine molecule is substituted for a charged glutamic acid in the beta chain. The resulting abnormal haemoglobin is called haemoglobin S. At low oxygen concentrations the haemoglobin S molecules adhere together and polymerize, producing long tubular fibres which make the red cells rigid and sickle shaped.

The gene responsible for haemoglobin S occurs throughout tropical Africa as well as in blacks in the USA and in other countries. It is also found in parts of the Middle East and India. The mode of inheritance is autosomal recessive. In some parts of Africa up to 45% of the population are carriers of the sickle cell gene.

Heterozygotes with one gene for haemoglobin A and one for haemoglobin S are defined clinically as having *sickle cell trait.* Their red cells contain between 20% and 45% haemoglobin S, the rest being haemoglobin A, and the cells do not sickle until the oxygen saturation falls below 40%.

Homozygotes for haemoglobin S have *sickle cell disease* (sickle cell anaemia). Almost all the haemoglobin in the red cells is haemoglobin S; they sickle at the oxygen tension normally found in venous blood. The increased rigidity of sickled red cells causes them to move slowly or even to become jammed in capillaries.

Renal changes

Several forms of renal abnormality are liable to develop in association with sickle cell trait or sickle cell disease.[125,126]

Rupture of venules in the pelvic mucosa Patients with sickle cell trait may have episodes of gross haematuria as a result of rupture of venules in the lamina propria of the pelvic mucosa that have become greatly engorged with sickled erythrocytes. The low venous oxygen pressure and the relatively high interstitial pressure in the renal medulla, which tends to impede the local venous circulation, probably favour aggregation of sickle cells in the venules of this region.

Papillary necrosis[127] The conditions in the medulla that predispose to venous engorgement and bleeding in these patients also predispose to necrosis of renal papillae. The necrosis is slow to develop and does not tend to cause acute renal failure.

Glomerular lesions In children with sickle cell disease the most constant effect on the kidney is distension of the glomerular and peritubular capillaries by masses of sickled red cells. This may be accompanied by proliferation of mesangial cells giving *diffuse mesangial proliferative glomerulonephritis* (Fig. 4.27; see p. 153).

In older children *focal segmental glomerulosclerosis* appears.[128] This may be due to glomerular hyperfiltration (see p. 28);[125] such an interpretation is supported by the finding that there is glomerular enlargement, most marked in the juxtamedullary region, in children with sickle cell disease.[129] The gradual decrease in renal function as the patients age and the frequent proteinuria can be explained by a hyperfiltration-mediated glomerulosclerosis.

Sometimes a *mesangiocapillary glomerulonephritis type I* (Fig. 4.28; see p. 166) develops.[130] Antigen derived from proximal tubular epithelium and antibody to that antigen have been identified in the deposits. There may be aggregates of iron and protein in the mesangium and in the tubular epithelium. These patients usually have proteinuria and they may develop the nephrotic syndrome. Immune complexes that contain renal tubular antigen have been described in the circulation. Death from renal failure occasionally occurs. The glomerular lesions appear to be mediated by immune complexes containing antigen from the proximal tubular cells. The complexes probably arise as a result of recurrent episodes of sickling that cause ischaemic damage to the tubular epithelium and release of antigen.[131]

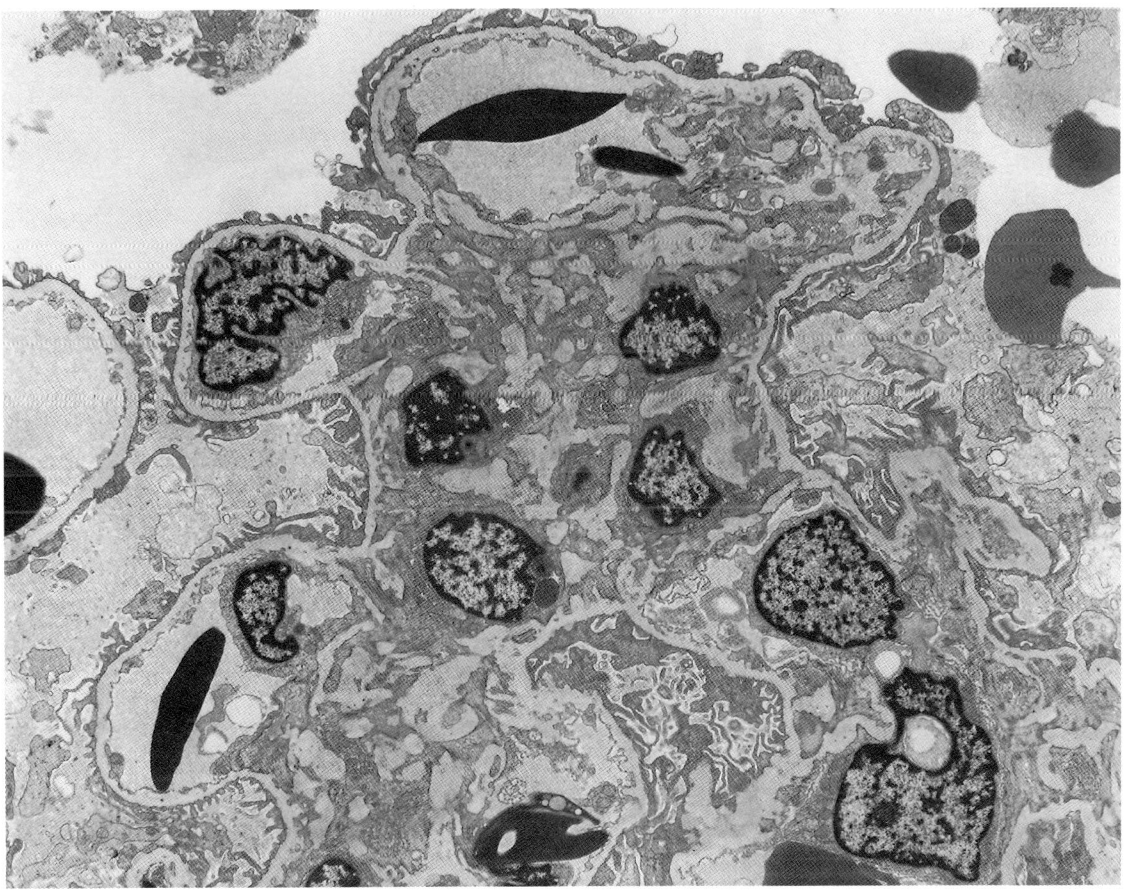

Fig. 4.27 Sickle cell disease. Electron micrograph of part of a glomerulus. There is a diffuse mesangial proliferative glomerulonephritis with expansion of the mesangium and an increase in the number of mesangial cells. There are sickled red cells in the capillary lumens.
× 8000

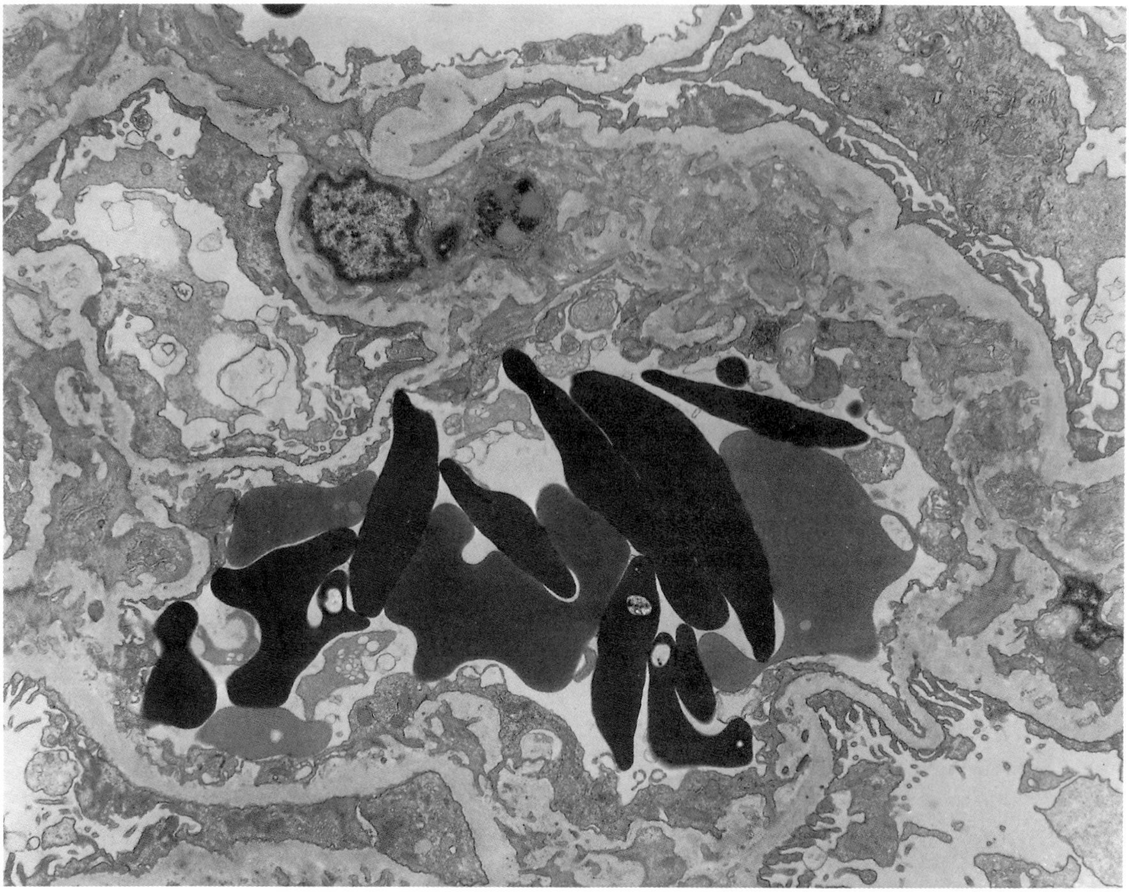

Fig. 4.28 Sickle cell disease. Electron micrograph of part of a glomerular capillary loop. There is a mesangiocapillary glomerulonephritis with marked thickening of the capillary wall by mesangial cell interposition. The capillary lumen contains sickled red cells.
× 11 250

Renal infarction[132] Gross cortical infarcts are seen occasionally, although it is unusual to find a thrombus in any large vessel. Infarcts of the renal papillae are a well-recognized complication of the sickle cell trait in those who undertake high altitude flying.

Slowing of medullary circulation by sickle cells The circulatory slowing that results from the effects of the distortion of the red cells on the local haemodynamics disturbs the countercurrent mechanism and leads to inability to concentrate the urine.

Pyelonephritis The kidneys are unusually prone to bacterial lodgement and proliferation in cases of sickle cell disease. Pyelonephritis is a correspondingly frequent complication: it is usually acute but may be chronic.

Acute renal failure This is rare. Indirect evidence suggests that it may sometimes be caused by released myoglobin or haemoglobin (see p. 492).[133]

DISORDERS OF IMMUNE SYSTEM

Hereditary deficiencies of complement components

Inherited deficiencies of components of the complement system, consisting of either the absence of the protein or the presence of a dysfunctional molecule, have been described for 15 of the 19 complement components and regulator proteins.[134] Most of the deficiencies are the result of autosomal recessive mutations, with the heterozygote relatives having 50% of the normal serum level of the relevant component. Exceptions are C1 esterase inhibitor (C1 Inh) deficiency, which is inherited as an autosomal dominant trait, and properdin (P) deficiency, which appears to be X-linked. Apart from C2 deficiency, in which it is calculated that 1.2% of the general population are heterozygotes and one in 28 000 individuals is homozygous, and C1 Inh deficiency, homozygous deficiencies are very rare.

Most hereditary deficiencies of complement components are associated with a high frequency of infections and some with an increased incidence of immune complex disorders, such as glomerulonephritis, systemic lupus erythematosus (SLE), SLE-like syndromes and various forms of vasculitis. The most common hereditary complement deficiency, C1 Inh deficiency, gives rise to hereditary angioneurotic oedema; it is also occasionally associated with SLE and type I mesangiocapillary glomerulonephritis.[135]

The immune complex disorders are particularly associated with deficiencies of those components involved in the classical pathway of complement activation (C1, C2, C4) and within this group patients with deficiencies of C1 subcomponents (C1q, C1r, C1s) or of C4 have a greater predisposition to immune complex disease than those with C2 deficiency.[134,136] A predilection to immune complex disease occurs even in the heterozygous state. SLE and sometimes glomerulonephritis have been reported in the following percentages of homozygotes deficient in a particular complement component: C1 77%, C4 62%, C2 35%, C3 36%, C5 8%, C6 6%, C7 5% and C8 6%.[134] These diseases have not been recorded with deficiencies of the other complement components or regulator proteins. Various morphological patterns of glomerulonephritis occur: the commonest is diffuse mesangiocapillary type 1, but diffuse mesangial proliferative is fairly common and diffuse endocapillary proliferative, diffuse membranous and focal and segmental glomerulosclerosis have been recorded.[137–143]

It has been proposed that deficiency of any complement component needed to form the classical pathway C3 convertase compromises the ability of the individual to eliminate antigens, so leading to immune complex disease.[136] Because the genes coding for C2 and C4 are closely linked to the major histocompatibility complex on chromosome 6, the possibility has been raised that the complement deficiency is not itself the cause of the immune complex disease but may be merely a marker for a closely linked genetic locus which causes a predisposition to the disease. However, this would not explain the susceptibility to immune complex disease of subjects with deficiencies of C1 and C3 in whom the genes concerned are not linked with the major histocompatibility complex.

MISCELLANEOUS DISORDERS

Hereditary systemic amyloidosis

Familial amyloid polyneuropathy

Familial amyloid polyneuropathy comprises a group of rare autosomal dominant diseases characterized by the inheritance of systemic amyloidosis. It is usually divided into four types. Type I familial amyloid polyneuropathy affects many families in Portugal, Sweden and certain parts of Japan;[144] the other types are all very rare. Symptoms do not occur until the third or fourth decade of life.

Renal involvement is confined to types I, III and IV; it is signalled by proteinuria. Type III affects families of British origin. In all types peripheral neuropathy is an early sign. Progression of the disease is rapid in type I, with death from renal failure often occurring in the fourth and fifth decades; progression is variable in types III and IV.

The subunits of amyloid fibrils from individuals with type I familial amyloid polyneuropathy are composed of a mixture of normal and variant prealbumen (transthyretin) with the variant predominating. The variant prealbumen differs from the normal by a single amino acid substitution of methionine for valine at position 30 on the prealbumen molecule. The amyloid fibril subunit in type III familial amyloid polyneuropathy is not known. In type IV disease it is a protein related to gelsolin, which is an actin-modulating protein.[145] What causes the variant prealbumen and the gelsolin-like protein to be deposited as amyloid fibrils is not at all clear. Both prealbumens and gelsolin are derived from the plasma.[146] The prealbumen mutation can be detected prenatally by a recombinant DNA method.[147]

Renal changes These often do not differ from those seen in other forms of amyloidosis (see p. 346),[148] but sometimes the amyloid is predominantly in the medulla.

Familial Mediterranean fever

Familial Mediterranean fever is a serious autosomal recessive disorder characterized by recurrent attacks of abdominal pain and fever which may be associated with polyserositis, arthritis and skin rashes. The disease affects preferentially Jews, Arabs, Armenians and Turks but may affect subjects of any ethnic group. More than 90% of the Jewish patients are of either Sephardic or Iraqi origin.

The frequency of the gene responsible for the disease in Sephardic Jews is about one in 45 persons. In one series of 418 Sephardic Jews carrying the gene, with a mean age of 22 years, 156 (37%) had shown evidence of amyloid and 101 of these had died of it, most from renal failure.[149] As Sephardic Jews constitute half Israel's population, patients with familial Mediterranean fever and amyloidosis form a substantial proportion of those requiring dialysis and transplantation in that country.

The subunits of amyloid fibrils from these individuals are composed of amyloid A protein (AA) derived from serum amyloid A protein, an acute-phase reactant. Presumably this is the result of the long-standing inflammatory processes that occur in these patients. However, Armenian patients and Ashkenazi Jews, in whom the clinical manifestations of familial Mediterranean fever are indistinquishable from those of the Sephardic Jews, almost never develop amyloidosis.

Colchicine treatment appears to ameliorate the effect of amyloidosis in familial Mediterranean fever and prophylactic colchicine seems to prevent its appearance.[150] How it does this is not known. In experimental mice colchicine inhibits the production of serum amyloid A protein by hepatocytes but in patients with familial Mediterranean fever it does not seem to affect the abrupt rise in serum amyloid A protein that accompanies the recurrent episodes of fever.[151]

Renal changes These are the same as those that occur in AA amyloidosis brought about by other causes (see p. 346).[152]

Renal transplantation This is usually combined with colchicine treatment. The results are similar to those in other forms of systemic amyloidosis (see p. 670).[153] Amyloid deposition occurs in about 20% of the grafts, usually between 2.5 and 4 years after transplantation, but occasionally as early as 6 months.[153] Deterioration of renal function is frequently slow; progression of extrarenal amyloidosis is the greater problem.

Other forms of hereditary systemic amyloidosis

Numerous other extremely rare types of hereditary systemic amyloidosis are characterized by renal involvement, e.g those described by Ostertag, by Maxwell and Kimball and by Muckle and Wells. These and the others have been reviewed.[154] The subunits of the amyloid fibrils in the Muckle and Wells type are composed of AA protein. The composition of the others is not yet known. The renal amyloid deposits are variable in quantity and distribution in these forms of hereditary systemic amyloidosis. In Ostertag's autosomal dominant type glomerular giant cells may be a feature.[155]

α_1-Antitrypsin deficiency

Severe deficiency of the protease inhibitor α_1-antitrypsin is closely linked with the development of emphysema and liver disease. Its association with renal disease, however, is less clear. Two patients with α_1-antitrypsin deficiency, phenotype PiZZ, developed microscopic polyarteritis with crescentic glomerulonephritis,[156,157] and in another three patients with the same phenotype diffuse mesangiocapillary glomerulonephritis type I occurred.[158] In one of these cases subendothelial deposits of α_1-antitrypsin, immunoglobulin and complement were demonstrated by immunofluorescence on the glomerular capillary walls. The sixth patient who had a PiSZ phenotype developed diffuse membranous glomerulonephritis.[159] With such small numbers of patients the association of glomerulonephritis and polyarteritis with the α_1-antitrypsin deficiency state may be simply due to chance.

RENAL INVOLVEMENT IN OTHER HEREDITARY DISEASES

NEUROFIBROMATOSIS TYPE 1 (VON RECKLINGHAUSEN'S DISEASE)

Neurofibromatosis type 1 (NF-1) is one of the most common autosomal dominant hereditary diseases; it affects 1 in about 3000 people. The spontaneous mutation rate is high, with 30–50% of cases representing new mutations. The gene responsible for the disease is located on the long arm of chromosome 17; it has recently been cloned.[160] The NF-1 gene is expressed in a wide variety of tissues, including many not of neural crest origin. The specificity of the NF-1 mutation is at present unexplained; it might involve tissue-specific modification or interaction of the NF-1 gene product with other proteins. The protein coded for by the NF-1 gene is closely related to another protein, GAP, so called because it activates guanosine triphosphatase. GAP downregulates or turns off *ras* protein which signals cells to grow. Possibly the NF-1 gene ordinarily holds a *ras*-like protein in check, and when both copies of the NF-1 gene are inactivated by a mutation, uncontrolled cell growth occurs.[161]

Clinical features

The disorder is characterized by skin lesions resembling large freckles (*café au lait* spots), multiple benign neurofibromas and hamartomas of the iris (Lisch nodules). In children with neurofibromatosis, defects of the skull and facial bones, kyphoscoliosis, optic gliomas, focal gigantism of a limb, and tumours of the renal pelvis and lower urinary tract may also occur.

Vascular lesions associated with neurofibromatosis have been recognized for more than half a century. Arteries and arterioles in the kidneys, endocrine glands, heart and gastrointestinal tract are usually affected; arterial stenosis and circulatory obstruction may result. Lesions in the abdominal aorta have been described.[162]

Changes in the renal vasculature are usually symptomless. In some cases, especially when the main renal artery is stenotic, they are associated with hypertension. This is particularly true in children; in adults, phaeochromocytoma – which also is of greater frequency in cases of neurofibromatosis – is the likelier cause of hypertension.[163]

Occasionally involvement of the renal vasculature leads to infarction and renal insufficiency.[164]

Renal changes

Vascular lesions

Arteries and arterioles are narrowed by an intimal thickening that consists of concentric layers of smooth muscle cells and increased amounts of mucinous ground substance (Figs 4.29, 4.30). There is rupture of the internal elastic lamina, atrophy of the media, formation of aneurysms and fibrous thickening of the adventitia.[165–167] The vascular changes are often focal. Morphologically, it can be difficult to distinguish these changes from the lesions that result from healed or 'burnt-out' polyarteritis: the presence of nodular collections of smooth muscle cells in the thickened intima and adventitia in the lesions accompanying neurofibromatosis is a distinguishing feature (Fig. 4.30).

Fusiform fibrous nodules in the interstitium

Multiple elliptical to fusiform nodules composed of laminae of fibrous tissue have been described in the cortex of three patients (Fig. 4.31).[160] The nodules appear to start around tubules. It has been suggested that they may be hamartomas[168] (hamartoma is defined in the section on 'Tuberous Sclerosis', below).

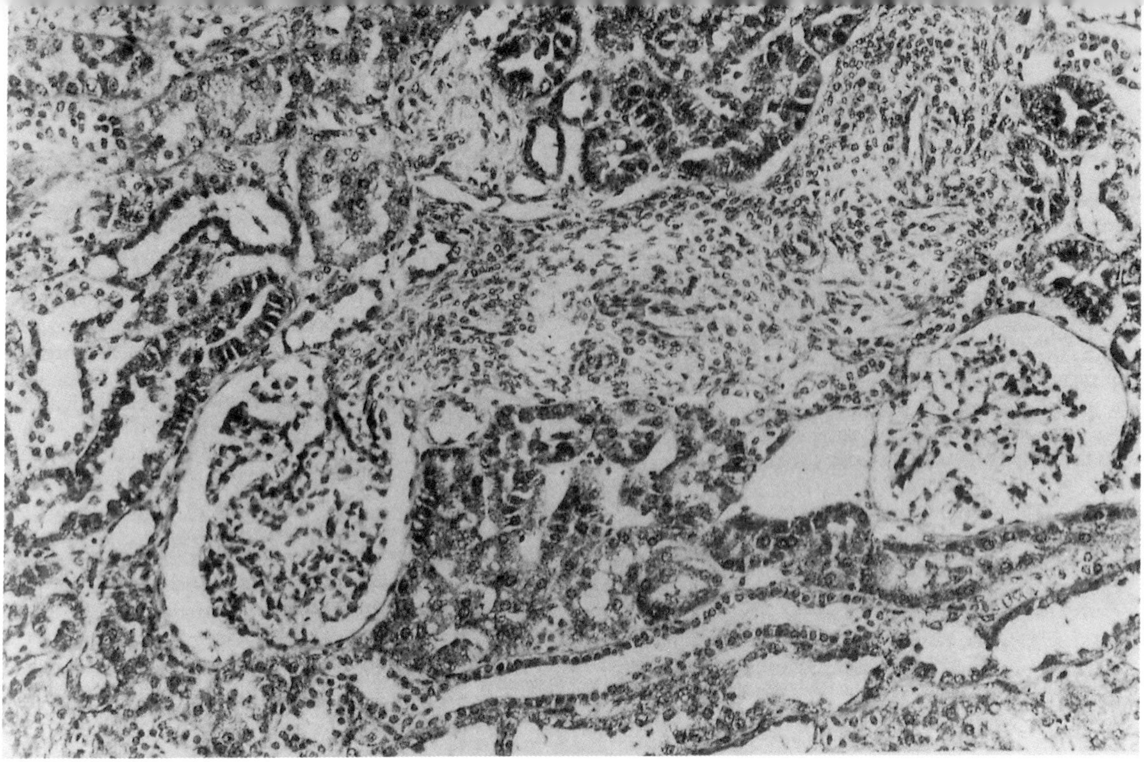

Fig. 4.29 Neurofibromatosis type 1. Smooth muscle proliferation involving an afferent arteriole. Haematoxylin-eosin × 100
Reproduced by permission from: Finley JL, Dabbs DJ. Hum Pathol 1988; 19: 107 (Fig. 1A)

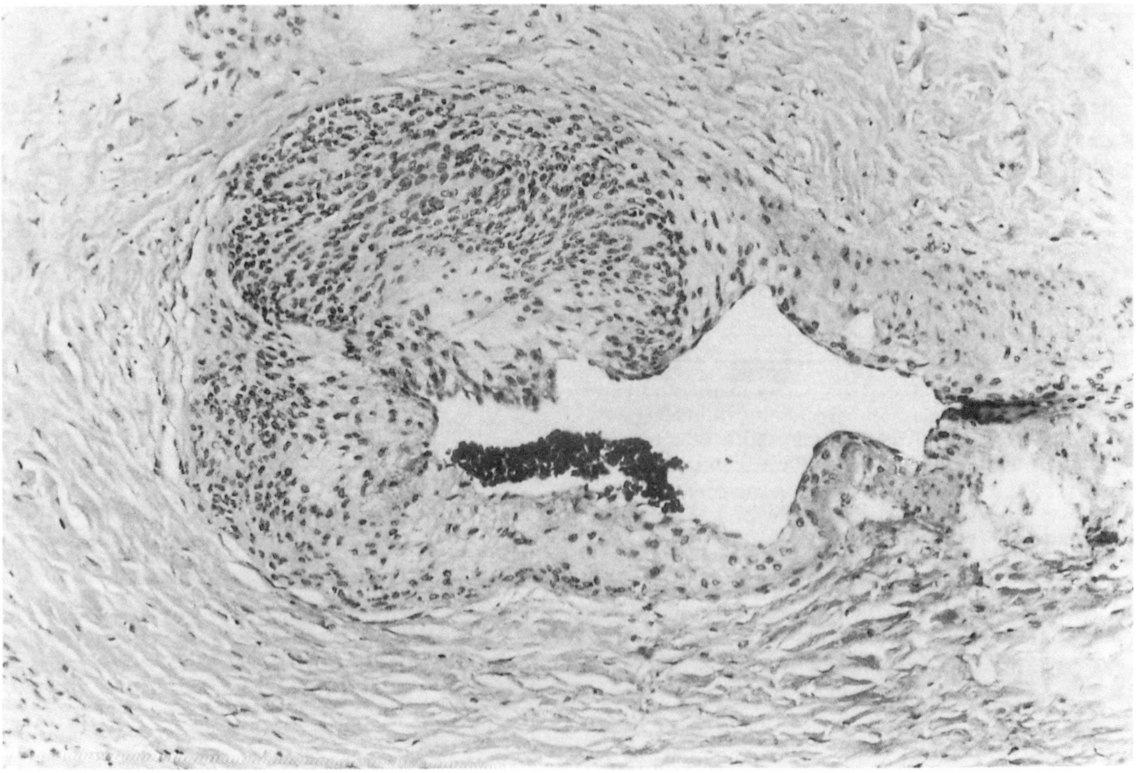

Fig. 4.30 Neurofibromatosis type 1. Section of an interlobular artery. The intima is thickened by smooth muscle cells and increased amounts of ground substance; some of the smooth muscle cells are in nodules. There is marked thinning of the media. Haematoxylin-eosin × 200
Reproduced by permission from: Finley JL, Dabbs DJ. Hum Pathol 1988; 19: 704 (Fig. 1B)

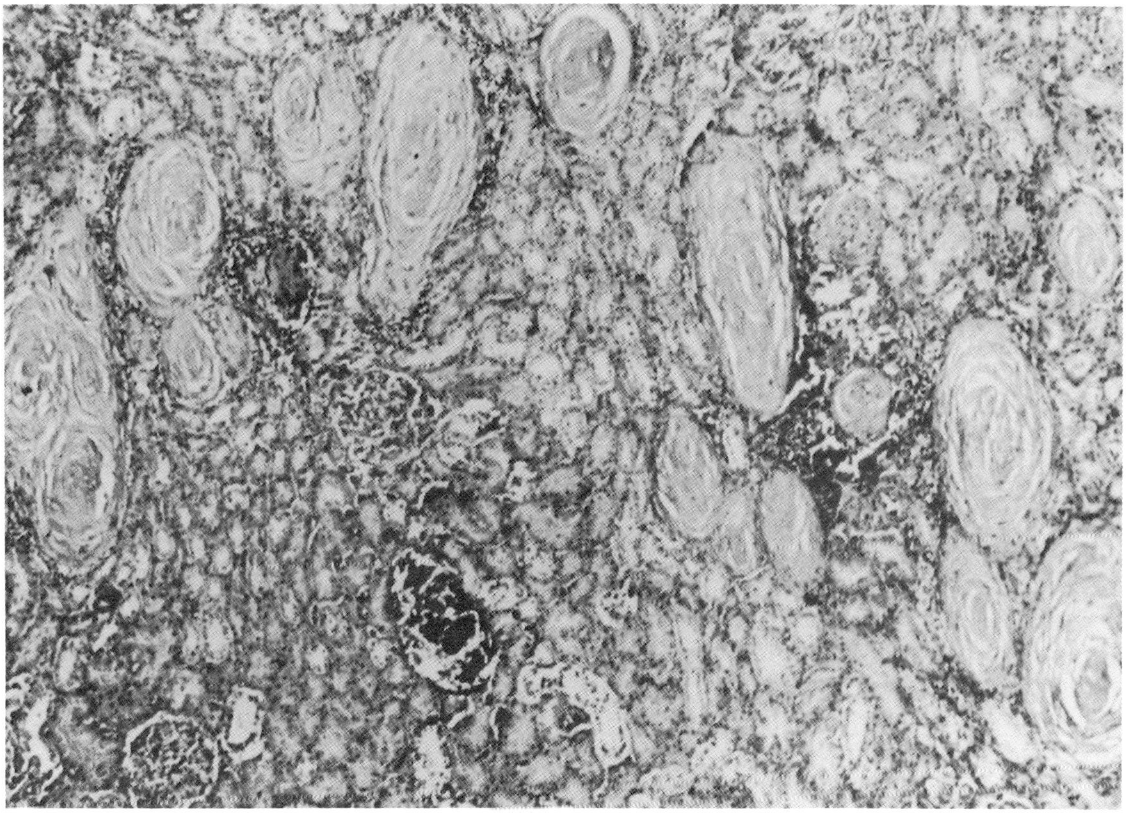

Fig. 4.31 Neurofibromatosis. The renal cortex contains elliptical and fusiform fibrous nodules of various sizes. Haematoxylin-eosin × 56
Reproduced by permission from: Mandybur TI, Weiss MA. Hum Pathol 1981; 12: 704 (Fig. 1)

Schwannomas of the renal pelvis

Malignant schwannomas occasionally occur in the renal pelvis (see p. 615).[169]

TUBEROUS SCLEROSIS

Tuberous sclerosis is characterized by the occurrence of hamartomas of the brain, retina, skin, heart, bone, lung and kidney. Hamartomas are congenital tumours composed of tissues that normally are present in a given organ but that are abnormal in quantity, arrangement or degree of maturation and that may grow and behave as benign neoplasms.[170] Clinically the brain hamartomas produce convulsions in 80% of affected individuals and mild to severe mental retardation in half the patients. Hypopigmented macules occur on the skin of almost all the patients and adenoma sebaceum in 60–70%.

Tuberous sclerosis is an autosomal dominant condition with high penetrance but considerable variability in expression. Linkage analysis suggests that the gene responsible for the disease is on the distal long arm of chromosome 9.[171] The reported frequency in Great Britain is one case in 15 000 persons,[172] but in other countries it may be more frequent. For example, in Rochester, Minnesota, the incidence is one case in 9407 persons.[173]

Renal changes are common in tuberous sclerosis. The most frequent lesions are hamartomas composed of blood vessels, smooth muscle and fat (usually called angiomyolipomas) and renal cysts.[174] Generally they are asymptomatic but in a few patients the number and size of the lesions cause renal failure. Occasionally an angiomyolipoma will bleed either chronically or suddenly and massively; intrarenal bleeding will produce flank pain. Mild proteinuria is common. Angiomyolipoma and renal cysts are best detected by computerized tomography or ultrasound.

Angiomyolipomas

These hamartomas occur in the kidneys in 50–80% of patients with tuberous sclerosis. Often they are bilateral and multiple but they may be unilateral and solitary.

Gross appearances[175]

The tumours are round or oval, 3–20 cm in diameter, and occur in both the renal cortex and the medulla. When in the superficial cortex they elevate the renal capsule producing a bulging smooth bosselated mass (Fig. 4.32). The cut surface is yellow to grey depending upon the proportion of fat to smooth muscle that is present in the hamartoma; there may be evidence of recent or old focal haemorrhage. About 25% of angiomyolipomas extend through the renal capsule, about 5% adhere to the perirenal tissues and rarely regional lymph nodes are diffusely replaced by the hamartomatous tissue (Fig. 4.33).[176,177]

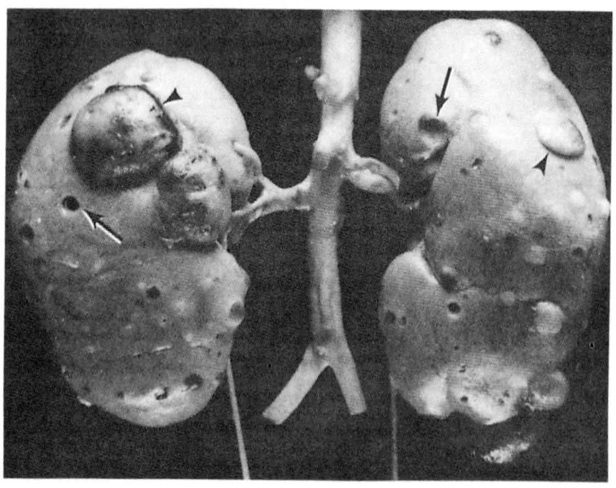

Fig. 4.32 Tuberous sclerosis. Multiple bilateral angiomyolipomas (arrowheads). There are also scattered renal cysts (arrows).
Reproduced by permission from: Farrow GM, Harrison EG, Utz DC, Jones DR. Cancer 1968; 22: 564 (Fig. 2C)

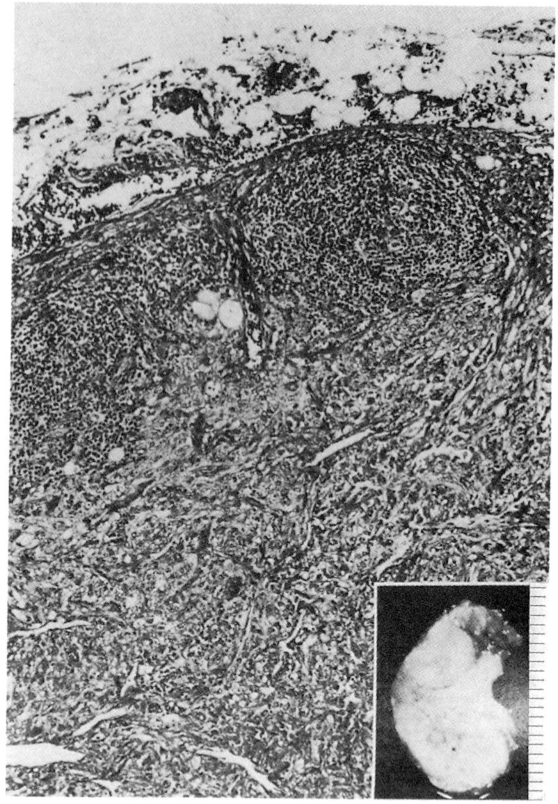

Fig. 4.33 Angiomyolipoma in tuberous sclerosis. Inset: Bisected lymph node from hilum of kidney; much of the node is replaced by lighter angiomyolipomatous tissue (one division = 1 mm). Main photograph: Lymph node diffusely replaced by angiomyolipomatous tissue; small lymphoid follicles remain beneath the capsule.
Haematoxylin-eosin × 100
Reproduced by permission from: Dao AH, Pinto AC, Kirchner FK, Halter SA. Arch Pathol Lab Med 1984; 108: 612 (Fig. 1)

Light microscopy[178]

The hamartomas are composed of a mixture of mature adipose tissue, tortuous, poorly formed, often thick-walled blood vessels, and sheets of smooth muscle (Fig. 4.34). The amount of each of these three components varies in different parts of the tumour and from patient to patient. The smooth muscle sometimes forms mantles around the blood vessels (Fig. 4.35); their nuclei may be hyperchromatic and moderately pleomorphic and mitoses may be present. Frequently the blood vessels are imperfect with walls of varying thickness and absence of normal elastic laminae.

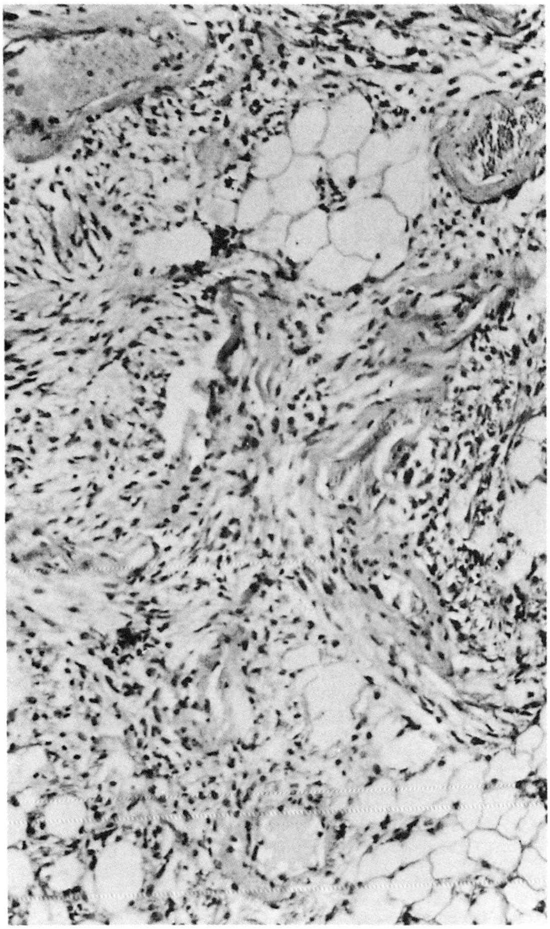

Fig. 4.34 Angiomyolipoma in tuberous sclerosis. Numerous small poorly formed blood vessels are surrounded by adipose tissue and sheets of smooth muscle.
Haematoxylin-eosin × 95
Reproduced by permission from: Bennington JL, Beckwith JB Atlas of tumor pathology, 2nd series, Fascicle 12. Washington, Armed Forces Institute of Pathology, 1983; p 201 (Fig. 163)

Sometimes bizarre giant cells are present. Tubules and calcified spicules also occur in the tumours.

Flow cytometric analysis

DNA flow cytometric analysis in three cases of angiomyolipoma of the kidney with lymph node involvement showed that the tumours, including those in lymph nodes, contained diploid DNA.[177]

Renal transplantation

The few results that have been published have

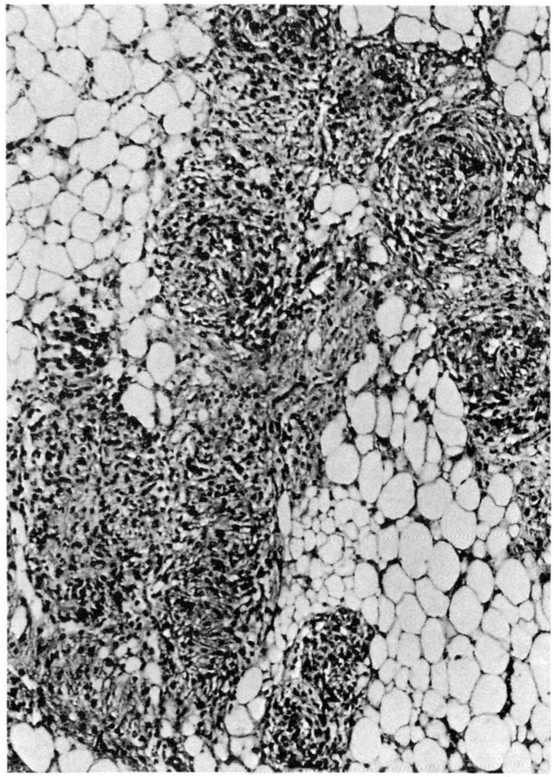

Fig. 4.35 Angiomyolipoma in tuberous sclerosis. Small blood vessels surrounded by whorls of smooth muscle and embedded in adipose tissue.
Haematoxylin eosin × 112
Reproduced by permission from: Bennington JL, Beckwith JB. Atlas of tumor pathology, 2nd series, Fascicle 12. Washington: Armed Forces Institute of Pathology, 1983; p 201 (Fig . 164)

been satisfactory. Because of the small risk of neoplastic transformation in the patients' own kidneys, these should be closely monitored by computerized tomography scan.[179]

Prognosis

Despite the sometimes worrying microscopic appearance, the extension outside the renal capsule and even involvement of local lymph nodes, angiomyolipomas behave in a benign fashion. No distant metastases have been recorded. This is important because conservative treatment with preservation of functional renal parenchyma is the treatment of choice in most cases.[176] The lymph node involvement probably represents a multicentric growth pattern; in follow-up studies on 11 cases the patients were alive and well 1–15 years (median follow-up 3 years) after operation.[177] The lack of aneuploidy in these angiomyolipomas supports their benign and multifocal nature.[177]

In the past angiomyolipomas have been misdiagnosed as liposarcoma, leiomyosarcoma, malignant mesenchymoma and fibrosarcoma. However, a renal cell carcinoma may occur in patients with tuberous sclerosis and produce metastases; several such cases have been reported.[175] There is also a suggestion that patients with tuberous sclerosis may be at greater risk of developing a malignant tumour when they are young.[178]

Renal cysts[177]

The incidence of renal cysts in tuberous sclerosis is not known but in one series it was about 30%.[174] Cysts and angiomyolipomas often coexist. Like the latter, cysts are commonly multiple and bilateral; occasionally they are diffuse and resemble adult type polycystic disease (see p. 62). The cysts in tuberous sclerosis are lined with a characteristically hyperplastic and hypertrophic epithelium. The abnormal epithelium is often piled into small nodules.

ALAGILLE'S SYNDROME (ARTERIOHEPATIC DYSPLASIA)

In Alagille's syndrome there is congenital absence or diminution in number and size of the intrahepatic interlobular bile ducts accompanied by peripheral pulmonary artery stenosis, cardiac, ocular and skeletal anomalies and characteristic facies. The mode of inheritance is consistent with an autosomal dominant gene exhibiting reduced penetrance and variable expression.[180]

The hepatic disorder causes jaundice and very high levels of lipids in the blood, especially cholesterol and phospholipids. Lipids are deposited in various tissues including the kidney. In long-surviving cases this may lead to proteinuria and progressive renal failure in adolescence or early adult life.[181]

The light microscopic and ultrastructural changes in the kidney are the same as those seen in familial lecithin-cholesterol acyltransferase deficiency (see p. 98).

FAMILIAL HAEMOLYTIC URAEMIC SYNDROME

The condition of haemolytic anaemia with fragmented red cells, thrombocytopenia and acute renal failure, known as the haemolytic uraemic syndrome, rarely occurs in a familial form. There have been reports of 28 families.[182] In the majority the disease seems to be inherited as an autosomal recessive trait; in seven families it appeared to be inherited as an autosomal dominant.[183]

Familial haemolytic uraemic syndrome develops insidiously in older children or adults with no seasonal variation in incidence and with no prodromal illness. More than a year separates the onset of the disease in individual siblings. The mortality is about 70% if treatment with dialysis or renal transplantation is not available.

Renal changes

The renal lesions are the same as those seen in the epidemic variety of haemolytic uraemic syndrome (see p. 283).

Renal transplantation

In many patients renal transplanation will be the treatment of choice although the risk of recurrence of the haemolytic uraemic syndrome is considerable (see p. 669).[184]

Pathogenesis

Familial haemolytic uraemic syndrome may be caused by an inherited fault in prostacyclin metabolism. In some patients there is a persistent deficiency of prostacyclin (PGI_2).[185] This may occur either because of lack of a plasma factor needed for PGI_2 production by endothelial cells, or because of the presence in the plasma of an inhibitor of PGI_2 production, or because of excessively rapid degradation of PGI_2.

CYSTIC FIBROSIS

Cystic fibrosis, a common autosomal recessive systemic disease of infancy or childhood, occurs in approximately one in 2000 whites; orientals and blacks are seldom affected. The carrier frequency is about 5%. The abnormal gene, which has been cloned, is on the long arm of chromosome 7 in band q31.[186] The disease is characterized by a defect in the secretory functions of the exocrine glands. Most importantly, the mucous glands produce abnormally viscid secretions. Inspissated mucus accumulates in the pancreatic ducts leading to fibrocystic disease, with loss of pancreatic secretion and consequent intestinal malabsorption. Accumulation of such mucus in the bronchioles and bronchi leads to chronic respiratory infections, chronic bronchitis, bronchiectasis and lung abscesses. In about a quarter of the patients inspissation of mucus within the bile ducts impairs excretion of bile; in a few cases biliary cirrhosis develops. Complications include cor pulmonale with cardiac failure. Diabetes mellitus may develop.

At autopsy renal lesions are common.[187] The most frequent is *glomerulomegaly*. In a series of 34 patients all the glomeruli were enlarged up to twice their normal size. *Focal segmental glomerulosclerosis* was also common. Both these changes are known to occur in association with cyanosis and chronic congestive cardiac failure (see p. 320). *Diffuse or segmental mesangial hypercellularity with increase of mesangial matrix* was also common and often associated with granular deposits of IgM and C3 and electron-dense deposits. Elution studies showed anti-pseudomonas antibodies in the renal deposits, suggesting that at least in some cases these might be due to immune complexes that are either filtered from the circulation or formed in situ. About half the cases showed *hyperplasia of the juxtaglomerular body*, probably secondary to reduced cardiac output. *Foci of tubular atrophy, interstitial fibrosis and chronic inflammatory cell infiltration* were present in about three-quarters of the patients and may be related to the aminoglycosides (see p. 517) that are used over long periods in patients with cystic fibrosis to treat their chronic infections. Large dense periodic acid-Schiff positive *casts of Tamm–Horsfall protein* are often present; they are perhaps caused by a basic defect in the production of Tamm–Horsfall protein by the ascending limb of Henle's loop. *Diabetic renal lesions* have also been recorded.[188] Recently *microscopic nephrocalcinosis* has been found in 92% of kidneys in cases of cystic fibrosis, including three that were examined close to the time of birth.[189] It has been suggested that there may be a primary abnormality of calcium metabolism in the kidney.

MISCELLANEOUS DISORDERS

Many other rare hereditary diseases and syndromes have been described in which there are histological changes in the kidney. Examples are Charcot–Marie–Tooth disease, mitochondrial cytopathy, Cockayne's syndrome, Kartagener's syndrome, epidermolysis bullosa, Meltzer's syndrome, Wiskott–Aldrich syndrome, hypothyroidism with deafness, hereditary osteolysis and Alström's syndrome (see p. 476). Information on these rare diseases and syndromes is available in specialist texts.[190,191]

There are also several hereditary disorders which affect the renal tubule but produce minimal or no histological changes. Examples are renal glycosuria, Hartnup's disease, iminoglycinuria, galactosaemia, Wilson's disease and tyrosinaemia. They are not discussed in this volume; details of the functional changes that occur in them are available in standard medical texts.[192]

REFERENCES

Introduction

1. Bernstein J. Hereditary renal disease. In: Churg J, Spargo BH, Mostofi FK et al, eds. Kidney disease: present status. Baltimore: Williams and Wilkins, 1979: 295–326.

Hereditary glomerular nephropathies

2. Guthrie LG. Idiopathic, or congenital, hereditary and family haematuria. Lancet 1902; 1: 1243–1246.
3. Hurst AF. Hereditary familial congenital haemorrhagic nephritis occuring in sixteen individuals in three generations. Guy's Hosp Rep 1923; 3: 368–370.
4. Alport AC. Hereditary familial congenital haemorrhagic nephritis. Br Med J 1927; 1: 504–506.
5. Perkoff GT, Stephens FE, Dolowitz DA, Tyler FH. A clinical study of hereditary interstitial pyelonephritis. Arch Intern Med 1951; 88: 191–200.
6. Wing AJ, Broyer M, Brunner FP, et al. Combined report on regular dialysis and transplantation in Europe, 1982. Proc Eur Dial Transplant Assoc 1983; 20: 5–75.
7. Feingold J, Bois E, Chompret A, Broyer M, Gubler M-C, Grünfeld J-P. Genetic heterogeneity of Alport's syndrome. Kidney Int 1985; 27: 672–677.
8. Govan JAA. Ocular manifestations of Alport's syndrome: a hereditary disorder of basement membranes? Br J Ophthalmol 1983; 67: 493–503.
9. Perrin D, Jungers P, Grünfeld J-P, Delons S, Noël L-H, Zenatti C. Perimacular changes in Alport's syndrome. Clin Nephrol 1980; 13: 163–167.
10. Gubler M, Levy M, Broyer M, et al. Alport's syndrome. A report of 58 cases and a review of the literature. Am J Med 1981; 70: 493–505.
11. Bernstein J. The glomerular basement membrane abnormality in Alport's syndrome. Am J Kidney Dis 1987; 10: 222–229.
12. Habib R, Gubler M-C, Hinglais N, et al. Alport's syndrome: experience at Hôpital Necker. Kidney Int 1982; 21: suppl 11, S20–28.
13. Savage COS, Reed A, Kershaw M, et al. Use of a monoclonal antibody in differential diagnosis of children with haematuria and hereditary nephritis. Lancet 1986; 1: 1459–1461.
14. Lubec G, Shabbir C. Non-invasive diagnosis of Alport's syndrome. Lancet 1984; 1: 1119.
15. Milliner DS, Pierides AM, Holley KE. Renal transplantation in Alport's syndrome. Anti-glomerular basement membrane glomerulonephritis in the allograft. Mayo Clin Proc 1982; 57: 35–43.
16. Querin S, Noël L-H, Grünfeld J-P, et al. Linear glomerular IgG fixation in renal allografts: incidence and significance in Alport's syndrome. Clin Nephrol 1986; 25: 134–140.
17. Boyce N, Holdsworth S, Atkins R, Dowling J. De-novo anti-GBM-antibody-induced glomerulonephritis in renal transplant. Clin Nephrol 1985; 23: 148–151.
18. Pochet J-M, Bobrie G, Landais P, Goldfarb B, Grünfeld J-P. Renal prognosis in Alport's and related syndromes: influence of the mode of inheritance. Nephrol Dial Transplant 1989; 4: 1016–1021.
19. Spear GS. Alport's syndrome: a consideration of pathogenesis. Clin Nephrol 1973; 1: 336–337.
20. Jeraj K, Kim Y, Vernier RL, Fish AJ, Michael AF. Absence of Goodpasture's antigen in male patients with familial nephritis. Am J Kidney Dis 1983; 2: 626–629.
21. Savage COS, Pusey CD, Kershaw MJ, et al. The Goodpasture antigen in Alport's syndrome: studies with a monoclonal antibody. Kidney Int 1986; 30: 107–112.
22. Melvin T, Kim Y, Michael AF. Amyloid P component is not present in the glomerular basement membrane in Alport-type hereditary nephritis. Am J Pathol 1986; 125: 460–464.
23. Barker DF, Hostikka SL, Zhou J, et al. Identification of mutations in the COL4A5 collagen gene in Alport syndrome. Science 1990; 248: 1224–1227.
24. Thorner PS, Baumal R, Eddy A, Marrano PM. A study by immunofluorescence microscopy of the NC1 domain of collagen type IV in glomerular basement membranes of two patients with hereditary nephritis. Virchows Arch [A] 1990; 416: 205–212.
25. Goyer RA, Reynolds J, Burke J, Burkholder P. Hereditary renal disease with neurosensory hearing loss, prolinuria and ichthyosis. Am J Med Sci 1968; 256: 166–179.
26. Parsa KP, Lee DBN, Zamboni L, Glassock RJ. Hereditary nephritis, deafness and abnormal thrombopoiesis. Study of a new kindred. Am J Med 1976; 60: 665–672.
27. McConville J, West C, McAdams A. Familial and non-familial benign haematuria. J Pediatr 1966; 69: 207–214.
28. Rogers PW, Kurzman NA, Bunn SM, White MG. Familial benign essential haematuria. Arch Intern Med 1973; 131: 257–262.
29. Dische FE, Weston MJ, Parsons V. Abnormally thin glomerular basement membranes associated with haematuria, proteinuria or renal failure in adults. Am J Nephrol 1985; 5: 103–109.
30. Abe S, Amagasaki Y, Iyori S, et al. Thin basement membrane syndrome in adults. J Clin Pathol 1987; 40: 318–322.
31. Tiebosch ATMG, Frederik PM, van Breda Vriesman PJC, et al. Thin-basement-membrane nephropathy in adults with persistent hematuria. N Engl J Med 1989; 320: 14–18.
32. Lang S, Stevenson B, Risdon RA. Thin basement membrane nephropathy as a cause of recurrent haematuria in childhood. Histopathology 1990; 16: 331–337.
33. Dische FE, Anderson VER, Keane SJ, Taube D, Bewick M, Parsons V. Incidence of thin membrane nephropathy: morphometric investigation of a population sample. J Clin Pathol 1990; 43: 457–460.
34. Yoshikawa N, Hashimoto H, Katayama Y, Yamada Y, Matsuo T, Okada S. The thin glomerular basement membrane in children with haematuria. J Pathol 1984; 142: 253–257.
35. Gauthier B, Trachtman H, Frank R, Valderrama E. Familial thin basement membrane nephropathy in children with asymptomatic microhematuria. Nephron 1989; 51: 502–508.
36. Aarons I, Smith PS, Davies RA, Woodroffe AJ, Clarkson AR. Thin membrane nephropathy: a clinico-pathological study. Clin Nephrol 1989; 32: 151–158.
37. Osawa G, Kimmelstiel P, Seiling V. Thickness of glomerular basement membrane. Am J Clin Pathol 1966; 45: 7–20.

38. Steffes MW, Barbosa J, Basgen JM, Sutherland DE, Najarian JS, Mauer SM. Quantitative glomerular morphology of the normal human kidney. Lab Invest 1983; 49: 82–86.
39. Basta-Jovanovic G, Venkataseshan VS, Gil J, Kim DU, Dikman SH, Churg J. Morphometric analysis of glomerular basement membranes (GBM) in thin basement membrane disease (TBMD). Clin Nephrol 1990; 33: 110–114.
40. Dische FE, Brooke IP, Cashman SJ, et al. Reactivity of monoclonal antibody P1 with glomerular basement membrane in thin-membrane nephropathy. Nephrol Dial Transplant 1989; 4: 611–617.
41. Simpson LO. Basement membranes and biological thixotropy: a new hypothesis. Pathology 1980; 12: 377–389.
42. Hoyer JR, Michael AF, Vernier Rl. Renal disease in nail-patella syndrome: clinical and morphologic studies. Kidney Int 1972; 2: 231–238.
43. Bennett WM, Musgrave JE, Campbell RA, et al. The nephropathy of the nail–patella syndrome. Am J Med 1973; 54: 304–319.
44. Renwick JH, Lawler SD. Genetical linkage between the ABO and nail-patella loci. Ann Hum Genet 1955; 19: 312–331.
45. Schleutermann DA, Bias WB, Murdoch JL, et al. Linkage of the loci for the nail–patella syndrome and adenylate kinase. Am J Hum Genet 1969; 21: 606–630.
46. Uranga VM, Simmons RL, Hoyer JR, Kjellstrand CM, Buselmeier TJ, Najarian JS. Renal transplantation for the nail patella syndrome. Am J Surg 1973; 125: 777–779.
47. Sutcliffe NP, Cashman SJ, Savage COS, Fox JG, Boulton-Jones JM. Variability of the antigenicity of the glomerular basement membrane in nail–patella syndrome. Nephrol Dial Transplant 1989; 4: 262–265.
48. Sabnis SG, Antonovych TT, Argy WP, Rakowski TA, Gandy DR, Salcedo JR. Nail–patella syndrome. Clin Nephrol 1980; 14: 148–153.
49. Dombros N, Katz A. Nail–patella like renal lesions in the absence of skeletal abnormalities. Am J Kidney Dis 1982; 1: 237–240.
50. Norio R. Heredity in the congenital nephrotic syndrome; a genetic study of 57 Finnish families with a review of reported cases. Ann Paediatr Fenn 1966; 12: suppl 27, 1–94.
51. Giles HMcC,Pugh RCB, Darmady EM, Stranack F, Woolf LI. The nephrotic syndrome in early infancy: a report of three cases. Arch Dis Child 1957; 32: 167–180.
52. Huttunen N-P. Congenital nephrotic syndrome of Finnish type: a study of 75 patients. Arch Dis Child 1976; 51: 344–348.
53. Hallman N, Norio R, Rapola J. Congenital nephrotic syndrome. Nephron 1973; 11: 101–110.
54. Mathias R, Stecklein H, Guay-Woodford L, Harmon WE, Harris HW. Gamma globulin deficiency in newborns with congenital nephrotic syndrome. N Engl J Med 1989; 320: 398–399 (letter).
55. Aula P, Rapola J, Karjalainen O, Lindgren J, Hartikainen AL, Seppala M. Prenatal diagnosis of congenital nephrosis in 23 high-risk families. Am J Dis Child 1978; 132: 984–987.
56. Spritz RA, Soiffer SJ, Siegel NJ, Mahoney MJ. False-negative AFP screen for congenital nephrosis Finnish type. Lancet 1978; 2: 1251.
57. Rapola J, Sariola H, Ekblom P. Pathology of fetal congenital nephrosis: immunohistochemical and ultrastructural studies. Kidney Int 1984; 25: 701–707.
58. Huttunen NP, Rapola J, Vilska J, Hallman N. Renal pathology in congenital nephrotic syndrome of Finnish type: a quantitative light microscopic study on 50 patients. Int J Pediatr Nephrol 1980; 1: 10–16.
59. Rapola J, Savilahti E. Immunofluorescent and morphological studies in congenital nephrotic syndrome. Acta Pediatr Scand 1971; 60: 253–263.
60. Martul EV, Cuesta MG, Churg I. Histopathologic variability of the congenital nephrotic syndrome. Clin Nephrol 1987; 28: 161–168.
61. Mahan JD, Mauer SM, Sibley RK, Vernier RL. Congenital nephrotic syndrome: evolution of medical management and results of renal transplantation. J Pediatr 1984; 105: 549–557.
62. Vernier RL, Klein DJ, Sisson SP, Mahan JD, Oegema TR, Brown DM. Heparin sulphate rich anionic sites in the human glomerular basement membrane. Decreased concentration in congenital nephrotic syndrome. N Engl J Med 1983; 309: 1001–1009.
63. Holmberg C, Jalanko H, Koskimies O, et al. Renal transplantation in children with congenital nephrotic syndrome of the Finnish type. Transplant Proc 1990; 22: 158–159.
64. Habib R, Bois E. Hétérogénéité des syndromes néphrotiques à début précoce du nourrisson (syndrome néphrotique 'infantile'). Helv Paediatr Acta 1973; 28: 91–107.
65. Kaplan BS, Bureau MA, Drummond KN. The nephrotic syndrome in the first year of life: is a pathologic classification possible? J Pediatr 1974; 85: 615–621.
66. Seelig HP, Seelig R, Scharer K. Immunohistologische Untersuchungen bei der diffusen mesangialen Sklerose mit nephrotischem Syndrom in Säuglingsalter. Z Kinderheilk 1975; 120: 111–120.
67. Rumpelt HJ, Bachmann HJ. Infantile nephrotic syndrome with diffuse mesangial sclerosis: a disturbance of glomerular basement membrane development? Clin Nephrol 1980; 13: 146–150.

Renal involvement in hereditary metabolic disorders

68. Fabry J. Ein Beitrag zur Kenntniss der purpura haemorrhagica nodularis (purpura papulosa haemorrhagica Hebrae). Arch Dermatol Syphilis 1898; 44: 187–200.
69. Anderson W. A case of angiokeratoma. Br J Dermatol 1898; 10: 113–117.
70. Desnick RJ, Sweeley CC. Fabry's disease: alpha-galactosidase A deficiency. In: Stanbury JB, Wyngaarden JB, Fredrickson DS, Goldstein JL, Brown MS, eds. The metabolic basis of inherited disease, 5th edn. New York: McGraw-Hill, 1983: 906–944.
71. Bernstein HS, Bishop DF, Astrin KH, et al. Fabry disease: six gene rearrangements and an exonic point mutation in the α-galactosidase gene. J Clin Invest 1989; 83: 1390–1399.
72. Desnick RJ, Allen KY, Desnick SJ, et al. Fabry's disease: enzymatic diagnosis of hemizygotes and heterozygotes. J Lab Clin Med 1973; 81: 157–171.

73. Faraggiana T, Churg J. Renal lipidoses: a review. Hum Pathol 1987; 18: 661–679.
74. Faraggiana T, Churg J, Grishman E et al. Light and electron microscopic histochemistry of Fabry's disease. Am J Pathol 1981; 103: 247–262.
75. Friedlaender MM, Kopolovic J, Rubinger D et al. Renal biopsy in Fabry's disease eight years after successful renal transplantation. Clin Nephrol 1987; 27: 206–211.
76. Spranger JW, Wiedeman HR. The genetic mucolipidoses: diagnosis and differential diagnosis. Humangenetik 1970; 9: 113–139.
77. Leroy JG, De Mars RI, Opitz JM. 'I cell' disease. Birth Defects 1969; 5(4): 174–185.
78. Hickman S, Neufeld EF. A hypothesis for I cell disease: defective hydrolases that do not enter lysosomes. Biochem Biophys Res Commun 1972; 49: 992–999.
79. Terashima Y, Tsuda K, Isomura S, Sugiura Y, Nogami H. I cell disease. Report of three cases. Am J Dis Child 1975; 129: 1083–1090.
80. Riches WG, Smuckler EA. A severe infantile mucolipidosis. Clinical, biochemical and pathologic features. Arch Pathol Lab Med 1983; 107: 147–152.
81. Wolfe HJ, Pietra GG. The visceral lesions of metachromatic leukodystrophy. Am J Pathol 1964; 44: 921–930.
82. MacFaul R, Cavenagh N, Lake BD et al. Metachromatic leukodystrophy: review of 38 cases. Arch Dis Child 1982; 57: 168–175.
83. Rodriques-Soriano J, Rivera JM, Vallo A et al. Proximal renal tubular acidosis in metachromatic leukodystrophy. Helv Paediatr Acta 1978; 33: 45–52.
84. Hirsch TV, Pfeiffer J. A histochemical study of the pre-lipid and metachromatic degenerative products in leucodystrophy. In: Van Bogaert L, Cummings JN, Lowenthal A, eds. Cerebral lipidoses. Oxford: Blackwell Scientific, 1957: 68–76.
85. Volk BW, Adachi M, Schneck L. The gangliosidoses. Hum Pathol 1975; 6: 555–569.
86. Molz G. Farbersche Krankheit: pathologisch-anatomische Befunde. Virchows Arch [A] 1968; 344: 86–99.
87. Marshall WC, Ockenden BG, Fosbrooke AS et al. Wolman's disease. A rare lipidosis with adrenal calcification. Arch Dis Child 1969; 44: 331–341.
88. Shimamura K, Hakozaki H, Takahashi K et al. Sanfilippo B syndrome – a case report. Acta Pathol Jpn 1976; 26(6): 739–764.
89. Gahl WA, Bashan N, Tietze F, Bernardini I, Schulman JD. Cystine transport is defective in isolated leukocyte lysosomes from patients with cystinosis. Science 1982; 217: 1263–1265.
90. Schulman JD. Cystinosis – a review. Scott Med J 1975; 20: 5–18.
91. Jablonski S. Illustrated dictionary of eponymic syndromes and diseases and their synonyms. Philadelphia: WB Saunders, 1969: 101–102.
92. Spear GS, Slusser RJ, Tousimis AJ, Taylor CG, Schulman JD. Cystinosis. An ultrastructural and electron-probe study of the kidney with unusual findings. Arch Pathol 1971; 91: 206–221.
93. Spear GS, Slusser RJ, Schulman JD, Alexander F. Polykaryocytosis of the visceral glomerular epithelium in cystinosis with description of an unusual clinical variant. Johns Hopkins Med J 1971; 129: 83–99.
94. Barnes BA, Bergan JJ, Braun WE et al. Renal transplantation in congenital and metabolic diseases. A report from the ASC/NIH Renal Transplant Registry. JAMA 1975; 232: 148–153.
95. Langlois RP, O'Regan S, Pelletier M, Robitaille P. Kidney transplantation in uremic children with cystinosis. Nephron 1981; 28: 273–275.
96. Proesmans W, Baten E, Hoogmartens J, Bruyneel P. Nephropathic cystinosis: effect of long term cysteamine therapy. Clin Nephrol 1987; 27: 309–312.
97. Segal S, Thier SO. Cystinuria. In: Stanbury JB, Wyngaarden JB, Fredrickson DS, Goldstein JL, Brown MS, eds. The metabolic basis of inherited disease, 5th edn. New York: McGraw-Hill, 1983: 1774–1791.
98. Bartter FC, Pronave P, Gill JR, MacCardle RC. Hyperplasia of the juxtaglomerular complex with hyperaldosteronism and hypokalemic alkalosis. Am J Med 1962; 33: 811–828.
99. Barajas L, Salido EC, Smolens P, Hart D, Stein JH. Pathology of the juxtaglomerular apparatus including Bartter's syndrome. In: Tisher CC, Brenner BM, eds. Renal pathology with clinical and functional correlations. Philadelphia: Lippincott, 1989; 1: 877–912.
100. Stein JH. The pathogenetic spectrum of Bartter's syndrome. Kidney Int 1985; 28: 85–93.
101. Gjone E, Norum KR. Familial serum cholesterol ester deficiency: clinical study of a patient with a new syndrome. Acta Med Scand 1968; 180: 107–112.
102. Teisberg P, Gjone E, Olaisen B. Genetics of LCAT (lecithin cholesterol acyltransferase) deficiency. Ann Hum Genet 1975; 38: 327–331.
103. Myhre F, Gjone F, Flatmark A et al. Renal failure in familial lecithin-cholesterol acyltransferase deficiency. Nephron 1977; 18: 239–248.
104. Borysiewicz LK, Soutar AK, Evans DJ, Thompson GR, Rees AJ. Renal failure in familial lecithin-cholesterol acyltransferase deficiency. Q J Med 1982; 51: 411–426.
105. Ohta Y, Yamamoto S-I, Tsuchida H et al. Nephropathy of familial lecithin-cholesterol acyltransferase deficiency: report of a case. Am J Kidney Dis 1986; 7: 41–46.
106. Stokke KT, Bjerve KS, Blomhoff JP et al. Familial lecithin-cholesterol acyltransferase deficiency. Studies on lipid composition and morphology of tissues. Scand J Clin Lab Invest 1974; 33: suppl 137, 93–100.
107. Armstrong D, Koppang N, Rider JA, eds. Ceroid lipofuscinosis (Batten's disease). Amsterdam: Elsevier Biomedical, 1982.
108. Buia LM, Kovanen PT, Bilheimer DW. Cellular pathology of homozygous familial hypercholesterolemia. Am J Pathol 1979; 97: 327–345.
109. Amatruda JM, Margolis S, Hutchins GM. Type III hyperlipoproteinemia with mesangial foam cells in renal glomeruli. Arch Pathol 1974; 98: 51–54.
110. Pabico RC, Gruebel BJ, McKenna BA et al. Renal involvement in Refsum's disease. Am J Med 1981; 70: 1136–1143.
111. Chen Y-T, Coleman RA, Scheinman JI, Kolbeck PC, Sidbury JB. Renal disease in type I glycogen storage disease. N Engl J Med 1988; 318: 7–11.
112. Von Gierke E. Hepato-nephromegalia glykogenica (Glykogenspeicherkrankheit der Leber und Nieren). Beitr Pathol Anat 1929; 82: 497–513.
113. Baker L, Dahlem S, Goldfarb S et al. Hyperfiltration and renal disease in glycogen storage disease, type I. Kidney Int 1989; 35: 1345–1350.

114. Pompe JC. Over idiopatische hypertrofie van her hart. Ned Tijdschr Geneeskd 1932; 76: 304–311.
115. Hug G, Schubert WK. Glycogenosis type II. Glycogen distribution in tissues. Arch Pathol 1967; 84: 141–152.
116. Verani R, Bernstein J. Renal glomerular and tubular abnormalities in glycogen storage disease type I. Arch Pathol Lab Med 1988; 112: 271–274.
117. Jonas AJ, Verani RR, Howell RR, Conley SB. Hypertension in a child with type IA glycogen storage disease. Am J Kidney Dis 1988; 11: 264–266.
118. Danpure CJ, Jennings PR, Watts RWE. Enzymological diagnosis of primary hyperoxaluria type I by measurement of hepatic alanine: glyoxylate aminotransferase activity. Lancet 1987; 2: 289–291.
119. Williams HE, Smith LH. Primary hyperoxaluria. In: Stanbury JB, Wyngaarden JB, Fredrickson DS, Goldstein JL, Brown MS, eds. The metabolic basis of inherited disease, 5th edn. New York: McGraw-Hill, 1983: 204–228.
120. Scowen EF, Stansfeld AG, Watts RWE. Oxalosis and primary hyperoxaluria. J Pathol Bacteriol 1959; 77: 195–205.
121. Scheinman JI, Najarian JS, Mauer SM. Successful strategies for renal transplantation in primary oxalosis. Kidney Int 1984; 25: 804–811.
122. Watts RWE, Calne RY, Rolles K et al. Successful treatment of primary hyperoxaluria type I by combined hepatic and renal transplantation. Lancet 1987; 2: 474–475.
123. McDonald JC, Landreneau MD, Rohr MS, Devault GA. Reversal by liver transplantation of the complications of primary hyperoxaluria as well as the metabolic defect. N Engl J Med 1989; 321: 1100–1103.
124. Wyngaarden JB, Kelly WN. Gout. In: Stanbury JB, Wyngaarden JB, Fredrickson DS, Goldstein JL, Brown MS, eds. The metabolic basis of inherited disease, 5th edn. New York: McGraw-Hill, 1983: 1043–1114.
125. De Jong PE, Statius van Eps LW. Sickle cell nephropathy: new insights into its pathophysiology. Kidney Int 1985; 27: 711–717.
126. Allon M. Renal abnormalities in sickle cell disease. Arch Intern Med 1990; 150: 501–504.
127. Eckert DE, Jonutis AJ, Davidson AJ. The incidence and manifestations of urographic papillary abnormalities in patients with S hemoglobinopathies. Radiology 1974; 113: 59–63.
128. Tejani A, Phadke K, Adamson O, Nicastri A, Chen CK, Sen D. Renal lesions in sickle cell nephropathy in children. Nephron 1985; 39: 352–355.
129. Buckalew VM, Someren A. Renal manifestations of sickle cell disease. Arch Intern Med 1974; 133: 660–669.
130. Pardo V, Strauss J, Kramer H et al. Nephropathy associated with sickle cell anemia: an autologous immune complex nephritis. II. Clinicopathologic study of seven patients. Am J Med 1975; 59: 650–659.
131. Strauss J, Pardo V, Koss MN, Griswold W, McIntosh RM. Nephropathy associated with sickle cell anemia: an autologous immune complex nephritis. I. Studies on nature of glomerular bound antibody and antigen identification in a patient with sickle cell disease and immune deposit glomerulonephritis. Am J Med 1975; 58: 382–387.
132. Femi-Pearse D, Odunjo EO. Renal cortical infarcts in sickle cell trait. Br Med J 1968; 3: 34.
133. Kelly CJ, Singer I. Acute renal failure in sickle cell disease. Am J Kidney Dis 1986; 8: 146–150.
134. Ross SC, Densen P. Complement deficiency states and infection: epidemiology, pathogenesis and consequences of neisserial and other infections in an immune deficiency. Medicine (Baltimore) 1984; 63: 243–273.
135. Hory B, Haultier JJ. Glomerulonephritis and hereditary angioedema: report of 2 cases. Clin Nephrol 1989; 31: 259–263.
136. Schifferli JA, Peters DK. Complement, the immune complex lattice, and the pathophysiology of complement-deficiency syndromes. Lancet 1983; 2: 957–959.
137. Leyva-Cobian F, Moneo I, Mampaso F, Sanchez-Bayle M, Ecija JL, Bootello A. Familial Clq deficiency associated with renal and cutaneous disease. Clin Exp Immunol 1981; 44: 173–180.
138. Kim Y, Friend PS, Dresner IG et al. Inherited deficiency of the second component of complement (C2) with membranoproliferative glomerulonephritis. Am J Med 1977; 62: 765–771.
139. Loirat C, Levy M, Peltier AP et al. Deficiency of the second component of complement. Its occurrence with membranoproliferative glomerulonephritis. Arch Pathol Lab Med 1980; 104: 467–472.
140. Genin C, Freyeon M-T, Berthoux FC et al. Glomérulonéphrite familiale et déficit héréditaire de la deuxième fraction du système complément. Arch Fr Pediatr 1978; 35: 1085–1095.
141. Berger M, Barlow JE, Wilson CB, Frank MM. Circulating immune complexes and glomerulonephritis in a patient with congenital absence of the third component of complement. N Engl J Med 1983; 308: 1009–1012.
142. Roord JJ, van Diemen-van Steenvoorde RAAM, Schuurman H-J et al. Membranoproliferative glomerulonephritis in a patient with congenital deficiency of the third component of complement: effect of treatment with plasma. Am J Kidney Dis 1989; 13: 413–417.
143. Coleman TH, Forristal J, West CD. Hereditary C6 deficiency in membranoproliferative glomerulonephritis type 1 (abstract). Pediatr Res 1979; 13: 446.
144. Anderson R. Hereditary amyloidosis with polyneuropathy. Acta Med Scand 1970; 188: 85–94.
145. Haltia M, Ghiso J, Prelli F et al. Amyloid in familial amyloidosis, Finnish type, is antigenically and structurally related to gelsolin. Am J Pathol 1990; 136: 1223–1228.
146. Cohen AS, Connors LH. The pathogenesis and biochemistry of amyloidosis. J Pathol 1987; 151: 1–10.
147. Sasaki H, Sasaki Y, Takagi Y et al. Presymptomatic diagnosis of heterozygosity for familial amyloidotic polyneuropathy by recombinant DNA techniques. Lancet 1985; 1: 100 (letter)
148. Andrade C. A peculiar form of peripheral neuropathy. Familial atypical generalized amyloidosis with special involvement of the peripheral nerves. Brain 1952; 75: 408–427.
149. Pras M, Bronspigel N, Zemer D, Gafni J. Variable incidence of amyloidosis in familial Mediterranean fever among different ethnic groups. Johns Hopkins Med J 1982; 150: 22–26.
150. Zemer D, Pras M, Sohar E, Modan M, Cabili S, Gafni J. Colchicine in the prevention and treatment of the

amyloidosis of familial Mediterranean fever. N Engl J Med 1986; 314: 1001–1005.
151. Knecht A, De Beer FC, Pras M. Serum amyloid A protein in familial Mediterranean fever. Ann Intern Med 1985; 102: 71–72.
152. Heller H, Sohar E, Gafni J, Heller J. Amyloidosis in familial Mediterranean fever. Arch Intern Med 1961; 107: 539–550.
153. Pras M, Gafni J, Jacob ET, Cabli S, Zemer D, Sohar E. Recent advances in Mediterranean fever. Adv Nephrol 1984; 13: 261–270.
154. Alexander F, Atkins EL. Familial renal amyloidosis. Case reports, literature review and classification. Am J Med 1975; 59: 121–128.
155. Weiss SH, Page DL. Amyloid nephropathy of Ostertag with special reference to renal glomerular giant cells. Am J Pathol 1973; 72: 447–460.
156. Miller F, Kuschner M. Alpha$_1$-antitrypsin deficiency, emphysema, necrotising angiitis and glomerulonephritis. Am J Med 1969; 46: 615–623.
157. Lewis M, Kallenbach J, Zaltzman M. Severe deficiency of alpha$_1$-antitrypsin associated with cutaneous vasculitis, rapidly progressive glomerulonephritis, and colitis. Am J Med 1985; 79: 489–494.
158. Moroz SP, Cutz E, Williamson Balfe J, Sass-Kortsak A. Membranoproliferative glomerulonephritis in childhood cirrhosis associated with alpha$_1$-antitrypsin deficiency. Pediatrics 1976; 57: 232–238.
159. Rodriquez-Soriano J, Fidalgo I, Camarero C, Vallo A, Oliveros R. Juvenile cirrhosis and membranous glomerulonephritis in a child with alpha$_1$-antitrypsin deficiency PiSZ. Acta Paediatr Scand 1978; 67: 793–796.

Renal involvement in other hereditary diseases

160. Wallace MR, Marchuk DA, Andersen LB et al. Type 1 neurofibromatosis gene: identification of a large transcript disrupted in three NF1 patients. Science 1990; 249: 181–186.
161. Xu G, O'Connell P, Viskochil D et al. The neurofibromatosis type I gene encodes a protein related to GAP. Cell 1990; 62: 599–608.
162. Reubi F. Les vaisseaux et les glandes endocrines dans la neurofibromatose. These Genève. Rev Suisse Pathol 1944; 7: 168–236.
163. Tilford DL, Kelsch RC. Renal artery stenosis in childhood neurofibromatosis. Am J Dis Child 1973; 126: 665–668.
164. DiPrete DA, Abuelo JG, Abuelo DN, Cronan JJ. Acute renal insufficiency due to renal infarctions in a patient with neurofibromatosis. Am J Kidney Dis 1990; 15: 357–360.
165. Habib R, Habib EC. Les lésions vasculaires de la neurofibromatose de von Recklinghausen. Arch d'anat pathol 1962; 10: 47–53.
166. Greene JF, Fitzwater JE, Burgess J. Arterial lesions associated with neurofibromatosis. Am J Clin Pathol 1974; 62: 481–487.
167. Finley JL, Dabbs DJ. Renal vascular smooth muscle proliferation in neurofibromatosis. Hum Pathol 1988; 19: 107–110.
168. Mandybur T, Weiss MA. Sclerosing peritubular nodules: a hereditary renal abnormality in von Recklinghausen's disease. Hum Pathol 1981; 12: 704–712.
169. Fein RL, Hamm FC. Malignant schwannoma of the renal pelvis: a review of the literature and a case report. J Urol 1965; 94: 356–361.
170. Albrecht E. Ueber Hamartome. Verh Dtsch Pathol Ges 1904; 7: 153–157.
171. Fryer AE, Chalmers A, Connor JM et al. Evidence that the gene for tuberous sclerosis is on chromosome 9. Lancet 1987; 1: 659–660.
172. Hunt A, Lindenbaum RH. Tuberous sclerosis: a new estimate of prevalence within the Oxford region. J Med Genet 1984; 21: 272–277
173. Wiederholt WC, Gomez MR, Kurland LT. Incidence and prevalance of tuberous sclerosis in Rochester, Minnesota, 1950 through 1982. Neurology 1985; 35: 600–603.
174. Stillwell TJ, Gomez MR, Kelalis P. Renal lesions in tuberous sclerosis. J Urol 1987; 138: 477–481.
175. Farrow GM, Harrison EG, Utz DC, Jones DR. Renal angiomyolipoma: a clinicopathologic study of 32 cases. Cancer 1968; 22: 564–570.
176. Dao AH, Pinto AC, Kirchner FK, Halter SA. Massive nodal involvement in a case of renal angiomyolipoma. Arch Pathol Lab Med 1984; 108: 612–613.
177. Ro JY, Ayala AG, El-Naggar A, Grignon DJ, Hogan SF, Howard DR. Angiomyolipoma of kidney with lymph node involvement. Arch Pathol Lab Med 1990; 114: 65–67.
178. Bernstein J, Robbins TO, Kissane JM. The renal lesions of tuberous sclerosis. Semin Diagn Pathol 1986; 3: 97–105.
179. Balligand J-L, Pirson Y, Squifflet J-P, Cosyns J-P, Alexandre GPG, van Ypersele de Strihou C. Outcome of patients with tuberous sclerosis after renal transplantation. Transplantation 1990; 49: 515–518.
180. Mueller RF. The Alagille syndrome (arteriohepatic dysplasia). J Med Genet 1987; 24: 621–626.
181. Chung-Park M, Petrelli M, Tavill AS, Hall PW, Henoch MS, Dahms BB. Renal lipidosis associated with arteriohepatic dysplasia (Alagille's syndrome). Clin Nephrol 1982; 18: 314–320.
182. Pirson Y, Lefebvre C, Arnout C, van Ypersele DE, Strihou C. Hemolytic uremic syndrome in three adult siblings: a familial study and evolution. Clin Nephrol 1987; 28: 250–255.
183. Fong JSC, de Chaderevian JP, Kaplan BS. Hemolytic-uremic syndrome: current concepts and management. Pediatr Clin North Am 1982; 29: 835–856.
184. Hebert D, Sibley RK, Mauer SM. Recurrence of hemolytic uremic syndrome in renal transplant recipients. Kidney Int 1986; 30: S51–S58.
185. Turi S, Beattie TJ, Belch JJF, Murphy AV. Disturbances of prostacyclin metabolism in children with hemolytic-uremic syndrome and in first degree relatives. Clin Nephrol 1986; 25: 193–198.
186. Rommens JM, Iannuzzi MC, Kerem B-S et al. Identification of the cystic fibrosis gene: chromosome walking and jumping. Science 1989; 245: 1059–1065.
187. Abramowsky CR, Swinehart GL. The nephropathy of cystic fibrosis. Hum Pathol 1982; 13: 934–939.
188. Oppenheimer EH. Glomerular lesions in cystic fibrosis: possible relation to diabetes mellitus, acquired cyanotic heart disease and cirrhosis of the liver. Johns Hopkins Med J 1972; 131: 351–366.

189. Katz SM, Krueger LJ, Falkner B. Microscopic nephrocalcinosis in cystic fibrosis. N Engl J Med 1988; 319: 263–266.
190. Gilbert E, Optiz J. Renal involvement in genetic-hereditary malformation syndromes. In: Hamburger J, Crosnier J, Grünfeld J-P, eds. Nephrology. New York: Wiley-Flammarion, 1979: 909–944.
191. Gilli G, Berry AC, Chantler C. Syndromes with a renal component. In: Holliday MA, Barratt TM, Vernier RL, eds. Pediatric nephrology, 2nd edn. Baltimore: Williams and Wilkins, 1987: 384–404.
192. Weatherall DJ, Ledingham JGG, Warrell DA, eds. Oxford textbook of medicine, 2nd edn. Oxford: Oxford University Press, 1987.

5

K. A. Porter

Primary glomerulonephritis 1

INTRODUCTION

The glomerulus may be damaged by many different agents and in the course of numerous diseases. In some of the disorders the kidney seems to be the only or predominant organ involved and the glomerular damage appears to be more important than any change in the tubules, interstitium, blood vessels or renal pelvis. Diseases satisfying these two not very precise criteria constitute the various types of primary glomerulonephritis and are considered in this and the next two chapters. The original requirement for the glomerulus to show signs of inflammation has long been ignored. The only indication of unease with this situation has been the use of the term 'disease' (e.g. minimal change disease), 'nephropathy' (e.g. IgA nephropathy) or 'glomerulosclerosis' (e.g. focal segmental glomerulosclerosis) for those conditions that lack any obvious inflammatory element.

Glomerular lesions in conditions other than primary glomerulonephritis are discussed under the appropriate disease (e.g. systemic lupus erythematosus, antiglomerular basement membrane disease, Henoch–Schönlein purpura, microscopic polyarteritis).

Primary glomerulonephritis is a major cause of morbidity and death from renal disease, accounting for over one-third of patients with terminal renal failure requiring dialysis or renal transplantation. The incidence of renal failure from glomerulonephritis in Britain and the USA is approximately 70 per million of the total population per year for males and 45 for females; there is little doubt that the incidence is higher in tropical areas of the world and in many underdeveloped countries, but statistical evidence to support this contention is fragmentary.

CLINICAL MANIFESTATIONS OF GLOMERULAR DISEASE

The ways in which glomerular disease can present clinically are very limited and not unique to primary glomerulonephritis.[1] Damage to the glomerulus may:

1. Alter the permeability of the capillary wall allowing leakage of abnormal quantities of plasma proteins into the urine giving *proteinuria*.
2. Reduce or otherwise alter the filtering surface of the capillary wall leading to *reduction in the glomerular filtration rate*.
3. Disturb the regulation of sodium and water excretion causing retention of NaCl and water which may become apparent as either *oedema* or *hypertension* or both.
4. Allow the passage of red cells across the capillary basement membrane giving *haematuria*.

Each fundamental disturbance may appear either alone or in combination with one or more of the other three manifestations but there are six common ways in which patients with primary glomerulonephritis can present clinically. These are: acute nephritic syndrome, nephrotic syndrome, asymptomatic haematuria, asymptomatic proteinuria, acute renal failure and chronic renal failure. The syndromes frequently overlap and during its course a particular glomerular disease may initially cause one clinical syndrome, then evolve into another, or develop features of two or more syndromes.

ACUTE NEPHRITIC SYNDROME

The acute nephritic syndrome consists of haematuria, proteinuria, hypertension, decreased glomerular filtration rate and mild oedema, all occurring abruptly.

NEPHROTIC SYNDROME

The nephrotic syndrome consists of clinically detectable oedema, heavy proteinuria (more than 3.0 g/24 hours in adults or more than 0.05 g/kg body weight/24 hours in children) and hypoalbuminaemia (less than 30 g/l). Usually there is also hyperlipidaemia and oval fat bodies are found in the urine but neither is an essential part of the syndrome.

Complications of the nephrotic syndrome[2]

Thrombosis

Patients with the nephrotic syndrome arising from membranous glomerulonephritis (see p. 191) are particularly likely to develop renal venous thrombosis. Angiography shows that up to 44% of these patients have renal venous thrombi that are usually small and clinically silent (see p. 200)[3].

Extrarenal thrombosis is common in adults with the nephrotic syndrome, but not in children. Almost a quarter of the adults have deep venous thrombosis in the legs[4] associated with pulmonary emboli, detectable in 15% by ventilation/perfusion isotope scanning.[5]

In children arterial thromboses are more common, intracardiac and pulmonary arterial thrombosis being particularly frequent.

The reason for this extraordinary tendency to thrombosis is not understood. Although there are complex changes in the humoral factors associated with coagulation in the nephrotic syndrome these do not seem to be the main cause; various abnormalities of platelet function are probably more important.[2] The lipid abnormalities in the nephrotic syndrome also affect coagulation.

Infections

Children with the nephrotic syndrome are particularly susceptible to infections with *Streptococcus pneumoniae* (pneumococcus) and primary peritonitis caused by this organism is still a problem.[6]

Hyperlipidaemia

There are complex alterations of lipoproteins in

nephrotic patients, with a rise in the low density and the very low density lipoprotein fractions. The high density lipoprotein, however, is usually normal. The total plasma cholesterol is raised in proportion to the reduction in plasma albumin. It is still not clear whether patients with the nephrotic syndrome are more susceptible to vascular disease because of these changes. The small number of cases available in epidemiological terms and the lack of adequate controls have invalidated some studies.[2]

Acute renal failure

This unusual complication is commonest in patients with the nephrotic syndrome caused by minimal change disease (see p. 135) or focal segmental glomerulosclerosis (see p. 204). Hypovolaemic shock and circulatory collapse account for many cases, particularly those patients with an accompanying septicaemia; in some older patients hypovolaemia does not seem to be the mechanism and increased renal interstitial pressure from oedema has been suggested as a factor.[7]

ASYMPTOMATIC HAEMATURIA

The haematuria may be microscopic or macroscopic, persistent or recurrent. Renal function is normal and hypertension is absent. There are no clinical symptoms specifically referable to the urinary tract.

Erythrocytes gaining access to the urine across the glomerular capillary wall become distorted and fragmented. Such dysmorphic erythrocytes are smaller than normal, have an irregular and bizarre shape and have often lost much of their haemoglobin.[8,9] These changes are best seen by phase contrast microscopy or by supravital staining of urinary sediment.[10–12] They can be quantitated by flow cytometry of urinary cells.[11] By contrast, red cells entering the urine distal to the glomerulus (e.g. from a bleeding tumour of the bladder or from bleeding in the renal pelvis due to trauma of the epithelium by a stone) retain their normal appearance.[8,9] A knowledge of this difference can prevent unnecessary testing and invasive procedures and lead to prompt recognition of glomerular disease.[13]

ASYMPTOMATIC PROTEINURIA

The amount of protein in the urine is increased but is less than the quantity needed to produce the nephrotic syndrome. Renal function is normal and hypertension absent. The patient does not have any symptoms specifically referable to the urinary tract. The proteinuria may be persistent or recurrent.

ACUTE RENAL FAILURE

The clinical syndrome of acute renal failure is characterized by a sudden fall in the glomerular filtration rate. This is always associated with an increase in the plasma urea and plasma creatinine concentration; oliguria (a total daily urine output of less than 400 ml) is frequent but not invariable. Other abnormalities, such as metabolic acidosis, hyperphosphataemia and hyperkalaemia, occur with varying frequency.

CHRONIC RENAL FAILURE

As renal function becomes impaired, the concentrating power of the kidney is lost and eventually only a urine of fixed osmolality and specific gravity can be formed. There is an osmotic mild polyuria more marked at night. The plasma urea, creatinine and uric acid concentrations rise. Metabolic acidosis develops because of retention of hydrogen ions. There is excessive loss of sodium in the urine. Often there is a moderate degree of potassium retention. Once the glomerular filtration rate falls below about 10% of normal the clinical syndrome of uraemia is produced (see (p. 33).

PATHOGENESIS OF GLOMERULONEPHRITIS

There are three main postulated mechanisms of

glomerular injury that appear relevant to the pathogenesis of glomerulonephritis – immune mechanisms, loss of glomerular polyanion and hyperfiltration.

IMMUNE MECHANISMS

Immune mechanisms seem to be responsible for initiating most cases of primary glomerulonephritis. Experimental work in animals has shown that the immune mechanisms can be divided into two major categories, in one of which antibodies react with antigens situated in the glomerulus (in situ immune complex formation) while in the other antigen–antibody complexes formed in the circulation are deposited in the kidney (circulating immune complex formation). These mechanisms are not mutually exclusive and in humans both seem to play a role. Cell-mediated immunity does not seem to be important. Attempts to induce glomerulonephritis in experimental animals by activation of complement by the alternative pathway have been unsuccessful.

In situ immune complex formation

Antibodies entering the glomerulus may react either with insoluble fixed (intrinsic) glomerular antigens that are part of the glomerular structure or with non-glomerular antigens that have previously entered the glomerulus from the circulation and become attached to or planted on to some structure within the glomerulus.

Fixed intrinsic glomerular antigens

The antigen may be part of the glomerular capillary basement membrane or part of one of the cellular components of the glomerulus.

Glomerular capillary basement membrane antigen If sheep or goats are immunized by multiple injections of preparations of glomerular basement membrane (from their own or some other species) in Freund's adjuvant, the animals form antibodies which react with their own glomerular capillary basement membranes and produce a nephritis (Steblay's nephritis).[14] This autoimmune disease progresses rapidly and is characterized by breaks in the continuity of the basement membrane, crescents, numerous granulocytes and monocytes. Immunofluorescence or immunoperoxidase microscopy demonstrates that the antibody is attached to the subendothelial aspect of the glomerular capillary basement membrane and this produces linear staining for IgG. In Steblay's nephritis the antibody reacts with intrinsic antigen scattered diffusely throughout the lamina rara interna of the glomerular capillary basement membrane.

The similarities between Steblay's nephritis and human crescentic glomerulonephritis are very striking and led to the suggestion that one of the causes of the latter might be an anti-basement-membrane antibody. This has now been established (see p. 217).

gp 330 antigen Injection of rats with preparations of proximal tubular brush border (from rats) in Freund's adjuvant results in the animals forming antibodies to brush border antigens and developing a chronic nephritis (Heymann's nephritis) characterized by the nephrotic syndrome. The histology of the glomerular lesions bears a striking resemblance to human idiopathic membranous glomerulonephritis (see p. 191) and immunofluorescence or immunoperoxidase micro scopy reveals granular subepithelial deposits of IgG and C3 on the glomerular capillary basement membranes. The antigen responsible for this lesion is a glycoprotein with a molecular weight of 330 KDa named gp 330. It is distributed not only in the proximal tubular brush border but also on the surface of the glomerular visceral epithelial cells in coated pits (see p. 12). The autoantibody first encounters gp 330 on the soles of the epithelial foot processes; the immune complexes are subsequently shed on to the lamina rara externa of the capillary basement membrane and into the slit pores producing subepithelial granules.[15]

Other fixed antigens Another example of a glomerulonephritis due to an antibody reacting with an epithelial cell antigen that is not gp 330 has been reported in rabbits.[16]

Planted antigens (non-glomerular antigens attached to some component of the glomerulus)

When an isolated rabbit kidney is perfused with cationic protein (e.g. bovine serum albumin chemically modified to increase the isoelectric point from 4.5 to greater than 9.0), the protein antigen binds to anionic sites on the subepithelial side of the glomerular capillary basement membrane (see p. 10). If this procedure is then followed by perfusion of antibody to that antigen, immune complexes are formed at the site of the planted antigen, giving subepithelial deposits.[17] Cationic antigens have been identified in the glomeruli of patients early in the course of poststreptococcal endocapillary proliferative glomerulonephritis (see p. 153). Experimentally, large cationic antigens such as ferritin may first localize along the subendothelial surface of the capillary wall and secondary fixation of antibody leads to the formation of large latticed subendothelial deposits. These complexes subsequently can dissolve and individual components can cross the capillary wall or reform as larger immune complex aggregates in the subepithelial space.[18]

Anionic antigens such as bovine serum albumin and DNA can also act as planted antigens and produce both experimental and clinical immune complex glomerulonephritis.[19] Other planted antigens include viral, parasitic and bacterial products, such as endostreptosin (see p. 152), drugs and large aggregated proteins which deposit in the mesangium because of their size. These antigens may bind by mechanisms independent of electrical charge. Finally, because subendothelial and mesangial deposits, whether formed locally or from trapping of circulating immune complexes, are in direct contact with the circulation, rheumatoid factors or anti-idiotypic antibodies may bind to the deposited IgG and cause further glomerular injury.[19]

Circulating immune complex formation

Antibody combines with antigen in the circulation to form antigen–antibody complexes. Sometimes the preformed immune complexes are then trapped in their passage through the glomerulus. The antigen may be either exogenous (e.g. a foreign protein) or endogenous (e.g. DNA).

Injections of bovine serum albumin into a rabbit will result in circulating soluble complexes composed of the bovine albumin with rabbit antibody to the albumin. Complexes than appear in the glomeruli and cause serum sickness nephritis. The lesions produced in the rabbit are similar to those seen in humans with the glomerular lesions associated with bacterial endocarditis (see p. 373). The assumption is often made that the glomerular appearances are caused by the circulating immune complexes becoming trapped in the glomerulus. However, evidence to support this claim is not strong.[20]

Numerous studies have shown that preformed immune complexes injected intravenously are passively trapped in the glomerular mesangium and on the subendothelial side of the capillary basement membrane. This trapping, however, produces a transitory influx of scavenging mononuclear cells but little other histological or functional evidence of glomerular disease. It does not produce serum sickness nephritis. The primary role of trapping of circulating immune complexes in the induction of glomerulonephritis therefore remains controversial. The disease in which the importance of circulating immune complexes is perhaps most widely acknowledged is lupus nephritis (see p. 225), but as anti-DNA antibodies can react with cell surface antigens, the possibility that in situ formation of immune complexes can occur even in this disease has to be considered.[21]

Factors regulating the glomerular localization of preformed complexes from the circulation include systemic factors, glomerular factors and properties of the immune complexes themselves.[19] Systemic factors are renal blood flow,[22] functioning of the mononuclear phagocyte system[23] and erythrocyte complement receptor systems.[24] Glomerular factors include hydrostatic pressure and filtration fraction, mesangial function and electrical charge of the capillary wall.[19] Properties of the immune complexes themselves are particularly their size, charge and ability to fix complement. Highly cationic complexes tend to cross the glomerular capillary basement membrane to reach its subepithelial aspect. Highly anionic complexes are excluded from crossing the membrane and tend to stay on its subendothelial side. More neutral complexes tend to accumulate in the mesangium. Very large, lattice-like, insoluble complexes are cleared rapidly by the mononuclear phagocyte system (reticuloendothelial system) or are deposited in small amounts in the mesangium; they do not usually enter the glomerular basement membrane.

In humans there is little correlation between the level of circulating immune complexes and the presence or severity of glomerulonephritis. The measurement of circulating immune complexes is of little value in the investigation and treatment of patients' illnesses.

Cell-mediated immunity

There is evidence that cell mediated mechanisms can induce glomerular injury in experimental animals.[25] For example, when rats are injected with a small amount of soluble immune complexes, this leads to glomerular localization without apparent injury; if the rats are then injected with lymphocytes from donors sensitized against a component of the complexes, this results in glomerular hypercellularity, due principally to mononuclear cell infiltration.[26] In neonatally bursectomized chickens, with severely depressed humoral immunity but with unimpaired cellular immunity, proliferative glomerulonephritis develops following immunization with glomerular basement membrane preparations, in the absence of antiglomerular basement membrane antibodies.[27]

There is no direct evidence that T lymphocytes mediate any form of glomerulonephritis in humans. Indirect evidence for a role of delayed-type hypersensitivity has been obtained in some patients with antiglomerular basement membrane nephritis through the demonstration that their blood lymphocytes react in vitro to glomerular basement membrane.[28]

Mediators of immune glomerular injury

The formation of antigen–antibody complexes within the glomerulus does not directly injure tissue. Damage occurs as a consequence of activation of other systems.

Complement

One mechanism is the activation of complement which generates chemotactic peptides, primarily C5a, which results in the attraction of neutrophil granulocytes to the site of immune deposition.[29] The granulocytes release proteases and other enzymes as well as oxygen-derived free radicals, which damage the glomerular cells and basement membrane. Degranulating neutrophil granulocytes displace endothelial cells to abut directly on denuded glomerular capillary basement membrane which becomes increasingly permeable to tracer molecules. Neutrophil-derived proteolytic enzymes and fragments of glomerular basement membrane appear in the urine.[30] But this mechanism applies only to a few forms of glomerulonephritis, in particular that following the deposition of antiglomerular basement membrane antibody. Many types of human glomerulonephritis show very few neutrophil granulocytes in the glomeruli.

Another mechanism involves complement activation by the classic and alternative pathways to form the membrane attack complex (C5b-9) but does not involve inflammatory cells. In Heymann's nephritis (see p. 202) the membrane attack complex is necessary if the deposits of immune complex on the subepithelial aspect of the glomerular capillary basement membrane are to cause proteinuria. Without the participation of C5b-9 the deposits are symptomless. C5b-9 produces some alteration in the way in which the glomerular filtration barrier handles macromolecules; the exact nature of that alteration is not known. In Heymann's nephritis it may involve insertion of the membrane attack complex into the plasma membrane of the epithelial foot processes. This results in epithelial cell damage with increased permeability caused by either loss of the sialoglycoproteins on the cell surface or detachment of the cell itself from the basement membrane (see p. 202).[30] At present there is no direct evidence that this mechanism operates in humans. However, the presence of the membrane attack complex in immune deposits and at other sites in a variety of human renal diseases suggests that this mechanism may be important in man as well as in animals.

Macrophages

Macrophages participate in immune complex

disease independently of complement. They are prominent in the glomeruli in several forms of experimental immune complex nephritis in animals as well as in human disease.[19,31] Activated macrophages release many biologically active molecules and it is probable that some of these participate in the evolution of glomerulonephritis. In particular, interleukin-1 stimulates mesangial cells to proliferate and form matrix (see p. 14). Some studies suggest that macrophages are recruited primarily by immune adherence mechanisms; others indicate that macrophages follow an earlier T lymphocyte infiltrate. The capacity of specifically sensitized cells to cause glomerular disease has been referred to under cell-mediated immunity (see p. 130).

Arachidonic acid metabolites, reactive oxygen species and interleukin-1

Intrinsic mesangial cells (see p. 14) may participate in some types of immune complex-mediated glomerular disease. Mesangial cells can produce a variety of potential inflammatory mediators, including prostaglandins, acidic and neutral proteases, reactive oxygen species and interleukin-1. The mesangial cells may be stimulated to produce these substances by exposure to, or endocytosis of, immune complexes, complement components (including the membrane attack complex) and platelet activating factor.

Thromboxane B_2 is greatly increased in patients with lupus nephritis and in animals with nephrotoxic serum nephritis. *Hydroxyeicosate-traenoic acid* and *leukotriene* production is also raised. The role of these arachidonic acid metabolites in the development of glomerular injury and in the alteration of glomerular function is not yet clear.[32] *Reactive oxygen species* are released from both activated neutrophil granulocytes and macrophages within the glomerular capillaries and mesangium and from the mesangial cells themselves. They have been referred to earlier under the role of complement (see p. 130). The complement membrane attack complex, immune complexes and platelet activating factor will also all stimulate the release of reactive oxygen species by cultured mesangial cells.[32]

Mesangial cells produce *interleukin-1*, an autocrine growth factor, which stimulates both cultured human and rat mesangial cells to proliferate.[33] This suggests that the release of interleukin-1 and other growth factors, such as *transforming growth factor β1 (TGF-β1)*,[34] either by infiltrating leucocytes or by activated mesangial cells, may initiate the mesangial proliferation and matrix expansion that characterize many forms of glomerulonephritis.

Platelets

Platelet-derived factors can also be implicated as possible mediators of glomerular injury and mesangial proliferation. In most types of glomerular disease, however, platelets are not detectable by morphological methods, making it unlikely that the release of factors from platelets, particularly growth factors, is a main mechanism.

LOSS OF GLOMERULAR POLYANION

The glomerular capillary wall is rich in sialoproteins coating the endothelial and epithelial cell surfaces and there are heparin sulphate proteoglycan anionic sites in the lamina rara interna and externa of the basement membrane (see p. 10). These polyanionic sites contribute to the glomerular filter an electrical charge-selective permeability barrier that facilitates the filtration of cationic proteins and restricts anionic molecules. Removal of heparin sulphate proteoglycan by specific degrading enzymes results in loss of charge selectivity and leakage of anionic molecules such as albumin.[35]

There is evidence of loss of charge selectivity in human minimal change disease (see p. 142), congenital nephrotic syndrome of Finnish type (see p. 84) and in diabetic glomerulosclerosis (see p. 337). The cause of the reduction in glomerular anionic sites is unknown.

HYPERFILTRATION

Once sufficient nephrons have been destroyed in a kidney to reduce the glomerular filtration rate to 30–50% of normal, inexorable progression to end-stage renal failure occurs, even if the original cause of renal injury is removed (see p. 26).[36–38] As surviving glomeruli undergo hypertrophy the single nephron glomerular filtration rate, the glomerular blood flow and the capillary pressure all rise; these haemodynamic changes are often collectively referred to as hyperfiltration. Although hyperfiltration is an adaptive response it injures the glomerular endothelial and epithelial cells, increasing glomerular permeability to protein with the result that proteins accumulate in the mesangial matrix. The injury is followed by the development of segmental glomerular sclerosis which progresses to global sclerosis.

TERMINOLOGY

In the past there was great variation in usage of terms describing the distribution of glomerular lesions. Since 1982 there has been a general acceptance of the terms recommended by the World Health Organization's Working Party on the classification of glomerular diseases[39] and these are used throughout this volume.

Diffuse indicates involvement of more than 80% of the glomeruli.
Focal implies a process affecting some but not more than 80% of the glomeruli.
Global indicates that the injury uniformally involves the whole of each affected glomerulus.
Segmental denotes that the lesion is confined to only part of each affected glomerulus.

A term that sometimes causes confusion is *sclerosis*. This is a lesion consisting of fibrillar material resulting from either an increase in the amount of mesangial matrix or collapse and condensation of the glomerular capillary basement membrane or both. The sclerotic material stains with eosin and periodic acid-Schiff. It is to be distinguished from *fibrosis* which is a lesion consisting of collagen fibres that do not stain with periodic acid-Schiff but stain red with Van Gieson's stain.

Hyalinosis and *hyaline change* are synonyms widely used to denote changes that commonly occur in arteriolar walls in benign phase hypertension and in diabetes mellitus. In this volume they will also be used to describe glomerular collections of similar acellular material (structureless by light microscopy) consisting of glycoproteins and sometimes incorporating lipids. The hyaline material stains intensely with eosin and periodic acid-Schiff.

CLASSIFICATION OF GLOMERULONEPHRITIS

The classification of glomerulonephritis may be based on pathogenesis, morphology or clinical presentation. An aetiological or pathogenetic classification would be particularly useful but for the present there is too little information for either to be practical. In contrast, a good deal of evidence supports the belief that we can identify certain crude patterns of structural damage that in at least some instances are associated with a consistent clinical evolution. These histopathological patterns represent the balance between injurious stimuli and host response. The classification used in this volume is based on this premise. It was proposed by the World Health Organization in 1982 and has been widely accepted (Table 5.1).[39] The patterns described do not usually represent disease entities but they do provide a rough guide to the degree of tissue damage and its likelihood of reversibility. The morphological diagnosis is not an end in itself, but if used in conjunction with clinical and immunological data gives the nephrologist a useful framework for determining therapy and prognosis.[40]

Table 5.1 Major categories of primary glomerulonephritis[39]

A Minor glomerular abnormalities or no lesion
- a. Minimal change disease

B Diffuse glomerulonephritis
- a. Proliferative glomerulonephritis
  - Endocapillary proliferative glomerulonephritis
  - Mesangial proliferative glomerulonephritis
    - IgA nephropathy
  - Mesangiocapillary glomerulonephritis
  - Dense deposit disease
  - Crescentic glomerulonephritis
- b. Membranous glomerulonephritis
- c. Sclerosing glomerulonephritis

C Focal and/or segmental lesions with no or only minor lesions in other glomeruli
- a. Focal segmental glomerulosclerosis
- b. Focal glomerulonephritis

D Unclassified

REFERENCES

Clinical manifestations of glomerular disease

1. Glassock RJ. Clinical aspects of glomerular diseases. Am J Kidney Dis 1987; 10: 181–185.
2. Cameron JS. The nephrotic syndrome and its complications. Am J Kidney Dis 1987; 10: 157–171.
3. Wagoner RD, Stanson AW, Holley KE, Winter CS. Renal vein thrombosis in idiopathic membranous glomerulopathy and nephrotic syndrome: incidence and significance. Kidney Int 1983; 23: 368–374.
4. Andrassy K, Ritz E, Bommer J. Hypercoagulability in the nephrotic syndrome. Klin Wochenschr 1980; 58: 1029–1036.
5. Cameron JS. Thrombosis and thromboembolic complications of the nephrotic syndrome. Adv Nephrol 1984; 13: 75–114.
6. Krensky AM, Ingelfinger JR, Grupe WE. Peritonitis in childhood nephrotic syndrome. Am J Dis Child 1982; 136: 732–736.
7. Lowenstein J, Schacht RG, Baldwin DS. Renal failure in minimal change nephrotic syndrome. Am J Med 1981; 70: 227–233.
8. Fairley KF, Birch DR. Haematuria: a simple method for identifying glomerular bleeding. Kidney Int 1982; 21: 105–108.
9. Fassett RG, Horgam B, Grove D et al. Scanning electron microscopy of glomerular and non–glomerular red blood cells. Clin Nephrol 1983; 20: 11–16.
10. Hauglustaine D, Bollens W, Michielson P. Detection of glomerular bleeding using a simple method for light microscopy. Lancet 1982; 2: 761–762.
11. Shichiri M, Dowada A, Nishio Y et al. Use of autoanalyzer to examine urinary red cell morphology in the diagnosis of glomerular haematuria. Lancet 1986; 2: 781–782.
12. Rizzoni G, Braggion F, Zachello G. Evaluation of glomerular and non-glomerular haematuria by phase-contrast microscopy. J Pediatr 1983; 103: 370–374.
13. Schramek P, Schuster FX, Georgopoulos M, Porpaczy P, Maier M. Value of urinary erythrocyte morphology in assessment of symptomless microhaematuria. Lancet 1989; 2: 1316–1319.

Pathogenesis of glomerulonephritis

14. Steblay RW. Antiglomerular basement membrane glomerulonephritis. Am J Pathol 1979; 96: 875–878.
15. Kerjaschki D, Miettinen A, Farquhar MG. Initial events in the formation of immune deposits in passive Heymann nephritis. gp 330-anti-gp 330 immune complexes form in epithelial coated pits and rapidly become attached to the glomerular basement membrane. J Exp Med 1987; 163: 109–128.
16. Neale TJ, Woodruffe AJ, Wilson CB. Spontaneous glomerulonephritis in rabbits. Role of a glomerular capillary antigen. Kidney Int 1984; 26: 701–711.
17. Ward HJ, Cohen AH, Border WA. In situ formation of subepithelial immune complexes in the rabbit glomerulus: requirement of a cationic antigen. Nephron 1984; 36: 257–264.
18. Vogt A, Rohrbach R, Shimizu F, Takamiya H, Batsford S. Interaction of cationized antigen with rat glomerular basement membrane: in situ immune complex formation. Kidney Int 1982; 22: 27–35.
19. Couser WG. Mechanisms of glomerular injury in immune-complex disease. Kidney Int 1985; 28: 569–583.
20. McCluskey RT. Immunopathogenetic mechanisms in renal disease. Am J Kidney Dis 1987; 10: 172–180.
21. Jacob L, Letty M, Howard D et al. Binding of a monoclonal anti-DNA autoantibody to identical protein(s) present at the surface of several human cell types involved in lupus pathogenesis. J Clin Invest 1985; 75: 315–317.
22. Herbert LA, Allhiser CL, Koethe SM. Some haemodynamic determinants of immune complex trapping by the kidney. Kidney Int 1978; 14: 452–465.
23. Barcelli U, Rabbmacher R, Ooi YM, Ooi BS. Modification of glomerular immune complex deposition in mice by activation of the reticuloendothelial system. J Clin Invest 1981; 67: 20–27.
24. Cornacoff JB, Herbert LA, Smead WL, Van Aman ME, Birmingham DJ. The primate erythrocyte-immune complex clearing mechanism. J Clin Invest 1983; 71: 236–247.
25. McCluskey RT, Bhan AK. Cell-mediated immunity in renal disease. Hum Pathol 1986; 17: 146–153.
26. Bhan AK, Collins AB, Schneeberger EE, McCluskey RT. A cell mediated reaction against glomerular-bound immune complexes. J Exp Med 1979; 150: 1410–1420.
27. Bolton WK, Tucker FL, Sturgill BC. New avian model of experimental glomerulonephritis consistent with mediation by cellular immunity. J Clin Invest 1984; 73: 1263–1276.
28. Rocklin RE, Lewis EJ, David JR. In vitro evidence for cellular hypersensitivity to glomerular basement membrane antigens in human glomerulonephritis. N Engl J Med 1970; 283: 497–501.
29. Schreiber RD, Muller-Eberhard HJ. Complement and renal disease. Contemp Issues Nephrol 1978; 3: 67–105.
30. Couser WG, Baker PJ, Adler S. Complement and the direct mediation of immune glomerular injury: a new perspective. Kidney Int 1985; 28: 879–890.
31. Ferrario F, Castiglione A, Colasanti G et al. The detection of monocytes in human glomerulonephritis. Kidney Int 1985; 28: 513–519.
32. Ardaillou R, Baud L, Sraer J. Role of arachidonic acid metabolites and reactive oxygen species in glomerular immune-inflammatory process. Springer Semin Immunopathol 1987; 9: 371–385.
33. Lovett DH, Szamel M, Ryan JL, Sterzel RB, Gemsa D, Resch K. Interleukin I and the glomerular mesangium. 1.Purification and characterization of a mesangial cell-derived autogrowth factor. J Immunol 1986; 136: 3700–3705.
34. Border WA, Okuda S, Languino LR, Sporn MB, Ruoslahti E. Suppression of experimental glomerulonephritis by antiserum against transforming growth factor β1. Nature 1990; 346: 371–374.
35. Kanwar YS, Farquhar MG. Role of glycosaminoglycans in the permeability of the glomerular basement membrane. Fed Proc 1980; 39: 344 (abstr).
36. Hostetter TH, Olson JL, Rennke HG, Venkatachalam MA, Brenner BM. Hyperfiltration in remnant nephrons: a potentially adverse response to renal ablation. Am J Physiol 1981; 241: F85–F93.

37. Olson JL, Heptinstall RH. Biology of disease. Nonimmunologic mechanisms of glomerular injury. Lab Invest 1988; 59: 564–578.
38. Anderson S, Diamond JR, Karnovsky MJ, Brenner BM. Mechanisms underlying transition from acute glomerular injury to late glomerular sclerosis in a rat model of nephrotic syndrome. J Clin Invest 1988; 82: 1757–1768.

Terminology

39. Churg J, Sobin LH. Renal disease; classification and atlas of glomerular disease. Tokyo. Igaku-Shoin 1982.

Classification of glomerulonephritis

40. Seymour AE. Glomerulonephritis: approaches to classification. Pathology 1985; 17: 225–238.

6

K. A. Porter

Primary glomerulonephritis 2

MINIMAL CHANGE DISEASE (EPITHELIAL CELL DISEASE; LIPOID NEPHROSIS; MINIMAL CHANGE SYNDROME)

In minimal change disease the patient presents with the nephrotic syndrome. When a renal biopsy is examined by light microscopy the glomeruli apppear normal, but by electron microscopy the foot processes of the visceral epithelial cells are seen to be obliterated. Minimal change disease is the most frequent single cause of the nephrotic syndrome; it occurs most commonly in children, but it is also encountered in adults of all ages. In most instances it responds dramatically to treatment with corticosteroids. The outlook for the majority of patients is favourable.

Clinical features

Minimal change disease is mainly a disease of young children, 50% presenting by the age of 3 years and 80% by the age of 6 years.[1] The overall annual incidence rate is about two cases in every 100 000 children under 16 years of age.[2] In infants and children between the ages of 12 weeks and 16 years minimal change disease accounts for 76% of all cases of the nephrotic syndrome.[1] The incidence of minimal change disease in children may vary in different populations with, for example, a higher than the overall incidence rate in Arab children in Libya[3] and a lower than the overall incidence rate in black children in South Africa;[4] in several of these studies, however, a steroid-responsive nephrotic syndrome in children was being studied and not all cases were biopsy-proved minimal change disease. Minimal change disease also occurs in adults, but much less frequently, being responsible for 20–30% of cases of the nephrotic syndrome in patients over the age of 15 years; the annual incidence is only 0.6 per 100 000 adults.[5] The disease is seen at all ages; in one series 25% of the patients were over 60 years old.[6] In children minimal change disease is twice as common in boys as in girls;[1] in adults the sex incidence is equal.[6]

The onset of the disease is rapid, oedema being the usual presenting sign. Occasionally ascites is prominent; rarely there is acute renal failure. A non-specific infection of the upper respiratory tract, a bee-sting, contact with poison ivy or routine prophylactic immunization may precede the attack by a few days. Some patients have a history of atopy (see p. 141).[7]

The proteinuria is heavy and in 85% of children the urine contains molecules the size of albumin and smaller ('selective proteinuria' – the result of a highly selective process of filtration in the kidney); in adults larger molecules are often excreted ('non-selective proteinuria' – the result of a poorly selective process of filtration in the kidney). In children occasional microscopic haematuria is present in 23%, and hypertension and some impairment of renal function are each present in 14%.[1] In adults with minimal change disease there is a higher incidence of hypertension and impairment of renal function. Urinary excretion of the vasoconstrictor thromboxane (Tx) B_2 is raised in both children and adults.

The condition tends to remit spontaneously, but relapses occur in the majority of cases, usually after a few months. Sometimes relapse is postponed for many years. If untreated, patients with minimal change disease are at risk from the many complications of the nephrotic syndrome, particularly septicaemia, peritonitis, hypovolaemia, acute renal failure and venous thrombosis. In the period before the introduction of treatment with antibiotics and steroids only about one-third of the patients survived 5 years from the onset of oedema. Intercurrent infection with measles may lead to remission.

Minimal change disease responds very well to steroid therapy, 93% of children and 60% of adults losing their proteinuria during an 8-week course of prednisolone.[6,8] About 70% relapse, almost all within 1–2 years of the onset of the disease; relapse frequently follows an intercurrent infection. Most of those relapsing respond to further treatment with prednisolone. The frequency of relapse tends to decrease as the child gets older. Those not responding to steroids ('steroid resistant') and those who respond but have frequent relapses ('steroid dependent') or suffer from the side-effects of prednisolone, often benefit from treatment with short courses of cyclophosphamide or, if very resistant, of chlorambucil.[9]

Tissue typing

There is an increased incidence of class II major histocompatibility antigen HLA-DR7 in children with steroid-responsive minimal change disease[10] and of HLA-DRW8 and DQW3 in patients in Japan with adult-onset minimal change disease.[11]

Serology

The serum level of the third component of complement (C3) is almost always normal, only about 1.5 per cent having low levels.[1] Circulating immune complexes containing IgG are found in a proportion of patients even in remission.[12] There are no complexes that bind Clq.

Peripheral blood lymphocytes

The lymphocytes of a patient with minimal change disease do not function normally, but these abnormalities are not specific being found in other disorders causing the nephrotic syndrome (see p. 141).

Renal changes

Light microscopy

Characteristically the light microscope discloses no abnormality in the glomeruli (Fig. 6.1).[13] In about 4% of patients there is a mild focal and segmental mesangial hypercellularity with a few glomeruli containing three mesangial cells in one or two peripheral mesangial areas (Fig.6.2). A mesangial area is the tissue between a group of

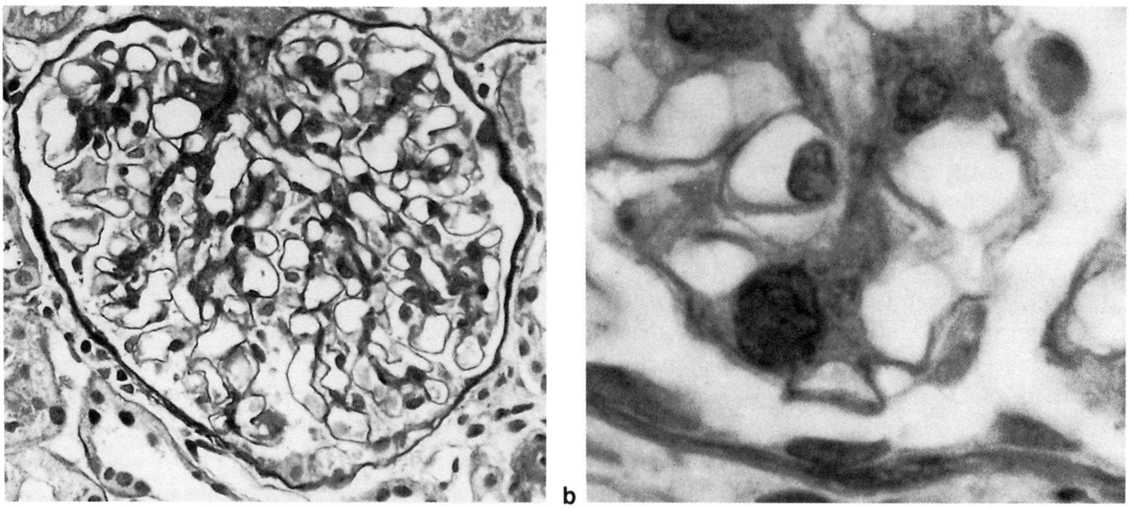
a b

Fig. 6.1 Minimal change disease. The glomerulus appears normal by light microscopy. (**a**) Whole glomerular tuft. (**b**) Part of glomerular tuft showing a mesangial area containing one mesangial cell.
Periodic acid-Schiff: (**a**) × 200; (**b**) × 600

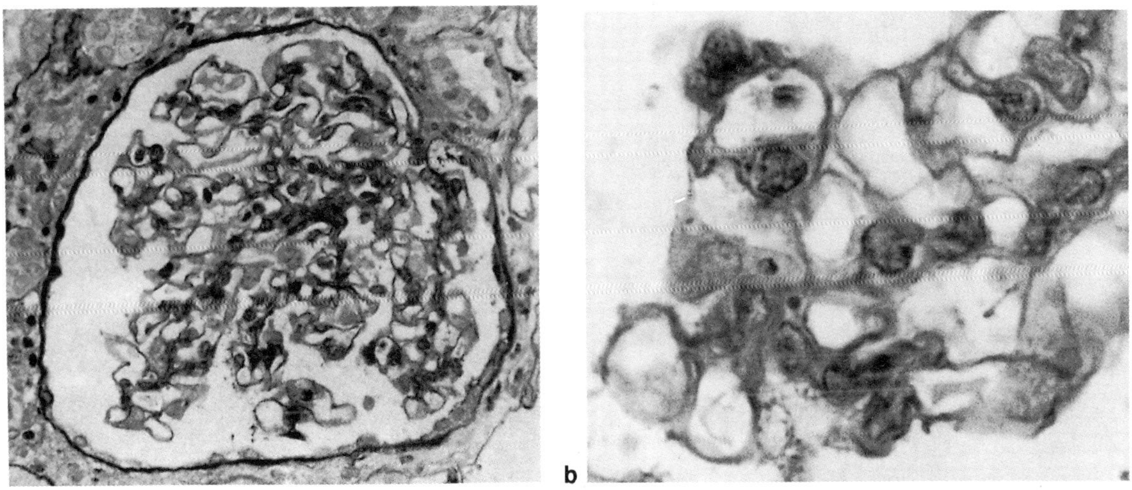
a b

Fig. 6.2 Minimal change disease. The glomerulus shows mild segmental mesangial hypercellularity. (**a**) Whole glomerular tuft. (**b**) Part of glomerular tuft showing a mesangial area containing three mesangial cells.
Periodic acid-Schiff: (**a**) × 200; (**b**) × 600

capillaries at the periphery of a glomerular tuft (Fig. 6.2); the normal number of mesangial cells is one or two per mesangial area in paraffin wax sections 2 μm thick. The mesangium may be expanded up to twice normal in the areas of increased cellularity; the expansion is caused by an increase in the amount of matrix. In about 1% of patients the mild degree of mesangial hypercellularity and expansion is diffuse, affecting more than 80% of glomeruli, and global, involving 75% or more of the peripheral mesangial areas in each glomerulus[14]. Focal or diffuse mesangial hypercellularity of this degree does not seem to affect the patient's survival[13–15]; one study of 521 children, however, indicates that it is associated with a higher proportion of patients who do not initially respond to corticosteroid treatment,[11] and two other studies suggest that it might be associated with more frequent relapse.[16,17] In adults there will be a few globally sclerosed glomeruli but the numbers must be within the limits recognized as normal for the patient's age (see p. 25).

Hyalin (reabsorbed protein) and droplets of lipid are often present in the cytoplasm of the tubular epithelial cells and hyaline casts are sometimes seen in the tubular lumen. In about 5% of children with minimal change disease there is also slight focal tubular atrophy or dilatation.[13] If tubular atrophy is present then a glomerular lesion must be sought, in particular focal and segmental glomerulosclerosis. Unexplained slight focal tubular changes are associated with a higher rate of failure to respond to an initial course of corticosteroids.[13] In adults, as the result of glomerular obsolescence during ageing, atrophy of a few nephrons is inevitable, but even so a careful search should always be made to verify the cause. There may be patchy interstitial oedema but any interstitial scarring or cellular infiltration is highly suggestive of some other disease. Occasionally there are small groups of foam cells in the interstitium.

Electron microscopy

The foot processes of the visceral epithelial cells of the glomeruli are totally obliterated so that each capillary basement membrane is covered by a sheet of epithelial cytoplasm (Fig. 6.3). The cytoplasm of the visceral epithelial cells usually contains a zone of electron-dense fibrillar material adjacent to the capillary basement membrane; there are also increased numbers of organelles, vacuoles and lipid droplets. Numerous microvilli

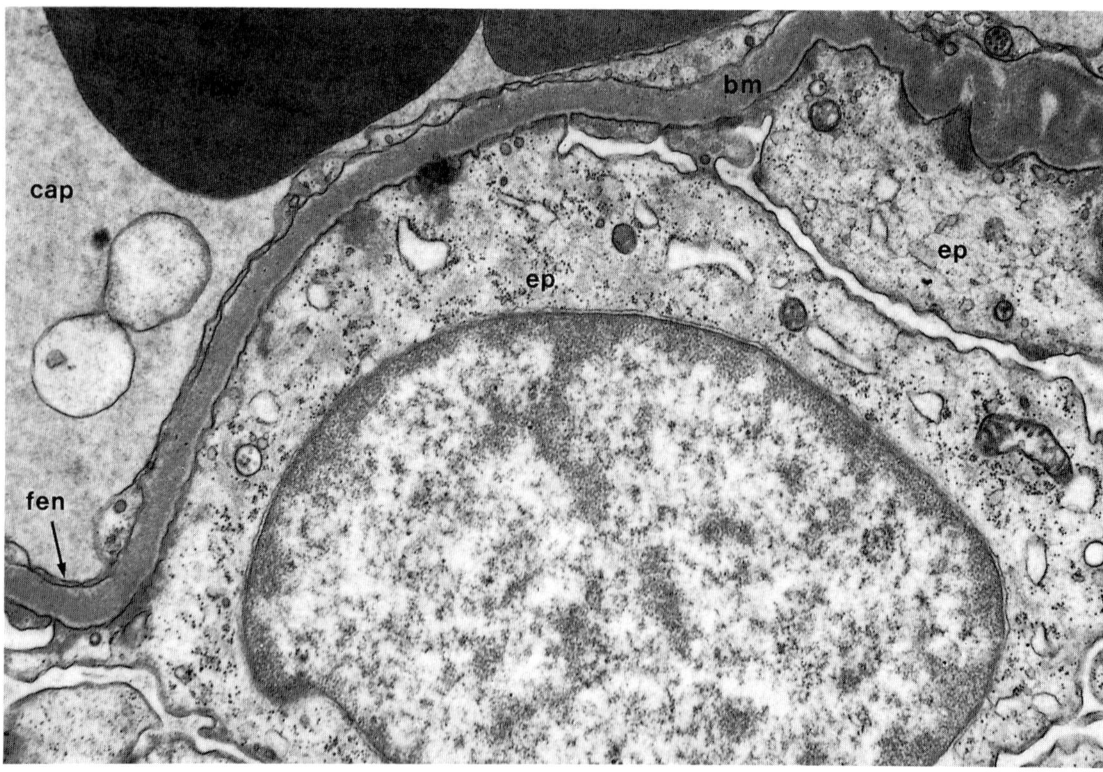

Fig. 6.3 Minimal change disease. Electron micrograph of part of a glomerular capillary. The epithelial foot processes are retracted and appear fused. The basement membrane (bm) is normal. cap, capillary lumen; fen, fenestrated endothelium; ep, visceral epithelial cell; rbc, red blood cell in capillary lumen.
× 10 000

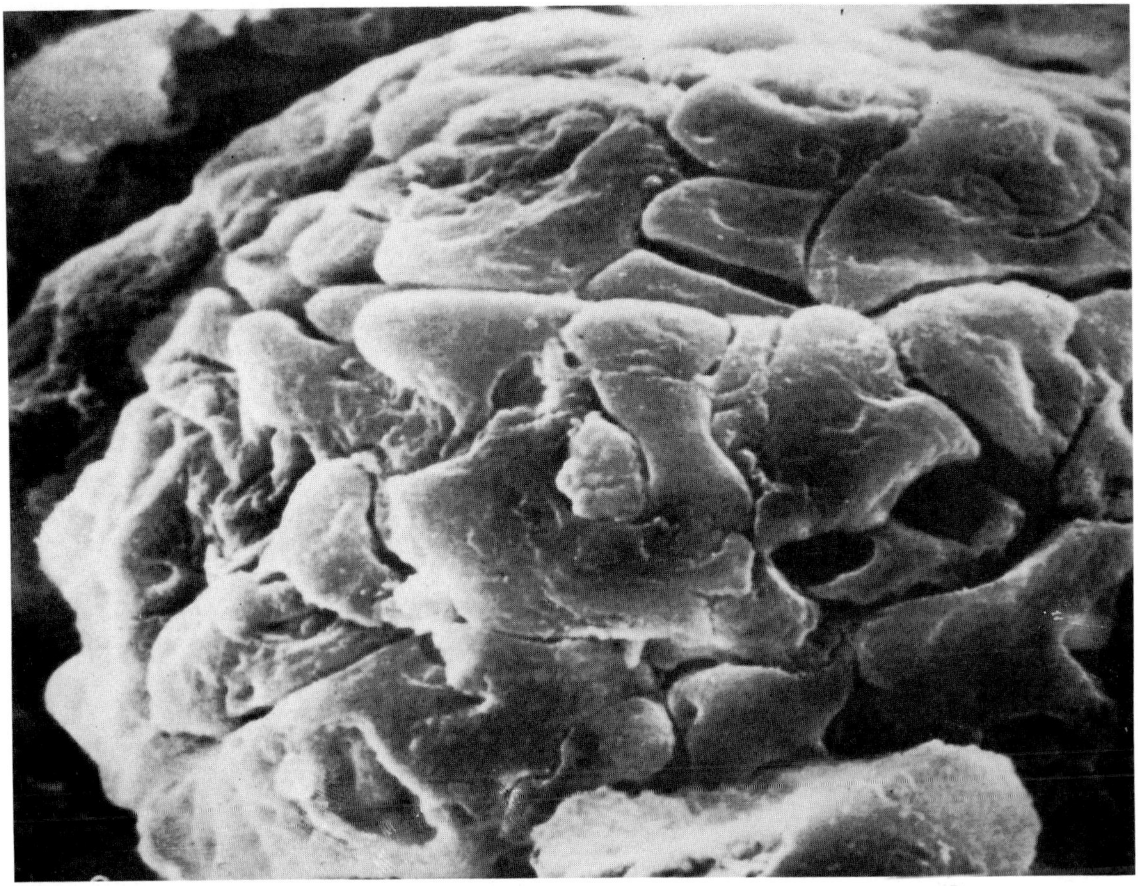

Fig. 6.4 Minimal change disease. Scanning electron micrograph of a glomerulus. The visceral epithelial cells are swollen and their foot processes have retracted and disappeared (compare with Fig.1.9, p. 12).
× 5400
Reproduced by permission from: Arakawa M. Lab Invest 1970; 23: 489 (Fig. 8)

protrude from the surface of the epithelial cells. Scanning electron micrographs show that the visceral epithelial cells are swollen and that obliteration of the foot processes is due to their retraction into the body of the cell (Fig. 6.4).[18] In most cases the capillary basement membrane is normal; sometimes the lamina rara interna is irregularly widened. The endothelial and mesangial cells usually appear normal. Rarely, isolated small clumps of platelets may be seen in some capillary lumina. In minimal change disease there are usually no electron-dense deposits in the mesangium or on the glomerular capillary basement membranes. Electron-dense deposits are occasionally found in the mesangium of the 18% of patients with mesangial deposits of IgM or C3.

When natural remission of the disease occurs the epithelial foot processes reappear. A diagnosis of minimal change disease can therefore only be made if the biopsy is taken in a period of proteinuria. During remission induced by treatment with corticosteroids the restitution of the foot processes is only partial.

Immunofluorescence/immunoperoxidase microscopy

In most cases there are no deposits of immunoglobulin or complement in the glomeruli. In about 18% there may be IgM in the mesangium; occasionally this is accompanied by C3.[19] The clinical features, response to corticosteroid treatment and long-term course are the same whether there is

IgM in the mesangium or not.[19] Segmental IgM and C3 in occasional glomeruli, involving capillary walls as well as mesangium, is not a feature of minimal change disease and if present is most likely to be a first sign of focal and segmental glomerulosclerosis (see below).

Differential diagnosis

The major problems are to recognize diffuse mesangial proliferative glomerulonephritis and to exclude focal and segmental glomerulosclerosis.

Diffuse mesangial proliferative glomerulonephritis

In any case thought to be minimal change disease it is important to count the number of mesangial cells per mesangial area using a standard semi-quantitative system of grading.[20] Mesangial area is defined on page 136. Thus, if there are three or less glomerular mesangial cells per mesangial area then it is currently accepted that this is compatible with a diagnosis of minimal change disease; if 75% or more of the peripheral mesangial areas of 80% or more of the glomeruli contain four or more mesangial cells then the diagnosis is diffuse mesangial proliferative glomerulonephritis (see p. 153). In many published reports the two diseases are lumped together under the heading of minimal change nephrotic syndrome. Where this has been done it has often been noted that those patients whose kidneys show diffuse mesangial hypercellularity, i.e. diffuse mesangial proliferative glomerulonephritis, have a higher incidence of relapse after treatment with steroids, are more likely to be resistant to treatment with steroids and sometimes have a poorer long-term prognosis than those cases in which the kidneys show normal glomerular mesangial cellularity.[14–16]

As even mild mesangial hypercellularity (three mesangial cells per peripheral mesangial area) is associated with a higher rate of failure to respond promptly to corticosteroids,[13] there is a strong argument for ceasing to regard these cases as variants of minimal change disease and to reclassify them as diffuse mesangial proliferative glomerulonephritis (see p. 156).

Focal segmental glomerulosclerosis (see p. 204)

Biopsies from cases thought to be minimal change disease should be examined at many levels because if segmental lesions characteristic of focal segmental glomerulosclerosis are present they may be very sparse. Particular care should be taken if there are mesangial expansion, mesangial hypercellularity, sclerotic glomeruli, segmental collections of immunoglobulin or complement, interstitial scarring or tubular atrophy.[21,22] Small segmental lesions are easily overlooked.

Other problems

Even the most careful light microscopic examination of paraffin wax and epoxy resin sections will miss some early cases of membranous glomerulonephritis and amyloidosis. Electron microscopy and immunofluorescence or immunoperoxidase microscopy are necessary to avoid this pitfall.

Complications

Focal segmental glomerulosclerosis

This often appears in patients whose clinical course is marked by frequent relapses.

It is not always a true complication; the original diagnosis of minimal change disease may have been incorrect because the renal biopsy did not include any glomeruli from the deep cortex where the lesions of focal segmental glomerulosclerosis are first found (see p. 208).

Nevertheless, in many instances the disease does seem to be a true late complication. In one series of 48 children diagnosed as minimal change disease, focal segmental glomerulosclerosis was present in 26 (45%) on a second or third renal biopsy taken over the next 5–18 years; of the 26 who developed focal segmental glomerulosclerosis, 12 (46%) progressed to chronic renal failure and either died, went on to dialysis or received a renal transplant.[23] Most of the children in this series were black or hispanic.[24] A recent study, yet to be confirmed, suggests that patients who have glomerular hypertrophy when first diagnosed as minimal change disease are more likely to develop focal segmental glomerulosclerosis.[25]

Complications of the nephrotic syndrome

These are discussed on page 126. Of particular importance in children with minimal change disease are *acute renal failure*, which is usually due to hypovolaemia, and *pneumococcal peritonitis; venous thrombosis* is the most important complication of the nephrotic syndrome in adults.

Occurrence of minimal change disease in association with systemic disease

Minimal change disease is sometimes associated with Hodgkin's disease and other lymphomas and with atopy.

Hodgkin's disease and other lymphomas

Occasionally minimal change disease develops early in the course of Hodgkin's disease (see p. 617). The nephrotic syndrome disappears when the tumour is treated and in some patients recurs when the tumour reappears.[26,27] The association seems to be specific because remissions of the minimal change disease occur not only when the treatment is with cytotoxic agents but also when the tumour is treated with local ionizing radiation. The renal disease is usually not progressive. Rarely minimal change disease is associated with other lymphomas[26,27] and with lymphoid hamartomas.[28]

Atopy

Minimal change disease is sometimes associated with grass pollen allergy, cow's milk hypersensitivity and other food allergy,[29] mould-sensitive allergic rhinitis and eczema. In one study 38% of children with minimal change disease gave a history of atopy (a tendency to synthesize IgE antibody after contact with one or more environmental antigens) compared with 18% of age-matched controls.[7]

Renal transplantation

End-stage steroid-resistant minimal change disease is often complicated by focal and segmental glomerulosclerosis. A kidney transplant in these circumstances runs the risk of developing recurrent focal segmental glomerulosclerosis (see p. 209).

Prognosis

The outlook for most white patients with minimal change disease is favourable; about 3–6% die and another 6–8% continue to have relapses in adult life.[9,30] In adults relapses are less frequent and stable remission is more commonly attained after cyclophosphamide treatment.[6] The prognosis is probably similar for ethnically Indian children.[31] Blacks and hispanics, however, seem to have a poorer outlook; in one study with a follow-up ranging from 5 to 18 years, 25% progressed to end-stage renal failure as the result of complicating focal segmental glomerulosclerosis.[23,24]

Pathogenesis

This is not known. Some clinical features of minimal change disease point to an immune-mediated mechanism. For example, the response to steroids and immunosuppressive drugs; the association with atopy and the fact that the disease sometimes remits following desensitization;[32] an increased incidence of class II major histocompatibility antigen HLA-DR7 in children with steroid-responsive minimal change disease[33] and HLA-DRW8 and DQW3 with adult-onset minimal change disease in Japanese;[10] and the increased incidence of minimal change disease in patients with Hodgkin's disease in whom defects in T-cell-mediated immunity are well recognized.

In addition, the lymphocytes of a patient with minimal change disease function abnormally. There is, for example, reduced transformation of the patient's lymphocytes by mitogens during relapse, reduced transformation of normal lymphocytes by patient's sera, sensitization of patient's lymphocytes to renal tissue, lymphokine production causing increased capillary permeability, and decrease in suppressor cell activity.[34] However, these abnormalities of lymphocyte function are not specific for minimal change disease, being found in other disorders causing the nephrotic syndrome, such as focal segmental glomerulosclerosis and membranous glomerulonephritis. It seems most likely that the malfunctioning of the lymphocytes in minimal change disease is secondary to the nephrotic state.[34]

There is now considerable evidence that the increased albumin excretion in minimal change disease is due to loss of the charge selective function of the glomerulus (see p. 131).[35] Histochemical studies with cationic markers have shown a reduction in glomerular anionic sites in patients with minimal change disease.[36] This reduction in negative charge is also found in the congenital nephrotic syndrome of Finnish type (see p. 84); it leads to a greatly increased clearance of albumin through the glomerulus. The cause of the reduction in glomerular anionic sites is not known. It is probable that there is either a metabolic defect in the visceral epithelial cells leading to decreased production of anionic sugar residue or a circulating factor blocking the exposed anionic charges.

It is claimed that in patients with minimal change disease, but not in nephrotic patients with other conditions, the peripheral blood mononuclear cells release some substance or substances that cause brief changes in glomerular permeability in rats, with resulting proteinuria.[37] This work remains to be confirmed. Thromboxane (Tx) B_2, which is raised in the urine, may contribute to the altered glomerular permeability.[38]

The flattening and retraction of the glomerular epithelial foot processes is a non-specific finding common in proteinuria. It indicates altered selectivity of the glomerular capillary basement membrane but there is no correlation between the degree of proteinuria and the extent of the foot process effacement.[39]

The infrequent occurrence of IgM in the mesangium of patients with minimal change disease could be caused by impairment of the mechanism for clearing macromolecules through the mesangium.

On several occasions it has been questioned whether minimal change disease, diffuse mesangial proliferative glomerulonephritis and focal segmental sclerosis are entities or whether they represent a spectrum of a single disease. Several pieces of evidence have been used to support the latter view. Firstly, some cases that appear to be minimal change disease on a couple of renal biopsies become unresponsive to steroids after many years and then, when rebiopsied, show focal segmental sclerosis.[14] Secondly, other cases that are minimal change disease on an initial biopsy develop over the years mesangial hypercellularity and finally focal segmental glomerulosclerosis.[40] Thirdly, focal segmental sclerosis is not a specific lesion; it occurs in other diseases complicated by the nephrotic syndrome and in conditions in which the glomerular filtration rate is raised in individual nephrons (see p. 205). It may be a stage in progression to glomerular obsolescence. Fourthly, focal segmental glomerulosclerosis recurs in renal transplants, but the initial histological changes in the grafts are those of minimal change disease (see p. 209). Persuasive though this evidence may be it is circumstantial and insufficient to resolve the relationship between these conditions.

DIFFUSE ENDOCAPILLARY PROLIFERATIVE GLOMERULONEPHRITIS (ACUTE PROLIFERATIVE GLOMERULONEPHRITIS)

Diffuse endocapillary glomerulonephritis is characterized by marked hypercellularity of 80% or more of the glomerular tufts. The hypercellularity is partly due to an increase in the number of mesangial cells and partly to neutrophil granulocytes and monocytes in the capillary lumina and mesangium. The glomerular tufts appear bloodless because the capillary lumina are narrowed or occluded by expansion of the mesangium, swelling of the endothelial cells and accumulation of neutrophil granulocytes and monocytes. The typical ultrastructural feature of diffuse endocapillary proliferative glomerulonephritis is scattered large dome-shaped electron-dense deposits (‘*humps*’) on the subepithelial aspect of the capillary basement membranes. Immunofluorescence or immunoperoxidase microscopy reveals granules of IgG and C3 along the capillary walls and in the mesangium.

Diffuse endocapillary proliferative glomerulonephritis usually follows an infection. Patients typically present with an acute nephritic syndrome (see p. 126); many, however, do not show all the features and the clinical picture may be very mild. In some the condition is detectable only by microscopic examination of the urine. The majority of patients regain normal renal function and blood pressure within a year; a few are left with permanent functional impairment and in a few the condition progresses. In the long-term a small number of children and a larger percentage of adults develop diffuse sclerosing glomerulonephritis.

Diffuse endocapillary proliferative glomerulonephritis is seen most often in school-age children but no age group is exempt; the disease tends to be more severe in adults. Males are affected twice as frequently as females. It occurs in all parts of the world, sometimes in epidemics. The incidence of diffuse endocapillary proliferative glomerulonephritis has declined in developed countries and it is now rare in Britain[41] (as in Europe generally) and the USA. It remains common in Africa, the Caribbean, South America, the Middle East, the Indian subcontinent and the Far East (with the exception of Japan). It accounts for 2–5% of all admissions of African and Indian children to the paediatric wards in Durban, South Africa[42]. In the Caribbean[43] and in Venezuela[44] it is endemic and epidemic; in China about one out of every 300 children develops the clinical features of diffuse endocapillary proliferative glomerulonephritis each year.

An infection often precedes the onset of diffuse endocapillary proliferative glomerulonephritis by about 1–2 weeks. This latent period between infection and the onset of renal symptoms and signs is characteristic when the infection is streptococcal; it is less noticeable with other infections. In most cases in Britain the infection is in the throat or tonsils, but the skin, upper respiratory tract and middle ear are also common sites. Scarlet fever was formerly a frequent initiating factor. In hot countries the disease is often a complication of infections of the skin, occurring particularly in association with impetigo but also with notable frequency in cases of septic scabies.

The infection is often with a Lancefield type A beta-haemolytic streptococcus of one of a limited number of 'nephritogenic' serotypes. The principal serotypes implicated have been M protein types 1, 2, 12, 49, 55, 57 and 60 (M protein is a fibrillar structure on the cell surface of group A streptococci; it functions as an antiphagocytic determinant).[45] Throat infections are usually associated with M type 12; impetigo is particularly associated with M types 49, 55 and 57. Even within a given nephritogenic type, only certain strains cause nephritis; these strains probably secrete a unique streptokinase.[46]

Occasionally diffuse endocapillary proliferative glomerulonephritis is associated with a Lancefield type C or G beta-haemolytic streptococcus.[47] The risk of glomerulonephritis after skin infections with M type 49 group A streptococci in children younger than 6½ years of age is about 43%;[48] it is less in older children and adults. Before the advent of antibiotics streptococci were isolated in up to 80% of cases; today the frequency of positive cultures is much lower. However, indirect evidence of streptococcal disease may be found. Glomerulonephritis may not be prevented by prompt treatment of clinical infection,[49] but treatment will reduce spread of the streptococcus to others.

Serum antibodies to streptococcal antigens, such as antistreptolysin O (ASO), antistreptokinase, antihyaluronidase (ANase) and antideoxyribonuclease B (ADNase-B) may be raised. Antibodies to a streptococcal cytoplasmic antigen, endostreptosin, are detectable in the serum of approximately 95% of cases of poststreptococcal glomerulonephritis at the very beginning of the disease.[50] The upper limit of normal for the ASO titre in children 5–12 years old is 333 international units/ml; above that age the limit is 200 international units/ml. The upper limit of normal for both antihyaluronidase and antideoxyribonuclease is 80 units/ml. The ASO titre usually begins to rise within a few days of infection by type A streptococci, reaches a peak after several weeks, and then slowly falls. Since certain strains of type 12 group A streptococci do not produce streptolysin O, the ASO titre is only of value in about two-thirds of patients with pharyngeal infection. The ASO titre often does not rise significantly after an attack of streptococcal impetigo, though high titres of antideoxyribonuclease and antihyaluronidase are usual after this disease. The administration of antibiotics sometimes inhibits the development of these antibodies.

Since not all group A beta-haemolytic streptococci are nephritogenic, an increased titre of antibodies to their antigens does not prove that the glomerulonephrits was caused by this organism. Also, as the antibody response may persist for many months after acute infection has subsided it might relate to an earlier infection and not the one immediately preceding the attack of glomerulonephritis. Type-specific antibodies develop very slowly after streptococcal infection but persist for many years. Because of this long-lasting immunity second attacks of diffuse endocapillary proliferative glomerulonephritis are rare.

Sometimes the preceding infection is caused by organisms other than beta-haemolytic streptococci. Instances of infection with staphylococci, meningococci, pneumococci, mycoplasmas, leprosy, salmonella and various viruses have been reported.

Clinical features

During the latent period the symptoms of the infection wane and the patient's temperature falls. Then, classically, 1–2 weeks after the onset of the infection the urine suddenly becomes scanty and coffee coloured, and the face becomes puffy from oedema. The urine is found to contain some protein (usually less than 5 g/24 hours), many red blood cells and polymorphonuclear leucocytes, and granular, red cell and hyaline casts. The urine is brown because the red cells undergo haemolysis and the released haemoglobin becomes transformed into haematin. When the urine is shaken the sediment of red cells, leucocytes and casts swirls up to give a smoky appearance. There is generally a moderate degree of hypertension and sometimes indications of early cardiac failure. In a few patients these cardiovascular signs predominate and urinary changes are relatively minor. Glomerular filtration and the filtration fraction are reduced. In a minority of cases the patient presents with the nephrotic syndrome; an occasional patient is anuric when first seen. In recent years the severity of the disease seems to be diminishing.[51]

There is increasing evidence from studies during epidemics, from prospective studies after group A streptococcal infections, and from examination of sibling contacts, that poststreptococcal glomerulonephritis can be symptomless and that many subclinical cases are overlooked. In one such survey more than 50% of patients with poststreptococcal glomerulonephritis remained asymptomatic and were detected only by routine screening for microscopical haematuria followed by renal biopsy when haematuria was found. In the patients who were biopsied light microscopy revealed focal mesangial proliferative glomerulonephritis in 35%, diffuse mesangial proliferative glomerulonephritis in 45% and diffuse endocapillary proliferative glomerulonephritis in only 15%.[52]

The acute nephritic syndrome is not confined to cases of diffuse endocapillary proliferative glomerulonephritis (see p. 126). It may occur in patients with diffuse mesangiocapillary glomerulonephritis, diffuse crescentic glomerulonephritis, IgA nephropathy and some systemic diseases such as Henoch–Schönlein purpura.

Tissue typing

Although it has been suggested that there may be a genetic predilection towards developing acute endocapillary proliferative glomerulonephritis, most investigators have observed no difference in HLA distribution in affected family members and the general population. The exception is a study from Venezuela which found HLA DRW4 to be more frequent in patients compared to controls.[53]

Serology

The serum level of the third component of complement (C3) is reduced in most patients in the first 1–2 weeks after the onset of the acute nephritic syndrome; the level returns to normal within the next 8 weeks.[54] A level of less than 800 mg/l is almost diagnostic. The serum levels of C1q, C2 and C4 remain normal or are mildly or transiently depressed. Persistent, markedly depressed levels of C3 are not associated with endocapillary proliferative glomerulonephritis: they suggest mesangiocapillary glomerulonephritis or lupus nephritis. Circulating cryoglobulins and immune complexes are nearly always present in the early phase of diffuse endocapillary proliferative glomerulonephritis. Antibodies against all the major macromolecular components of glomerular capillary basement membrane are also found in the serum.[55] Antibodies to a range of streptococcal antigens may be present in patients in whom the preceeding infection was due to that organism (see p. 153).

Renal changes

Gross appearances

The kidneys are enlarged. The glomeruli may be easily visible on the cut surface as grey dots.

Light microscopy

At the time of the acute attack all the glomerular tufts are enlarged and excessively cellular (Fig. 6.5). Each enlarged tuft appears bloodless; it often fills Bowman's space and the normal lobular pattern is exaggerated. The increased cellularity is due to the presence of more cells in the mesangium and in the capillary lumens. Mesangial hypercellularity usually predominates and is caused by proliferation of intrinsic mesangial cells and infiltration of the mesangium by monocytes and neutrophil granulocytes. The capillary lumens contain neutrophil granulocytes, monocytes, a few eosinophils and increased numbers of endothelial cells. Irrefutable evidence of endothelial proliferation is rarely obtained but in one light microscopy study counts on 1.0 μm thick sections of resin-embedded material showed that the number of endothelial nuclei per grid square of glomerular tuft (using an eyepiece graticule) was significantly greater in diffuse endocapillary proliferative glomerulonephritis than in controls.[56] The glomeruli appear bloodless because the capillary lumens are narrowed or occluded by mesangial expansion, swelling of the endothelial cells and accumulation in the lumen of granulocytes and monocytes. The amount of mesangial matrix is slightly increased. The basement membrane of the glomerular capillaries appears normal in silver-impregnated sections 2 μm thick, but Masson's trichrome stain or azocarmine may sometimes reveal minute red dots on the epithelial side of the membrane. In 1μm thick sections of resin-embedded material the dots are seen to be large scattered subepithelial deposits (Fig. 6.6).

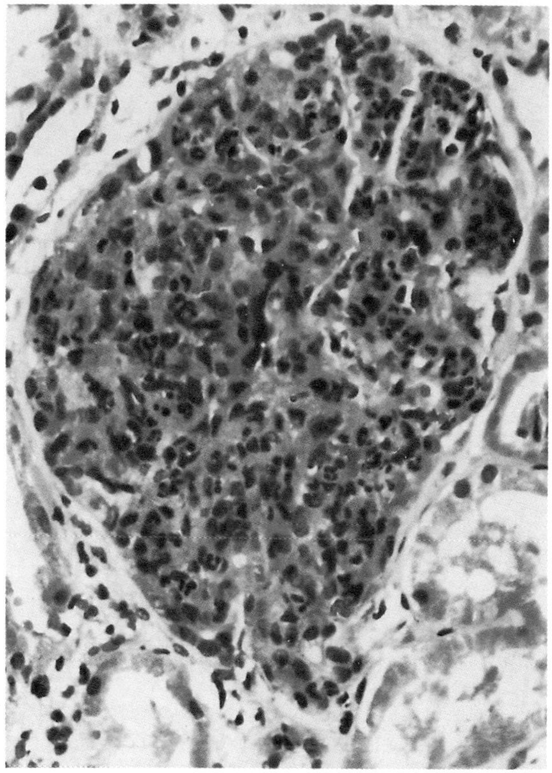

Fig. 6.5 Diffuse endocapillary proliferative glomerulonephritis. The glomerular tuft is swollen reducing Bowman's space. The tuft is also much more cellular than is normal; this is because of the increase in the number of mesangial cells and of the presence of some granulocytes and monocytes. The capillary lumens are narrowed or obliterated, causing the tufts to appear bloodless. Haematoxylin-eosin × 250

Although endocapillary proliferative glomerulonephritis is diffuse, there is often variation in the degree of hypercellularity between glomeruli and between segments within a glomerulus. The number of granulocytes in the glomeruli varies greatly from patient to patient; they tend to be present in the largest numbers in the first few days after the onset of the acute nephritic syndrome[57] and to be sparse in patients with mild signs and symptoms. Occasionally cellular capsular crescents are seen in a few glomeruli; rarely they may be diffuse (see p. 152).[58]

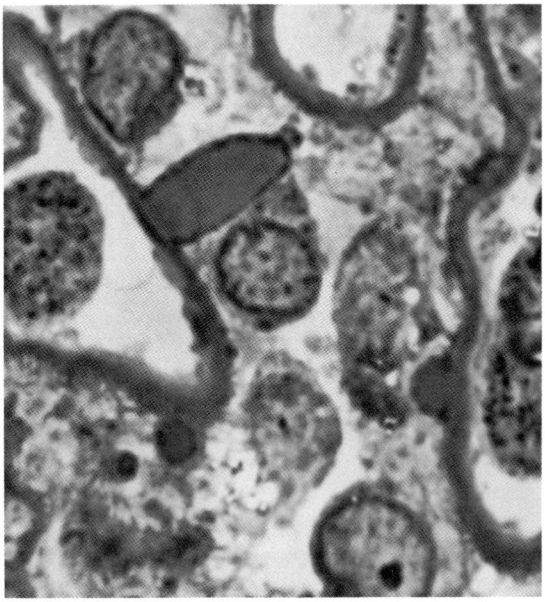

Fig. 6.6 Diffuse endocapillary proliferative glomerulonephritis. Resin-embedded section of part of a glomerular tuft showing scattered large subepithelial deposits. Azur II × 600

Hyaline droplets are usually present in the epithelial cells lining the proximal convoluted tubules. Red cells, red cell casts and sometimes granulocytes are found in the lumen of the tubules.

There is usually some interstitial oedema and focal infiltration by mononuclear cells and neutrophils.

The arteries and arterioles are generally normal. Very rarely there may be a necrotizing arteritis; this has been reported as only involving the renal vessels and not affecting the prognosis.[59]

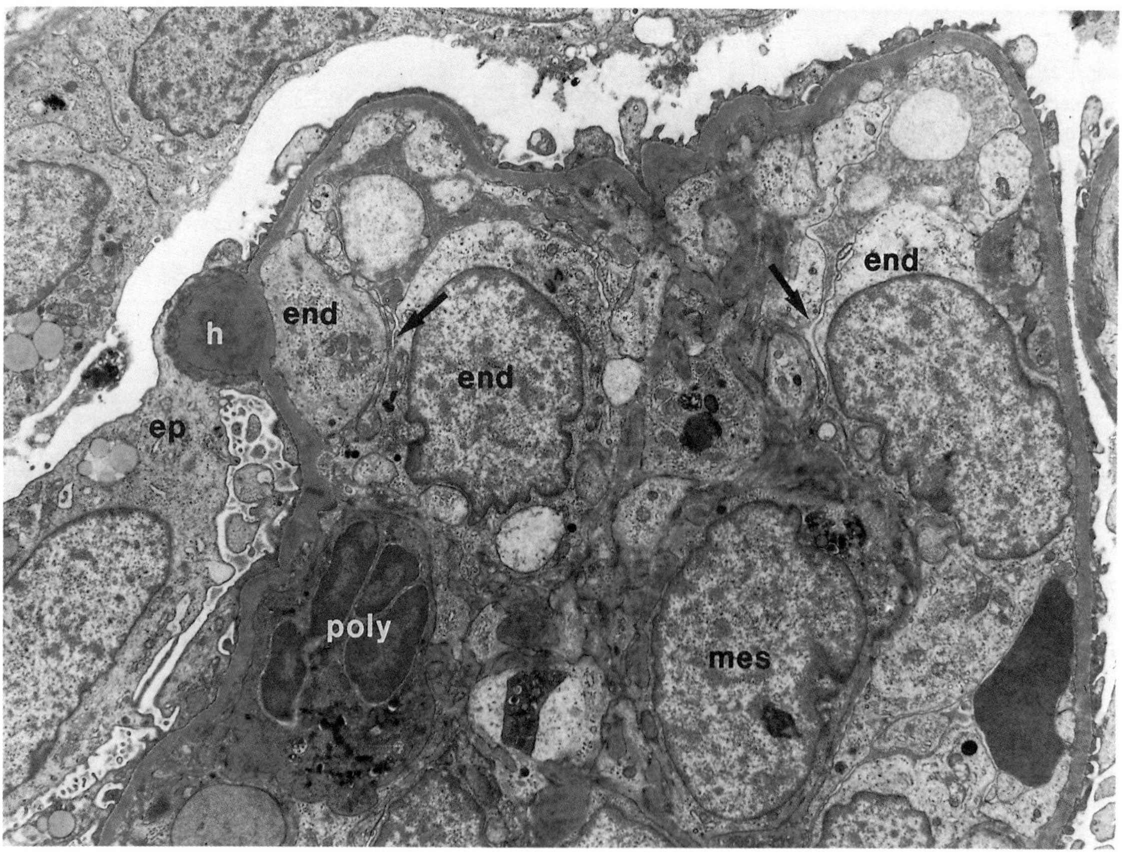

Fig. 6.7 Diffuse endocapillary proliferative glomerulonephritis. Electron micrograph of part of a glomerulus. The capillary lumen (arrows) is obliterated by swollen endothelial cells (end) and encroaching mesangial cells (mes). There is a subepithelial hump (h) and a neutrophil polymorphonuclear leucocyte (poly) lying in contact with the basement membrane. The epithelial foot processes (ep) are obliterated over the hump.
× 5350

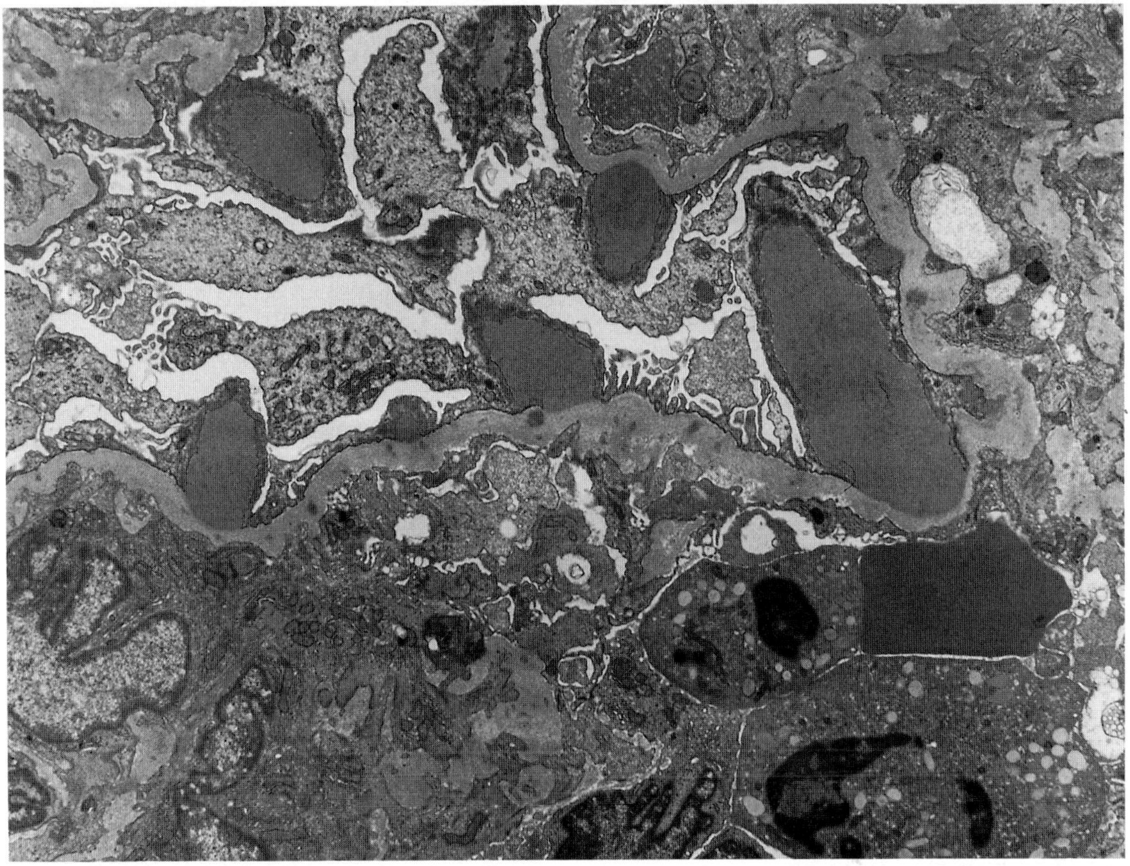

Fig. 6.8 Diffuse endocapillary proliferative glomerulonephritis. Electron micrograph of part of a glomerulus. There are several subepithelial humps of different sizes.
× 8000

Electron microscopy

Large, dome-shaped deposits of homogeneous, electron-dense material ('*humps*') are frequently present on the epithelial side of the glomerular capillary basement membrane (Figs 6.7, 6.8). They are often accompanied by smaller, variably shaped subepithelial, mesangial, intramembranous and subendothelial deposits of similar electron-dense material; intramembranous deposits may be linear (Fig. 6.9). Small amounts of fibrin are sometimes present on the subendothelial aspect of the capillary basement membranes. In approximately 45% of cases the lamina densa of the basement membranes in the vicinity of the electron-dense deposits is thinner than normal and split;[60] occasionally the basement membrane is ruptured (Fig. 6.10).[58] The foot processes of the epithelium overlying the humps are retracted and their cytoplasm contains a corona of fine, electron-dense granules. In cases where humps are sparse they are usually located over mesangial areas (Fig. 6.9) and these are the sites that should be carefully searched when diffuse endocapillary proliferative glomerulonephritis is suspected.[61]

The expanded mesangium contains enlarged and proliferating intrinsic mesangial cells and infiltrating monocytes and granulocytes (Figs 6.7, 6.10). The endothelial cells lining the glomerular capillaries are generally hypertrophic but in certain places, particularly adjacent to subepithelial deposits, the endothelium is replaced by granulocytes which lie in direct contact with the capillary basement membrane (Fig. 6.11). The capillary lumens contain variable numbers of granulocytes and monocytes (Figs 6.7, 6.10).

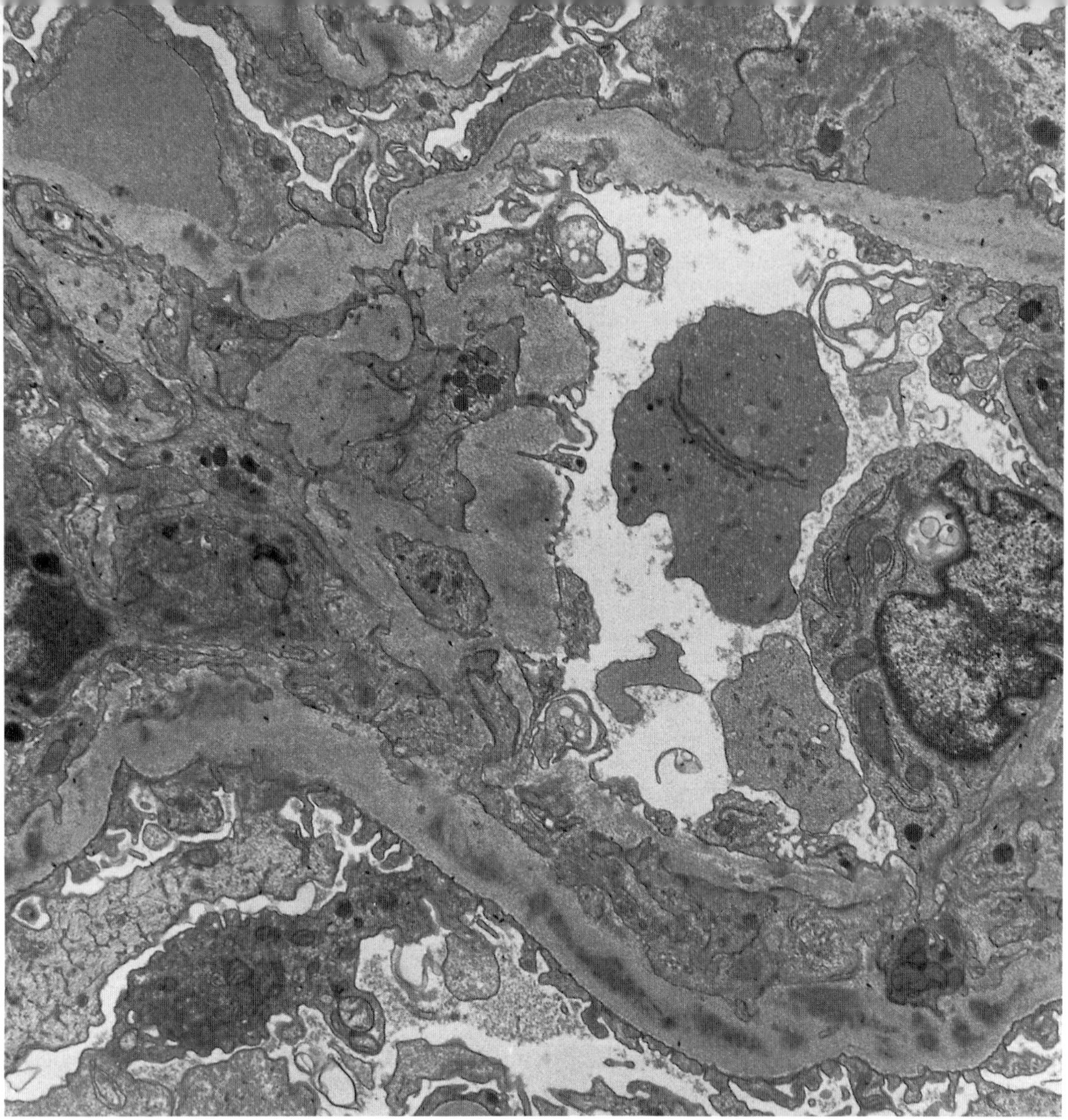

Fig. 6.9 Diffuse endocapillary proliferative glomerulonephritis. Electron micrograph of part of a glomerulus. A hump is present over the mesangial area and there is another on the adjacent capillary basement membrane. There are some linear deposits of electron-dense material in the basement membrane.
× 5350

Fig. 6.10 Diffuse endocapillary proliferative glomerulonephritis. Part of a glomerulus showing a capillary and the adjacent expanded mesangium. The capillary lumen is occluded by neutrophil granulocytes, swollen endothelial cells and monocytes. The mesangium contains increased numbers of enlarged mesangial cells. There are two humps: one on the capillary wall, the other over the mesangium. The basement membrane is ruptured beneath the hump on the capillary wall.
× 8000

Fig. 6.11 Diffuse endocapillary proliferative glomerulonephritis. Part of a glomerular capillary loop showing a hump and a neutrophil granulocyte in direct contact with the basement membrane which has been denuded of its endothelial lining. There is a corona of fine electron-dense granules in the cytoplasm of the epithelium overlying the hump. There are also some intramembranous and subendothelial electron-dense deposits.
× 17 100

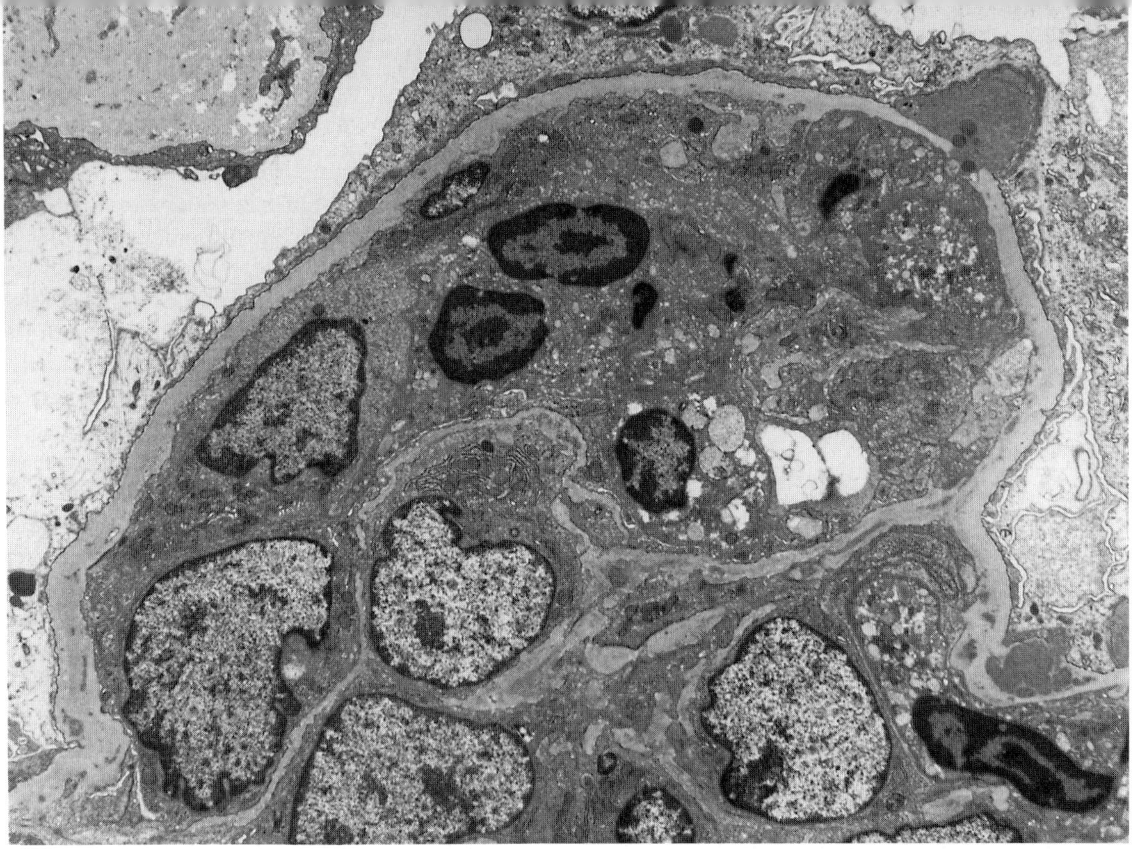

Fig. 6.10

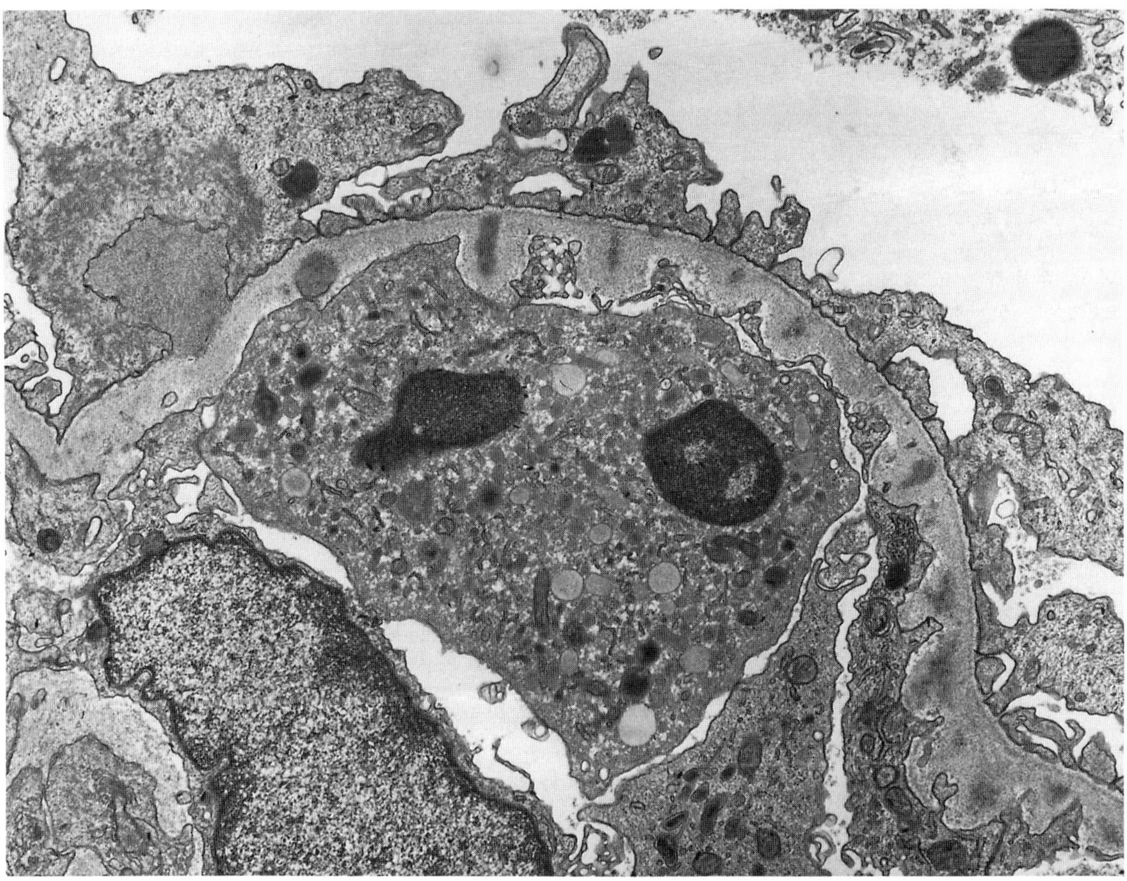

Fig. 6.11

Immunofluorescence/immunoperoxidase microscopy

Biopsies taken in the first 2 weeks after the onset of the disease usually have irregular, granular deposits of IgG and C3 along the capillary walls and sometimes in the mesangium (Fig. 6.12). Properdin is also often present but the early acting complement components C1q, C2 and C4 are absent. IgM and IgA are either absent or present in only trace amounts. Later in the disease there may be no deposits of IgG but prominent granules of C3 remain. In approximately 25% of patients the deposits of IgG and C3 are densely arranged along the walls of the capillaries at the periphery of the glomeruli producing what is sometimes called a *garland pattern.*[62] This pattern is often associated with heavy proteinuria and a poor prognosis. In the first few days of poststreptococcal disease various streptococcal antigens can sometimes be demonstrated; a cytoplasmic protein antigen, endostreptosin, and a plasma membrane antigen have been identified in the mesangium and in the wall of glomerular capillaries[63,64] and cationic extracellular streptococcal antigens have been found in the mesangium.[65]

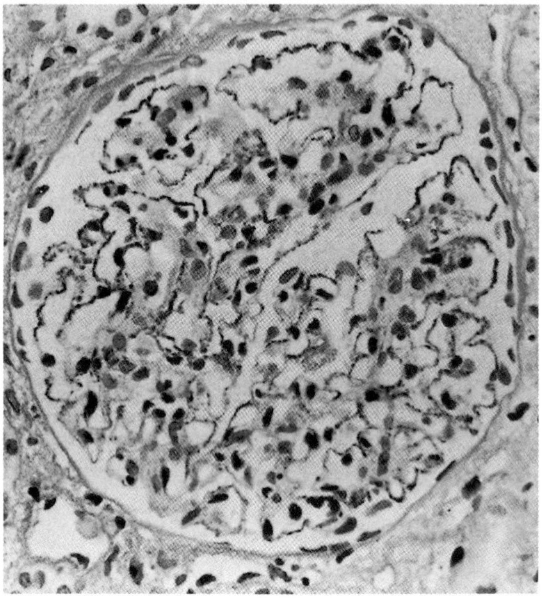

a

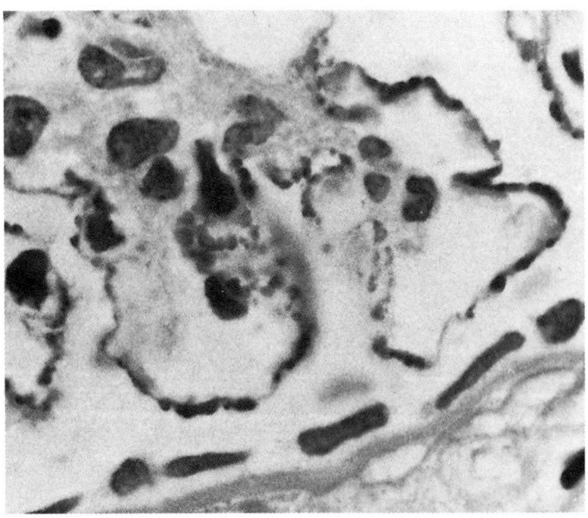

b

Fig. 6.12 Diffuse endocapillary proliferative glomerulonephritis. (**a**) Glomerulus showing global distribution of granular deposits of IgG along the capillary walls. (**b**) Part of glomerulus with granular subepithelial deposits of IgG.
Immunoperoxidase: (**a**) × 450; (**b**) × 1000

Ferritin-labelled antibody studies

This method has demonstrated IgG, C3 and streptococcal antigens in the subepithelial humps, in the mesangium and in the subendothelial and intramembranous deposits.[66] Endostreptosin has been shown by ferritin-labelled antigen studies to be on the subendothelial side of the glomerular basement membranes .[63]

Resolution of lesions

The acute changes continue for some 4–6 weeks after the onset of haematuria and oliguria. The reaction then gradually subsides, the polymorphonuclear leucocytes and subepithelial humps disappear, and the deposits of IgG and C3 diminish in amount and lose their distinctive granular distribution in the capillary walls. The endothelial cells return to normal and the patency of the capillaries is largely restored. Subepithelial humps are rarely seen after 8 weeks from the onset of the disease; their resolution leaves irregularities of the basement membrane and sometimes areas of electron-lucency within the membrane (Fig. 6.13).

The number of mesangial cells and the amount of mesangial matrix often remain increased for many months or years, even when clinical remission has occurred, giving a pattern of either diffuse or focal mesangial proliferative glomerulonephritis (see p. 153). In a few cases changes persist for as

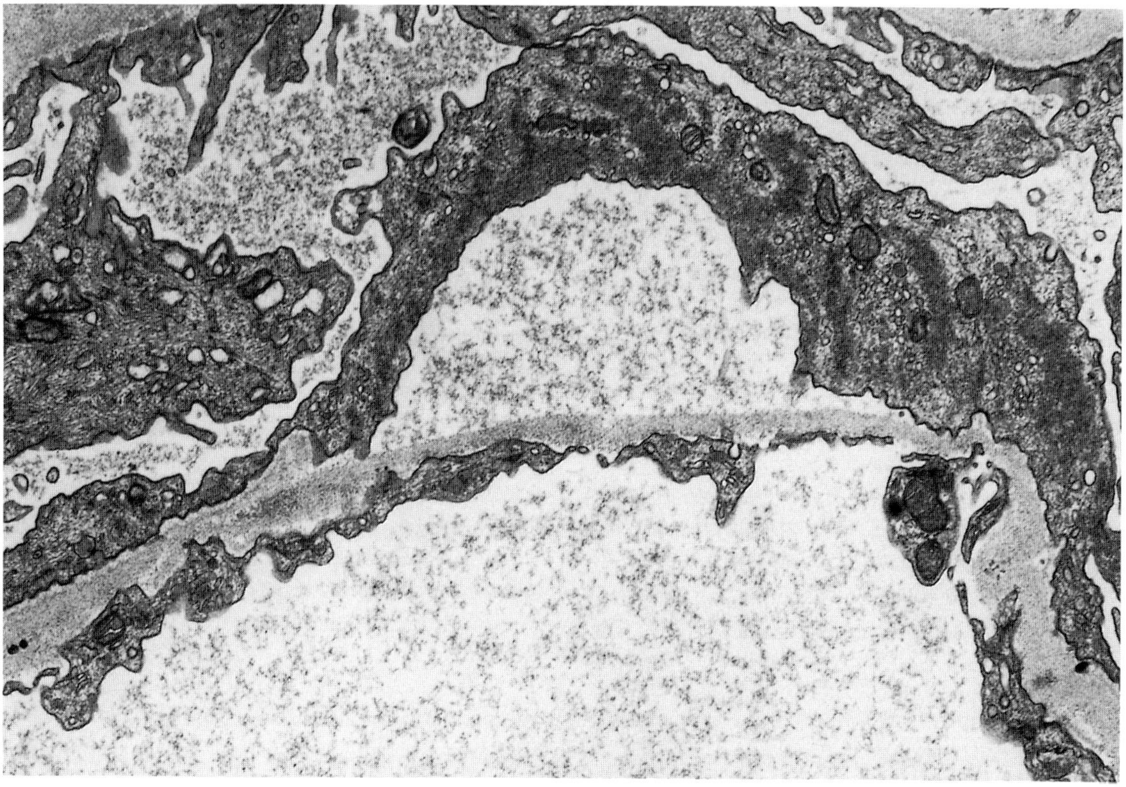

Fig. 6.13 Resolving post-streptococcal diffuse endocapillary proliferative glomerulonephritis. Electron micrograph of part of a glomerular capillary. A large subepithelial deposit has become electronlucent. × 17120

long as 10 years, with eventual healing. In a study in which renal biopsy was performed on children with sporadic acute poststreptococcal nephritic syndrome at the outset of the illness and at specific intervals during the next 5 years, residual excessive cellularity and increased mesangial matrix were found in half the cases 2 years after the acute attack;[67] by 5 years healing had taken place in all but one of the group of 40 children who had been shown by the first biopsy to have classic diffuse endocapillary proliferative glomerulonephritis.[68]

Differential diagnosis

During the resolution of diffuse endocapillary proliferative glomerulonephritis into diffuse or focal mesangial proliferative glomerulonephritis, difficulties will at times arise in deciding into which category to place a particular case because there will be a stage in which a biopsy will show features of two patterns of glomerulonephritis.[56] This is inevitable but fortunately in practice morphological separation of the two categories is readily made in most instances; in one study only 6% of cases caused disagreement between two observers.[56] Biopsies early in the disease usually show the glomerular capillary lumens filled with cells and irregular subepithelial deposits of both IgG and C3 in the capillary walls. Once resolution is well under way the cells in the capillary lumens and the subepithelial deposits disappear and the capillary wall deposits of IgG and C3 are replaced by mesangial C3 alone.

Complications

Focal segmental glomerulosclerosis

Progression of the disease is quite often accompanied by focal segmental sclerosis (see p. 204).

This may occasionally progress to focal global sclerosis and rarely to diffuse sclerosing glomerulonephritis.

Crescentic glomerulonephritis

Small numbers of crescents are occasionally seen, but crescents affecting more than 50% of the glomeruli are rare and associated with a poor prognosis (see p. 185).

Prognosis

There is still uncertainty about the eventual fate of patients with diffuse endocapillary proliferative glomerulonephritis. The issue remains unsettled because many studies lack the bacteriological, serological and histological criteria required for exact diagnosis and determination of outcome; even when these data are available the periods of follow-up are often relatively short. Bearing these difficulties in mind, present evidence suggests that in children and adults recovery occurs in practically all cases of poststreptococcal diffuse endocapillary proliferative glomerulonephritis observed during epidemic conditions.[69] The few exceptions are those patients with diffuse epithelial crescents; they occasionally develop residual renal damage with persistent proteinuria and hypertension or they may very rarely go into chronic renal failure and need dialysis or renal transplantation. The outlook for children with poststreptococcal diffuse crescentic glomerulonephritis is much better than for other forms of crescentic glomerulonephritis.[70]

Among sporadic cases of poststreptococcal and other forms of postinfectious diffuse endocapillary proliferative glomerulonephritis, persistent disease ensues in a small number of children and rather more adults. In adults, clinical studies indicate that chronic disease follows acute glomerulonephritis in about 50% of cases;[71,72] renal biopsy shows partial or complete sclerosis of some glomeruli in 70% of cases in spite of what had seemed to be complete resolution of the clinical manifestations and urinary abnormalities following the acute stage in some of these.[71] However, the actual proportion showing continuing renal disease is uncertain: the figures quoted may be an overestimate because most reports are based on special groups of referred patients, and usually it is only severe cases of acute glomerulonephritis that are sent to hospital and submitted to biopsy. The percentage developing terminal renal failure after 10–12 years of follow-up is about 3%.[72]

Pathogenesis

The presence of deposits of immunoglobulin and complement in diffuse endocapillary proliferative glomerulonephritis has led to the hypothesis that the disease is caused by an immune complex-mediated mechanism. It is not known which antigen or antigens might be responsible for triggering such an immune reaction. Possible candidates in the poststreptococcal form of the disease are the streptococcal cytoplasmic antigen endostreptosin,[63] one of the cationic streptococcal antigens[65] or one of the other extracellular streptococcal antigens.[64] Certainly all these streptococcal antigens have been detected in the glomeruli in renal biopsies obtained from patients seen after the onset of poststreptococcal diffuse endocapillary proliferative glomerulonephritis. Also antibody to each of these antigens is present in the serum of patients with diffuse endocapillary proliferative glomerulonephritis. During the latent period after the infection, but before the onset of glomerulonephritis, circulating antibodies to the various components of the streptococcus appear in rather small amounts so there is still an excess of streptococcal antigen.

That the antibodies react with the streptococcal antigen in the circulation to form soluble antigen–antibody complexes which become trapped in the glomerulus seems unlikely to be the main mechanism;[51] the evidence increasingly suggests that the antibodies react with insoluble streptococcal antigen that has left the circulation and become fixed or planted in the glomerulus. A currently favoured view is that endostreptosin is deposited at a very early stage on the subendothelial side of the glomerular basement membranes and is rapidly covered by newly formed specific antibody and complement with resultant immune damage to the glomeruli.[73] The formation of this in situ complex may reduce the anionic charge of the glomerular basement membrane and facilitate the migration of the immune complex into the subepithelial space.[63] An alternative is that the planted antigen may be a cationic streptococcal antigen. Antigens of this type have been identified in the mesangium and glomerular capillary walls in early biopsies of patients with endocapillary proliferative glomerulonephritis.[65] Also, in experimental animals, cationized antigen can penetrate the glomerular capillary basement membrane and reach the subepithelial area by electrostatic attraction; it there binds circulating antibody, resulting in in-situ formation of immune complexes and prominent subepithelial deposits.[74]

The in-situ formed immune complexes are seen by electron microscopy as electron-dense humps, by immunofluorescence or immunoperoxidase microscopy as granules, and occasionally by light microscopy in trichrome-stained preparations as minute red dots.

Following the appearance of immune complexes in the glomeruli complement is activated. This activation does not seem to occur by the classical pathway; it is thought to involve the alternative pathway because in diffuse endocapillary proliferative glomerulonephritis there are reduced serum levels of C3 but not of C1 and C4, and the glomerular immune deposits contain alternative pathway components, including properdin, factor H and factor B, but not classical pathway components C1 and C4. Complement activation involving the alternative pathway could be initiated in diffuse endocapillary proliferative glomerulonephritis in several ways, one of which could be by plasmin; this is produced when plasminogen reacts with streptokinase secreted by nephritogenic strains of streptococci.

As a result of the complement activation chemotactic agents (mainly C5a) are generated and these attract granulocytes. The granulocytes release proteases and other enzymes which degrade the glomerular capillary basement membrane; they also release oxygen-derived free radicals which damage the endothelial cells. Although C5a is also chemotactic for monocytes, experiments using complement depletion and $F(ab^1)_2$ fragments suggest that complement plays only a small role in attracting monocytes in diffuse endocapillary proliferative glomerulonephritis.[75] It seems more probable that Fc immune adherence mechanisms or possibly sensitized T lymphocytes are involved.

The monocytes that infiltrate the glomerulus become activated macrophages and release a wide range of biologically active molecules, including interleukin-1, a polypeptide which stimulates mesangial cells to proliferate (see p. 131). The intensity and duration of local production of interleukin 1 by monocytes and intrinsic mesangial cells may be important determinants controlling the extent of mesangial cell proliferation and mesangial matrix production during the course of diffuse endocapillary proliferative glomerulonephritis.

It is also possible that the formation of autologous immune complexes might play a role. According to this hypothesis neuraminidase from the streptococci removes sialic acid from immunoglobulins which then become autoantigenic. The finding of anti-IgG antibodies in the circulation and fixed in the glomeruli in diffuse endocapillary proliferative glomerulonephritis is compatible with this hypothesis.[76] The complex initially formed between antigen and specific antibody might also be enlarged by binding of rheumatoid-like antibodies to altered IgG.

DIFFUSE MESANGIAL PROLIFERATIVE GLOMERULONEPHRITIS

Diffuse mesangial proliferative glomerulonephritis is characterized by an increase in the number of mesangial cells and in the amount of mesangial matrix in over 80% of the glomeruli. It is generally accepted that in a paraffin wax section 2 μm thick the degree of glomerular hypercellularity needed to make a diagnosis of diffuse mesangial proliferative glomerulonephritis is four mononuclear cells or more in each peripheral mesangial area.[77] Mesangial area is defined on page 136. A lesser degree of hypercellularity (three cells per mesangial area) may occur in a number of conditions, including minimal change disease (see p. 136).

Diffuse mesangial proliferative glomerulonephritis usually occurs as part of a recognized systemic disease or associated with another form of glomerulonephritis. Examples of systemic diseases in which mesangial hypercellularity is a common feature are systemic lupus erythematosus (see p. 225), Henoch–Schönlein purpura (see p. 252) and infective endocarditis (see p. 373). Diffuse mesangial proliferative glomerulonephritis is often the morphological form taken by resolving diffuse endocapillary proliferative glomerulonephritis (see p. 142) and occasionally it is the predominant pattern in a mild case of postinfectious glomerulonephritis (see p. 381). Diffuse mesangial proliferative glomerulonephritis is frequently associated with focal segmental glomerulosclerosis (see p. 204) and IgA nephropathy (see p. 157); it sometimes accompanies membranous glomerulonephritis (see p. 191).

Occasionally diffuse mesangial proliferative glomerulonephritis occurs independently of the conditions mentioned above. The account which follows deals solely with this idiopathic form of mesangial hypercellularity; the other forms are considered with the associated systemic disorder on the pages noted above.

Clinical features

Idiopathic diffuse mesangial proliferative glomerulonephritis is commonest in children but may occur in adults. Its exact incidence is not known but it accounts for about 4.5% of cases of the nephrotic syndrome in children[13] and probably it is no more frequent in adults. Diffuse mesangial proliferative glomerulonephritis often presents with combined proteinuria and haematuria. The proteinuria may be severe enough to give a nephrotic syndrome. Less frequently idiopathic diffuse mesangial proliferative glomerulonephritis produces isolated proteinuria or isolated gross or microscopic haematuria. Hypertension occurs in about a third of the patients. About 45% of children with diffuse mesangial proliferative glomerulonephritis fail to respond to treatment

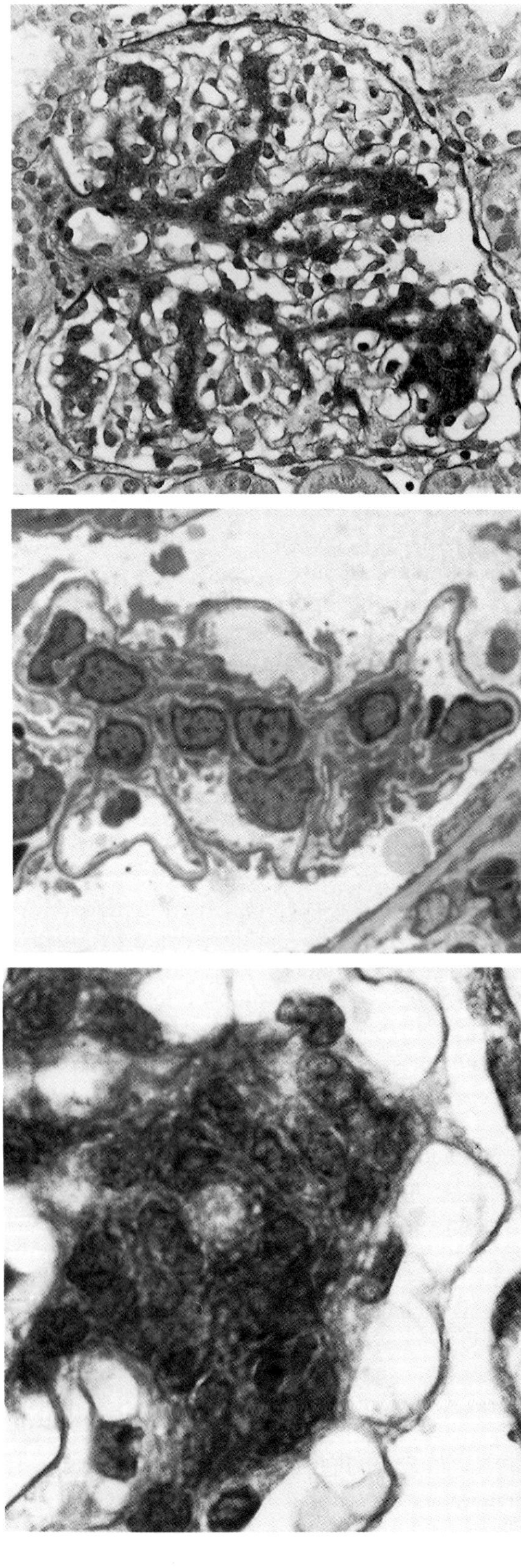

a

b

c

Fig. 6.14 Diffuse mesangial proliferative glomerulonephritis. There are four or more mononuclear cells and an increase in the amount of mesangial matrix in each of the peripheral mesangial areas. The capillary walls appear normal.
(**a**) Whole glomerular tuft. (**b**) Part of a glomerular tuft showing a mesangial area containing five mesangial cells. Resin-embedded section. (**c**) Part of a glomerular tuft showing a mesangial area containing numerous mesangial cells and much matrix.
(**a**) Periodic acid-Schiff × 200; (**b**) Azur II × 600; (**c**) Periodic acid-Schiff × 600

with prednisolone within 8 weeks;[13] this is in contrast to minimal change disease in which approximately 90% of children and 60% of adults lose their proteinuria during an 8-week course of prednisolone.[6,8]

Renal changes

Light microscopy

The glomerular mesangium is expanded and contains clusters of four or more mononuclear cells in each peripheral mesangial area. The mesangial hypercellularity is global, i.e. uniform throughout the glomerulus, and diffuse, i.e. involves over 80% of the glomeruli (Fig. 6.14). The amount of mesangial matrix is increased. The glomerular capillary wall is normal. Characteristically the capillary lumens are normal but occasionally when mesangial expansion is marked they may show some narrowing. The tubules and interstitium are usually normal. There may be hyalin in the arteriolar walls.

Electron microscopy

Electron microscopy confirms the increase in the number of mesangial cells and the amount of mesangial matrix (Fig. 6.15). In those cases in which immunoglobulin or complement can be detected by immunofluorescence or immuno-

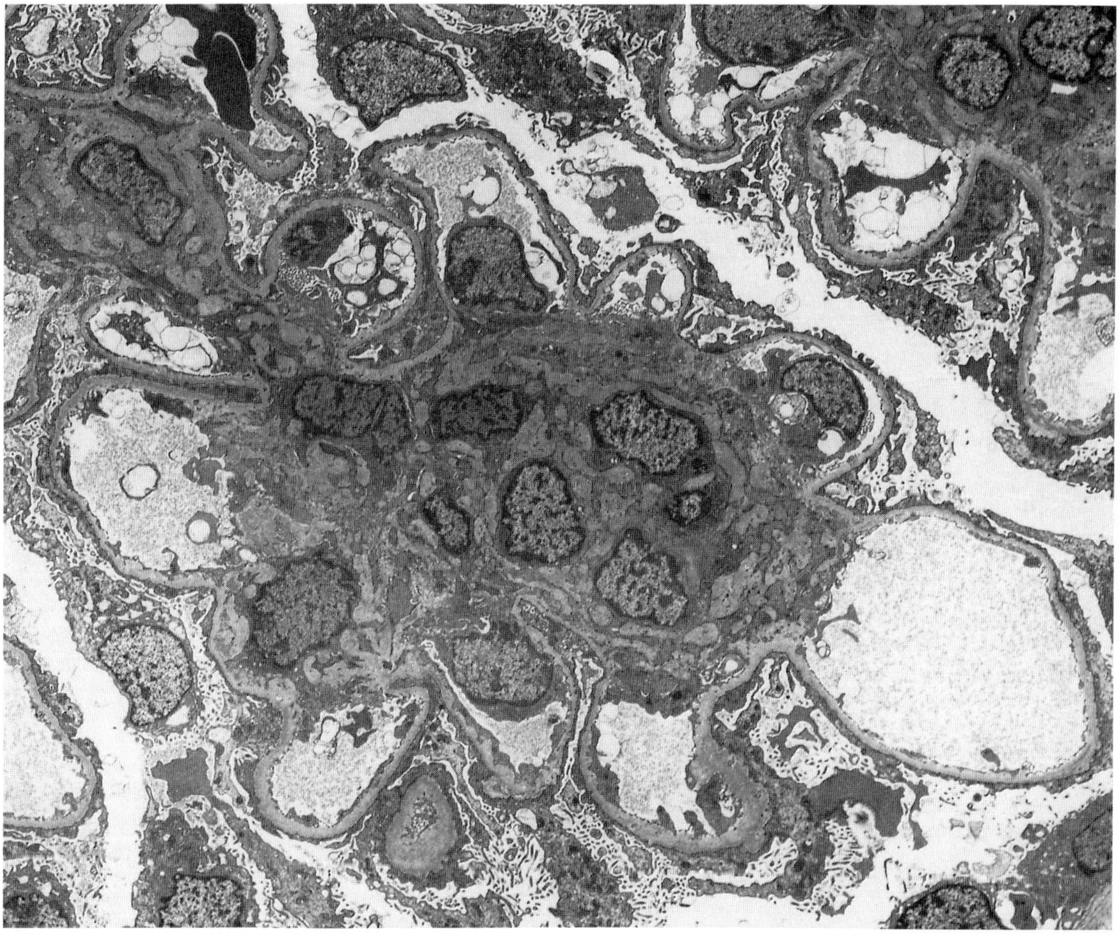

Fig. 6.15 Diffuse mesangial proliferative glomerulonephritis. Electron micrograph of part of the glomerulus shown in Figure. 6.14. The increase in the number of mesangial cells and amount of mesangial matrix is confirmed. There are no electron-dense deposits in the mesangium. The capillary basement membrane is shown to be normal. × 8000

peroxidase there may be electron-dense deposits in the mesangium and in the paramesangial region (see p. 17). The capillary basement membranes are normal.

Immunofluorescence/immunoperoxidase microscopy

Most often these studies are negative in idiopathic diffuse mesangial proliferative glomerulonephritis. Some patients, however, have mesangial deposits predominantly of IgM with or without C3 (Fig. 6.16); these cases have been considered a distinct group by some authors and the syndrome of mesangial hypercellularity and IgM deposits has been designated mesangial IgM nephropathy. In a few cases there are isolated deposits of C3 in the mesangium. It has been suggested that these patients have isolated C3 mesangial proliferative glomerulonephritis.

Mesangial IgM nephropathy[78,79] As experience with diffuse mesangial proliferative glomerulonephritis associated with IgM has accumulated it has become increasingly difficult to sustain the argument that these cases represent a distinctive clinicopathological group; there do not appear to be any significant differences in response to treatment or prognosis between patients with IgM deposits and those without.[80]

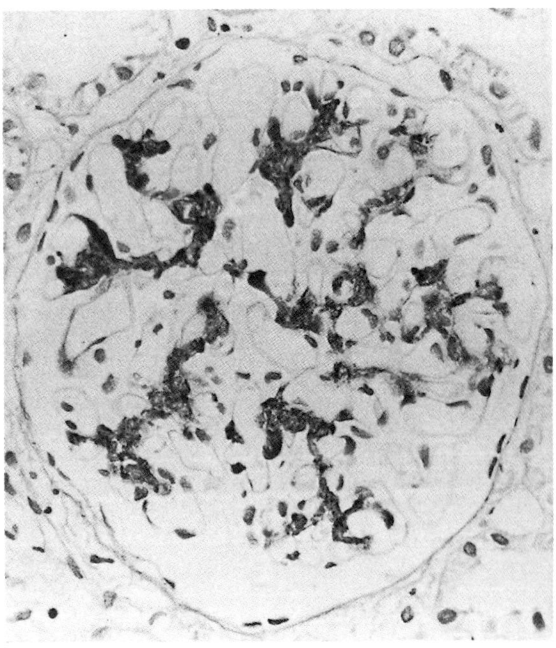

Fig. 6.16 Diffuse mesangial IgM nephropathy. Glomerulus with granular IgM in the mesangium. Immunoperoxidase × 350

Isolated C3 mesangial proliferative glomerulonephritis A few patients have isolated deposits of C3 in the mesangium. It has been reported that they present with microscopical haematuria and do well. There are insufficient data at present to know whether this claim can be sustained.[81]

Differential diagnosis

The distinction between diffuse mesangial proliferative glomerulonephritis and '*mild mesangial hypercellularity*' relies entirely upon good quality sections and a careful count of the number of mesangial cells in the peripheral glomerular mesangial areas. In 'mild mesangial hypercellularity' there are three cells per mesangial area and in diffuse mesangial proliferative glomerulonephritis four cells per mesangial area. As discussed previously (see p. 140) it would be more logical to classify 'mild mesangial hypercellularity' as diffuse mesangial proliferative glomerulonephritis and in one widely respected textbook of renal pathology this has been done.[82] Most pathologists, however, value the stability regarding nomenclature that has followed international acceptance of the World Health Organization's classification of glomerular diseases[77] and are reluctant to move away from this classification and risk returning to chaos.

IgA nephropathy is easily distinguished on immunofluorescence or immunoperoxidase microscopy (see p. 157).

Renal transplantation

A recurrent nephrotic syndrome has been described in a patient with diffuse mesangial proliferative glomerulonephritis and IgM deposits who was given a renal transplant. The details provided of histopathological changes in the biopsy of the graft are insufficient to assess whether the disease had recurred.[83]

Prognosis

The prognosis of idiopathic mesangial proliferative glomerulonephritis is uncertain. Most cases are thought to do well but data to support this impression are lacking. A few cases are known to progress to focal segmental glomerulosclerosis and renal failure.[84]

Pathogenesis

The pathogenesis of idiopathic diffuse mesangial proliferative glomerulonephritis is unknown.

Due to high hydraulic pressures in the glomerular capillaries and the absence of a limiting endothelial basement membrane, the mesangium is continually exposed to plasma constituents, including immune complexes, complement components and platelet products. All of these substances are capable in experimental animals of stimulating mesangial cell proliferation and matrix expansion and they may be important in initiating diffuse mesangial proliferative glomerulonephritis. As mesangial proliferative glomerulonephritis is a heterogeneous group of conditions, different stimuli and combinations of stimuli probably operate in individual patients. The local production of interleukin-1 by the mesangial cells may be an important determinant controlling the extent of cellular proliferation and matrix formation.[85]

A specific immunological mechanism has been proposed for those cases with IgM and C3 in the mesangium but the results of IgM elution and heterologous complement fixation to frozen sections of biopsies do not support this claim.[80]

Variants

Claims that *mesangial IgM nephropathy* and *isolated C3 mesangial proliferative nephritis* should be considered separate entities have already been discussed (see p. 156).

IgA NEPHROPATHY (IgA NEPHRITIS; BERGER'S DISEASE)

IgA nephropathy is characterized by deposits consisting predominantly of IgA and usually also C3 in the mesangium of almost all the glomeruli. There may be accompanying small amounts of either IgG or IgM or both; Clq is found less often and C4 is rarely observed. Nearly three-quarters of the cases show some increase in the number of mesangial cells and segmental lesions, particularly sclerosis and hyalinosis. A few crescents are often present.

In most patients no cause is apparent, but in some the IgA nephropathy is part of a systemic disease, usually Henoch–Schönlein purpura (see p. 252). IgA nephropathy is also associated with chronic alcoholic liver disease (see p. 513), coeliac disease, inflammatory bowel disease,[86] dermatitis herpetiformis,[87] adenocarcinoma,[88] IgA monoclonal gammopathy,[89] episcleritis[90] ankylosing spondylitis (see p. 251) and mycosis fungoides.[91] Familial IgA nephropathy occurs but is rare.[92] Clinical manifestations are usual in idiopathic and familial IgA nephropathy and in the nephritis associated with Henoch–Schönlein purpura, but are uncommon in the other forms of the disease.

Idiopathic IgA nephropathy (Berger's disease)[93] is in the majority of patients a slowly progressive condition leading to a gradual decline in renal function so that only half the patients have functioning kidneys at 20 years. It is most common in young adults, particularly males. The commonest clinical findings are episodic macroscopic haematuria, asymptomatic proteinuria and microscopic haematuria and, in adults, hypertension. During periods of macroscopic haematuria the serum IgA concentration is usually increased and circulating immune complexes containing IgA are often found. Serum complement levels are generally normal.

In many countries idiopathic IgA nephropathy is now recognized as the commonest form of glomerulonephritis in adults, but there is striking variation world wide in the reported frequency of the disease (see below). The account that follows is concerned with the idiopathic form of the disease.

Incidence

IgA nephropathy is the commonest form of primary glomerulonephritis in France, Spain, Germany, Singapore, Australia, South Korea and

Japan and in American Indians in New Mexico; it is apparently less frequent in other parts of the USA and in Canada, the Netherlands and Britain.[94] Detection of the nephropathy in 43.3% of renal biopsies for primary glomerular disease in Japan[95] contrasts with a frequency of 10% in Britain.[96] However, the incidence in Britain is rising as a result of an increase in the numbers of patients attending nephrology clinics with microscopic haematuria and proteinuria.[97]

Biopsy policy and urinalysis screening are important influences in determining these rates.[94,98] In Britain and the USA, two countries in which routine urinalysis of school children is not done and patients with microscopic haematuria or mild proteinuria are seldom biopsied, only 10–20% of patients described as primary glomerulonephritis have IgA nephropathy. In Japan, where school children have their urine screened and where those with microscopic haematuria and proteinuria are usually biopsied, over 40% of patients with primary glomerulonephritis have IgA nephropathy.

The annual number of cases of IgA nephropathy detected in military conscripts in Finland is 22 per 100 000 men aged 19–20 years.[99] Idiopathic IgA nephropathy appears to be rare in American blacks and has not yet been reported in African blacks.[100] But these figures refer to particular sections of each community; the incidence of IgA nephropathy in the general population of different countries is still not known.

Bearing in mind the size of the population of Asia and those parts of Europe where IgA nephropathy is the most prevalent form of glomerulonephritis, and the likely under-recognition of IgA nephropathy in most of the USA, Canada and Britain, IgA nephropathy is probably the commonest form of glomerulonephritis in the world.[98]

Clinical features

Patients range in age from 4 to 80 years, with a mean age of 33 years. Those over the age of 40 years comprise less than 15% of all patients. Males are affected three times more often than females in most parts of the world, the exception being Japan.

Most patients are discovered because either they present with an acute reversible episode of gross haematuria or asymptomatic microscopic haematuria is detected during routine urinalysis.[101,102] About 10% of patients present with nephrotic range proteinuria, severe hypertension or chronic renal insufficiency.[103]

Patients presenting with gross haematuria

The episode of gross haematuria generally occurs 24–48 hours after or concomitant with an upper respiratory tract or, much less frequently, a gastro-intestinal or urinary tract infection; occasionally it follows vaccination or strenuous physical effort. It may be accompanied by fever, malaise and sometimes severe loin pain. The duration of the haematuria varies from a few hours to many days. In about two-thirds of patients episodes of gross haematuria recur at intervals of a few months to many years; the recurrent attacks are often associated with the same precipitating factor as before. In Europe and North America gross haematuria is the presenting clinical sign in approximately 80% of children, 65% of adolescents, 55% of young adults and 25% of those older than 45 years. In Japan, where urinary specimens from school children are regularly screened, the percentages of children presenting with gross haematuria are considerably lower. Between attacks of gross haematuria microscopic haematuria is usual.

Patients with asymptomatic microscopic haematuria

The microscopic haematuria is usually persistent and is often accompanied by proteinuria and occasional casts. The proteinuria is less than 1 g/day in approximately 60% of patients. Hypertension is present at the time of diagnosis in about 35% of these patients; it is accompanied by decreased renal function in 25%. Some of the patients with asymptomatic microscopic haematuria at the time of diagnosis later develop episodes of gross haematuria.

Tissue typing

There is a family predisposition to idiopathic IgA nephropathy; the underlying abnormality responsible for this phenomenon is not known. Several large studies of patients with this disease have noted significantly increased frequencies of certain HLA antigens, most commonly C4-null, B35, B12 and DR4, but these observations have not been confirmed in other studies.[92] They may simply reflect linkage disequilibrium.[104] Recently evidence has been produced suggesting that a gene or genes within or adjacent to the HLA DQB locus may be important in conferring susceptibility to the disease;[105] these findings have not yet been confirmed.

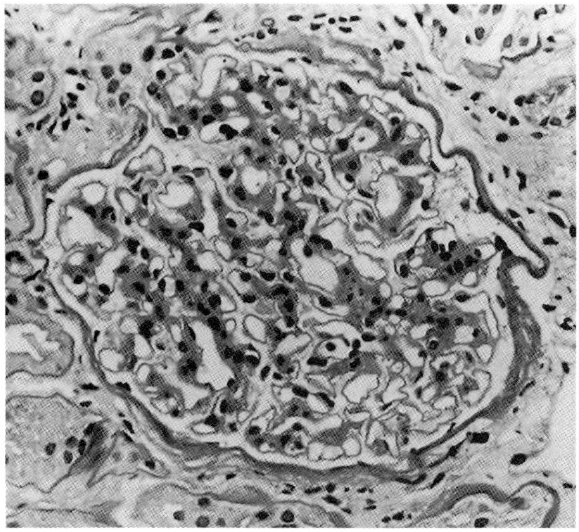

Fig. 6.17 IgA nephropathy. There is mild global increase in the number of mesangial cells and in the amount of mesangial matrix, i.e. the appearance is that of mesangial proliferative glomerulonephritis.
Periodic acid-Schiff × 350

Serology

The serum level of IgA is frequently raised, especially during episodes of infection or gross haematuria. IgA exists in two molecular forms in the body: monomeric IgA which predominates in the serum, and polymeric IgA, consisting of dimer and higher polymers, which is produced at mucosal surfaces in response to antigenic challenge. The increase in serum IgA in idiopathic IgA nephropathy is particularly in the levels of dimer and higher IgA polymers.[106] IgA rheumatoid factor is common in the serum.

Circulating immune complexes containing IgA are found; some groups report an association between levels of circulating immune complexes and episodes of gross haematuria, others do not.[106]

Levels of serum complement components C3, C4, C1q and factor B are normal during both remissions and periods of relapse.

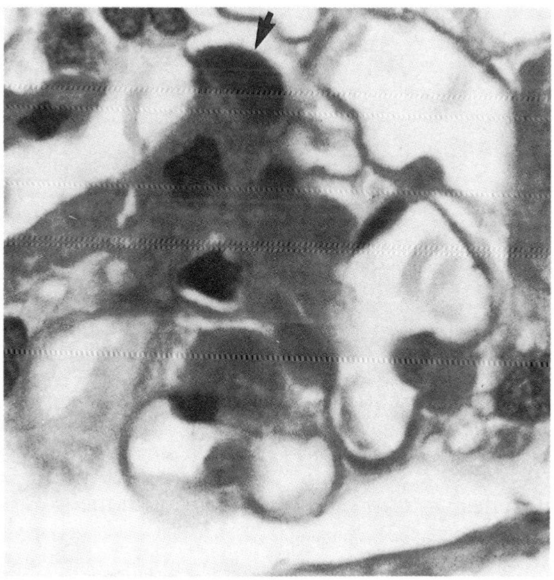

Fig. 6.18 IgA nephropathy. Part of mildly hypercellular glomerulus with a paramesangial hyaline nodule (arrow).
Periodic acid-Schiff × 600

Peripheral blood lymphocytes

During periods of gross haematuria there are rises in the number of IgA-bearing B lymphocytes, in the ratio of T-helper lymphocytes to T-suppressor lymphocytes and in the amount of mitogen-induced IgA production by lymphocytes.[106]

Renal changes

Light microscopy[103]

The characteristic changes in the glomeruli are a mild increase in the number of mesangial cells (three or more per mesangial area) and in the amount of mesangial matrix, segmental lesions and paramesangial hyaline nodules (Figs 6.17–6.19). All three changes each occur in approximately 70% of cases but not always together. The mesangial expansion and hypercellularity are diffuse in a little over half the patients and focal in the others: these changes may be global or seg-

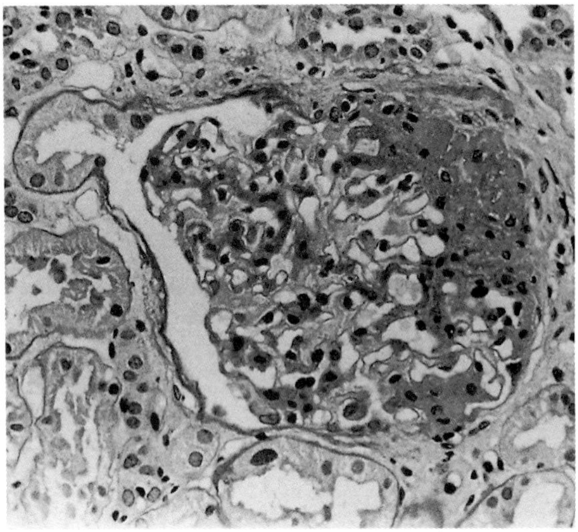

Fig. 6.19 IgA nephropathy. Glomerulus with segmental hyalinosis and sclerosis and mild global mesangial hypercellularity.
Periodic acid-Schiff × 350

mental. Mesangial proliferation is least in children (Fig. 6.20). The segmental lesions (in addition to segmental mesangial hypercellularity) are focal and consist of sclerosis and hyalinosis in most (Fig. 6.19), necrosis with fibrin exudation in some and mesangial interposition in a few. Hyaline nodules protrude from paramesangial areas (Fig. 6.18). They stain red with Masson's trichrome. Crescents affecting small numbers of glomeruli are present in approximately half the cases and are usually cellular; diffuse crescentic glomerulonephritis is rare (1%).

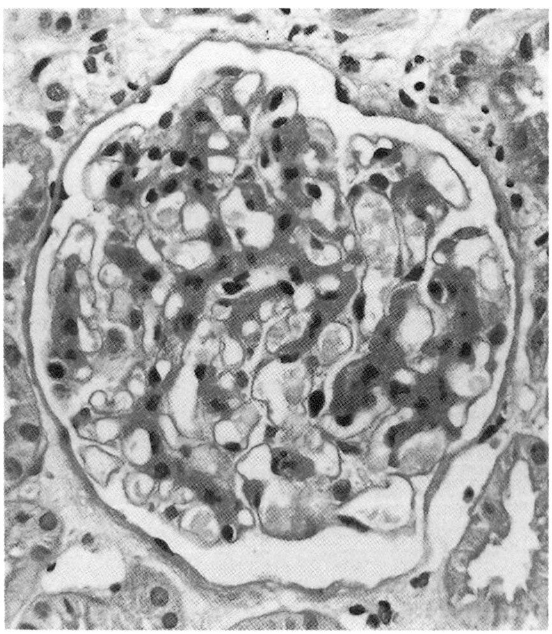

Fig. 6.20 IgA nephropathy in a child. Glomerulus with mesangial expansion but minimal segmental increase in cellularity.
Periodic acid-Schiff × 350

If there is mesangial hypercellularity but no segmental lesions and no nodules, the appearance is that of mesangial proliferative glomerulonephritis (see p. 155). Normal glomeruli are seen in approximately 7% of cases.[103] The segmental sclerotic and hyaline areas are indistinguishable from those seen in idiopathic focal segmental glomerulosclerosis (see p. 204).

In adults small foci of tubular atrophy and interstitial fibrosis are common. Arteriolar hyalinosis is also common and often appears nodular; it bears little relationship to whether the patient is hypertensive or not.

Various schemes for grading the degree of histological damage have been proposed. None are widely used because good correlation between the histological grade and prognosis is only obtained for the low and high grades.[107]

Electron microscopy[103]

The expanded and hypercellular mesangium contains large electron-dense deposits which lie mainly under the basement membrane (Figs 6.21, 6.22). The deposits are often nodular, protruding into Bowman's space. Deposits are also very common in the paramesangium, sometimes appearing as strips rather than nodules. In approximately 20% of cases occasional deposits are also found in subepithelial, intramembranous and subendothelial sites. The subepithelial aspect of the glomerular capillary basement membrane is irregular, sometimes with spikey projections, in about 30% of cases – a change referred to as 'etching'. In some glomerular segments the capillary basement membrane is thinner than normal (less than 200 nm in thickness), may be laminated and may contain electron-lucent areas.[108] Segments of mesangial interposition are occasionally present. As the disease advances the amount of mesangial matrix increases, collagen fibrils appear in in-

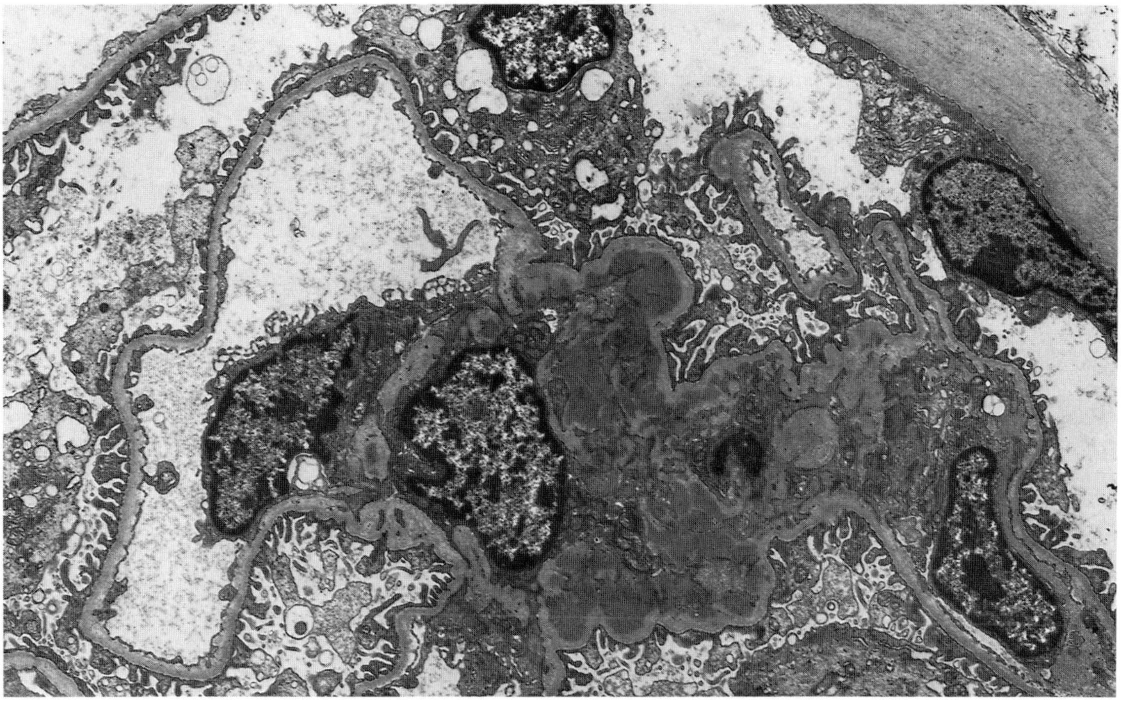

Fig. 6.21 IgA nephropathy. Electron micrograph of part of a glomerulus. The mesangium is expanded by large electron-dense deposits.
× 6500

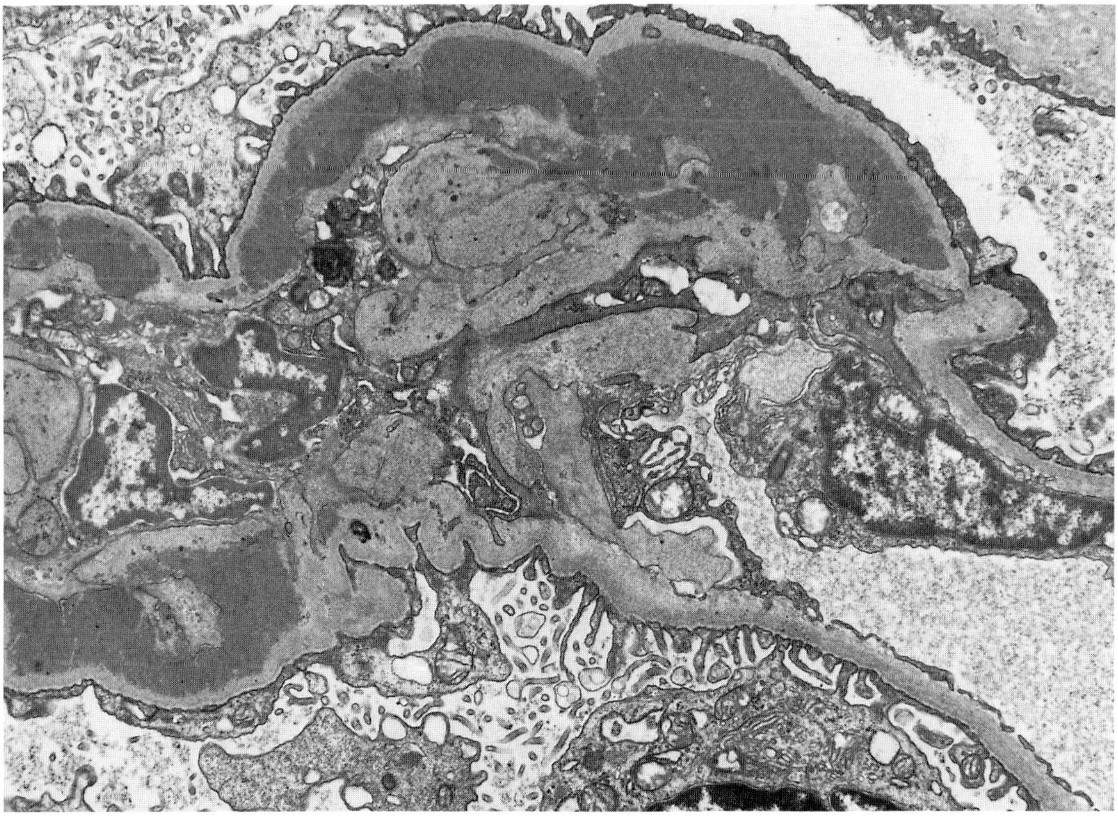

Fig. 6.22 IgA nephropathy. Electron micrograph of part of the mesangium. The large electron-dense deposits lie mainly under the basement membrane.
× 8000

creasing numbers and the electron-dense deposits cease to be nodular and become dispersed and small.

Immunofluorescence/immunoperoxidase microscopy

By definition over 80% of the glomeruli contain fine or coarse granular deposits of IgA in the mesangium and in the paramesangium and sometimes in the adjacent capillary walls (Fig. 6.23). In most patients the mesangial IgA is predominantly of the IgA_1 subclass; IgA_1 is the major constituent of circulating IgA, representing approximately 90% of serum IgA. The deposits are able to bind free secretory component; many show a predominance of lambda light chains.[109] In 80–90% of cases there is a similar distribution of granular C3 in the mesangium.

In children IgG is present in half the cases and IgM is infrequent; in adults the opposite is true, IgM being present in approximately 60% of kidneys and IgG in only a quarter. C1q occurs in the mesangium of 10–25% of all patients but in small quantities; C4 is infrequent (13%). C9 and S protein, which are regulatory components of the membrane attack complex, have been detected in the mesangium of approximately 70% of cases.[110]

Elution studies

After acid elution of renal biopsies 64% of the mesangial IgA is found to be composed of polymeric and dimeric IgA with affinity for secretory component.[111] The eluted IgA is predominantly anionic (isoelectric point pI 4.5–5.6), suggesting that electrostatic binding may play a role in the deposition of IgA in the mesangium. Indirect evidence indicates that IgA is antibody (either anti-antigenic or anti-idiotypic) forming part of an immune complex. It has been reported that the eluted IgA binds to nuclear regions of tissue-cultured cells infected with an extract from the same patient's tonsils;[112] this suggests a possible role of viral antigens in producing a complex.

Changes in other organs: skin and skeletal muscle[113,114]

IgA has been demonstrated by immunofluorescence in the walls of small vessels in the dermis and in the muscles of 30–100% of patients with IgA nephropathy. However, in these studies IgA was also found in the skin vessels of, on average, 33% of patients with other renal disease and even

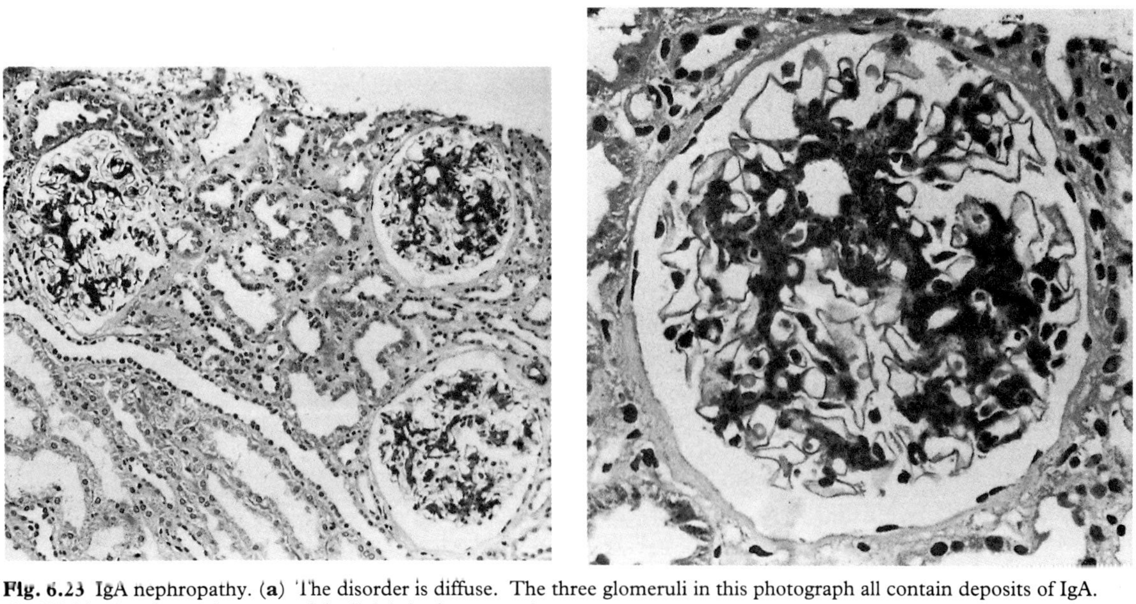

a

Fig. 6.23 IgA nephropathy. (**a**) The disorder is diffuse. The three glomeruli in this photograph all contain deposits of IgA. (**b**) Within the glomerulus most of the IgA is in the mesangium.
Immunoperoxidase: (**a**) × 150; (**b**) × 400

in healthy controls; it has been suggested that there may have been difficulties with non-specific or trace staining. Other investigators have found that only 5% of patients have IgA deposits in their dermal vessels. Based on these studies it would seem that a skin biopsy is of little use and no substitute for a renal biopsy in making a diagnosis of IgA nephropathy.

Differential diagnosis

Although on light microscopy alone idiopathic IgA nephropathy might sometimes be mistaken for *minimal change disease, diffuse mesangial proliferative glomerulonephritis* or *focal segmental glomerulosclerosis*, the finding of predominantly IgA in the mesangium by immunofluorescence or immunoperoxidase microscopy removes any difficulty. *Lupus nephritis* occasionally presents with predominant IgA in the mesangium but this is always accompanied by Clq and C4 which make IgA nephropathy unlikely – in this circumstance estimation of the serum DNA-binding level should always be done. The presence of 2 + or greater staining for C1q (on a scale of 0–4+) rules out IgA nephropathy.[115] At times it can be impossible on a biopsy alone to distinguish *Henoch–Schönlein nephritis* from IgA nephropathy, but usually focal necrotizing lesions and crescents are more frequent and more prominent in Henoch–Schönlein. *In alcoholic liver disease* the renal lesion is more likely to be a mesangiocapillary glomerulonephritis; also serum levels of C3 are often depressed (see p. 513).

Complications

Diffuse crescentic glomerulonephritis

A small number of crescents are commonly found in idiopathic IgA nephropathy but involvement of 80% or more of the glomeruli (diffuse crescentic glomerulonephritis) is rare. In one large series of patients with idiopathic IgA nephropathy diffuse crescentic glomerulonephritis occurred in 1%.[103] The patients with this complication usually have hypertension and renal insufficiency that progresses to end-stage renal disease within 2 years.[116]

Renal transplantation

Idiopathic IgA nephropathy recurs in the renal allograft of approximately 50–75% of patients within 2 months to 4 years after transplantation; the mean time of onset is 1 year (see p. 667). The first clinical indication of recurrence is microscopic haematuria, sometimes accompanied by proteinuria; initially the IgA deposits do not necessarily produce changes in the urine and are only detectable by routine biopsy. The recurrent disease is generally slow in reducing renal function and does not constitute a contraindication to transplantation as a form of treatment in end-stage IgA nephropathy.[117,118]

Prognosis

Accumulated data now show that idiopathic IgA nephropathy is a persistent disease which begins in childhood or early adult life and does not resolve. Spontaneous clinical remissions occur but are rare. Eighty per cent of patients survive for 10 years, but progression to end-stage renal failure continues, with the result that only 50% of patients are alive with functioning kidneys at 20 years.[119] In 1984 idiopathic IgA nephropathy accounted for 21% of patients with end-stage glomerulonephritis diagnosed by biopsy in Australia.[120] In the majority of patients the decline in renal function is very gradual; a few individuals progress to end-stage renal failure in a few years.

It is difficult to predict how individual patients are going to behave. Unfavourable clinical features are thought to be absence of gross haematuria, persisting high urinary erythrocyte counts (above 10^5/ml), persisting heavy proteinuria, hypertension, and being age 40 years or over at the time of discovery of the disease. Unfavourable morphological features are interstitial scarring, marked mesangial proliferation, glomerulosclerosis (either global or segmental), IgA in the capillary walls and narrowing of arteries and arterioles by intimal fibrosis and deposition of hyalin.[104,107,121]

There is no proven specific treatment for idiopathic IgA nephropathy. There have been no cases where repeat biopsies have shown morphological improvement in the glomerular tuft abnormalities, but the number of crescents may reduce between episodes of gross haematuria. Immunoglobulin A deposits have only been shown to disappear from affected kidneys that have been inadvertently transplanted (see p. 626).

Pathogenesis

The aetiology and pathogenesis of idiopathic IgA nephropathy are unknown. Current hypotheses[98,107,122,123] present four ideas.

First, it is suggested that there is a primary, probably genetic, abnormality in the regulation of IgA production which leads to either increased synthesis or reduced clearance of IgA or both. This would explain the increased level of polymeric IgA in the blood. It is known that cultured peripheral lymphocytes of patients with idiopathic IgA nephropathy produce more IgA than those of normal individuals and that this IgA is partially polymeric. Also more IgA antibodies are produced by patients with IgA nephropathy after stimulation with influenza and poliomyelitis vaccine. The number of IgA-specific CD8 (suppressor) T lymphocytes is reduced and the number of IgA-specific CD4 (helper) T lymphocytes is increased in the peripheral blood in idiopathic IgA nephropathy. Tonsils of patients with IgA nephropathy have a greater than normal percentage of IgA-bearing B lymphocytes which after stimulation produce greater than normal amounts of polymeric IgA. In nearly half the patients there is a circulating IgA rheumatoid factor which is partially polymeric. Members of the families of some patients, while asymptomatic, have several of these changes, including increased production of IgA. There is also evidence that in addition there is a defect in mononuclear phagocytosis in idiopathic IgA nephropathy and that this leads to impaired clearance of polymeric IgA.

Second, it is proposed that the increased IgA synthesis is in response to stimulation of migratory lymphocytes in the mucosa of the respiratory, gastrointestinal or urinary tract by bacteria, viruses or some antigen in the diet. This would explain why some patients develop recurrent bouts of gross haematuria following tonsillar and upper respiratory tract infections. Other patients with IgA nephropathy have high levels of IgA antibodies to food antigens such as gliadin.[124] These antibodies could be responsible for a continuous formation of IgA immune complexes.

Third, it is suggested that IgA immune complexes are formed and that the aggregated polymeric IgA and IgA immune complexes then become trapped in the mesangium where they activate the alternative complement pathway. Some defect in mesangial function may contribute by impairing the clearing of the complexes. The IgA deposited in the mesangium may be an abnormal polymeric IgA of mucosal or secretory origin. Elution studies show that IgA deposited in the glomeruli of patients is composed of polymeric IgA. Claims that cytomegalovirus antigen can be demonstrated in the mesangium of cases of IgA nephropathy have not been confirmed.

Fourth, it is proposed that activation of the complement cascade and other mediators of inflammation leads to proliferation of mesangial cells and mesangial sclerosis. This is discussed under diffuse mesangial proliferative glomerulonephritis (see p. 157).

How the accumulation of IgA and complement in the mesangium causes haematuria is unknown.

DIFFUSE MESANGIOCAPILLARY GLOMERULONEPHRITIS (MEMBRANOPROLIFERATIVE GLOMERULONEPHRITIS TYPES I AND III; MESANGIOCAPILLARY GLOMERULONEPHRITIS TYPES I AND III)

Diffuse mesangiocapillary glomerulonephritis is characterized by expansion of the mesangium and thickening of the glomerular capillary walls. The mesangial expansion is usually accompanied by an increase in the number of mesangial cells. The capillary wall is thickened by mesangial cell interposition and subendothelial electron-dense deposits; when stained by the periodic acid-Schiff technique the capillary basement membrane appears duplicated. Granular deposits of the third component of complement (C3) and often IgG are present in the glomerular capillary wall and mesangium.

Diffuse mesangiocapillary glomerulonephritis is a chronic progressive disease particularly affecting older children and young adults. It usually presents with proteinuria and the nephrotic syndrome but haematuria is common and hypertension and impairment of renal function are frequent. Depression of the serum level of C3 develops in the majority of patients. The clinical course is characterized by periods of remission and exacerbation. Chronic renal failure occurs in approximately 40% of patients in 10 years; most patients need dialysis or renal transplantation within 20 years of the clinical onset of the disease.

In the majority of patients no cause is apparent, but a few cases are associated with chronic infections, e.g. infective endocarditis (p. 374), infective ventriculoatrial shunts (see p. 381), chronic suppuration (see p. 380), schistosomiasis (see p. 421), hepatitis B (see p. 395) and malaria (see p. 418). Effective treatment of these conditions sometimes leads to resolution of the glomerular lesions. Occasionally patients are found to have an epithelial tumour (see p. 616), leukaemia or malignant lymphoma (see p. 616), macroglobulinaemia (see p. 361) or cryoglobulinaemia (see p. 352). Diffuse mesangiocapillary glomerulonephritis is often associated with the rare complement deficiencies (see p. 107) and sometimes with alpha$_1$-antitrypsin deficiency (see p. 110), sickle cell disease (see p. 107) and heroin abuse (see p. 509). Systemic lupus erythematosus occasionally develops the morphological picture of diffuse mesangiocapillary glomerulonephritis (see p. 230). The account that follows is concerned with the idiopathic form of the disease.

Clinical features

Idiopathic diffuse mesangiocapillary glomerulonephritis occurs at any age but is seen most frequently between 5 and 30 years. There is a slight predominance of female patients.[125] There are no reliable data on the incidence of the disease; there is a suggestion that its frequency has decreased in France and Spain during recent years.[126]

In children, haematuria and oedema are equally frequent first symptoms; in adults, the disease usually presents with the nephrotic syndrome or with symptomless proteinuria. In many patients it is the chance discovery of proteinuria and microscopical haematuria that leads to the diagnosis. Almost all the patients have microscopical haematuria but at the onset 35% of the children have gross haematuria, either as part of an acute nephritic illness or as recurrent haematuria. The adults are less likely to have gross haematuria but more likely to be hypertensive and have a lower glomerular filtration rate at diagnosis.[127] The differential clearance of plasma proteins shows moderate to severe impairment of renal selectivity. About 30% of the patients give a history of a preceding infection of the upper respiratory tract and have an antistreptolysin-O titre of above 200 international units per millilitre (see p. 143).

The clinical course is usually slowly progressive, punctuated sometimes by episodes of gross haematuria or the nephrotic syndrome. Occasionally there is rapid deterioration associated with diffuse crescentic glomerulonephritis (see p. 185). A few patients go into remission which may last for years, with hypocomplementaemia as the only laboratory manifestation of the disease.

Serology

About 40% of patients with diffuse mesangiocapillary glomerulonephritis have a reduced level of C3 in the serum at presentation.[127] Those patients that are initially normocomplementaemic may later become hypocomplementaemic. There may be marked variations in the serum level of C3 in individual patients during the course of the disease; there may even be periods when the level is raised.[128] The amounts of C1q and C4 are also sometimes reduced.[129]

In about 20% of patients with diffuse mesangiocapillary glomerulonephritis the serum contains an IgG autoantibody, *C3-nephritic factor* (NeF),[127] capable of activating the complement system and producing a breakdown of C3; it does this by the alternative pathway of complement activation, which is essentially a feedback mechanism in which C3b, a principal breakdown product of C3, generates more C3-converting enzyme (C3bBb). The C3 nephritic factor is specifically directed against C3bBb; it binds to and acts as a stabilizer of C3bBb, prolonging the half-life of C3bBb and as a result bringing about continuing C3 activation.[129] Not all C3 nephritic factors are the same; some activate C3 strongly without any activation of the terminal pathway (probably because they bind to C3bBb in a way that inhibits generation of C5 convertase), whereas other nephritic factors activate both the early and late phases of the complement cascade.[130]

C4 nephritic factor (C4NeF) is also found in some of these patients. C4NeF is an autoantibody; it is specifically directed against and stabilizes the classical complement pathway C3 convertase, C4b2a.[131]

Circulating immune complexes have been detected in 20–50% of patients with diffuse mesangiocapillary glomerulonephritis, depending on the techniques used. There is no correlation between levels of circulating complexes and disease activity.[132]

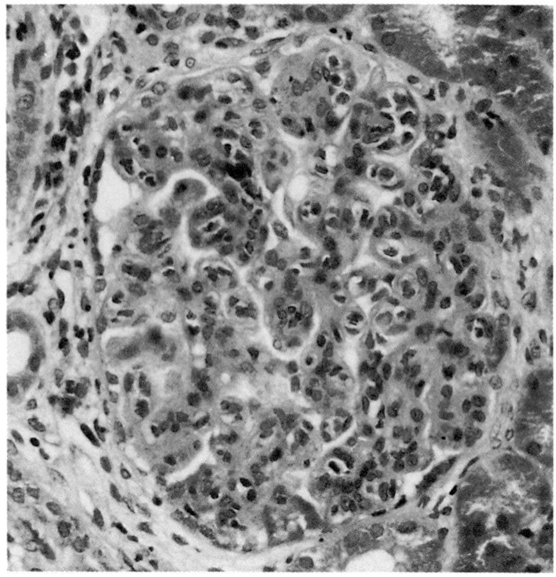

Fig. 6.24 Diffuse mesangiocapillary glomerulonephritis. The lobular pattern of the swollen glomerular tuft is accentuated by the expanded mesangium which contains an increased number of mesangial cells and more matrix than normal. The walls of the capillaries are thickened and the capillary lumens narrowed.
Haematoxylin-eosin × 280

Renal changes

Light microscopy

All the glomeruli are enlarged and their lobular pattern is accentuated. The tufts are more cellular than normal because of an increase in the number of mesangial cells and, sometimes, the presence of small numbers of neutrophil granulocytes. The mesangial matrix is increased in amount. The walls of the capillaries are thickened and the basement membranes appear to have split: this is best seen by the periodic acid-Schiff or periodic acid-silver methenamine methods and has been referred to as the '*tram track*' or '*double contour*' appearance (Figs 6.24, 6.25).[125] The stained basement membrane has the appearance of two dark lines separated by a pale zone. For a diagnosis of diffuse mesangiocapillary glomerulonephritis several loops in over 80% of the glomeruli must show this basement membrane change. Within the double contours deposits of hyaline material (corresponding to subendothelial electron-dense deposits) are often seen; because of their shape the deposits are often referred to as '*slugs*' (Fig. 6.26). As the disease progresses the glomerular capillary lumens become smaller because of encroachment by the expanding mesangium and the thickening capillary walls. The proportion of cells to matrix in the mesangium gradually diminishes; in advanced cases the lobular centres become sclerosed (Fig. 6.27), simulating the Kimmelstiel–Wilson nodules of diabetes mellitus.

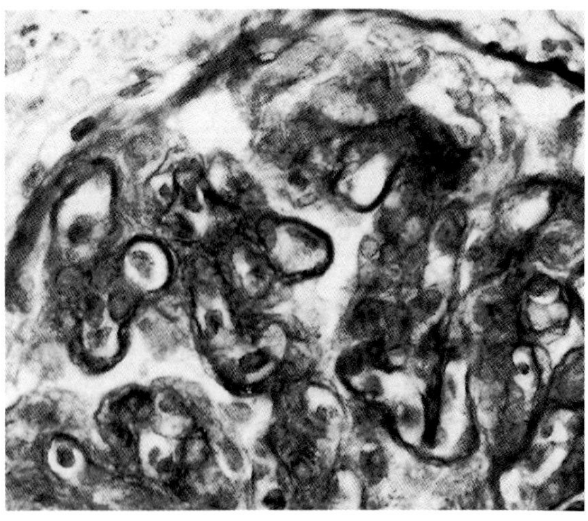

Fig. 6.25 Diffuse mesangiocapillary glomerulonephritis. Part of a glomerular tuft. The capillary walls have double contours.
Periodic acid-Schiff × 500

A few small capsular crescents occur in about half the cases but in about 7% they are large and

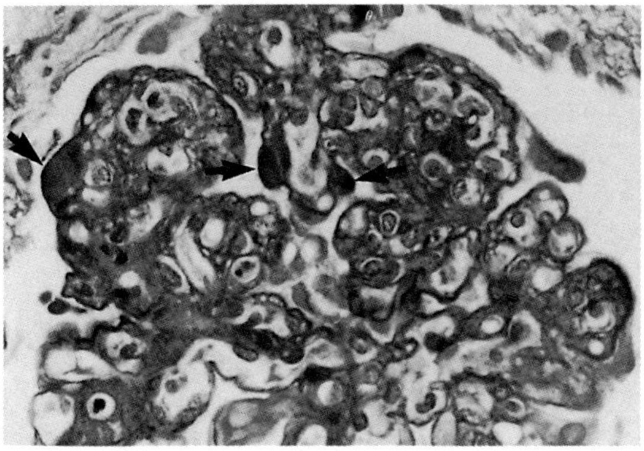

Fig. 6.26 Diffuse mesangiocapillary glomerulonephritis. Part of a glomerular tuft. 'Slugs' of hyaline material (arrows) are present within some of the thickened capillary walls. Periodic acid-Schiff × 500

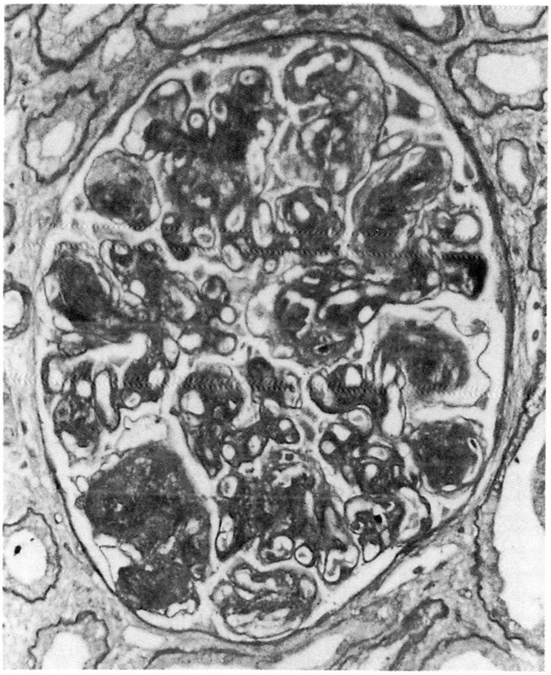

Fig. 6.27 Advanced diffuse mesangiocapillary glomerulonephritis with sclerosis of glomerular lobules. Periodic acid-Schiff × 300

numerous.[127,133] The crescents may be all cellular or all fibrous or there may be a mixture of the two forms. In cases of long duration a few glomeruli may come to contain a few mesangial foam cells with or without segmental sclerosis.

Biopsy evidence suggests that in some cases the disease starts focally and only later becomes diffuse. In one study in which a group of six patients who presented with focal mesangiocapillary glomerulonephritis was followed up and repeat biopsies performed, four of the cases progressed to diffuse mesangiocapillary glomerulonephritis over 2½ years.[134]

Electron microscopy

The greatly increased bulk of the mesangium consists of mesangial cells embedded in abundant matrix that often contains electron-dense deposits; there may also be a few neutrophil granulocytes (Fig. 6.28). The nodules in the glomeruli in long surviving cases of diffuse mesangiocapillary glomerulonephritis consist of mesangial matrix (Fig. 6.29).

The capillary walls are thickened by an extension of mesangial cell cytoplasmic processes, and matrix formed by them, along the subendothelial aspect of the basement membrane. Immediately beneath the endothelium there is a thin layer of new basement membrane formed by the endothelial cells (Figs 6.28, 6.30). This combined inner layer of matrix and new basement membrane stains purple with periodic acid-Schiff and creates an impression of a second irregular glomerular capillary basement membrane in sections examined by light microscopy; the mesangial cell cytoplasm remains unstained and is seen as a clear layer between the true basement membrane and the new combined layer of matrix and basement membrane. This phenomenon is known as *mesangial cell interposition.*[135] It occurs, although to a much lesser extent, in many other renal diseases.

Deposits of electron-dense homogeneous material are common in the subendothelial layer of mesangium and new basement membrane. Some of the deposits may be massive and elongated; these are the 'slugs' seen by light microscopy. Large deposits may extend into the basement membrane. Subepithelial deposits are present in about 15–20% of cases;[125] sometimes these take the form of humps as in diffuse endocapillary proliferative glomerulonephritis (see p. 147) or they may be numerous and uniform as in membranous glomerulonephritis (see p. 194). In patients with marked proteinuria the foot processes of the visceral epithelial cells are retracted and obliterated.

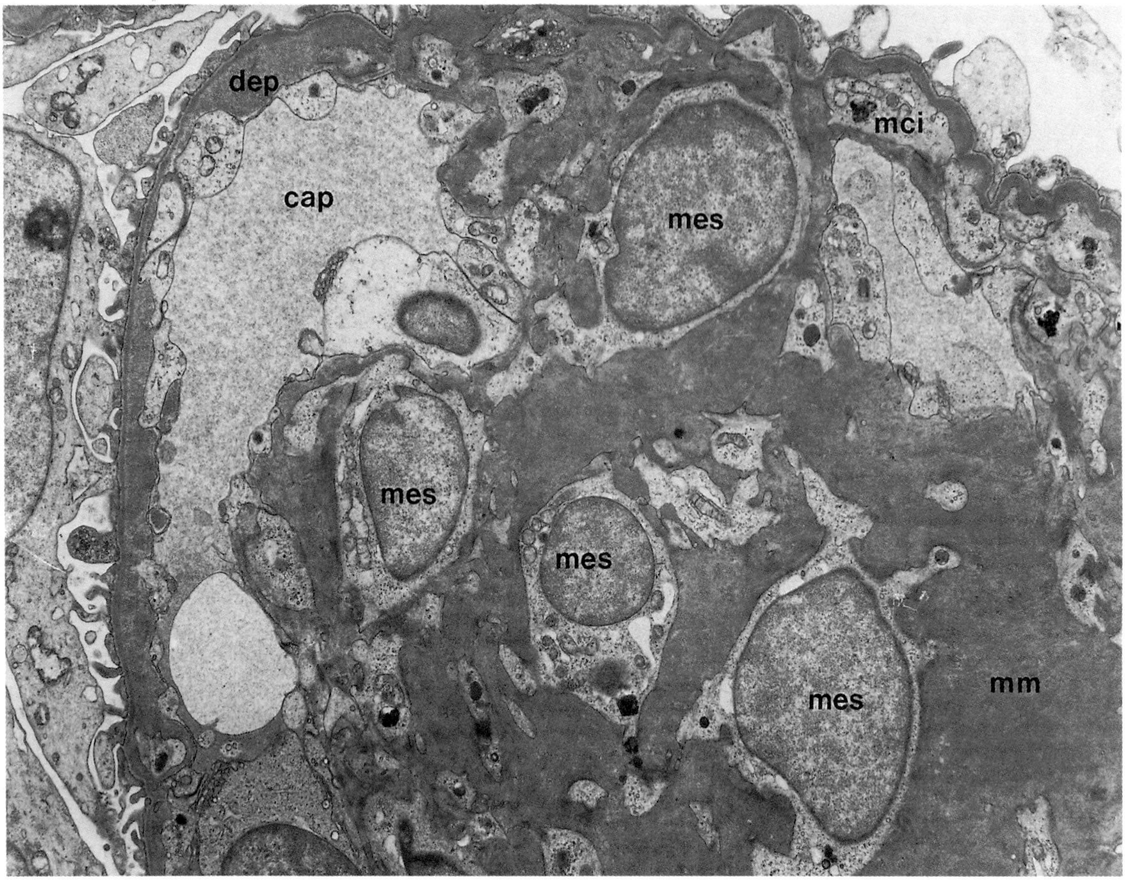

Fig. 6.28 Diffuse mesangiocapillary glomerulonephritis. Electron micrograph of part of a glomerulus. The capillary wall is thickened by mesangial cell interposition (mci) and by subendothelial deposits (dep). The number of mesangial cells (mes) and the amount of mesangial matrix (mm) are increased. cap, capillary lumen
× 4030

Fig. 6.29 Advanced diffuse mesangiocapillary glomerulonephritis. Electron micrograph of part of a glomerulus. There is a marked increase in the amount of mesangial matrix in the centre of the lobule.
× 6200

Fig. 6.30 Diffuse mesangiocapillary glomerulonephritis. Electron micrograph of part of a glomerulus. Mesangial cell processes and mesangial matrix extend along the subendothelial aspect of the capillary basement membrane. Subendothelial electron-dense deposits are also present.
× 8000

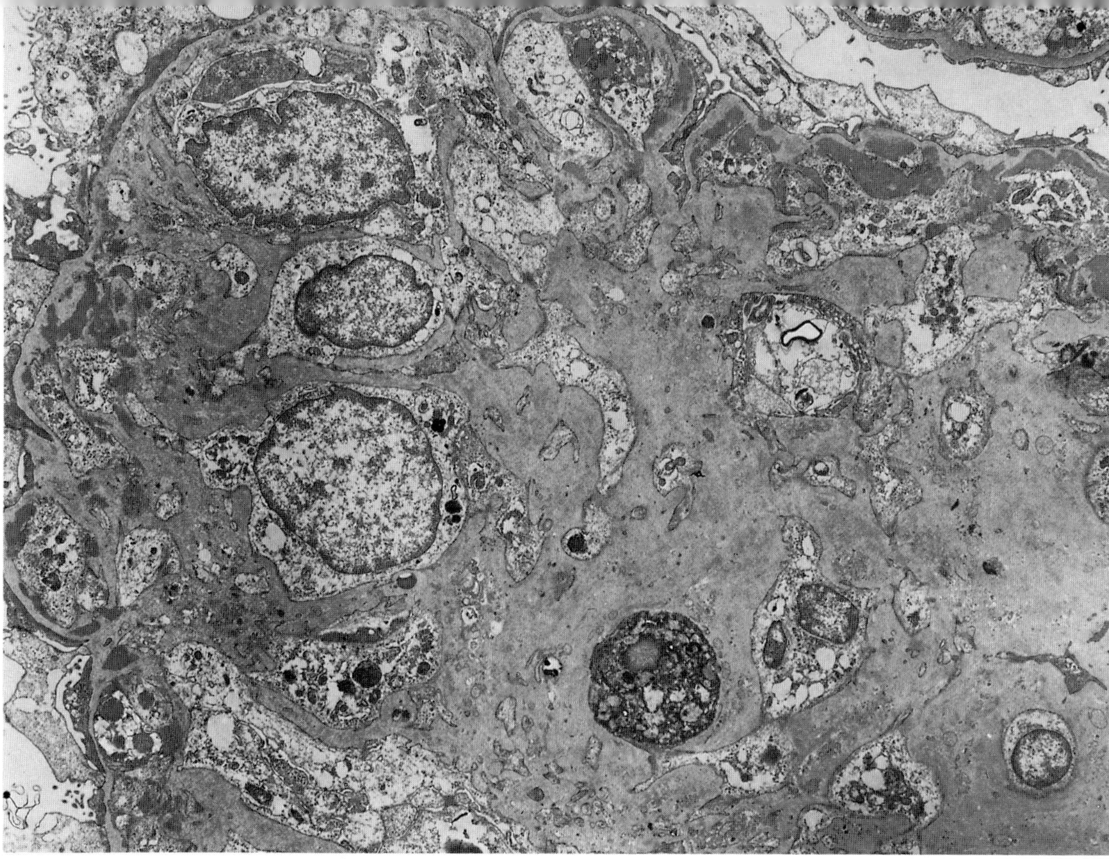

Fig. 6.29

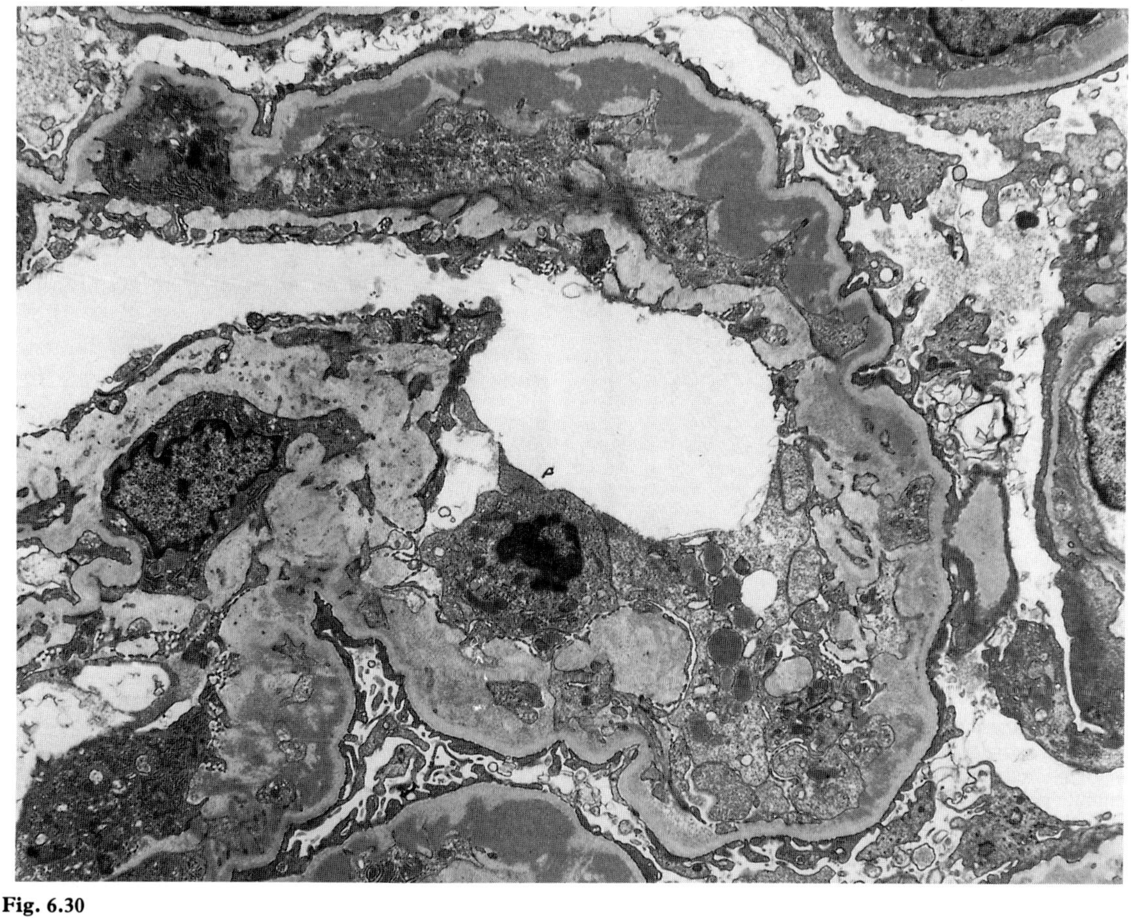

Fig. 6.30

Immunofluorescence/immunoperoxidase microscopy

Diffuse mesangiocapillary glomerulonephritis is characterized in almost all cases by the presence of coarse and fine granules and short linear slugs of C3 in the walls of the glomerular capillaries and, to a lesser extent, in the mesangium (Fig. 6.31). The C3 is accompanied by IgG and properdin in about 60% of patients and IgM and C1q in about 50%; IgA and C4 are present in about 30%.[127] In advanced diffuse mesangiocapillary glomerulonephritis the mesangium often contains very few deposits, giving a distinctive lobular pattern of predominantly C3 deposition in the walls of the peripheral glomerular capillaries (Fig. 6.32).

The predominant IgG subclass in the glomerular deposits is IgG_3 which makes up only 7% of total serum IgG.[136]

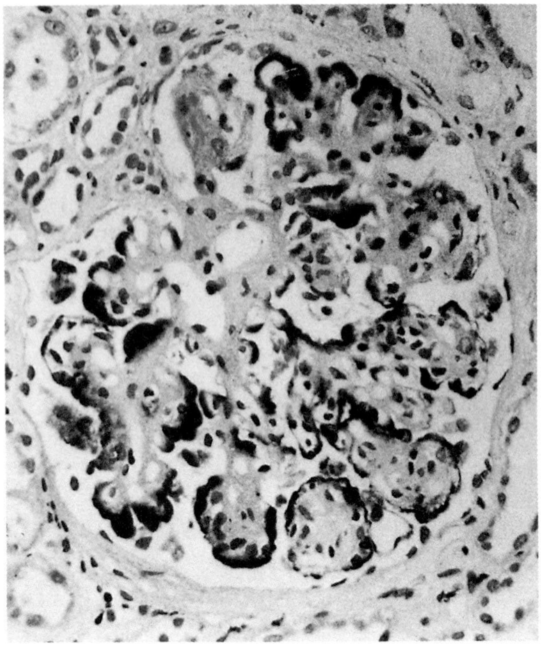

Fig. 6.32 Advanced mesangiocapillary glomerulonephritis. There are granular deposits of C3 in the peripheral capillary walls; the mesangium is spared. Immunoperoxidase × 250

Differential diagnosis

Mesangial expansion producing centrilobular nodules also occurs in *diabetic glomerulosclerosis* (see p. 333) and in *kappa light chain disease* (see p. 363), but the electron microscopic changes in these conditions are quite different from those seen in diffuse mesangiocapillary glomerulonephritis.

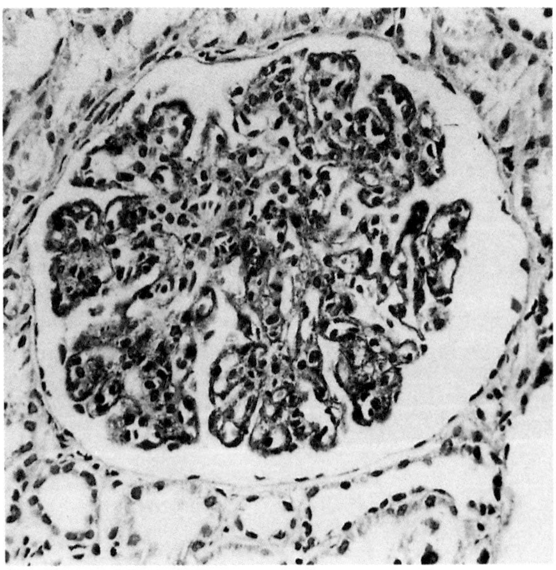

Fig. 6.31 Diffuse mesangiocapillary glomerulonephritis. There are granular deposits of C3 in the glomerular capillary walls and in the mesangium. Immunoperoxidase × 250

Circumferential mesangial cell interposition and subendothelial deposits are often encountered in *pre-eclampsia* (see p. 557) but the ultrastructure of the deposits is different and immunofluorescence or immunoperoxidase microscopy shows a preponderance of IgM with relatively small amounts of C3. Small quantities of segmental mesangial cell interposition are common in a few glomeruli in several renal conditions,[135] but this should not pose any problem because for a diagnosis of diffuse mesangiocapillary glomerulonephritis the majority of the glomeruli must show mesangial cell interposition.

Renal transplantation

Diffuse mesangiocapillary glomerulonephritis affects transplanted kidneys and occasionally develops de novo. The frequency is difficult to establish because of the similar morphological changes that occur in transplant glomerulopathy, a form of chronic rejection. A recurrence rate of 40% has been reported (see p. 664). When recurrence occurs it is usually many years before renal function is impaired. The possibility of recurrence, therefore, should not act as a deterrent to using renal transplantation as a treatment for end-stage renal failure in diffuse mesangiocapillary glomerulonephritis.

Prognosis

Approximately 40% of patients affected by this progressive disease either die or undergo dialysis or renal transplantation within 10 years after diagnosis. After 20 years about 90% of patients have renal failure.[127] Children with diffuse mesangiocapillary glomerulonephritis initially fare better than adults, but after 10 years their survival rate becomes as poor as that of adults. The presence of a nephrotic syndrome at any time in the course of the disease, or the finding of sclerosed glomeruli or crescents in the initial renal biopsy, is associated with a poorer prognosis.[127] There is no specific proved treatment for diffuse mesangiocapillary glomerulonephritis, although there is some evidence that dipyridamole and aspirin slow the deterioration of renal function.[137] These agents, which interfere with platelet aggregation, are used because in some forms of experimental glomerulonephritis intra-glomerular coagulation is responsible for the progression of the disease.

Pathogenesis

Many of the systemic diseases associated with secondary diffuse mesangiocapillary glomerulonephritis are immune complex disorders and specific antigens have been detected in the glomerular deposits of several of these conditions (see p. 422). It may well be that some cases of idiopathic diffuse mesangiocapillary glomerulonephritis are also mediated by immune complexes but that masking of reactive sites or some other problem has prevented detection of an exogenous or endogenous antigen in the deposits.

It has been suggested that the low serum levels of C3 encountered in a number of these patients may lead to defective clearance of antigen by antibody and the persistence of an acquired viral or bacterial infection; this would promote the continuous formation of immune complexes either in the blood stream or in the kidney.[138] However, this explanation of the pathogenesis of idiopathic mesangiocapillary glomerulonephritis presupposes that hypocomplementaemia precedes the development of the renal lesions, a sequence that is not yet proven; also, it does not explain cases that present identical clinical and morphological features but with normal C3 levels.

C3 nephritic factor (NeF) does not seem to be a primary factor in the pathogenesis of diffuse mesangiocapillary glomerulonephritis. It has been suggested that the formation of NeF is induced by the presence in the circulation of immune complexes bearing C3bBb and having certain characteristics that favour induction of this autoantibody.

Genetic factors may be important in some patients with idiopathic diffuse mesangiocapillary glomerulonephritis. Evidence for this is the rarity of the disease in blacks in the USA,[139] the report of a family in which diffuse mesangiocapillary glomerulonephritis was inherited as an X-linked recessive disorder,[140] and the occurrence of a particular major histocompatibility complex extended haplotype (a combination of alleles that tend to occur together) in 13% of patients with diffuse mesangiocapillary glomerulonephritis compared with 1% of controls.[141]

Variants

Diffuse mesangiocapillary glomerulonephritis type III[142]

In a few cases of diffuse mesangiocapillary glomerulonephritis the electron-dense deposits in the glomerular capillary walls are found in a markedly disrupted lamina densa and on the epithelial side of the capillary basement membrane in addition to their usual location in the subendothelial mesangium (Fig. 6.33). Mesangial cell proliferation is less severe and IgG less prominent in the deposits than in most examples of diffuse mesangiocapillary glomerulonephritis.

On the basis of these differences it has been suggested that these patients comprise a distinct

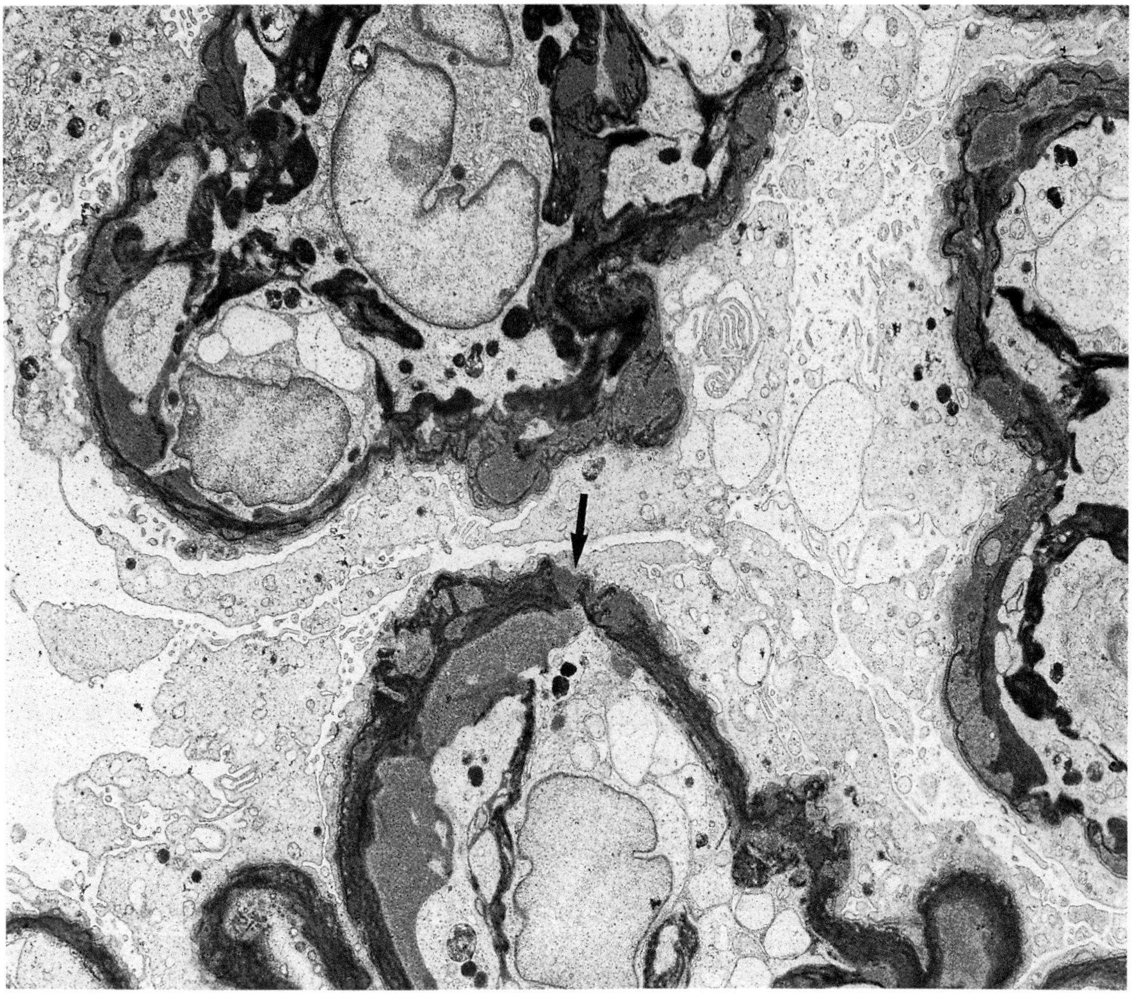

Fig. 6.33 Diffuse mesangiocapillary glomerulonephritis Type III variant. Electron micrograph of part of a glomerulus. The lamina densa of the capillary basement membrane has been stained black with silver. The capillary walls are thickened by lighter stained subendothelial and subepithelial electron-dense deposits and by mesangial cell interposition. There has been irregular laying down of new lamina densa-like material. In one of the capillary loops the basement membrane is ruptured (arrow).
Silver impregnation × 71 680
Reproduced by permission from: Strife CF, McEnergy PT, McAdams AJ, West CD. Clin Nephrol 1977;7:65 (Fig. 3b)

subgroup which has been referred to as mesangiocapillary glomerulonephritis type III (type I is the usual form of diffuse mesangiocapillary glomerulonephritis that has been described in the preceding account, and type II is dense deposit disease, which is described on p. 179).

The clinical features and prognosis in these patients are broadly similar to those in the usual form of diffuse mesangiocapillary glomerulonephritis, although a higher proportion are first detected by a chance discovery of microscopic haematuria or proteinuria in an otherwise healthy individual. Nephritic factor is rarely detected and serum levels of C4 are more commonly normal than in the usual form of diffuse mesangiocapillary glomerulonephritis.

To many pathologists these distinctions do not seem sufficient to justify a separate category of glomerulonephritis and in the World Health Organization classification of glomerular disease these cases are considered under the general grouping of diffuse mesangiocapillary glomerulonephritis.

Focal segmental mesangiocapillary glomerulonephritis

A few patients who initially show diffuse mesangiocapillary glomerulonephritis convert after a few years to a combination of mild to moderate increase in the number of mesangial cells and in the amount of mesangial matrix in all the glomeruli, with segmental mesangial cell interposition, marked mesangial hypercellularity and subendothelial deposits in a minority of the glomeruli. This combination is sometimes confusingly referred to as focal segmental mesangiocapillary glomerulonephritis even though it is essentially a diffuse change; it seems to be associated with a good outcome.[143]

Focal and segmental mesangiocapillary glomerulonephritis as the first manifestation of renal disease is described on page 167.

REFERENCES

Minimal change disease

1. International Study of Kidney Disease in Children. Nephrotic syndrome in children: prediction of histopathology from clinical and laboratory characteristics at time of diagnosis. Kidney Int 1978; 13: 159–165.
2. Schlesinger ER, Sultz HA, Mosher WE, Feldman JG. The nephrotic syndrome. Its incidence and implications for the community. Am J Dis Child 1968; 116: 623–632.
3. Elzouki AY, Amin F, Jaiswal OP. Primary nephrotic syndrome in Arab children. Arch Dis Child 1984; 59: 253–255.
4. Adhikari M, Coovadia HM, Loening WEK. The nephrotic syndrome in children. S Afr Med J 1976; 50: 39–45.
5. Tiebosch ATMG, Wolters J, Frederik PFM et al. Epidemiology of idiopathic glomerular disease: a prospective study. Kidney Int 1987; 32: 112–116.
6. Nolasco F, Cameron JS, Heywood EF, Hicks J, Ogg C, Williams DG. Adult-onset minimal change nephrotic syndrome: a long-term follow up. Kidney Int 1986; 29: 1215–1223.
7. Thomson PD, Barratt TM, Stokes CR, Turner MW, Soothill JF. HLA antigens and atopic features in steroid-responsive nephrotic syndrome. Lancet 1976; 2: 765–768.
8. International Study of Kidney Disease in Children. The primary nephrotic syndrome in children. Identification of patients with minimal change nephrotic syndrome from initial response to prednisone. J Pediatr 1981; 98: 561–564.
9. Trompeter RS, Lloyd BW, Hicks J, White RHR, Cameron JS. Long-term outcome for children with minimal change nephrotic syndrome. Lancet 1985; 1: 368–370.
10. Alfiler CA, Roy LP, Doran T, Sheldon A, Bashir H. HLA-DRW7 and steroid responsive nephrotic syndrome of childhood. Clin Nephrol 1980; 14: 71–74.
11. Kobayashi Y, Chen X-M, Hiki Y, Fujii K, Kashiwagi N. Association of HLA-DRW8 and DQW3 with minimal change nephrotic syndrome in Japanese adults. Kidney Int 1985; 28: 193–197.
12. Cairns SA, London A, Mallick NP. Immune complexes in minimal change glomerulopathy. N Engl J Med 1980; 302: 1033 (letter).
13. International Study of Kidney Disease in Children. Primary nephrotic syndrome in children: clinical significance of histopathologic variants of minimal change and of diffuse mesangial hypercellularity. Kidney Int 1981; 20: 765–771.
14. Southwest Pediatric Nephrology Study Group. Childhood nephrotic syndrome associated with diffuse mesangial hypercellularity. Kidney Int 1983; 23: 87–94.
15. Churg J, Habib R, White RHR. Pathology of the nephrotic syndrome in children. A report for the International Study of Kidney Disease in Children. Lancet 1970; 1:1299–1302.
16. Allen WR, Travis LB, Cavallo T, Brouhard BH, Cunningham RJ. Immune deposits and mesangial hypercellularity in minimal change nephrotic syndrome: clinical relevance. J Pediatr 1982; 100: 188–191.
17. Waldherr R, Fydryk J, Scharer K. Mesangial cellularity in steroid-responsive nephrotic syndrome. J Pediatr 1982; 101: 794.
18. Arakawa M. A scanning electron microscope study of the human glomerulus. Am J Pathol 1971; 64: 457–462.
19. Vilches AR, Turner DR, Cameron JS, Ogg CS, Chantler C, Williams DG. Significance of mesangial IgM deposition in 'minimal change' nephrotic syndrome. Lab Invest 1982; 46: 10–15.
20. Murphy WM, Jukkola AF, Roy S. Nephrotic syndrome with mesangial cell proliferation in children – a distinct entity? Am J Clin Pathol 1979; 72: 42–47.
21. Siegel NJ, Kashgarian M, Spargo BH et al. Minimal change and focal sclerotic lesions in lipoid nephrosis. Nephron 1974; 13: 125–137.
22. Habib R. Focal glomerular sclerosis. Kidney Int 1973; 4: 355–361.
23. Tejani A. Morphological transition in minimal change nephrotic syndrome. Nephron 1985; 39: 157–159.
24. Ingulli E, Gonzalez R, Rajpoot D, Tejani A. Nephrotic syndrome: from toddlers to twenties. Lancet 1989; 1: 674 (letter).
25. Fogo A, Hawkins EP, Berry PL et al. Glomerular hypertrophy in minimal change disease predicts subsequent progression to focal glomerular sclerosis. Kidney Int 1990; 38: 115–123.
26. Eagen JW, Lewis EJ. Glomerulopathies of neoplasia. Kidney Int 1977; 11: 297–306.
27. Gagliano RG, Costanzi JJ, Beathard GA, Sarles HE, Bell JD. The nephrotic syndrome associated with

neoplasia: an unusual paraneoplastic syndrome. Report of a case and review of the literature. Am J Med 1976; 60: 1026–1031.
28. Humphreys SR, Holley KE, Smith LH, McIlrath DC. Mesenteric angiofollicular lymph node hyperplasia (lymphoid hamartoma) with nephrotic syndrome. Mayo Clin Proc 1975; 50: 317–321.
29. Lagrue G, Laurent J, Rostoker G. Food allergy and idiopathic nephrotic syndrome. Kidney Int 1989; 36: suppl 27, S147–151.
30. Lewis MA, Baildom EM, Davis N, Houston IB, Postlethwaite RJ. Nephrotic syndrome: from toddlers to twenties. Lancet 1989; 1: 255–259.
31. Coovadia HM, Adhikari M. Outcome of childhood minimal-change disease. Lancet 1989; 1: 1199–1200.
32. Richards W, Olsen D, Church JA. Improvement of idiopathic nephrotic syndrome following allergy therapy. Ann Allergy 1977; 39: 332–334.
33. Mouzon-Cambon A de, Bouissou F, Dutau G et al. HLA-DR7 in children with idiopathic nephrotic syndrome. Correlation with atopy. Tissue Antigens 1981; 17: 518–524.
34. Taube D, Brown Z, Williams DG. Impaired lymphocyte and suppressor cell function in minimal change nephropathy, membranous nephropathy and focal glomerulosclerosis. Clin Nephrol 1984; 22: 176–182.
35. Carrie BJ, Salyer WR, Myers BD. Minimal change nephropathy: an electrochemical disorder of the glomerular membrane. Am J Med 1981; 70: 262–268.
36. Blau EB, Haas JE. Glomerular sialic acid and proteinuria in human renal disease. Lab Invest 1973; 28: 477–481.
37. Yoshizawa N, Kusumi Y, Matsumoto K et al. Studies of a glomerular permeability factor in patients with minimal-change nephrotic syndrome. Nephron 1989; 51: 370–376.
38. Benigni A, Rizzoni G, Antolini A, Piccinelli A, Remuzzi G. Preliminary report: renal thromboxane A_2 synthesis in children with frequent relapsing nephrotic syndrome. Lancet 1990; 336: 533– 534.
39. Fries JWU, Rumpelt H-J, Thoenes W. Alterations of glomerular podocytic processes in immunologically mediated glomerular disorders. Kidney Int 1987; 32: 742–748.
40. Waldherr R, Gubler M, Levy M, Broyer M, Habib R. The significance of pure diffuse mesangial proliferation in idiopathic nephrotic syndrome. Clin Nephrol 1978; 10: 171–179.

Diffuse endocapillary proliferative glomerulonephritis

41. Meadow SR. Poststreptococcal glomerulonephritis – a rare disease? Arch Dis Child 1975; 50: 379–382.
42. Hallett AF, Adhikari M, Cooper R et al. Post-streptococcal glomerulonephritis in African children. Trans R Soc Trop Med Hyg 1977; 71: 241–246.
43. Poon-King T, Potter EV, Svartmen M et al. Epidemic acute nephritis with reappearance of M-type 55 streptococci in Trinidad. Lancet 1973; 1: 475–479.
44. Rodriguez-Iturbe B, Castillo L, Valbuena R, Cuenca L. Acute post-streptococcal glomerulonephritis. A review of recent developments. Pediatrician 1979; 8: 307–324.
45. Stollerman GH. Rheumatogenic and nephritogenic streptococci. Circulation 1971; 43: 915–921.
46. Johnston KH, Zabriskie JB. Purification and partial characterisation of the nephritis strain-associated protein from *Streptococcus pyogenes*, group A. J Exp Med 1986; 163: 697–712.
47. Barnham M, Thornton TJ, Lange K. Nephritis caused by *Streptococcus zooepidemicus* (Lancefield group C). Lancet 1983; 1: 945–948.
48. Anthony BF, Kaplan EL, Wannamaker LW, Briese FW, Chapman SS. Attack rates of acute nephritis after type 49 streptococcal infection of the skin and of the respiratory tract. J Clin Invest 1969; 48: 1697–1704.
49. Weinstein L, Le Frock J. Does antimicrobial therapy of streptococcal pharyngitis or pyoderma alter the risk of glomerulonephritis? J Infect Dis 1971; 124: 229–231.
50. Seligson G, Lange K, Majeed H, Deol H, Cronin W, Bovie R. Significance of endostreptosin antibody titers in poststreptococcal glomerulonephritis. Clin Nephrol 1985; 24: 69–75.
51. Tejani A, Ingulli E. Poststreptococcal glomerulonephritis. Current clinical and pathologic concepts. Nephron 1990; 55: 1–5.
52. Sagel I, Treser G, Ty A et al. Occurrence and nature of glomerular lesions after group A streptococci infections in children. Ann Intern Med 1973; 79: 492–499.
53. Layrisse Z, Rodriguez-Iturbe B, Garcia-Ramirez R, Rodriguez A, Tiwari J. Family studies of the HLA system in acute poststreptococcal glomerulonephritis. Hum Immunol 1983; 7: 177–185.
54. Lewis EJ, Carpenter CB, Schur PH. Serum complement component levels in human glomerulonephritis. Ann Intern Med 1971; 7 5: 555–560.
55. Kefalides NA, Pegg MT, Ohno N, Poon-king T, Zabriskie J, Fillit H. Antibodies to basement membrane collagen and to laminin are present in sera from patients with poststreptococcal glomerulonephritis. J Exp Med 1986; 163: 588–602.
56. Pound SE, MacDonald MK, Thomson D. Diffuse proliferative glomerulonephritis – how many types? Histopathology 1987; 11: 227–243.
57. Sorger K, Gessler U, Hubner FK et al. Subtypes of acute post-infectious glomerulonephritis. Synopsis of clinical and pathological features. Clin Nephrol 1982; 17: 114–128.
58. Fairley C, Mathews DC, Becker GJ. Rapid development of diffuse crescents in post-streptococcal glomerulonephritis. Clin Nephrol 1987; 28: 256–260.
59. Ingelfinger JR, McCluskey RT, Schneeberger EE, Grupe WE. Necrotizing arteritis in acute poststreptococcal glomerulonephritis. Report of a recovered case. J Pediatr 1977; 91: 228–232.
60. Lee HS, Choi Y, Oh HY, Koh HI. Abnormalities of glomerular basement membrane in acute postinfectious glomerulonephritis. Clin Nephrol 1990; 33: 220–226.
61. Lewy JE, Salinas-Madrigal L, Herdson PB, Pirani CL, Metcoff J. Clinico-pathologic correlations in acute poststreptococcal glomerulonephritis. Medicine (Baltimore) 1971; 50: 453–501.
62. Sorger K, Balun J, Hubner FK et al. The garland type of acute post-infectious glomerulonephritis: morphological characteristics and follow-up studies. Clin Nephrol 1983; 20: 17–26,
63. Lange K, Seligson G, Cronin W. Evidence for the in situ origin of poststreptococcal glomerulonephritis: glomerular localization of endostreptosin and the

clinical significance of the subsequent antibody response. Clin Nephrol 1983; 19: 3–10.
64. Tresner G, Semar M, McVicar M et al. Antigenic streptococcal components in acute glomerulonephritis. Science 1969; 163: 676.
65. Vogt A, Batsford S, Rodriguez-Iturbe B, Garcia R. Cationic antigens in poststreptococcal glomerulonephritis. Clin Nephrol 1983; 20: 271–279.
66. Andres GA, Accinni L, Hsu KC, Zabriskie JB, Seegal BC. Electron microscopic studies of human glomerulonephritis with ferritin conjugated antibody. Localisation of antigen–antibody complexes in glomerular structures of patients with acute glomerulonephritis. J Exp Med 1966; 123: 399–412.
67. Dodge WF, Spargo BH, Bass JA, Travis LB. The relationship between the clinical and pathologic features of poststreptococcal glomerulonephritis. A study of the early natural history. Medicine (Baltimore) 1968; 47: 227–267.
68. Dodge WF, Spargo BH, Travis LB et al. Poststreptococcal glomerulonephritis. A prospective study in children. N Engl J Med 1972; 286: 273–278.
69. Potter EV, Lipschultz SA, Abidh S, Poon-King T, Earle DP. Twelve to seventeen year follow up of patients with poststreptococcal acute glomerulonephritis in Trinidad. N Engl J Med 1982; 307: 725–729.
70. Southwest Pediatric Nephrology Study Group. A clinicopathologic study of crescentic glomerulonephritis in 50 children. Kidney Int 1985; 27: 450–458.
71. Baldwin DS, Gluck MC, Schacht RG, Gallo G. The long term course of poststreptococcal glomerulonephritis. Ann Intern Med 1974; 80: 342–358.
72. Vogl W, Renke M, Mayer Eichberger D, Schmitt H, Bohle A. Long-term prognosis for endocapillary glomerulonephritis of poststreptococcal type in children and adults. Nephron 1986; 44: 58–65.
73. Cronin W, Deol H, Azadegan A, Lange K. Endostreptosin: isolation of the probable immunogen of acute post-streptococcal glomerulonephritis. Clin Exp Immunol 1989; 76: 198–203.
74. Vogt A, Rohrbach R, Shimizu F, Takamiya H, Batsford S. Interaction of cationized antigen with rat glomerular basement membrane: in situ immune complex formation. Kidney Int 1982; 22: 27–35.
75. Holdsworth SR. Fc dependence of macrophage accumulation and subsequent injury in experimental glomerulonephritis. J Immunol 1983; 130: 735–739.
76. McIntosh RM, Garcia R, Rubio L, Rabideau D, Rodriguez-Iturbe B. Evidence for an autologous immune complex pathogenic mechanism in acute post-streptococcal glomerulonephritis. Kidney Int 1978; 14: 501–510.

Diffuse mesangial proliferative glomerulonephritis

77. Churg J, Sobin LH. Renal disease. Classification and atlas of glomerular disease. Tokyo: Igaku-Shoin, 1982.
78. Bhasin HK, Abuelo JG, Nayak R, Esparza AR. Mesangial proliferative glomerulonephritis. Lab Invest 1978; 39: 21–29.
79. Lawler W, Williams G, Tarpey P, Mallick NP. IgM associated primary diffuse mesangial proliferative glomerulonephritis. J Clin Pathol 1980; 33: 1029–1038.
80. Pardo V, Riesgo I, Zilleruelo G, Strauss J. The clinical significance of mesangial IgM deposits and mesangial hypercellularity in minimal change nephrotic syndrome. Am J Kidney Dis 1984; 3: 264–269.
81. Grekas D, Morley AR, Wilkinson R, Kerr DNS. Isolated C3 deposition in patients without systemic disease. Clin Nephrol 1984; 21: 270–274.
82. Spargo BH, Seymour AE, Ordonez NG. Renal biopsy pathology with diagnostic and therapeutic implications. New York: John Wiley. 1980: 71.
83. Soloman LR, Cairns SA, Lawler W, Johnson RWG, Mallick NP. Reduction of post-transplant proteinuria due to recurrent mesangial proliferative (IgM) glomerulonephritis following plasma exchange. Clin Nephrol 1981; 16: 44–50.
84. Hirszel P, Yamase HT, Carney WR et al. Mesangial proliferative glomerulonephritis with IgM deposits. Clinicopathologic analysis and evidence for morphologic transitions. Nephron 1984; 38: 100–108.
85. Lovett DH, Szamel M, Ryan JL, Sterzel RB, Gemsa D, Resch K. Interleukin I and the glomerular mesangium. I. Purification and characterisation of a mesangial cell-derived autogrowth factor. J Immunol 1986; 136: 3700–3705.

IgA nephropathy

86. Makdassy R, Beaufils M, Meyrier A et al. Conditions associated with IgA mesangial nephropathy: preliminary results. Contrib Nephrol 1984; 40: 292–295.
87. Pape JF, Mellbye OJ, Oystese B, Brodwall EK. Glomerulonephritis in dermatitis herpetiformis. Acta Med Scand 1978; 203: 445–448.
88. Sinniah R. Mucus secreting cancer with mesangial IgA deposits. Pathology 1982; 14: 303–308.
89. Dosa S, Cairns SA, Mallick NP et al. Relapsing Henoch–Schönlein syndrome with renal involvement in a patient with an IgA monoclonal gammopathy. Nephron 1980; 26: 145–148.
90. BénéMC, De Ligny BH, Sirbat D, Faure G, Kessler M, Duheille J. IgA nephropathy: dimeric IgA-secreting cells are present in episcleral infiltrate. Am J Clin Pathol 1984; 82: 608–611.
91. Ramirez G, Stinson JB, Zawada ET, Moatamed F. IgA nephritis associated with mycosis fungoides. Report of two cases. Arch Intern Med 1981; 141: 1287–1291.
92. Julian BA, Quiggins PA, Thompson JS, Woodford SY, Gleason K, Wyatt RJ. Familial IgA nephropathy. Evidence of an inherited mechanism of disease. N Engl J Med 1985; 312: 202–208.
93. Berger J, Hinglais N. Les dépots intracapillaires d'IgA-IgG. J Urol Nephrol 1968; 74: 694–695.
94. Levy M, Berger J. Worldwide perspective of IgA nephropathy. Am J Kidney Dis 1988; 12: 340–347.
95. Nakamoto Y, Asano Y, Dahi K et al. Primary IgA glomerulonephritis and Schönlein–Henoch purpura nephritis: clinicopathological and immunohistological characteristics. Q J Med 1978; 47: 495–516.
96. Davison AM. Idiopathic IgA nephropathy in the United Kingdom: findings from the UK Medical Research Council's glomerulonephritis registry. Ninth. International Congress of Nephrology 1984: 81A (abstr).
97. Ballardie FW, O'Donoghue DJ, Feehally J. Increasing frequency of adult IgA nephropathy in the UK? Lancet 1987; 2: 1205 (letter).

98. Emancipator SN, Lamm ME. IgA nephropathy: pathogenesis of the most common form of glomerulonephritis. Lab Invest 1989; 60: 168–183.
99. Pettersson E, von Bonsdorff M, Törnroth T, Lindholm H. Nephritis among young Finnish men. Clin Nephrol 984; 22: 217–222.
100. Jennette JC, Wall SD, Wilkman AS. Low incidence of IgA nephropathy in blacks. Kidney Int 1985; 28: 944–950.
101. D'Amico G. Clinical features and natural history in adults with IgA nephropathy. Am J Kidney Dis 1988; 12: 353–357.
102. Hogg RJ. IgA nephropathy: clinical features and natural history – a pediatric perspective. Am J Kidney Dis 1988; 12: 358–361.
103. Lomax-Smith JD, Woodroffe AJ, Clarkson AR, Seymour AE. IgA nephropathy – accumulated experience and current concepts. Pathology 1985; 17: 219–224.
104. Berthoux FC, Genin C, Le Petit JC, Laurent B. Immunogenetics of mesangial IgA nephritis. Contrib Nephrol 1984; 40: 118–123.
105. Moore RH, Hitman GA, Lucas EY et al. HLA DQ region gene polymorphism associated with primary IgA nephropathy. Kidney Int 1990; 37: 991–995.
106. Feehally J, Beattie J, Brenchley PEC, Coupes BM, Mallick NP, Postlethwaite RJ. Sequential study of the IgA system in relapsing IgA nephropathy. Kidney Int 1986; 30: 924–931.
107. Emancipator SN, Gallo GR, Lamm ME. IgA nephropathy: perspectives on pathogenesis and classification. Clin Nephrol 1985; 24: 161–179.
108. Morita M, Sakaguchi H. A quantitative study of glomerular basement membrane changes in IgA nephropathy. J Pathol 1988; 154: 7–18.
109. Lai K-N, Chui SH, Lai FM-M, Lam CWK. Predominant synthesis of IgA with lambda light chain in IgA nephropathy. Kidney Int 1988; 33: 584–589.
110. Tomino Y, Yagame M, Eguchi K, Nomoto Y, Sakai H. Immunofluorescent studies on S-protein in glomeruli from patients with IgA nephropathy. Am J Pathol 1987; 129: 402–406.
111. Monteiro RC, Halbwachs-Mecarelli L, Roque-Barreira MC, Noël L-H, Berger J, Lesavre P. Charge and size of mesangial IgA in IgA nephropathy. Kidney Int 1985; 28: 666–671.
112. Tomino Y, Sakai H, Miura M, Nomoto Y, Umehara K, Hashimoto K. Detection of antigenic substances in patients with IgA nephropathy. Contrib Nephrol 1984; 40: 69–73.
113. Tomino Y, Nomoto Y, Endoh M, Sakai M. Deposition of IgA dominant immune complexes in muscular vessels from patients with IgA nephropathy. Acta Pathol Jpn 1981; 31: 361–365.
114. Hasbargen JA, Copley JB. Utility of skin biopsy in the diagnosis of IgA nephropathy. Am J Kidney Dis 1985; 6: 100–102.
115. Jennette JC. The immunohistology of IgA nephropathy. Am J Kidney Dis 1988; 12: 348–352.
116. Abuelo JG, Esparza AR, Matarese RA, Endreny RG, Carvalho JS, Allegra SR. Crescentic IgA nephropathy. Medicine (Baltimore) 1984; 63: 396–406.
117. Habib R, Antignac C, Hinglais N, Gagnadoux M-F, Broyer M. Glomerular lesions in the transplanted kidney in children. Am J Kidney Dis 1987; 10: 198–207.
118. Berger J. Recurrence of IgA nephropathy in renal allografts. Am J Kidney Dis 1988; 12: 371–372.
119. Droz D. Natural history of primary glomerulonephritis with mesangial deposits of IgA. Contrib Nephrol 1976; 2: 150–157.
120. Disney APS, ed. Australian and New Zealand Dialysis and Transplant Registry. Seventh report. Adelaide: Queen Elizabeth Hospital, 1984.
121. Gallo GR, Katafuchi R, Neelakantappa K, Baldwin DS. Prognostic pathologic markers in IgA nephropathy. Am J Kidney Dis 1988; 12: 362–365.
122. Bene MC, Faure G. IgA nephropathy. Springer Semin Immunopathol 1987; 9: 387–394.
123. D'Amico G. The commonest glomerulonephritis in the world: IgA nephropathy. Q J Med 1987; 64: 709–727.
124. Rostoker G, Laurent J, Andre C, Cholin S, Lagrue G. High levels of IgA antigliadin antibodies in patients who have IgA mesangial glomerulonephritis but not coeliac disease. Lancet 1988; 1: 356–357 (letter).

Diffuse mesangiocapillary glomerulonephritis

125. Habib R, Kleinknecht C, Gubler MC, Levy M. Idiopathic membranoproliferative glomerulonephritis in children. Report of 105 cases. Clin Nephrol 1973; 1: 194–214.
126. Gonzalo A, Matesanz R, Teruel JL, Ortuno J. Incidence of membranoproliferative glomerulonephritis in a Spanish population. Clin Nephrol 1986; 26: 161.
127. Cameron JS, Turner DR, Heaton J et al. Idiopathic mesangiocapillary glomerulonephritis. Comparison of types I and II in children and adults and long term prognosis. Am J Med 1983; 74: 175–192.
128. Kim Y, Michael AF. Idiopathic membranoproliferative glomerulonephritis. Ann Rev Med 1980; 31: 273–288.
129. Scott DM, Amos N, Sissons JGP, Lachmann PJ, Peters DK. The immunological nature of nephritic factor. Clin Exp Immunol 1978; 32: 12–24.
130. Mollnes TE, Ng YC, Peters DK, Lea T, Tschopp J, Harboe M. Effect of nephritic factor on C3 and on the terminal pathway of complement *in vivo* and *in vitro*. Clin Exp Immunol 1986; 65: 73–79.
131. Tanuma Y, Ohi H, Watanabe S, Seki M, Hatano M. C3 nephritic factor and C4 nephritic factor in the serum of two patients with hypocomplimentaemic membranoproliferative glomerulonephritis. Clin Exp Immunol 1989; 76: 82–85.
132. Davis CA, Marder H, West CD. Circulating immune complexes in membranoproliferative glomerulonephritis. Kidney Int 1981; 20: 728–732.
133. Korzets Z, Bernheim J, Bernheim J. Rapidly progressive glomerulonephritis (crescentic glomerulonephritis) in the course of Type I idiopathic membranoproliferative glomerulonephritis. Am J Kidney Dis 1987; 10: 56–61.
134. Taguchi T, Bohle A. Evaluation of change with time of glomerular morphology in membranoproliferative glomerulonephritis: a serial biopsy study of 33 cases. Clin Nephrol 1989; 31: 297–306.
135. Arakawa M, Kimmelstiel P. Circumferential mesangial interposition. Lab Invest 1969; 21: 276–284.
136. Bannister KM, Howarth GS, Clarkson AR, Woodroffe AJ. Glomerular IgG subclass distribution in human glomerulonephritis. Clin Nephrol 1983; 19: 161–165.

137. Donadia JV, Anderson CF, Mitchell JC et al. Membranoproliferative glomerulonephritis. A prospective clinical trial of platelet-inhibitor therapy. N Engl J Med 1984; 310: 1421–1426.
138. Peters DK, Williams DG, Charlesworth JA, et al. Mesangiocapillary glomerulonephritis, partial lipodystrophy and hypocomplementaemia. Lancet 1973; 2: 535–538.
139. Mandalenakis N, Mendoza N, Pirani CL, Pollak VE. Lobular glomerulonephritis and membranoproliferative glomerulonephritis: a clinical and pathologic study based on renal biopsies. Medicine (Baltimore) 1971; 50: 319–355.
140. Stutchfield PR, White RHR, Cameron AH, Thompson RA, Mackintosh P, Wells L. X-linked mesangiocapillary glomerulonephritis. Clin Nephrol 1986; 26:150–156.
141. Welch TR, Beischel L, Balakrisknan K, Quinlan M, West CD. Major-histocompatibility-complex extended haplotypes in membranoproliferative glomerulonephritis. N Engl J Med 1986; 23: 1476–1481.
142. Jackson EC, McAdams AJ, Strife CF, Forristal J, Welch TR, West CD. Differences between membranoproliferative glomerulonephritis types I and III in clinical presentation, glomerular morphology, and complement perturbation. Am J Kidney Dis 1987; 9: 115–120.
143. Watson AR, Poucell S, Thorner P, Arbus GS, Rance CP, Baumal R. Membranoproliferative glomerulonephritis type I in children: correlation of clinical features with pathologic subtypes. Am J Kidney Dis 1984; 4: 141–146.

7

K. A. Porter

Primary glomerulonephritis 3

DENSE DEPOSIT DISEASE (MESANGIOCAPILLARY GLOMERULONEPHRITIS TYPE II)

The distinguishing feature of dense deposit disease is a unique replacement of long lengths of the glomerular, tubular and splenic basement membranes and of Bowman's capsule by material of exceptional electron density when examined in tissue fixed in osmium tetroxide. This electron-dense material does not react with labelled antisera to immunoglobulins. The replacement of the basement membrane by electron-dense material usually causes thickening of the glomerular capillary walls; mesangial interposition with apparent duplication of the basement membrane is only occasionally present. The basement membrane thickening is accompanied by a variable amount of expansion of the mesangium and increase in the number of mesangial cells.

Dense deposit disease is a chronic progressive condition affecting older children and young adults. It often presents with a nephrotic syndrome, an acute nephritic syndrome, or an episode of macroscopic haematuria. Most patients with dense deposit disease show a persistent and profound depletion of serum C3, with normal values for the early acting components. In about 70% of cases the serum contains C3 nephritic factor (NeF). About half of those affected need dialysis or renal transplantation within 10 years. A further third become uraemic within the same period.[1]

In the majority of patients no cause is apparent; in about 10% the disease is associated with partial lipodystrophy (see p. 260).Very occasionally it occurs with infections such as pneumococcal pneumonia,[2] streptococcal pharyngitis,[3] systemic candidosis[4] and tuberculosis.[5] One patient had disseminated melanoma.[6] It has also been recorded in association with an inherited defect of the protein H (beta-1H-globulin) which is important in the control of the alternative pathway of complement activation.[7] The following account deals with the idiopathic form of the disease.

Clinical features

Dense deposit disease occurs most frequently in children over the age of 3 years and in young adults. It is a rare condition but there are no reliable data on its incidence. There is a slight predominance of male patients.[8] Clinical signs and symptoms often follow an upper respiratory tract infection. About half the patients present with the nephrotic syndrome, 20% with an acute nephritic syndrome and the others with either persistent proteinuria or recurrent haematuria. Microscopic haematuria is present in 90%; isolated macroscopic haematuria (not part of an acute nephritic syndrome) occurs in about a third of the patients.[1] Rapidly progressive renal failure may occur at any stage of the disease due to the development of diffuse crescentic glomerulonephritis (see p. 185); this occurs more frequently in dense deposit disease than in diffuse mesangiocapillary glomerulonephritis.

Serology

Approximately 65% of all patients with dense deposit disease have a reduced level of C3 in the serum at presentation; in children the proportion is about 75%.[1] In most cases the depression of the C3 level is persistent and results from both an increase in catabolism of this complement component and a decrease in its synthesis. The levels of the early acting components of complement, C1q and C4, are usually normal. The IgG autoantibody, C3 nephritic factor (NeF) (see p. 165), is commonly present. In one series NeF was discovered in 71% of children with dense deposit disease and in 57% of those who developed the disease in adult life.[1] Circulating immune complexes are found in some patients.[9]

Renal changes

Light microscopy[10–12]

In the majority of cases all the glomeruli show marked eosinophilic ribbon-like thickening of the capillary walls. The eosinophilic membranes stain red with periodic acid-Schiff, green with Masson trichrome and light brown (not black) with silver. The membranes are also slightly birefringent and fluoresce brightly with thioflavine T. Although these membrane changes are characteristic they are not pathognomonic: occasionally they are simulated by other conditions in which there are extensive basement membrane deposits. In approximately 60% of cases the number of mesangial cells and the amount of mesangial matrix are diffusely increased, usually mildly to moderately but sometimes more markedly, with accentuation of the lobularity of the glomerular tuft (Fig. 7.1). Eosinophilic material is also present as nodules in the mesangium and as interrupted

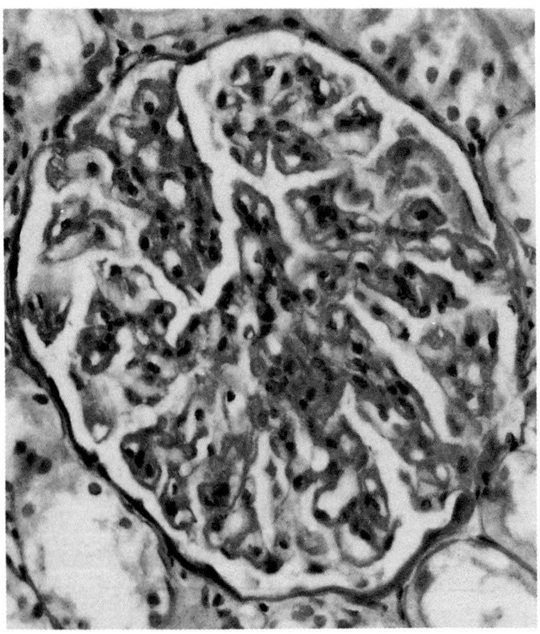

Fig. 7.1 Dense deposit disease. The glomerular tuft lobularity is accentuated, the number of mesangial cells and the amount of mesangial matrix are increased and there is continuous ribbon-like thickening of the capillary walls and Bowman's capsule by PAS-positive material. There are also PAS-positive granules in the mesangium.
Periodic acid-Schiff × 500

linear masses of different lengths in Bowman's capsule, on the proximal convoluted tubular basement membranes and in the membranes of peritubular capillaries and in the walls of arterioles. In about 60% of patients there are also some glomerular capsular crescents; in one study 20% or more of the glomeruli were affected in 36% of the patients. Variable numbers of sclerosed glomeruli are present in about 40% of patients.[1] Focal segmental fibrinoid necrosis in the glomerular tufts and an increase in the number of neutrophil granulocytes within glomerular capillaries occurs in approximately 30% of cases.[12] There may also be segmental duplication of capillary basement membranes. Mild focal mononuclear cell infiltration of the interstitium and focal tubular atrophy are common.

About 10% of patients when first biopsied only show a mild focal and segmental mesangial proliferative glomerulonephritis and the membrane changes may be so slight that they are easily missed by light microscopy.[12]

Electron microscopy is necessary in all cases, firstly to detect the disease in its early stages and secondly to confirm the diagnosis in those with obvious eosinophilic refractile basement membrane thickening.

Electron microscopy

The lamina densa of the glomerular capillary basement membranes is replaced by linear or fusiform masses of homogeneous material of exceptional electron density which appear almost black in electron micrographs (Figs 7.2, 7.3). The width of the thickened basement membranes is usually between 500 and 1500 nm (normal 250–350 nm). In most patients the extremely

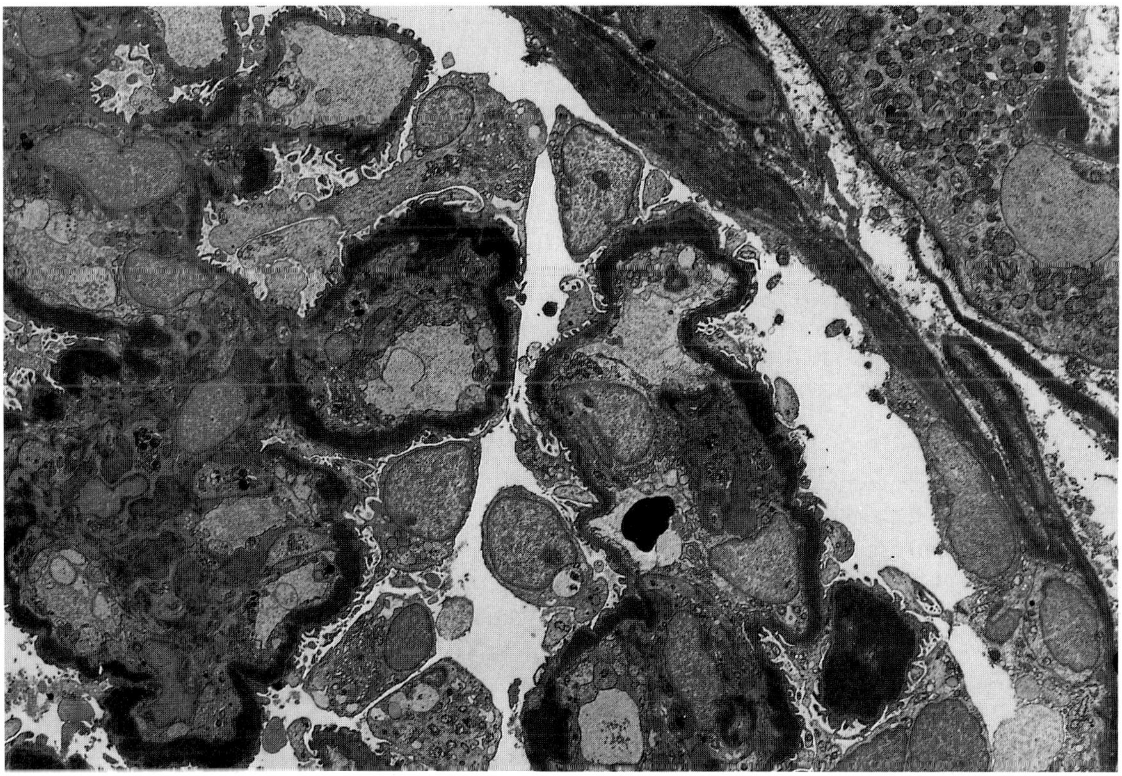

Fig. 7.2 Dense deposit disease. Electron micrograph of part of a glomerular tuft. The lamina densa of the capillary basement membranes is replaced and thickened by homogeneous extremely electron-dense material. Similar material is also present on the outer aspect of Bowman's capsule and on the basement membranes of a peritubular capillary and a tubule. ×1770

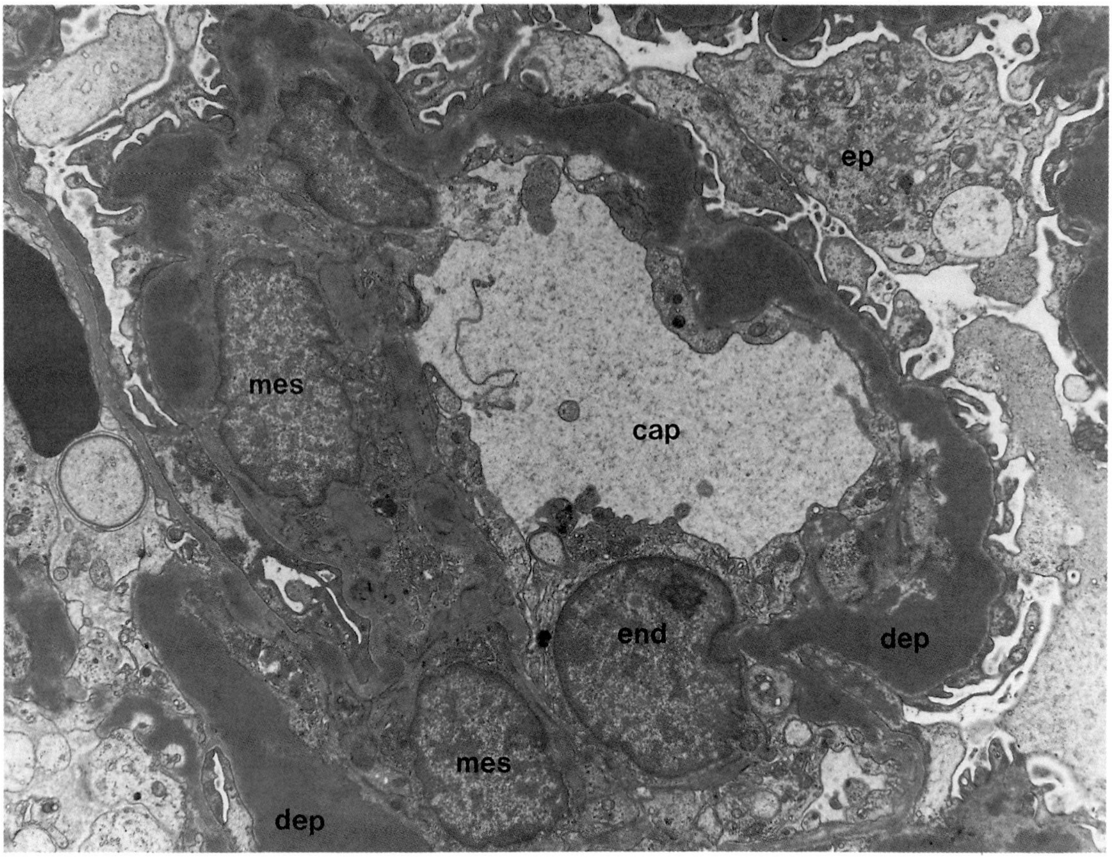

Fig. 7.3 Dense deposit disease. Electron micrograph of part of a glomerulus. Segments of the lamina densa of the capillary basement membranes are replaced by a wide irregular band of osmiophilic material (dep) that is much more electron dense than normal lamina densa. Small nodules of similar material are also present in the mesangial matrix. There is some mesangial cell interposition. The foot processes of the epithelial cells are partially retracted. cap, capllary lumen; end, endothelial cell; ep, epithelial cell; mes, mesangial cell.
×3370

electron-dense material is present in the majority of the capillary loops in many of the glomeruli.[10,11] In a few patients the changes are segmental and affect predominantly the lamina densa adjacent to the mesangium.[11] Similar very electron-dense material is often present as nodules in the mesangial matrix (Fig. 7.3) and as segmental linear deposits on the external side of Bowman's capsule, on the basement membranes of the proximal convoluted tubules and peritubular capillaries (Fig. 7.2), and on the internal elastic lamina of arterioles.[11] Subepithelial humps (see p. 147), composed of the less electron-dense finely granular material that is usual in immune deposits, are sometimes found. Occasionally there are also flattened subepithelial immune deposits flanked on either side by spikes of new basement membrane. Obliteration of visceral epithelial foot processes and small amounts of mesangial interposition are usually present.

Immunofluorescence/immunoperoxidase microscopy[11,12]

In the glomeruli of many of the patients C3 is present, coating the collections of very electron-dense material. This gives the appearance under low power magnification of strongly stained

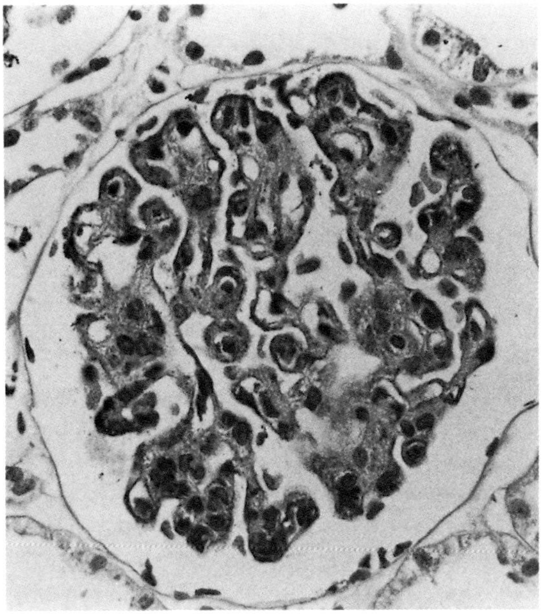

Fig. 7.4 Dense deposit disease. Glomerulus showing staining for C3 along the capillary walls and fine granules of the same complement component in the mesangium.
Immunoperoxidase × 250

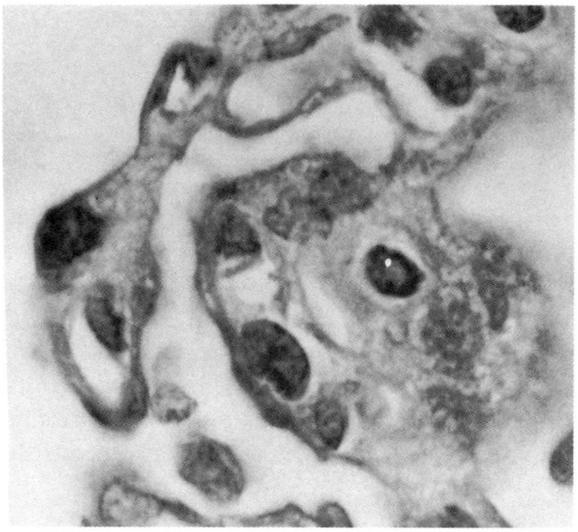

Fig. 7.5 Dense deposit disease. Part of a glomerulus showing staining for C3 on either side of the very electron-dense material in the capillary walls. In the mesangium on each nodule of deposit an outer ring of C3 surrounds an unstained core.
Immunoperoxidase × 600

coarse and fine granules in the mesangium and faint continuous or interrupted linear staining of the capillary walls (Fig. 7.4). Deposits of C3 are also often present as segments of variable thickness in Bowman's capsule and on the basement membranes of the proximal tubules. Under higher magnification the staining of the glomerular capillary wall appears as parallel thin strips of C3 on either side of the unstained very electron-dense material. Similarly, the mesangial granules appear as rings of C3 with unstained centres (Fig. 7.5).

In about a quarter of the cases, superimposed on this pattern there are scattered granules of C3 and IgM in the glomerular capillary walls, corresponding to the subepithelial humps. Staining for IgG or IgA is less common. In some patients, more than a third in one series[1], there is no staining for any immunoglobulins or complement components.

Changes in other organs

Spleen

Accumulations of extremely electron-dense material, similar to that in renal basement membranes, occur in the basement membranes of the sinusoids of the spleen, but not in other organs.[13]

Differential diagnosis

So long as electron microscopy is undertaken there is little difficulty in the diagnosis of dense deposit disease. *Light chain deposition disease* is superficially similar but the very electron-dense material lies principally in the lamina rara interna, is distinctly granular and on immunofluorescence or immunoperoxidase microscopy contains predominantly kappa or lambda light chains (see p. 362). Intramembranous deposits are found in the *type III variant of mesangiocapillary glomerulonephritis*, but these are not exceptionally electron dense, they are associated with disruption of the basement membrane and they contain immunoglobulins and complement (see p. 171).

Complications

Diffuse crescentic glomerulonephritis

The development of diffuse crescentic glomerulonephritis may occur at any time during the course of dense deposit disease. It leads to the rapid onset of renal failure.[11]

Renal transplantation

Dense deposit disease almost always recurs in transplanted kidneys (see p. 666).[14] The appearance of dense material in the basement membranes of the renal allograft has been observed as early as 20 days after transplantation.[15] It has also been known to affect two sequential allografts in the same patient. The dense material first appears near the vascular pole of the glomerulus in that part of the lamina densa that overlies the mesangium; from there it spreads to the peripheral capillary walls. The clinical manifestations of recurrence are usually moderate proteinuria with or without haematuria. Progressive renal failure is unusual; only about 10% of patients develop severe disease that leads to loss of the graft. Because so few grafts are lost through recurrent disease, the presence of dense deposit disease in a patient should not deter one from using renal transplantation in treatment.

Prognosis

About 50% of patients with dense deposit disease need dialysis or renal transplantation within 10 years[1,11] but the prognosis is not uniform. Some patients have a rapidly progressive course and develop end-stage renal disease within 2 years, whereas a number, varying from 28% to 63% in different series,[8] pursue a relatively benign course and show no evidence of renal insufficiency 10 years after the onset of dense deposit disease. It has been suggested that the focal segmental variety of dense deposit disease is more likely to follow this benign course.[16] Spontaneous remission is very rare. Partial regression of the lesion occasionally occurs.[17] A persistent nephrotic syndrome, gross haematuria and the presence of sclerosis or capsular crescents in the initial renal biopsy appear to indicate a poor outcome.[1,18]

The role of steroid therapy in patients with dense deposit disease remains controversial but most reports show no significant benefit.[8] A recent study, however, suggests that after 6–11 years of continuous alternate-day treatment with prednisone, the amount of mesangial cell proliferation may decrease and the patency of the glomerular capillaries improve. This may be accompanied by a change in position of the dense deposit in the glomerular basement membranes from the lamina densa to the lamina rara interna. Occasionally the dense material disappears from the capillary basement membranes, but deposits usually remain in the mesangium.[19]

Pathogenesis

The pathogenesis of dense deposit disease is unknown. The occasional association with streptococcal, pneumococcal and other infections might suggest that it is an unusual form of immune complex disease, but the very electron-dense material does not contain immunoglobulin and only its surface appears to bind C3.

Originally it was thought that dense deposit disease was due to a primary metabolic abnormality of basement membrane synthesis.[10] The highly osmiophilic component of the deposit can be extracted with lipid solvents; it is most likely to be a compound rich in unsaturated fatty acids.[20] Biochemical studies have shown that the altered basement membranes quantitatively contain more sialic acid and less cystine than normal basement membranes.[10] The basement membranes also selectively bind the lecithin wheat germ agglutinin or its succinylated derivative, indicating that the dense material contains appreciable quantities of internally linked *N*-acetylglucosamine.[21] However, the rapid appearance of the very electron-dense material in renal allografts indicates that some circulating factor is responsible and this observation seems incompatible with the notion that dense deposit disease is due to a primary metabolic abnormality of basement membrane synthesis.

The unifying feature of all of the conditions associated with dense deposit disease, and in most of the patients with the idiopathic condition, is a low level of serum C3 with normal C1 and C4 levels, which indicates activation of the alternative complement pathway although it is difficult to see how this might interfere with basement membrane metabolism. Also, a few patients with idiopathic dense deposit disease have normal serum levels of C3,[11] and prolonged systemic activation of the alternative complement pathway in rabbits has not produced glomerular disease.[22] There is no evidence that the C3 nephritic factor (NeF) plays a primary role in the pathogenesis of dense deposit disease.

The subepithelial humps often seen in patients with dense deposit disease may be due to superimposed immune complex disease because of impaired clearance of circulating immune complexes secondary to depletion of C3.

DIFFUSE CRESCENTIC GLOMERULONEPHRITIS

Diffuse crescentic glomerulonephritis is a rare condition characterized by the presence in the majority of glomeruli of large collections of proliferating cells on the inside of Bowman's capsule. The cell collections, which protrude into the urinary space, are called *crescents* because, when cross sectioned and viewed by light microscopy, they often look like a quarter moon. A crescent probably forms in response to a sudden release of a large quantity of plasma into Bowman's space following a rupture in the glomerular capillary basement membrane.

Most patients present with the acute nephritic syndrome and the clinical course is often fulminant. This, together with recent therapeutic advances which may alter that course, makes it imperative that an accurate diagnosis is achieved as soon as possible and treatment started.

There is no agreement on the number and size of crescents that are necessary before a patient is included in the diagnostic category of diffuse crescentic glomerulonephritis; in the World Health Organization classification of glomerular disease it is suggested that at least 50% and usually 80% of the glomeruli should contain large occluding crescents.[23] The arbitrary figure of 80% is used by many pathologists in defining diffuse crescentic glomerulonephritis. Only those crescents that cover 60% or more of the circumference of the glomerulus are counted.

In approximately 60% of patients the condition develops as a complication during the course of some other disease such as microscopic polyarteritis (see p. 273), Wegener's granulomatosis (see p. 277), antiglomerular basement membrane disease (see p. 221), Goodpasture's syndrome (see p. 224), diffuse endocapillary proliferative glomerulonephritis (see p. 152), Henoch–Schönlein purpura (see p. 256), systemic lupus erythematosus (see p. 230) and dense deposit disease (see p. 183). In other cases either there is no evidence of a primary disease or the crescents are so florid that it is not possible to detect any underlying lesion. The account in this chapter is confined to the idiopathic form of diffuse crescentic glomerulonephritis.

Smaller numbers of crescents are encountered in many conditions, including essential mixed cryoglobulinaemia (see p. 352), diffuse mesangiocapillary glomerulonephritis (see p. 166), systemic lupus erythematosus (see p. 230), the haemolytic uraemic syndrome (see p. 283), subacute infective endocarditis (see p. 375) and other forms of postinfectious nephritis (see p. 380), malignant hypertension (see p. 312), membranous glomerulonephritis (see p. 200), alpha-1-antitrypsin deficiency (see p. 110), hereditary nephritis (see p. 75), IgA nephropathy (see p. 163), various types of cancer (see p. 616), relapsing polychondritis (see p. 257) and relapsing pancreatitis. In these diseases it is rare for the number of glomeruli with crescents to reach 80% but this can happen.

As crescent formation in the glomerulus is fast and leads to permanent scarring of the tuft, it is essential to rapidly diagnose the underlying disease that is causing the capillary walls to rupture before a large number of glomeruli are irreparably damaged. Patients in whom more than 70% of the glomeruli contain crescents rarely recover any renal function.[24]

Examination of a renal biopsy is the single most important procedure in distinguishing between the various causes of crescentic glomerulonephritis.

Clinical features

Idiopathic diffuse crescentic glomerulonephritis is commonest in adults, particularly the middle aged and elderly (mean age 58 years); it is rare in children. Males are affected more than females.

Most patients present with acute or rapidly progressive renal failure but sometimes the onset is more insidious.[24-26] Oliguria is frequent. The blood pressure is usually normal. All have at least moderate microscopic haematuria (more than 100 red cells/μl) and some have macroscopic haematuria. Most have proteinuria, occasionally in excess of 3.5 g/day, but the nephrotic syndrome is unusual. About half the patients give a preceding history of pain in muscles, joints, loins, back or abdomen with fever and malaise.[25] In a few the prodromal symptoms last for several weeks or months.[26] Progression to end-stage renal failure often occurs within 1–2 weeks.[25]

Serology

To exclude antiglomerular-basement-membrane-antibody disease these antibodies must be sought (see p. 218); if the diffuse crescentic glomerulonephritis is idiopathic they should be absent from the serum. In microscopic polyarteritis and Wegener's granulomatosis the serum usually contains antibodies to neutrophil cytoplasmic antigen (see p. 272); in idiopathic diffuse crescentic glomerulonephritis these antibodies should not be present.[27] The antinuclear factor (ANF) is negative in the idiopathic disease, and the antistreptolysin (ASO) titres are not raised. The serum complement levels are normal. Assays for circulating immune complexes are generally negative.[25]

Renal changes

Gross appearance of the kidneys

The kidneys are enlarged. Their subcapsular surface is smooth and there may be petechial haemorrhages.

Light microscopy

The most striking change is cellular proliferation, more than two cells thick and confined to Bowman's space, in 80% or more of the glomeruli (Fig. 7.6). The cells composing the crescent range from spindle to oval in form. Most have abundant clear cytoplasm but some are small and dark. There may be groups of macrophage-like cells

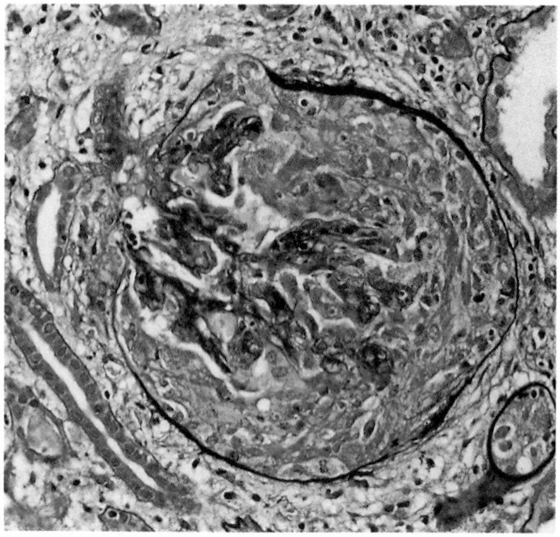

Fig. 7.6 Idiopathic diffuse crescentic glomerulonephritis. Glomerulus with large cellular crescent that fills Bowman's space. The tuft is compressed.
Periodic acid-Schiff × 350

clustered around fragments of basement membrane.[28] Mitotic figures are frequently found in the proliferating cells. The crescent may cover a part or the whole of the glomerular circumference and in some cases may almost fill Bowman's space. Neutrophil granulocytes, fibrin and red cells are frequently found amongst the proliferating cells. Occasionally multinucleate giant cells are present. Cellular crescents sometimes resolve but more often strands of PAS-positive basement-membrane-like material and collagen soon appear among the cells, transforming the cellular crescents into fibrocellular crescents.[28] Staining with monoclonal antibodies shows the presence of types IV and V collagen and of laminin and fibronectin.[29] Eventually the crescents become largely fibrous. This progression is rapid, occurring in the course of 3–4 weeks. Cellular, fibrocellular and fibrous crescents often coexist in the same kidney. In some glomeruli with fully circumferential crescents there is rupture of Bowman's capsule and the glomerulus becomes surrounded by mononuclear cells (Fig. 7.7). Sometimes this is followed by the disappearance of Bowman's capsule, collapse and obliteration of the tuft and periglomerular fibrosis and mononuclear cell infiltration (Fig. 7.8).

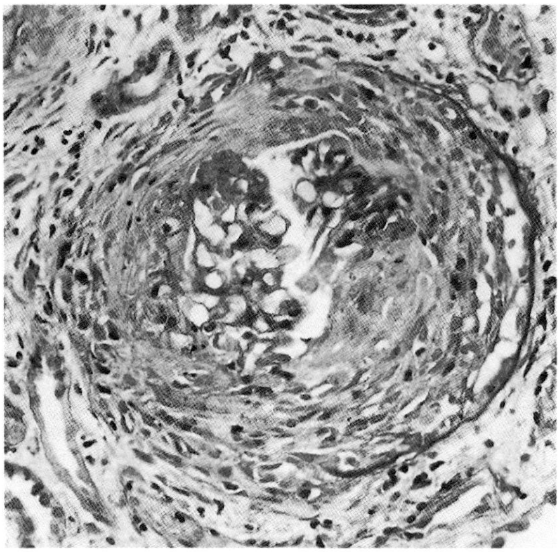

Fig. 7.7 Idiopathic diffuse crescentic glomerulonephritis. A collapsed glomerular tuft is surrounded by a large circumferential fibrocellular crescent. Bowman's capsule is ruptured.
Periodic acid-Schiff × 330

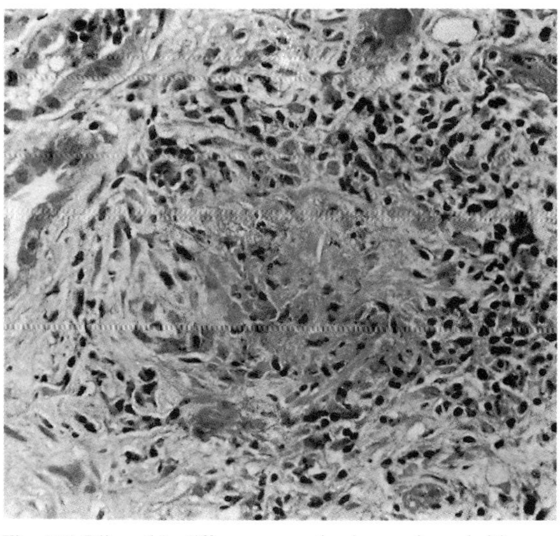

Fig. 7.8 Idiopathic diffuse crescentic glomerulonephritis. Obsolete glomerulus surrounded by an area of fibrosis and mononuclear cell infiltration. Bowman's capsule has disappeared.
Periodic acid-Schiff × 350

In idiopathic diffuse crescentic glomerulonephritis the glomerular tufts are often collapsed. Segmental lesions, consisting of rupture of the glomerular capillary basement membrane surrounded by fibrin and neutrophil granulocytes, and thrombi in a few capillary loops, are usually present but often in only a few glomeruli. There is little if any proliferation of mesangial or endothelial cells.

The tubules frequently contain red blood cells and red cell casts; tubular atrophy develops very rapidly. The arterioles and arteries may show changes brought about by hypertension and ageing. The interstitium is oedematous and there is a focal infiltration with lymphocytes, plasma cells, macrophages and sometimes granulocytes. Later there is fibrosis.

Electron microscopy

Cellular crescents are composed of multiple layers of cells. Some of the cells have a light staining nucleus and voluminous cytoplasm that contains only a few scattered profiles of endoplasmic reticulum and small mitochondria; others have dark staining nuclei and dark cytoplasm filled with rough endoplasmic reticulum and ribosomes.[28] Macrophages and fibroblasts are sometimes recognizable. Between the groups of cells are strands of fibrin and a few red cells.

As the crescent matures the cells flatten and arrange themselves into concentric layers parallel to Bowman's capsule and fine collagen fibrils and basement-membrane-like material appear. Eventually collagen replaces the cells and only small fragments of cytoplasm remain.[28]

The visceral epithelial cells enlarge and their foot processes become obliterated focally or diffusely. In the glomerular tuft segments of some capillary loops are thrombosed and there are breaks in the capillary basement membrane with fibrin extravasation into Bowman's space (Fig. 7.9). The perforations in the capillary basement membrane are beautifully shown in scanning electron microscopy of preparations in which the cells have been digested away from the glomerular capillary wall leaving only the basement membrane. The perforations are round or oval, vary greatly in size, tend to cluster within an affected lobule and have edges that curl slightly into the capillary lumen (Fig. 7.10).[30] In idiopathic diffuse crescentic glomerulonephritis there are no capillary wall or mesangial electron-dense deposits.

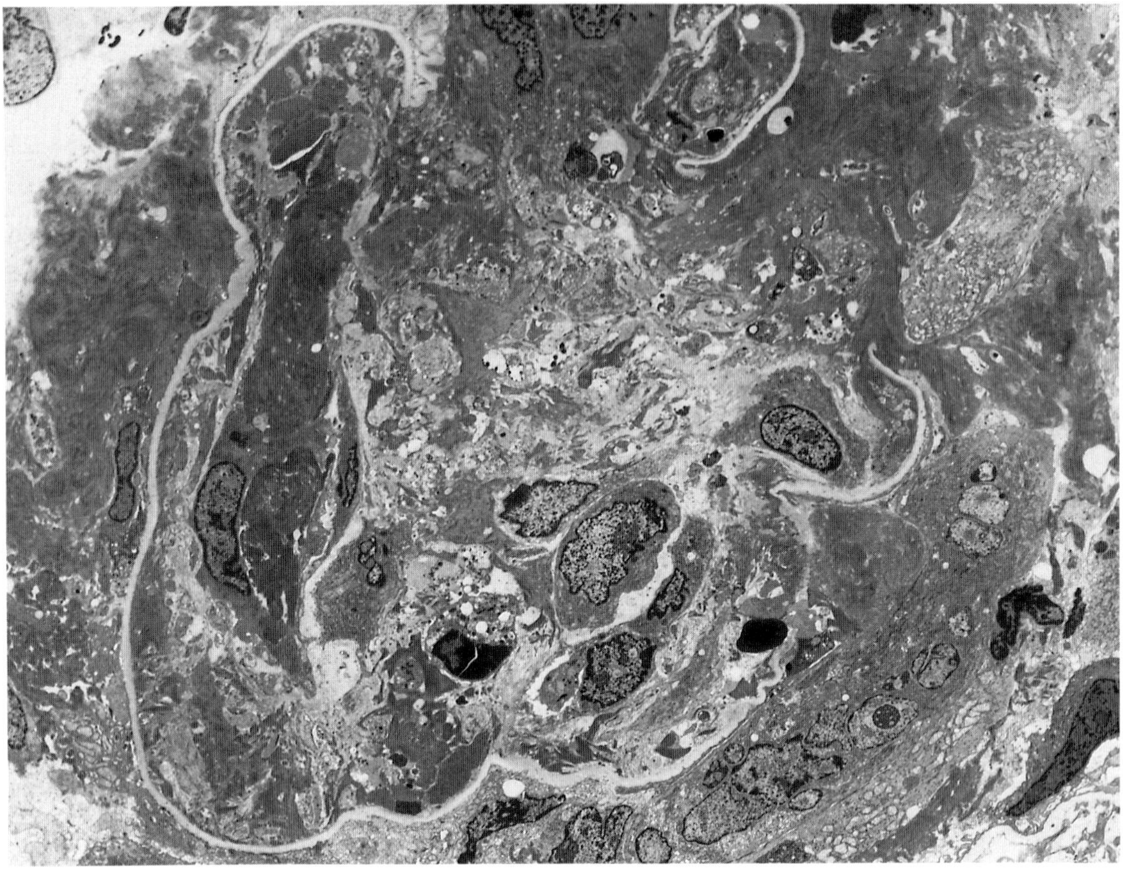

Fig. 7.9 Idiopathic diffuse crescentic glomerulonephritis. Electron micrograph of part of a glomerulus. The basement membrane of a capillary loop (which appears as a white line) is disrupted in two places. The gaps are filled with fibrin and the urinary space contains fibrin in different stages of polymerization.
× 2020

Immunofluorescence/immunoperoxidase microscopy

Immunofluorescence and immunoperoxidase studies are usually negative in idiopathic diffuse crescentic glomerulonephritis. Sometimes there is segmental localization of small quantities of C3, C4 and occasionally IgM or IgG in capillary walls and mesangium.[26]

Immunohistochemistry

Phenotyping, using monoclonal antibodies, reveals that large numbers of macrophages are present in the crescents. The glomerular tufts contain increased numbers of both macrophages and T lymphocytes; the lymphocytes are predominantly cluster designation 4 (CD4) positive. The numbers of T lymphocytes infiltrating the glomeruli diminish as the disease progresses. The cells infiltrating the interstitium are mostly a mixture of CD4+ and CD8+ T lymphocytes with the CD4+ cells being twice as common as the CD8+. Some B lymphocytes are also present.[31]

Differential diagnosis

Crescent formation is always a complication of some underlying disease and for two reasons it is most important to establish the primary diagnosis as quickly as possible. First, the type of treatment selected depends on that diagnosis; no one form

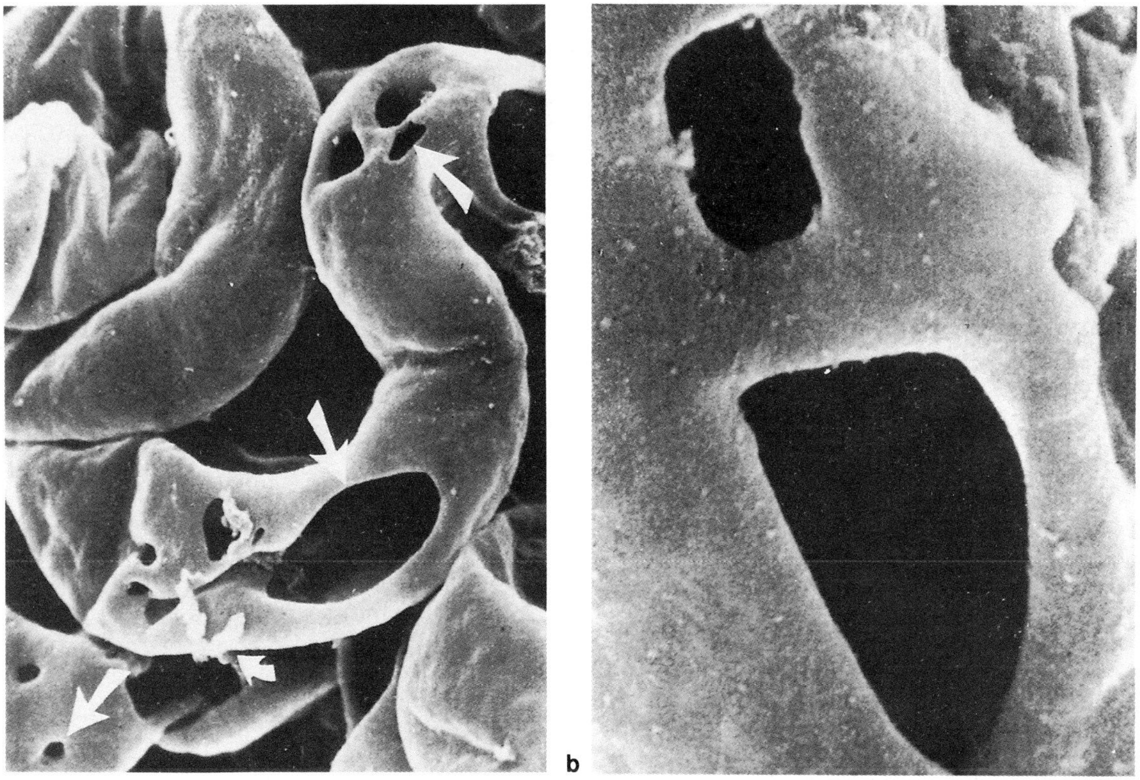

a b

Fig. 7.10 Diffuse crescentic glomerulonephritis. (**a**) Scanning electron micrograph of a glomerular capillary loop after digestion of the cells leaving only the basement membrane. There are multiple perforations (arrows) of variable sizes in the membrane. The curved arrow indicates residual tissue debris. (**b**) Two perforations in a glomerular capillary. The sharply demarcated edges curl slightly into the capillary lumen.
(**a**) × 2000; (**b**) × 6000
Reproduced by permission from: Bonsib SM. Am J Pathol 1985; 119: 357 (Figs 2B, C)

of therapy is effective for all the diseases that may present with crescents. Second, unless appropriate treatment is started promptly the prognosis is poor.

Differentiation between the various primary underlying diseases cannot be made on the basis of light microscopy alone; both electron microscopic and immunofluorescence studies must be included.[32]

The findings on immunofluorescence or immunoperoxidase microscopy are a useful starting point in the differential diagnosis: these are indicated in the following paragraphs.

Linear deposits of IgG with or without complement

If there are diffuse linear deposits of IgG and linear or irregular C3 outlining the glomerular capillary walls the diagnosis is most probably *antiglomerular-basement-membrane disease* (see p. 217). This diagnosis can be confirmed by finding antiglomerular basement membrane antibodies in the serum using radioimmune assay (RIA) or an enzyme-linked immunosorbent assay (ELISA).[33]

No deposits of immunoglobulin or complement

Should immunofluorescence reveal only minor focal and segmental deposits or no deposits of immunoglobulin or complement, *microscopic polyarteritis* (see p. 272) and *Wegener's granulomatosis* (see p. 275) should be considered. If light microscopy shows no mesangial proliferation but segmental glomerular capillary thromboses with fibrin this is strong presumptive evidence for a vasculitis. A search for foci of fibrinoid necrosis in the walls of arterioles and small arteries should be made but these lesions are often very difficult to find. If there are pronounced interstitial mononuclear cell infiltration and small necrotizing granulomas then Wegener's granulomatosis is the most probable diagnosis. Confirmation should be sought by looking for antibodies to neutrophil cytoplasmic antigen in the serum (see p. 272).[27]

Granular deposits of immunoglobulin and/or complement

If most of the glomeruli contain definite granules of either immunoglobulin or complement or both then a number of possibilities arise.

A combination of granular IgG and C3 accompanied by diffuse increase in glomerular tuft cellularity, with swelling and proliferation of endothelial cells and subepithelial humps on electron microscopy, suggests *diffuse endocapillary proliferative glomerulonephritis* (see p. 142).

If the increase in tuft cellularity is accompanied by thickening of the glomerular capillary walls then *diffuse mesangiocapillary glomerulonephritis* (see p. 164) or *dense deposit disease* (see p. 179) are possibilities. Mesangiocapillary glomerulonephritis is confirmed by finding extensive mesangial interposition and subendothelial deposits on electron microscopy. Dense deposit disease is confirmed by the ultrastructural finding of black ribbons of material replacing the lamina densa.

If the deposits are predominantly IgA and mesangial then *Henoch–Schönlein purpura* (see p. 252) or *IgA nephropathy* (see p. 157) are the most likely conditions.

Should the IgA be accompanied by a wide range of immunoglobulins or complement components and electron microscopy showing subendothelial and mesangial deposits, *systemic lupus erythematosus* (see p. 225) should be suspected. Confirmation should be sought by looking for antinuclear and anti-double-stranded-DNA antibodies in the serum (see p. 226). If the deposits are highly organized with annular and cylindrical structures, *mixed essential cryoglobulinaemia* (see p. 351) is probably the diagnosis and cryoglobulins should be looked for in the serum.

Renal transplantation

Idiopathic diffuse crescentic glomerulonephritis only rarely recurs in renal allografts. When it does, the rapidity with which the renal failure progresses follows closely the course of the original disease.[34]

Prognosis

Those patients in whom more than 70% of the glomeruli contain crescents or who have oliguria, resistant to diuretics, at presentation, rarely recover any renal function.[24] Patients without oliguria when first seen may show substantial recovery. There is a close correlation between the eventual glomerular filtration rate and the degree of tubular and interstitial damage at the time of the initial renal biopsy. Prompt treatment with large intravenous doses of corticosteroids or plasma exchange, sometimes accompanied by azathioprine and anticoagulants, contributes to recovery.[24] About 40% of patients who achieve stable renal function for longer than 2 years following treatment, have a relapse; most respond again to treatment.[35]

Pathogenesis

Rupture of the glomerular capillary wall is the initiating event in the formation of a glomerular crescent. By definition, in idiopathic diffuse crescentic glomerulonephritis the underlying process causing this injury is unknown. Increasingly it is suspected that idiopathic diffuse crescentic glomerulonephritis is closely allied to polyarteritis – it has even been described as a renal-limited variant of polyarteritis.[36] Certainly the renal changes in idiopathic diffuse crescentic glomerulonephritis are immunopathologically and ultrastructurally indistinguishable from those in microscopic polyarteritis. Antibodies to antigens in the cytoplasm of neutrophil granulocytes[27] are present in most cases of microscopic polyarteritis and have been detected in the majority of patients thought to have idiopathic diffuse crescentic glomerulonephritis,[37,38] placing these two disorders within the same category.

The events that follow rupture of the glomerular capillary wall are the same whatever the cause. The release of plasma into Bowman's space is followed by coagulation and fibrin deposition. The formation of fibrin is an important signal for the accumulation in Bowman's space of monocytes and macrophages that constitute the beginning of a crescent. The mechanism of this development is not known, but thrombin is an effective chemotaxin for monocytes.[39] In rabbits with antiglomerular-basement-membrane nephritis, if fibrin deposition is prevented by administration of ancrod (a fibrinogen splitting enzyme from viper venom) crescents do not form;[40] enhancing fibrin deposition with antifibrinolytic drugs increases crescent formation.[41] Fibrin deposition also seems to play a key role in inducing crescent formation in humans.[42] The next change to develop in the glomeruli in diffuse crescentic glomerulonephritis is proliferation of the parietal epithelial cells. The signal responsible for stimulating this proliferation has not been identified but it could be a growth factor produced by the macrophages.

Studies in man using monoclonal antibodies to various cells,[43] and experiments in rabbits using tritiated thymidine as a label,[44] indicate that within a short while most of the cells in the crescent are derived from parietal epithelial cells. These results are supported by the finding that up to 50% of cells in cellular crescents stain positively for cytokeratin, an intermediate filament found exclusively in the cytoskeleton of epithelial cells.[45] The exception to the epithelial derivation is when Bowman's capsule ruptures; in these circumstances macrophages become the major cellular component.[43] As the crescent matures either the local cells secrete collagen or fibroblasts infiltrate the crescent through breaks in Bowman's capsule. In vitro, glomerular epithelial cells are known to be able to secrete types IV and V collagen, laminin and fibronectin.

DIFFUSE MEMBRANOUS GLOMERULONEPHRITIS

Diffuse membranous glomerulonephritis is characterized by a uniform thickening of the glomerular capillary walls which may range from minimal to marked. It is caused by subepithelial deposits of predominantly IgG and usually C3 on the capillary basement membranes. A cup of new basement membrane forms around each deposit; on section the cups appear as silver staining spikes. In time the basement membrane grows over the deposits and on section the joined spikes take on the appearance of a chain. The mesangium is usually not expanded and tuft cellularity is often normal.

Diffuse membranous glomerulonephritis is a chronic progressive disease but its course may be interrupted by spontaneous remissions. It is most common in adult men and usually presents with the nephrotic syndrome. Serum complement levels are normal in the idiopathic disease. Hypertension often develops at some stage. There is slow deterioration in renal function and about 25% of those in whom the onset was in adult life need dialysis or renal transplantation within 15 years; in children the prognosis is much better and permanent remissions occur.

In 70% of patients in Britain and the USA no cause is apparent, but some cases may be associated with a variety of systemic infections such as those due to hepatitis B virus (see p. 393), syphilis (see p. 388), schistosomiasis (see p. 421), filariasis (see p. 423), malaria (see p. 417) and leprosy (see p. 387). These infective associations are very rare in Britain, Europe and the USA, but some are frequent elsewhere in the world. For example, associations with hepatitis B virus in Japan and Zimbabwe (see p. 393), and malaria in Nigeria (see p. 417). An association with neoplasms, particularly carcinomas of the bronchus and large gut, is found in up to 10% of adult patients in Britain and the USA (see p. 616).

Diffuse membranous glomerulonephritis occasionally follows exposure to various drugs, such as gold and penicillamine, used in the treatment of rheumatoid arthritis (see pp. 515, 523), and to mercury, once used by black people in Kenya to lighten the colour of their skin (see p. 505). Drug addicts (see p. 510) and possibly those chronically exposed to volatile hydrocarbons (see p. 192) are more likely to develop membranous glomerulonephritis, as are those treated with captopril (see p. 523) and probenecid.

Membranous glomerulonephritis sometimes occurs in systemic lupus erythematosus (lupus nephritis class V; see p. 230) and mixed connective tissue disease (see p. 247). An association with Guillain–Barré syndrome and diabetes mellitus (see p. 336) has also been reported. De novo diffuse membranous glomerulonephritis also occurs in renal allografts (see p. 671).

The account that follows is concerned with the idiopathic form of the disease.

Clinical features

Idiopathic diffuse membranous glomerulonephritis occurs at any age but most often affects adults between the ages of 30 and 50 years. In one large series of cases the mean age at the time of recognition of the disease was 37.6 years.[46] The condition is uncommon in childhood. There is a male predominance of about 2:1. There are few data on the incidence of the disease; in Edinburgh there are 3.9 cases per 100 000 per 20 years, but some of these may be secondary to exposure to organic solvents.[47]

The onset is insidious. About 75% of the patients present with the nephrotic syndrome; the remainder are found by chance to have symptomless proteinuria. Microscopic haematuria is detectable in half the patients; gross haematuria is rare. Hypertension is present in a quarter of the patients when they are first seen and develops at some time during the course of the disease in up to half the patients.[46,48,49]

In adults the clinical course is usually very slowly progressive, but individuals may periodically remit for short or long periods; permanent complete remissions are reported in 20–25% of patients.[46,48] In those with only proteinuria at the onset, the nephrotic syndrome commonly develops at some time in the course of the disease.

In children many cases have an indolent and apparently unprogressive course and permanent remission occurs in about 50%.[50]

Tissue typing

The phenotype frequencies of some of the antigens of the major histocompatibility complex are raised in idiopathic membranous glomerulonephritis, but there are geographical differences. HLA-DR3 is significantly increased in patients in Britain, Germany, Spain, France and China, whereas in Japan the increase is in HLA-DR2.[51] There is also an increase in the frequency of HLA-B8 in patients in Newcastle, England and Germany, and of HLA-B18 in Manchester, England and Spain. An increase in the rare Bf allele (Bf*F1) has been reported but this has not yet been confirmed. The association between HLA-DR3 and idiopathic membranous glomerulonephritis has been confirmed at the level of DNA; it is suggested that in Caucasians the DR3 and DR5 DQA1 allele is an important factor conferring susceptibility to the disease.[52]

Serology

Serum complement levels are normal, cryoglobulins are usually absent and tests for circulating immune complexes are generally negative.[53]

Renal changes

Gross appearance of the kidneys

In the case of patients who die early, before the development of renal failure, the kidneys are enlarged and have a pale, smooth subcapsular surface. Later in the course of the disease the size of the kidneys is normal or reduced and the subcapsular surface appears finely granular.

Light microscopy

In the very early stages the capillary wall is so slightly thickened that the abnormality is easily missed. Silver stains do not help because spikes of new basement membrane have not yet formed.

With progression of the lesion the capillary wall thickening becomes obvious. There is fairly uniform, eosinophilic (but not usually refractile) thickening of the capillary basement membrane. The change affects all the capillaries in each tuft (Fig. 7.11): the process is both global and diffuse. When sections 2 μm thick are stained by the periodic acid-Schiff: methenamine silver method the true glomerular capillary basement membrane appears within the thickened capillary walls as a thin, silver-positive (that is, black) line from which numerous silver-positive *spikes* with club-shaped ends protrude (Fig. 7.12). The thickening of the membrane is due to the presence of material on its surface, between the spikes, that does not take up

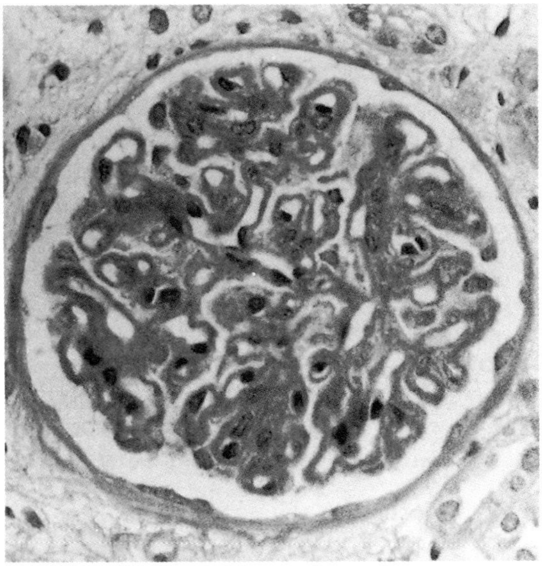

Fig. 7.11 Idiopathic membranous glomerulonephritis. Glomerulus showing widespread (global) thickening of the basement membrane of the capillaries. Tuft cellularity appears normal.
Periodic acid-Schiff × 320

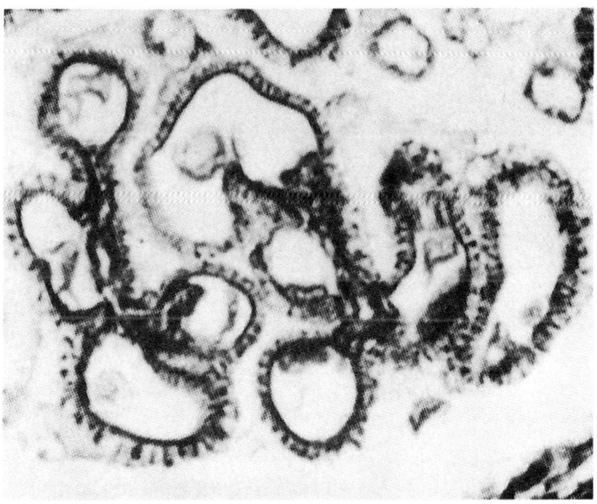

Fig. 7.12 Idiopathic membranous glomerulonephritis. Group of glomerular capillaries stained with silver. Black spikes project outwards from the basement membrane.
Periodic acid-Schiff: methenamine silver × 1200

silver but is stained red by Masson's trichrome method. The lumen of the capillaries is widely patent and there is usually no obvious increase in the cellularity of the tufts or in the amount of mesangial matrix. However, quantitative analysis reveals in many cases mild increase in the number of mesangial cells and in the amount of mesangial matrix.

As the disease progresses the thickening of the capillary wall increases and the capillary lumen becomes progressively smaller. As new basement membrane grows over the deposits a double-layered membrane is formed, the residua of the original spikes appearing as transverse bands between the two layers. After staining with silver the thickened membrane looks like a chain (Fig.7.13). Segmental sclerosis and hyalinosis develop in some of the glomeruli.

Finally, most of the glomeruli become sclerotic, giving the histological appearance known as diffuse sclerosing glomerulonephritis (see p. 203). Usually there is no increase in lobulation of the tuft at any stage of the disease.

During prolonged periods of remission there may be remarkable restoration to normal of the glomeruli that have not developed segmental sclerosis and hyalinosis.

In the early stages of the disease the proximal convoluted tubules contain lipid, and hyaline casts are common, particularly in the collecting tubules. Later, there is atrophy of the tubules, and focal fibrosis and scattered small accumulations of mononuclear cells appear in the interstitium. In-

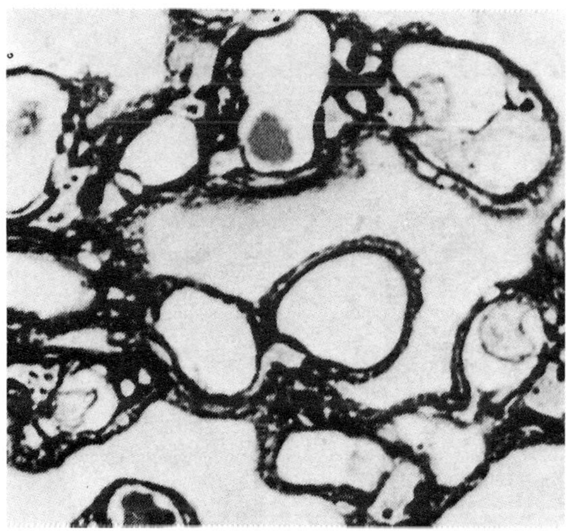

Fig. 7.13 Idiopathic membranous glomerulonephritis. Later state of disease than in Figure 7.12. Group of glomerular capillaries stained with silver. The thickened capillary walls look like chains.
Periodic acid-Schiff: methenamine silver × 1200

terstitial collections of cells with foamy cytoplasm (due to lipids) are often seen, as in all forms of chronic proteinuria, and there may be cholesterol granulomas.

Electron microscopy

The changes in the capillary wall are usually divided into four stages.[54]

Stage I Initially, small scattered subepithelial electron-dense homogeneous deposits appear along the glomerular capillary walls (Fig. 7.14). The distribution is often segmental, some capillary loops being spared. The deposits may be dome-shaped or irregularly flattened, and the underlying basement membrane is either normal or there are occasional small protrusions extending between a few of the deposits. The foot processes of the visceral epithelial cells are retracted and obliterated over the deposits. Immunogold labelling has shown that the subepithelial deposits contain IgG.[55]

Stage II The subepithelial deposits are larger and more numerous and involve almost all the capillary loops. The deposits (Fig. 7.15) are each surrounded by a cup of basement membrane material which has grown up from the original basement membrane. This is best seen in scan-

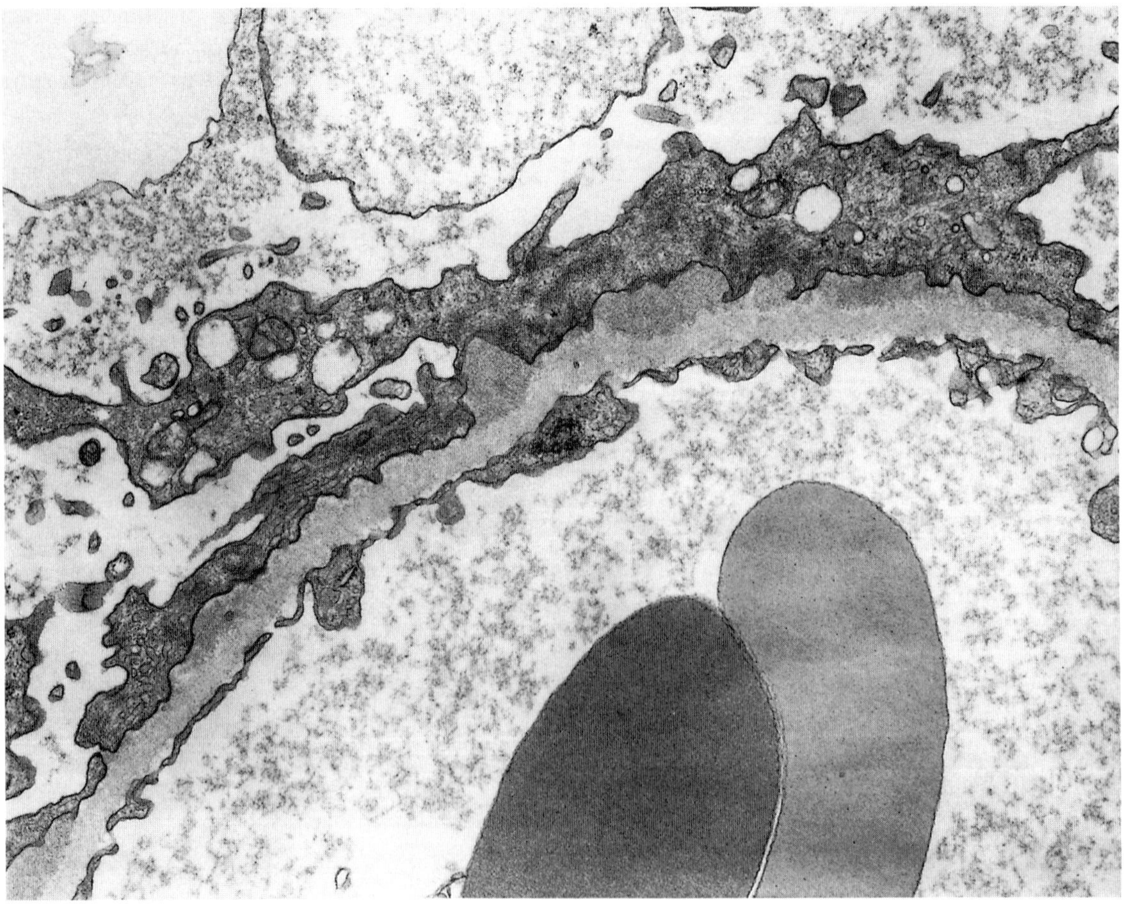

Fig. 7.14 Idiopathic membranous glomerulonephritis stage I. Electron micrograph of part of a glomerular capillary loop. Small, scattered deposits are present on the basement membrane. The visceral epithelial foot processes are obliterated. × 20 000

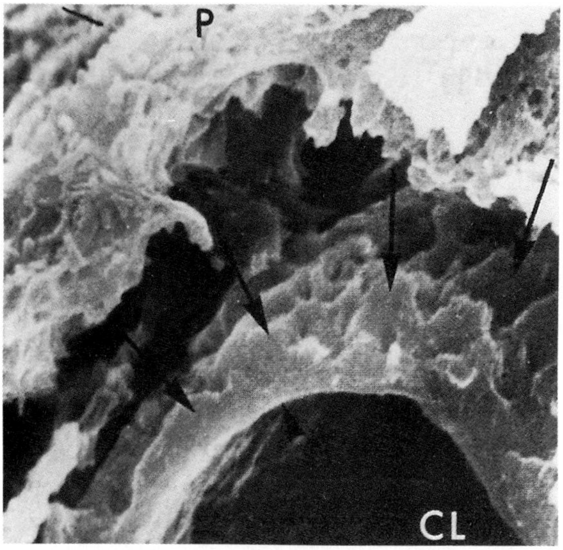

Fig. 7.15 Idiopathic membranous glomerulonephritis stage II. Scanning electron micrograph of cross-section of a glomerular capillary. The immune deposits (arrows) protrude from the epithelial surface of the capillary. CL, capillary lumen; P, epithelial cell (podocyte); arrowhead, capillary basement membrane.
× 8600
Reproduced by permission from: Jao W, Horn T. Am J Kidney Dis 1986; 7: 35 (Fig. 7)

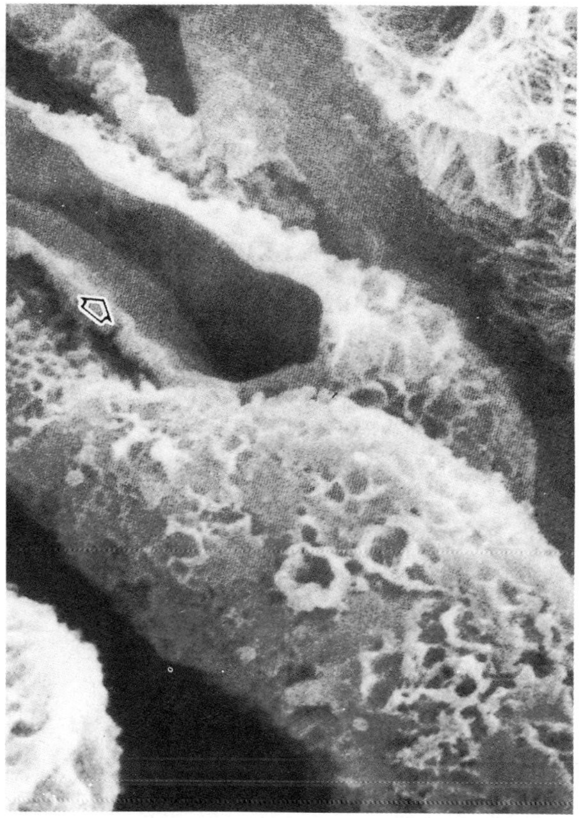

Fig. 7.16 Idiopathic membranous glomerulonephritis stage II. Scanning electron micrograph of part of a glomerular capillary from which the cells and deposits have been removed by digestion leaving only the basement membrane. On the outer (epithelial) surface of the membrane numerous cups of new basement membrane have produced structures that resemble volcano craters. The inner (endothelial) surface of the membrane (arrow) is smooth.
× 4750
Reproduced by permission from: Weidner N, Lorentz WB. Lab Invest 1986; 54: 84 (Fig. 2A)

ning electron micrographs of preparations of the glomerulus in which all the cells and immune deposits have been digested away leaving only the capillary basement membrane. The outer (epithelial) side of the basement membrane is studded with raised structures looking like volcano craters (Fig. 7.16).[56] On section the electron-dense deposits appear to be separated from one another by spikes of basement membrane, the spikes being the sides of the cups or 'volcanoes' (Figs 7.17, 7.18). The spikes differ from normal basement membrane in containing laminin but not type IV collagen.[57] The epithelial foot processes are diffusely retracted and obliterated at this stage.

Stage III The cups of new basement membrane gradually extend to enclose the subepithelial deposits. This does not happen in a uniform way and capped and uncapped deposits are found in different parts of the capillary basement membrane. Scanning electron microscopy of the denuded capillary basement membranes shows the caps as plaques among the craters.[56] On section the thickened capillary wall then appears to consist of the original basement membrane, a central layer of deposits separated by transverse strands of basement membrane material (the residua of the cup walls or spikes) and an outer irregular layer of new basement membrane capping the deposits and separating them from the visceral epithelial cells. Some of the deposits may show irregular loss of their electron density (Fig. 7.19).

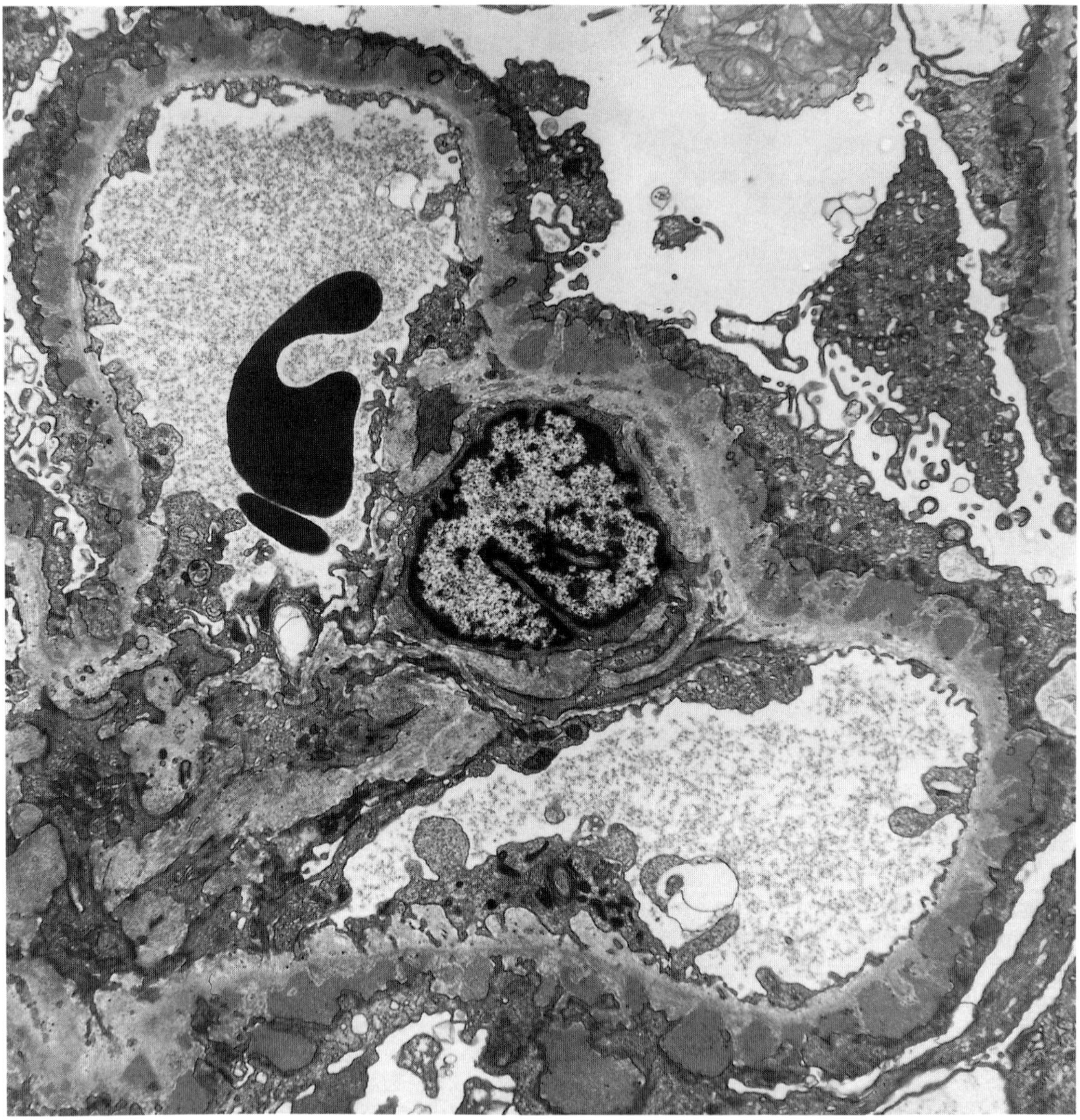

Fig. 7.17 Idiopathic membranous glomerulonephritis stage II. Electron micrograph of two glomerular capillary loops. There are multiple large subepithelial deposits. The sides of the cups of new basement membrane material surrounding each deposit appear in section as projections from the basement membrane. These projections are the spikes seen by light microscopy after silver staining of paraffin sections.
× 8000

Fig. 7.19 Idiopathic membranous glomerulonephritis stage III. Electron micrograph of part of a glomerular capillary loop. The multiple subepithelial deposits have become capped by new basement membrane and some of the deposits appear moth-eaten because of irregular loss of their electron density.
× 17 000

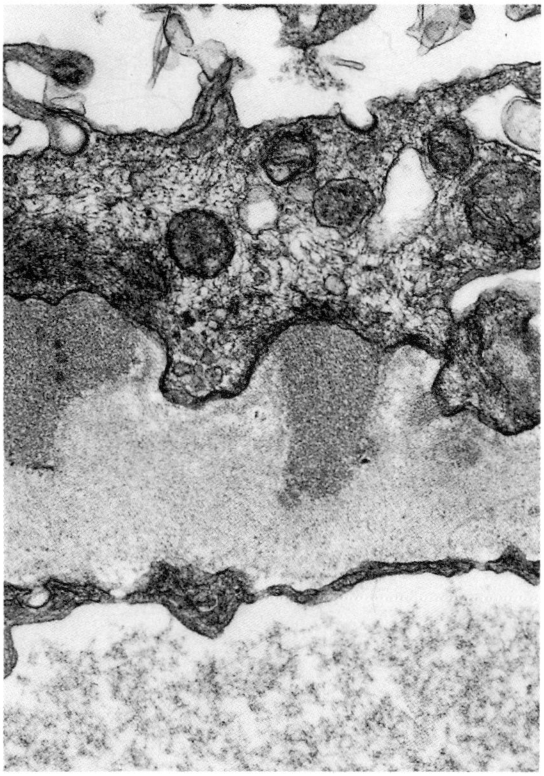

Fig. 7.18 Idiopathic membranous glomerulonephritis stage II. Electron micrograph of part of a glomerular capillary. Two subepithelial deposits are flanked by spikes of basement membrane. The epithelial foot processes are retracted above the deposits.
× 29 800

Stage IV The glomerular capillary basement membranes are greatly thickened and distorted. Most of the deposits have disappeared leaving only a few irregular electron-lucent areas (Fig. 7.20).

Mixture of stages Frequently the distribution of the deposits and the apparent stage of the changes vary between glomeruli and within individual capillary loops, and fresh subepithelial deposits may be found even in stage IV lesions (Fig. 7.20).

Mesangial deposits Rarely in idiopathic diffuse membranous glomerulonephritis deposits are also present in the mesangium, but before these cases can be accepted as idiopathic, causes such as systemic lupus erythematosus, syphilis and

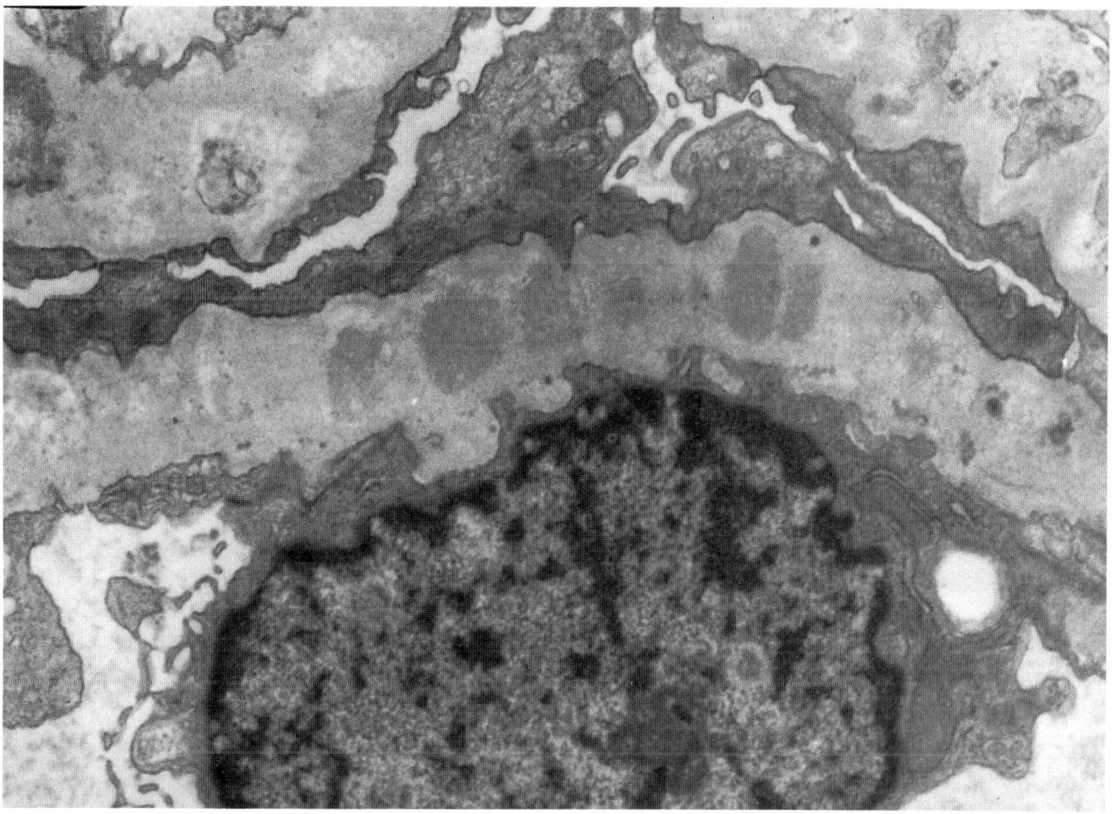

Fig. 7.19

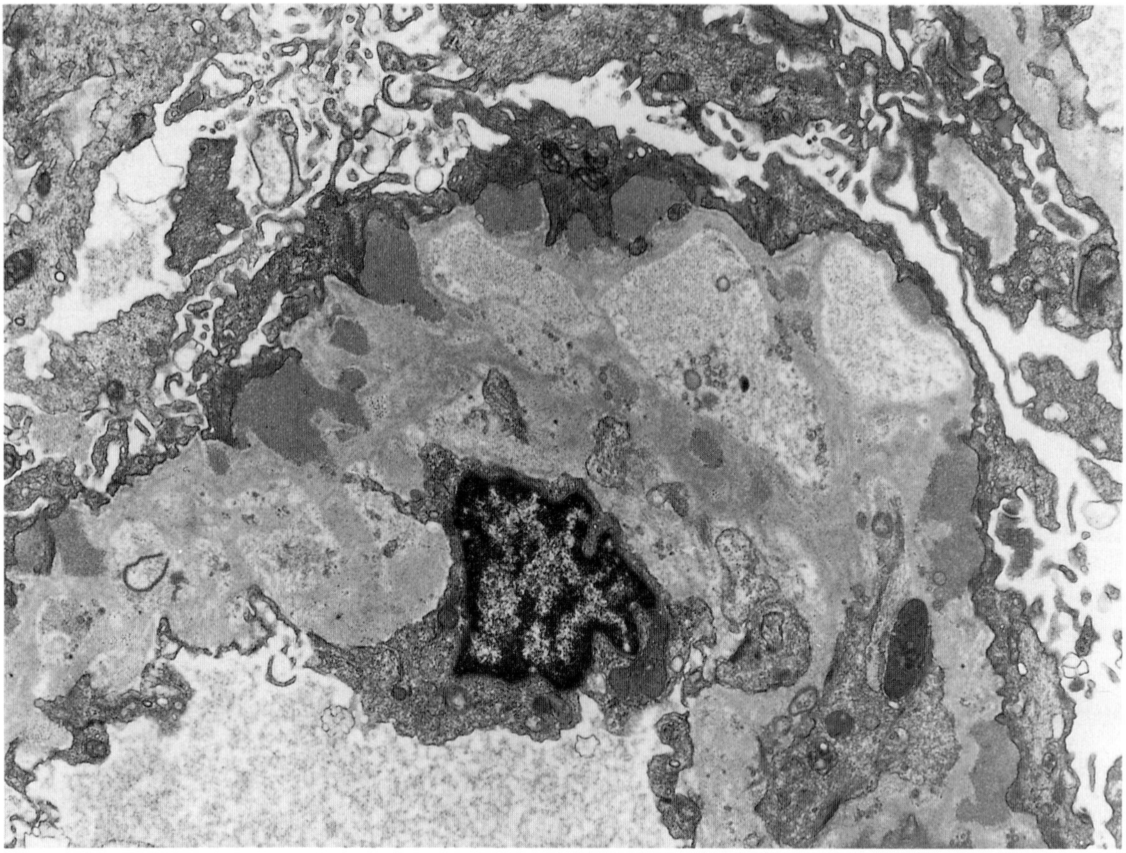

Fig. 7.20 Idiopathic membranous glomerulonephritis stage IV. Electron micrograph of part of a glomerular capillary loop. The basement membrane is greatly and irregularly thickened. There are several electronlucent areas. Scattered small stage I deposits are present beneath the epithelium indicating that the disease is still active.
× 17 000

hepatitis B virus infection must be rigorously excluded.

Remission In patients who enter a prolonged period of remission the deposits become electronlucent and gradually disappear (Fig.7.21). Discrete epithelial foot processes return and eventually the only remaining abnormalities may be small subendothelial irregularities of the basement membrane.[58,59]

Immunofluorescence/immunoperoxidase microscopy

Closely packed granular deposits of IgG and C3 are usually present in the walls of the glomerular capillaries (Fig. 7.22). When the granules are small and numerous low power examination may suggest a linear distribution but this is usually resolved by examination under higher power. IgA, IgM, C1q and C4 are often absent; if they are present they are usually only scattered small granules. Mesangial deposits are rare in idiopathic membranous glomerulonephritis. If there are prominent capillary wall deposits of IgA, IgM, C1q and C4 and mesangial deposits lupus nephritis must be excluded.

The predominant IgG subclasses in the granular deposits are IgG_3 and IgG_4. These IgG subclasses make up only 7% and 4% of total serum IgG respectively. The reason for this subclass distribution in the immune deposits is not yet clear.[60]

Immunohistochemistry Phenotypic analysis, using monoclonal antibodies, shows that the cells that appear in the interstitium as the disease

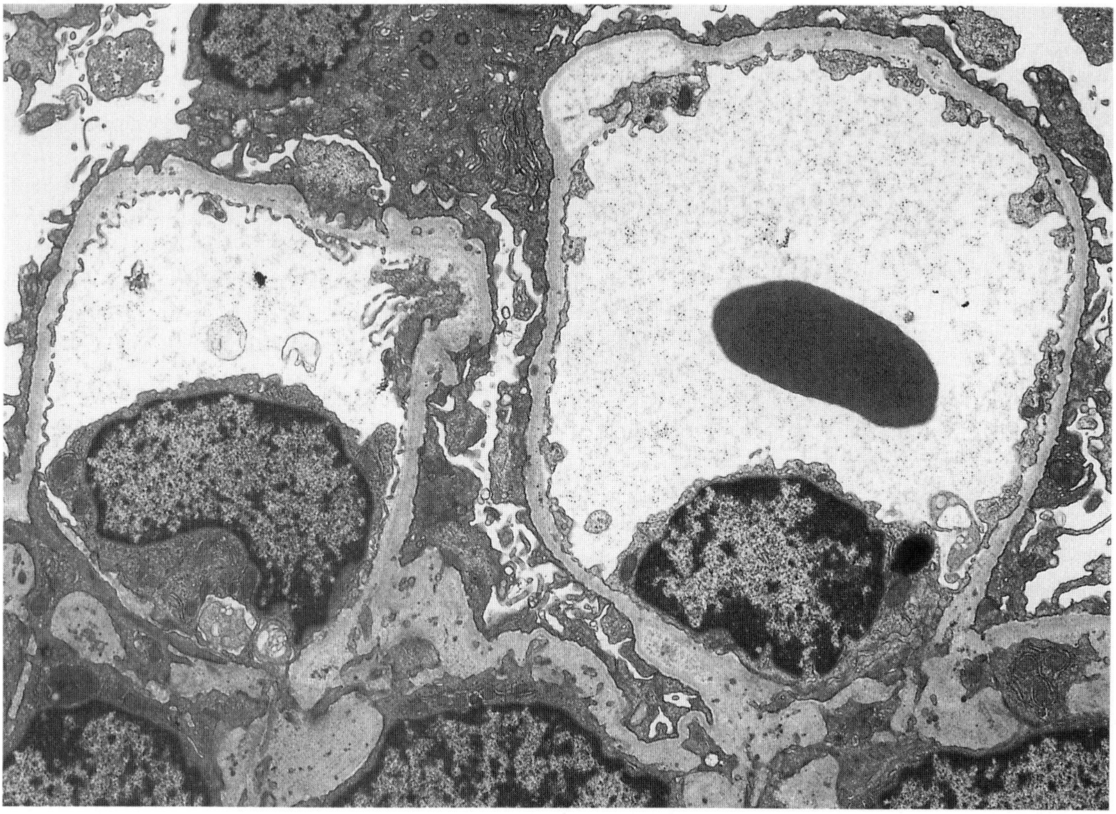

Fig. 7.21 Idiopathic membranous glomerulonephritis during remission. Electron micrograph of two glomerular capillary loops. In one capillary there is a subepithelial electronlucent area where a deposit has been absorbed. In the other capillary the basement membrane is segmentally irregular. There is still effacement (retraction) of the epithelial foot processes.
× 6550

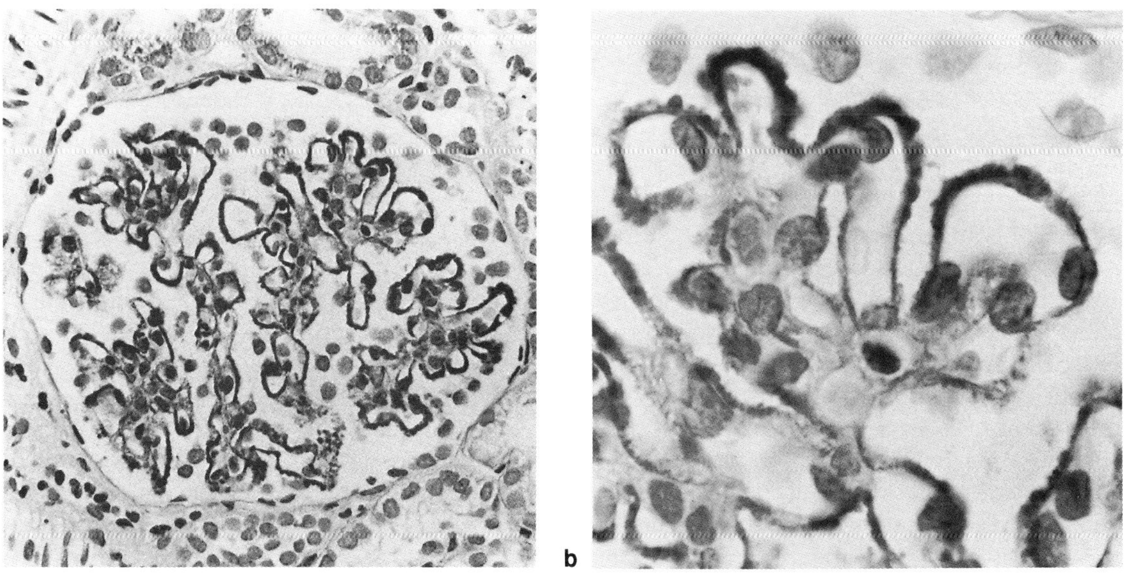

a b

Fig. 7.22 Idiopathic membranous glomerulonephritis. Glomerulus with closely packed granular deposits of IgG along the capillary wall. (**a**) Whole glomerulus. (**b**) Higher power view of glomerular capillary walls.
Immunoperoxidase: (**a**) × 280; (**b**) × 950

progresses are largely macrophages and T lymphocytes; among the T lymphocytes CD4+ cells predominate.[61]

Differential diagnosis

As long as immunofluorescence or immunoperoxidase microscopy and electron microscopy are used as well as light microscopy there should be no difficulty in diagnosing membranous glomerulonephritis. Difficulties only arise when reliance is placed solely upon light microscopy and the methenamine silver stain. Stage I lesions in membranous glomerulonephritis will frequently be missed and the presence of silver-positive spikes in amyloidosis (see p. 346) may be misinterpreted.

Once the presence of diffuse membranous glomerulonephritis has been established it is then very important, particularly with stage I lesions, to attempt to exclude associated and potentially reversible conditions. Lupus nephritis WHO class V should be suspected if there are many deposits of IgA, IgM, C1q and C4 and if there are mesangial or subendothelial deposits. Tubuloreticular bodies in endothelial cells and deposits on the tubular basement membranes should be sought (see p. 232).[61] If gold nephropathy seems a possibility then the characteristic inclusions should be looked for in the tubular cells (see p. 515).

Complications

Renal vein thrombosis (see p. 293)

This complication of the nephrotic syndrome occurs some time during the course of approximately half the cases of idiopathic membranous glomerulonephritis.[62] The extent of venous involvement ranges from occlusion of a small peripheral venous radical to partial occlusion of both main renal veins. In most patients neither proteinuria nor renal function are influenced by the presence of renal venous thrombi. Interstitial oedema and margination of neutrophil granulocytes in glomerular capillaries may occur in acute renal vein thrombosis but are absent in other cases.[63]

Crescentic glomerulonephritis (see p. 185)

Rarely diffuse crescentic glomerulonephritis complicates idiopathic diffuse membranous glomerulonephritis.[64] In two cases antiglomerular basement membrane antibodies were found in the serum and similar antibodies were eluted from the glomeruli of a third case. The onset of crescentic glomerulonephritis is usually accompanied by haematuria and a rapid fall in renal function.

Interstitial nephritis (see pp. 458, 467).

Occasionally acute hypersensitivity interstitial nephritis occurs secondary to the use of diuretics in the treatment of idiopathic diffuse membranous glomerulonephritis.

Renal transplantation

Membranous glomerulonephritis seldom recurs in a renal allograft (see p. 668). De novo membranous glomerulonephritis is more frequent (see p. 671).[65] The patients develop marked proteinuria, often with the nephrotic syndrome, and their subsequent clinical course is the same as for idiopathic membranous glomerulonephritis.

Prognosis

There is relatively little information on untreated adults with idiopathic membranous glomerulonephritis. In three studies 19, 28 and 51% of the patients showed a steady deterioration in renal function in the first 2 years.[46,66,67] The remainder retained normal renal function, some of them for long periods. Between 15 and 20% developed spontaneous complete remission of proteinuria and in an additional 20% there was reduction in the amount of proteinuria within 1–2 years of the discovery of the disease.

In long-term studies of untreated patients and those treated with steroids or cytotoxic drugs or both, approximately 50% are likely to enter into lasting complete or partial remission and approximately 40% will develop end-stage renal disease during a period of 15 years. The remainder of the patients will die from incidental disease.[68]

Better results than these have been reported from Japan with approximately 80% of treated patients surviving for 15 years.[69] One of several possible explanations for this difference is that many more of the Japanese patients were not nephrotic when first discovered; patients presenting with asymptomatic proteinuria are known to have a better prognosis.[48] Another possibility is that idiopathic diffuse membranous glomerulonephritis is a more benign disease in Japan; the strong association with HLA-DR2 in Japan compared with HLA-DR3 in Britain and Europe might indicate that the difference is a consequence of some genetic factor. Some investigators have shown a higher prevalence of HLA-B18, Bf*F1, DRW3 haplotype in patients with idiopathic diffuse membranous glomerulonephritis who develop progressive disease.

The outcome of diffuse membranous glomerulonephritis is always said to be much better in children than in adults with only 10% developing renal failure by 5 years and an actuarial renal survival rate of 90% at 10 years after discovery of the disease.[50] Two more recent reports on smaller series have been less optimistic with 21 and 27% of the patients progressing to renal failure.[70,71]

Several other factors seem to affect the long-term prognosis of idiopathic membranous glomerulonephritis. Women appear to fare better than men. Impaired renal function at the time of diagnosis presages terminal renal failure. Some investigators have claimed a correlation between histological staging of the glomerular lesions and the clinical course[46] but this is denied by others.[53] Interstitial and vascular changes are seen more frequently in those patients who later develop renal insufficiency.[68]

The tendency for spontaneous remission in idiopathic membranous glomerulonephritis makes the evaluation of treatment difficult. A claim that prednisone 125 mg every other day for 2 months appears to be beneficial, slowing the progression of the disease,[67] has not been confirmed.[72]

Pathogenesis

The pathogenesis of idiopathic diffuse membranous glomerulonephritis is not known. In animals lesions closely resembling human membranous glomerulonephritis can be produced in several ways. On the basis of these experiments it has been suggested that the three mechanisms described below might be relevant in the human disease. At present there is no proof that any of them operate in human membranous glomerulonephritis.

Deposition of circulating immune complexes in the glomeruli

In rabbits the clinical and histological manifestations of membranous glomerulonephritis can be induced by injections of bovine serum albumin.[73,74] Immune deposits of bovine albumin and antibody develop on the glomerular capillary basement membranes coincident with the appearance of circulating, soluble immune complexes of the same antigen and antibody; but it is only the poor antibody producers, or animals repeatedly reinjected with small doses of bovine albumin to maintain antigen excess, that develop subepithelial deposits with no glomerular inflammation. The glomerular lesions regress when antigen administration ceases.

Because isolated antigen or antibody are not detected in the glomeruli, it was initially concluded that the granular deposits appear because soluble immune complexes formed in the circulation became trapped in the glomerulus, which acts as a passive filter.

Although circulating immune complexes are found in 10–20% of patients with idiopathic membranous glomerulonephritis there is no direct evidence that they are involved in the production of the disease. At present it is generally felt that circulating immune complexes do not play the initiating role in human membranous glomerulonephritis, although they could be responsible for the amplification of glomerular subepithelial deposits that have been formed in some other way.

In situ formation of glomerular immune complexes

In situ formation of glomerular immune complexes can occur either by circulating autoantibody binding to an insoluble, intrinsic glomerular antigen or by circulating antibody binding to a soluble extrinsic, non-glomerular antigen attached to the subepithelial aspect of the glomerular capillary basement membrane.

Insoluble intrinsic glomerular antigens In rats membranous glomerulonephritis can be induced by active or passive immunization against an antigen which is present in both the brush border of proximal tubular cells and in glomerular visceral epithelial cells (Heymann's nephritis). The antigen is a glycoprotein with a molecular weight of about 330 kDa (gp 330). On the epithelial foot processes gp 330 is found mainly in the clathrin-coated pits (see p. 12) that are present all along the surface of the visceral epithelial cells.[75] The circulating divalent autoantibodies to gp 330 cross the glomerular capillary basement membrane and first encounter this antigen on the soles of the foot processes; this induces redistribution of the antigen and the formation of coarse caps on the cell surface. Immune complexes are then shed into the underlying lamina rara externa of the glomerular capillary basement membrane and into slit pores. Complement fixation, probably including insertion of the membrane attack complex of the complement system (C5b-C9) into the plasma membrane of the foot processes, appears to cause the damage that leads to proteinuria.[76] The presence of the membrane attack complex has been detected by immunofluorescence in the glomeruli of 50% of patients with idiopathic membranous glomerulonephritis.[77]

Searches for evidence of a brush border antigen or of antibody to such an antigen have been made in human idiopathic membranous glomerulonephritis. With rare exceptions these studies have been negative. But few attempts have been made to find an antibody directed against an epithelial cell antigen other than one shared with tubular brush border. There is still a strong suspicion that an autoimmune mechanism similar to that operating in Heymann's membranous glomerulonephritis in the rat is probably responsible for human idiopathic membranous glomerulonephritis.[78] Preliminary studies indicate that autoantibodies against an epithelial cell glycoprotein may be involved;[79] 3 years later these findings have still not been confirmed by other investigators. However, a monoclonal antibody against cultured human glomerular epithelial cells has been raised, which recognizes a 60 kDa protein, and forms small transient subepithelial immune deposits when injected into monkeys or perfused through isolated human kidneys.[80]

Planted non-glomerular antigens Chronic serum sickness can be induced in rabbits with cationic bovine serum albumin (albumin chemically modified to increase the pI from 4.5 to greater than 9.0). The cationic albumin binds to the epithelial side of the glomerular capillary basement membrane. When antibody is produced against the albumin it binds to the antigen on the capillary basement membrane producing subepithelial deposits.[81] However, some deposits also occur in subendothelial and mesangial sites, which is not seen in idiopathic membranous glomerulonephritis but may occur in some of the secondary forms of the disease such as lupus nephritis WHO class V or nephritis in infections with hepatitis B virus.

Variants of membranous glomerulonephritis

Focal segmental membranous glomerulonephritis

Cases in which there are subepithelial electron-dense or partly electron-lucent deposits in the walls of a few capillaries of only some glomeruli are uncommon. When this focal segmental glomerulonephritis occurs it is usually in the absence of other glomerular lesions and is generally considered to be either an early or resolving stage of idiopathic diffuse membranous glomerulonephritis. It is commonest in children and associated with mild proteinuria and a favourable clinical course.[82]

Sometimes, however, focal segmental membranous glomerulonephritis is not isolated but associated with some previously existent glomerular disease such as diabetic glomerulosclerosis, minimal change disease or hereditary nephritis. In these cases there is no evidence of evolution into diffuse membranous glomerulonephritis and the focal segmental membranous glomerulonephritis is most probably a transient phenomenon of limited clinical significance.[83]

DIFFUSE SCLEROSING GLOMERULONEPHRITIS

Diffuse sclerosing glomerulonephritis is characterized by global sclerosis of almost all the glomeruli with evidence that the basic process is of glomerular origin, although the type of glomerular disease can no longer be identified precisely.[23] Diffuse sclerosing glomerulonephritis is not a specific entity, it is the end result of a variety of glomerular diseases.

Clinical features

Patients with diffuse sclerosing glomerulonephritis usually present with chronic renal failure. There is often proteinuria, haematuria and hypertension.

Renal changes

Gross appearances

The kidneys are usually reduced in size. The capsule is adherent and the subcapsular surface is firm and finely granular (Fig. 7.23). The cortex is narrowed. The arcuate arteries have thickened walls and are conspicuous. Because of the loss of renal substance, the amount of fat in the hilum is increased. The calyces and renal pelvis are normal.

Light microscopy

The glomeruli are crowded and reduced in

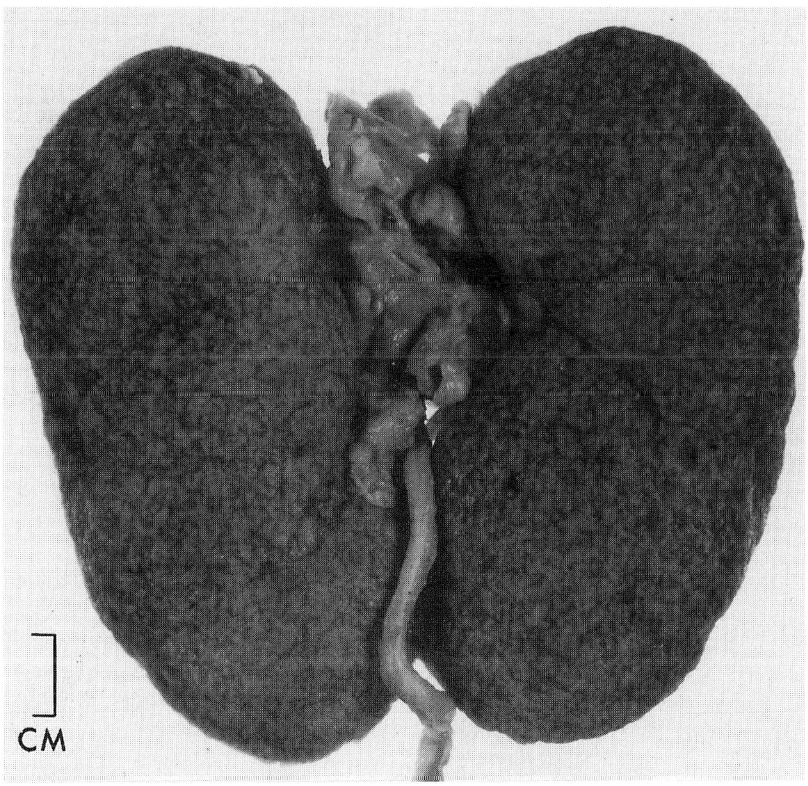

Fig.7.23 Diffuse sclerosing glomerulonephritis. External aspect of bisected kidney. The organ is reduced in size and has a finely granular subcapsular surface.
Reproduced by permission of Professor RH Heptinstall from: Systemic pathology, 1st edn London: Longman, 1966.

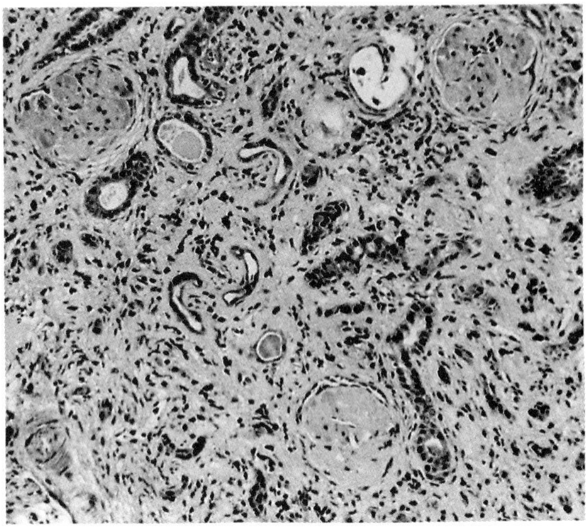

Fig. 7.24 Diffuse sclerosing glomerulonephritis. Section of renal cortex showing three sclerosed glomeruli. There is widespread tubular atrophy.
Haematoxylin-eosin × 100

number. Most of them consist of small sclerotic nodules but there are usually a few survivors (Fig.7.24). Several of them are partly sclerosed; occasional glomeruli appear normal. In the partly sclerosed glomerular tufts there may be collections of hyalin (Fig. 7.25). Atrophy of tubules is widespread but there are collections of dilated hypertrophic tubules scattered throughout the cortex. The dilated tubules form the granules that are seen on the subcapsular surface of the kidneys with the naked eye. Interstitial fibrosis and focal collections of mononuclear cells, mostly small lymphocytes, are also features. The arterioles often show hyaline change in their walls and the arteries moderate to severe fibrous thickening of the intima and multiplication of the internal elastic lamina.

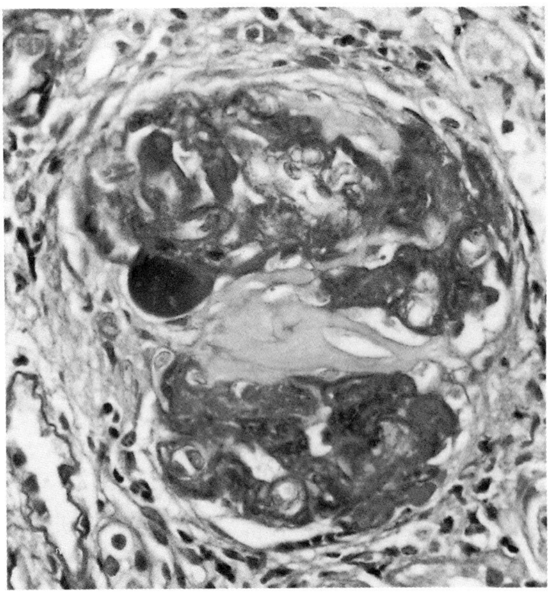

Fig. 7.25 Diffuse sclerosing glomerulonephritis. Sclerosed glomerulus containing collections of hyalin.
Periodic acid-Schiff × 450

Electron microscopy

The obsolete glomeruli consist of collapsed and wrinkled capillary basement membranes, denuded of cells; there are variable amounts of mesangial matrix. Less damaged tufts show segmental or diffuse increase in the mesangial matrix and in the number of mesangial cells. The capillary basement membrane is often thickened by a mostly electron-lucent subendothelial layer which contains collections of granular material and cell fragments. Electron-dense deposits are sometimes present on the endothelial side of the basement membrane and in the mesangium. Subepithelial deposits are unusual. Circumferential mesangial cell interposition is common, but not as extensive as in mesangiocapillary glomerulonephritis (see p. 167).

Immunofluorescence/immunoperoxidase microscopy

Focal and segmental coarse granular deposits of IgM and C3 are sometimes seen coinciding with the hyaline material visible by light microscopy. This pattern is often interpreted as non-specific trapping of immunoglobulins and complement.

Prognosis

Patients slowly progress to uraemia. Once this stage is reached terminal renal failure usually occurs within 6 months to 2 years.

FOCAL SEGMENTAL GLOMERULOSCLEROSIS

Focal segmental glomerulosclerosis is characterized by segmental glomerular lesions consisting initially of collections of intracapillary foam cells or subendothelial deposits of hyalin which later progress to segmental sclerosis or hyalinosis. The lesions often stain for IgM and C3.

These distinctive but non-specific lesions occur in many different renal diseases, such as reflux nephropathy (see p. 443), hypertension (see p. 305), Alport's syndrome (see p. 73), nail–patella syndrome (see p. 80), heroin addiction (see p. 510), acquired immune deficiency syndrome (see p. 398) and diabetic glomerulosclerosis (see p. 336). They are also found in the glomerulomegaly associated with chronic lung and heart disease (see p. 320), obesity (see p. 321) and hepatic cirrhosis (see p. 513). They occur in the single kidney in some patients with unilateral agenesis and in the remaining kidney after unilateral nephrectomy (see p. 26). They are seen as a complication in minimal change disease (see p. 140), membranous glomerulonephritis (see p. 193), IgA nephropathy (see p. 160), diffuse mesangial proliferative glomerulonephritis (see p. 153) and diffuse endocapillary proliferative glomerulonephritis (see p. 151). Focal segmental glomerulosclerosis also occasionally occurs as a familial disease.[84]

Idiopathic focal segmental glomerulosclerosis occurs most frequently in children and adolescents and affects males slightly more frequently than females. It is probably commoner in black people than in white.[85] The patients usually present with persisent proteinuria or the nephrotic syndrome and often also have microscopic haematuria. Although remissions do occur the disease is generally progressive; the rate of deterioration is extremely variable.

The account that follows is concerned with the idiopathic form of the disease.

Clinical features

Focal segmental glomerulosclerosis is commoner in children than in adults. The onset in children is usually before the age of 6 years. Boys are affected more often than girls up to the age of 3 years; beyond that age the frequency in the two sexes is similar.[86]

The onset of the disease is manifested by persistent heavy proteinuria which may exceed 15 g in 24 hours. The proteinuria is non-selective, i.e. molecules larger than albumin are being excreted as the result of a poorly selective process of filtration in the kidney. This is in contrast to minimal change disease in which the process is highly selective (see p. 136). The proteinuria is often sufficient to produce the nephrotic syndrome, particularly in children, 80% of whom present with the syndrome and almost all of whom develop it at some time during the clinical course. Microscopic haematuria is present in approximately 60% of children and hypertension in about 35%. The glomerular filtration rate is reduced in half the children.[86] Hypertension and renal insufficiency are more common in adults.

Tissue typing

In familial focal segmental glomerulosclerosis there appears to be a highly significant increase in the incidence of HLA-DRW8 in the patients.[84] In the idiopathic disease it is claimed that the frequency of HLA-DR4 is significantly increased in white and black people, the association being strongest in those who develop the disease as adults. There is also an increase in the incidence of HLA-A28 in blacks but not whites with the disease. These data suggest that there may also be a genetic predisposition to idiopathic focal segmental glomerulosclerosis.[87]

Serology

The serum levels of the various complement components are normal. Circulating immune complexes are found in about one-third of the patients.

Renal changes

Light microscopy[88,89]

In early lesions a group of capillary loops in a segment of the glomerular tuft is filled either by foam cells, each with a small nucleus and a large amount of vacuolated, lipid-laden cytoplasm, or by subendothelial collections of hyaline, an acellular structureless material that stains in-

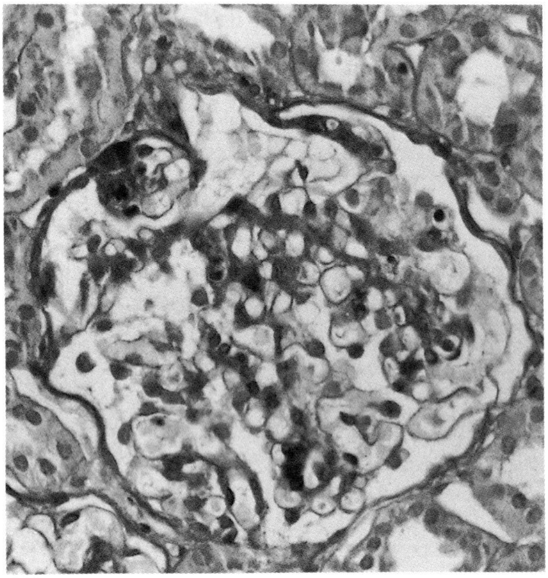

Fig. 7.26 Focal segmental glomerulosclerosis. Glomerulus with early lesion. A few capillaries near the hilum are obstructed by hyaline and cells.
Periodic acid Schiff × 490

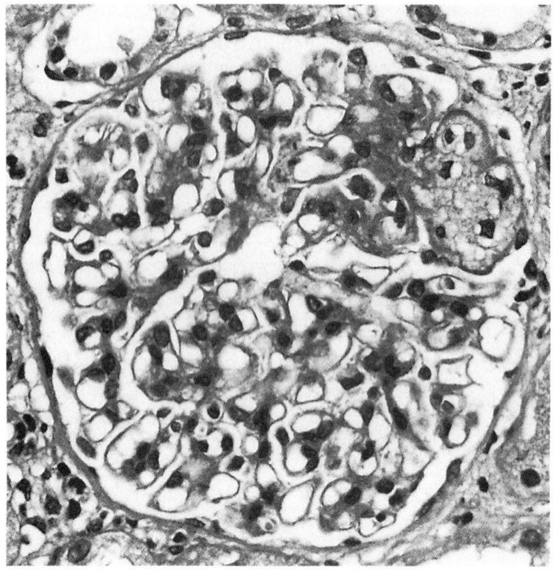

Fig. 7.27 Focal segmental glomerulosclerosis. Glomerulus with segment of sclerosis. The capillaries in the lesion contain cells with foamy cytoplasm.
Van Gieson × 490

tensely with periodic acid-Schiff but not with silver (Fig. 7.26). The adjacent visceral epithelial cells also have vacuolated cytoplasm and frequently contain large PAS-positive droplets. The affected part of the glomerulus is adherent to Bowman's capsule. The lesions are slightly more common near the hilum of the glomerulus. Initially they may be very sparse and preferentially affect the juxtamedullary glomeruli.

As the lesion progresses the affected segment appears to collapse and consolidate and the hyaline masses become larger; groups of foam cells remain in the solidified segment (Fig.7.27). Diffuse mesangial proliferation is a common accompanying feature. If there are four or more mesangial cells per mesangial area then the focal segmental glomerulosclerosis should be regarded as a complication of diffuse mesangial proliferative glomerulonephritis.[90]

In those cases in which the disease progresses the sclerosis and hyalinosis may spread to involve the whole tuft or new segmental lesions may arise. Later the lesions become sclerotic (Fig. 7.28). Eventually there is global sclerosis but it is often still possible to find small segments of hyalinosis.

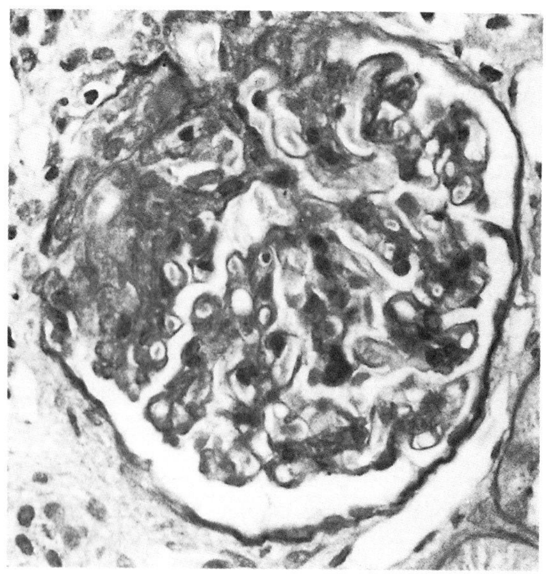

Fig. 7.28 Advanced focal segmental glomerulosclerosis. The segmental lesion in the glomerulus is predominantly sclerotic; it is adherent to Bowman's capsule.
Periodic acid-Schiff x 490

Additionally more and more glomeruli become affected and in cases which have progressed to end-stage renal failure global sclerosis is found in most glomeruli.

Groups of tubules atrophy and disappear and this is accompanied by interstitial fibrosis. Small foci of tubular interstitial damage and a few infiltrating mononuclear cells are found even in cases with apparently very few scarred glomeruli. The tubules often contain haem casts. Collections of lipid-filled foam cells are often present in the interstitium as in all cases with prolonged severe proteinuria.

Hyalin deposits in the walls of the afferent arterioles are common in adults whether or not hypertension is present. Frequently there is continuity between the arteriolar hyalin lesions and the hyalin in the segmental glomerular lesions.[91] In children vascular changes are uncommon.

Electron microscopy

The sclerotic foci are characterized by irregular collapse of glomerular capillaries, increase in the amount of mesangial matrix and an accumulation of finely granular electron-dense material, often forming a nodule. The electron-dense masses frequently contain lipid vacuoles and, in more advanced lesions, abundant collagen fibrils. Sometimes there are more discrete mesangial or subendothelial deposits. Over the sclerotic lesions the visceral epithelial cells are often damaged and detached from the capillary basement membrane (Fig. 7.29).[92] The space between the epithelial cell and the denuded membrane may appear empty or filled with fibrillar material. The foot processes of the visceral epithelial cells are retracted and obliterated in all the glomeruli, whether or not they contain sclerotic lesions. The epithelial cells

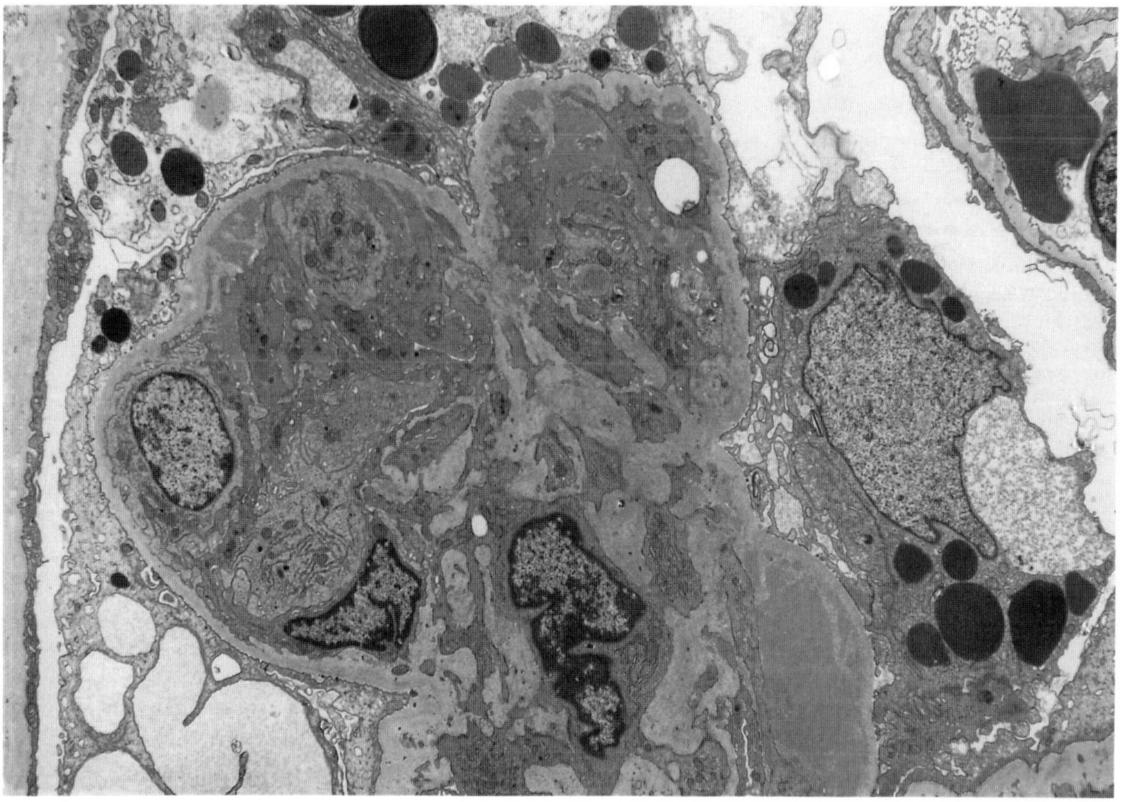

Fig. 7.29 Focal segmental glomerulosclerosis. Electron micrograph of early lesion in a glomerulus. The capillary lumens contain cellular and finely granular electron-dense material; there are also mesangial and subendothelial deposits. The visceral epithelial cells over the lesion are damaged and their cytoplasm is filled with vacuoles and osmiophilic lipid droplets. × 8000

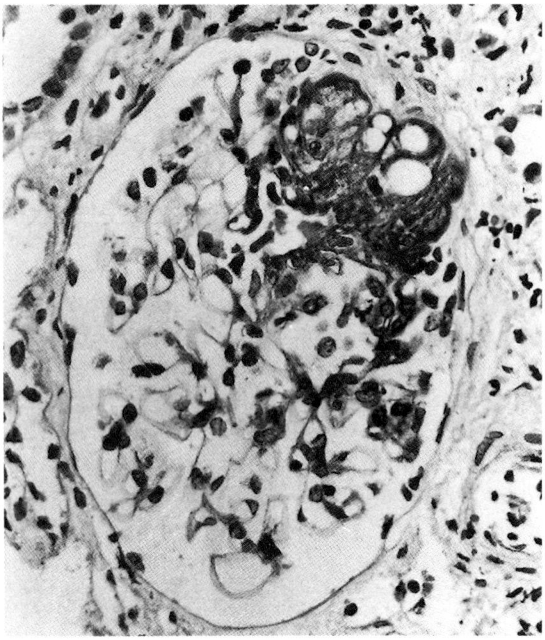

Fig. 7.30 Focal segmental glomerulosclerosis. Glomerulus with segmental depositon of IgM. Immunoperoxidase × 350

are hypertrophied and their cytoplasm contains many cysts and lysosomes. Non-specific villous hyperplasia is common on those surfaces of the visceral epithelial cells that do not abut on to the capillary basement membrane.

Immunofluorescence/immunoperoxidase microscopy

The subendothelial and nodular masses of hyaline usually stain for IgM or C3 or both (Fig. 7.30). Occasionally there is also some staining for IgG, C1q and non-specific reagents such as albumin or weak staining for IgM in the mesangium of most glomeruli. Sometimes there is no staining for immunoglobulins or complement components. Focal and segmental staining for IgM or C3 or both may precede the appearance of lesions recognizable on light microscopy.

Differential diagnosis

On encountering the lesions of focal segmental glomerulosclerosis the important need is to consider, and exclude where possible, all the secondary forms of focal segmental glomerulosclerosis. In most instances the secondary forms are usually distinguished either by their clinical dissimilarity or by the characteristic findings on light, immunofluorescence/immunoperoxidase and electron microscopy, or on both of these grounds. The significance of secondary focal segmental glomerulosclerosis varies from disease to disease. In some it may lead to more rapid progression into renal failure; in others it may have little prognostic significance. The two conditions that are likely to cause most difficulty in differential diagnosis are minimal change disease and diffuse mesangial proliferative glomerulonephritis.

Minimal change disease

It may be impossible to distinguish focal segmental glomerulosclerosis from minimal change disease early in the course of the disease because the biopsy may not contain any of the segmentally sclerosed glomeruli. This usually happens because affected glomeruli are sparse and are particularly found in the corticomedullary region that is often not sampled in a needle biopsy. If the biopsy does sample the juxtamedullary glomeruli and a few globally (as distinct from segmentally) sclerotic glomeruli are found this does not help in the distinction. In a child the globally sclerotic glomeruli can be congenitally sclerotic (see p. 53); in an adult they may be glomeruli that have become sclerotic as a result of ageing (see p. 25). The finding of globally sclerotic glomeruli should make one search very carefully at different levels in the biopsy for glomeruli with segmental lesions. Only the presence of segmental lesions enables one to make the diagnosis of focal segmental glomerulosclerosis.

Diffuse mesangial proliferative glomerulonephritis

It is generally accepted that if in a paraffin wax section 2 μm thick the glomeruli contain four mesangial cells or more in each peripheral mesangial area, in addition to showing segmental sclerosis, then this constitutes diffuse mesangial proliferative glomerulonephritis complicated by focal segmental glomerulosclerosis. A lesser degree of hypercellularity (three cells per mesangial area) combined with segmental lesions is compatible with idiopathic focal segmental glomerulosclerosis.

Complications

The complications encountered in focal segmental glomerulosclerosis are those associated with the nephrotic syndrome. They are discussed on page 126.

Renal transplantation

Focal segmental glomerulosclerosis recurs in approximately 30% of renal allografts, with a higher incidence of recurrence in second grafts (see p. 663). Patients develop heavy proteinuria, sometimes within hours of transplantation. In this early stage segmental lesions are not present and immunofluorescence is negative. Only later do the typical lesions develop. Most patients with recurrent disease do not respond to steroids and in one large series[15] approximately half the cases with recurrent disease progressed to failure of the graft after 5 months to 3 years. A further 30% continued with heavy proteinuria and the nephrotic syndrome in all but one; the urine became protein free in only 20%.

Prognosis

Focal segmental glomerulosclerosis is a progressive disease but deterioration may occur at a very variable rate. Complete remissions are uncommon; when they occur it is usually associated with treatment. In the 1985 report of the Southwest Pediatric Nephrology Study Group (based in Texas, USA) it was found that of 75 children presenting with focal segmental glomerulosclerosis and the nephrotic syndrome, and subsequently treated, 21% had reached end-stage renal failure within 5 years and a further 23% had developed a decrease in the glomerular filtration rate; 11% were in remission.[86] A study of 46 adults with focal segmental glomerulosclerosis followed up for the same length of time showed very similar results.[93]

The uncertain outlook for these patients has led to many attempts to define which pathological and clinical features of the disease can be used as guides in predicting prognosis. It has been suggested that histopathological indicators of a poor outcome are mesangial hypercellularity, the relative percentage of global versus segmental sclerotic lesions, the presence of segmental hyalinosis, the amount of tubulointerstitial scarring and the presence of arteriolar hyalinosis. Clinical indicators of a poor prognosis that have been suggested are hypertension, the nephrotic syndrome and haematuria. However, the data supporting most of these suggestions are inconclusive. The Southwest Pediatric Nephrology Study Group's data show that arteriolar hyalinosis and tubulointerstitial disease tend to be more frequent in the initial biopsy from patients who subsequently develop renal failure but these associations did not reach statistical significance. There was an increase in the percentage of globally sclerotic glomeruli in follow-up biopsies from the kidneys of those patients with a decreasing glomerular filtration rate.[86] None of the other suggested indicators emerged as of any value. The suggestion that it is possible to predict the clinical outcome in patients with focal segmental glomerulosclerosis on the basis of the location of the segmental sclerotic lesion within the glomerular tuft is discussed on page 211. A recent retrospective analysis of 250 cases has suggested that the amount of interstitial fibrosis and the presence of the nephrotic syndrome at the time of renal biopsy are the only variables with significant independent value in predicting the prognosis.[94]

Pathogenesis

The fact that massive proteinuria may immediately follow the transplantation of a normal kidney into a patient suffering from focal segmental glomerulosclerosis strongly suggests that at least in some patients the disease is caused by a circulating factor or factors that increase glomerular permeability. To test this hypothesis serum from a patient who had had recurrence of the nephrotic syndrome and focal segmental glomerulosclerosis after two renal allografts was infused into the aorta of anaesthetized rats.[95] During the infusion the amount of protein excreted in the urine approximately doubled and this excretion persisted for an hour after the infusion was stopped. Control studies in which serum from patients with the nephrotic syndrome secondary to other glomerular diseases was infused into the rats produced no changes in urinary protein excretion. Infusion of serum from a patient whose focal segmental glomerulosclerosis did not recur after transplantation also produced no change in the rats' urine. The increases in urinary protein were independent of changes in glomerular filtration rate, urinary volume or fractional excretion of sodium. The serum was heated at 56°C for 30 minutes prior to use and did not contain any antiglomerular basement membrane antibody. Some of the sera used in the control tests came from patients receiving prednisolone and azathioprine in doses similar to those received by the patients with recurrent focal segmental glomerulosclerosis. The results of this study are most interesting and should stimulate further more sophisticated searches for a circulating factor in patients in whom focal segmental glomerulosclerosis has recurred in a renal allograft. No long-term studies have been performed and no histological renal lesion has been induced because of the problems of prolonged administration of human protein to rats and the probability of inducing immunological glomerular injury.

It has been claimed that the circulating factor can be partially removed by plasma exchange and completely absorbed on a protein A column. Preliminary studies of column eluates suggest that the factor is a protein but not an immunoglobulin.[96] When idiopathic focal segmental glomerulosclerosis recurs in renal allografts the earliest pathological change is diffuse obliteration of the foot processes of the visceral epithelial cells; this is seen at the onset of the heavy proteinuria. Later the epithelial cells begin to show focal separation from the capillary basement membrane and necrosis. Hyaline and sclerotic segmental lesions do not develop for several weeks or months. One hypothesis to explain these facts is that the postulated circulating factor alters the function of the visceral epithelial cells and ultimately injures these cells. Failure of the visceral epithelial cells to maintain normal capillary wall function, possibly as a consequence of loss of epithelial polyion, then leads to increased trapping of serum macromolecules in the mesangium and segmental collapse of the capillary tuft and scarring.

The initial occurrence of idiopathic focal segmental glomerulosclerosis in the juxtamedullary glomeruli in humans could be because these glomeruli have the highest filtration rate. Any circulating factor would then tend to localize preferentially in the glomeruli of this region.

Single nephron hyperfiltration (see p. 131) in rats leads to focal segmental glomerulosclerosis. This haemodynamic mechanism is probably not relevant in idiopathic focal segmental glomerulosclerosis in the human. On the other hand, adaptive hyperfiltration is a very likely explanation for several of the forms of secondary focal segmental glomerulosclerosis, particularly those in which there is a reduction in functioning renal tissue, as occurs, for example, in unilateral renal agenesis (see p. 55).

Variant

The glomerular tip lesion

In 1984 attention was drawn to a segmental glomerular lesion found in 20 young adults who presented with heavy proteinuria or the nephrotic syndrome.[97] The lesion was present in all the glomeruli and its most distinctive feature was its position in the glomerular tuft. It occurred in the part of the tuft that is opposite the hilum and it consisted of obliteration of a group of glomerular capillaries, initially by cells with foamy cytoplasm and later by hyaline. Apart from the segmental lesion, which was adherent to Bowman's capsule immediately adjacent to the origin of the proximal tubule, the glomerular tuft was normal. Immunohistopathological studies were undertaken in only five of the cases; in two the segmental lesions contained IgM with or without C3 (Fig. 7.31) and in three no immunoglobulins or complement components were detected. Sixteen of the patients were treated with steroids with lessening of their proteinuria. In a later paper, in which additional cases are discussed, it is mentioned that one patient who received a renal allograft afterwards developed almost immediate recurrence of proteinuria.[98] It has been claimed that this segmental glomerular lesion, in association with an otherwise normal glomerular tuft, constitutes a specific clinicopathological entity with a good prognosis after treatment with steroids.

Basically, the report does not deal with a new

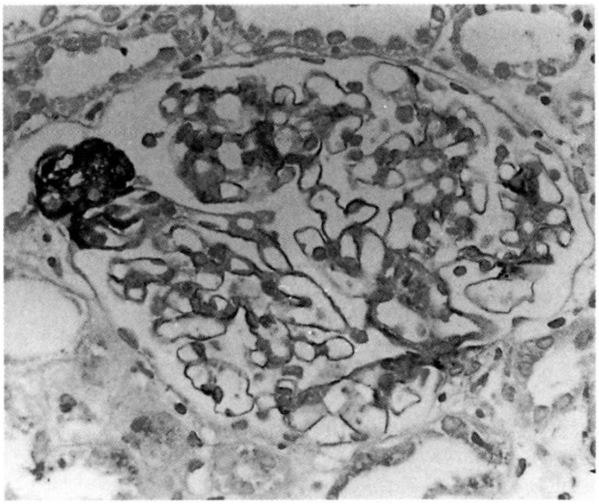

Fig. 7.31 Focal segmental glomerulosclerosis. Variant sometimes called the glomerular tip lesion. The segment of glomerulosclerosis is opposite the hilum of the glomerulus and adherent to Bowman's capsule immediately adjacent to the origin of the proximal tubule. The lesion contains IgM. Immunoperoxidase × 350

entity. In effect, it claims that it is possible to predict the clinical outcome in patients with focal segmental glomerulosclerosis from the location of the segmental lesions within the glomeruli in the initial renal biopsy specimen (providing there is no mesangial hypercellularity).

Another paper making this claim also appeared in 1984; it was demonstrated that in children with focal segmental glomerulosclerosis in whom the segment of sclerosis was peripheral, i.e. away from the glomerular hilum, the prognosis was very good, while in those with hilar or hilar plus peripheral sclerosis the prognosis was poor.[99]

These findings have yet to be confirmed by others. One recent study has detected no significant difference in outcome between hilar and peripheral focal segmental glomerulosclerosis; the investigators make the point that over the course of the follow-up (mean 9.3 years), transitions occurred from one type to another in most cases.[100]

FOCAL GLOMERULONEPHRITIS

Focal glomerulonephritis is the presence of segmental, or less frequently global, lesions in some of the glomeruli. The remaining glomeruli are normal. The lesions may be an increase in the number of mesangial cells and amount of mesangial matrix, an area of necrosis or a focus of sclerosis. Almost always it is a manifestation of some systemic disease, e.g. Henoch–Schönlein purpura (see p. 252), microscopic polyarteritis (see p. 272), Wegener's granulomatosis (see p. 275), systemic lupus erythematosus (see p. 225), bacterial endocarditis (see p. 375), antiglomerular basement membrane disease (see p. 217), IgA nephropathy (see p. 159), hereditary nephritis (see p. 75), resolving endocapillary proliferative glomerulonephritis (see p. 150) or hypertension (see p. 310). Occasionally, even after the most careful electron microscopy and immunofluorescence/immunoperoxidase microscopy, cases remain in which no underlying cause can be detected. The following account is concerned with these idiopathic cases of focal glomerulonephritis.

Clinical features

A few elderly patients develop an influenza-like illness followed by an acute nephritic syndrome. This may progress to renal failure. Other patients have a nephrotic syndrome.

Renal changes

Light microscopy

Various numbers of glomeruli contain usually segmental areas of mesangial cell proliferation, necrosis or sclerosis (Figs 7.32, 7.33). Occasionally these changes are global rather than segmental. The number and proportion of glomeruli showing one or more of these lesions vary greatly between cases. Sometimes there are crescents.

Electron microscopy

The findings by electron microscopy confirm those identified by light microscopy.

Immunofluorescence/immunoperoxidase microscopy

There are usually no deposits of immunoglobulins or complement.

Differential diagnosis

The glomerular changes in idiopathic focal glom-

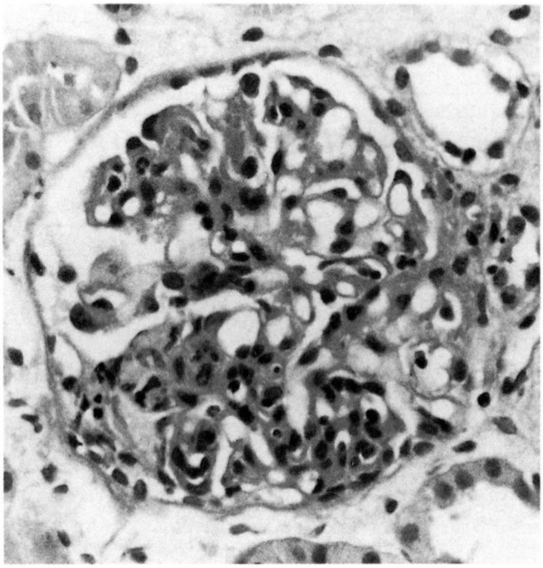

Fig. 7.32 Focal glomerulonephritis. The glomerulus contains a segment of mesangial cell proliferation with excess mesangial matrix.
Periodic acid-Schiff × 260

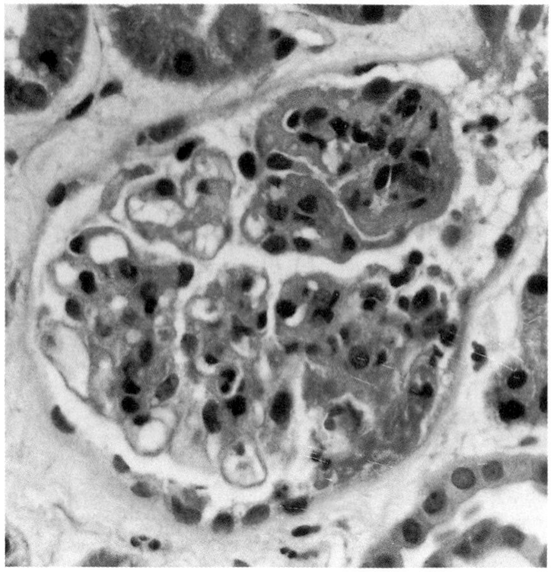

Fig. 7.33 Focal glomerulonephritis. The glomerulus contains a segment of necrosis.
Haematoxylin-eosin × 260

erulonephritis are indistinguishable from those in *microscopic polyarteritis* (see p. 272). The *secondary forms of focal glomerulonephritis* can be distinguished by their distinctive light microscopic, immunofluorescence/immunoperoxidase microscopic or electron microscopic appearances.

Prognosis

Patients with idiopathic focal glomerulonephritis behave in the same way as those in whom microscopic polyarteritis has been proven. They respond to steroids and should be treated as though the diagnosis is microscopic polyarteritis.

REFERENCES

Dense deposit disease

1. Cameron JS, Turner DR, Heaton J et al. Idiopathic mesangiocapillary glomerulonephritis. Comparison of types I and II in children and adults and long term prognosis. Am J Med 1983; 74: 175–192.
2. Hyman LR, Jenis EH, Hill GS, Zimmerman SW, Burkholder PM. Alternate C3 pathway activation in pneumococcal glomerulonephritis. Am J Med 1975; 58: 810–814.
3. Jenis EH, Sandler P, Hill GS, Kneiser MR, Jensen GE, Roskes SD. Glomerulonephritis with basement membrane dense deposits. Arch Pathol Lab Med 1974; 97: 84–91.
4. Chesney RW, O'Regan S, Guyda HJ, Drummond KN. Candida endocrinopathy syndrome with membranoproliferative glomerulonephritis: demonstration of glomerular candida antigen. Clin Nephrol 1976; 5: 232–238.
5. Hariprasad MK, Dodelson R, Eisinger RP, Gary NE. Dense deposit disease in tuberculosis. NY State J Med 1979; 79: 2084–2085.
6. Olson JL, Philips TM, Lewis MG, Solez K. Malignant melanoma with renal dense deposits containing tumour antigens. Clin Nephrol 1979; 12: 74–82.
7. Levy M, Halbwachs-Mecarelli L, Gubler M-C et al. H deficiency in two brothers with atypical dense intramembranous deposit disease. Kidney Int 1986; 30: 949–956.
8. Southwest Pediatric Nephrology Study Group. Dense deposit disease in children: prognostic value of clinical and pathologic indicators. Am J Kidney Dis 1985; 6: 161–169.
9. Ooi YM, Vallota EH, West CD. Serum immune complexes in membranoproliferative and other glomerulonephritides. Kidney Int 1977; 11: 275–283.
10. Galle P, Mahieu P. Electron dense alteration of kidney basement membranes. A renal lesion specific of a systemic disease. Am J Med 1975; 58: 749–764.
11. Habib R, Gubler M-C, Loirat C, Ben Maiz H, Levy M. Dense deposit disease: a variant of membranoproliferative glomerulonephritis. Kidney Int 1975; 7: 204–215.
12. Sibley RK, Kim Y. Dense intramembranous deposit

disease: new pathologic features. Kidney Int 1984; 25: 660–670.
13. Thorner P, Baumal R. Extraglomerular dense deposits in dense deposit disease. Arch Pathol Lab Med 1982; 106: 628–631.
14. Cameron JS. Glomerulonephritis in renal transplants. Transplantation 1982; 34: 237–245.
15. Habib R, Antignac C, Hinglais N, Gagnadoux M-F, Broyer M. Glomerular lesions in the transplanted kidney in children. Am J Kidney Dis 1987; 10: 198–207.
16. Kashtan CE, Burke B, Burch G, Fisher SG, Kim Y. Dense intramembranous deposit disease: a clinical comparison of histological subtypes. Clin Nephrol 1990; 33: 1–6
17. Kher KK, Makker SP, Aikawa M, Kirson IJ. Regression of dense deposits in type II membranoproliferative glomerulonephritis, case report of clinical course in a child. Clin Nephrol 1982; 17: 100–103.
18. Bennett WM, Fassett RG, Walker RG, Fairley KF, d'Apice AJF, Kincaid-Smith P. Mesangiocapillary glomerulonephritis type II (dense deposit disease): clinical features of progressive disease. Am J Kidney Dis 1989; 13: 469–476.
19. McEnery PT, McAdams AJ. Regression of membranoproliferative glomerulonephritis type II (dense deposit disease): observations in six children. Am J Kidney Dis 1988; 12: 138–146.
20. Muda AO, Barsotti P, Marinozzi V. Ultrastructural histochemical investigations of a 'dense deposit disease'. Pathogenetic approach to a special type of mesangiocapillary glomerulonephritis. Virchows Arch [A] 1988; 413: 529–537.
21. Nevins TE. Lectin binding in membranoproliferative glomerulonephritis. Evidence for *N*-acetylglucosamine in dense intramembranous deposits. Am J Pathol 1985; 118: 325–330.
22. Verroust PJ, Wilson CB, Dixon FJ. Lack of nephritogenicity of systemic activation of the alternate complement pathway. Kidney Int 1974; 6: 157–169.

Diffuse crescentic glomerulonephritis

23. Churg J, Sobin LH. Renal disease. Classification and atlas of glomerular diseases. New York: Igaku-Shoin, 1982: 9.
24. Neild GH, Cameron JS, Ogg CS et al. Rapidly progressive glomerulonephritis with extensive glomerular crescent formation. Q J Med 1983; 52: 395–416.
25. Couser WG. Idiopathic rapidly progressive glomerulonephritis. Am J Nephrol 1982; 2: 57–69.
26. Baldwin DS, Neugarten J, Feiner HD, Gluck M, Spinowitz B. The existence of a protracted course in crescentic glomerulonephritis. Kidney Int 1987; 31: 790–794.
27. Savage COS, Winearls CG, Jones S, Marshall PD, Lockwood CM. Prospective study of radioimmunoassay for antibodies against neutrophil cytoplasm in diagnosis of systemic vasculitis. Lancet 1987; 1: 1389–1393.
28. Morita T, Suzuki Y, Churg J. Structure and development of the glomerular crescent. Am J Pathol 1973; 72: 349–368.
29. Yoshioka K, Takemura T, Akano N, Miyamoto H, Iseki T, Maki S. Cellular and non-cellular compositions of crescents in human glomerulonephritis. Kidney Int 1987; 32: 284–291.
30. Bonsib SM. Glomerular basement membrane discontinuities. Scanning electron microscopic study of acellular glomeruli. Am J Pathol 1985; 119: 357–360.
31. Markovic-Lipkovski J, Muller CA, Risler T, Bohle A, Muller GA. Association of glomerular and interstitial mononuclear leukocytes with different forms of glomerulonephritis. Nephrol Dial Transplant 1990; 5: 10–17.
32. Spargo BH, Ordonez NG, Ringus JC. The differential diagnosis of crescentic glomerulonephritis. The pathology of specific lesions with prognostic implications. Hum Pathol 1977; 8: 187–204.
33. Wheeler J, Simpson J, Morley AR. Routine and rapid enzyme linked immunosorbent assays for circulating anti-glomerular basement membrane antibodies. J Clin Pathol 1988; 41: 163–170.
34. Turney JK, Adu D, Michael J, McMaster P. Recurrent crescentic glomerulonephritis in renal transplant recipient treated with cyclosporin. Lancet 1986; 1: 1104.
35. Bruns FJ, Adler S, Fraley DS, Segel DP. Long-term follow-up of aggressively treated idiopathic rapidly progressive glomerulonephritis. Am J Med 1989; 86: 400–406.
36. Croker BP, Lee T, Gunnells JC. Clinical and pathologic features of polyarteritis nodosa and its renal limited variant: primary crescentic and necrotizing glomerulonephritis. Hum Pathol 1987; 18: 38–44.
37. Jayne DRW, Marshall PD, Jones SJ, Lockwood CM. Autoantibodies to GBM and neutrophil cytoplasm in rapidly progressive glomerulonephritis. Kidney Int 1990; 37: 965–970.
38. Tervaert JWC, Goldschmeding R, Elema JD et al. Autoantibodies against myeloid lysosomal enzymes in crescentic glomerulonephritis. Kidney Int 1990; 37: 799–806.
39. Bar-Shavit R, Kahn A, Wilner GD, Fenton JW. Monocyte chemotaxis: stimulation by specific exosite region in thrombin. Science 1983; 220: 728–731.
40. Naish P, Penn GB, Evans DJ, Peters DK. The effect of defibrination on nephrotoxic serum nephritis in rabbits. Clin Sci 1972; 42: 643–646.
41. Watanabe T, Tanaka K. The role of coagulation and fibrinolysis in the development of rabbit Masugi nephritis. Acta Pathol Jpn 1976; 26: 147–165.
42. Foster GR, Carmichael DJS, Kermode A, Hulme B, Gabriel JRT, Cattell V. Extensive crescent formation with antifibrinolytic therapy in a case of diffuse endocapillary glomerulonephritis. Nephrol Dial Transplant 1990; 5: 152–154.
43. Boucher A, Droz D, Adafer E, Noel L-H. Relationships between the integrity of Bowman's capsule and the composition of cellular crescents in human crescentic glomerulonephritis. Lab Invest 1987; 56: 526–533.
44. Cattell V, Jamieson SW. The origin of glomerular crescents in experimental nephrotoxic serum nephritis in the rabbit. Lab Invest 1978; 39: 584–590.
45. Magil AB. Histogenesis of glomerular crescents. Am J Pathol 1985; 120: 222–229

Diffuse membranous glomerulonephritis

46. Noël LH, Zanetti M, Droz D. Long-term prognosis of idiopathic membranous glomerulonephritis. Study of 116 untreated patients. Am J Med 1979; 66: 82–90.

8

K. A. Porter

The kidneys in some selected systemic diseases

INTRODUCTION

Renal disease complicates many systemic conditions. Some of these systemic diseases and syndromes are hereditary, or have a major vascular, cardiac, metabolic or infectious component, or are associated with pregnancy: these are considered in other chapters on a purely arbitrary basis. The remainder, including those with a predominantly immunological basis and those often referred to as 'collagen diseases', are discussed in this chapter.

ANTIGLOMERULAR BASEMENT MEMBRANE DISEASE

Antiglomerular basement membrane disease is a rare condition characterized by linear deposition of IgG on the glomerular capillary basement membrane, the presence of antiglomerular basement membrane antibodies in the circulation and focal segmental necrotizing glomerular lesions. There are usually also glomerular crescents and diffuse crescentic glomerulonephritis is frequent. The patients often develop rapidly progressive renal failure, with or without haemoptysis. Almost none of the patients who are dependent on dialysis at presentation recovers any renal function. Of the others, up to 70% recover or maintain renal function after treatment with various combinations of steroids, azathioprine or cyclophosphamide (to suppress antiglomerular basement membrane antibody synthesis) and plasma exchange (to remove circulating antibodies).

Clinical features

Antiglomerular basement membrane antibody-mediated disease is rare but data on its incidence in the population are not available. It is encountered in less than 5% of renal biopsies. Men are affected more than women in a ratio of approximately 4 : 3. The overall mean age at onset of clinical signs and symptoms is 47.8 years with a range from 17 to 75 years; the age distribution is bimodal with a peak in young adult life (with men predominating) and a second peak in the 60–69-year age group (with women predominating).[1] The disease has a seasonal incidence with most cases occurring in spring or early summer.[2]

At presentation approximately 70% of patients are in renal failure and dependent on dialysis. Most of the others have the acute nephritic syndrome. Occasionally the disease is detected in patients being investigated for isolated haematuria or proteinuria. Approximately 35% of the patients also have haemoptysis: antiglomerular basement membrane disease is a common cause of Goodpasture's syndrome (see p. 224). Most of the patients who present with this syndrome are men in their twenties.[1] Haemoptysis sometimes precedes evidence of renal disease by up to 1 year. Subclinical pulmonary haemorrhage is more common and can be detected by serial measurements of carbon monoxide uptake.[3] Pulmonary haemorrhage is accompanied by an acute, transient increase in the diffusing capacity for carbon monoxide. This occurs because the gas becomes bound to the haemoglobin in the extravasated blood. Taken together subclinical and clinical pulmonary haemorrhage occurs at some time in almost two-thirds of patients with antiglomerular basement membrane disease.

Tissue typing

There is a strong association between HLA-DR2 and antiglomerular basement membrane disease.[4]

Serology

By definition the serum contains raised titres of autoantibodies against human glomerular basement membrane; they are detected by solid phase radioimmunoassay[5] or enzyme-linked immunosorbent assay.[6] The antibodies are directed against epitopes located on the carboxyl terminal propeptides of type IV procollagen in the basement membrane of the kidney, lung and choroid plexus. The type IV procollagen molecule is composed of several domains. One of these domains is globular and resists collagenase digestion. It is referred to as the non-collagen I (NCI) domain. Antiglomerular basement membrane antibodies react with the monomeric and dimeric components of the NCI of the glomerular, alveolar and choroidal basement membranes. NCI is sometimes known as the Goodpasture antigen but it is not yet determined whether molecules other than procollagen IV are also involved in the induction of antiglomerular basement membrane antibodies.[7] The antibody titre correlates with the plasma creatinine concentration in patients who at presentation are not dependent on dialysis; there is no correlation in patients who require dialysis. There is no simple relationship between circulating levels of antiglomerular basement membrane antibodies and the occurrence or severity of pulmonary haemorrhage;[8] this suggests that the nature of the antibody and local factors also are important in determining whether lung injury occurs.

All patients have IgG antibodies to glomerular basement membrane; approximately 30% also have autoantibodies to neutrophil cytoplasmic antigens,[9] 20% have IgA antibodies, 8% have IgM antibodies and 3% have both IgA and IgM antibodies. There are no obvious clinical features associated with the presence of IgA and IgM antiglomerular basement membrane antibodies. The antibodies to neutrophil cytoplasmic antigens are associated with systemic vasculitis; patients with these antibodies in addition to anti-GBM antibody have a different prognosis from those patients with only anti-GBM antibody.[9] The IgG subclasses of the antiglomerular basement membrane antibodies are restricted to IgG_1 and IgG_4. A predominance of IgG_1 antibody, which can fix complement and bind to macrophages, is associated with clinical manifestations of disease. A predominance of IgG_4, which does not fix complement or have the facility for binding to macrophages through the Fc receptor, does not seem to be harmful, perhaps because it masks antigen and halts tissue injury set in train by IgG_1 antibody. The interplay between IgG_1 and IgG_4 may partly account for the varying degree of disease expression seen in patients who have very similar overall levels of antiglomerular basement membrane antibody.[10]

In patients treated only by dialysis the titres of antiglomerular basement membrane antibodies decline gradually and spontaneously and evidence of antibodies disappears in most patients within 2 years of the clinical onset of the disease.[11] Treatment by plasma exchange and with immunosuppressive drugs almost always causes the circulating antiglomerular basement membrane antibodies to disappear within 8 weeks, irrespective of the initial antibody titre.[1]

More than half the patients with antiglomerular basement membrane disease also have circulating antitubular basement membrane antibodies (see p. 446).

Complement components are generally normal. Immune complexes are sometimes present.

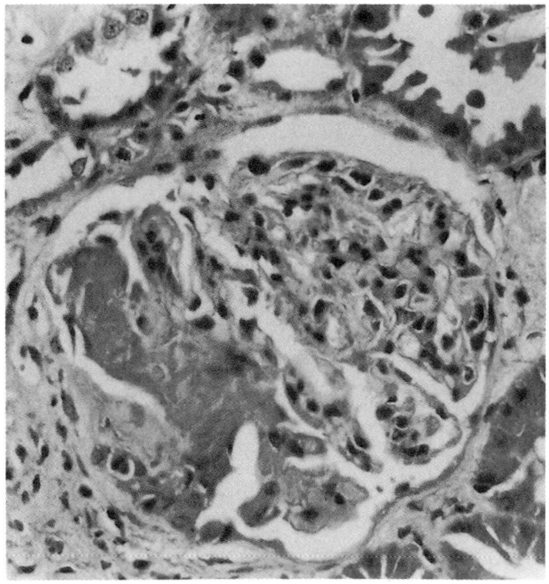

Fig. 8.1 Antiglomerular basement membrane disease. Glomerulus showing segment of necrosis in capillary tuft. There is proliferation of epithelial cells adjacent to the lesion. Haematoxylin-eosin × 335

Peripheral blood lymphocytes

In a patient with untreated antiglomerular basement membrane glomerulonephritis and haemoptysis, serial determination of T-lymphocyte subsets revealed a persistent but variable deficiency of T-suppressor (cluster of differentiation number 8 – CD8)[12] lymphocytes during the period of active disease. As the percentage of CD8 cells returned to normal levels, antibasement membrane autoantibody production decreased and finally ceased.[13]

Renal changes

Light microscopy

A variable number of the glomeruli contain a segment of necrosis (Fig. 8.1). In the lesion the capillaries are disrupted and surrounded by fibrin. There is also fibrin in the adjacent part of Bowman's space associated with local proliferation of epithelial cells with crescent formation (Fig. 8.2). Neutrophil granulocytes are often abundant in the lesion and the number of mesangial cells may

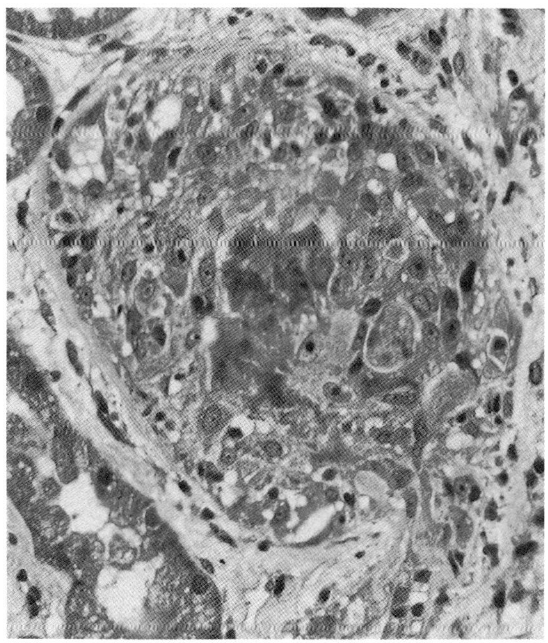

Fig. 8.2 Antiglomerular basement membrane disease. Glomerulus with crescent formation. The glomerular tuft is collapsed and shows segmental necrosis. Haematoxylin-eosin × 350

be increased; there is no swelling or proliferation of the endothelial cells and monocytes are not prominent. In approximately 5% of cases there is just segmental mesangial cell hypercellularity with a few granulocytes; segmental necrosis and crescents are rare or absent in these cases. In roughly 70% of cases the necrotic lesions are common and 80% or more of the glomeruli contain crescents (diffuse crescentic glomerulonephritis). The segmental lesions often show different degrees of organization; there may be segmental or global sclerosis and fibrocellular or fibrous crescents in some glomeruli. Occasionally the crescents contain multinucleate giant cells or cells in mitosis.

The interstitium is oedematous and there is often a patchy dense infiltration with mononuclear cells. Among the lymphocytes in this infiltrate CD4 (T-helper) cells are much more common than CD8 (T-suppressor) cells; B lymphocytes and natural killer (NK) cells are rare.[13]

The arterioles and arteries are usually normal. Rarely there is a necrotizing arteritis or arteriolitis.[14]

Electron microscopy

The lamina rara interna of the glomerular capillary basement membrane may be irregular, a little thicker and much less electron dense than normal but this change is found in many other renal conditions. Breaks in the capillary basement membrane are common in cases with many crescents (see p. 187).

Immunofluorescence/immunoperoxidase microscopy

Linear deposition of IgG is present along the capillary basement membranes of all the glomeruli in approximately 94% of the cases (Fig. 8.3); about half of these show concurrent C3, either in a continuous linear or in an interrupted, occasionally granular, pattern. In 2% there is linear IgA and C3 without IgG. Another 2% show linear IgM and C3 and in a further 2% linear C3 only is found.[1] As the disease progresses the linear deposits of immunoglobulin and complement become fainter and discontinuous. There are no differences in the clinical courses of patients with and without complement deposits in their glomeruli. Linear IgG deposits are also common on the tubular basement membranes (see p. 466) and Bowman's capsule.[15]

Changes in other organs

Lungs

About a third of the patients with antiglomerular

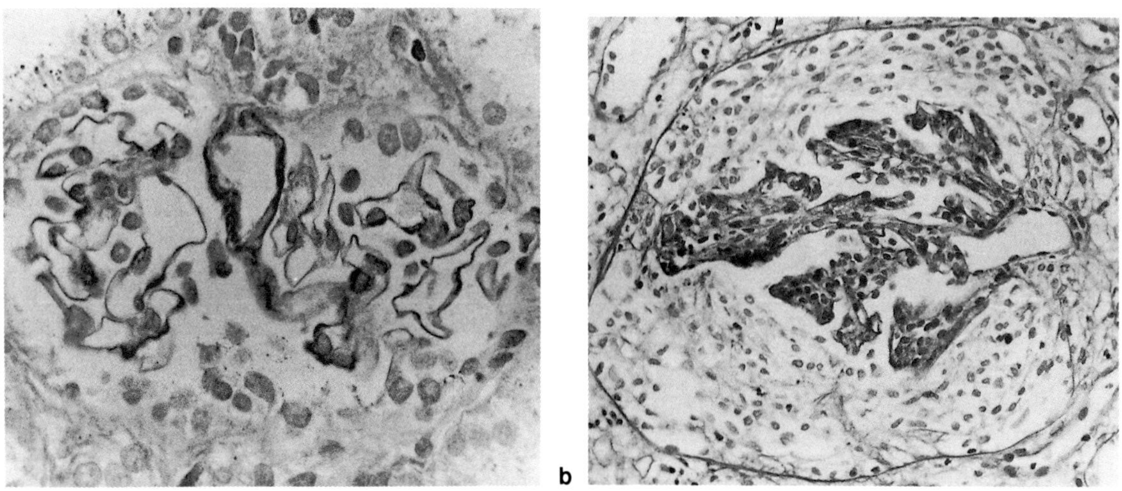

a b

Fig. 8.3 a, b Antiglomerular basement membrane disease. Glomeruli showing linear IgG deposits on the capillary basement membrane and Bowman's capsule. The glomerular tufts are compressed by epithelial crescents; compression is most severe in the glomerulus on the right. Immunoperoxidase: (**a**) × 360; (**b**) × 250

basement membrane disease have haemoptysis and more have evidence of fresh lung haemorrhage on serial carbon monoxide measurement.

Gross appearances The lungs are enlarged and firm and the pleural surface is mottled with purplish areas. On the cut surface there are red and brown areas of recent and old haemorrhage.

Light microscopy The dominant finding is diffuse alveolar haemorrhage: the alveoli contain large numbers of red blood cells, haemosiderin-laden macrophages and fibrin. Usually the alveolar septa are widened by oedema and infiltrated by neutrophil granulocytes. Sometimes there are perivascular mononuclear cell infiltrates. Fibrin thrombi are present in alveolar capillaries. There is evidence of alveolar damage including hyaline membranes. Hyperplasia of type II alveolar lining cells is prominent.[16]

Electron microscopy There are focal areas of mottling and deposition of electron-dense material on the alveolar septal basement membrane. Breaks in the basement membrane are frequent.[17]

Immunofluorescence/immunoperoxidase microscopy IgG is distributed in a linear manner and C3 in a granular pattern along the alveolar basement membrane.[16] The affected alveoli are usually clustered in the vicinity of haemorrhages.

Elution studies IgG eluted from the lungs binds specifically with alveolar and glomerular capillary basement membranes of fresh normal human lung and kidney.[18] The eluate does not become attached to basement membranes of other organs.

Choroidal plexus

Linear deposits of IgG and C3 are present on the basement membrane of the choroidal plexus in some patients.[19]

Differential diagnosis

Linear IgG is sometimes found on the glomerular capillary basement membranes in *diabetic glomerulosclerosis* (see p. 334), *lupus nephritis* (see p. 234) and in *kidneys examined at autopsy*. Circulating antiglomerular basement membrane antibodies are not present in these conditions. To diagnose antiglomerular basement membrane disease, therefore, the demonstration of linear IgG on the glomerular basement membrane is not enough. It is essential that the autoantibodies are sought in the blood at the earliest possible moment using either solid-phase radioimmunoassay[5] or enzyme-linked immunosorbent assay.[6] The rapid enzyme-linked immunosorbent assay, when necessary, can be performed in less than 4 hours.[6]

Complications

Diffuse crescentic glomerulonephritis

Diffuse crescentic glomerulonephritis (see p. 185) occurs in approximately 70% of cases of anti-glomerular basement membrane disease.

Infections

Infections such as varicella, herpes zoster and bacterial endocarditis caused by *Staphylococcus epidermidis* have been recorded.[11]

Pulmonary haemorrhage

Haemorrhages into the lungs may be very severe and patients have died from this complication.

Renal transplantation

If transplantation is delayed until solid-phase radioimmunoassay or enzyme-linked immunosorbent assay no longer detect any antiglomerular basement membrane antibodies in the circulation, the operation can be carried out safely (see p. 668). On the rare occasion when antibodies return, they often fix to the graft without causing significant injury; only about 40% of the grafts with bound antibody are severely damaged by such recurrence.[20] The lack of renal injury in these cases could be explained by the small amount of antibody bound, or by its slow rate of deposition.

The risk of serious damage to the transplanted kidney by antiglomerular basement membrane disease is high if renal transplantation is performed while the patient still has large amounts of antiglomerular basement membrane antibody circulating.

Antiglomerular basement membrane disease occasionally occurs in renal allografts in patients suffering from Alport's syndrome, presumably because antibodies have been formed to the Goodpasture antigen which is present in the graft but was absent from the patients' own kidneys (see p. 77).[21]

De novo IgG linear deposits along the glomerular basement membranes of renal allografts occur in approximately 4.5% of patients whose original disease was not antiglomerular basement membrane antibody mediated.[22] These deposits are not associated with antiglomerular basement membrane antibodies in the circulation. In most cases the deposits produce no symptoms; a few patients develop transient proteinuria.

Prognosis

Patients with antiglomerular basement membrane disease who are dependent on dialysis when they are first diagnosed almost always fail to recover any renal function, even if they receive full treatment with plasma exchange and immunosuppressant drugs.[1] Exceptions who recover sufficient function to remain independent of dialysis are very rare.[23] Because of this poor outlook for renal recovery most nephrologists withhold potentially toxic immunosuppressive drug treatment and plasma exchange from patients dependent on dialysis unless their disease is accompanied by lung haemorrhage or early renal transplantation is required.

In contrast, up to 70% of patients who are not dependent on dialysis at diagnosis recover, or sustain no further deterioration in renal function after treatment with plasma exchange and immunosuppressive drugs.[1] It is for this reason that it is so important that the diagnosis of antiglomerular basement membrane disease is made at the earliest possible moment; if there are surviving glomeruli they can be conserved by prompt treatment. Delays will almost certainly condemn the patient to dialysis or renal transplantation.

Smoking appears to exacerbate injury to the lungs of patients with circulating antibasement membrane antibodies[24] and smoking should be forbidden once the diagnosis of antiglomerular basement membrane disease is suspected to avoid precipitating a life-threatening pulmonary haemorrhage.

A few patients with antiglomerular basement membrane disease have multiple recurrence of Goodpasture's syndrome over a period of many years; one patient was reported as still having episodes, mostly of haemoptysis, 14 years after he was first diagnosed.[25] In another patient circulating antiglomerular basement membrane antibody persisted throughout the course of the illness and the renal and lung tissue continued to demonstrate linear IgG even during periods when the disease was quiescent.[26]

Patients who have autoantibodies to both GBM and neutrophil cytoplasmic antigens are more likely to recover renal function even if they are dependent on dialysis at presentation; also the chance of disease recurring many months after remission is higher than in patients with only antibodies to GBM.[9]

Pathogenesis

Antiglomerular basement membrane disease is an autoimmune disorder caused by the production of antibodies that react with the renal basement membranes. They also frequently react with the pulmonary alveolar basement membranes and sometimes with the basement membrane of the choroid plexus. The disease appears analogous to the nephritis that can be produced in animals by active immunization with glomerular basement membrane (Steblay's nephritis; see p. 128). The role of antiglomerular basement membrane antibodies in human disease was firmly established in 1967 when it was shown that linear glomerular basement membrane deposits and nephritis could be induced in subhuman primates by passively transferring antibodies eluted from the kidneys of patients with antiglomerular basement membrane disease.[27]

Genetic susceptibility to develop autoantibodies to basement membrane has been demonstrated in Steblay's nephritis. The strong association between HLA-DR2 and antiglomerular basement membrane disease in man, together with the occurrence of the disease in siblings and twins, suggests that heredity is also important in humans.[4] Since the HLA-DR genes are thought to be the human equivalent of the major histocompatibility complex (MHC) linked immune response genes in animals, possession of the DR2 antigen may identify the genetic determinant of the autoimmune response initiated by the release of basement membrane.

The initial stimulus responsible for the formation of such antibodies is unknown. One possibility is that the patient's own glomerular basement membrane antigens are released into the circulation. Certainly following glomerular injury the quantity of glomerular basement membrane antigens released into the urine increases markedly. Injection of these antigens into experimental animals induces antiglomerular basement membrane glomerulonephritis. Perhaps under appropriate circumstances the released glomerular basement membrane antigens make contact with immunologically competent cells leading to autoimmunization and antibody formation. A variation on this hypothesis supposes that some toxic or infective episode leads to dissociation of the NCI hexamer in the glomerular basement membrane and exposure of the Goodpasture epitopes. This may stimulate autoantibody production. However, if this was a common mechanism, antiglomerular basement membrane disease superimposed upon other forms of glomerular injury should be frequent, whereas in fact it is very rare.

Another possibility would be the formation of cross-reactive antibodies following exposure to substances with a similar antigenic composition. The most popular hypothesis is that some infection or other form of injury results in release of pulmonary alveolar basement membranes into the circulation. Antibody formation follows and if the primary antipulmonary basement membrane antibodies were to cross react with glomerular basement membranes renal damage would result. This hypothesis is supported by experimental findings in rabbits, in which it has been shown that antibody to alveolar basement membrane cross reacts in the postulated way and produces immune-mediated damage to lungs and kidneys.[28] In humans, Goodpasture antigen has been identified in alveolar basement membrane.[29]

The suggestion that antiglomerular basement membrane production is triggered by solvent induced pulmonary alveolar injury has not been supported by epidemiological data.[30] Individual cases, nevertheless, continue to be recorded which suggest some link with chemical inhalation injury.[31] This link, however, may be a different one. Tissue damaging agents might facilitate the binding of antiglomerular basement membrane antibodies to Goodpasture antigen within the alveolar basement membrane, either by damaging the alveolar capillary endothelium or by exposing Goodpasture epitopes hidden within the globular domain of type IV collagen (see p. 218). This might explain the increased frequency of pulmonary haemorrhage in cigarette smokers, as well as the sporadic association between Goodpasture's syndrome and exposure to volatile solvents and viral infections.[8]

Capillaries other than those of the glomeruli are probably less susceptible to injury by circulating antibasement membrane antibodies because, in contrast to the highly fenestrated glomerular endothelium, alveolar and most other capillary endothelia lack open fenestrae and provide a very effective barrier to the passage of antibasement membrane antibodies.[8]

The possible role of cell-mediated injury in antiglomerular basement membrane disease has been mentioned earlier (see p. 130). The effect of antibody binding on the basement membrane has also been discussed (see p. 130). In many cases complement activation and inflammatory cell infiltration are clearly important, but only antibody deposition activates the renin–angiotensin system and induces vasoconstriction, reduction in the glomerular capillary ultrafiltration coefficient and a fall in the glomerular filtration rate.[32]

Variant

Concurrent antiglomerular basement membrane antibody and immune complex-mediated glomerulonephritis

Rarely, scattered subepithelial electron-dense deposits have been described in patients with antiglomerular basement membrane disease. Immunofluorescence has revealed fine diffuse global granular deposits of IgG and C3 external to the linear staining on the glomerular capillary basement membranes. In some of these cases the antiglomerular basement membrane disease seemed to be secondary to damage to the glomerular capillary basement membrane by a preceding immune complex glomerulonephritis. In others it appeared that the subepithelial deposits were due to antiglomerular basement membrane antibodies complexed with freed glomerular basement membrane antigens.[33]

GLOMERULONEPHRITIS WITH PULMONARY HAEMORRHAGE (GOODPASTURE'S SYNDROME)

The association of haemoptysis and glomerulonephritis in a young man thought to have severe influenza was described in 1919 by Goodpasture[34] and in 1958 the eponym Goodpasture's syndrome was coined to describe any patient presenting with clinical evidence of nephritis and pulmonary haemorrhage.[35]

Patients presenting with this syndrome may have a variety of underlying diseases. Many cases are due to systemic necrotizing vasculitis or to antiglomerular basement membrane disease (see p. 217). The vasculitis is most commonly polyarteritis (see p. 272) or that of Wegener's granulomatosis (see p. 275). Smaller numbers of cases are due to systemic lupus erythematosus (see p. 225), Henoch–Schönlein purpura (see p. 252), bacterial endocarditis (see p. 373), cryoglobulinaemia (see p. 351) and Behçet's disease (see p. 320). Rare causes are penicillamine toxicity (see p. 523) and mixed connective tissue disease (see p. 247). However, between 20 and 30% of cases have no identifiable cause and are usually referred to as idiopathic.

A suggestion in 1978 that the use of the eponym be restricted to patients with antiglomerular basement membrane disease and pulmonary haemorrhage[36] has been accepted by many nephrologists and histopathologists but not by all. This has led to confusion and it would be much better if the term Goodpasture's syndrome was no longer used.

The following account deals with those cases in which the underlying cause of nephritis with lung haemorrhage cannot be determined.

Clinical features

The syndrome is commonest in young adult males. Its onset is sometimes preceded by an influenza-like illness. Most patients are anaemic and all give either a history of haemoptysis or have evidence of lung haemorrhage on carbon monoxide uptake by the lungs (see p. 218). The pulmonary haemorrhage may be life threatening. Haemosiderin-laden macrophages are common in the sputum. Exertional dyspnoea is common and infiltrates are usually present on chest X-ray. Evidence of renal disease may precede the pulmonary haemorrhage, be present initially or only appear later. It may consist of the acute nephritic syndrome (see p. 126), acute renal failure, haematuria or proteinuria. Hypertension is mild or absent.

Serology

Serum complement levels are usually normal. Circulating immune complexes are occasionally present. There are no antiglomerular basement membrane antibodies in the serum. The antistreptolysin O titre is usually within normal limits.

Renal changes

Light microscopy

Generally there is a diffuse crescentic glomerulonephritis. The compressed glomerular tufts often contain increased numbers of mesangial cells and more mesangial matrix than normal. There is usually also segmental tuft thrombosis and necrosis. In milder cases only focal segmental lesions are present with small numbers of crescents.

Electron microscopy

There are often breaks in the capillary basement membranes of a variable number of glomeruli.

Subendothelial and mesangial electron-dense deposits are sometimes present; sparse subepithelial deposits occur very rarely.

Immunofluorescence/immunoperoxidase microscopy

Granular deposits of IgG and C3 may be present in a few or many of the glomerular capillary walls and in the mesangium. Frequently there is no staining for immunoglobulins or complement.

Changes in other organs

Lungs

The pulmonary changes are similar to those seen in antiglomerular basement membrane disease (see p. 220) with the exception that there are no linear deposits of immunoglobulin or complement. Occasionally there are granular deposits of IgG and C3 along alveolar septae.

Differential diagnosis

When a patient presents with pulmonary haemorrhage and evidence of nephritis it is essential that *antiglomerular basement membrane disease* is excluded as quickly as possible (see p. 221). After this the other possible causes of the syndrome (see p. 224) can usually be detected by the characteristic lesions found in a renal biopsy by light, electron and immunofluorescence/immunoperoxidase microscopy, together with serology and any other clinical manifestations.

Complications

The complications of glomerulonephritis with lung haemorrhage are the same as those encountered in antiglomerular basement membrane disease (see p. 221).

Renal transplantation

The recipient's original disease has not developed in the few kidneys that have been transplanted into patients with glomerulonephritis and lung haemorrhage of unknown origin.

Prognosis

As in antiglomerular basement membrane disease the prognosis depends very much upon whether the patient needs dialysis when first seen by the doctor. Those needing dialysis rarely regain any renal function; those not needing dialysis on presentation often respond to treatment with high doses of steroids.

Pathogenesis

By definition, the aetiology and pathogenesis of idiopathic glomerulonephritis with pulmonary haemorrhage are unknown.

SYSTEMIC LUPUS ERYTHEMATOSUS

Systemic lupus erythematosus is a multisystem disorder or group of disorders in the course of which the immune system produces immunoglobulins capable of binding to self components: most conspicuous among the autoantibodies are those which recognize nuclear antigens. Immune complexes often circulate in the blood and DNA-anti-DNA immune complexes are either deposited or form in the kidneys and other tissues. Subsequently these complexes fix complement and mediate inflammation and tissue destruction. There is also evidence of hyperactivity of B lymphocytes and abnormalities of T lymphocyte function.

The aetiology of systemic lupus erythematosus is not known; the syndromes comprising it may not be a single disease but represent a spectrum of autoimmune disorders produced by a variety of agents and pathogenetic mechanisms.

Systemic lupus erythematosus is a fairly common disease with an incidence rate of 7.4 and a prevalence rate of 50.8 per 100 000 persons in the USA for the period 1965–73.[37] It is nine times more common in females than males, and during the childbearing years this ratio rises to 15 : 1. There are racial differences in prevalence and severity. It is commoner in black women in Britain and the USA[37] and in women of Chinese origin rather than in Malay and Indian women in South East Asia.[38] Korean patients seem to have a more active and potentially more fulminating disease than blacks or whites in Britain and the USA.[39] The peak age at onset is in the age group 20–30 years.

The manifestations of systemic lupus erythematosus are variable and protean, with a course characterized by exacerbations and remissions. Renal involvement is very common and may lead to renal failure.

Clinical features[40–42]

Arthralgia or arthritis of non-deforming character, with tenosynovitis, occurs in 95% of patients with systemic lupus erythematosus. The joints most commonly involved are the small joints of the fingers, the wrists and the knees. Myalgia is also very common. Skin lesions, including discoid lupus and the classic facial butterfly rash, affect 80% of patients some time in the course of the illness. The cutaneous eruptions are often prompted or exacerbated by exposure to sun. Fever is present in approximately 77% of cases and neurological or psychiatric disorders such as epilepsy, chorea, thrombotic vascular episodes, peripheral neuropathy and disturbances of behaviour occur in about 60% of patients. Respiratory signs and symptoms such as dyspnoea, pleurisy and pleural effusion occur in nearly 50% of patients. Cardiovascular manifestations, in particular pericarditis and systolic murmurs, are found in approximately 40% of patients. Raynaud's phenomenon is common. A mild to moderate normochromic, normocytic anaemia is usual. A haemolytic anaemia, sometimes with a positive direct Coombs' test, is less frequent. A leucopenia with lymphopenia is found in 40–65% of patients. There is often a mild thrombocytopenia.

Clinical evidence of renal involvement is present in 40% of patients at presentation and later appears in up to 75%. However, almost all patients show immunohistopathological abnormalities on renal biopsy even when renal function and the urine are normal.

Renal manifestations

The most frequent presenting abnormality is proteinuria and in half the patients the protein loss is sufficient to give the nephrotic syndrome. Most patients have microscopic haematuria; gross haematuria is rare. The urine contains hyaline, granular and red cell casts. Mild hypertension is present in about a quarter of the patients when first seen. The acute nephritic syndrome or acute renal failure are occasional modes of presentation. Reduced glomerular filtration rate is characteristic of severe disease. At any time there may be a sudden exacerbation of symptoms. Spontaneous regression is uncommon.

Tissue typing[42,43]

Systemic lupus erythematosus is not associated with any one particular HLA antigen, but in white populations associations have been described most constantly with HLA-DR2 and -DR3 but also with HLA-A1, -B5, -B7 and -B8. The importance of these associations remains uncertain; one possibility is that they reflect linkage disequilibrium with other loci that determine risk factors.

Serology

Patients with systemic lupus erythematosus produce a remarkable range of antibodies to a wide variety of antigens; many are autoantibodies but some are directed against extrinsic antigens. The presence of so many antibodies causes hypergammaglobulinaemia. Among the autoantibodies the majority are not specific to any particular organ; organ-specific antibodies are uncommon.

Antibodies that are not organ specific

Antinuclear antibodies (ANA)[44] Antinuclear antibodies are present at some time during the course of the illness in about 95% of patients. The immunofluorescence test for ANA, with rat liver as substrate, still provides the screening test for systemic lupus erythematosus because it detects a wide range of antibodies to various nuclear components. However, it is not specific for systemic lupus erythematosus, being found in other autoimmune diseases and in 5% of the normal population.

The number of nuclear antigens now recognized is increasing rapidly. They fall into two groups: DNA and the histones, the structure of which are known chemically, and non-histone antigens which are mostly saline extracts of unknown chemical structure (extractable nuclear antigen, ENA).

Antibodies to double-stranded DNA are found in over 60% of patients, are highly specific and remain the diagnostic yardstick for systemic lupus erythematosus.

Antibodies to single-stranded DNA are non-specific, occurring in a wide variety of autoimmune conditions, but when present in systemic lupus erythematosus they fluctuate with disease activity.

Antibodies to histones are found in systemic lupus erythematosus and in virtually all cases of drug-induced systemic lupus erythematosus (see p. 240).

Antibodies to extractable nuclear antigens.[45] Over 20 extractable nuclear antigens are known. Of these, antibody to Smith antigen (*anti-Sm antibody*) occurs in the sera of about 30% of black and Chinese patients with systemic lupus erythematosus but only in 7% of white patients. *Anti-ribonucleoprotein (anti-RNP) antibodies* are found in 23% of patients with systemic lupus erythematosus and *anti-Ro antibody* (an antibody to another small ribonucleoprotein) is seen in 24% of cases of systemic lupus erythematosus. The presence of these antibodies may support the diagnosis of systemic lupus erythematosus when antibodies to DNA are absent. Anti-Ro antibodies are associated with the development of congenital heart block in babies born of patients with systemic lupus erythematosus. Anti-RNP antibodies are associated with Raynaud's phenomenon.

Antibodies to phospholipid[42] Antiphospholipid antibodies are present in approximately 20% of patients. *Anticardiolipin antibodies* are responsible for giving a false-positive VDRL (Venereal Disease Reference Laboratory) test for syphilis. The circulating *lupus anticoagulant* (a paradoxical term in that this inhibitor protein is neither specific for systemic lupus erythematosus nor primarily causes haemorrhage) is associated with an increased tendency to thrombosis of arteries and veins and a high incidence of recurrent abortion. Lupus anticoagulant interferes with the prothrombin activator complex and is found in 30–40% of patients with systemic lupus erythematosus. It may block the metabolism of arachidonic acid to prostacyclin, a potent inhibitor of platelet aggregation.

Rheumatoid factors Rheumatoid factors, autoantibodies directed against determinants on slightly altered IgG, are common in systemic lupus erythematosus.

Cytotoxic antibodies Antibodies cytotoxic to lymphocytes and neutrophil granulocytes are present in nearly half the patients. Antiplatelet antibodies, direct or indirect, or both, are found in over 80% of patients with systemic lupus erythematosus; their presence does not correlate with the platelet count.

Organ-specific antibodies

Antithyroid, antimitochondrial, antigastric parietal cell and antismooth muscle antibodies occur but are rare, being found in only approximately 2% of patients.

Antibodies to viruses

The titres of antibodies to various organisms, particularly viruses and rickettsiae, are elevated.

Circulating immune complexes

Immune complexes in the serum are frequent but only a small proportion are DNA related.

Acute-phase reactants

The levels of acute-phase reactants are usually elevated in periods of activity of systemic lupus erythematosus. The exception is C-reactive protein which remains normal or low except in the presence of infection.

Complement

Characteristically, serum levels of the classical

complement pathway components, C1, C2, C3, C4, C5, and factor B and whole complement activity (THC or CH_{50}) are reduced because of increased utilization.[46]

Both genetic and acquired deficiencies of the C1, C2 and C4 components are associated with systemic lupus erythematosus.[47] The prevalence of systemic lupus erythematosus is higher with C1 and C4 deficiencies than with C2 and with complete deficiencies compared to partial deficiencies. Some of the cases of systemic lupus erythematosus associated with early complement deficiencies are atypical (see p. 241).

Peripheral blood lymphocytes

Lymphocytes in systemic lupus erythematosus show hyperactivity of B cells, dysfunction of CD4+ helper T cells, hyperactivity of CD8+ suppressor T cells and a defect in cell communication.[48]

Renal changes

Gross appearance of the kidneys

There are no characteristic naked eye changes. The kidneys are usually normal in size, smooth and pale. Petechial haemorrhages are sometimes present.

Light microscopy

Almost any form of glomerulonephritis from the mildest to the most severe can occur in systemic lupus erythematosus. The World Health Organization in 1975 proposed a classification of lupus nephritis in which five main classes were recognized; this classification was modified and expanded to six classes in 1982[49] and it is this latest World Health Organization classification that is used in the following account.

Class I: minor glomerular abnormalities In this category are placed those cases that appear normal on light microscopy of renal biopsies. This lack of glomerular change on light microscopy is encountered in about 16% of renal biopsies from patients with systemic lupus erythematosus. Abnormalities are almost always detectable in these cases by electron microscopy and immunofluorescence or immunoperoxidase microscopy.

Class II: mesangial widening and or mesangial hypercellularity The mesangium is expanded due to a global increase in the number of mesangial cells (to three cells per mesangial area away from the vascular pole in 3 μm thick sections) and in the amount of mesangial matrix (Fig. 8.4). These changes affect more than 80% of the glomeruli. This morphological pattern is seen in about 16% of renal biopsies from patients with systemic lupus erythematosus and is common in patients with mild clinical disease or in remission.

Class III: focal segmental glomerulonephritis This category includes cases with segmental lesions of mesangial cell proliferation, inflammation, necrosis and sclerosis (Fig. 8.5). The number of involved glomeruli may vary from a few to 80%. Segmental inflammation is accompanied by exudation of neutrophil granulocytes; some of these will die and the lesion will come to contain their fragmented nuclei. Segmental necrosis is of fibrinoid type and usually contains a group of thrombosed glomerular capillaries. Segmental sclerosis consists of acellular scars that are often adherent to Bowman's capsule. The focal lesions are commonly superimposed upon one of the other categories of morphological change, usually on class II. Focal segmental glomerulonephritis is found in approximately 20% of renal biopsies from patients with systemic lupus erythematosus.

Class IV: diffuse proliferative glomerulonephritis In this category more than 80% of the glomeruli are involved by one or more of the following histological patterns:

1. *Proliferative, necrotizing and sclerosing glomerulonephritis.* This is the most common form. It is characterized by mesangial proliferative glomerulonephritis (four or more mononuclear cells per mesangial area away from the vascular pole in 2 μm thick sections – see p. 153) combined with variable degrees of necrosis and sclerosis (Fig. 8.6). The pattern is typically irregular with minimally altered segments alternating with areas

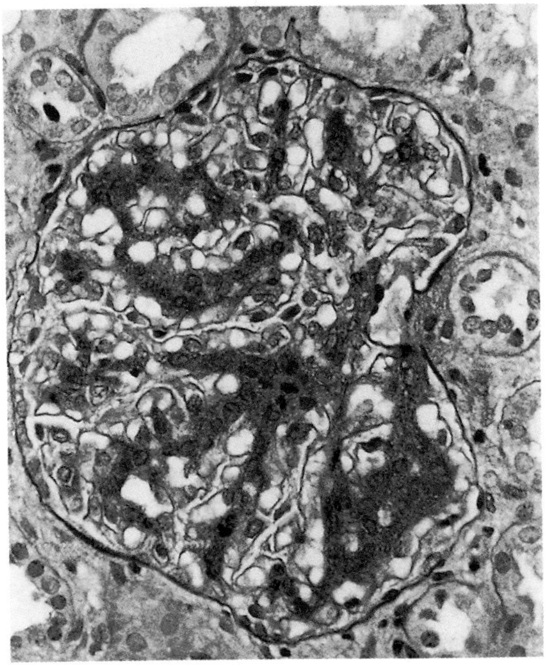

Fig. 8.4 Lupus nephritis – mesangial hypercellularity (class II).
Periodic acid-Schiff × 500

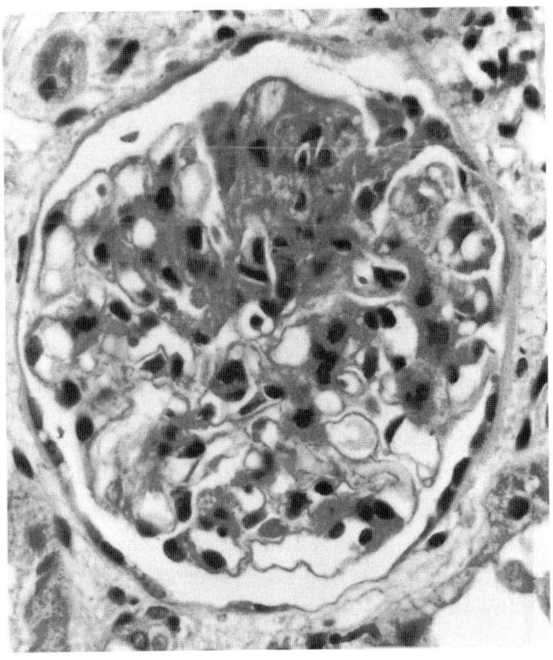

Fig. 8.5 Lupus nephritis – focal segmental glomerulonephritis (Class III). The segmental necrotic lesion in the upper part of the glomerulus is adherent to Bowman's capsule.
Haematoxylin-eosin × 335

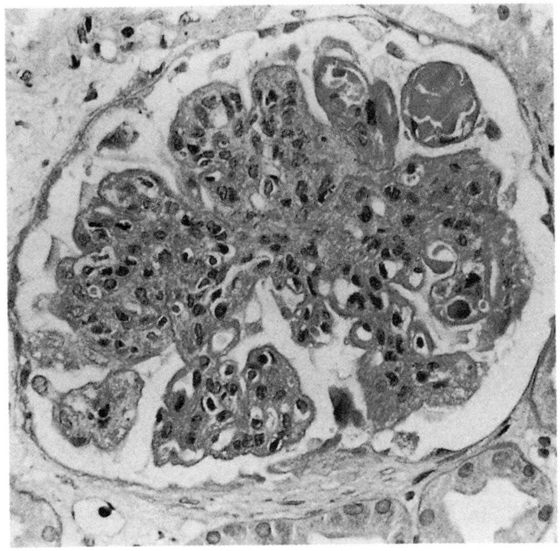

Fig. 8.6 Lupus nephritis – diffuse proliferative glomerulonephritis (Class IV). Glomerulus in which mesangial proliferation involves several lobules. There is also segmental thickening of capillary walls and a few hyaline thrombi.
Periodic acid-Schiff × 400

of proliferation, necrosis, wire loops and occlusion of capillary lumens by hyaline material – *hyaline thrombi* (Fig. 8.7). *Wire loops* are greatly thickened eosinophilic segments of glomerular capillary wall; the thickening is caused by subepithelial

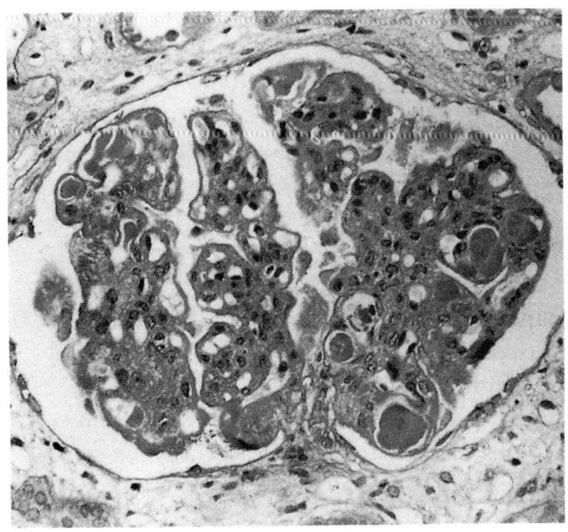

Fig. 8.7 Lupus nephritis – glomerulus with several hyaline thrombi in capillary lumina. There is also segmental thickening of capillary walls and segmental mesangial cell proliferation.
Periodic acid-Schiff × 350

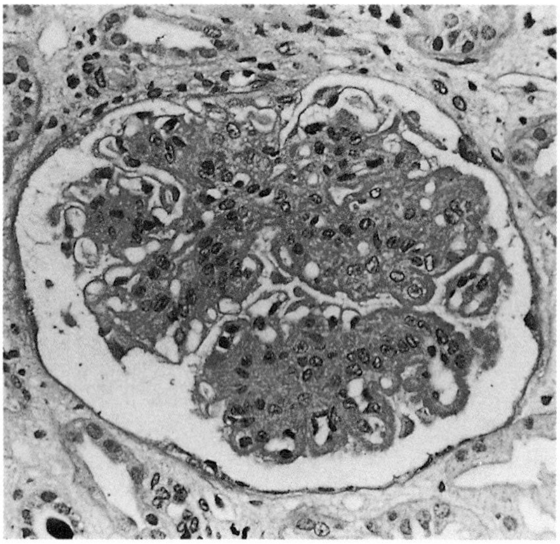

Fig. 8.8 Lupus nephritis – glomerulus showing several capillaries at bottom right of picture with segmental thickening of their walls producing wire loop lesions. Periodic acid-Schiff × 350

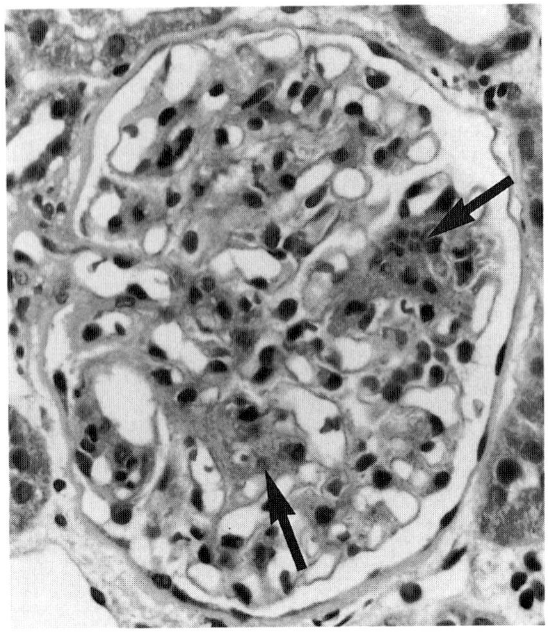

Fig. 8.9 Lupus nephritis – glomerulus with two segmental lesions containing scattered haematoxyphil bodies (arrows). Haematoxylin-eosin × 400

immune deposits (Fig. 8.8). In the necrotic areas some of the nuclear fragments stain lilac with haematoxylin and are called *haematoxyphil* or *haematoxylin bodies*. These bodies range in size from tiny fragments to irregularly rounded masses roughly the size of a nucleus (Fig.8.9). Occasionally they are found in the cytoplasm of macrophages. Haematoxyphil bodies are rarely obvious but they can be found in the majority of cases if a careful search is made through many sections. They are considered to be pathognomonic of lupus nephritis.

Because lupus nephritis is subject to exacerbations and periods of relative quiescence, active proliferation may coexist with focal segmental sclerosis from previous damage.

2. *Diffuse endocapillary proliferative glomerulo-nephritis*. By light microscopy this may occasionally be difficult to distinguish from the postinfectious and other forms of diffuse endocapillary proliferative glomerulonephritis (see p. 145). However, there are usually other changes such as wire loops, hyaline thrombi and segments of necrosis. Also the subendothelial deposits can sometimes be detected.

3. *Diffuse mesangiocapillary proliferative glomerulonephritis*. Focal and segmental areas of mesangial interposition are common in lupus nephritis. Infrequently, the changes are diffuse and produce a pattern that may be indistinguishable by light microscopy from other forms of diffuse mesangiocapillary proliferative glomerulonephritis (see p. 166)

4. *Diffuse crescentic glomerulonephritis*. Occasionally this is superimposed upon the other forms of diffuse lupus glomerulonephritis. The presence of only small numbers of crescents is commoner.

Diffuse proliferative glomerulonephritis is found in approximately 38% of renal biopsies from patients with systemic lupus nephritis.

Class V: diffuse membranous glomerulonephritis In this category more than 80% of the glomeruli are involved. The capillary walls are uniformally thickened and there are often spikes of new basement membrane between the deposits (Fig. 8.10). If this type of lupus nephritis occurs in pure form it may be indistinguishable by light microscopy from idiopathic diffuse membranous glomerulonephritis (see p. 192), although often the distribution of the capillary wall thickening is less uniform than in the idiopathic disease. Some-

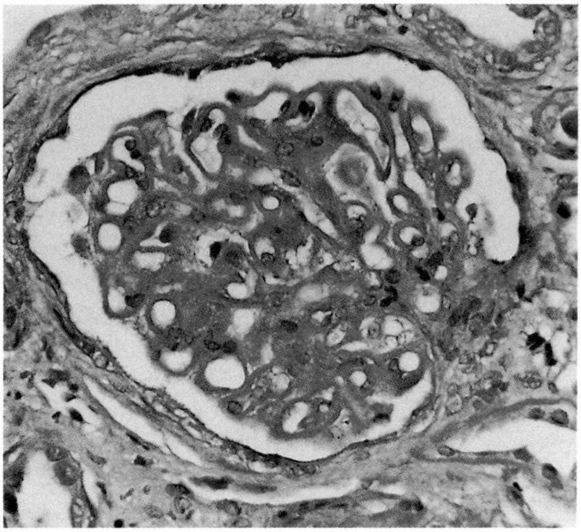

Fig. 8.10 Lupus nephritis – diffuse membranous glomerulonephritis (Class V). The capillary wall is diffusely thickened.
Periodic acid-Schiff × 625

times the membranous change is focal. Both focal and diffuse membranous change are often combined with other categories of lupus nephritis. Membranous lupus nephritis, either in its pure form or mixed with other lupus changes, is seen in approximately 10% of renal biopsies from patients with systemic lupus erythematosus.

Class VI: Sclerosing glomerulonephritis As diffuse proliferative lupus nephritis progresses the glomerular tufts become less cellular, with decrease in the number of mesangial cells and disappearance of neutrophil granulocytes, and segmental and global glomerular sclerosis increases. Eventually the appearances are difficult to distinguish from idiopathic sclerosing glomerulonephritis (see p. 203).

Interstitial changes (see p. 464) The inter-

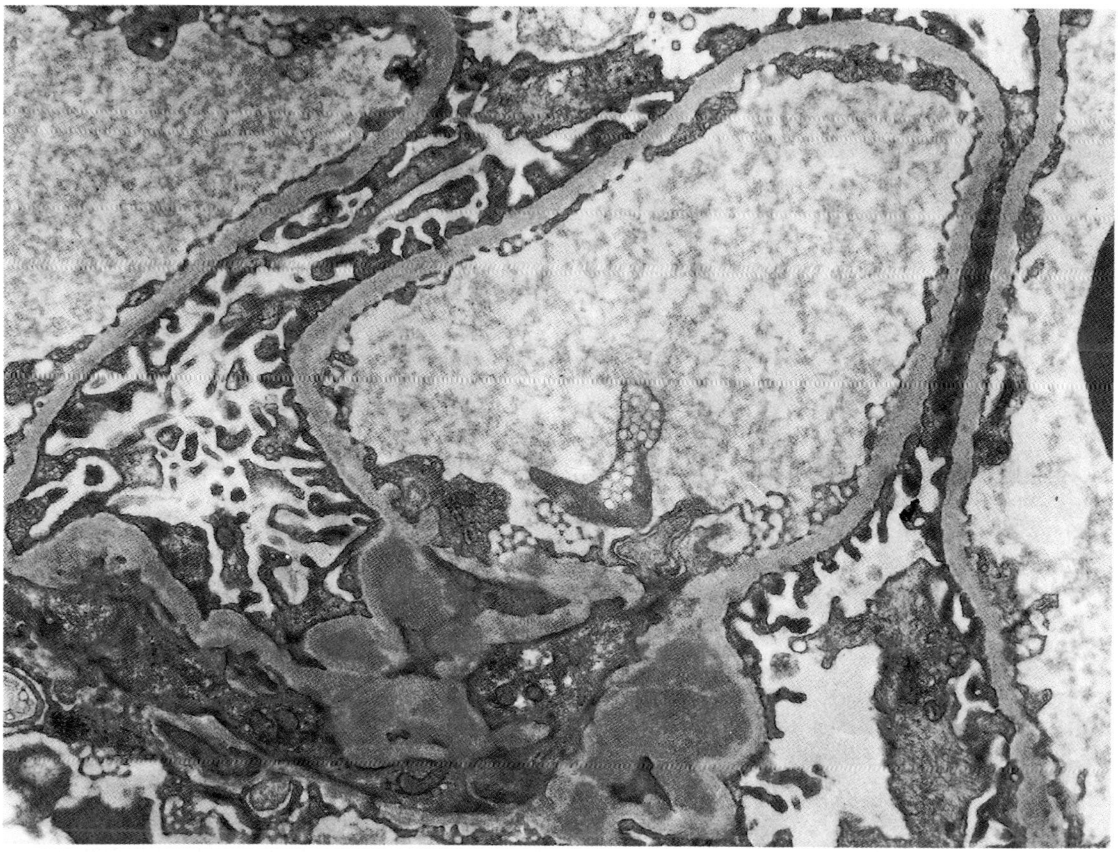

Fig. 8.11 Lupus nephritis – mesangial hypercellularity (class I). Electron micrograph of part of a glomerulus showing mesangial deposits but normal capillary walls. No significant glomerular changes were seen by light microscopy.
× 13 800

stitium is almost always infiltrated by mononuclear cells. Most of these are activated CD4+ helper T lymphocytes.[50,51] Occasionally the interstitial cellular infiltrate, together with interstitial fibrosis and extensive tubular damage and atrophy, are the dominant morphological changes in the kidney, the glomerular changes being minor.

Changes in small arteries and arterioles Lesions in the small arteries and arterioles, apart from those accompanying hypertension (see p. 306) and ageing (see p. 25), are sometimes seen in lupus nephritis. The vascular lesions may consist of fibrin in the walls, with mural or occluding thrombus, but minimal cellular infiltration of the arterial wall.[52] Occasionally, the vascular lesions are indistinguishable from those seen in polyarteritis[53] (see p. 267) or thrombotic microangiopathy[54]; necrotizing lesions are more likely to be seen in kidneys at autopsy than in renal biopsies.

Tubular changes Hyaline droplets are common in epithelial cells of the proximal convoluted tubules. Occasionally eosinophilic deposits can be discerned along the tubular basement membranes. As the disease progresses tubular atrophy occurs and in advanced cases this is often extensive.

Electron microscopy

Electron-dense deposits are found in the mesangium in almost all cases. These are usually the only deposits in patients whose glomeruli look normal by light microscopy (class I) (Fig. 8.11) and in those with various degrees of mesangial hypercellularity (class II). Subendothelial, as well as mesangial, electron-dense deposits are usually found in patients with focal segmental lupus nephritis (class III). In kidneys showing diffuse proliferative lupus nephritis (class IV) by light microscopy, conspicuous and frequent mesangial and subendothelial deposits usually predominate (Fig. 8.12) but variable numbers of subepithelial and intramembranous deposits are often also present. Subendothelial deposits may be large, sometimes blocking capillary lumens. The intracapillary hyaline thrombi seen by light microscopy are these large subendothelial deposits cut tangentially. Glomerular capillaries with massive subendothelial deposits appear as wire loops on light microscopy. The haematoxyphil bodies of light microscopy consist of degenerate nuclear chromatin and cytoplasmic organelles within membrane sacs.[55] In some patients mesangial interposition, subendothelial deposits and small numbers of subepithelial deposits produce a picture indistinguishable from that sometimes seen in idiopathic diffuse mesangiocapillary glomerulonephritis. Subepithelial electron-dense deposits predominate in membranous lupus nephritis (class V). They are usually accompanied by mesangial deposits and often a few subendothelial deposits; there are generally cups of new basement membrane (Fig. 8.13) separating the subepithelial deposits from one another as in the idiopathic disease (see p. 194).[56]

Deposits are also commonly found along tubular basement membranes and in the walls of peritubular capillaries. Sometimes deposits are present in the arteriolar walls in addition to collections of hyalin and rarely fibrin.

The electron-dense deposits are generally finely granular but in approximately 10% of cases some or all of them exhibit an organized structure.[57] This may take the form of either a whorled finger print pattern or arrays of straight microtubules (Fig.8.14). Deposits with an organized pattern are highly characteristic of systemic lupus erythematosus but not diagnostic.

Another common but not diagnostic feature is the presence of *tubuloreticular bodies*: these are usually found in the cytoplasm of the glomerular and peritubular capillary endothelial cells, and rarely in mesangial and visceral epithelial cells. They consist of fine interlacing tubular structures and vesicles (Fig. 8.15). Small numbers of tubuloreticular bodies are found in many renal diseases but the presence of large numbers should suggest the possibility of systemic lupus erythematosus or infection with the human immunodeficiency virus (see p. 398). It has been postulated that tubuloreticular bodies arise from distorted profiles of endoplasmic reticulum.[58]

Proliferation of mesangial cells and proliferation and swelling of endothelial cells account for the increased cellularity of the tufts. Focal retrac-

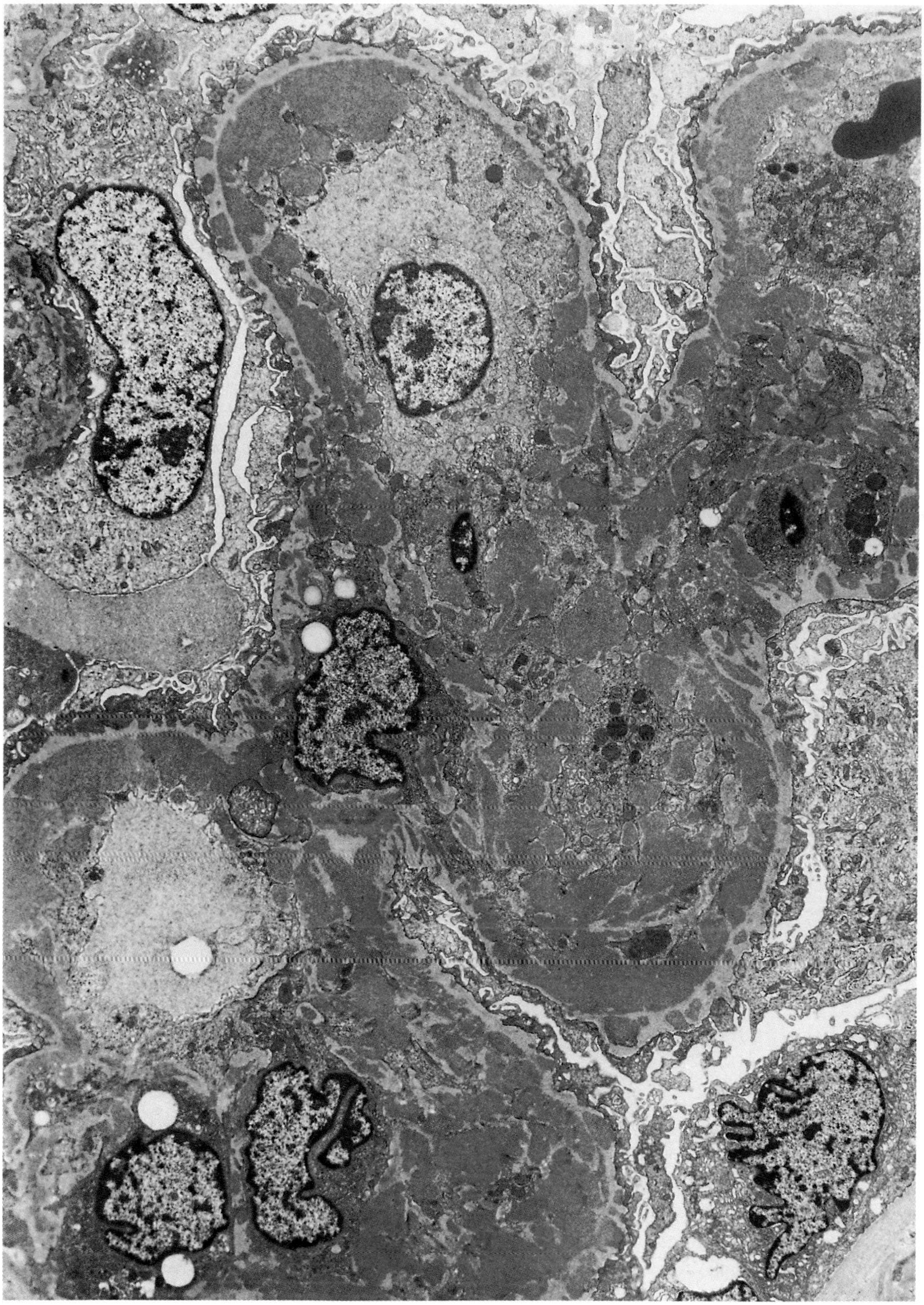

Fig. 8.12 Lupus nephritis – diffuse proliferative glomerulonephritis (class IV). Electron micrograph of part of a glomerulus showing large subendothelial and mesangial deposits. There are also scattered small subepithelial and intramembranous deposits.
× 7200

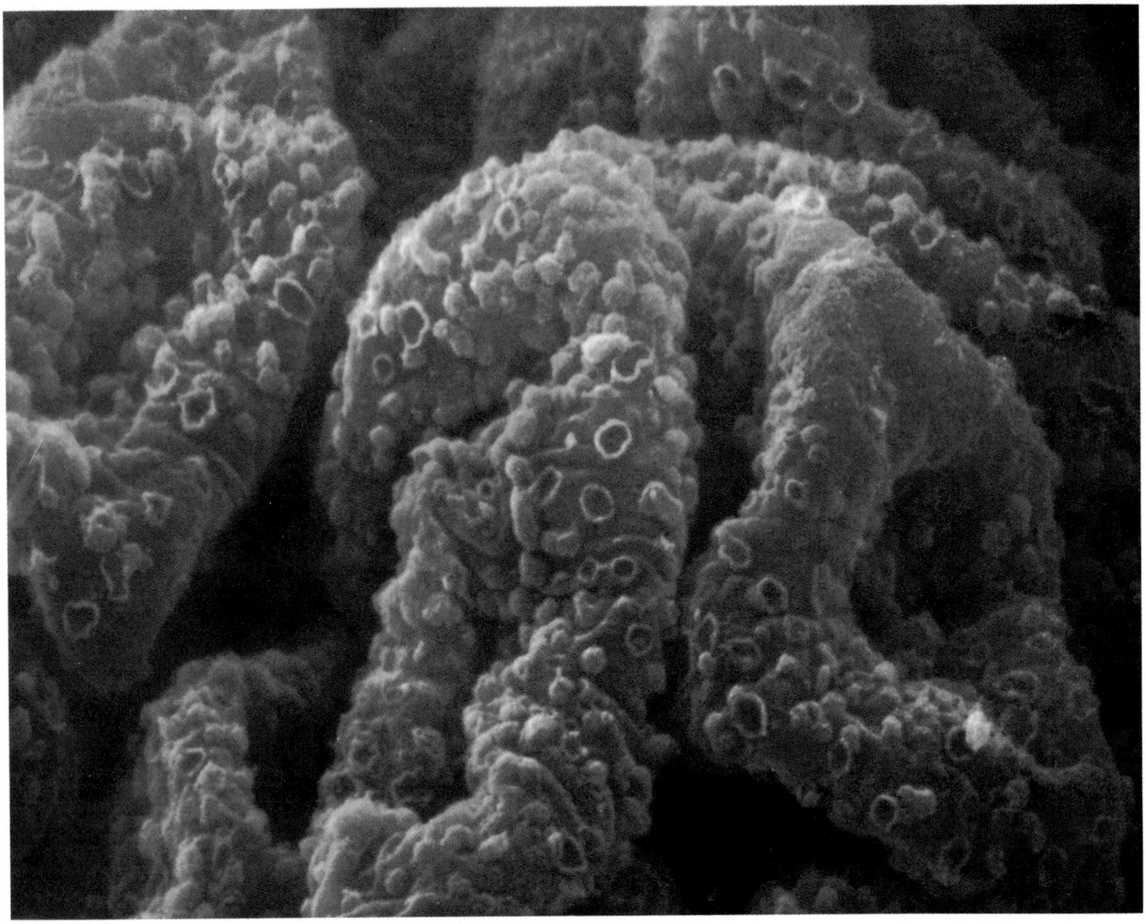

Fig. 8.13 Lupus nephritis – diffuse membranous glomerulonephritis (class V). Scanning electron microscopic view of part of a glomerulus showing numerous crater- or cup-like abnormalities of the glomerular capillary basement membrane.
× 1400
Reproduced by permission from: Weidner N, Lorentz WB. Am J Clin Pathol 1986; 85: 135 (Fig. 7)

tion and obliteration of the foot processes of the visceral epithelial cells are common.

Immunofluorescence/immunoperoxidase microscopy

Granular deposits of immunoglobulin and complement are found in almost all cases of systemic lupus erythematosus; linear deposits are very rare. The composition of the deposits varies. The predominant immunoglobulin is usually IgG and this is often accompanied by abundant IgA and IgM. Occasionally either IgA or IgM is present in the greatest amount. C3 and the early acting components C1q and C4 are generally present; C1q is often abundant. The simultaneous presence of all the immunoglobulins and complement components mentioned is particularly characteristic of lupus nephritis.

The patterns of immunoglobulin and complement deposits correlate with the light microscopic changes. Those cases that by light microscopy either appear normal or show mesangial hypercellularity (classes I and II) usually show only mesangial deposits (Fig. 8.16). Focal segmental glomerulonephritis (class III) is associated with granular deposits in segments of capillary wall in addition to the mesangium. In diffuse proliferative glomerulonephritis (class IV) deposits are found in the mesangium and along all the capillary walls of most glomeruli (Fig. 8.17). Some of the capil-

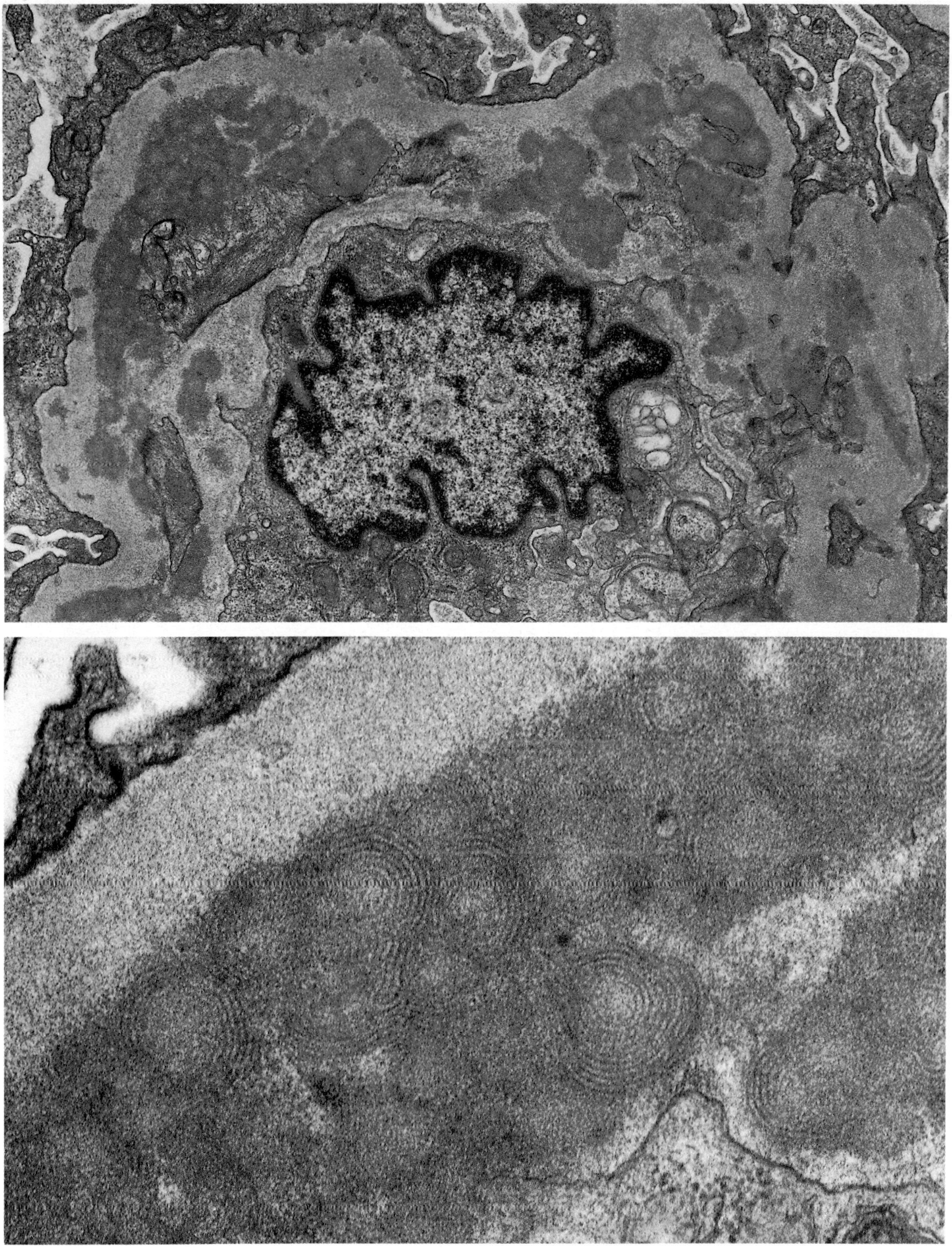

a

b

Fig. 8.14 a, b Lupus nephritis. Electron micrographs of part of a glomerular capillary showing subendothelial electron-dense deposits with finger print configuration.
(**a**) × 13 800; (**b**) × 53 000

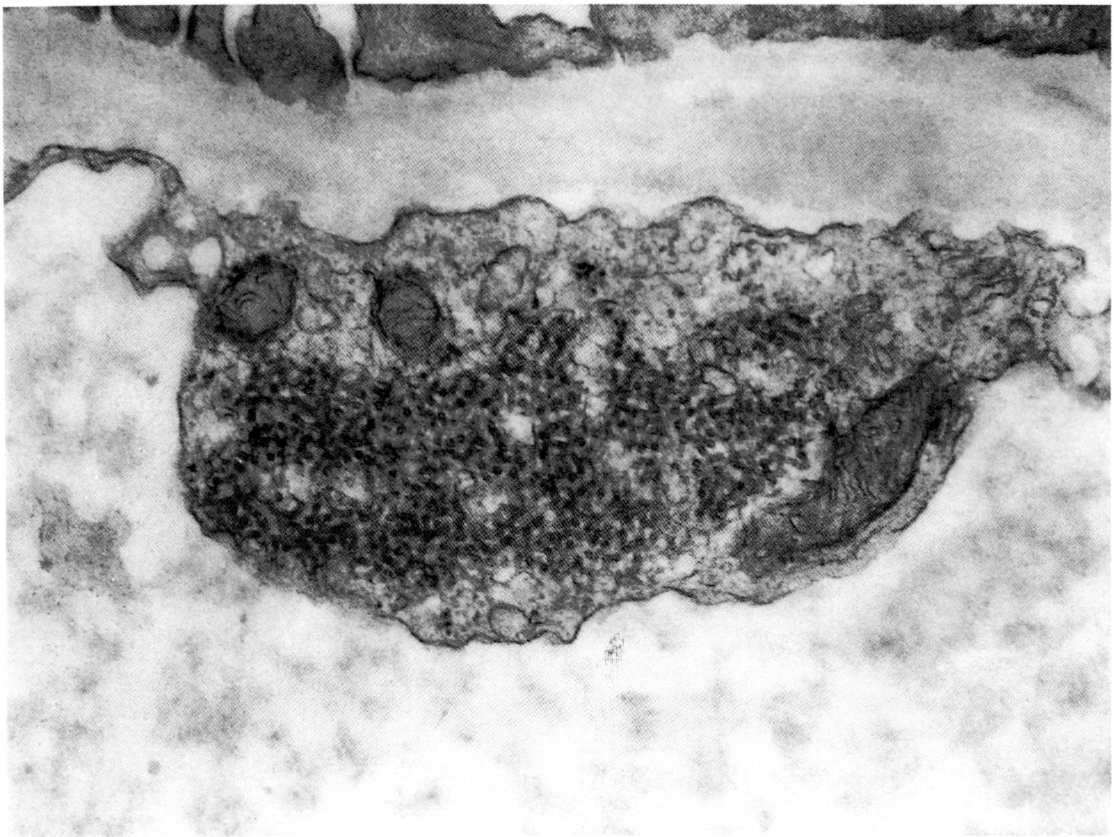

Fig. 8.15 Lupus nephritis. Electron micrograph of part of a glomerular capillary. An endothelial cell contains clusters of tubuloreticular bodies.
× 50 200

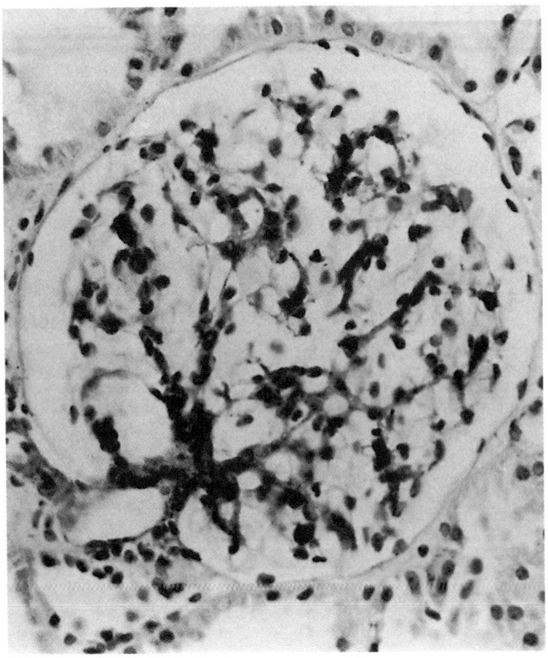

lary deposits take the form of broad sausage-like strips which correspond to the wire loops seen by light microscopy. The diffuse membranous pattern (class V) is associated with multiple small granular deposits along all the glomerular capillary walls with glomerular mesangial deposits (Fig. 8.18).

Discrete granular deposits of IgG and C3 are also common along the tubular basement membranes, in the thickened basement membranes of the peritubular capillaries, in the interstitium and sometimes in the media of the interlobular arteries and in Bowman's capsule.[59] Tubular, vascular, interstitial and capsular deposits are most frequent in association with class IV lupus nephritis and rare in class V.

Fig. 8.16 Lupus nephritis – mesangial proliferative glomerulonephritis (Class II). Immunoperoxidase showing deposits of IgG in mesangium.
× 350

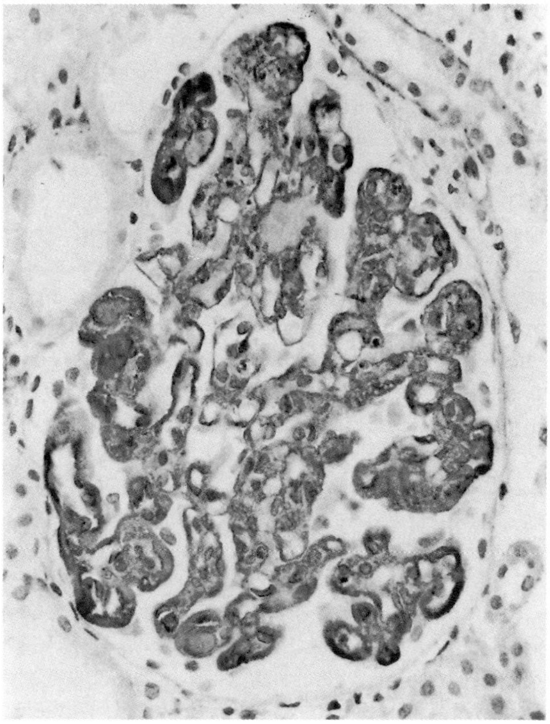

Fig. 8.17 Lupus nephritis – diffuse proliferative glomerulonephritis (Class IV). Immunoperoxidase staining showing coarse subendothelial and mesangial deposits of IgG in a glomerulus.
× 350

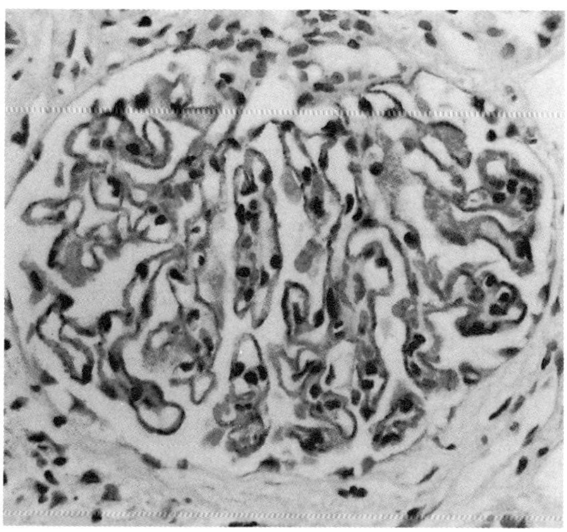

Fig. 8.18 Lupus nephritis – diffuse membranous glomerulonephritis (Class V). Immunoperoxidase showing granular deposits of IgG along capillary walls.
× 340

Renal transplantation

Many patients with lupus nephritis have received renal allografts but only in five has the disease developed in the transplanted kidney (see p. 671). Recurrence is usually marked by proteinuria occurring without signs of rejection.[60,61]

The activity of systemic lupus erythematosus dies out when end-stage renal failure occurs, probably because of the immunosuppressive effect of uraemia (see p. 37). The rarity of recurrence of lupus nephritis might be due to immunosuppressive treatment preventing reactivation of the disease after the return of good renal function. Another possibility is that the immune responsiveness of the recipient continues to be depressed by the effect of the blood transfusions received in preparation for renal transplantation.

The graft and patient survival rates are comparable with those of non-diabetic patients under the age of 55 years with renal allografts. Systemic lupus erythematosus activity of any sort is rare in such patients.[61,62]

Prognosis

Although the better use of corticosteroids and cytotoxic agents has increased the survival of patients with severe disease, renal failure eventually causes the death of approximately 20% of patients with systemic lupus erythematosus. The other major causes of mortality are infection and involvement of the central nervous system, each of which accounts for the death of approximately 13% of patients.[63]

The mean 5-year survival rates for the different histological classes of lupus nephritis are: mesangial proliferative (class II) 100%; focal segmental (class III) 73%; diffuse proliferative (class IV) 60% and membranous (class V) 90%. Diffuse proliferative glomerulonephritis, therefore, is the glomerular lesion in lupus nephritis with the most serious prognosis, but the variable clinical outcomes of individual patients reduce the predictive value of the World Health Organization classification.

An attempt to overcome this weakness has been to introduce a semiquantitative histological scoring system which produces activity and

Table 8.1 Indices of activity and chronicity of lupus nephritis

	Maximum score
Index of activity of lupus nephritis[64]	
Glomerular karyorrhexis and fibrinoid necrosis	6
Cellular crescents	6
Wire loops and hyaline thrombi	3
Granulocyte infiltration of glomeruli	3
Glomerular mononuclear cellularity	3
Interstitial mononuclear cell infiltration	3
	24
Index of chronicity of lupus nephritis[64]	
Glomerular sclerosis	3
Fibrous crescents	3
Tubular atrophy	3
Interstitial fibrosis	3
	12

chronicity indices (Table 8.1).[64] This approach has won a fair degree of support and the indices are used quite widely to augment the prognostic information derived from the World Health Organization classification. A high composite chronicity index is a good indicator that an individual patient is likely to develop renal failure within 5 years. Particularly striking is the predictive value of tubular atrophy. The simultaneous occurrence of tubular atrophy, glomerular sclerosis and cellular crescents identifies a very high risk group within the category of patients showing World Health Organization class IV changes on light microscopy in their kidneys. In one series nearly 70% of such patients progressed to end-stage renal failure within 4 years of diagnosis.[64]

The value of the activity and chronicity indices remains controversial. A recent investigation by the Lupus Collaborative Study group in the USA found that, in patients with systemic lupus erythematosus and diffuse proliferative glomerulonephritis (class IV lupus nephritis), the indices did not improve the predictive value of the standard histological classification.[65] In contrast, another study in the same period confirmed the predictive importance of the activity and chronicity indices.[66]

Combinations of histological categories of lupus nephritis seem to be prejudicial. In a follow-up of 85 patients with lupus nephritis those with a combination of membranous glomerulonephritis and either severe focal segmental glomerulonephritis or diffuse proliferative glomerulonephritis had a poorer prognosis than those with only one category of lesion.[67]

Pathogenesis

Family and twin studies provide clear evidence that a predisposition to systemic lupus erythematosus is inherited.[68] The disease occurs in the relatives of patients several hundred times more frequently than in the general population. Supporting evidence for a genetic element comes from the association of systemic lupus erythematosus with HLA antigens, particularly DR2 and DR3, and with inherited deficiencies of complement components, particularly C2 and C4. The genes that impart susceptibility to develop systemic lupus erythematosus and allow polyclonal B lymphocyte activation need not be HLA or complement genes but may be sited near to them on chromosome 6, so that they are inherited in linkage disequilibrium.

Patients with systemic lupus erythematosus have a highly significant increase in the prevalence of null (silent) alleles for C4 compared with normal controls. There is a strong linkage disequilibrium between HLA-DR3 and the null alleles, suggesting a directly inherited partial or complete deficiency of complement in this disease.[69] A homozygous or heterozygous deficiency of complement may result in abnormal handling of immune complexes with greater tissue damage; it may also allow an infectious agent to persist, causing a prolonged immunological stimulus.

Sex hormones influence the development and course of systemic lupus erythematosus. In the reproductive years the incidence of the disease is nine times greater in women than men, but before puberty the ratio of affected girls to boys is 3 : 1 and after the menopause the ratio of women to men is 1 : 1. The signs and symptoms of the disease are exacerbated in the 10 days before menstruation.[70] Oral contraceptives adversely affect the disease.[70] Oestrogen receptors exist on CD8+ suppressor T lymphocytes and the sex hormones may modulate the immune system in some way. The effect of pregnancy on systemic lupus erythematosus is considered on page 553.

A variety of immunological abnormalities affecting both T and B lymphocytes occurs in systemic lupus erythematosus, resulting in chronic autoantibody production. The B lymphocytes are polyclonally hyperactive; this could be a genetically determined intrinsic defect in the B lymphocytes and not a consequence of CD8 suppressor T lymphocyte abnormalities. Alternatively, the B lymphocytes could become polyclonally a target of CD4+ helper T lymphocytes because they harbour a virus or because of mutations that lead to quantitative or qualitative alterations of the major histocompatibility complex or other molecules.[71]

There are also abnormalities in factors that concern the handling of immune complexes. For example, there is a reduction in erythrocyte complement receptor numbers and the Fc receptor mediated uptake of circulating immune complexes by the monocyte–phagocyte system (reticuloendothelial system) is markedly impaired. Production of immune mediators, particularly interleukin-1 and -2, and expression of interleukin-2 receptors on T lymphocytes, are also deficient in systemic lupus erythematosus. Immune interferon levels, however, are high. These mediators influence the function of lymphocytes and may play a role in the pathogenesis of some of the lesions of systemic lupus erythematosus.

Environmental factors may also be involved in the pathogenesis of some cases of systemic lupus erythematosus. Drugs such as hydralazine, procainamide and penicillamine can induce a response that resembles systemic lupus erythematosus (see p. 240). Viruses have long been suggested to be the cause of systemic lupus erythematosus in humans because type C-RNA oncornaviruses play a part in the production of tissue damage in a spontaneous disease closely resembling systemic lupus erythematosus that occurs in New Zealand Black mice and the F1 hybrid produced by mating of New Zealand Black with New Zealand White mice.[72] However, despite claims that type C-RNA oncornavirus antigens have been identified in tissues from patients with systemic lupus erythematosus, these results have not been widely confirmed and there is little to suggest that viruses play a primary role in the pathogenesis of systemic lupus erythematosus. Attempts to isolate a virus from human systemic lupus erythematosus tissue have not been successful.

DNA–anti-DNA immune complexes are found in the glomerular deposits of most patients with active lupus nephritis.[73] However, circulating DNA–anti-DNA complexes are infrequent.[74] It seems probable that at least some of the deposits arise by local (in situ) binding of anti-DNA antibody to receptors for DNA on the membranes of the various glomerular cells and also to exposed nuclear material (see p. 129); other deposits arise from immune complexes filtered out from the circulation (see p. 129).

Although immune complex systems involving rheumatoid factors, nuclear antigens other than DNA, or viral antigens do sometimes participate in the pathogenesis of lupus nephritis, present evidence supports the view that in most patients DNA–anti-DNA complexes play the major role in its development[74] In a few patients elution of the renal deposits has shown that they contain anti-Ro antibodies but no detectable anti-DNA antibodies.[75] Idiotype–anti-idiotype immune complexes are also sometimes deposited; in one study cross-reactive anti-DNA antibody idiotypes were identified on immunoglobulins bound to tissue in about half the renal biopsies from patients with systemic lupus erythematosus.[76]

The factors that lead to the formation of anti-DNA antibodies in patients with systemic lupus erythematosus are not known. Purified autologous DNA is a very poor immunogen; anti-DNA antibody production is probably triggered by some of the products of the catabolism of nuclei from dead cells, particularly by the chromatin itself.[74] Since cytolysis occurs in many conditions but is not followed by the production of anti-DNA antibodies, it has been speculated that in systemic lupus erythematosus there is either a genetic predisposition to make such antibodies, or there is a defect in the catabolism of chromatin.[74]

Once immune complexes have been deposited or have formed in the glomeruli several different events may occur. In some kidneys activation of C5a causes the recruitment of neutrophil granulocytes which release proteases and other enzymes that degrade the glomerular capillary basement membrane; they also release oxygen-derived free radicals which damage cells (see p. 131). In other kidneys the membrane attack complex (C5b-9) is activated and damages the capillary wall (see p. 130). Sometimes monocytes infiltrate the glomerulus and produce many biologically active substances which lead to damage and inflammation; they also release interleukin-1, which stimulates mesangial cell proliferation (see

p. 131), and coagulation factors which convert fibrinogen to fibrin locally.

Variants

Late-onset systemic lupus erythematosus[42]

Late-onset disease is seen in people aged 50 years or older and comprises 6–12% of cases of systemic lupus erythematosus. About a quarter of the patients are men and there is a striking increase in circulating anti-Ro antibodies and an increased association with HLA-DR3 and HLA-DR2 in this group of patients. Hypocomplementaemia and the presence of antibodies to double-stranded DNA are less common. Pulmonary lesions are more frequent than in classical systemic lupus erythematosus and clinical nephritis is less frequent. When nephritis occurs it does not seem to differ either in form or in distribution of classes from the disease that occurs in younger age groups.

Neonatal lupus[42]

Mothers of HLA-DR3 phenotype with circulating anti-Ro antibodies are at increased risk of producing a baby with either lupus skin lesions, congenital heart block or congenital heart lesions. The anti-Ro antibodies cross the placenta and are detectable in the infant's circulation for several months. Occasionally there are other systemic lesions but these are mild and short lived. No renal changes have been reported in neonatal lupus.

Discoid lupus

In discoid lupus there is little if any extra-cutaneous or systemic involvement and renal disease is not a feature.

Subacute cutaneous lupus erythematosus and ANA-negative systemic lupus erythematosus

Extreme photosensitivity is the dominant feature of this variant. The skin lesions are similar to those in neonates with lupus. Polyarthritis is seen in about one-third of the patients. Nephritis is uncommon, affecting about 12% of patients: when it occurs there are no unusual features.

Drug-induced systemic lupus erythematosus

Long-term administration of certain drugs, in particular, hydralazine, procainamide and isoniazid, is associated with the appearance of antinuclear antibodies, antihistone antibodies and antibodies to single-stranded DNA. Antibodies to double-stranded DNA, Sm and RNP are not found and frequently the serum complement levels are normal. Some of the patients later develop a syndrome resembling systemic lupus erythematosus; in a proportion of these the kidney is involved.[77] Hydralazine, procainamide and isoniazid are acetylated by the liver *N*-acetyl transferase and many, but not all, patients who develop systemic lupus erythematosus while taking any of these drugs are genetically slow acetylators.[78] The unacetylated drugs react with nuclear antigens and may produce an immunogenic drug–antigen complex. Hydralazine and isoniazid may inhibit the covalent binding of C4 to antigen–antibody complexes and thereby predispose to immune deposits in the tissues.[79]

Hydralazine The peripheral vasodilator hydralazine is commonly added to antihypertensive treatment when a combination of a beta blocker and a thiazide diuretic has failed to control the blood pressure. After 3 years' treatment with hydralazine the incidence of the systemic lupus erythematosus syndrome is 6.7%; the disease is rarely seen with less than 3 months' treatment. The incidence is dose dependent, with no cases recorded in patients taking 50 mg daily, an incidence of 5.4% with 100 mg daily and 10.4% with 200 mg daily. The induction of systemic lupus erythematosus is commoner in women (11.6%) than in men (2.8%). In women taking 200 mg daily the 3-year incidence is 19.4%.[80] Predisposition to the toxic effect is associated with HLA-DR4.[81] Most patients are elderly, the mean age being 58 years. In many cases the criteria for full-blown systemic lupus erythematosus are not fulfilled; joint lesions are common but fever, skin lesions, lymphadenopathy and disorders of the nervous system are unusual.[42]

Renal involvement has been demonstrated in

20–50% of patients with systemic lupus erythematosus induced by hydralazine.[78,82] Microscopic haematuria is an early sign of renal disease and there may be proteinuria and impaired renal function. The renal abnormalities may be difficult to separate from those due to the severe hypertension or primary renal disease, or both, for which the patient was given hydralazine. The renal changes are usually class III focal segmental lupus nephritis. They are often accompanied by necrosis and crescent formation.[83–85] Recognition of the disease and immediate withdrawal of hydralazine results in improvement of renal function but complete recovery is uncommon.

Procainamide Procainamide, which is used to control cardiac arrhythmias, is associated in approximately 30% of patients with a systemic lupus erythematosus syndrome similar to that seen after treatment with hydralazine. The patients are often elderly men. They have received procainamide for at least 1½ months and usually much longer and the total dose given has been at least 90 g.

Renal involvement is rare. The histological findings in the kidney vary: classes I–V lupus nephritis have all been recorded, including one case with crescentic glomerulonephritis; class III focal segmental changes are slightly commoner than the others.[86,87] Withdrawal of the drug has been followed in most cases by improvement in renal function.

Systemic lupus erythematosus associated with hereditary deficiencies of complement (see p. 108)[47]

Lupus diseases have been associated for the most part with deficiencies of the early complement components C1, C4 and C2, but there have been occasional reports of cases with each of the other components.

C1q deficiency All but one of the 10 reported cases have had lupus or a lupus-like disease but only one fulfilled the criteria for systemic lupus erythematosus. All the affected cases had skin involvement and eight of the nine had glomerulonephritis, usually mesangiocapillary type I. Antinuclear antibodies were weakly positive in five patients; anti-DNA antibodies were present in only one case. Men are affected more than women. The C1q deficiency is not linked to the HLA complex.

C1r and C1s deficiency Eight of the 10 reported cases have had systemic lupus erythematosus or disease resembling systemic lupus. In five of the cases the antinuclear antibodies were negative. Four of the seven cases had glomerulonephritis. The C1r and C1s deficiencies always occur together and are not linked to the HLA complex.

C4 deficiency The prevalence of systemic lupus erythematosus among individuals with complete C4 deficiency is very high. Twelve of 15 patients had systemic lupus erythematosus or a similar syndrome; eight of these cases fulfilled the criteria for systemic lupus erythematosus, but five of the eight did not have antinuclear antibodies and six did not have antibodies to DNA. Instead some had anti-Ro antibodies.

C2 deficiency C2 deficiency is the most common homozygous complement component deficiency. Approximately 34% of patients with this deficiency have lupus. It occurs predominantly in females and does not commonly affect the kidneys.

Systemic lupus erythematosus associated with acquired deficiencies of complement[47]

Persistent complement depression over prolonged periods, due to either C1 esterase inhibitor deficiency, selective C4 deficiency or chronic hypocomplementaemic cutaneous vasculitis, is associated with lupus-like diseases.

C1 esterase inhibitor deficiency A genetic deficiency of C1 esterase inhibitor is associated with hereditary angioneurotic oedema. Fifteen patients with lupus disease have been reported; five fulfilled the criteria for systemic lupus erythematosus. A few have lupus nephritis, usually class III.

Selective C4 deficiency This is associated only with discoid lupus erythematosus. Renal lesions have not been reported.

Chronic hypocomplementaemic cutaneous vasculitis Marked depression of C1q, C2 and C4 and moderate depression of C3 occur in the syndrome of chronic hypocomplementaemic cutaneous vasculitis. Most cases do not have anti-nuclear antibodies or anti-DNA antibodies but anti-Ro antibodies are common. Patients with this syndrome do not fulfil the diagnostic criteria for systemic lupus erythematosus but have many features of that disease. Approximately 56% of the patients have lupus nephritis, usually of classes I or II.

SYSTEMIC SCLEROSIS

Systemic sclerosis is characterized by vascular disease and excessive collagen deposition affecting many organs in the body. It is predominantly a disease of women aged 20–50 years but it may occur in males and at all ages. There are few reports on the incidence of systemic sclerosis but the average annual incidence of new cases in Tennessee, USA, in 1947–68 was 2.7 new patients per million population.[88] In other populations an annual incidence as high as 12 cases per million has been recorded. Systemic sclerosis is distributed widely both geographically and racially; its apparent rarity in some African and Asian countries may be due to differences in clinical features.[89] There have been a number of familial cases. An increased incidence has been reported in stone masons, coal miners and gold miners. Systemic sclerosis is usually subdivided into two groups on the basis of its clinical course: acrosclerosis and diffuse or progressive systemic sclerosis.

Acrosclerosis

Acrosclerosis is the most common form. The skin of the fingers and the face becomes first oedematous, then fibrotic and finally atrophic. This form of the disease is usually associated with *c*alcinosis, *R*aynaud's phenomenon, *o*esophageal dysfunction, *s*clerodactyly and *t*elangiectasia, the so-called CREST syndrome.[90] Involvement of the viscera is limited and occurs late and the disease tends to pursue a very slow course. The kidneys are only occasionally involved.

Diffuse or progressive systemic sclerosis

Diffuse or progressive systemic sclerosis is less common. There is widespread skin involvement at the onset and early manifestations of changes in the kidneys, heart, lungs, gastrointestinal tract and musculoskeletal system. This form of the disease runs a rapidly progressive course and is often fatal. The kidneys are commonly affected.

Clinical features

Most patients first develop Raynaud's phenomenon, then swelling of the hands and thickening and stiffening of the skin. The progressive dermal fibrosis eventually leads to immobilization of the joints. Muscular weakness and atrophy, difficulty in swallowing and gastrointestinal symptoms appear. Dyspnoea and cough occur as the lungs become involved. Myocardial fibrosis produces arrhythmias, conduction defects, angina and cardiac failure.

Renal disease is the principal fatal complication of systemic sclerosis. The reported incidence of involvement of the kidneys is 5–45%.[91,92] This wide variation between centres receiving referred cases is largely because of the different percentage of cases of progressive systemic sclerosis compared with acrosclerosis seen at each centre, and of the use of different criteria to define renal involvement. Reports from dermatologists usually show a relatively low incidence of kidney disease while those from nephrologists emphasize the frequency of renal involvement. The onset of renal disease is usually in the first 6 years after the clinical recognition of systemic sclerosis.[93]

About half the patients develop hypertension. Of these approximately 25% have an abrupt onset of malignant-phase hypertension associated with rapid deterioration of renal function causing renal failure (scleroderma renal crisis). Papilloedema, cardiac failure, encephalopathy, elevated plasma renin levels and a microangiopathic haemolytic anaemia are frequent accompaniments.[94] The remaining 75% with raised blood pressure have benign phase hypertension which may remain uncomplicated by proteinuria or azotaemia for long periods.

Azotaemia occurs in about a quarter of the patients; it develops both in normotensive and hypertensive patients and in many cases leads to death or necessitates dialysis or renal transplantation within 3 years.

Mild proteinuria (less than 0.5 g/24 hours) is also common, being present in about a quarter of the patients; sometimes it is the first sign of renal involvement by systemic sclerosis.

Tissue typing

There is an increased incidence of HLA-DR5 and -DRw8. The association with HLA-DR5 appears to be strongest in patients with the CREST syndrome.[95]

Peripheral blood lymphocytes

The number of circulating T lymphocytes is reduced in systemic sclerosis; the depression is particularly marked in the CD8 subset.[95]

Serology

Antinuclear antibodies are present in 96% of cases but bear little or no correlation with disease severity or outcome. Two of these antibodies seem to be specific for systemic sclerosis. One, called Scl-70, is an antibody to the abundant nuclear enzyme DNA topoisomerase 1; it is present in 30–40% of patients with progressive systemic sclerosis.[96] The other, an antibody to centromeres, is found in 50–70% of patients with the CREST syndrome.[97] Hypergammaglobulinaemia is present in 50% of cases and rheumatoid factor in 25%. Circulating immune complexes are frequent. The levels of complement fragments C3d and C4d in the plasma are raised in about half the patients with progressive systemic sclerosis.[98] These fragments are generated during complement activation. The levels of C3, C4 and other complement components are usually normal.

Renal changes

Gross appearance of the kidneys

The kidneys are normal in size. In many cases

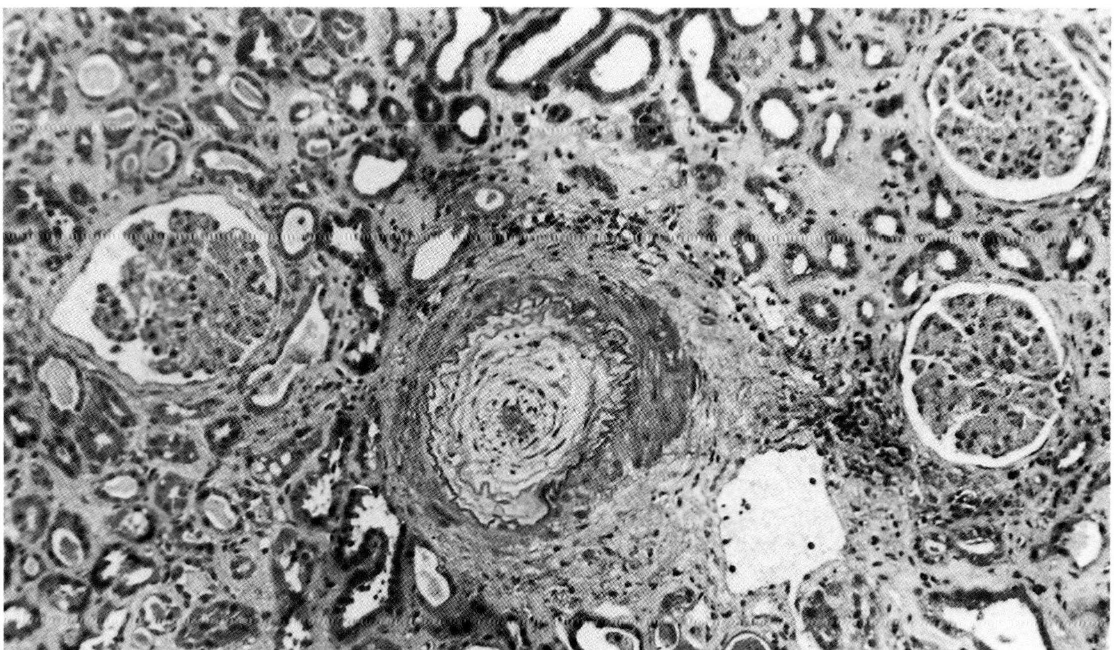

Fig. 8.19 Progressive systemic sclerosis. Interlobular artery showing massive loose-textured thickening of the intima with obliteration of the lumen. The nuclei in the thickened intima are arranged concentrically.
Haematoxylin-eosin × 300

there are numerous, minute, wedge-shaped cortical infarcts on the cut surface.

Light microscopy

The most striking changes are found in the interlobular arteries. These are greatly narrowed by marked thickening of the intima by loose-textured tissue that stains diffusely for acid mucopolysaccharides with the alcian blue and colloidal iron methods. The nuclei in the thickened intima are arranged concentrically (Fig. 8.19).[99] Occasionally there are small haemorrhages and deposits of fibrin in the intima. The internal elastic lamina may be duplicated, the media is thinner than normal and there is periarterial fibrosis.[92] The arcuate and interlobar arteries show few changes in patients with acute rapidly progressive systemic sclerosis associated with malignant hypertension. In the chronic forms of progressive systemic sclerosis these arteries develop fibrous intimal thickening and reduplication or multiplication of the internal elastic lamina (Fig. 8.20).

There is fibrinoid necrosis of the walls of the

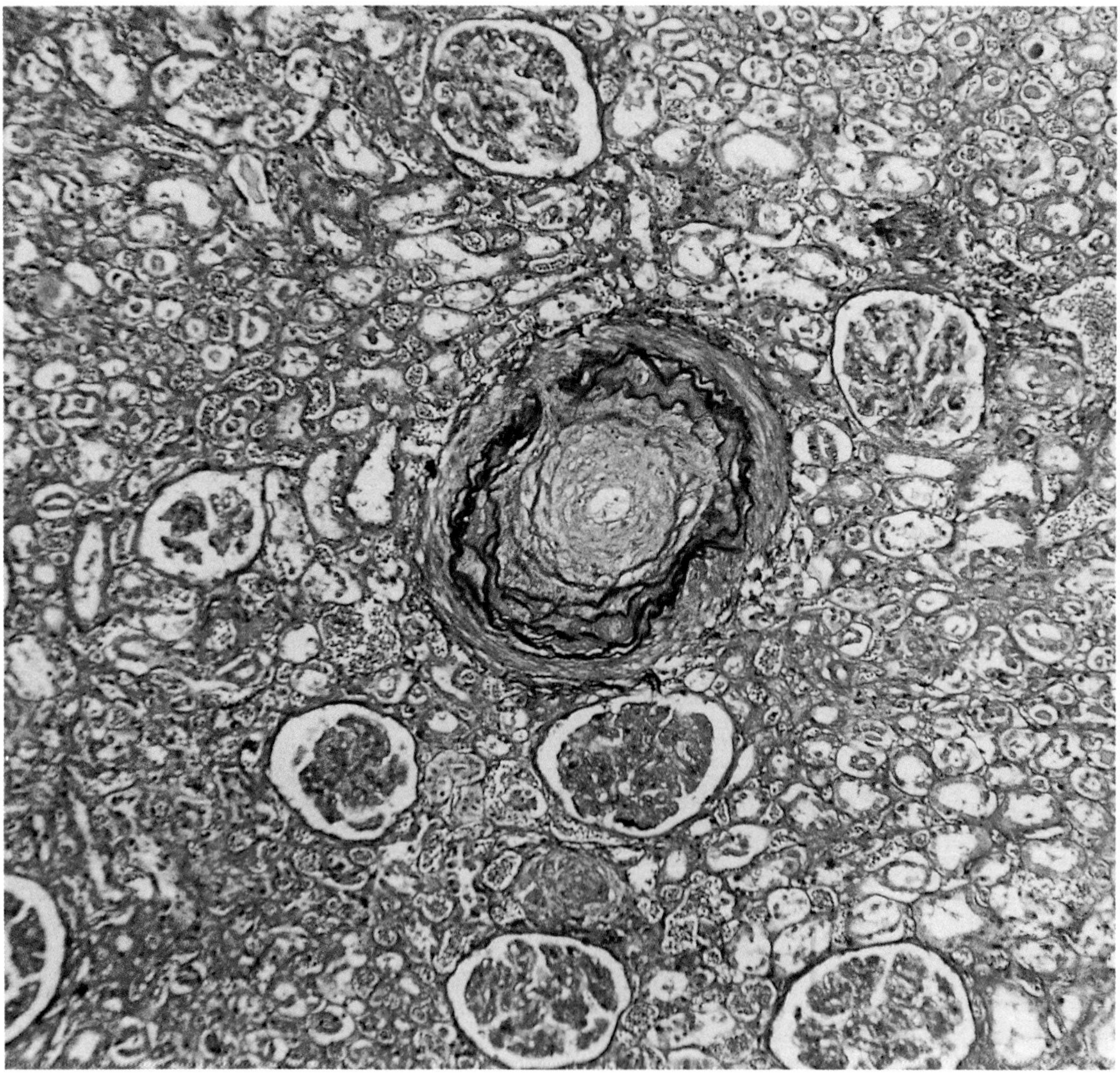

Fig. 8.20 Chronic forms of systemic sclerosis. Interlobular artery showing fibrous intimal thickening and reduplication of the internal elastic lamina.
Elastic-van Gieson × 300

afferent arterioles. The necrosis is not usually accompanied by cellular infiltration; it often extends into the glomerulus.

The glomeruli typically show ischaemic changes with irregular wrinkling and collapse of the capillary basement membranes. Occasionally there is also segmental sclerosis or segmental fibrinoid necrosis. The juxtaglomerular bodies are sometimes enlarged in those patients with malignant hypertension and high levels of plasma renin.

Thrombosis of arterioles and small arteries, producing multiple small cortical infarcts, are common in those cases with rapidly progressive disease associated with malignant hypertension.[100] In the chronic cases atrophy of tubules and interstitial fibrosis are frequent features, and there may be focal accumulation of mononuclear cells.

Electron microscopy

The interstitial space in the thickened arterial intima contains amorphous electron-lucent material (Fig. 8.21). The extent of this change correlates with the pallor of the intima as seen in

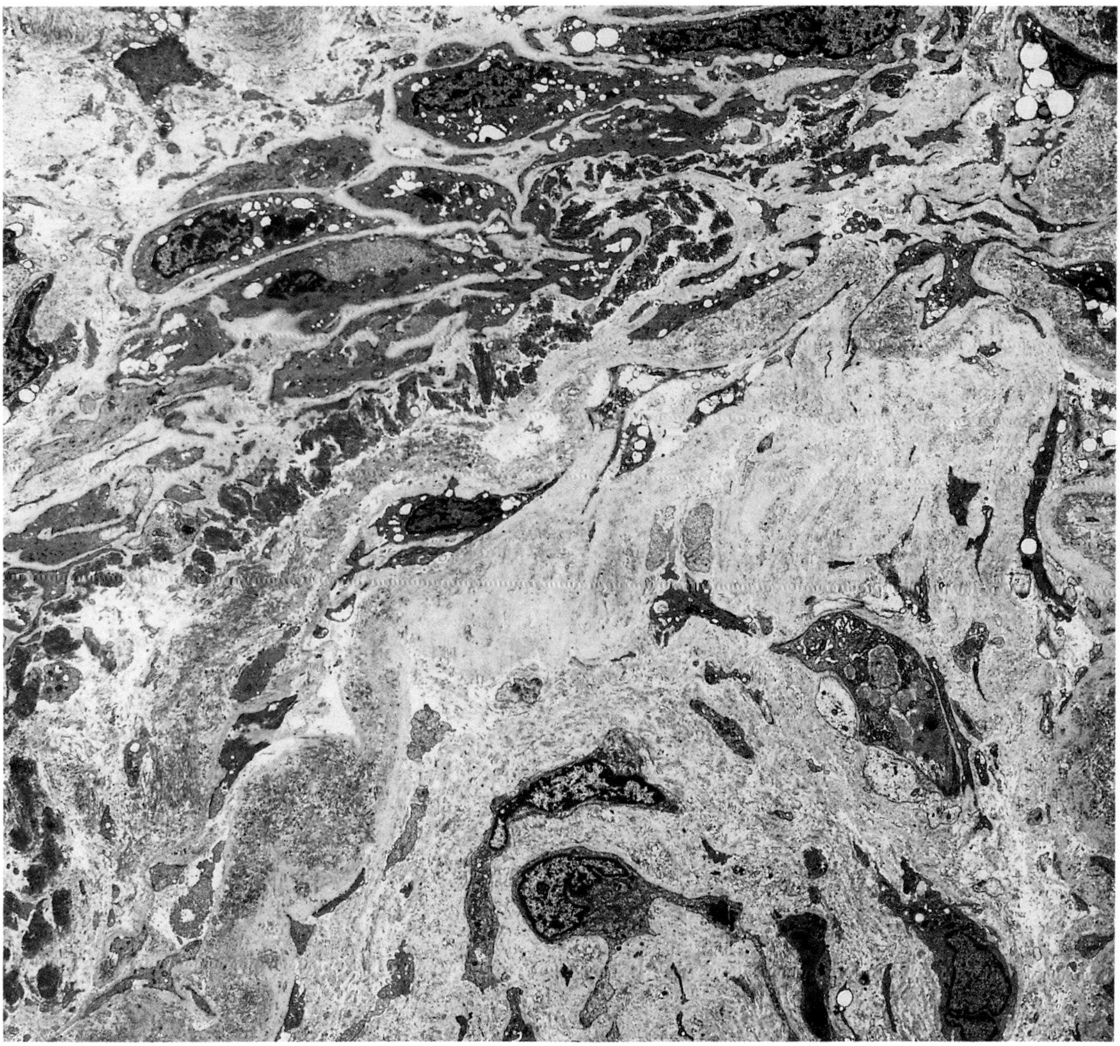

Fig. 8.21 Progressive systemic sclerosis. Electron micrograph of part of wall of interlobular artery. There are myointimal cells in an electron-lucent amorphous matrix. The adventitia is in the upper part of the photograph. ×550

haematoxylin and eosin stained sections viewed by light microscopy. In this matrix there are frequent smooth muscle cells (often called myointimal cells).[99] Strands of basement membrane are also present and with time the intima may become increasingly occupied by concentric layers of this material. The lining endothelial cells are often swollen, contributing to the vascular narrowing. Individual smooth muscle cells in the media are often atrophic. In patients with chronic disease and mild hypertension the thickened intima of the interlobular and arcuate arteries contains numerous bundles of collagen and smooth muscle cells but little interstitial electron-lucent material.[99] The glomeruli show extensive wrinkling and folding of the capillary basement membranes and, in many instances, broad bands of electron-lucent material lying between the endothelium and the basement membranes. These glomerular changes are caused by ischaemia and are non-specific.

Immunofluorescence/immunoperoxidase microscopy

The thickened arterial intima usually contains IgM and C1q and occasionally other immunoglobulins and complement components. The staining for immunoglobulins and complement is strongest in acute progressive cases with malignant hypertension. Fine granular staining with the same immunoglobulins and complement components is sometimes seen in the glomerular capillary walls and mesangium.

Differential diagnosis

The intimal thickening seen in systemic sclerosis is indistinguishable by light, electron or immunofluorescence/immunoperoxidase microscopy from that seen in *malignant phase hypertension* (see p. 311) or the *haemolytic uraemic syndrome* (see p. 283).[99] The presence of cortical infarcts favours systemic sclerosis but is not diagnostic.[92]

To differentiate systemic sclerosis from malignant phase hypertension a knowledge of the level of the blood pressure in the period preceding the onset of renal disease is needed. To distinguish the haemolytic uraemic syndrome it is necessary to know if the patient had an angiopathic haemolytic anaemia at the time the renal signs and symptoms appeared.

Renal transplantation

Few individuals with systemic sclerosis have been given a renal allograft because only 0.05% of all the patients who are on dialysis awaiting renal transplantation have systemic sclerosis. After renal transplantation 64% of graft kidneys function for at least 1–1½ years. In explanation of the rapid destruction of two grafts it has been suggested that the arterial lesions they contained were due to systemic sclerosis (see p. 671). However, the vascular changes of systemic sclerosis are indistinguishable from those that occur in chronic rejection so it is not known whether systemic sclerosis affects the graft. Progression of systemic sclerosis in other organs, particularly the oesophagus and lung, remains the main prognostic problem after renal transplantation.

Prognosis

The course of systemic sclerosis is extremely variable, but the majority of patients survive for prolonged periods. In a study of 727 cases in the USA, the 5-year survival rate was 70.3% and the 10-year survival rate was 58.9%.[101] Similar figures were obtained in a prospective study in Australia.[102] Patients with the CREST syndrome have a much better prognosis than those with diffuse progressive systemic sclerosis. The prognosis is largely determined by how quickly and extensively the kidneys, heart and lungs are involved. Any evidence of renal disease indicates a poor prognosis; 60% of patients with signs of involvement of the kidneys died over a period of 20 years in one series compared with 10% of those without such signs.[92] The mean time from the onset of evidence of renal disease to death in this group of patients was 7 months for proteinuria, 13 months for benign phase hypertension and 1 month for acute renal failure with malignant hypertension. The advent of renal dialysis, more effective treatment of severe hypertension, and renal transplantation have improved survival in recent years.

Pathogenesis

The aetiology of systemic sclerosis is unknown. Two possible causes that are commonly considered are an autoimmune disturbance and an alteration in collagen synthesis.

Following the observation that an IgM antibody, eluted from the kidney in a case of diffuse progressive systemic sclerosis, bound to smooth muscle and elastic in small arteries, it has been suggested that the vascular lesions of systemic sclerosis are mediated by complement-fixing antibodies.[103] Other studies have indicated that a circulating cytotoxic factor causes recurrent injury to the endothelium of the capillaries.[104] The hypothesis is that the autoimmune injury leads to platelet aggregation and release of factors that cause intimal thickening and induce perivascular fibrosis.

The collagen in systemic sclerosis is not abnormal but cultured fibroblasts from patients with this disease synthesize twice as much collagen as normal fibroblasts.[105] What induces the fibroblasts to generate more collagen is not known. Growth factors released by macrophages and lymphocytes have been suggested. Another possibility is that Scl-70 may accelerate collagen gene transcription by virtue of its activity as a topoisomerase 1, a DNA template-modifying enzyme.[106]

Variants

Drug- and chemical-induced systemic sclerosis

Systemic sclerosis-like conditions have developed following exposure to vinyl chloride, other chlorinated hydrocarbons and epoxy resins. The drugs bleomycin, tryptophan and carbidopa also occasionally produce systemic sclerosis-like conditions. Renal changes occasionally occur; they are identical to those seen in typical systemic sclerosis.

Eosinophilic fasciitis

This syndrome of sclerodermatous change in the skin of the limbs and trunk, but not hands, is not associated with renal or other visceral complications. There may be eosinophilia and hypergammaglobulinaemia.

MIXED CONNECTIVE TISSUE DISEASE

Mixed connective tissue disease was first described in 1972.[107] Patients with this disease show many overlapping features of systemic sclerosis, systemic lupus erythematosus and polymyositis. Characteristic features are arthritis, a puffy sausage-shaped appearance of the fingers, Raynaud's phenomenon, oesophageal hypomotility and myositis. The patients also have very high titres of circulating anti-ribonucleoprotein (RNP; see p. 227), particularly during remissions of the disease; the antibody titres may fall during exacerbations.[108] This may happen because of massive organ deposition of antigen–antibody complexes leaving low levels of antibody in the serum or, more probably, the massive proteinuria during exacerbations of the disease results in loss of antibody in the urine. Females are affected more than males.

Sometimes there are difficulties in separating mixed connective tissue disease and systemic lupus erythematosus because a small proportion of patients with systemic lupus may exhibit antibodies to RNP, but in lupus there are also anti-DNA or anti-Sm antibodies which are not present in mixed connective tissue disease. Serum complement levels are usually within the normal range.

Nephritis occurs in approximately 20% of patients with mixed connective tissue disease.[109] It is relatively more common in children. In the majority of cases the nephritis has been diffuse membranous glomerulonephritis (see p. 192), but diffuse mesangiocapillary glomerulonephritis (see p. 166), diffuse endocapillary proliferative glomerulonephritis (see p. 145), and diffuse mesangial proliferative glomerulonephritis (see p. 155) have also been reported.[110] In all the forms of glomerulonephritis that occur in mixed connective tissue disease, electron-dense deposits have been recorded in the mesangium. Immune complex mediated tubulointerstitial disease, which occurs in systemic lupus erythematosus (see p. 464), has also been reported in mixed connective tissue disease.[108] The arteries and arterioles are normal apart from any hypertensive or ageing changes.

Pulmonary haemorrhage and neurological and psychiatric problems may occur as complications underlining the overlap between mixed connective tissue disease and systemic lupus erythematosus.

The majority of patients with mixed connective tissue disease have a good prognosis, but those with renal complications have a less certain outlook. Some appear to be responsive to steroids but in others the renal disease may be slowly progressive, with remissions and exacerbations. Often there is a stable nephrotic syndrome for years. Acute renal failure occurred in one reported case.[108]

The renal lesions appear to be mediated by immune complexes but even less is known about their pathogenesis than is known about those that occur in lupus nephritis (see p. 238).

SJØGREN'S SYNDROME

Sjøgren's syndrome is characterized by dry eyes (keratoconjunctivitis sicca), dry mouth (xerostomia) and recurrent swelling of the parotid[111] resulting from a chronic immunologically mediated inflammatory process involving the lacrimal and salivary glands. Sjøgren's syndrome occurs most frequently in women over the age of 40 years. In 40% of patients it occurs as an isolated disorder (sicca syndrome); in 60% it is associated with rheumatoid arthritis, systemic lupus erythematosus, systemic sclerosis, polymyositis, vasculitis, or thyroiditis.[112] Renal disease is common in patients with Sjøgren's syndrome.

Clinical features

In addition to the dryness and secondary changes in the eyes and mouth, some patients have mild arthritis, neuropathy and Raynaud's phenomenon. Patients with tubulointerstitial nephritis have hyposthenuria, a renal tubular acidification defect with or without acidaemia and renal tubular acidosis, uricosuria, phosphaturia and generalized aminoaciduria (de Toni–Fanconi syndrome). The few patients who develop glomerulonephritis usually present with proteinuria and microscopic haematuria; occasionally there is a nephrotic syndrome.

Tissue typing

There is an increased incidence of HLA-DR3 among patients with the primary form of the disease and HLA-DR4 among these with associated rheumatoid arthritis.

Serology

Approximately 50–80% of patients have circulating antinuclear antibodies. In addition about 70% also have anti-Ro (SS-A) antibodies and 60% anti-La (SS-B) antibodies; the anti-La antibodies are particularly associated with Sjøgren's syndrome and are uncommon in other autoimmune diseases.[113] Antibodies are also found to many other antigens including thyroglobulin, thyroid microsomal antigens, gastric parietal cells, mitochondria and salivary duct cells. There is always hypergammaglobulinaemia and most patients have rheumatoid factor. Antibodies to double-stranded DNA, Sm antigen, Scl-70 antigen and Jo-1 antigen occur in less than 5% of patients. Circulating immune complexes are found in 85% of patients.

Renal changes

Approximately one-third of the patients develop a focal tubulointerstitial nephritis; rarely a glomerulonephritis occurs either alone or in association with a tubulointerstitial nephritis; exceptionally vasculitis occurs.

Focal tubulointerstitial nephritis (see p. 466)

The interstitium contains foci of lymphocytes, plasma cells and macrophages, and there is marked fibrosis around the tubules (Fig. 8.22). There is also patchy tubular atrophy. These changes may affect the medulla as well as the cortex.[114] In the mononuclear cell infiltrate T lymphocytes predominate, most are CD4 (helper) cells but a few are CD8 cells. There are also rare isolated collections of B lymphocytes.[115]

In some patients electron-dense deposits are present in the tubular basement membranes; these correspond to the coarse granules and ribbons of IgG and C3 which are sometimes seen by immunofluorescence or immunoperoxidase microscopy in those membranes.[116]

Glomerulonephritis

Glomerulonephritis is rare in primary Sjøgren's syndrome and only a few cases have been reported.

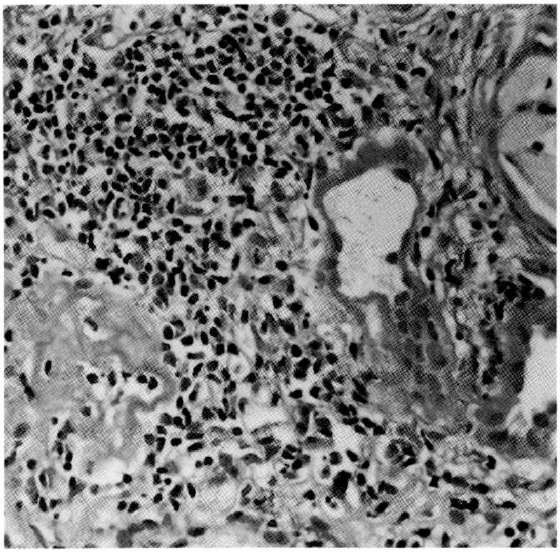

Fig. 8.22 Sjøgren's syndrome. The interstitium is focally infiltrated by mononuclear cells and there is some tubular atrophy.
Van Gieson-elastic × 240

Diffuse membranous and diffuse mesangiocapillary glomerulonephritis have been the commonest forms but focal glomerulonephritis has been described in one case. The membranous glomerulonephritis reported differed from the idiopathic form in that most glomeruli showed a moderate swelling and proliferation of endothelial cells and the subepithelial deposits contained large amounts of C1q.[117] The mesangiocapillary glomerulonephritis did not differ from the idiopathic disease.

Pathogenesis

The pathogenesis of Sjøgren's syndrome is unknown. As in systemic lupus erythematosus there is a polyclonal B lymphocyte hyperactivity, but there is no evidence to indicate what might be inducing that hyperactivity. Immune complex formation, either in situ or by filtration from the circulation, has been suggested to account for the tubular and glomerular lesions. However, the interstitial cellular infiltration raises the possibility that some of the lesions could be the consequence of cellular immunity. It has been speculated that the CD4+ T lymphocytes in the infiltrate aid both local formation of antibodies and activation of CD8+ T lymphocytes.

Variants

Vasculitis

Approximately 12% of patients with primary Sjøgren's syndrome have a vasculitis of small or medium sized vessels or both.[118] These changes are usually in the vessels of the skin or gastrointestinal tract; rarely they occur in vessels elsewhere including those in the kidneys. The renal vasculitis affects small and medium sized arteries producing lesions similar to those seen in the acute phase of polyarteritis but without aneurysm formation.[118]

POLYMYOSITIS AND DERMATOMYOSITIS

Polymyositis is a chronic inflammatory myopathy of unknown cause. When a skin rash is also present it is called dermatomyositis. The disease can occur at any age but there are two peaks, one in the age group 5–15 years and the other in the age group 50–60 years. There is a female preponderance under the age of 50 years. The incidence has been estimated in the USA as 0.5 per 100 000 population; in north-east England a prevalence of eight per 100 000 has been reported

Antibodies to the Jo-1 antigen, which is a subunit of transfer RNA, are found in the circulation of 30–50% of patients with polymyositis and dermatomyositis. They occur in less than 5% of patients with systemic lupus erythematosus, systemic sclerosis or Sjøgren's syndrome.[113]

In children, and in some acute cases in adults, widespread necrotizing vasculitis may be present involving many organs, including the kidney. The vascular lesions resemble those seen in polyarteritis nodosa.[119] Acute tubular necrosis with myoglobin casts occurs rarely. Approximately 60% of patients with polymyositis and dermatomyositis recover with immunosuppressive treatment.[120] The widespread vasculitis seems to be mediated by immune complex formation.

RHEUMATOID ARTHRITIS

Rheumatoid arthritis is a systemic, chronic inflammatory disease that affects principally the joints; other tissues may be involved, including the kidney. The frequency with which the kidney is damaged in rheumatoid arthritis is difficult to assess; estimates vary widely depending upon the sensitivity of the criteria used for diagnosis and the specialty of the investigators. Four main types of kidney damage have been reported: amyloid deposition, glomerulonephritis, vascular changes and chronic interstitial nephritis.

Renal changes

Amyloid deposition

In the past amyloid was found in approximately 15% of cases of rheumatoid arthritis at autopsy,[121] but nowadays the incidence is nearer 7%,[122] perhaps because secondary infections are fewer Amyloid is found much more frequently in biopsies because they are only performed on those patients with evidence of renal disease; [123] if the nephrotic syndrome is the criterion for performing the biopsy then amyloid may be found in as many as 71%.[124]

Amyloid deposition is associated with proteinuria; this is often heavy enough to produce the nephrotic syndrome. Usually there is progression to renal failure. Occasionally the amyloid deposition will cease after treatment with prednisone and cyclophosphamide; [125] the existing deposits are then reabsorbed leaving electron-lucent areas in the glomerular capillary basement membrane similar to those seen in resolving membranous glomerulonephritis.[126]

The amyloid affects predominantly the glomeruli, small arteries and arterioles. It is AA in type (see p. 344).

Glomerulonephritis

Membranous glomerulonephritis Membranous glomerulonephritis is found in 23–30% of patients biopsied because of urinary abnormalities.[127,128] In about two-thirds of the cases the glomerular lesions are focal; in the others they are diffuse.[129] The subepithelial deposits are stage I (see p. 194) in about half the cases and stage II or rarely stage III in the others. The usual clinical manifestation is proteinuria and sometimes the nephrotic syndrome. Most rheumatoid patients with membranous glomerulonephritis have been treated with gold (see p. 515) or penicillamine (see p. 523) before biopsy. These are therapeutic agents known to cause glomerular injury. However, there are now several cases on record in which this type of glomerulonephritis has occurred in the absence of these forms of therapy and in patients without evidence of antinuclear antibodies, cryoglobulins or hepatitis B antigenaemia.[128,130]

Mesangial proliferative glomerulonephritis
Mesangial proliferative glomerulonephritis is present in approximately 20-30% of rheumatoid arthritis cases biopsied because of urinary abnormalities.[127,129] There is a global or segmental increase in the amount of mesangial matrix and in the number of mesangial cells; the changes are usually mild and diffuse. Mesangial electron-dense deposits are rare. The usual clinical manifestation is isolated haematuria. In one series less than half the patients had received gold or penicillamine treatment before biopsy.[129]

IgA nephropathy IgA nephropathy has been found in a few patients with rheumatoid arthritis who have been biopsied because of haematuria.[127] The association may be fortuitous but IgA nephropathy is linked to ankylosing spondylitis, another rheumatic disease (see p. 25).

Necrotizing glomerulonephritis A few cases with diffuse endocapillary proliferation, segmental capillary occlusion by mononuclear cells, fibrin, infiltrating neutrophil granulocytes and karyorrhectic debris, fibrin in Bowman's space and segmental proliferation of epithelial cells, have been recorded in rheumatoid arthritis.[131] In these cases fibrinoid necrosis was not present in the arterioles and small arteries. The necrotic glomerular segments contained non-specific scanty amounts of various immunoglobulins and complement components. The patients were biopsied because they had the nephritic syndrome. Half responded to treatment with cyclophosphamide and prednisone.

Vascular changes

Necrotizing arteriolitis and arteritis Necrotizing arteriolitic and arteritic changes, similar to those seen in polyarteritis nodosa, are found in various organs at autopsy in approximately a quarter of patients with rheumatoid arthritis.[132] The kidneys are only affected in 9%.[122]

Intimal thickening of small arteries Non-specific intimal thickening of small arteries is common, being found in approximately half the cases of rheumatoid arthritis at autopsy. It occurs even in the absence of hypertension, but many of these patients are elderly and ageing changes have to be taken into account. In fact, arterial intimal thickening is about as common in age-matched controls.[122]

Chronic interstitial nephritis

Interstitial fibrosis is very common at autopsy in patients with rheumatoid arthritis but not in age-matched controls.[122] This may be due to the analgesics taken by these patients (see p. 458) or to various other non-steroidal anti-inflammatory agents used in the treatment of rheumatoid arthritis (see p. 474). Papillary necrosis (see p. 473) may also occur in these patients; it has been recorded in 3–30% of different autopsy series.[122]

Variant

Juvenile chronic arthritis
Renal amyloidosis is one of the major complications of this variant of rheumatoid arthritis. In one series it was present in 61% of renal biopsies in patients with juvenile chronic arthritis who had proteinuria with or without the nephrotic syndrome.[133] *Chronic interstitial nephritis* is also found.

ANKYLOSING SPONDYLITIS

Ankylosing spondylitis is an inflammatory arthritis which mainly involves the spine. The sacroiliac joints are always affected and sometimes the hip and shoulder joints. Occasionally it is associated with ocular, cardiac and pulmonary lesions. The overall mean prevalence in Britain and the USA is approximately one per 1000 of the population. It predominantly affects young men, the peak age of onset being 18–25 years. There is a strong association between ankylosing spondylitis and HLA-B27; approximately 90% of patients with this disease are of this tissue type compared with 5% of the general population. Serum IgA concentrations are usually elevated in ankylosing spondylitis and there seems to be a correlation between the IgA level and disease activity.[134] Circulating immune complexes are common.

Kidney involvement is uncommon in ankylosing spondylitis but four forms of renal lesion can occur: amyloidosis, glomerulonephritis, vasculitis and chronic interstitial nephritis.

Renal changes

Amyloidosis

Renal amyloidosis is found at autopsy in 5% of cases of ankylosing spondylitis.[135] As in rheumatoid arthritis it mainly affects the glomeruli, arteries and arterioles. It is AA in type (see p. 344).

Glomerulonephritis

Glomerulonephritis has been reported at autopsy in 2% of patients with ankylosing spondylitis.[135] However, the investigators did not look for IgA or mild glomerular mesangial proliferative changes and in recent years the great majority of cases of glomerulonephritis reported in association with ankylosing spondylitis have been IgA nephropathy.[136–140] It is difficult to estimate the true prevalence of IgA nephropathy in ankylosing spondylitis because most reports refer to renal biopsies on very small numbers of cases. Uraemia has been reported as the cause of death in 46.2% of patients with ankylosing spondylitis;[141] it is not clear whether IgA nephropathy plays any appreciable part in producing this renal failure. The assumption is that the renal dysfunction is almost entirely due to renal amyloidosis.[141]

The changes in the IgA nephropathy that occurs in ankylosing spondylitis are the same as those described under the idiopathic disease (see p. 159). Some are complicated by focal segmental sclerosis and hyalinosis.[136] The clinical presentation is usually with proteinuria and microscopic haematuria rather than episodes of macroscopic haematuria.

The pathogenesis of IgA nephropathy in ankylosing spondylitis is unclear. Possible mechanisms have been described under idiopathic IgA nephropathy (see p. 164). As in the idiopathic disease it is probable that in ankylosing spondylitis there is a genetic abnormality in the regulation of IgA production which leads to either increased synthesis in response to infection or reduced clearance or both. In ankylosing spondylitis inflammation is common at IgA-producing mucosal sites such as ocular, oral, enteric and genitourinary. The IgA immune complexes formed become trapped in the mesangium, activating the alternative complement pathway and other mediators of inflammation which cause mesangial cell proliferation and mesangial sclerosis.

Isolated examples of membranous glomerulonephritis, and mesangial proliferative glomerulonephritis with IgM deposits in one case and C3 in another have also been reported.[137]

Vascular changes

Subintimal fibrinoid changes in the arterioles and small arteries have been described.[142] They are not accompanied by cellular infiltration of the vessel wall or the perivascular tissues.

Chronic tubulointerstitial nephritis

Interstitial fibrosis and tubular atrophy occur in ankylosing spondylitis but nowhere near as frequently as in rheumatoid arthritis. The changes seem to be related mainly to the vascular alterations, although some are probably caused by drugs used in treatment. Papillary necrosis has been recorded but only rarely.

HENOCH–SCHÖNLEIN PURPURA

The Henoch–Schönlein syndrome consists of a purpuric rash, painful joints and various abdominal disturbances.[143,144] The underlying lesion is a systemic vasculitis of leucocytoclastic type. The condition is most frequent in children, particularly boys.

Renal involvement, as shown by proteinuria with or without haematuria, occurs in approximately 30% of patients under 16 years of age and in about 50% of patients over that age.[145] The prognosis is largely determined by the severity of the renal disease and by the gastrointestinal complications. In the majority of patients with renal involvement the disease follows a relatively benign course, but this is not always the case and Henoch–Schönlein purpura is a significant cause of end-stage renal failure, accounting for 15% of children entering dialysis programmes.[146]

The disease is associated with elevated serum IgA levels. IgA is also present in the capillaries of the skin and is the predominant immunoglobulin in the mesangium of those patients with renal involvement.

Clinical features

The great majority of cases of Henoch–Schönlein purpura appear between the ages of 2 and 11 years. Children under 2 years are infrequently affected and tend to have a comparatively mild disease with fewer renal manifestations. Henoch-Schönlein purpura is rare in adults; in a review of 1599 cases, only 100 (0.06%) patients were over 16 years of age.[145] The disease is more common in boys, in a ratio of approximately 2 : 1.

The rash is the most typical manifestation of the syndrome, consisting of recurrent crops of palpable purpuric lesions distributed symmetrically over the extensor surfaces of the lower legs, especially around the ankles, and on the buttocks and the elbows. Arthralgia or arthritis occurs in about 70% of cases and particularly affects the ankles and knees. Colicky abdominal pain, vomiting, gastrointestinal haemorrhage and intussusception are also frequent.

Renal manifestions usually appear within 3 months after the initial skin or visceral signs; infrequently they are the first indication of the disease. The most common evidence of renal involvement is haematuria accompanied by proteinuria. The haematuria is usually microscopic but may be macroscopic. In about 40% of patients referred to hospital the proteinuria is of sufficient severity to cause the nephrotic syndrome.[147] Sometimes there is an acute nephritic syndrome; typically this occurs within 6 weeks of the onset of the disease and it is frequently associated with a nephrotic syndrome. Renal involvement may occur even when the skin, joint or abdominal manifestations are very mild and there is no consistent relationship between the severity of the nephritis and the severity of the extrarenal manifestations.[148] An infection of the upper respiratory tract often precedes the illness but no specific organism has been consistently isolated.

Tissue typing

There does not seem to be an undue frequency of any particular HLA antigen in patients with Henoch–Schönlein purpura.[148]

Serology

Circulating IgA immune complexes[149] and cryoglobulins[150] are found in Henoch–Schönlein purpura. Serum complement levels are usually normal.[148]

Peripheral blood lymphocytes

Increased numbers of IgA-bearing peripheral blood lymphocytes have been described in children during the acute phase of Henoch–Schönlein purpura.[151] There is also some evidence that unstimulated B lymphocytes spontaneously produce increased amounts of IgG, IgA and IgM, as occurs in systemic lupus erythematosus, suggesting that there are increased numbers of circulating immunoglobulin secreting B lymphocytes in both conditions.[152] Excessive CD4+ (helper) T lymphocyte activity with or without insufficient CD8+ (suppressor) T lymphocyte activity has also been observed.[152] Serum IgA concentrations are often raised; these tend to return to normal when the activity of the disease subsides.[148] The antistreptolysin O titre is elevated in up to a third of patients, but the frequency is no greater than in control populations.[153]

Renal changes

Gross appearance of the kidneys

In the cases with a rapid course the kidneys are usually enlarged and pale, and are often speckled with petechial haemorrhages.

Light microscopy

Changes that range from mild mesangial proliferation alone to diffuse crescentic glomerulonephritis may be encountered.

Minor glomerular alterations In some patients there is only mild mesangial hypercellularity (no more than three mononuclear cells per mesangial area; see p. 136); this may be focal and segmental or global, or diffuse and segmental or global. Rarely no glomerular changes are seen by light microscopy. There are no abnormalities in the tubules, interstitium or blood vessels.

Focal segmental glomerulonephritis Focal segmental glomerulonephritis (see p. 211) is a common lesion. In some of the glomeruli there is a segment containing four or more mesangial cells. The focus of proliferation is often restricted to the peripheral part of one or two lobules (Fig. 8.23) and it is sometimes adherent to the parietal epithelial cells lining Bowman's capsule.

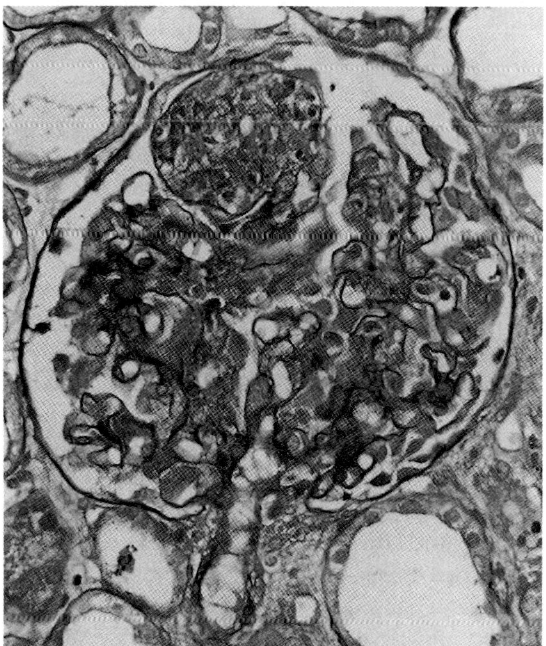

Fig. 8.23 Henoch–Schönlein purpura. Glomerulus showing focus of mesangial proliferation in lobule.
Periodic acid-Schiff × 420

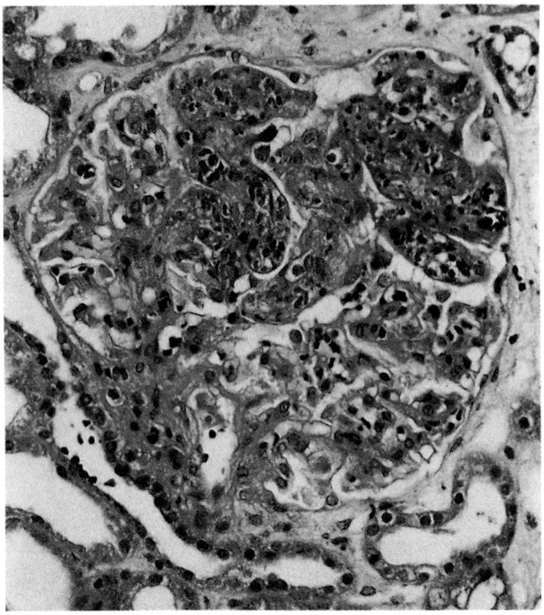

Fig. 8.24 Henoch–Schönlein purpura. Shortly after onset of haematuria and proteinuria. Glomerulus showing segmental focus of mesangial proliferation and fibrinoid necrosis. Haematoxylin-eosin × 420

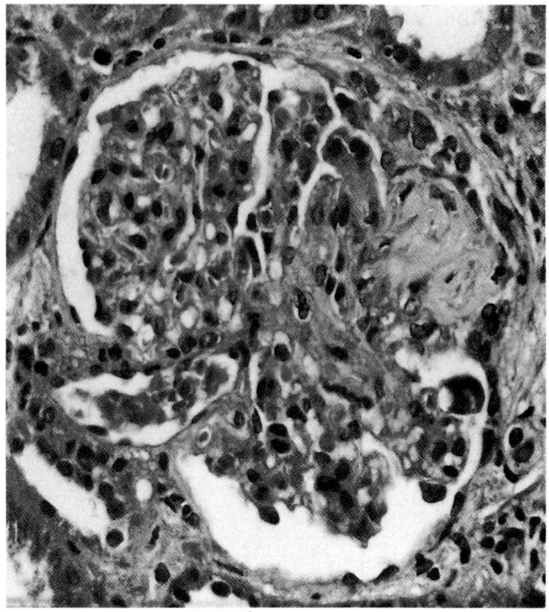

Fig. 8.25 Henoch–Schönlein purpura. The same case as in Figure 8.24, some 3 months later. Glomerulus showing segmental sclerosis following healing. Haematoxylin-eosin × 420

The focus may also contain an area of fibrinoid change, or intracapillary thromboses may be visible (Fig. 8.24). In patients biopsied at intervals during the course of their disease the focal segmental lesions may heal to give foci of glomerular sclerosis (Fig. 8.25). Focal segmental glomerulonephritis may be accompanied by crescents but these are usually small.[148] In the milder forms only minor degrees of tubular atrophy and interstitial fibrosis are present. Those with severe glomerular lesions show greater tubular and interstitial damage. Rarely there may be fibrinoid necrosis of the walls of arterioles and small arteries, with or without inflammatory cell infiltration.

Diffuse mesangial proliferative glomerulonephritis Diffuse mesangial proliferative glomerulonephritis (see p. 155) is common and often accompanied by variable numbers of crescents. In one large series of cases of Henoch–Schönlein purpura in children with renal lesions, 56% showed diffuse mesangial proliferative glomerulonephritis; of these 95% also had crescents. Amongst the cases with crescents, 38% had diffuse crescentic glomerulonephritis (see p. 186).[148] The crescents vary in size and degree of evolution. In addition to the diffuse mesangial proliferation, areas of mesangial sclerosis and segments of glomerular capillary wall with double contours (see p. 166) are often found, particularly in those parts of the glomerular tuft adjacent to crescents.[148] Serial renal biopsies usually show diminution of the mesangial proliferation and healing or reduction in number of the crescents. Those cases with many crescents have marked tubular damage and the interstitium is oedematous and contains infiltrating mononuclear cells, particularly plasma cells. A vasculitis is sometimes present; this may be morphologically indistinguishable from polyarteritis (see p. 268).

Diffuse mesangiocapillary glomerulonephritis Occasionally diffuse mesangiocapillary glomerulonephritis (see p. 166) occurs in Henoch–Schönlein purpura. It differs from the idiopathic form in the predominance of IgA in the mesangium.[154]

Electron microscopy

A common feature is the presence of electron-dense deposits in the mesangial matrix and often in the paramesangial region. Additionally in some cases there are subendothelial and, less frequently, subepithelial deposits.[154] Subepithelial etching, similar to that seen in IgA nephropathy (see p. 160), is occasionally seen and the capillary basement membrane may be irregularly thickened. Usually there is also an increase in the amount of mesangial matrix and in many cases there is an increase in the number of mesangial cells.

Immunofluorescence/immunoperoxidase microscopy

All the glomeruli contain intensely staining deposits of IgA in the mesangium (Fig. 8.26). Sometimes the IgA extends a little on to the capillary walls, and it may occasionally be present in the afferent and efferent arteriolar walls. Deposits of IgG and IgM are also often present but the IgA deposits predominate. There is usually C3 in the mesangium, but the early acting complement components C1q and C4 are absent.

Changes in other organs

Skin

Skin biopsies in Henoch–Schönlein purpura usually

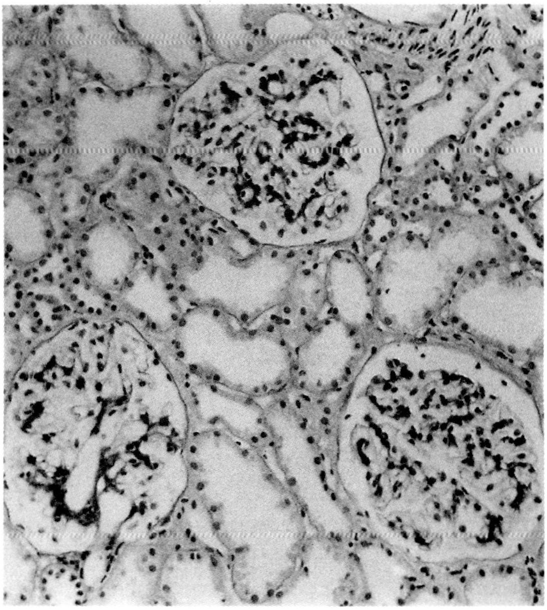

Fig. 8.26 Henoch–Schönlein purpura. Three glomeruli showing heavy deposition of IgA in the mesangium. Immunoperoxidase × 150

show a perivascular accumulation of neutrophil granulocytes and a few mononuclear cells around the arterioles, venules and capillaries in the dermis. A prominent feature is often the presence among the cellular infiltrate of many scattered nuclear fragments resulting from the disintegration of neutrophil granulocytes. The term *leucocytoclastic vasculitis* is often used to describe these changes.[155] Extravasation of erythrocytes is usually present. Deposits of IgA and C3, together sometimes with smaller amounts of other immunoglobulins, are found in the walls of the small dermal blood vessels, both in the areas of the skin showing purpura and in apparently unaffected areas as well.[156,157] Electron-dense deposits are present beneath the endothelial cell basement membranes of these vessels.[158]

Intestinal and other tissues

Similar vasculitic lesions are encountered in the intestine and sometimes in other tissues such as pancreas and gall bladder.[158]

Differential diagnosis

Many conditions can mimic the light microscopic changes seen in the kidney in Henoch–Schönlein purpura. However, only *IgA nephropathy* (see p. 157) and the occasional case of *lupus nephritis* (see p. 225) will show a predominance of IgA in the mesangium of all the glomeruli. The absence of a rash and of joint or gut lesions will usually distinguish IgA nephropathy from Henoch–Schönlein purpura. Raised titres of antibody to double-stranded DNA in the circulation and often the presence of early acting complement components C1q and C3 in the renal deposits will in most cases distinguish systemic lupus erythematosus from Henoch–Schönlein purpura. Immunofluorescence or immunoperoxidase microscopy is essential in making the important decision whether one is dealing with Henoch–Schönlein purpura or *polyarteritis*. The diagnosis of Henoch–Schönlein purpura should be viewed with great caution in older patients unless there is clear evidence of IgA deposition in isolation or as the predominant immunoglobulin in the glomeruli in a renal biopsy or in the small dermal blood vessels in a skin biopsy. There have been a number of instances in which adult patients labelled as Henoch–Schönlein purpura without this supporting evidence have been allowed to deteriorate dangerously with loss of renal function before the correct diagnosis of microscopic polyarteritis has been made and the appropriate treatment started (see p. 272).

Complications

The main renal complication is the development of *diffuse crescentic glomerulonephritis* (see p. 185).

Renal transplantation

Henoch–Schönlein purpura can affect the graft (see p. 669). The usual manifestation is the appearance of IgA in the mesangium. This probably occurs very frequently; in one series eight of nine patients were affected.[159] The accumulation of IgA is usually symptomless. Only one of the eight patients in the series referred to developed focal segmental glomerulonephritis in the renal allograft, with haematuria and proteinuria, and progressed to chronic renal failure with the nephrotic syndrome and death 9 years after transplantation.[159] It is thought that the risk of losing a graft because of recurrent disease might be increased if transplantation is performed before, or too soon after, the active purpura has subsided.[160]

Prognosis

In the majority of cases of Henoch–Schönlein purpura the course is relatively benign and spontaneous remissions are frequent.[148,161,162] In a group of 135 patients, all aged less than 20 years, the 10-year survival was approximately 90%.[163] If renal failure is going to occur it usually appears within 3 years of the onset of the disease.[148,162,163] However, renal failure after as long as 15 years has been recorded.[161] The course is characteristically difficult to predict but certain clinical and histological features have been shown to help.

Patients with only microscopic haematuria at presentation seldom develop progressive disease, while 50% of those with the nephrotic syndrome, complicated by renal insufficiency or hypoproteinaemia when first seen, progress to end-stage renal failure. Patients with an uncomplicated nephrotic syndrome have a relatively favourable prognosis.[148,161–163] High levels of IgA in the serum are also associated with a more benign course.[164]

Renal histology at presentation is moderately useful in predicting outcome. Almost all patients with minimal lesions on light microscopy are likely to be normal or have only minor urinary abnormalities 6½ years later.[160,162] In those with more severe disease the prognosis is most closely associated with the percentage of glomeruli affected by crescents. If in the initial biopsy less than 50% of the glomeruli exhibit crescents then approximately 4% of those patients progress to chronic renal failure; with 50–70% of the glomeruli bearing crescents the risk of uraemia rises to 25%; if more than 75% of the glomeruli contain crescents approximately 65% of the patients go on to terminal renal failure.[148,162,163] In one series no patient with diffuse mesangial proliferative glomerulonephritis and crescents in 100% of the glomeruli regained any renal function – all progressed to end-stage renal failure.[148]

Corticosteroid and immunosuppressive therapy is widely used and may favourably affect soft tissue swelling, joint and gastrointestinal symptoms but it has yet to be demonstrated that any form of treatment alters the outcome of Henoch-Schönlein nephritis.[147]

Pathogenesis

The clinical and pathological similarities between Henoch–Schönlein purpura and IgA nephropathy are close and suggest a common pathogenesis. It may be that IgA nephropathy represents a limited clinical expression of Henoch–Schönlein purpura in which only the renal features are apparent.[156,157]

Present evidence suggests that IgA immune complexes are responsible for Henoch–Schönlein purpura. As in the case of IgA nephropathy (see p. 164), it is proposed that there is a primary genetic abnormality in the regulation of IgA production which leads either to increased synthesis of IgA or to its reduced clearance or to both. The stimulus that initiates the IgA synthesis may be some infective agent involving the respiratory or gastrointestinal mucosa. The IgA antibodies then form immune complexes with the antigen of the infecting organism; the complexes become trapped in the mesangium where they activate the alternative complement pathway. Activation of the complement cascade leads to proliferation of mesangial cells and in some circumstances to activation of the coagulation mechanism. Why the accumulation of IgA and complement in the mesangium should be followed by haematuria is not understood. These hypotheses are discussed under IgA nephropathy on page 164.

Food allergens, various drugs, insect bites, vaccination and exposure to cold have all been suggested as factors in the pathogenesis of Henoch–Schönlein purpura, but there is little to support these claims.

RELAPSING POLYCHONDRITIS

Relapsing polychondritis is a systemic disorder characterized by inflammation and destruction of cartilage throughout the body. The pinnae, nasal septum, larynx, tracheobronchial tree, articular surfaces and audiovestibular apparatus are particularly affected. The vitreous, nuclei pulposi and aorta are also involved. The disease is associated with the presence of circulating IgA and IgG antibodies to type II collagen, an immunologically and biochemically distinct collagen that is found predominantly in cartilage, vitreous, aorta and notochord. Circulating IgG and IgA immune complexes are also present.

Serum creatinine levels are elevated in about 10% of patients with relapsing polychondritis but reports of biopsy-proven renal disease are rare. In the nine cases so far reported, there was diffuse crescentic glomerulonephritis in six, mesangial proliferative glomerulonephritis with occasional crescents in one and IgA nephropathy in two.[165] These lesions are probably mediated by lodging of circulating immune complexes in the glomerulus; type II collagen does not occur in glomeruli and this makes in situ formation of the complexes improbable.

ACUTE RHEUMATIC FEVER

Rheumatic fever is an acute, recurrent, inflammatory disease that usually follows several weeks after a throat infection with group A beta-haemolytic streptococci. It is commonest in children aged 6–16 years but about one-fifth of first attacks occur in adults. Many tissues and organs are affected but characteristically there is a migratory inflammation of the large joints and carditis: subcutaneous nodules, erythema marginatum and chorea are less frequent manifestations. Arteritis is sometimes found, and rarely pneumonitis and pleurisy.

Renal complications are common and consist of glomerular lesions, interstitial nephritis, arteritis, arteriolitis and infarction.

Glomerular lesions

Glomerular abnormalities occur in about 65% of cases of acute rheumatic fever.[166] In most instances they are manifested by microscopical haematuria or proteinuria, or both. Occasionally, there are no accompanying signs of functional disturbance.

Light microscopy

The commonest type of lesion is a mild mesangial hypercellularity (three mesangial cells per peripheral mesangial area). In a little over half the cases the hypercellularity is diffuse and global; in the others it is focal and segmental. Occasionally there is diffuse mesangial proliferative glomerulonephritis (see p. 153).[167] Focal segmental necrotizing lesions have also been described. Diffuse endocapillary proliferative glomerulonephritis is rare.[168]

Electron microscopy

Deposits of electron-dense material are usually present in the mesangium or within the glomerular capillary basement membranes.[167] In severe cases there are extensive subendothelial deposits. Subepithelial deposits and humps are rare.[168]

Immunofluorescence/immunoperoxidase microscopy

Fine granular deposits of IgG and C3 are present in the walls of the glomerular capillaries and in the mesangium.

Pathogenesis

The glomerular lesions are probably caused by immune complexes. It is not know whether they come from the circulation and impact in the glomeruli or are formed in situ. The antigen is probably derived from the streptococci responsible for the acute rheumatic fever. The rarity of diffuse endocapillary proliferative glomerulonephritis in acute rheumatic fever may be partly accounted for by the fact that whereas rheumatic fever may be caused by most, if not all, group A beta-haemolytic streptococci, only a few strains can produce diffuse endocapillary proliferative glomerulonephritis (see p. 143).

Interstitial nephritis

Foci of chronic inflammatory cells are frequently found in the interstitium of patients with acute rheumatic fever. Infrequently there is marked diffuse oedema of the interstitium accompanied by variable numbers of infiltrating lymphocytes.[168]

Arteritis and arteriolitis

Acute arteritis and arteriolitis manifested by inflammatory cell infiltration in the walls of small arteries and arterioles is seen in about 10% of cases.[167]

Infarction

The myocarditis in acute rheumatic fever may cause atrial fibrillation with the development of auricular thrombi and sometimes the release of emboli. The emboli occasionally lodge in the kidneys, producing infarcts (see p. 301).

SARCOIDOSIS

Sarcoidosis is a systemic disorder characterized by the formation of non-caseating granulomas in almost any organ of the body. Lymph nodes are most commonly affected, particularly those in the hilar regions of the lungs and in the mediastinum. When the disease is active it is marked by hypercalciuria, usually with hypercalcaemia. There is also usually hypergammaglobulinaemia, a raised level of angiotensin-converting enzyme in the serum and a positive Kveim skin test to a saline suspension of human sarcoid tissue. The disease is most frequent in young adults, particularly women. It is common in the USA, Britain, Scandinavia and the Caribbean countries. The highest reported incidence is in Sweden. Blacks are more likely to be affected than whites and tend to have more chronic disease. The cause of the condition is unknown.

Impairment of renal function, which is rare, is usually due to hypercalcaemia, nephrocalcinosis or renal stone formation caused by hypercalciuria. A much less common cause is a granulomatous interstitial nephritis or glomerulonephritis.

Hypercalcaemia, nephrocalcinosis and renal calculi

Hypercalcaemia

Hypercalcaemia occurs in 10–20% of cases of sarcoidosis; it is caused by increased 1,25-dihydroxy vitamin D_3 (calcitriol) synthesis which occurs, at least in part, in the sarcoid tissue.[169,170] The rise in circulating 1,25-dihydroxy vitamin D_3 results in increased calcium absorption and an elevation in the level of calcium in the blood. Hypercalcaemia may sometimes have a direct depressant action on renal function, without causing structural changes in the kidneys.[171]

Nephrocalcinosis or nephrolithiasis

In other patients *nephrocalcinosis* and *nephrolithiasis* are found (see p. 531). Clinically these forms of renal injury may be either asymptomatic or follow a slowly progressive course manifested initially by polyuria due to a defect in urinary concentration.

Granulomatous interstitial nephritis

Characteristic granulomatous lesions are found post-mortem in the interstitium of the kidneys in 20% of patients with sarcoidosis[172] but clinical manifestations are rare and most often caused by accompanying nephrocalcinosis, hypercalcaemia or glomerular disease. There are, however, an increasing number of reports of rapidly progressive or acute renal failure caused by isolated sarcoid granulomatous interstitial nephritis.[173–175] Because these patients do not have the classical features of sarcoidosis when they present in renal failure, diagnosis may be delayed.

Renal changes

The granuloma consists of a circumscribed focus of large epithelioid cells, often with occasional multinucleate Langhans giant cells, surrounded by a moderate number of lymphocytes and macrophages (Fig. 8.27). There is no caseation although there may be a little central necrosis. The cytoplasm of the giant cells may contain inclusions of two types – *Schaumann bodies*, which are very large (25–200 μm), concentrically laminated and composed of a mucopolysaccharide matrix impregnated with calcium salts and some iron, and *asteroid bodies* which are smaller (5–30 μm), star shaped, refractile and composed of microfilaments and other organelles embedded in an amorphous matrix.

Immunohistochemical analysis with monoclonal antibodies shows that the lymphocytes in sarcoid granulomas are predominantly activated CD4+ T cells; the macrophages are also activated and producing interleukin-1.[176]

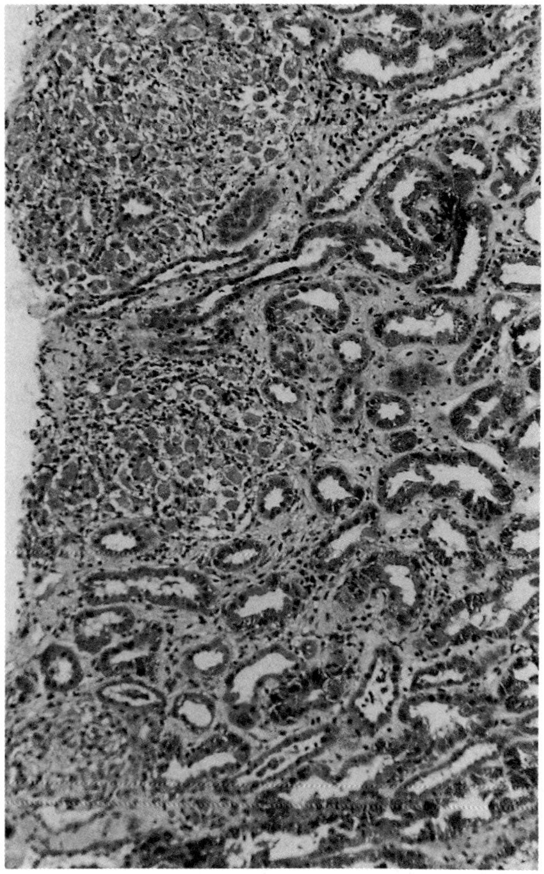

Fig. 8.27 Granulomatous interstitial nephritis in sarcoidosis. Haematoxylin-eosin × 200

Differential diagnosis

Although the granulomas are characteristic and highly suggestive of sarcoidosis, they are not diagnostic; in the kidney identical lesions may be caused by *reactions to drugs* such as methicillin, phenytoin, sulphonamides and other substances (see p. 454). Very similar lesions are also found in *tuberculosis, leprosy, fungal infections* and *brucellosis* (see pp. 384, 387, 392, 409, 414). Confusion with *Wegener's granulomatosis* should not occur because in this disease there are large areas of necrosis, the cellular infiltrate often also contains acute inflammatory cells and the glomeruli will almost always show segmental necrotizing lesions (see p. 277). Occasionally non-caseating granulomas are found in the renal interstitium in patients who show no evidence of sarcoid elsewhere in the body, have a negative Kveim test and nothing to suggest any other cause. It is unwise to label these lesions as sarcoid.

Prognosis

Most cases of granulomatous interstitial nephritis in sarcoidosis respond to treatment with steroids.

Disappearance of the granulomas may be followed by interstitial fibrosis.

Glomerulonephritis

Focal segmental glomerulosclerosis, membranous glomerulonephritis, mesangial proliferative glomerulonephritis, mesangiocapillary glomerulonephritis, IgA nephropathy and crescentic glomerulonephritis have all been described in patients with sarcoidosis.[177,178] The commonest form has been membranous glomerulonephritis and this has occurred more frequently than might be expected by chance alone. It is often associated with the nephrotic syndrome. The pathogenetic mechanisms are not known.

PARTIAL LIPODYSTROPHY

Lipodystrophy is an uncommon condition in which there is loss of subcutaneous fat.[179] In *total lipodystrophy* the fat over the whole of the body is lost; this condition may be present at birth or it may appear later. *Partial lipodystrophy* usually commences in childhood; it is commoner in girls. It occurs in two forms. In the more frequent form there is symmetrical loss of fat from the face and sometimes from the arms, chest, abdomen and hips; fat is retained on the legs. In the other form the subcutaneous fat of the face is normal or increased while that of the limbs and trunk is lost.[180]

Patients with lipodystrophy, whether total or partial, may present other abnormalities, including diabetes mellitus, enlargement of the liver and hypertriglyceridaemia.

Patients with partial lipodystrophy, but not those with total lipodystrophy, usually have abnormalities of complement.[181] In the commoner form of partial lipodystrophy, with loss of fat from the face, the concentration of C3 in the serum is low and C3 nephritic factor is often present. The serum concentration of C1q, C2 and C4 is usually normal. About a third of these patients develop either *dense deposit disease* (see p. 179) or, less frequently, *mesangiocapillary glomerulonephritis* (see p. 164). In the rarer form of partial lipodystrophy, with loss of fat confined to the limbs and trunk, the concentration of C1q, C2 and C4 in the serum is sometimes low; glomerulonephritis has not been recorded as a complication of this form of the disease.

When glomerulonephritis is associated with lipodystrophy the latter always precedes the development of the nephritis. It is not known whether the abnormalities of complement always precede the nephritis, but if they do they may predispose to its development by allowing persistent infection and chronic immune complex formation. The reason for the association between partial lipodystrophy and complement activation is also unknown. Possibly the complement deficiency induced by the C3 nephritic factor predisposes to chronic viral infections that lead to lipodystrophy or glomerulonephritis or both.

REFERENCES

Antiglomerular basement membrane disease

1. Savage COS, Pusey CD, Bowman C, Rees AJ, Lockwood CM. Antiglomerular basement membrane antibody mediated disease in the British Isles 1980–4. Br Med J 1986; 292: 301–304.
2. Davison AM.Seasonal incidence of glomerulonephritis: findings of UK Medical Research Council's glomerulonephritis registry. Proc Ninth Int Congress Nephrol 1984; 84A (abstr).
3. Ewan PW, Jones HA, Rhodes CG, Hughes JM. Detection of intrapulmonary haemorrhage with carbon monoxide uptake. Application in Goodpasture's syndrome. N Engl J Med 1976; 295: 1391–1396.
4. Rees AJ, Peters DK, Compston DAS, Batchelor JR. Strong association between HLA-DRW2 and antibody-mediated Goodpasture's syndrome. Lancet1978; 1: 966–968.
5. Bowman C, Lockwood CM. Clinical application of a radioimmunoassay for autoantibodies to glomerular basement membrane. J Clin Lab Immunol 1985; 17: 197–202.
6. Wheeler J, Simpson J, Morley AR. Routine and rapid enzyme linked immunosorbent assays for circulating anti-glomerular basement membrane antibodies. J Clin Pathol 1988; 41: 163–170.
7. Kefalides NA. The Goodpasture antigen and basement membranes: the search must go on. Lab Invest 1987; 56: 1–2 (editorial).

8. Salant DJ. Immunopathogenesis of crescentic glomerulonephritis and lung purpura. Kidney Int 1987; 32: 408–425.
9. Jayne DRW, Marshall PD, Jones SJ, Lockwood CM. Autoantibodies to GBM and neutrophil cytoplasm in rapidly progressive glomerulonephritis. Kidney Int 1990; 37: 965–970.
10. Bowman C, Ambrus K, Lockwood CM. Restriction of human IgG subclass expression in the population of auto-antibodies to glomerular basement membrane. Clin Exp Immunol 1987; 69: 341–349.
11. Flores JC, Taube D, Savage COS et al. Clinical and immunological evolution of oligoanuric anti-GBM nephritis treated by haemodialysis. Lancet 1986; 1: 5–8.
12. McMichael AJ, ed. Leucocyte typing III: white cell differentiation antigens. Oxford: Oxford University Press, 1987.
13. Bolton WK, Innes DJ, Sturgill BC, Kaiser DL. T cells and macrophages in rapidly progressive glomerulonephritis: clinicopathologic correlations. Kidney Int 1987; 32: 869-876.
14. Wu MJ, Rajaram R, Shelp WD, Beirne GJ, Burkholder PM. Vasculitis in Goodpasture's syndrome. Arch Pathol Lab Med 1980; 104: 300–302.
15. Andres G, Brentjens J, Kohli R et al. Histology of human tubulointerstitial nephritis associated with antibodies to renal basement membranes. Kidney Int 1978; 13: 480–491.
16. Lombard CM, Colby TV, Elliott CG. Surgical pathology of the lung in anti-basement membrane antibody-associated Goodpasture's syndrome. Hum Pathol 1989; 20: 445–451.
17. Donald KJ, Edwards RL, McEvoy JDS. Alveolar capillary basement membrane lesions in Goodpasture's syndrome and idiopathic pulmonary hemosiderosis. Am J Med 1975; 59: 642–649.
18. Koffler D, Sandson J, Carr R, Kunkel HG. Immunologic studies concerning the pulmonary lesions in Goodpasture's syndrome. Am J Pathol 1969; 42: 293–304.
19. McIntosh RM, Copack P, Chernack WB, Griswold WR, Weil R, Koss MN. The human choroid plexus and autoimmune nephritis. Arch Pathol 1975; 99: 48–50.
20. Wilson CB, Dixon FJ. Anti-glomerular basement membrane induced glomerulonephritis. Kidney Int 1973; 3: 74–89.
21. Querin S, Noël L-H, Grünfeld J-P et al. Linear glomerular IgG fixation in renal allografts: incidence and significance in Alport's syndrome. Clin Nephrol 1986; 25: 134–140.
22. Habib R, Antignac C, Hinglais N, Gagnadoux M-F, Broyer M. Glomerular lesions in the transplanted kidney in children. Am J Kidney Dis 1987; 10: 198–207.
23. Briggs WA, Johnson JP, Teichman S et al. Antiglomerular basement membrane antibody mediated glomerulonephritis and Goodpasture's syndrome. Medicine (Baltimore) 1979; 58: 348–361.
24. Donaghy M, Rees AJ. Cigarette smoking and lung haemorrhage in glomerulonephritis caused by autoantibodies to glomerular basement membrane. Lancet 1983; 2: 1390–1393.
25. Mehler PS, Brunvand MW, Hutt MP, Anderson RJ. Chronic recurrent Goodpasture's syndrome. Am J Med 1987; 82: 833–835.
26. Teichman S, Briggs WA, Kneisser MR, Enquist RW. Goodpasture's syndrome: two cases with contrasting early course and management. Am Rev Respir Dis 1976; 113: 223–232.
27. Lerner R, Glassock R, Dixon F. The role of antiglomerular basement membrane antibody in the pathogenesis of human glomerulonephritis. J Exp Med 1967; 126: 989–1004.
28. Willoughby WF, Dixon FJ. Experimental hemorrhagic pneumonitis produced by heterologous anti-lung antibody. J Immunol 1970; 104: 28–37.
29. Yoshioka K, Iseki T, Okada M, Morimoto Y, Eryu N, Maki S. Identification of Goodpasture antigens in human alveolar basement membrane. Clin Exp Immunol 1988; 74: 419–426.
30. Churchill DN, Fine A, Gault MH. Association between hydrocarbon exposure and glomerulonephritis: an appraisal of the evidence. Nephron 1983; 33: 169–172.
31. Bernis P, Hamels J, Quoidbach A, Mahieu PH, Bouvy P. Remission of Goodpasure's syndrome after withdrawal of an unusual toxin. Clin Nephrol 1985; 23: 312–317.
32. Boyce NW, Holdsworth SR. Intrarenal hemodynamic alterations induced by anti-GBM antibody. Kidney Int 1987; 31: 8–14.
33. Jennette JC, Lamanna RW, Burnette JP, Wilkman AS, Iskander SS. Concurrent antiglomerular basement membrane antibody and immune complex mediated glomerulonephritis. Am J Clin Pathol 1982; 78: 381–386.

Glomerulonephritis with pulmonary haemorrhage (Goodpasture's syndrome)

34. Goodpasture EW. The significance of certain pulmonary lesions in relation to the etiology of influenza. Am J Med Sci 1919; 158: 863–870.
35. Stanton MC, Tange JD. Goodpasture's syndrome (pulmonary haemorrhage associated with glomerulonephritis). Aust NZ J Med1958; 7: 132–144.
36. Glassock RJ. A clinical and immunopathologic dissection of rapidly progressive glomerulonephritis. Nephron 1978; 22: 253–264.

Systemic lupus erythematosus

37. Fessel WJ. Systemic lupus erythematosus in the community: incidence, prevalence, outcome and first symptoms. Arch Intern Med 1974; 134: 1027–1035.
38. Frank AO. Apparent predisposition to systemic lupus erythematosus in Chinese patients in West Malaysia. Ann Rheum Dis 1980; 39: 266–269.
39. Lee HS, Spargo BH. A renal biopsy study of lupus nephropathy in the United States and Korea. Am J Kidney Dis 1985; 5: 242–250.
40. Estes D, Christian CL. The natural history of systemic lupus erythematosus by prospective analysis. Medicine (Baltimore) 1971; 50: 85–95.
41. Hochberg MC, Boyd RE, Ahearn JM et al. Systemic lupus erythematosus: a review of clinico-laboratory features and immunogenetic markers in 150 patients

with emphasis on demographic subsets. Medicine (Baltimore) 1985; 64: 285–295.
42. Stevens MB. Systemic lupus erythematosus clinical issues.Springer Semin Immunopathol 1986; 9: 251–270.
43. Walport MJ, Black CM, Batchelor JR. The immunogenetics of SLE. Clin Rheum Dis 1982; 8: 2–21.
44. Cohen SA, Hughes GRV, Christian CL. AntiDNA activity in systemic lupus erythematosus. A diagnostic and therapeutic guide. Ann Rheum Dis 1971; 3 0: 259–261.
45. Hughes GRV. Autoantibodies in lupus and its variants: experience in 1000 patients. Br Med J 1984; 289: 339–342.
46. Schur PH. Complement and lupus erythematosus. Arthritis Rheum 1982; 25: 793–798.
47. Agnello V. Lupus diseases associated with hereditary and acquired deficiencies of complement. Springer Semin Immunopathol 1986; 9: 161–178.
48. Zubler RH, Huang Y-P, Miescher PA. Mechanisms of physiologic B cell responses and B cell hyperactivity in systemic lupus erythematosus. Springer Semin Immunopathol 1986; 9: 195–217.
49. Churg J, Sobin L. Renal disease. Classification and atlas of glomerular diseases. Tokyo: Igaku-Shoin, 1982: 128.
50. Caligaris-Cappio F, Bergui L, Tesio L, Ziano R, Camussi G. HLA-DR+ T cells of the Leu 3 (helper) type infiltrate the kidneys of patients with systemic lupus erythematosus. Clin Exp Immunol 1985; 59: 185–189.
51. Alexopoulos E, Séron D, Hartley RB, Cameron JS. Lupus nephritis: correlation of interstitial cells with glomerular function. Kidney Int 1990; 37: 100–109.
52. Bhathena DB, Sobel BJ, Migdal SD. Noninflammatory renal microangiopathy of systemic lupus erythematosus ('lupus vasculitis'). Am J Nephrol 1981; 1: 144–159.
53. Tsumagari T, Fukumoto S, Kinjo M, Tanaka K. Incidence and significance of intrarenal vasculopathies in patients with systemic lupus erythematosus. Hum Pathol 1985; 16: 43–49.
54. Magil AB, McFadden D, Rae A. Lupus glomerulonephritis with thrombotic microangiopathy. Hum Pathol 1986; 17: 192–194.
55. Cohen AH, Zamboni L. Ultrastructural appearance and morphogenesis of renal glomerular haematoxylin bodies. Am J Pathol1977; 89: 105–118.
56. Weidner N, Lorentz WB. Scanning electron microscopy of the acellular glomerular and tubular basement membrane in lupus nephritis. Am J Clin Pathol 1986; 85: 135–145.
57. Churg J, Grishman E. Ultrastructure of immune deposits in renal glomeruli. Ann Intern Med 1972; 76: 479–486.
58. Hruban Z, Wong T-W, Itabashi M et al. Glomiform and fibrillar cytoplasmic inclusions. Virchows Arch [B] 1976; 20: 91–102.
59. Park MH, D'Agati V, Appel GB, Pirani CL. Tubulointerstitial disease in lupus nephritis: relationship to immune deposits, interstitial inflammation, glomerular change, renal function and prognosis. Nephron 1986; 44: 309–319.
60. Kumano K, Sakai T, Mashimo S et al. A case of recurrent lupus nephritis after renal transplantation. Clin Nephrol 1987; 27: 94–98.
61. Mejia G, Zimmerman SW, Glass NR, Miller DT, Sollinger HW, Belzer FO. Renal transplantation in patients with systemic lupus erythematosus. Arch Intern Med 1983; 143: 2089–2092.
62. Bumgardner GL, Mauer SM, Payne W et al. Single center 1–15 year results of renal transplantation in patients with systemic lupus erythematosus. Transplantation 1988; 46: 703–709.
63. Rosner S, Ginzler EM, Diamond HS et al. A multicenter study of outcome in systemic lupus erythematosus. II. Causes of death. Arthritis Rheum 1982; 25: 612–617.
64. Austin HA, Muenz LR, Joyce KM, Antonovych TT, Balow JE. Diffuse proliferative lupus nephritis: identification of specific pathologic features affecting renal outcome. Kidney Int 1984; 25: 689–695.
65. Schwartz MM, Bernstein J, Hill GS et al. Predictive value of renal pathology in diffuse proliferative lupus glomerulonephritis.Kidney Int 1989; 36: 891–896.
66. Esdaile JM, Levinton C, Federgreen W, Hayslett JP, Kashgarian M. The clinical and renal biopsy predictors of long-term outcome in lupus nephritis: a study of 87 patients and review of the literature. Q J Med 1989; 72: 779–833.
67. Schwartz MM, Lan S-P, Bonsib SM et al. Clinical outcome of three discrete histological patterns of injury in severe lupus glomerulonephritis. Am J Kidney Dis 1989; 13: 273–283.
68. Shen HH, Winchester RJ. Susceptibility genetics of systemic lupus erythematosus. Springer Semin Immunopathol 1986; 9: 143–159.
69. Fielder AHL, Walport MJ, Batchelor JR et al. Family study of the major histocompatibility complex in patients with systemic lupus erythematosus: importance of null alleles of C4A and C4B in determining disease susceptibility. Br Med J 1983; 286: 425–428.
70. Lahita RG. The influence of sex hormones on the disease systemic lupus erythematosus. Springer Semin Immunopathol 1986; 9: 305–314.
71. Zubler RH, Huang Y-P, Miescher PA. Mechanisms of physiologic B cell responses and B cell hyperactivity in systemic lupus erythematosus. Springer Semin Immunopathol 1986; 9: 195–217.
72. Theofilopoulos AN, Kofler R, Noonan D, Singer P, Dixon FJ. Molecular aspects of murine systemic lupus erythematosus. Springer Semin Immunopathol 1986; 9: 121–142.
73. Andres GA, Accinni L, Beiser SM et al. Localisation of fluorescein-labelled antinucleoside antibodies in glomeruli of patients with active systemic lupus erythematosus nephritis. J Clin Invest 1970; 49: 2106–2118.
74. Fournie GJ. Circulating DNA and lupus nephritis. Kidney Int 1988; 33: 487–497.
75. Maddison PJ, Reichlin M. Deposition of antibodies to a soluble cytoplasmic antigen in the kidneys of patients with systemic lupus erythematosus. Arthritis Rheum 1979; 22: 858–863.
76. Isenberg DA, Collins C. Detection of cross-reactive anti-DNA antibody idiotypes on renal tissue-bound immunoglobulins from lupus patients. J Clin Invest 1985; 76: 287–294.
77. Harpey JP. Drugs and disseminated lupus erythematosus. Adverse Drug React Bull 1973; 43: 140–143.

78. Perry HM. Late toxicity to hydralazine resembling systemic lupus erythematosus or rheumatoid arthritis. Am J Med 1973; 54: 58–72.
79. Sim E, Gill EW, Sim RB. Drugs that induce systemic lupus erythematosus inhibit complement component C4. Lancet 1984; ii: 422–424.
80. Cameron HA, Ramsay LE. The lupus syndrome induced by hydralazine: a common complication with low dose treatment. Br Med J 1984; 289: 410–412.
81. Batchelor JR, Welsh KI, Mansilla Tinoco R et al. Hydralazine-induced systemic lupus erythematosus: influence of HLA-DR and sex on susceptibility. Lancet 1980; 1: 1107–1109.
82. Alarcon-Segovia D, Wakim KG, Worthington JW et al. Clinical and experimental studies on the hydralazine syndrome and its relationship to SLE. Medicine (Baltimore) 1967; 46: 1–33.
83. Shapiro KS, Pinn VW, Harrington JJ, Levey AS. Immune complex glomerulonephritis in hydralazine-induced SLE. Am J Kidney Dis1984; 3: 270–274.
84. Ihle BU, Whitworth JA, Dowling JP, Kincaid-Smith P. Hydralazine and lupus nephritis. Clin Nephrol 1984; 22: 230–238.
85. Bjorck S, Westberg G, Svalander C. Hydralazine-induced glomerulonephritis. Lancet 1985; 1: 392 (letter).
86. Foucar E, Erickson DG, Tung KSK. Glomerulonephritis in procainamide induced lupus erythematosus: report of a case and review of the literature. J Clin Lab Immunol 1979; 2: 79–84.
87. Sheikh TK, Charron RC, Katz A. Renal manifestations of drug induced systemic lupus erythematosus. Am J Clin Pathol 1981; 75: 755–762.

Systemic sclerosis

88. Medsger TA, Masi AT. Epidemiology of systemic sclerosis (scleroderma). Ann Intern Med 1971; 74: 714–721.
89. Barnett AJ. Scleroderma. Springfield, Illinois: Thomas, 1974.
90. Medsger TA. Systemic sclerosis (scleroderma), eosinophilic fasciitis, and calcinosis. In: McCarty DJ, ed. Arthritis and allied conditions. Philadelphia: Lea and Febiger, 1985: 994.
91. Medsger TA, Masi AT. Survival with scleroderma. II. A life table analysis of clinical and demographic factors in 358 male US veteran patients. J Chron Dis 1973; 26: 647–660.
92. Cannon PJ, Hassar M, Case DB, Casarella WJ, Sommers SC, LeRoy EC. The relationship of hypertension and renal failure in scleroderma (progressive systemic sclerosis) to structural and functional abnormalities of the renal cortical circulation. Medicine (Baltimore) 1974; 53: 1–46.
93. Oliver JA, Cannon PJ. The kidney in scleroderma. Nephron 1977; 18: 141–150.
94. Traub YM, Shapiro AP, Rodnan GP et al. Hypertension and renal failure (scleroderma renal crisis) in progressive systemic sclerosis. Review of 25-year experience with 68 cases. Medicine (Baltimore) 1983; 62: 335–352.
95. Barnett AJ, Tait BD, Barnett MA, Toh BH. T lymphocyte subset abnormalities and HLA antigens in scleroderma (systemic sclerosis). Clin Exp Immunol 1989; 76: 24–29.
96. Shero JH, Bordwell N, Rothfield NF, Earnshaw WC. High titers of autoantibodies to topoisomerase I (Scl-70) in sera from scleroderma patients. Science 1986; 231: 737–740.
97. Tan EM, Rodnan GP, Garcia I, Moroi Y, Fritzler MJ, Peebles C. Diversity of antinuclear antibodies in progressive systemic sclerosis. Anti-centromere antibody and its relationship to CREST syndrome. Arthritis Rheum 1980; 23: 617–625.
98. Senaldi G, Vergani D, McWhirter A, Black CM. Complement activation in progressive systemic sclerosis. Lancet 1987; 1: 1143–1144 (letter).
99. Sinclair RA, Antonovych TT, Mostofi FK. Renal proliferative arteriopathies and associated glomerular changes. A light and electron microscopic study. Hum Pathol 1976; 7: 565–588.
100. Gouge SF, Wilder K, Welch P, Sabnis SG, Antonovich T. Scleroderma renal crisis prior to scleroderma. Am J Kidney Dis 1989; 14: 236–238.
101. Tuffanelli DL, Winklemann RK. Systemic scleroderma. A clinical study of 727 cases. Arch Dermatol 1961; 84: 359–371.
102. Barnett AJ. Scleroderma (progressive systemic sclerosis): progress and course based on a personal series of 118 cases. Med J Aust 1978; 2: 129–134.
103. Evans DJ, Cashman SJ. Walport M. Progressive systemic sclerosis: autoimmune arteriopathy. Lancet 1987; 1: 480–482.
104. Kahaleh MB, Sherer GK, LeRoy EC. Endothelial injury in scleroderma. J Exp Med 1979; 149: 1326–1335.
105. Jayson MIV. Collagen changes in the pathogenesis of systemic sclerosis. Ann Rheum Dis 1977; 36: suppl 2, 26–28.
106. Douvas A. Does Scl-70 modulate collagen production in systemic sclerosis? Lancet 1988; 2: 475–477.

Mixed connective tissue disease

107. Sharp GC, Irvin WS, Tan EM et al. Mixed connective tissue disease. An apparently distinct rheumatic disease syndrome associated with a specific antibody to an extractable nuclear antigen (ENA). Am J Med 1972; 52: 148–159.
108. Germain MJ, Davidman M. Pulmonary haemorrhage and acute renal failure in a patient with mixed connective tissue disease. Am J Kidney Dis 1984; 3: 420–424.
109. Bennett RM, Spargo BH. Immune complex nephropathy in mixed connective tissue disease. Am J Med 1977; 63: 534–541.
110. Jones MB, Osterholm RK, Wilson RB et al. Fatal pulmonary hypertension and resolving immune complex glomerulonephritis in mixed connective tissue disease. Am J Med 1978; 65: 855–863.

Sjøgren's syndrome

111. Sjøgren H. Zur Kenntnis der Keratoconjuctivitis sicca (Keratitis filiformis bei Hypofunction der Tränendrüsen). Acta Ophthalmol (KBH) 1933; 2: suppl, 1–151.
112. Moutsopoulos HM, Chused TM, Mann DL et al. Sjøgren's syndrome (sicca syndrome): current issues. Ann Intern Med 1980; 92: 212–226.

113. McCarty GA. Autoantibodies and their reaction to rheumatic diseases. Med Clin North Am 1986; 70: 237–261.
114. Tu WH, Shearn MA, Lee JC et al. Interstitial nephritis in Sjøgren's syndrome. Ann Intern Med 1968; 69: 1163–1170.
115. Rosenberg ME, Schendel PB, McCurdy FA, Platt JL. Characterization of immune cells in kidneys from patients with Sjøgren's syndrome. Am J Kidney Dis 1988; 11: 20–22.
116. Winer RL, Cohen AH, Sawhney AS, Gorman JT. Sjøgren's syndrome with immune-complex tubulointerstitial renal disease. Clin Immunol Immunopathol 1977; 8: 494–503.
117. Moutsopoulos HM, Balow JE, Lawley TJ, Stahl NI, Antonovych TT, Chused TM. Immune complex glomerulonephritis in sicca syndrome. Am J Med 1978; 64: 955–960.
118. Tsokos M, Lazarou SA, Moutsopoulos HM. Vasculitis in primary Sjøgren's syndrome. Am J Clin Pathol 1987; 88: 26–31.

Polymyositis and dermatomyositis

119. Callen JP. Dermatomyositis. Int J Dermatol 1979; 18: 423–433.
120. Ansell BM. Inflammatory disorders of muscle. Clin Rheum Dis 1984; 10: 1–216.

Rheumatoid arthritis

121. Missen GAK, Taylor JD. Amyloidosis in rheumatoid arthritis. J Pathol Bacteriol 1956; 71: 179–192.
122. Ramirez G, Lambert R, Bloomer HA. Renal pathology in patients with rheumatoid arthritis. Nephron 1981; 29: 124–126.
123. Pollak VE, Pirani CL, Steck IE, Kark RM. The kidney in rheumatoid arthritis: studies by renal biopsy. Arthritis Rheum 1962; 5: 1–9.
124. Ennevaara K, Oka M. Rheumatoid arthritis with amyloidosis. Ann Rheum Dis 1964; 2: 131–138.
125. Hajzok O, Tomik F, Hajzokova M. Amyloidosis in rheumatoid arthritis: a study of 48 histologically confirmed cases. Z Rheumatol 1976; 35: 356–362.
126. Falck HM, Törnroth T, Skrifvars B, Wegelius O. Resolution of renal amyloidosis secondary to rheumatoid arthritis. Acta Med Scand 1979; 205: 651–656.
127. Helin H, Korpela M, Mustonen J, Pasternack A. Mild mesangial glomerulopathy – a frequent finding in rheumatoid arthritis patients with haematuria or proteinuria. Nephron 1986; 42: 224–230.
128. Evers J, Statz T, Dickmans A, Renner E. Membranous glomerulonephritis in rheumatoid arthritis unrelated to gold or penicillamine treatment. Clin Nephrol 1985; 24: 159 (letter).
129. Sellars L, Siamopoulos K, Wilkinson R, Leohapand T, Morley AR. Renal biopsy appearances in rheumatoid disease. Clin Nephrol 1983; 20: 114–120.
130. Heaney DJ, Kupor LR, Györkey F, Weinman EJ, Schloeder FX. Membranous nephropathy associated with rheumatoid arthritis. South Med J 1978; 71: 467–469.
131. Kuznetsky KA, Schwartz MM, Lohmann LA, Lewis EJ. Necrotizing glomerulonephritis in rheumatoid arthritis. Clin Nephrol 1986; 26: 257–264.
132. Cruickshank B. The arteritis in rheumatoid arthritis. Ann Rheum Dis 1954; 13: 136–145.
133. Levy M, Prieur A-M, Gubler M-C et al. Renal involvement in juvenile chronic arthritis: clinical and pathologic features. Am J Kidney Dis 1987; 9: 138–146.

Ankylosing spondylitis

134. Franssen MJ, van de Putte LBA, Gribneau FWJ. IgA serum levels and disease activity in ankylosing spondylitis: a prospective study. Ann Rheum Dis 1985; 44: 766–771.
135. Cruickshank B. Pathology of ankylosing spondylitis. Clin Orthop 1971; 74: 43–58
136. Veis JH, Hammond WS, Teitelbaum I. Hematuria and proteinuria in a patient with ankylosing spondylitis. Am J Kidney Dis 1988; 11: 196–198.
137. Shu K-H, Lian J-D, Yang Y-F et al. Glomerulonephritis in ankylosing spondylitis. Clin Nephrol 1986; 25: 169–174.
138. Saba SR, Ramirez G, Espinoza LR, Brueggemeyer CD. Ankylosing spondylitis and glomerulonephritis. Nephron 1985; 40: 227–229.
139. Lagrue G, Bruneau C, Intrator L, Laurent J. IgA nephropathy associated with seronegative spondylarthropathies: efficacy of non-steroidal anti-inflammatory drugs (NSAIDS). Clin Nephrol1985; 23: 107–108 (letter).
140. Méry J-P, Kenouch S, Dard S. More on IgA nephropathy in a patient with ankylosing spondylitis and a solitary kidney. Clin Nephrol 1984; 22: 267 (letter).
141. Lehtineh K. The mortality and causes of death of patients with 'hypergamma type' of ankylosing spondylitis. Scand J Rheumatol1983; 12: 3–4.
142. Pasternack A, Tallqvist G, Martio J. Renal vascular changes in ankylosing spondylitis. Acta Med Scand 1970; 187: 519–523.

Henoch–Schönlein purpura

143. Schönlein JL. Allgemeine und specielle Pathologie und Therapie, 3rd edn, vol 2. Freyburg: St Gallen, 1837: 48.
144. Henoch EH. Über eine eigentumliche Form von Purpura. Berl klin Wschr 1874; 11: 641–643.
145. Crumb CK. Renal involvement in Schönlein-Henoch syndrome. In: Suki WN, ed. The kidney in systemic disease. New York: Wiley,1976: 43.
146. Chantler C, Donckerwolcke RA, Brunner FP et al. Combined report on regular dialysis and transplantation of children in Europe,1977. In: Robinson BHB, Hawkins JB eds. Proceedings of the European Dialysis and Transplant Association. London: Pitman, 1978: 77.
147. Austin HA, Barlow JE. Henoch–Schönlein nephritis: prognostic features and the challenge of therapy. Am J Kidney Dis 1983; 2: 512–520.
148. Levy M, Broyer M, Arsan A, Levy-Bentolila D, Habib R. Anaphylactoid purpura nephritis in childhood: natural history and immunopathology. Adv Nephrol 1976; 6: 183–228.
149. Kauffmann RH, Herrmann WA, Meyer CJLM, Daha MR, van Es LA. Circulating IgA-immune complexes in Henoch–Schönlein purpura. A longitudinal study of their relationship to disease activity and vascular deposition of IgA. Am J Med 1980; 69: 859–866.
150. Garcia-Fuentes M, Chantler C, Williams DG.

Cryoglobulinaemia in Henoch–Schönlein purpura. Br Med J 1977; 2: 163–165.
151. Kuno-Sakai H, Sakai H, Nomoto Y et al. Increase of IgA-bearing peripheral blood lymphocytes in children with Henoch–Schönlein purpura. Pediatrics 1979; 64: 918–922.
152. Beale MG, Nash GS, Bertovich MJ et al. Similar disturbances in B cell activity and regulatory T cell function in Henoch–Schönlein purpura and systemic lupus erythematosus. J Immunol 1982; 128: 486–491.
153. Ayoub EM, Hoyer J. Anaphylactoid purpura: streptococcal antibody titres and beta C1 globulin levels. J Pediatr 1969; 75: 193–201.
154. Heaton JM, Turner DR, Cameron JS. Localisation of glomerular 'deposits' in Henoch–Schönlein nephritis. Histopathology 1977; 1: 93–104.
155. Sams WM, Thorne EG, Small P et al. Leukocytoclastic vasculitis. Arch Dermatol 1976; 112: 219–226.
156. Baart DE, La Faille-Kuyper EH, Kater L, Kooiker CJ, Dorhout Mees EJ. IgA deposits in cutaneous blood-vessel walls and mesangium in Henoch–Schönlein syndrome. Lancet 1973; 1: 892–893 (letter).
157. Baart DE, La Faille-Kuyper EH, Kater L, Kuijten RH et al. Occurrence of vascular IgA deposits in clinically normal skin of patients with renal disease. Kidney Int 1976; 9: 424–429.
158. Stevenson JA, Leong LA, Cohen AH, Border WA. Henoch–Schönlein purpura. Simultaneous demonstration of IgA deposits in involved skin, intestine and kidney. Arch Pathol Lab Med 1982; 106: 192–195.
159. Habib R, Antignac C, Hinglais N, Gagnadoux M-F, Broyer M. Glomerular lesions in the transplanted kidney in children. Am J Kidney Dis 1987; 10: 198–207.
160. Cameron JS, Glomerulonephritis in renal transplants. Transplantation 1982; 34: 237–245.
161. Counahan R, Winterborn MH, White RHR et al. Prognosis of Henoch–Schönlein nephritis in children. Br Med J 1977; 2: 11 14.
162. Koskimies O, Mir S, Rapola J. Henoch–Schönlein nephritis: long term prognosis of unselected patients. Arch Dis Child 1981; 56: 482–484.
163. Cameron JS. The nephritis of Schönlein–Henoch purpura: current problems. In: Kincaid-Smith P, d'Apice AJF, Atkins RC, eds. Progress in glomerulonephritis. New York: Wiley, 1979; 15: 283.
164. Fogazzi GB, Pasquali S, Moriggi M et al. Long-term outcome of Schönlein–Henoch nephritis in the adult. Clin Nephrol 1989; 31: 60–66.

Relapsing polychondritis

165. Dalal BI, Wallace AC, Slinger RP. IgA nephropathy in relapsing polychondritis. Pathology 1988; 20: 85–89.

Acute rheumatic fever

166. Cohen S, Salomon M, Grishman E, Gribetz D, Churg J. The kidney in acute rheumatic fever. Arch Intern Med 1971; 127: 245–249.
167. Grishman E, Cohen S, Salomon MI, Churg J. Renal lesions in acute rheumatic fever. Am J Pathol 1967; 51: 1045–1061.
168. Gibney R, Reineck HJ, Bannayan GA, Stein JH. Renal lesions in acute rheumatic fever. Ann Intern Med 1981; 94: 322–326.

Sarcoidosis

169. Barbour GL, Coburn JW, Slatopolsky E, Norman AW, Horst RL. Hypercalcemia in an anephric patient with sarcoidosis: evidence for extrarenal generation of 1,25-dihydroxy vitamin D. N Engl J Med 1981; 305: 440–443.
170. Sandler LM, Winearls CG, Fraher LJ, Clemens TL, Smith R, O'Riordan JLH. Studies of the hypercalcaemia of sarcoidosis: effect of steroids and exogenous vitamin D_3 on the circulating concentrations of 1,25-dihydroxy vitamin D_3. Q J Med 1984; 53: 165–180.
171. Benabe JE, Martinez-Maldonado M. Hypercalcemic nephropathy. Arch Intern Med 1978; 138: 777–779.
172. Longcope WT, Freiman DG. Study of sarcoidosis based on combined investigation of 160 cases including 30 autopsies from Johns Hopkins Hospital and Massachusetts General Hospital. Medicine (Baltimore) 1952; 31: 1–132.
173. Singer DRJ, Evans DJ. Renal impairment in sarcoidosis: granulomatous nephritis as an isolated cause (two case reports and review of the literature). Clin Nephrol 1986; 26: 250–256.
174. McCurley T, Salter J, Glick A. Renal insufficiency in sarcoidosis. A clinical and pathologic study. Arch Pathol Lab Med 1990; 114: 488–492.
175. Hannedouche T, Grateau G, Noël LH et al. Renal granulomatous sarcoidosis: report of six cases. Nephrol Dial Transplant1990; 5: 18–24.
176. Chilosi M, Menestrina F, Capelli P et al. Immunohistochemical analysis of sarcoid granulomas. Evaluation of Ki67+ and interleukin-1+ cells. Am J Pathol 1988; 131: 191–198.
177. Goldszer RC, Galvanek EG, Lazarus JM. Glomerulonephritis in a patient with sarcoidosis. Report of a case and review of the literature. Arch Pathol Lab Med 1981; 105: 478–481.
178. Chung-Park M, Lam M, Yazdy AM. IgA nephropathy associated with sarcoidosis. Am J Kidney Dis 1990; 15: 601–602.

Partial lipodystrophy

179. Senior B, Gellis SS. The syndromes of total lipodystrophy and of partial lipodystrophy. Pediatrics 1964; 33: 593–612.
180. Dunningham MG, Cochrane MA, Kelly A et al. Familial lipoatrophic diabetes with dominant transmission. Q J Med 1974; 43: 33–48.
181. Sissons JGP, West RJ, Fallows J et al. The complement abnormalities of lipodystrophy. N Engl J Med 1976; 294: 461–465.

9

K. A. Porter

The kidneys in vascular diseases

CLASSICAL POLYARTERITIS

Classical polyarteritis is an uncommon disease characterized by necrotizing inflammation of the walls of predominantly medium-sized arteries. It often leads to medial injury and the formation of aneurysms that produce nodular swellings on the vessels. The arteritis is focal and episodic. Granuloma formation is not a feature of this condition; infarcts are common. Practically any organ may be affected but the lungs and the spleen are almost always spared. The renal vessels are very commonly involved and in one reported case were the only vessels showing the disease.[1] Renal failure is the single most important cause of morbidity and mortality. Because the vascular lesions are not confined to the kidneys, patients are often referred initially to general physicians, dermatologists, rheumatologists or gastroenterologists. The natural history is of progression to death over months or years with a 5-year survival rate of 10%[2,3] but treatment with cyclophosphamide and steroids can give a 5-year survival of 80%.[4] The aetiology and pathogenesis of classical polyarteritis are uncertain.

Clinical features

Classical polyarteritis affects men twice as frequently as women; it may occur at any time in life but its incidence increases with age. The clinical presentation is extremely varied. Commonly there is general ill-health, myalgia, flitting arthralgia, loss of weight and a fever. The patient has a moderate leucocytosis and a high erythrocyte sedimentation rate. Depending on which organs are affected, there may be abdominal pain, gastrointestinal bleeding, ulceration of the skin, muscle pain with wasting and weakness, loss of reflexes and peripheral neuropathy with irregularly distributed sensory impairment, or other signs and symptoms. Renal involvement may be manifested by attacks of loin pain, dysuria or gross haematuria; sometimes there is only proteinuria and microscopic haematuria. Hypertension is common and may rapidly enter a malignant phase. Most cases pursue a protracted course, with recurrent acute exacerbations.

Tissue typing

The incidence of the various HLA types in classical polyarteritis is normal.

Serology

Serum complement levels are usually normal or raised. Serum C-reactive protein concentrations are raised during exacerbations and are useful for monitoring disease activity.[5] In some cases there are circulating immune complexes, which do not always reflect disease activity, and cryoglobulinaemia. A few cases have hepatitis B antigenaemia and in some of these the complexes have been shown to contain hepatitis B antigen and immunoglobulin.[6] Autoantibodies against neutrophil cytoplasmic antigens have not been found in the small number of cases of classical polyarteritis that have been studied so far.[7]

Renal changes

Gross appearances

The kidneys are often smaller than normal. The subcapsular surfaces show evidence of infarction, which may be recent or old, the latter in the form of depressed scars. The cortex may be thinner than normal over large areas. The arcuate arteries are often very prominent; there may be thrombosis of some of them. Occasionally small aneurysms are present on the segmental and arcuate arteries.

Light microscopy

Changes are present in some of the segmental, arcuate and large interlobular arteries. The disease affects only short segments of the vessels, leaving the intervening areas unchanged. The lesions do not all develop at the same time: it is common to see acute, healing and healed lesions together.

Acute arterial lesions The whole or a part of the circumference of the arterial wall is destroyed and replaced by fibrin (*fibrinoid necrosis*). This change often involves the entire thickness of the wall of arcuate arteries; in larger vessels it is sometimes confined to the intima and media. The internal elastic lamina is ruptured, fragmented or destroyed. The necrotic area is surrounded by an accumulation of neutrophil granulocytes, mononuclear cells, and a variable number of eosinophils; this cellular reaction extends into the tissues round the vessel (Fig. 9.1). The lumen of the damaged part of the artery may become obliterated by thrombosis, with consequent death of the tissues supplied by the vessel. The pressure of the blood circulating through the vessel may cause the damaged part of the wall to bulge and form an aneurysm. Haemorrhage may result from rupture of an aneurysm or from simple leakage of blood.

Healing arterial lesions Inflammatory cells are fewer in number and the necrotic areas and thrombi are invaded by fibroblasts (Fig. 9.2). The intima becomes much thickened by proliferation of smooth muscle cells, which characteristically tend to assume a concentric disposition.

Healed arterial lesions The necrotic muscle of the vessel wall is replaced by fibrous tissue. The disrupted internal elastic lamina does not regenerate (Fig. 9.3). All that is left of the extravasated red blood cells is a little haemosiderin in the wall of the vessel or its vicinity. The intima is thickened and fibrous, and the lumen of the artery is reduced. The narrowing results in ischaemic atrophy of the tissues supplied by the vessels; this ischaemia initiates the hypertension that so frequently occurs. Any occlusive thrombi undergo organization and recanalization (Fig. 9.4).

The smaller interlobular arteries and the arterioles are normal or may show hypertensive changes. There are infarcts of varying ages. The

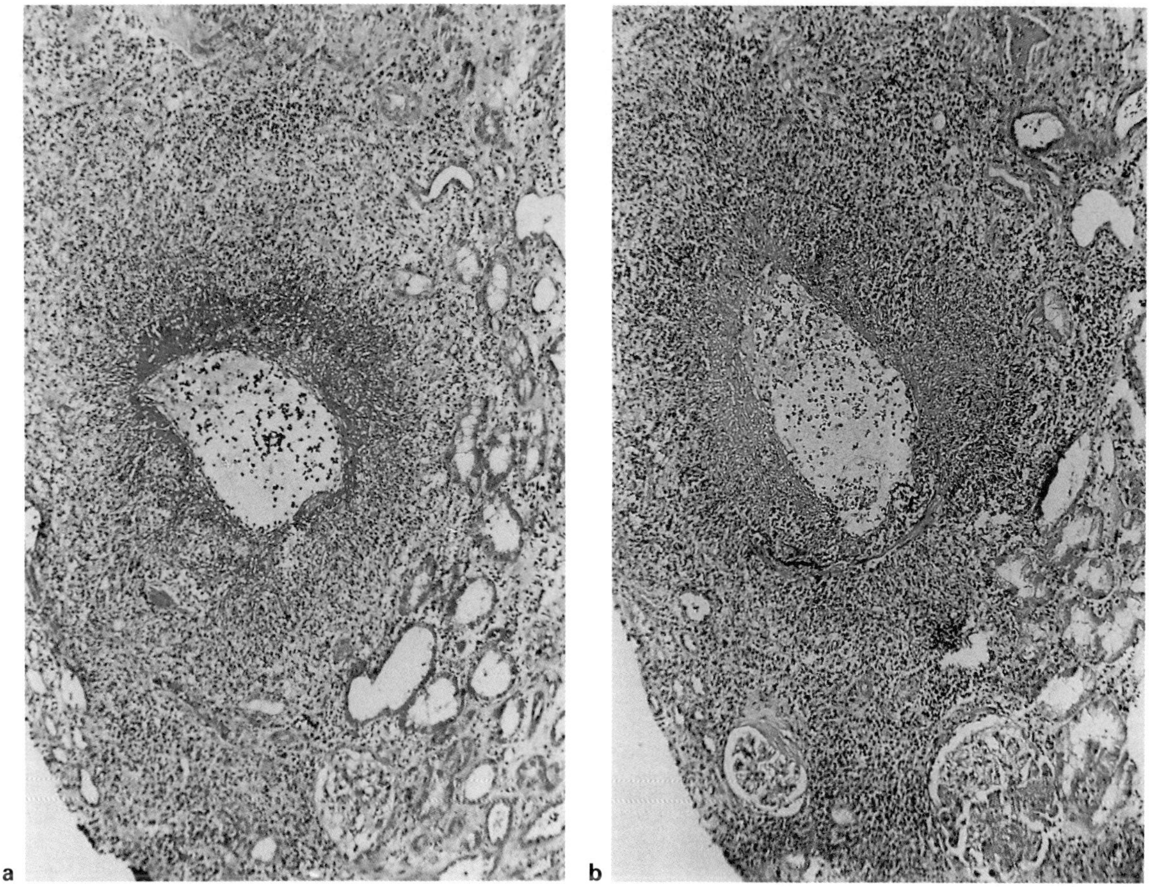

Fig. 9.1 a, b Classical polyarteritis. Acute arterial lesions. The whole of the circumference of a large interlobular artery is destroyed and replaced by fibrin. The necrotic area is surrounded and infiltrated by an accumulation of neutrophil granulocytes, mononuclear cells and a few eosinophils. The cellular reaction extends into the interstitium round the vessel. The elastic laminae are destroyed except for a small fragment at the bottom of (**b**).
(**a**) Haematoxylin-eosin × 100; (**b**) Elastic-Van Gieson × 100

rest of the kidney tissue is normal or shows ischaemic atrophy, affecting particularly the proximal tubules and accompanied by conspicuous fibrosis of the interstitium.

Electron microscopy

The changes confirm the light microscopy evidence. Electron-dense deposits are not usually found in the artery walls. Endothelial injury and subendothelial fibrin deposits are the earliest detectable changes.[8]

Immunofluorescence/immunoperoxidase microscopy

Immunoglobulin deposits in the affected parts of the vessel walls are infrequent and scanty. C3 is more common and fibrinogen is consistently found when lesions are recent.

Differential diagnosis

Necrotizing arteritis occasionally complicates *systemic lupus erythematosus* (see p. 232), *polymyositis* and *dermatomyositis* (see p. 249), *Henoch–Schönlein purpura* (see p. 254), *rheumatoid arthritis* (see p. 250), *infective endocarditis* (see p. 373), *Behçet's disease* (see p 320), *acute rheumatic fever* (see p. 258) and, very rarely, *antiglomerular basement membrane disease* (see p. 220) and *Sjøgren's syndrome* (see p. 249). The vascular lesions in these conditions may be indistinguishable from those

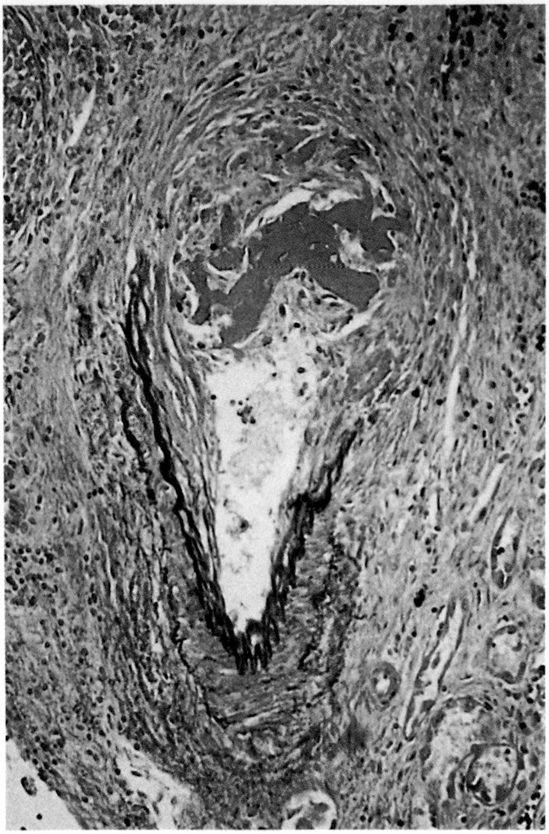

seen in classical polyarteritis and the only way of differentiating them is by the recognition of other characteristic associated clinical, serological or pathological features.

Renal complications

Hypertension

Hypertension occurs in approximately 70% of patients with classical polyarteritis.[9] It is commonest in those cases in which the segmental arteries are affected in the healing or healed stage of polyarteritis. Hypertension also seems to be particularly common in those cases associated with hepatitis B antigenaemia.[10]

Fig. 9.2 Classical polyarteritis. Healing phase of arteritis in arcuate vessel. There is organizing mural thrombus over the damaged area. The internal elastic lamina is ruptured. Inflammatory cells are few in number.
Elastic-Van Gieson × 72

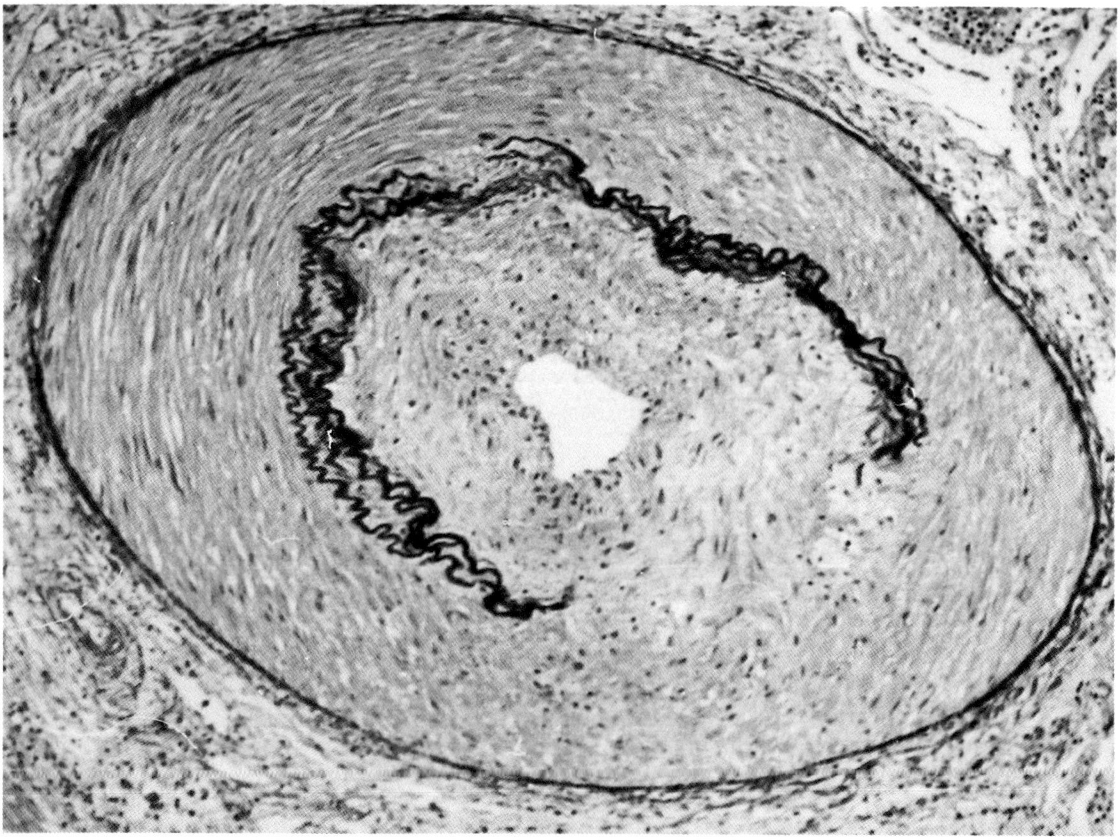

Fig. 9.3 Classical polyarteritis. Healed arterial lesion. The disrupted internal elastic lamina has not regenerated. The intima is thickened and fibrous. The lumen of the artery is greatly reduced.
Elastic-Van Gieson × 100

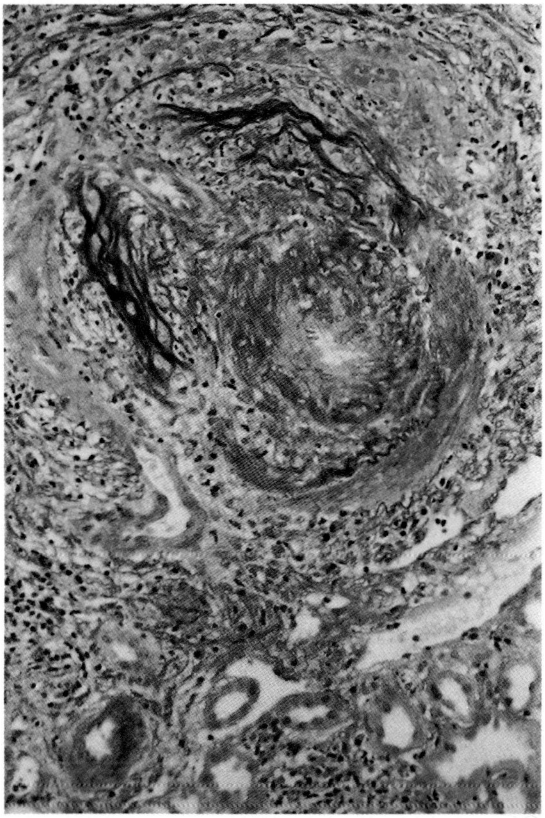

Fig. 9.4 Classical polyarteritis. Healed lesion. The lumen of a large interlobular artery is obliterated by fibrous tissue containing a few new tiny vessels as a result of organization and recanalization of an occlusive thrombus. Only fragments of the elastic laminae persist.
Elastic-Van Gieson × 100

Infarcts

Infarcts are common and have been mentioned under gross appearances and under light microscopy.

Perirenal haemorrhage

Rarely there is massive subcapsular or perirenal haemorrhage caused by rupture of a peripheral renal artery.

Renal transplantation

There have been a few reports of successful renal transplantation with no clinical or biopsy evidence of polyarteritis affecting the graft up to 5 years after the operation.[11]

Prognosis

When untreated 90% of patients with classical polyarteritis die within 5 years from renal failure, or as a direct result of vasculitis in some organ other than the kidney, or from the complications of benign or malignant phase hypertension. Patients with severe renal impairment or malignant hypertension at presentation do particularly badly. Treatment with cyclophosphamide and steroids is beneficial and in one series resulted in 80% of the patients still being alive at 5 years.[4] The major cause of death after treatment is sepsis, which is a particular hazard in any immunosuppressed patient. Patients with classical polyarteritis have the advantage that the disease is often associated with an overt clinical presentation including visceral infarction or haemorrhage or mononeuritis and this leads to early diagnosis and treatment before there is appreciable impairment of renal function.[12]

Pathogenesis

Classical polyarteritis is often presumed to have an immunological basis, usually because it has long been known that a necrotizing vasculitis occurs in the immune elimination phase of experimental acute serum sickness.[13] However, the morphological lesion of necrotizing vasculitis is non-specific and there is very little evidence to support the presumption of an immune origin in polyarteritis. Low levels of complement components are rare, deposits of immune material in vascular lesions are infrequent, small and scanty, and there is no correlation between the presence of circulating immune complexes and the finding of immune deposits in patients with classical polyarteritis.

Various microbial agents have been implicated but the strongest candidate for human immune complex vasculitis is hepatitis B surface antigen (HBsAg) which has been found in the serum of between 6 and 40% of patients with classical polyarteritis.[14] HBsAg has also been demonstrated in circulating immune complexes and in the vascular lesions of some patients.[15] However, the simultaneous presence of antibodies to HBsAg has not been shown in the vessel walls and there is no proof that the circulating immune complexes are implicated in the genesis of the arterial lesions. The best evidence that hepatitis B has an aetiological role comes from a longitudinal study of 266 patients undergoing haemodialysis who were chronic carriers of HBsAg.[16] Necrotizing vasculitis developed in three, whereas no cases occurred among 348 similarly dialysed patients who were not carriers.

Direct endothelial injury by viruses or other organisms and a reaction to various drugs have also been suggested as precipitants of classical polyarteritis but the evidence is circumstantial. There is nothing to indicate that cell-mediated injury is important in the pathogenesis.

MICROSCOPIC POLYARTERITIS

Microscopic polyarteritis is a commoner disease than classical polyarteritis and is characterized by necrotizing inflammation of small arteries, arterioles, capillaries and venules.[17] It is not associated with the formation of aneurysms and infarcts are uncommon. Typically the skin, mucous membranes, lungs, spleen, brain, heart, gastrointestinal tract, kidneys and muscle are involved. It has been suggested that primary necrotizing and crescentic glomerulonephritis is a renal limited form of microscopic polyarteritis.[18] There is often an initial acute non-specific illness followed by vasculitic rashes, musculoskeletal symptoms and impaired renal function with microscopic haematuria and proteinuria. Usually the renal failure progresses rapidly and, if treatment is not instituted, ends in death after several months in most patients. The disease responds to steroids and cyclophosphamides but less well than does classical polyarteritis.[19] Autoantibodies against antigens present in the cytoplasm of neutrophil granulocytes can be demonstrated in the circulation of patients with microscopic polyarteritis. Similar autoantibodies are also detected by immunofluorescence in Wegener's granulomatosis (see p. 276) and in the Churg–Strauss syndrome (see p. 279) but the antibodies in microscopic polyarteritis show a diffuse pattern of staining which contrasts with the granular pattern seen in Wegener's granulomatosis.[20] The aetiology and pathogenesis of microscopic polyarteritis are uncertain.

Clinical features

Microscopic polyarteritis is commoner in men than in women and although the average age is 40–50 years the disease can occur at any time in life.[14,19] Most patients notice some non-specific systemic signs and symptoms which are often followed by arthralgia, myalgia, skin purpura, haemoptysis and abdominal pain.[19] Initially there is almost always microscopic haematuria, proteinuria is common and in about half the patients the serum creatinine level is over 500 µmol/l. During the next few weeks the renal function deteriorates rapidly, highlighting the need for urgent diagnosis. A few patients present with acute renal failure and no obvious systemic signs or symptoms. Hypertension is not so common as in classical polyarteritis but is found in about 30%.[19] An elevated erythrocyte sedimentation rate and a normochromic normocytic anaemia are found in almost all the patients. Leucocytosis is a common finding, usually with neutrophilia.

Tissue typing

The incidence of HLA tissue types is normal, unlike Wegener's granulomatosis in which there is an increased frequency of HLA-DR2.

Serology

As in classical polyarteritis, serum complement levels are usually normal or raised; serum C reactive protein concentrations are raised during exacerbations and in about 45% of patients there are circulating immune complexes. Hepatitis B surface antigen (HBsAg) is not usually found. Autoantibodies against neutrophil cytoplasmic antigens are present during the initial acute phase of the illness.[20] Present evidence suggests that this is a specific and highly sensitive diagnostic test.[21]

Renal changes

Gross appearances

The kidneys are of normal size or enlarged. The subcapsular surface is smooth and often speckled with petechial haemorrhages. The arcuate arteries appear normal.

Light microscopy

Focal and segmental glomerulonephritis In contrast to classical polyarteritis the glomeruli bear the brunt of microscopic polyarteritis. There is usually a focal and segmental glomerulonephritis that is often necrotizing in type. Anything from 5–90% of the glomeruli contain areas of fibrinoid necrosis accompanied by minimal mesangial cell and endothelial proliferation (Fig. 9.5). Occasionally the necrotizing lesions are global (that is, involving the whole or almost the whole glomerulus). Initially there appears to be capillary thrombosis with destruction and collapse of the capillary wall at the periphery of the tuft. Release of red cells and fibrin into Bowman's space is followed by the formation of crescents, which are found in 80–90% of renal biopsies in microscopic polyarteritis. In about half the cases crescents are present in over 60% of the glomeruli.[17] The segmental lesions often differ in age and varying degrees of scarring may coexist with fresh necrotic areas (Fig. 9.6). The crescents likewise may differ in age.

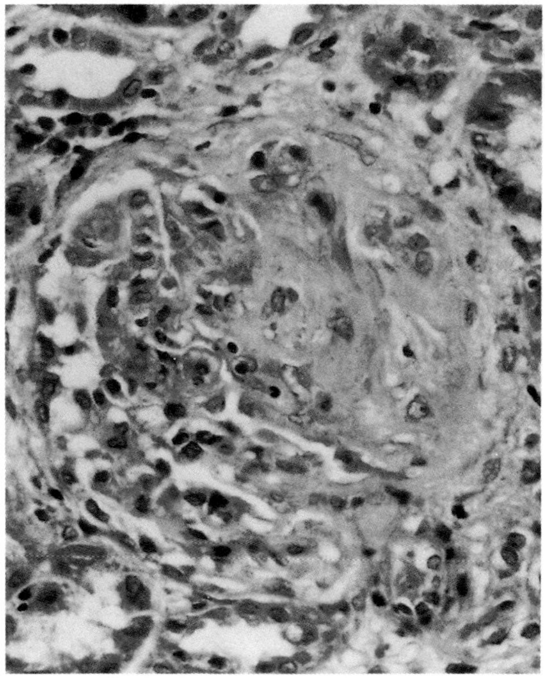

Fig. 9.6 Microscopic polyarteritis. Glomerulus with a sclerosed segment at the periphery of the tuft. Haematoxylin-eosin × 350

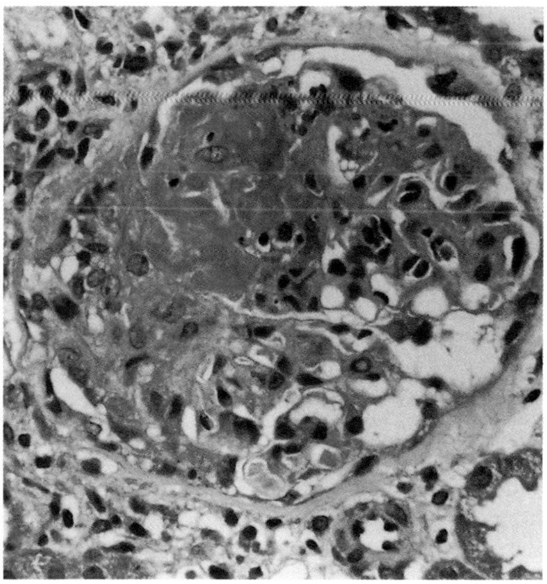

Fig. 9.5 Microscopic polyarteritis. Glomerulus with segmental area of fibrinoid necrosis and minimal cellular proliferation. Haematoxylin-eosin × 350

Vasculitis In 20% or less of biopsies in microscopic polyarteritis there is an arteritis or arteriolitis or both. Venules and peritubular capillaries are also sometimes affected. The walls of the smaller interlobular arteries and of the arterioles may be completely or segmentally replaced by fibrin; an infiltrate of neutrophil granulocytes, eosinophils and mononuclear cells often surrounds the affected vessels (Fig. 9.7). The vasculitic lesions tend to be of similar age but healed lesions with breaching of the internal elastic lamina are sometimes present. In the majority of cases the

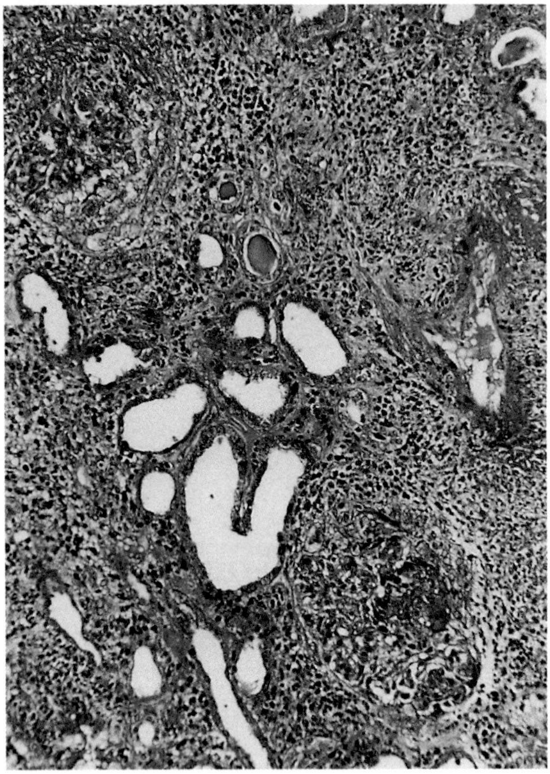

Fig. 9.7 Microscopic polyarteritis. A necrotic arteriole is surrounded by an inflammatory infiltrate. The upper glomerulus contains a cellular crescent; the lower glomerulus contains a segment of necrosis.
Haematoxylin-eosin × 240

glomerular lesions are the only evidence of vasculitis within the kidney.[22]

Tubulointerstitial changes There is often mild atrophy of the tubules and a mild to severe infiltration of the interstitium by mononuclear cells and eosinophils. Granulomatous foci of epithelioid cells may occur in the interstitium.

Electron microscopy

Swelling of the glomerular and vascular endothelial cells, with focal subendothelial fibrin deposits, are the earliest changes. Later the endothelium degenerates and is lost; in the glomerular capillaries thrombosis occurs and gaps appear in the basement membranes. Electron-dense deposits are occasionally seen in the glomeruli but not in the arterial and arteriolar walls.[8]

Immunofluorescence/immunoperoxidase microscopy

C3, C1q and fibrinogen are frequently detected in areas of necrosis or sclerosis in glomerular tufts and arterial or arteriolar walls. Immunoglobulin deposits in the lesions are infrequent, scanty and ill defined.

Differential diagnosis

Focal segmental necrotizing glomerulonephritis is also found in Wegener's granulomatosis (see p. 276), Henoch–Schönlein purpura (see p. 253), systemic lupus erythematosus (see p. 228), anti-glomerular basement membrane disease (see p. 219) and bacterial endocarditis (see p. 376). *Henoch–Schönlein purpura* can be differentiated because the mesangium contains a predominance of IgA. The linear deposit of IgG in *antiglomerular basement membrane disease* is also distinctive. In *systemic lupus erythematosus* mesangial deposits of immunoglobulin and complement are present and there are often tubuloreticular structures in the cytoplasm. *Bacterial endocarditis* is also associated with abundant deposits of immunoglobulin and complement. *Wegener's granulomatosis* may be indistinguishable on morphological grounds but the autoantibodies to antigens in the cytoplasm of neutrophil granulocytes that are present in these patients appear to differ from those present in cases of microscopic polyarteritis.[21] In microscopic polyarteritis the circulating antibodies detected by indirect immunofluoresence produce diffuse staining localized to the perinuclear region when they bind to normal neutrophils; in Wegener's granulomatosis the pattern is granular and distributed throughout the cytoplasm.

Renal complications

Diffuse crescentic glomerulonephritis

Diffuse crescentic glomerulonephritis commonly complicates microscopic polyarteritis.

Hypertension

Although hypertension is present in less than a third of the patients at presentation, and is mild, after treatment of the arteritis it develops in the majority of patients and is severe enough to require antihypertensive treatment.[19]

Renal transplantation

There is little information about the outcome of renal transplantation. In a review paper it is mentioned that three patients with microscopic polyarteritis were given renal allografts. Two were said to be surviving with functional transplants.[23]

Prognosis

There is rapid response to a combination of steroids and cyclophosphamide; even so about 20% of patients die during the first 2 months. The relapse rate is high with nearly half the surviving patients having at least one recurrence. The 5-year survival rate is approximately 65% for patients and 55% for kidneys;[19] most of the deaths are due to lung haemorrhage and sepsis. The survival rate is improved when treatment is started before the serum creatinine level rises above 400 µmol/l. Prompt diagnosis is therefore essential and the test for autoantibodies against neutrophil cytoplasmic antigens and renal biopsy are the two investigations that enable this to be achieved without delay.

Pathogenesis

Most of the points made in the discussion on the pathogenesis of classical polyarteritis also apply to microscopic polyarteritis. However, hepatitis B surface antigen (HB_sAg) has not been reported in the vascular lesions of patients with microscopic polyarteritis[14] and hepatitis B antigenaemia is less frequent in these patients than in patients with classical polyarteritis.

It is not known whether the autoantibodies to antigens in the cytoplasm of neutrophils that are found in untreated patients in the active phase of microscopic polyarteritis play any part in causing the necrotizing vascular lesions. The antibodies appear to be directed against at least one epitope of the enzyme alkaline phosphatase.[24] The disappearance of the autoantibodies as the activity of the disease diminishes suggests that they may have a pathogenetic role. When a monoclonal antibody to a purified component of the autoantigen was applied to sections of vessel walls it appeared to cross-react with determinants in the endothelial cells. This raises the possibility that the antibodies may be involved in a direct attack on such cells.[7]

Variant

Overlap syndrome

Sometimes patients with polyarteritis have evidence of involvement of both small and medium-sized vessels. The term 'overlap syndrome' has been used to describe these cases.[25]

WEGENER'S GRANULOMATOSIS

This rare disorder was first described in 1936.[26] It is characterized by three features:

1. Necrotizing granulomas with vasculitis affecting the respiratory tract, including the nose and mouth, paranasal sinuses, larynx, tracheobronchial tree and lungs.
2. Systemic vasculitis involving both small arteries and veins which may affect almost any vessel in any organ of the body but with a particular predilection for the respiratory tract, kidneys and spleen.
3. Focal necrotizing glomerulonephritis.[27]

Patients tend to present with symptoms of sinusitis, otitis media or chest infection. In addition, they may have any of the clinical manifestations of microscopic polyarteritis. Later, renal failure develops and, in the absence of treatment, this usually leads to death within 1 year.[27] Treatment with cyclophosphamide combined with steroids has transformed the outlook: in one series 88% of patients were alive after an average follow-up of 4 years.[27] However, it is critical to start treatment before irrevocable renal damage has occurred. Early diagnosis has now been made much easier by the finding that the serum of patients with Wegener's granulomatosis contains antibodies against cytoplasmic antigens in neutrophil granulocytes. The antibodies have different specificities from those encountered in microscopic polyarteritis (see p. 272) and Kawasaki disease mucocutaneous lymph node; this is reflected in their pattern of binding to immobilized normal human neutrophils on indirect immunofluorescence.[20] The aetiology and pathogenesis of Wegener's granulomatosis are unclear.

Clinical features

Wegener's granulomatosis affects men slightly more than women, with a ratio of 1.6 : 1.0; it may occur at as early an age as 14 years but it is predominantly a disease of the middle aged and elderly, the mean age being about 44 years.[27] The early symptoms are often non-specific. The first specific signs and symptoms are usually related to severe and persistent rhinitis with deafness, epistaxis and sinus pain. There is also dyspnoea, cough and haemoptysis. When the chest is X-rayed patchy infiltrates are found in about 70% of patients.[27,28] Fever, arthralgia or arthritis and eye abnormalities are frequent. Anaemia and a mild leucocytosis are common. Eosinophilia is sometimes found in the peripheral blood. The erythrocyte sedimentation rate is invariably raised.

Renal involvement occurs in about 85% of cases. It is associated with proteinuria and gross or microscopic haematuria, and is followed by renal failure, which may develop very rapidly. The mean time from the first symptoms of Wegener's granulomatosis to the onset of renal failure is 7½ months.[28] Most patients are normotensive when first seen.

Tissue typing

It has been claimed that there is a significantly increased frequency of HLA-DR2 in patients with Wegener's granulomatosis.[29]

Serology

Autoantibodies against cytoplasmic components of neutrophil granulocytes are present in all patients with active extensive disease; they are often absent during remission.[24,30] These IgG antibodies are highly specific and when detected by indirect immunofluorescence produce a characteristic granular pattern of staining throughout the cytoplasm of the neutrophil granulocytes.[20] The levels of C reactive protein are usually elevated. Complement levels are normal. Circulating immune complexes are present in nearly half the patients. Hepatitis B surface antigen (HB_sAg) is not found with increased frequency in the blood of patients with Wegener's granulomatosis in contrast to its frequent presence in cases of classical polyarteritis (see p. 271).

Renal changes

Gross appearances

The kidneys are usually enlarged. The subcapsular surface is often studded with small petechial haemorrhages. On the cut surface the larger arteries appear normal.

Light microscopy

The changes are often indistinguishable from those seen in microscopic polyarteritis. Initially there is a focal and segmental necrotizing glomerulonephritis, associated with glomerular thrombosis with or without breaks in the capillary basement membrane and karyorrhexis (Fig. 9.8).

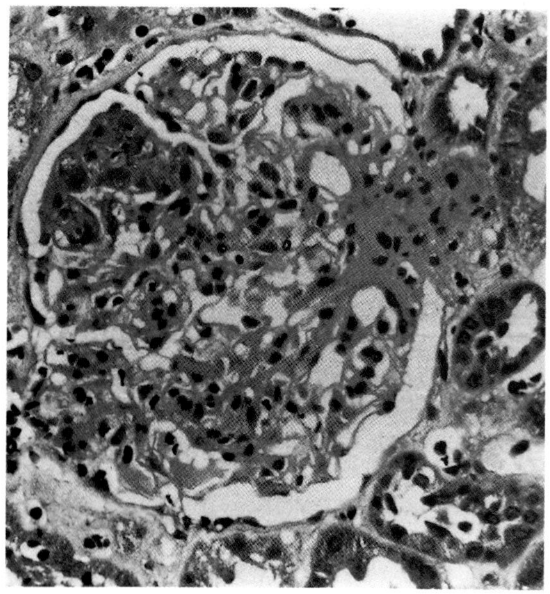

Fig. 9.8 Wegener's granulomatosis. Glomerulus showing a segment of necrotizing change at the periphery of the tuft. Haematoxylin-eosin × 350

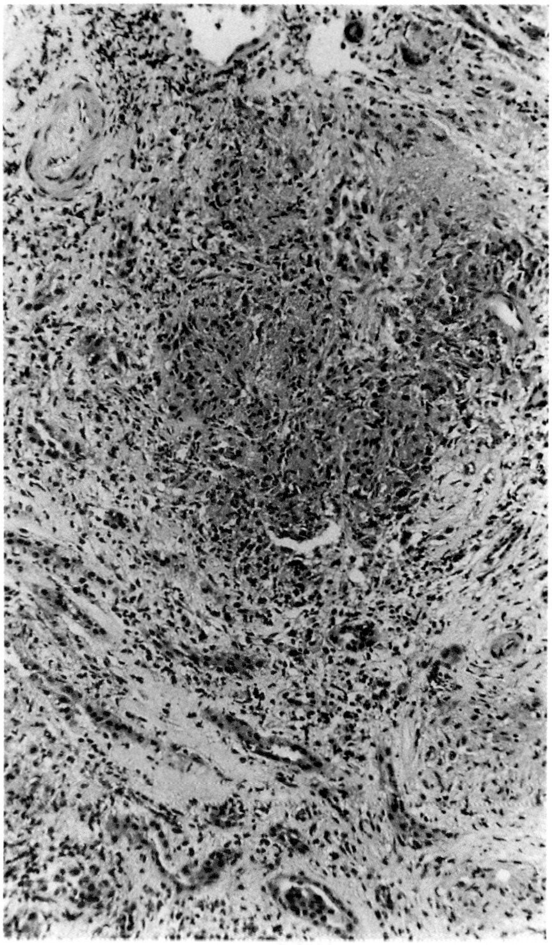

Fig. 9.9 Wegener's granulomatosis. Healed vasculitis involving interlobular artery (upper part of picture) with granulomatous reaction in adjacent interstitium. Haematoxylin-eosin × 100

Mesangial or endothelial proliferation or both are usually absent at this stage. There is extravasation of fibrin into Bowman's space and crescents are common. Occasionally there is disruption of Bowman's capsule with granulomatous inflammation. Vasculitis affecting small arteries and arterioles is only rarely seen in biopsy specimens (Fig. 9.9) although in one series it was found in about 25% of the specimens.[28] Interstitial inflammatory infiltrates tend to be mild; granulomas around glomeruli or vessels are sometimes present.

Later in the disease focal or diffuse mild mesangial hypercellularity is seen in about a third of the cases,[31] the number and size of crescents increases, and segmental sclerosis becomes common. In successfully treated cases many of the glomeruli show global and segmental scarring and crescents are fibrosed.

Electron microscopy

The findings on electron microscopy are similar to those encountered in microscopic polyarteritis (see p. 274).

Immunofluorescence/immunoperoxidase microscopy

In about a third of cases there is no staining for immunoglobulins or complement, but in the others tiny, sparse, focal and segmental deposits of C3 are present in the glomerular and vascular lesions, sometimes accompanied by equally small amounts of various immunoglobulins. Fibrinogen is common in the crescents.

Differential diagnosis

Focal segmental necrotizing glomerulonephritis is also found in microscopic polyarteritis (see p. 273), Henoch–Schönlein purpura (see p. 253), systemic lupus erythematosus (see p. 228), antiglomerular basement membrane disease (see p. 219) and bacterial endocarditis (see p. 376). As indicated when describing the differential diagnosis of microscopic polyarteritis (see p. 274), *Henoch–Schönlein purpura* and *antiglomerular basement membrane disease* each can be easily differentiated from Wegener's granulomatosis on immunofluorescence or immunoperoxidase microscopy by the predominance of IgA in the mesangium in Henoch–Schönlein purpura and the linear deposition of IgG in the glomerular capillary walls in antiglomerular basement membrane disease. *Systemic lupus erythematosus* usually shows much more obvious mesangial and subendothelial deposits of various combinations of immunoglobulin or complement and there are often tubuloreticular structures in the cytoplasm of the endothelial cells. *Bacterial endocarditis* is also associated with abundant deposits of immunoglobulin or complement. *Microscopic polyarteritis,* however, is usually indistinguishable on morphological grounds; the distinction has to be made on the clinical findings and on the specificity of the circulating autoantibodies to antigens in the cytoplasm of neutrophil granulocytes.[21] In Wegener's granulomatosis the antibodies produce on indirect immunofluorescence diffuse granules in the cytoplasm of the neutrophil; this contrasts with microscopic polyarteritis in which the antibodies produce diffuse staining in the perinuclear regions.[21]

Lymphomatoid granulomatosis[31a] is unlikely to be confused with Wegener's granulomatosis because the glomeruli remain normal, even though there are pulmonary lesions and the neoplastic cells may infiltrate the walls of renal vessels and simulate a vasculitis. *Kawasaki disease* too does not produce necrotizing glomerular lesions.

Complications

Diffuse crescentic glomerulonephritis is a common complication (see p. 185).

Renal transplantation

A significant proportion of treated patients in remission have end-stage renal failure because of damage done to their kidneys before treatment started. Renal transplantation in such patients can result in successful graft function for long periods.[27] In a few instances, however, the lesions of Wegener's granulomatosis either appear in the graft[32] or recur in the recipient's lower and upper respiratory tract. In the latter circumstance reintroduction of cyclophosphamide in the place of azathioprine or cyclosporin usually results in rapid remission without prejudicing the graft.[33]

Prognosis

The outlook for patients with Wegener's granulomatosis who have developed signs of renal disease, even if they are not in renal failure, is poor without treatment. The mean survival is 5 months and less than 10% survive 2 years.[27] With combined cyclophosphamide and steroid treatment almost all go into remission and in one series 75 out of 85 patients were alive after an average follow-up of 4 years.[27] The patients who do badly are those who are in renal failure when first seen.[28] After withdrawal of treatment, most patients remain in remission for long periods; late relapses usually respond to reinstitution of cyclophosphamide.

Pathogenesis

As with microscopic polyarteritis (see p. 275) the specific autoantibodies to neutrophil cytoplasmic antigens detected in the circulation may have a pathogenetic role. There is evidence that the antibodies cross react with determinants in the endothelial cells of the small blood vessels.[7] They also bind to antigens on the surfaces and in the cytoplasm of glomerular capillary endothelial cells and glomerular epithelial cells.[34] Some of the antineutrophil autoantibodies that stain cytoplasm are directed against proteinase 3 and some of the antineutrophil autoantibodies that give perinuclear staining react with myeloperoxidase.[35,36] It is possible that direct damage to such cells by the autoantibody may be important in the pathogenesis of the vasculitis and the focal segmental necrotizing glomerulonephritis.

Alternatively the antibodies may be taken up by neutrophil granulocytes and initiate a respiratory burst with release of proteases and oxygen-reactive species which induce glomerular and vascular injury.[35] Another suggestion is that the binding of antineutrophil cytoplasmic antibody to proteinase 3 does not inhibit its enzyme activity but prevents it being inactivated by its natural inhibitors. The uninhibited proteinase digests the elastic in the vessel walls leading to a necrotizing vasculitis.[37]

CHURG–STRAUSS SYNDROME

In 1951 Churg and Strauss[38] described a series of 13 patients with systemic vasculitis occurring in individuals with asthma, fever and eosinophilia. Six years later Rose and Spencer[39] divided a series of patients with systemic vasculitis into those with and without lung involvement; those with lung involvement represented essentially the same condition as the patients whose cases had been described earlier by Churg and Strauss. The condition has been infrequently reported but is probably not particularly rare.[40] The disease is commonly associated with diffuse infiltration of various tissues by eosinophils and sometimes by the formation of granulomas. The kidneys are frequently involved: granulomas and infiltration by eosinophils are often present but the commonest manifestation is a focal segmental necrotizing glomerulonephritis. The clinical effects of these renal lesions are often mild and renal failure is uncommon, in contrast to Wegener's granulomatosis and microscopic polyarteritis (see p. 278). Antineutrophil cytoplasmic antibodies are found in the serum of patients with active lesions. The disease responds well to steroids.

Clinical features

Individuals who develop this syndrome have often previously suffered for some years from allergic rhinitis and severe asthma. They have greatly increased numbers of eosinophils in their peripheral blood (usually higher than 1.5×10^9/l) and infiltration of various tissues by eosinophils occurs, producing a picture resembling Löffler's syndrome, chronic eosinophilic pneumonia or eosinophilic gastroenteritis. Pulmonary infiltrates are a central feature of Churg–Strauss syndrome, occuring in 72% of patients. After some years patients with Churg–Strauss syndrome develop signs and symptoms of systemic vasculitis which resemble those encountered in classical polyarteritis but severe renal disease is uncommon, renal failure being a cause of death in only 18% of patients. Cardiac involvement accounts for half the deaths. Hypertension is a common finding and may reflect the frequency of renal infarction in Churg–Strauss syndrome. The sex incidence is nearly equal and the mean age of onset of allergic rhinitis is 28 years, of asthma 35 years and of vasculitis 38 years.[40]

Tissue typing

No convincing association has been shown with any HLA tissue type.

Serology

Occasionally IgM-containing immune complexes are found in the circulation; usually they are absent. Complement levels are generally normal. Serum IgE levels are usually raised in the active vasculitic phase; this is not specific since elevated levels sometimes occur in Wegener's granulomatosis and in classical polyarteritis. Antibodies to antigens in the cytoplasm of neutrophil granulocytes are present in untreated Churg–Strauss syndrome.[41,42] At present it is not known whether these differ in immunoglobulin class or in specificity from those encountered in Wegener's granulomatosis (see p. 276) and microscopic polyarteritis (see p. 272).

Renal changes

The typical glomerular lesion is a focal segmental glomerulonephritis with necrotizing features.[43] Crescents are found in some cases. A necrotizing vasculitis involving mainly small vessels may also be present; occasionally this is granulomatous in type. Venous lesions have also been recorded. Interstitial disease is often present and may be characterized either by a diffuse infiltration by eosinophils (Fig. 9.10) or, infrequently, by necrotic granulomatous nodules. Each of the major histological features of Churg–Strauss syndrome may occur in isolation or they may coexist. Healed lesions predominate in cases with a long history. Infarcts are frequent.[38,40]

Differential diagnosis

The histological findings resemble those of both *Wegener's granulomatosis* and *microscopic polyarteritis*. If extensive infiltration of the interstitium by eosinophils is lacking then the three conditions may be indistinguishable on renal biopsy. However, in microscopic polyarteritis there is no lung involvment and Wegener's granulomatosis produces a more destructive process in the lungs, often with cavitation of pulmonary nodules. One further condition should also be mentioned: *sarcoidosis* is associated with interstitial granulomas and may be accompanied by peripheral eosinophilia and rarely vasculitis, but a focal segmental glomerulonephritis and diffuse infiltration of the interstitium by eosinophils are not found.

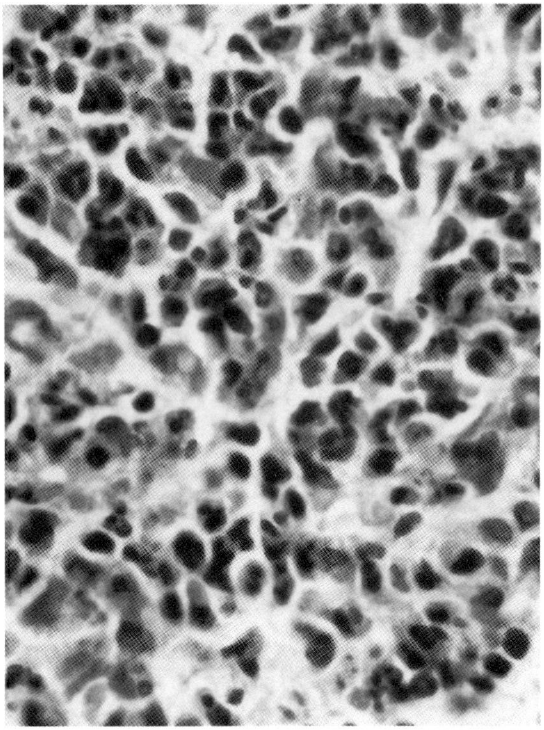

Fig. 9.10 Churg–Strauss' syndrome. The interstitium is densely infiltrated by eosinophils. Haematoxylin-eosin × 600

Prognosis

Without treatment very few patients survive, but the disease usually remits when high doses of prednisolone are given: in one series 62% of the treated patients were alive 5 years later and the median survival was 9 years.[44] Late relapse occurs in only a minority of cases. Although the histological findings in the kidneys resemble those of Wegener's granulomatosis, renal failure is uncommon in Churg–Strauss syndrome. The renal disease remits with steroids alone and even spontaneous remission has been observed. Hypertension is common and is often difficult to control.

Pathogenesis

Churg–Strauss syndrome seems to occur in a subset of atopic individuals whose allergy is atypical in that it commences later than usual, frequently in the absence of a family history, and is associated with severe upper respiratory disease and marked eosinophilia. It has been suggested that repeated antigenic stimulation in such individuals can trigger a self-perpetuating vasculitis and several instances have been recorded in which Churg–Strauss syndrome occurred during allergic hyposensitization treatment.[45] The role, if any, of the circulating antibodies to neutrophil cytoplasmic antigens that are present in these patients is not known.

GIANT CELL (TEMPORAL) ARTERITIS

Although giant cell arteritis characteristically affects the temporal arteries of the elderly, it is a systemic disease that may involve any large or medium sized artery. The kidneys are only rarely affected. In the few recorded cases the intrarenal arteries and arterioles have shown focal fibrinoid necrosis together with giant cells in the media.[46] The disease may produce terminal renal failure.

Occasionally, disseminated giant cell arteritis occurs in the absence of temporal artery involvement and may affect both glomeruli and renal arteries.[47]

TAKAYASU'S ARTERITIS

Takayasu's arteritis is an inflammatory and obliterative disease of the large and medium sized arteries.[48] It particularly affects the aorta and the origins of its main branches and, to a lesser extent, the pulmonary artery. The disease is most frequent in young women and the majority of the reports of this condition have come from Japan, Korea, China, South East Asia, India and Mexico. The disorder is not commonly recognized in Britain and the USA. However, the incidence of the disease in Olmsted, Minnesota, was 2.6 per million of the population per year in the period 1971–82 which is the same as that of Wegener's granulomatosis. Initially, there is a mononuclear cell infiltrate surrounding the vasa vasorum in the adventitia. Later, monocytes and neutrophil granulocytes invade the media and often giant cell granulomas form. There is disruption of the internal elastic lamina and aneurysms form. Slowly the intima, media and adventitia become thickened and fibrotic, narrowing the lumen of the vessel. Finally, the narrowed aortic branches become totally occluded by thrombus.

Clinically there are often general signs and symptoms such as arthralgia, fever and weight loss, and specific signs and symptoms of vascular stenosis such as arm claudication. There is weakening of the pulse in the upper part of the body, often accompanied by hypertension in the lower extremities. All patients have either multiple vascular bruits or absent pulses. Angiograms show that many arteries are involved. The erythrocyte sedimentation rate is greatly raised.

The kidneys are commonly affected. This is usually the result of renal artery stenosis and renovascular hypertension; infrequently there is a glomerulonephritis.

Renal artery stenosis and renovascular hypertension

The renal artery is often involved near its origin from the aorta. This leads to gradual narrowing of the lumen of the vessel and in the kidneys to progressive tubular atrophy, interstitial fibrosis and ultimately ischaemic collapse and sclerosis of the glomeruli (see p. 298).[49] It also often triggers hypertension and this produces additional renal damage (see p. 307). Uncontrolled hypertension can lead to death from cerebrovascular accident, cardiac failure and renal failure.[50] Renal autotransplantation has been successfully used to treat the hypertension.[51]

Glomerulonephritis

Glomerulonephritis is extremely rare in Takayasu's arteritis. Clinically there is usually microscopic haematuria and proteinuria. Focal segmental mesangial proliferative glomerulonephritis is the commonest pattern, usually with mesangial and sometimes also capillary wall deposits of IgG, IgM, IgA and C3. Serum complement levels are usually low. In the few cases reported the glomerulonephritis has been slowly progressive.[52]

HAEMOLYTIC URAEMIC SYNDROME

The haemolytic uraemic syndrome comprises microangiopathic haemolytic anaemia, a decrease in the number of circulating platelets and acute renal failure.[53] It is encountered most commonly in infants and young children as a sporadic, endemic or epidemic condition that often follows a gastrointestinal or respiratory tract infection. In this age group it is the most common cause of acquired acute renal failure in developed countries.[54] In adults the disease is sporadic and an infectious prodromal illness is less frequent. The haemolytic uraemic syndrome may also complicate pregnancy (see p. 565), the postpartum period (see p. 565) and the use of oestrogen preparations, including oral contraceptives. Occasionally it occurs after treatment with immunosuppressive and cytotoxic drugs. These include cyclosporin (see p. 670), mitomycin,[55] 5-fluorouracil and deoxycoformycin.[56] The syndrome is encountered as a secondary phenomenon in several other conditions, in particular malignant hypertension (see p. 310), thrombotic thrombocytopenic purpura (see p. 288), Addison's disease,[57] membranous glomerulonephritis (see p. 191), systemic sclerosis (see p. 242), acute irradiation nephritis (see p. 477), polyarteritis (see p. 267), renal allograft rejection (see p. 645) and bone marrow transplantation.[58] Some cases are familial (see p. 116).

Morphologically the syndrome is characterized by insudation of fibrin and red cells into the walls of the interlobular arteries, arterioles and glomerular capillaries. This may be accompanied by thrombosis and focal or confluent cortical necrosis. The damage to the vascular walls is followed by marked mucoid intimal thickening in the arteries and arterioles and subendothelial and mesangial accumulation of electron-lucent material in the glomeruli. The vasculature of organs other than the kidney may be involved as well but this occurs rarely.

The prognosis for the endemic or epidemic forms in childhood is moderately good with approximately 4.5–9% developing end-stage renal disease and 2.5–10% dying during the first admission.[59] In contrast, the outlook for adults is poor, the mortality rate ranging from 18 to 62%.[60]

Primary haemolytic uraemic syndrome in children is sometimes associated with infection by one of several strains of *Escherichia coli* that produce potent protein exotoxins.[61] The term verocytotoxin or verotoxin is used to denote this family of toxins because they kill a cultured cell line from monkey kidney called Vero. It is thought that the verotoxin causes endothelial damage and that this leads to release of unusually large von Willebrand factor multimers which induce platelet aggregation and thrombocytopenia.[62,63]

Clinical features

There are several clinical subgroups of the haemolytic uraemic syndrome.[64]

Childhood form of the haemolytic uraemic syndrome

This occurs mainly in infants under 2 years old, but may be seen at any time in childhood. The sexes are affected equally. It is commonest in the late summer and autumn and is preceded by an acute non-febrile gastroenteritis, often with vomiting and bloody diarrhoea. After about 5–7 days the patient becomes weak, lethargic and pale. At this stage a microangiopathic haemolytic anaemia can be detected with fragmented red cells, thrombocytopenia and a leucocytosis; there may also be purpura and hepatosplenomegaly. The onset of nephropathy is usually abrupt, with oliguria, proteinuria and microscopic haematuria. Hypertension is a feature in half the patients and anuria in 30%. A few patients develop gross haematuria or the nephrotic syndrome. Occasional patients have neurological involvement and may present with convulsions, transient hemiparesis or even coma.[65]

In Britain and North America the childhood form is the commonest subgroup of haemolytic uraemic syndrome; it occurs in about a third of the patients, usually as isolated cases or in small outbreaks. In Central America, South Africa and Bangladesh, where the incidence is higher, the childhood form of haemolytic uraemic syndrome appears to be endemic with occasional small and large epidemics.[66] The isolated cases or small outbreaks are often associated with infection by a verotoxin-producing strain of *E. coli*; in one series this organism was demonstrated in 75% of the patients.[61] Some of the epidemics are associated with salmonella infection or with shigella dysentery.[66,67] Childhood haemolytic uraemic syndrome has also been linked, usually inconsistently, to a number of other organisms.

Hereditary forms of the haemolytic uraemic syndrome

Haemolytic uraemic syndrome is familial in approximately 3% of patients. Both autosomal recessive and dominant forms are recognized. They usually develop insidiously in older children or adults with no seasonal variation in incidence and with no prodromal illness. Some forms are recurrent and hypertension is often severe. Familial haemolytic uraemic syndrome is discussed on page 116.

Adult form of the haemolytic uraemic syndrome

Adult haemolytic uraemic syndrome is commonest in women, particularly during the first few weeks or months after childbirth (see p. 565).[68] It may be preceded by a typical prodromal illness but more commonly develops abruptly with vaginal bleeding, purpura, oliguria and hypertension. The haemolytic uraemic syndrome may also develop during pregnancy or in women taking oral contraceptives, usually following an increase in oestrogen dosage (see p. 524). Occasional cases of the haemolytic uraemic syndrome occur in either sex with neither of these precipitating factors and often with no infectious prodromal illness.[69] Hypertension is especially common in adult haemolytic uraemic syndrome.

Haemolytic uraemic syndrome associated with systemic illnesses and other precipitating factors

The occasional occurrence of haemolytic uraemic syndrome in various systemic diseases and after treatment with immunosuppressive and cytotoxic drugs has already been mentioned.

Serology

Depending on the degree of haemolysis there will be an increase in unconjugated bilirubin and plasma lactic dehydrogenase and a decrease in haptoglobin levels. In some patients anti-endothelial cell antibodies are present.[70] Significant serological responses to verotoxin-producing *E. coli* and a rise in the levels of specific verotoxin-neutralizing antibody may occur. The plasma levels of von Willebrand factor are raised, reflecting endothelial injury.

Peripheral blood

The microangiopathic haemolytic anaemia is accompanied by the presence of fragmented and deformed red cells in the circulating blood. If there is sufficient haemolysis there will be an increase in reticulocytes. Thrombocytopenia (less than 100×10^9 platelets/l) occurs at some stage in the illness and lasts 7–14 days. Platelet survival is shortened, there is evidence of intravascular platelet activation and fibrin is formed in the microcirculation. The early complement components C3 and C4 may be reduced.

Renal changes

Gross appearance of the kidneys

The kidneys are usually a little enlarged in those cases in which death occurs in the acute phase of the illness. There may be many light yellow foci of necrosis in the cortex, which is pale and sometimes speckled with minute haemorrhages.

Light microscopy[71–74]

Glomerular changes The glomeruli typically show segmental or global thickening and the capillary walls have a double contour (Fig. 9.11). Thrombi are often found in the capillary lumens but are very variable in frequency and distribution (Fig. 9.12). Scattered crescents occur and sometimes there is irregular expansion of the mesangium and swelling of the capillary endothelial cells. The mesangium sometimes has a foamy appearance and the amount of mesangial matrix increases as the disease evolves. Superimposed on these changes are variable amounts of wrinkling, thickening and collapse of the capillary basement membrane as vascular narrowing progresses. Proliferation of mesangial cells is not a feature.

Vascular changes Focal damage occurs in the interlobular arteries and arterioles. The degree of

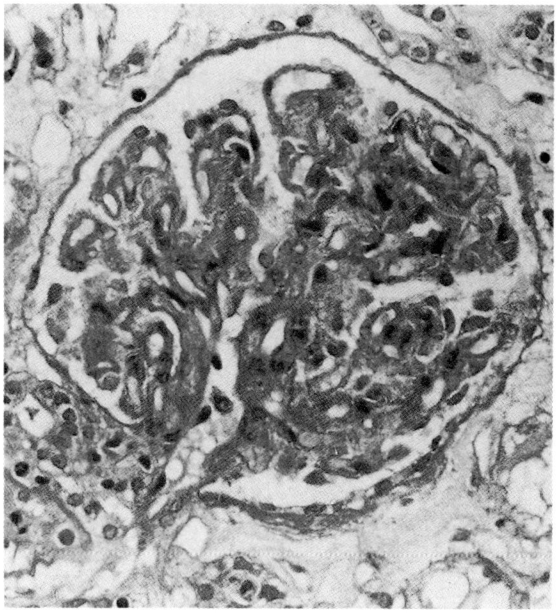

Fig. 9.11 Haemolytic uraemic syndrome. Glomerulus showing widespread thickening and reduplication of the capillary walls.
Periodic acid-Schiff × 375

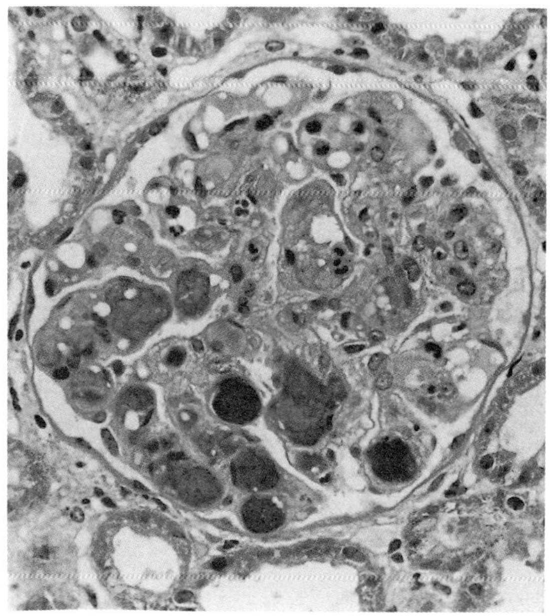

Fig. 9.12 Haemolytic uraemic syndrome. Glomerulus with thrombi in capillary lumens.
Martius scarlet blue x 375

involvement of these vessels is usually minimal in young children with haemolytic uraemic syndrome; it is most marked in adults. Insudation of fibrin and red cells occurs into the intima or throughout the vascular walls, often accompanied by thrombosis (Fig. 9.13). There may be sufficient damage to cause arteriolar microaneurysms (Fig. 9.14) and the occlusive vascular changes

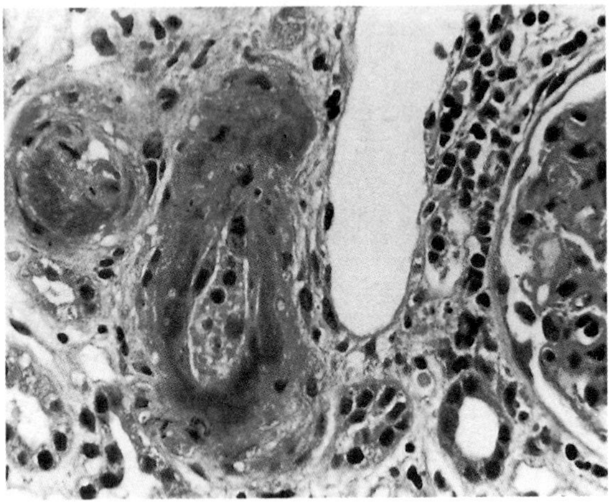

Fig. 9.13 Haemolytic uraemic syndrome. Arterioles showing insudation of fibrin and red cells into the intima.
Haematoxylin-eosin × 625

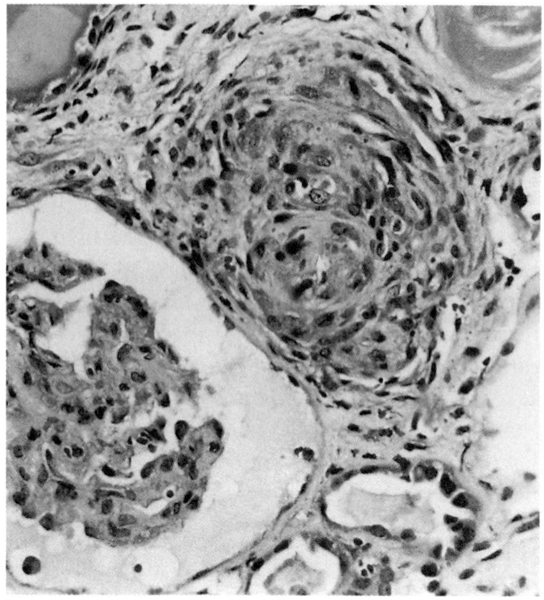

Fig. 9.15 Haemolytic uraemic syndrome. Endothelial proliferation in an afferent arteriole has produced a glomerulus-like structure.
Haematoxylin-eosin × 450

may result in either focal or extensive cortical necrosis. More commonly the vascular lesions are associated with tubular damage and oedema and

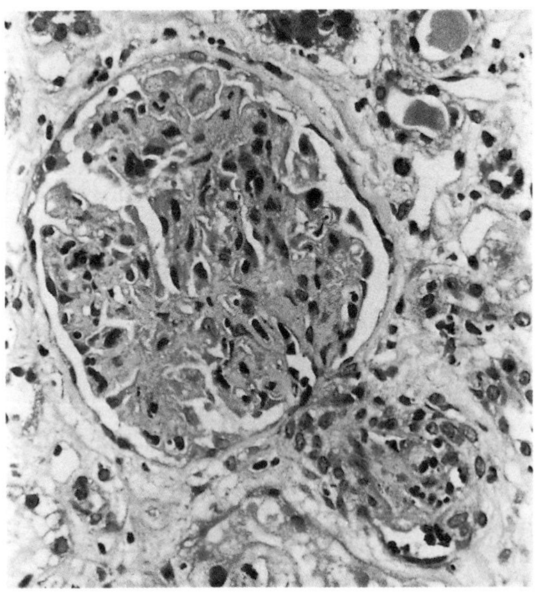

Fig. 9.14 Haemolytic uraemic syndrome. The afferent arteriole is aneurysmal.
Haematoxylin-eosin × 450

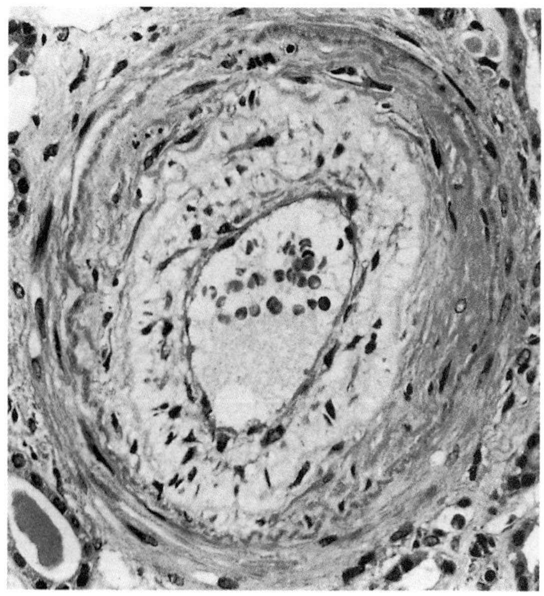

Fig. 9.16 Haemolytic uraemic syndrome. An interlobular artery is narrowed by mucoid intimal thickening.
Haematoxylin-eosin × 130

mononuclear cell infiltration of the interstitium. Endothelial proliferation in afferent arterioles may produce glomerulus-like structures (Fig. 9.15, see p. 289).

As the disease advances basophilic mucosal intimal thickening occurs in the affected vessels leading to progressive narrowing of their lumens (Fig. 9.16). Some of the cells in the intima may have foamy cytoplasm due to fat accumulation. Later the intimal thickening becomes fibrous and there may be reduplication or multiplication of the internal elastic lamina.

Electron microscopy[71,75]

Glomeruli In the glomeruli electron-lucent material accumulates in variable amounts between the lamina rara interna and the endothelium; large collections cause marked narrowing of the capillary lumen (Fig. 9.17). Within the subendothelial layer there are small irregular collections of finely particulate electron-dense material, scattered fibrils and sometimes red cells, fragments of fibrin and scattered cellular elements (Fig. 9.18). The electron-lucent deposit is separated from the endothelial cells by an irregular layer of basement membrane-like material which is possibly endothelial in origin. This layer, together with the original basement membrane, gives rise to the double contour seen by light microscopy. The mesangium is expanded by similar electron-lucent material. In some cases the mesangial structure

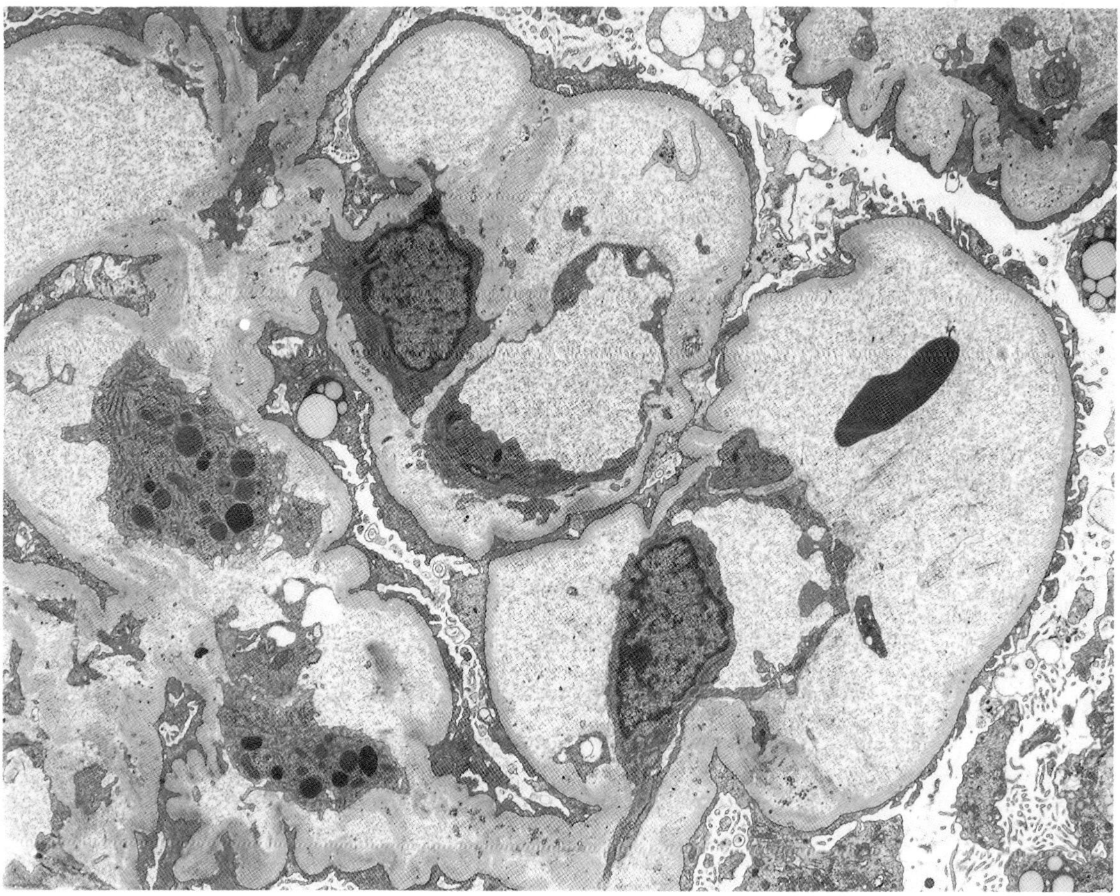

Fig. 9.17 Haemolytic uraemic syndrome. Electron micrograph of a glomerular capillary showing marked accumulation of predominantly electron-lucent material in the subendothelial space, with narrowing of the capillary lumen. × 8200

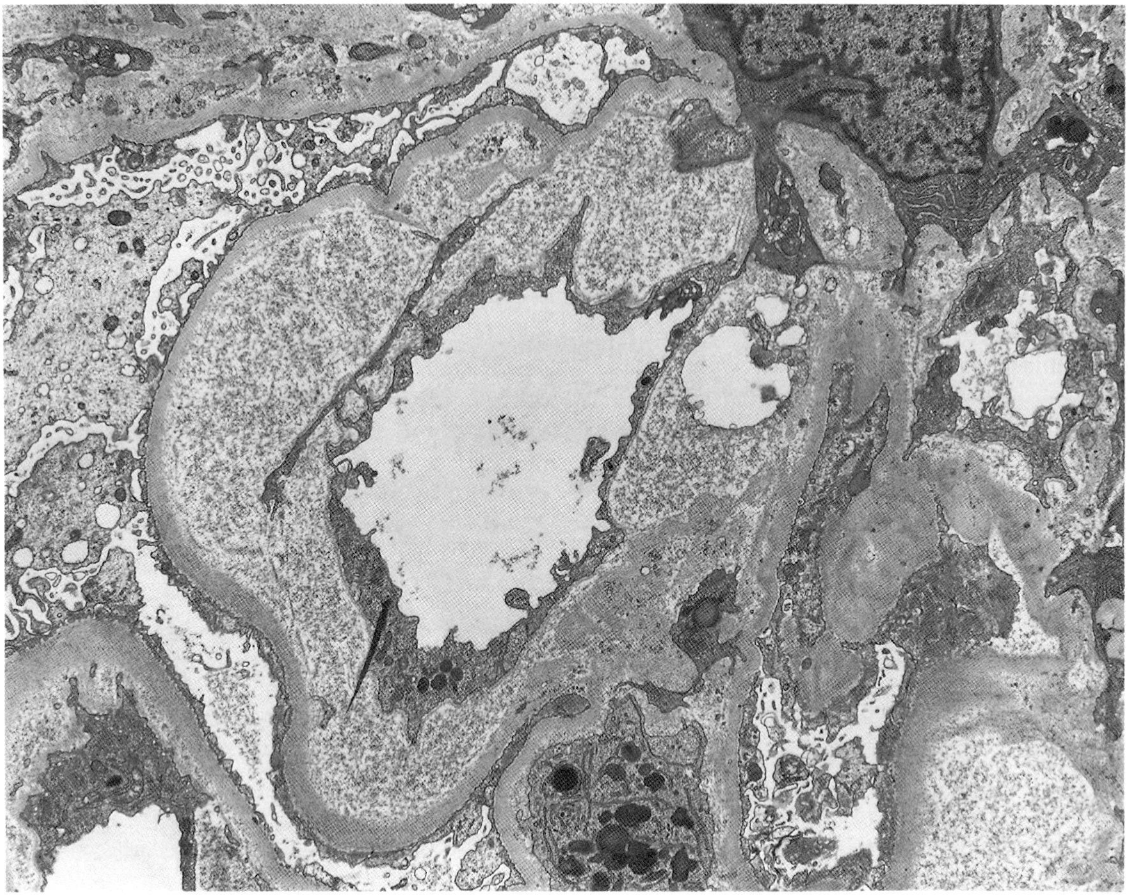

Fig. 9.18 Haemolytic uraemic syndrome. Electron micrograph of part of a glomerular capillary loop showing finely particulate electron-dense granules and fibrils in the predominantly electron-lucent subendothelial layer.
× 8200

appears completely disrupted – a condition described as mesangiolysis.[76] Later in the disease new basement membrane material is deposited in the subendothelial deposit causing massive irregular thickening of the basement membrane. The endothelial cells are swollen and often detached from the underlying glomerular capillary basement membrane; the mesangial cells are hypertrophied. In thrombosed capillaries the endothelial lining is focally denuded and the basement membrane thinned and occasionally ruptured. The epithelial cells are hypertrophic with extensive obliteration of foot processes.

Arterioles and small arteries The affected arterioles and interlobular arteries show endothelial swelling, expansion of the intima by electron-lucent material and disruption of the muscle by plasma and red cells. There is often mural or occluding thrombus.

Immunofluorescence/immunoperoxidase microscopy

Deposits of IgM, C3 and fibrin are often found in the walls of the arterioles and arteries. Similar deposits also occur in an irregular form in the glomerular mesangium and along the capillary walls.[77,78]

Changes in other organs

Occasionally small thrombi are found in vessels in

other organs. Small infarcts have been described in the liver and brain.[71]

Differential diagnosis

The differentiation of haemolytic uraemic syndrome from *thrombotic thrombocytopenic purpura* (see p. 289) is sometimes difficult because of overlapping clinical and pathological features. Indeed some observers consider the two conditions to be the same. In thrombotic thrombocytopenic purpura, however, thrombi are found in many organs, whereas in haemolytic uraemic sydrome the thrombi are usually limited to the kidney.

The differentiation of the lesions in haemolytic uraemic syndrome in adults from those caused by *malignant hypertension* (see p. 311) may be impossible. Distinguishing between haemolytic uraemic syndrome and *progressive systemic sclerosis* (see p. 243) may be very difficult, but the presence of widespread subendothelial electron-lucent deposits in the glomeruli favours haemolytic uraemic syndrome and review of the clinical data may decide the issue. Extensive arteriolar damage sometimes suggests *polyarteritis* (see p. 273) but the glomerular lesions of haemolytic uraemic syndrome, which are not present in polyarteritis, will usually distinguish the two conditions. The changes in the glomerular capillary wall in haemolytic uraemic syndrome may occasionally suggest *mesangiocapillary glomerulonephritis* but the absence of mesangial cell proliferation and mesangial interposition and the presence of arteriolar lesions should prevent confusion. The renal findings may resemble those seen in *disseminated intravascular coagulation* (see p. 291) but coagulation tests and estimation of the fibrinogen level in the peripheral blood will usually show only minimal changes in haemolytic uraemic syndrome whereas in disseminated intravascular coagulation there is a generalized activation of the clotting system.

Complications

The most serious renal complication is widespread *cortical necrosis*. Involvement of the colon may lead to pseudomembranous colitis, rectal prolapse or perforation of the gut with the production of peritonitis.[79,80]

Renal transplantation

Haemolytic uraemic syndrome is an uncommon cause of end-stage renal failure in children and in adults. When it occurs renal transplantation is frequently the treatment of choice but a problem is that the graft is quite likely to develop the lesions of haemolytic uraemic syndrome (see p. 669). In two recent series 50%[81] and 25%[82] of renal allografts were affected by haemolytic uraemic syndrome commencing 1 day to 15 months after transplantation, but mostly within 2 months. It is difficult to establish whether these lesions are the result of the original disease affecting the graft (so called recurrence) or whether the syndrome has been induced by severe acute rejection, malignant hypertension or the administration of cyclosporin. However, haemolytic uraemic syndrome rarely occurs in renal allograft patients other than those whose original disease was haemolytic uraemic syndrome. The figures appear to show that recurrence of the disease is only frequent in patients who have received a kidney from a living related donor but the small size of the patient groups does not allow any firm statement.[83]

Prognosis

In young children the use of blood transfusion, dialysis, control of hypertension and treatment of electrolyte and water imbalance have reduced the immediate mortality rate to between 2.5 and 10%.[59,83] Relapses are infrequent but not all children who survive the acute illness do well. In Argentina, where more patients per year are seen than in the rest of the world, approximately 18% develop a progressive deterioration of renal function.[65] In the USA and Western Europe 4.5–9% go on to end-stage renal failure;[59,83] additional cases develop hypertension and other late sequelae, leaving approximately 66% who make a complete recovery.[83]

In older children and young adults, however, haemolytic uraemic syndrome frequently still is a fatal disease; the recovery rate ranges from 18 to 62%[60] and is often higher when the syndrome is associated with mitomycin therapy[55] or is secondary to systemic disease. The prognosis usually depends on the degree of arterial involvement[73] and the severity of any underlying systemic disease.

A variety of specific treatments, such as fibrinolytic and antiplatelet agents, and non-specific manoeuvres, such as plasma infusion and plasma exchange, have been tried in haemolytic uraemic syndrome. None has yet been shown unequivocally to improve results.

Pathogenesis

Haemolytic uraemic syndrome probably has many causes, most of which initially act by injuring vascular endothelial cells. This damage either exposes thrombogenic subendothelial surfaces or effects the release from the Weibel–Palade bodies in the endothelium (see p. 5) of large von Willebrand factor multimers which induce or potentiate platelet aggregation.[84] In a small number of cases of haemolytic uraemic syndrome there is probably a primary inherited defect in one or more of the mechanisms that determine the non-thrombogenic properties of the vessel wall.

Infection with endotoxin-producing bacteria such as shigella and salmonella or exotoxin-producing strains of *Escherichia coli* have been proposed as a cause. The association between childhood haemolytic uraemic syndrome and infection by verotoxin-producing *E. coli* is now well recognized.[61] Evidence for outbreaks of such infection, mostly due to the most commonly reported serotype 0157-H7, indicates that the infection typically manifests itself as a diarrhoeal illness which is occasionally complicated by haemorrhagic colitis or haemolytic uraemic syndrome. In one outbreak in children about 7% of those with diarrhoea developed haemolytic uraemic syndrome;[85] in another outbreak, this time in adults, 22% with diarrhoea developed haemolytic uraemic syndrome.[86] The major source of *E. coli* 0157-H7 infection seems to be undercooked meat and unpasteurized milk. There is also some evidence that infection can be acquired through person-to-person transmission. The predisposing factors that determine susceptibility to verotoxin-producing *E. coli* infection and the risk factors for the development of haemolytic uraemic syndrome remain to be established. Susceptibility to infection may be related to the absence of specific immunity. Verotoxin-producing *E. coli* are best recovered in stool specimens obtained within 6 days of the onset of diarrhoea. Later, serology may help; a rise in specific verotoxin-neutralizing antibody levels occurs in about 60% of patients.

In other patients complement-fixing IgG and IgM antibodies that lyse endothelial cells have been found, suggesting that in those cases there may be an autoimmune pathogenesis for the haemolytic uraemic syndrome.[70] The antibodies are directed against an unknown antigen on the surface of the endothelial cell; the antigen is lost after treatment of the cell with gamma interferon which alters the structure or accessibility of the surface molecules.

Cyclosporin A and mitomycin, drugs that are associated with haemolytic uraemic syndrome, can directly cause endothelial damage.[87,88]

The endothelium of about 27% of childhood and some adult cases of haemolytic uraemic syndrome synthesizes diminished amounts of prostacyclin ($PG1_2$), a substance which inhibits activated platelets from adhering to endothelial cells.[89] Possible explanations for this phenomenon include lack of a normal factor required for $PG1_2$ synthesis, the presence of inhibitors and excessively rapid degradation. The presence of the same abnormality in relatives of some patients suggests that within certain families there may be an inherited defect that predisposes them to the development of haemolytic uraemic syndrome, triggered by different events.[90]

Why the vascular changes occur predominantly in the kidneys is unexplained. The anaemia of the haemolytic uraemic syndrome is almost certainly the result of structural damage to the red cells as they are forced past fibrin strands in the affected vessels.

THROMBOTIC THROMBOCYTOPENIC PURPURA

Thrombotic thrombocytopenic purpura is a rare disease first described in 1924 by Moschcowitz[91] in which there is sudden onset of fever, thrombocytopenia and microangiopathic haemolytic anaemia. Fluctuating signs of neurological disturbance are present in most cases. There is usually no history of a preceding acute infection and the disease does not occur in outbreaks.[92] Thrombotic thrombocytopenic purpura may occur at any age and in either sex but most of the patients are women in their thirties. Almost all patients have purpura or retinal, gastrointestinal or genitourinary bleeding. Renal disease occurs in 88% of the patients and is characterized by episodes of proteinuria, microscopic haematuria and impairment of renal function.[93]

There are many similarities between thrombotic thrombocytopenic purpura and haemolytic uraemic syndrome and some observers regard these conditions as variable expressions of a single disease.[94] The chief differences are that in thrombotic thrombocytopenic purpura the lesions are usually widespread throughout the body and there is less severe involvement of the kidneys. Acute anuria or oliguria is uncommon in thrombotic thrombocytopenic purpura.

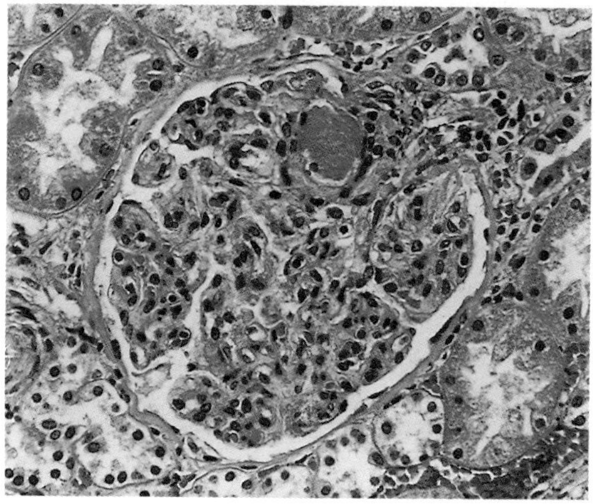

Fig. 9.19 Thrombotic thrombocytopenic purpura. Glomerulus showing thrombus in afferent arteriole as it enters glomerulus.
Haematoxylin-eosin × 225
Reproduced by permission from: Heptinstall RH. Pathology of the kidney, vol. 2, 3rd edn. Boston: Little, Brown 1983; 2: 935 (Fig. 18.20)

Renal changes

Light microscopy

Eosinophilic granular thrombi are conspicuous in the afferent arterioles, particularly at their junction with the glomerular tufts (Fig. 9.19). Thrombi are also found, but less frequently, in the interlobular arteries. Microaneurysms often develop from the dilated arterioles.[95] Endothelial proliferation in afferent arterioles may be florid, producing glomerulus-like structures (Fig. 9.20);[96] these are not specific for thrombotic thrombocytopenic purpura and may be found in haemolytic uraemic syndrome (Fig. 9.15) and in any patient with disseminated intravascular coagulation from any cause. Mucoid intimal thickening in the interlobular arteries is uncommon. Microthrombi are present in the glomerular tufts but subendothelial changes in the glomerular capillaries are only occasionally seen and are seldom extensive.

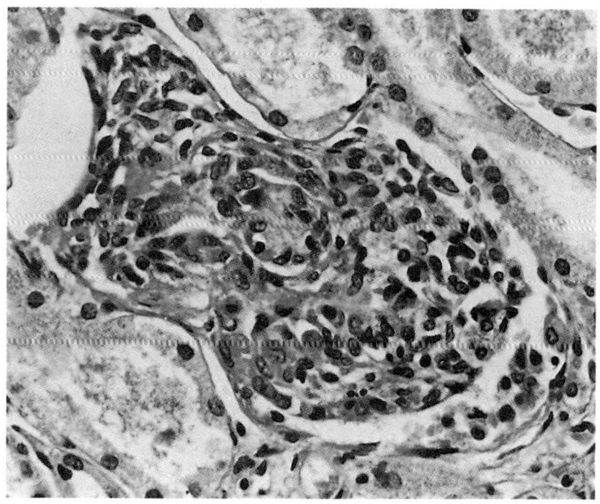

Fig. 9.20 Thrombotic thrombocytopenic purpura. Endothelial proliferation in afferent arteriole has produced a glomerulus-like structure.
Haematoxylin-eosin × 315
Reproduced by permission from: Heptinstall RH. Pathology of the kidney, vol 2, 3rd edn. Boston: Little, Brown 1983: 935 (Fig. 18.21)

Electron microscopy

The appearances do not differ from those seen in haemolytic uraemic syndrome (see p. 285). The arteriolar thrombi are composed predominantly of platelets.

Immunofluorescence/immunoperoxidase microscopy

In most studies there has been no localization of

immunoglobulins or complement in the arteriolar or capillary walls.

Changes in other organs

The most important distinction between the haemolytic uraemic syndrome and thrombotic thrombocytopenic purpura is in the distribution of the vascular lesions. In the former they are usually confined to the kidneys; in the latter they occur throughout the body, small microthrombi being particularly frequent in arterioles and capillaries in the brain, mycocardium, adrenals, pancreas and spleen.[92] Because of this wide distribution gingival and skin biopsies have been used to try to confirm the clinical diagnosis, but there is a high false-negative rate.

Differential diagnosis

The differential diagnosis of thrombotic thrombocytopenic purpura is the same as that for haemolytic uraemic syndrome (see p. 287).

Renal transplantation

Successful renal transplants have been performed in patients with thrombotic thrombocytopenic purpura but the numbers are small. A few grafts later developed thrombotic lesions.

Prognosis

For many years thrombotic thrombocytopenic purpura was regarded as a fulminant, almost invariably fatal disease. Since then increasing numbers of therapeutic successes have been reported. It is difficult to estimate the current rate of remission because of the lack of a central registry and the tendency to report favourable outcomes rather than other cases. However, approximately 88% of patients rapidly respond to intensive plasmapheresis and replacement with fresh frozen plasma; some patients relapse when therapy is discontinued and the infusions may have to be continued for periods of up to 2 years.[97]

Pathogenesis

The pathogenesis of thrombotic thrombocytopenic purpura remains unknown. Present evidence mainly supports the probability of a plasma abnormality causing platelet hyperaggregability and the initiation of thrombus formation.[97]

It has been shown that plasma from patients with thrombotic thrombocytopenic purpura lacks a factor which normally stimulates prostacyclin ($PG1_2$).[94] The factor, a stable substance with a molecular weight of 300–400 Da, protects the $PG1_2$-forming system from inactivation during chronic endothelial damage. Deficiency of this factor could explain the rapid beneficial effect of infusions of fresh plasma in many patients with thrombotic thrombocytopenic purpura. The discovery that normal serum binding of prostacyclin is reduced in patients with thrombotic thrombocytopenic purpura[98] further supports the concept of a reduction in the availability of $PG1_2$ at sites of vascular injury in this disease.

The plasma from patients with thrombotic thrombocytopenic purpura has also been found to contain a factor that aggregates both their own and normal platelets; the activity of this factor is inhibited by normal adult plasma or IgG concentrate.[99] There is some evidence that the inhibiting factor in adult plasma is an IgG antibody and that the aggregating factor may be some infectious agent.[100]

Unusually large multimers of von Willebrand factor, which could bind to and aggregate platelets, have been found in the plasma of some patients with thrombotic thrombocytopenic purpura and it has been suggested that in these cases the basic defect might be a primary abnormality of factor VIII synthesis.[101]

Immune complexes of the IgG subclass also bind to platelets and have been implicated in thrombotic thrombocytopenic purpura, especially when it has been associated with malignancy.[102]

DISSEMINATED INTRAVASCULAR COAGULATION

Disseminated intravascular coagulation occurs as a complication of a wide variety of conditions.[103] Common examples are retroplacental haemorrhage, amniotic fluid embolism, shock, septicaemia and liver failure. It is characterized by activation of the clotting cascade sequence that leads to fibrin deposition throughout the microcirculation. If this is sufficiently extensive there is depletion of the coagulation factors and platelets required for haemostasis (consumption coagulopathy). The fibrin formation also activates the fibrinolytic mechanism. The simultaneous activation of both clotting and fibrinolytic systems may give rise either to widespread tissue hypoxia and micro-infarcts caused by multiple microthrombi or to generalized haemorrhage, which varies from petechiae to copious bleeding into the gut or urinary tract. The widespread fibrin deposition also causes a microangiopathic haemolytic anaemia as the red cells become damaged while passing through the meshwork of fibrin strands. Acute renal failure is a common complication.

Renal changes

Fibrin microthrombi are found in the arterioles and in the glomerular capillaries in approximately 70% of patients.[104] There may also be glomeruloid changes in the arterioles (see p. 289) and expansion of the mesangium. In some cases the resultant ischaemia leads to cortical microinfarcts; rarely, it may even produce bilateral cortical necrosis (see p. 303).

Differential diagnosis

The renal findings may closely resemble those seen in *thrombotic thrombocytopenic purpura* but a coagulation screen and the fibrinogen level will usually show only minimal changes in thrombotic thrombocytopenic purpura, distinguishing the latter from disseminated intravascular coagulation. Also there is usually an obvious underlying disorder in patients with disseminated intravascular coagulation; this is exceptional in cases of thrombotic thrombocytopenic purpura. The striking subendothelial changes in the glomerular capillaries that are such a feature of the *haemolytic uraemic syndrome* are rarely seen in disseminated intravascular coagulation.

Prognosis

The prognosis is very variable, depending upon the underlying disorder as well as on the degree of renal ischaemic damage. If the provoking condition can be reversed and the disseminated intravascular coagulation halted, then even extensive fibrin thrombi in the glomerular capillaries can resolve within 7 days, with the return of good renal function. This has been dramatically shown in cases in which a kidney from a patient who has died with disseminated intravascular coagulation is transplanted.[105]

LOIN PAIN HAEMATURIA SYNDROME

The loin pain haematuria syndrome is a rare condition characterized by repeated episodes of severe flank pain accompanied by haematuria; it occurs predominantly, but not exclusively, in young women.[106] Renal function and blood pressure are normal, the urine is sterile and cystoscopy and intravenous urography reveal no abnormality. The pain may be unilateral or bilateral and the haematuria may be gross or microscopic. Flank tenderness is usually present and fever may occur. Arteriograms characteristically, but not invariably, demonstrate focal or generalized vascular lesions on the side or sides on which pain occurs; sometimes there are associated cortical infarcts.[107]

Renal changes

Light microscopy

There is focal eccentric thickening of the intima in the segmental, interlobar, arcuate and interlobular arteries. The widened intima is composed of fibrous tissue, smooth muscle cells and occasional small collections of fat. In the larger arteries the internal elastic lamina is intact but in a few of the interlobular arteries the intimal thickening is accompanied by rupture and reduplication of the internal elastic lamina and thinning of the media.[108] Parenchymal abnormalities vary from foci of subcapsular tubular atrophy and fibrosis to multiple areas of organized infarction. Arteries at the apex of the infarcts show evidence of previous occlusion and recanalization. These patchy vascular abnormalities, which correspond to those seen using radiological techniques, are often absent from the small samples obtained by needle biopsy.

Immunofluorescence/immunoperoxidase microscopy

In many cases there are uniform dense granular deposits of C3 in the walls of arterioles and interlobular arteries.[109]

Differential diagnosis

Flank pain and haematuria may occur in many other disorders such as *renal calculi* (see p. 532), *idiopathic hypercalciuria* (see p. 533), *IgA nephropathy* (see p. 158), *renal angiomyolipomas* (see p. 603), *renal vein thrombosis* (see p. 293) and *renal vein entrapment syndrome* (see below). All must be excluded before a diagnosis of loin pain haematuria syndrome can be entertained.

The changes in the renal arteries in loin pain haematuria syndrome are indistinguishable from those seen in *atherosclerosis* (arteriosclerosis); it is their presence in normotensive young women that is distinctive.

Renal transplantation

The pain may be so severe and incapacitating that opioid dependency becomes a hazard. Because of this, splanchnic nerve blockade, renal denervation or renal autotransplantation to the iliac fossa are sometimes used. Autotransplantation is followed by dramatic relief of pain, but this may be temporary.[110] In one case severe pain occurred at the site of the graft 1 year after transplantation, probably due to regeneration of the nerves that supply the kidney. It is known that axon-bearing nerves reach the interlobular arteries by 8 months after renal transplantation.[111]

Prognosis

The syndrome rarely, if ever, progresses to renal failure; it is the severe and disabling loin pain that is the problem.[112] After unilateral renal autotransplantation pain may recur in the other flank in relation to the previously unaffected kidney.[110]

Pathogenesis

The cause of the arterial lesions and the pathogenesis of the syndrome are unknown. It has been suggested that the syndrome may be initiated by platelet activation and fibrin deposition leading to microscopic intrarenal coagulation.[107] This hypothesis is supported by the finding that the heparin–thrombin clotting time is reduced,[107] there is increased availability of platelet factor 3 (PF3),[112] platelet life span is shortened,[112] plasma serotonin levels are raised[113] and high levels of fibrinopeptide A (a cleavage product of fibrin) are found in the venous effluent of the involved kidney.[114] Inability of the patient's serum to support normal prostacyclin (PGI_2) production by cultured endothelial cells has also been described and could represent a primary defect in the renal vascular endothelial cells.[114] In one patient an isolated deficiency of Hageman factor (factor XII) was found,[115] a condition known to predispose to thromboembolic disease. There appears to be a group of patients in whom the syndrome is caused or aggravated by oestrogen-containing oral contraceptives.[116] The pain of the syndrome seems to be mediated through the autonomic nervous system.

RENAL VEIN ENTRAPMENT SYNDROME

It is common on ultrasonography to find that the left renal vein is compressed as it passes between the superior mesenteric artery and the aorta.[117] This causes distension of the vein and an increase in renal venous pressure on the left side. In most cases there are no symptoms, but a few individuals with severe compression develop gross haematuria and loin pain (renal vein entrapment or 'nutcracker' syndrome). The bleeding is from the left kidney and the red cells are isomorphic, i.e. are not coming from the glomerulus (see p. 127). It is postulated that in these cases the venous hypertension has caused rupture of minute, thin-walled veins into the collecting system or renal fornix.[118]

Before diagnosing renal vein entrapment syndrome it is important to ensure that the patient's unilateral haematuria is not due to other causes such as *calculi* (see p. 532), *tumour* (see p. 569), *papillary necrosis* (see p. 458), *sickle cell nephropathy* (see p. 106) and other vascular abnormalities.

RENAL VEIN THROMBOSIS

Thrombosis of renal veins is a rare occurrence. It affects neonates and infants about as frequently as patients of all other ages put together. Haemorrhagic renal infarction usually results when the disease occurs in infancy but is exceptional in older patients, particularly adults.

Renal venous thrombosis in infancy

In most of the affected babies this condition develops during the first month of life, particularly in the first week, and is often a complication of acute gastroenteritis or of some systemic infection accompanied by dehydration. Other possible underlying causes are hydramnios and maternal toxaemia of pregnancy, maternal ingestion of thiazides for treatment of hypertension, diabetes in the mother, angiocardiography in the investigation of severe congenital heart disease, and cytomegalovirus infection of the child.[119,120] It may affect one side or both with equal frequency. If bilateral, it is generally asymmetrical and it may be accompanied by thrombosis of the inferior vena cava. Thrombosis starting in an arcuate or interlobular vein is much commoner than primary thrombosis of the main renal vein; in some cases the main renal vessel is not affected.[119]

Clinical features

The onset is acute with swelling in the loin, gross haematuria, thrombocytopenia and the finding on intravenous urography of an enlarged, poorly functioning or non-functioning kidney. Contrary to what occurs in adults, proteinuria may be minimal. The affected kidney or kidneys are readily palpable. There may be evidence of a consumptive coagulopathy with a rise in the quantity of degradation products of fibrin in the urine.

Renal changes

The extent of the damage depends on the size and number of veins involved. In severe cases the kidney is enlarged and deep purple. When thrombosis is confined to a few interlobular veins isolated dark red infarcts will be seen on the subcapsular surface and on section of the kidney. Microscopically, the picture is that of a haemorrhagic infarct. In patients who survive, the infarcted areas of the kidney undergo organization and sometimes calcification.

Prognosis

Over a third of affected individuals survive. There may be late sequelae; hypertension has been reported some months later, the nephrotic syndrome may occur and multiple tubular abnormalities have been found.

Renal vein thrombosis in older children and adults

In older children and adults renal venous thrombosis usually develops as a complication of the nephrotic syndrome; less often it is secondary to thrombosis of the inferior vena cava. The incidence of renal vein thrombosis in the nephrotic syndrome is variable but in one series it affected approximately 22% of such patients.[121] It is particularly likely to occur if the underlying cause of the nephrotic syndrome is membranous glomerulonephritis (see p. 200) or, less frequently, mesangiocapillary glomerulonephritis (see p. 164); renal vein thrombosis can be expected to occur at some time during the course of membranous glomerulonephritis in approximately 50% of the patients.[122]

Clinical features

Most patients remain asymptomatic, intravenous pyelograms disclose no abnormality and angiography is necessary to detect the renal vein thrombosis. A minority of younger patients present with sudden acute loin pain, marked tenderness in the costovertebral angle and gross haematuria.[121]

Renal changes

Gross appearance of the kidneys When renal vein thrombosis complicates membranous glomerulonephritis, the main renal vein and its tributaries usually contain organized thrombus;

occasionally the thrombus is confined to the tributaries. The kidney is normal in size and pale.

Light microscopy In addition to the changes associated with the underlying condition (e.g. membranous glomerulonephritis, diffuse mesangiocapillary glomerulonephritis, diabetes mellitus, focal glomerulosclerosis, minimal change disease, congenital nephrotic syndrome), there are thrombi of various ages in veins of different sizes; recanalization is present in older lesions. There is sometimes a greater degree of tubular atrophy and loss and consequent interstitial fibrosis (Fig. 9.21). Oedema of the interstitium and margination of neutrophil granulocytes on the glomerular capillary walls are occasionally found.

Electron microscopy & immunofluorescence/immunoperoxidase microscopy The changes are of the underlying condition; there are no findings unique to renal vein thrombosis.

Complications

The incidence of thromboembolic complications is high in untreated patients and they may die of pulmonary embolism.

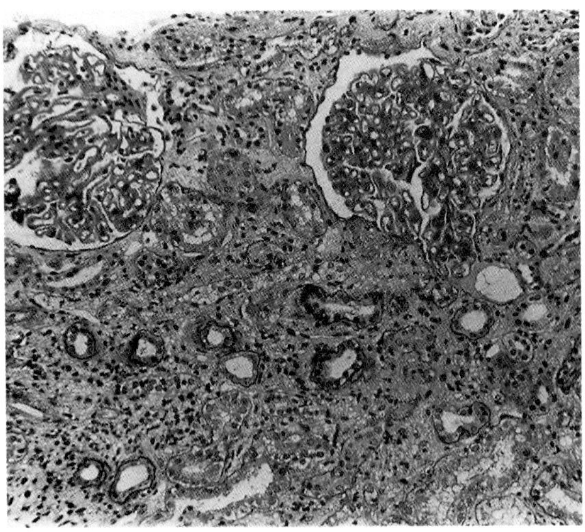

Fig. 9.21 Renal vein thrombosis in membranous glomerulonephritis. Tubular atrophy and interstitial fibrosis are more prominent than is usual in membranous glomerulonephritis uncomplicated by thrombosis of the renal vein.
Periodic acid-Schiff × 140

Prognosis

There is mild progressive deterioration of renal function which is not altered by anticoagulant drugs, but treated patients are much less likely to experience a new episode of thromboembolism than controls.[121]

Pathogenesis

The nephrotic syndrome is associated with a hypercoagulable state (see p. 126). Patients have an increase in the number of platelets and in blood levels of fibrinogen, factor V, combined factors VIII and X, accelerated thromboplastin generation, increased activation of Hageman factor (factor XII) and abnormal levels of procoagulant plasma proteins. It is likely that this hypercoagulable state is an important pathogenetic factor in the genesis of renal vein thrombosis, as well as other thromboembolic phenomena. However, no coagulation differences are noticed between patients with renal vein thrombosis and those without. Also, although membranous glomerulonephritis is complicated by renal vein thrombosis more frequently than any other renal disease, no reason for this has yet been discovered. Some evidence suggests that in patients with membranous glomerulonephritis the hypercoagulability, decreased fibrinolysis and reduction in plasma volume may be of greater magnitude than in other renal diseases, but this has yet to be confirmed.[123]

ATHEROSCLEROSIS

Atherosclerosis directly affects the renal arteries and their main branches less frequently than the aorta and coronary arteries.[124] It is commonest in patients with essential hypertension, diabetes mellitus or some genetic disorder of lipid metabolism, such as familial hypercholesterolaemia. Only rarely is it of sufficient degree to lead to changes in the renal parenchyma before the age of 35 years in males and 45 years in females. After this point in life the prevalence of damaging atherosclerosis slowly increases with each decade. The resulting renal ischaemic lesions are often asymptomatic;

hypertension is occasionally produced, usually as a result of severe renal artery stenosis (see p. 298). Infrequently the damaged and weakened atherosclerotic wall of the renal artery bulges to give one or more aneurysms which may rupture.

Atherosclerosis of the aorta may affect the kidneys in several ways: an atheromatous plaque in the abdominal aorta or an abdominal aortic aneurysm may compromise the origin of one or both renal arteries, and an embolus composed of fragments of atheromatous plaques from the aorta may lodge in the intrarenal arteries. Usually these changes have no functional significance but the narrowing of the orifice of the renal artery may cause hypertension and the emboli may occasionally precipitate renal failure.

Renal changes

Gross appearance of the kidneys

The kidneys are usually smaller than normal. On the subcapsular surface there are scars, some of which are large and coarse; the intervening areas may be smooth or coarsely granular. The pelvis and calyces are normal in contrast to chronic pyelonephritis in which the scars are related to an underlying dilated and distorted calyx. The wall of the main renal artery and of the segmental and arcuate arteries is thickened and the main renal artery may also contain atheromatous plaques. Thrombus may be superimposed on any of the lesions.

Light microscopy

In addition to the gross scars seen naked eye there are numerous tiny subcapsular scars. The glomeruli in the scars show ischaemic damage (see p. 306) of varying extent and severity, the tubules have either disappeared or are atrophic and the interstitium is fibrotic and contains collections of lymphocytes. The areas between the scars are normal or display minor ischaemic changes. The arteries show fibrous intimal thickening with reduplication of the internal elastic lamina. This is patchy and less pronounced in the interlobular arteries. Small collections of lipid are occasionally present in the intima in the main renal artery. There is focal hyalinization of the walls of afferent arterioles; this is more prominent in hypertensive patients.

Immunofluorescence/immunoperoxidase microscopy

Focal granular collections of C3 are often present in arteriolar walls in collections of hyaline; they are also occasionally found in the thickened intima in arteries.

Differential diagnosis

A scar in a kidney affected by atherosclerosis may be indistinguishable in a biopsy from one caused by *chronic infection*. The only certain way to separate the two is by gross examination of the kidney; atheromatous kidneys lack the dilated calyx in relation to the overlying scar seen in chronic pyelonephritis (see p. 440).

Cholesterol emboli

Emboli composed of fragments of atheromatous plaques are found at autopsy in patients over the age of 50 years in 4.7% of men and 2.7% of women.[125] They may occur spontaneously, but more commonly follow invasive arterial procedures, including arteriography, angiopathy, coronary artery bypass and repair of aortic aneurysms; they are particularly common after aortography, affecting one in four patients.[126] The lipid-containing atheromatous material, extruded from an atheromatous plaque in the aorta, acts as an embolus and usually becomes impacted in an interlobular artery; occasionally it involves an arcuate vessel. Cholesterol emboli are characterized in paraffin sections by the long needle-shaped clefts that remain after the lipid has been dissolved during histological processing. In recent lesions the cystals are surrounded by fibrin; in older emboli organization occurs and they become surrounded by fibrous tissue (Fig. 9.22). Infarction or ischaemic parenchymal atrophy results, depending on the completeness of the obstruction; on rare occasions hypertension or renal failure is produced.[127] The renal dysfunction is usually insidious in its development and may follow

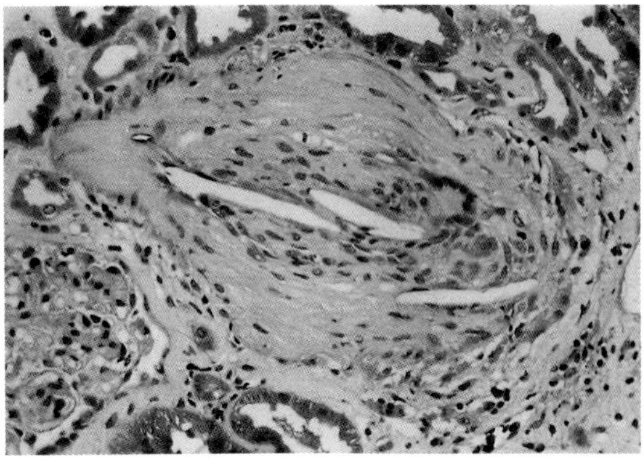

Fig. 9.22 Cholesterol embolization of a small interlobular artery. Needle-shaped clefts are present in the lumen of the vessel. The embolus is not recent because the clefts are surrounded by fibrous tissue; there is also a foreign body giant cell.
Haematoxylin-eosin × 140

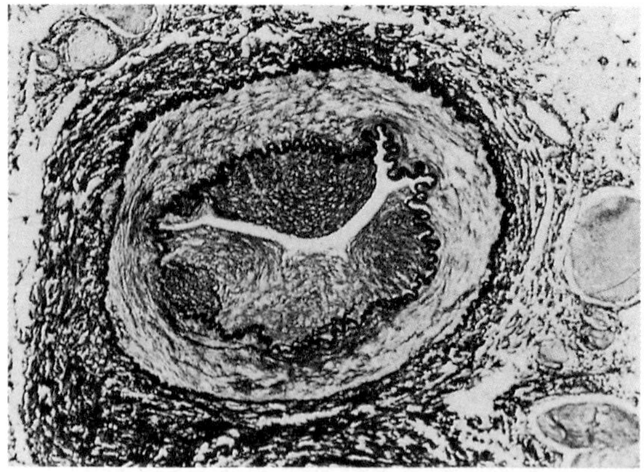

Fig. 9.23 Intimal fibroplasia of renal artery. The intima is greatly thickened by an accumulation of loose fibrous tissue. Elastic-Van Gieson × 25
Reproduced by permission from: Hunt JC, Harrison EG, Kincaid OW, Bernatz PE, Davis GD. Proc Staff Meet Mayo Clin 1962; 37: 181 (Fig. 7a)

the initial release of emboli by weeks or months. A case is described in which nephrotic range proteinuria occurred; there was focal segmental glomerulosclerosis in this patient as well as global sclerosis of just over a quarter of the glomeruli.[128]

DYSPLASIAS OF THE RENAL ARTERIES

The term 'dysplasia' has been given to a group of non-atherosclerotic fibrous and fibromuscular lesions that produce stenosis of one or both of the renal arteries.[129] They may occur as incidental pathological findings in asymptomatic patients, but when marked they produce functional stenosis of the renal artery and cause hypertension (see p. 298). They have been subdivided into intimal fibroplasia, medial dysplasia and periarterial fibroplasia according to the part of the arterial wall that is most affected.

Intimal fibroplasia

Intimal fibroplasia is uncommon. It is characterized by a circumferential or eccentric accumulation of loose, moderately cellular, fibrous tissue with no collections of lipid and no evidence of inflammation (Fig. 9.23). The internal elastic lamina may be reduplicated but the media and adventitia are normal. The intimal thickening involves segments of one or both main renal arteries or a segmental artery. Similar changes affect the arteries in the limbs and those supplying the intestinal tract.

Medial dysplasia

Medial dysplasia usually occurs in young women. It is divided into three categories according to the predominant histological finding.

Medial fibroplasia with aneurysms

This is the most common dysplasia of the renal arteries. It usually affects the distal two-thirds of the main renal artery and may extend into the segmental arteries. Thick fibromuscular ridges replace the normal structure of the intima and media of the artery and alternate with areas of great thinning of the wall that lack an internal elastic lamina and may become aneurysmal (Fig. 9.24). The external elastic lamina is usually intact. Medial fibroplasia with aneurysms gives rise to a characteristic 'string of beads' deformity on aortography. Although this condition is found predominantly in the renal arteries, it does occur in other branches arising from the aorta.

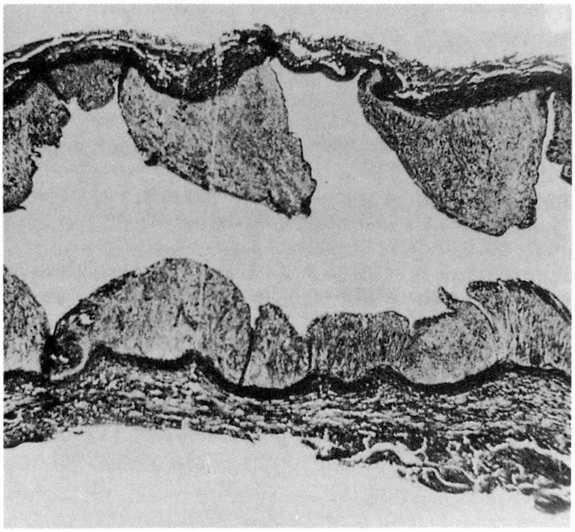

Fig. 9.24 Medial fibroplasia with aneurysms affecting the renal artery. Ridges of muscle and fibrous tissue alternate with areas of great thinning of the wall.
Elastic-Van Gieson × 20
Reproduced by permission from: Harrison EG, Hunt JC, Bernatz PE. Am J Med 1967; 43: 97 (Fig. 3c)

Medial hyperplasia

Medial hyperplasia is uncommon, although slightly more frequent than intimal fibroplasia. The number of smooth muscle cells in the media is greatly increased (Fig. 9.25) The intima, adventitia and internal elastic lamina are normal.

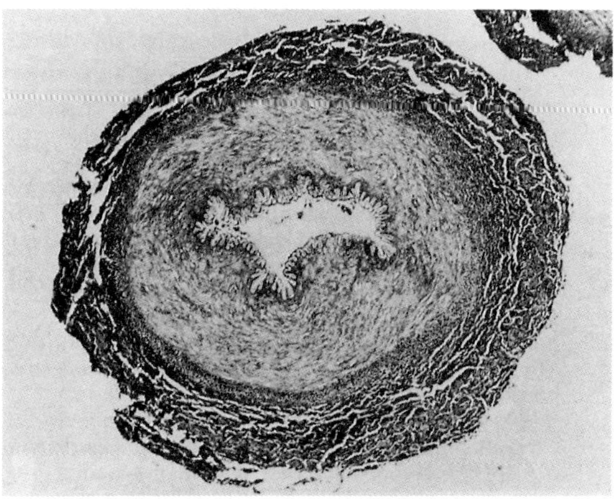

Fig. 9.25 Medial hyperplasia of renal artery. There is thickening of the media by excess muscle leading to narrowing of the lumen.
Mallory–Heidenhain × 25
Reproduced by permission from: Harrison EG, McCormack LJ. Mayo Clin Proc 1971; 46: 161 (Fig. 4b)

Perimedial fibroplasia

Perimedial fibroplasia is the second most common variant. The outer half to two-thirds of the media and usually the external elastic lamina are replaced by mature collagen (Fig. 9.26) The collagenous zone is of variable thickness resulting in an irregular beaded appearance on aortography but the beads are smaller than those produced by medial fibroplasia with aneurysms. Perimedial fibroplasia has not been recorded in arteries elsewhere in the body.

Medial dissection

Medial dissection is uncommon. A new channel, surrounded by fibrous tissue, is formed in the outer third of the media inside the external elastic lamina. Intimal fibroplasia may accompany the condition and completely obliterate the original lumen of the artery. Renal infarction may be produced.

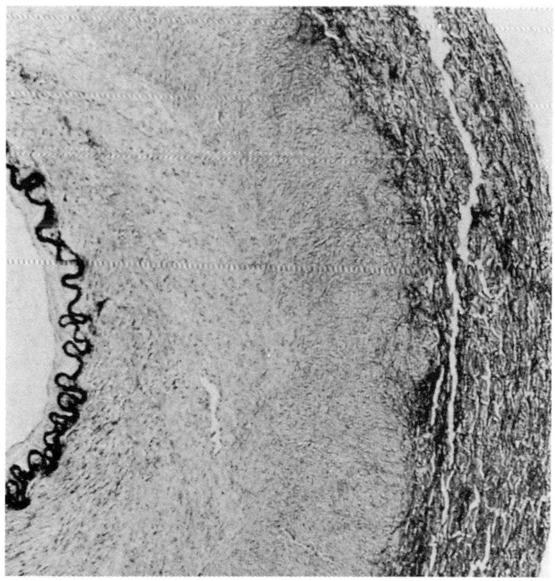

Fig. 9.26 Perimedial fibroplasia of renal artery. Part of vessel. The outer media and most of the external elastic lamina are replaced by dense fibrous tissue.
Elastic-Van Gieson × 60
Reproduced by permission from: McCormack LJ, Poutasse EF, Meaney TF, Noto TJ, Dustan HP. Am Heart J 1966; 72: 188 (Fig. 16)

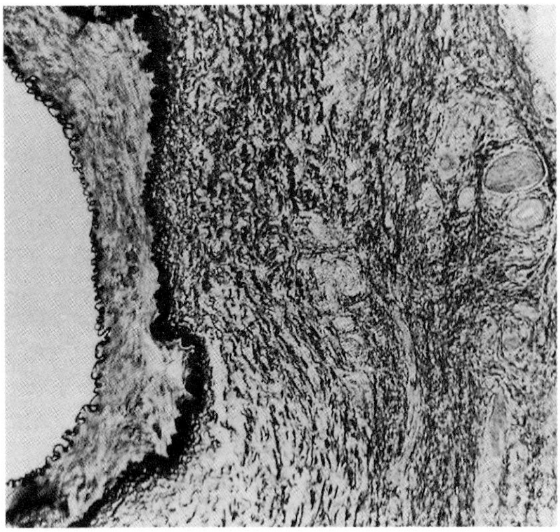

Fig. 9.27 Periarterial fibroplasia of renal artery. Part of vessel. Collagen encompasses the adventitia and extends into the surrounding fibrofatty tissue. The external elastic lamina is thickened and reduplicated.
Elastic-Van Gieson × 25
Reproduced by permission from: Hunt JC, Harrison EG, Kincaid OW, Bernatz PE, Davis GD. Proc Staff Meet Mayo Clin 1962; 37: 181 (Fig. 8a)

Periarterial fibroplasia

Periarterial fibroplasia is rare. Collagen encompasses the adventitia and extends into the fibrofatty tissue surrounding the artery (Fig. 9.27). The intima, media and elastic laminae are normal.

RENAL ARTERY STENOSIS

Clinical features[130]

The only clinical ground for suspecting the presence of stenosis of a renal artery is the discovery of an epigastric bruit. Bruits of continuous or systolic–diastolic duration are heard in about half the cases. The hypertension is often severe: it averaged 210/125 mmHg in one series. Renal angiography will usually locate the site of stenosis; comparison of the renin activity in blood taken from the two renal veins simultaneously and the response to angiotensin-converting enzyme inhibitors (e.g. captopril or enalapril) will help determine whether the lesion is a functional one. Renin activity is raised in the venous blood from a kidney with functional renal artery stenosis.

Renal changes

Pathological changes in the kidney with the obstructive arterial lesion

Gross appearance of the kidneys In those cases in which the obstructive lesion is confined to one artery in a kidney supplied by several arteries, or in which the lesion is in a segmental artery, the affected part of the kidney is depressed and the cortex in that area is reduced in width. When the single, main renal artery is involved the kidney is usually slightly and uniformly decreased in size and there is some fairly uniform reduction in cortical thickness.

Light microscopy In those kidneys in which shrinkage is visible grossly there is striking tubular atrophy, most marked in the superficial part of the cortex (Fig. 9.28). The diameter of the tubules is greatly reduced and they are lined by cubical

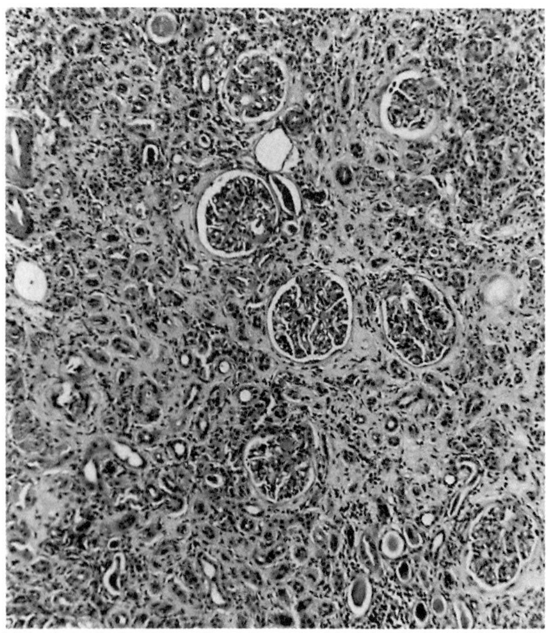

Fig. 9.28 Renal artery stenosis. There is much atrophy of the tubules, although the glomeruli are relatively little affected. Haematoxylin-eosin × 100

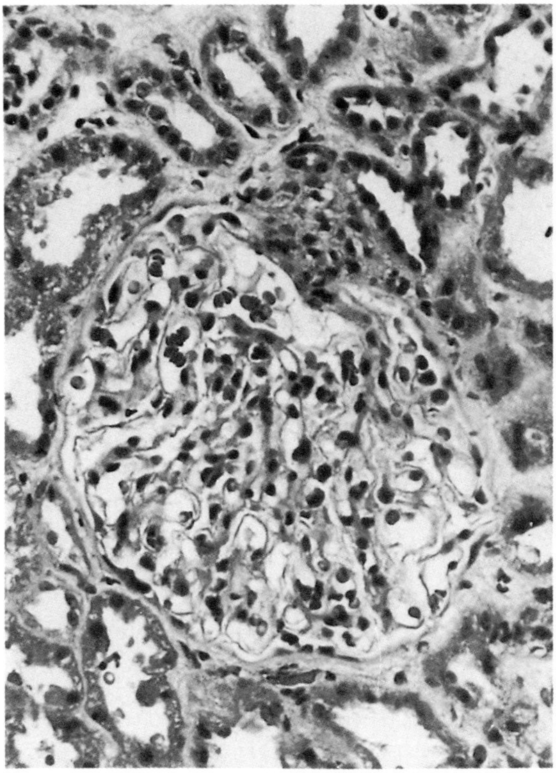

Fig. 9.29 Renal artery stenosis. The juxtaglomerular apparatus is hyperplastic. Haematoxylin-eosin × 240

epithelial cells. As a consequence of this atrophy the glomeruli are crowded together but structurally may appear surprisingly normal. Some show collagen formation internal to Bowman's capsule and collapse of the tuft. The interlobular and larger arteries may show some fibrous intimal thickening; the arterioles are normal. The interstitium is often fibrotic; there is no cellular infiltration. Hyperplasia of the juxtaglomerular apparatus is rarely found in such kidneys.

In other cases there is much less tubular atrophy. In these kidneys there is enlargement of the juxtaglomerular apparatus (Fig. 9.29), especially in the deeper, more normal parts of the cortex. The enlargement of the juxtaglomerular apparatus can be very marked, particularly when stenosis of a renal artery is associated not only with high blood pressure but also with a potassium-losing syndrome. The number of granular cells in the juxtaglomerular apparatus is increased; immunocytochemical methods show that the granules contain renin. The renin-secreting cells also extend their distribution proximally in the arterial tree as far as the interlobular arteries (Fig. 9.30).[131,132]

In kidneys in which there is no tubular atrophy the hyperplasia of the cells of the juxtaglomerular apparatus is greatest in the superficial third of the cortex.

When only one branch of a renal artery is stenotic the parts of the kidney that are not ischaemic may show hypertensive vascular changes.

Pathological changes in the opposite (non-ischaemic) kidney

Hypertensive vascular changes may be seen in the opposite, non-ischaemic, kidney if the stenosis of the renal artery is unilateral. Depending upon the duration of the hypertension and the gradient of blood pressure rise the changes will be those associated with either the benign or malignant phase of hypertension (see pp. 306 and 311). The juxtaglomerular bodies are normal.

Prognosis

A number of reconstructive operations, such as splenorenal arterial anastomosis in the case of stenosis of the left renal artery and a saphenous vein bypass graft from the aorta when the right renal artery is involved, cure the hypertension in over 50% of young patients with dysplasia of the renal artery. If the obstructive lesion is confined to the origin of a renal artery, autotransplantation of the affected kidney may be curative. Percutaneous transluminal angioplasty, an efficient and safe method of treating renal vascular stenoses without open surgery, appears to achieve success rates similar to those achieved by surgery.

ANEURYSMS OF THE RENAL ARTERIES

True aneurysms of the renal arteries are rare.[133] Most are atherosclerotic aneurysms. Less frequently there are the dissecting aneurysms and microaneurysms which are considered on pages 296 and 297 under dysplasias of the renal artery. Occasional causes are trauma, classical polyar-

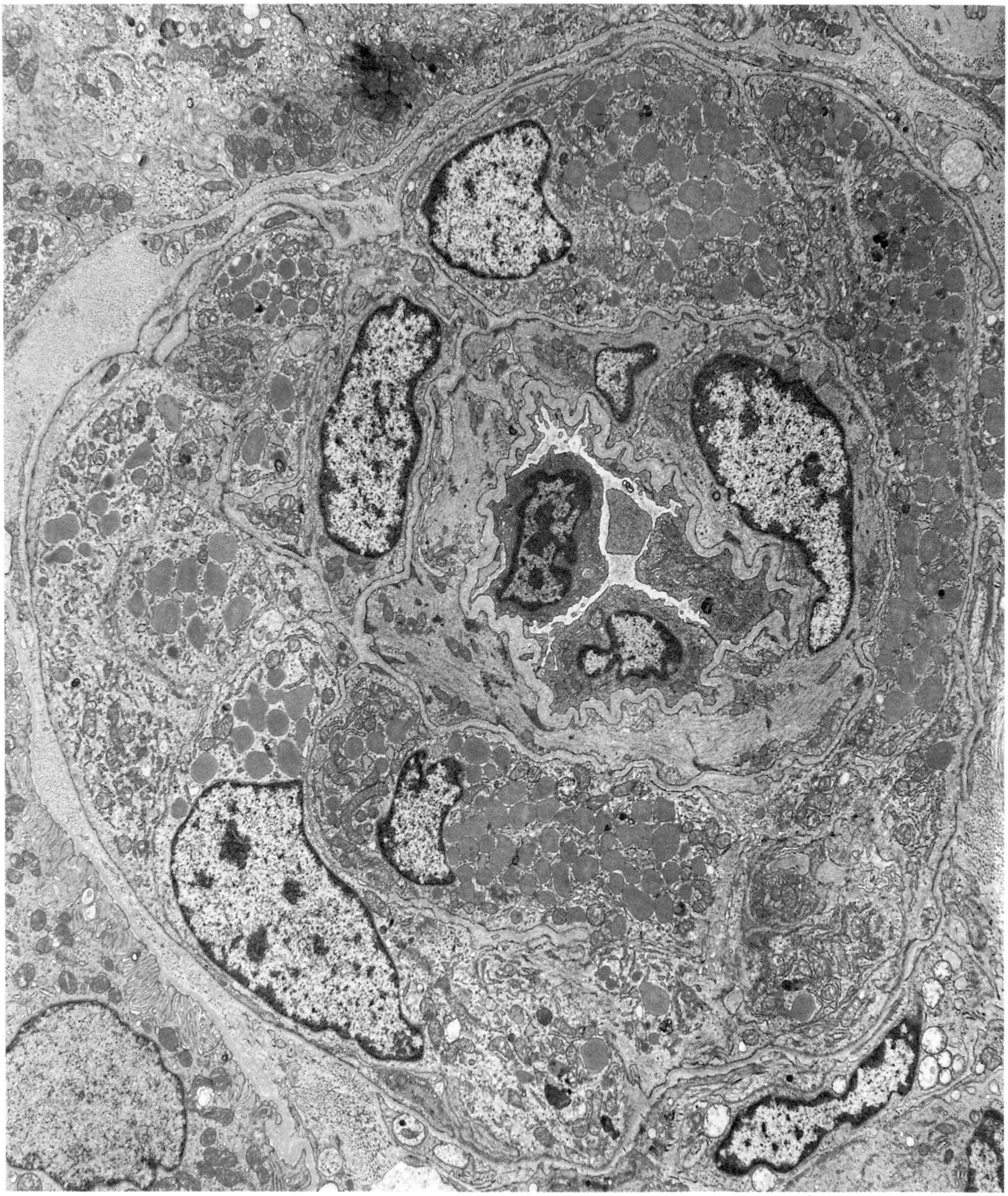

Fig. 9.30 Renal artery stenosis. Electron micrograph of a renal arteriole near its origin from an interlobular artery. Renin-secreting cells are abundant in the wall of the vessel. These granular cells are normally only present in afferent arterioles near the glomerular hilum. Following renal artery stenosis they extend their distribution proximally. × 6800

teritis and Takayasu's disease. In two cases there was medial agenesis and the aneurysms involved other visceral arteries.[134] Mycotic aneurysms, following impaction of infected emboli in cases of infective endocarditis, are also recorded.

Atherosclerotic aneurysms are generally small and saccular and they are often at or near the branching of the renal artery at the hilum of the kidney. They may be multiple and calcification is common in their walls.

False aneurysms also occur; they differ from true aneurysms in that their walls consist of organized blood clot instead of arterial media and adventitia. These aneurysms are almost always the result of trauma with rupture of the artery.

RENAL INFARCTION

Infarction of the kidney can result from blockage of arteries or veins. Arterial occlusion is the commoner cause.

Infarction from renal arterial occlusion

Renal arterial occlusion leading to infarction is fairly common, probably because approximately one-quarter of the cardiac output passes through the kidneys and the renal arteries have a segmental distribution with usually only a minimal alternative blood supply.

The majority of infarcts are caused by sudden, complete arterial blockage by emboli. These originate most commonly as thrombi within the chambers of the left side of the heart, as a complication of infarction of the wall of the left ventricle or of mitral stenosis. Less frequently the emboli arise from vegetations on heart valves in infective endocarditis; occasionally pieces of thrombus formed on atherosclerotic lesions in the aorta or in the main renal artery or lipid-laden material released from atherosclerotic plaques act as emboli and occlude the arteries within a kidney.

Less commonly, arterial obstruction is produced by thrombosis secondary to changes in the wall of the vessel associated with atherosclerosis, systemic sclerosis, malignant hypertension, polyarteritis, haemolytic uraemic syndrome, the loin pain haematuria syndrome, or aneurysm formation. In cases of sickle cell anaemia the small arterial branches in the kidneys may be occluded by the distorted red cells. Rarely, infarction is the result of injury to the main renal artery, even its avulsion, in accidents. Surgical ligation of aberrant arteries is another rare cause, most frequently seen in renal allografts.

Renal cortical necrosis (see p. 303) is an example of infarction due to arterial spasm followed by thrombosis.

Clinical findings

Many small infarcts go undetected and probably produce few if any symptoms. Large infarcts are usually associated with sudden pain in the loin, followed shortly by haematuria and proteinuria; transient hypertension with a peak at 3 days sometimes occurs. Bilateral obstruction of the main renal arteries ordinarily results in acute renal failure. In the newborn, acute renal failure may be induced even by unilateral occlusion of a renal artery by thrombosis.

Renal changes

Gross appearance of the kidneys The appearance of a renal infarct depends on its age, the size of vessel obstructed and the presence or absence of infection.

In the first hour, a sterile infarct is swollen, red and pyramidal, with the apex toward the obstructed artery. By 6 hours it has become greyish with a narrow red rim; the greyness is complete by 24 hours. At 4 days the infarct is yellowish-grey and no longer swollen (Fig. 9.31); by 7 days the red rim has disappeared and the infarct is depressed below the subcapsular surface. From then onwards the infarct shrinks; by 4 weeks the smaller infarcts have become V-shaped scars (Fig. 9.32). In large infarcts a central mass of inspissated, dead tissue persists; eventually calcification may occur.

Infarcts that are caused by emboli infected with pyogenic organisms, as in cases of acute bacterial endocarditis, rapidly become transformed into abscesses.

Light microscopy In the first hour the glom-

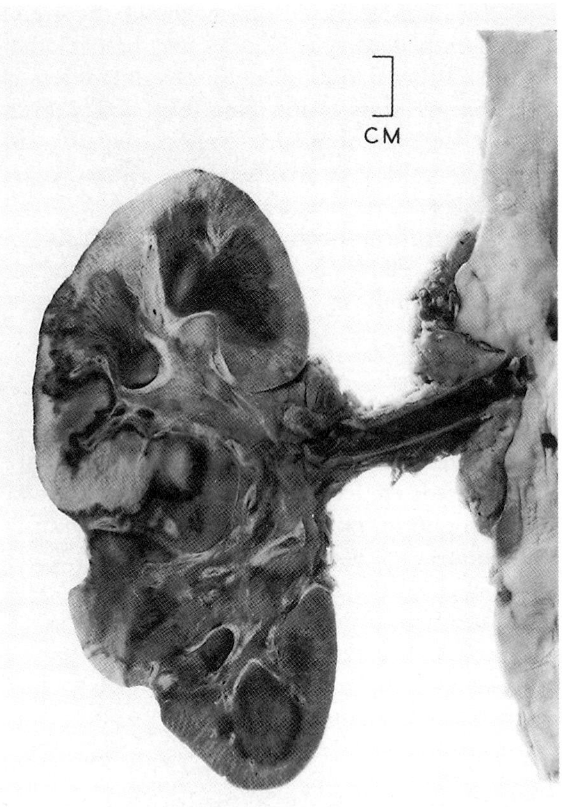

Fig. 9.31 Renal infarction of several days' duration. The dead tissue is pale; a dark rim of hyperaemia marks the junction between the infarction and the surviving tissue. A large embolus is seen in the main renal artery.
Specimen from the Pathology Museum, Charing Cross and Westminster Medical School, London, UK. Reproduced by permission of the Curator, Dr F. J. Paradinas.

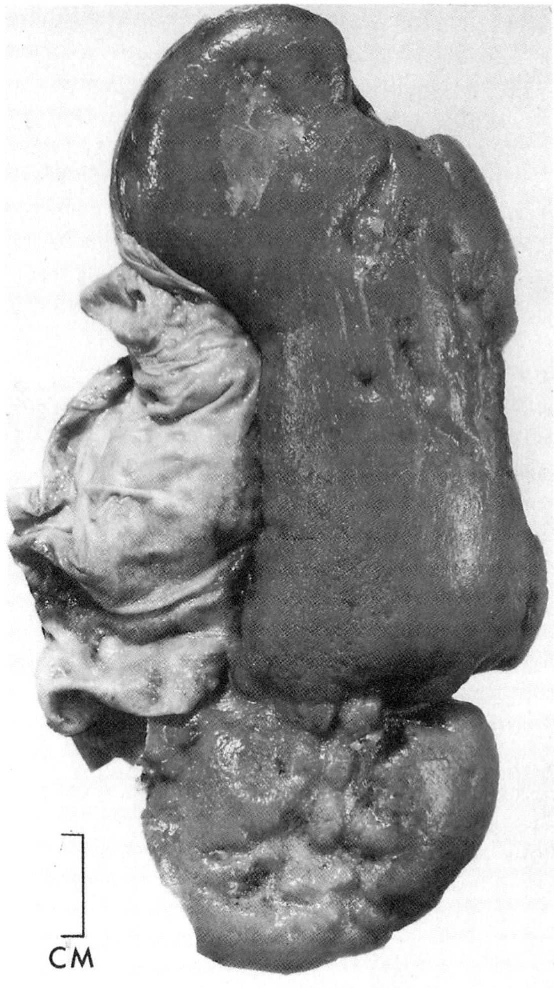

Fig. 9.32 Healed renal infarction. There are numerous scars, particularly at the lower pole, the outcome of infarcts resulting from multiple episodes of embolism.

erular and peritubular capillaries become filled with sludged red cells. Between 6 and 24 hours the red cells lose their haemoglobin, the tubular cells become pale, there is nuclear pyknosis and a zone of neutrophil granulocytes appears around the dead area. From 4 to 7 days the dead cells gradually lose their nuclei, the granulocytes undergo karyorrhexis and disappear, and organization, revascularization and regeneration become apparent at the periphery. The central dead area gradually collapses but glomerular capillary basement membranes can still be detected by the periodic acid-Schiff method up to 5 months later. At the margin of the infarcts the tubules atrophy and may disappear but the glomeruli persist and develop segmental necrosis and proliferation of parietal epithelial cells, sometimes with crescent formation; segmental and global sclerosis follows. The central dead area gradually shrinks. Eventually, the infarct is replaced by fibrous tissue.

Infarction from renal venous thrombosis

Renal vein occlusion is rare and almost always caused by thrombosis. In infants, particularly neonates, thrombosis of the renal veins causes haemorrhagic infarction. In adults infarction is unusual, the changes being confined to tubular atrophy and interstitial oedema followed by fibrosis. Renal vein thrombosis is considered in detail on page 293.

RENAL CORTICAL NECROSIS

Bilateral renal cortical necrosis is one of the rare causes of acute renal failure. There is death of a variable amount of the renal cortex; the medulla, the juxtamedullary cortex and sometimes a rim of cortex under the capsule are usually spared. It most commonly occurs in association with accidents of pregnancy (see p. 565) but may arise in cases of systemic sepsis, severe trauma or miscellaneous conditions such as pancreatitis, postoperative shock, diabetic ketoacidosis and snake venom or diethylene glycol poisoning.[135,136] Antepartum or postpartum haemorrhage associated with abruptio placentae, abortion or placenta praevia is responsible for 50–60% of all cases of acute bilateral renal cortical necrosis.[137] Overwhelming infections with bacterial shock account for 30–40%.[136] In children the precipitating event is often gastroenteritis with severe vomiting, diarrhoea and dehydration.[136] The prognosis in cases with extensive cortical destruction is poor; with less damage there may be sufficient recovery to allow survival without the necessity for chronic dialysis. Extensive cortical necrosis is a relatively common end-result of hyperacute or severe acute rejection in renal allografts (see p. 631).

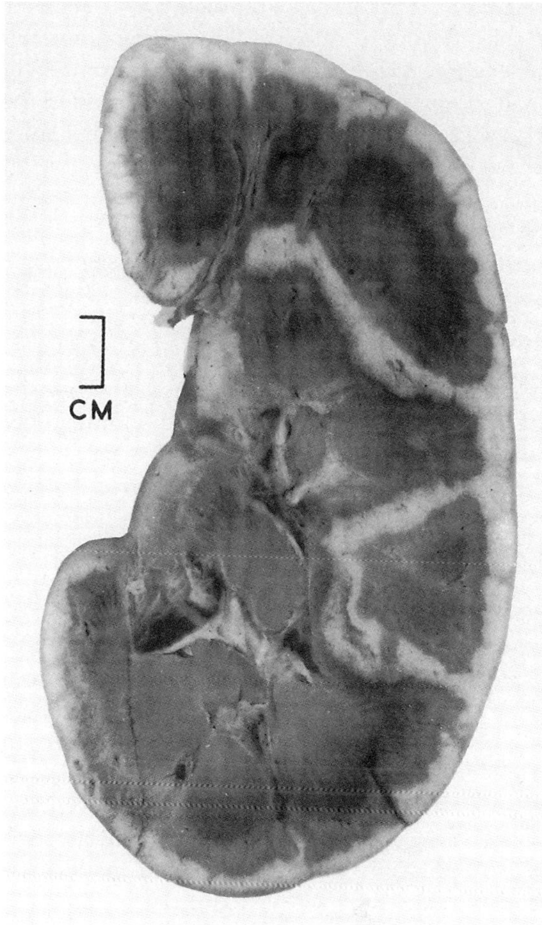

Fig. 9.33 Acute bilateral renal cortical necrosis. The necrotic areas are strikingly pale. There is a narrow zone just under the capsule and a wider surviving zone adjoining the medulla.
Reproduced by permission of the Curator of the Gordon Museum, Guy's Hospital, London, UK.

Clinical features

Initially, the clinical course is similar to that of acute tubular necrosis (see p. 492), except that oliguria is profound. However, diuresis fails to appear by the fourth week, and renal angiograms show attenuation of interlobular arteries, an increase in the subcapsular vessels and a negative nephrogram in the outer cortical zone. By about the sixth week calcification can sometimes be demonstrated radiologically in the cortex.[138]

Renal findings

Gross appearance

In severe cases the kidneys are usually moderately enlarged. Almost the entire cortex, including the columns of Bertin, is pale yellow, except for a fine rim of congested tissue immediately beneath the capsule and another at the corticomedullary junction (Fig. 9.33). In less severely affected cases the columns of Bertin are often spared. If the patient has survived for over a month the cortex will be reduced in thickness and may be patchily calcified.

Light microscopy

When the condition is severe most of the cortex

is necrotic. The tubules are lined by the remains of cells, devoid of nuclei. Many of the glomeruli are engorged with blood. A variable number of small groups of surviving nephrons is found in the otherwise dead tissue. The arteries and arterioles are necrotic and dilated, and contain thrombus in cases seen more than 2 days after the onset. In contrast, the parenchymal tissue in narrow subcapsular and corticomedullary zones is spared.

Other organ changes

Foci of necrosis have been described in the anterior lobe of the pituitary and in the tuber cinereum, and in the adrenals, spleen, lungs, gastrointestinal tract, liver, pancreas and uterus.[139,140]

Prognosis

Cortical necrosis varies in extent from patient to patient and in up to 50% of cases there is sufficient residual viable tissue to allow survival without the necessity for chronic dialysis. There is a direct correlation between the proportion of glomeruli destroyed and both the duration of oliguria and survival.[135] Patients who recover may develop a second, slower decline in renal function due to a progressive reduction in renal mass that is probably caused by a destructive rise in filtration rate within the individual surviving nephrons (see p. 26). There is also an increased incidence of malignant hypertension.[138]

Pathogenesis

Acute renal cortical necrosis is generally considered to be caused by vascular spasm that lasts for many hours, causing necrosis and secondary thrombosis of the arteries beyond the obstruction.[137] Experimental work on animals supports this concept. What causes the spasm is not known; probably many factors are involved.

HYPERTENSION

The term 'hypertension', used without qualification, implies elevation of systolic and diastolic pressure in the systemic arteries. The definition of what constitutes an elevation in pressure depends entirely upon what arbitrary limits are put on normality because the level of arterial pressure in a particular population is a continuously distributed variable. Hypertension represents the right end of a Gaussian curve for mean arterial pressure. It is not a disease, but because the heart and vessels in man have not evolved to withstand long-term pressure elevation, disease often ensues as a consequence of damage caused to the heart or to the arterial walls by a given level of blood pressure; this may lead to premature death.

Data are available on the morbidity and mortality for given levels of blood pressure related to age and sex from population studies,[141] and whether to define a particular level of blood pressure as abnormal or not is usually solved by reference to the degree of risk attached to that level. In studies on particular sections of the population a level of blood pressure that is associated with a morbidity twice to three times that of the general population is usually regarded as abnormal. For the general population a systolic pressure of 140 mmHg and a diastolic pressure of 90 mmHg are commonly taken as the arbitrary division between normal and abnormal.

Arterial blood pressure varies continuously in any one individual. Intra-arterial ambulatory monitoring of the blood pressure in normal individuals every 2 minutes over the 24 hours shows enormous fluctuations and a characteristic diurnal rhythm.[142] Also, when the blood pressure is measured in the arm by the conventional indirect method the defence reaction of the subject to the examiner can cause a spurious rise in the pressure. To overcome these difficulties it is usual to measure the pressure on several occasions over several weeks and to allow the subject plenty of time to become familiar with the surroundings and with the examiner.

No more than 5–10% of cases of hypertension are *secondary* to some demonstrable cause. When cases of secondary hypertension are excluded there remains a large group of patients whose hypertension has no apparent cause: this is the condition known as *essential hypertension* or primary hypertension.

When the gradient of the progressive rise in blood pressure in either essential or secondary hypertension is slow the patient is said to be in the *benign phase of hypertension.* Benign phase hypertension may go on for many years with few symptoms and little deterioration. The pressure rises are usually modest, although high levels may eventually occur and be sustained for long periods, particularly in women. If the condition causes death it usually terminates in cardiac failure or a cerebrovascular accident; only rarely is death due to renal failure.

When the gradient of the rise in blood pressure in either primary or secondary hypertension is very steep, the condition – if untreated – has a rapidly downhill course to a fatal outcome within a period of about 6 months to 2 years. This accelerated or *malignant phase of hypertension* is usually accompanied by papilloedema and commonly leads to renal failure. Malignant hypertension is often preceded by a variable period of benign phase hypertension.

It is often suggested that cardiovascular morbidity and mortality are more closely linked to the diastolic pressure than to the systolic pressure. This contention is not borne out by prospective epidemiological data obtained in the town of Framingham in Massachusetts, USA, where 5290 people were followed for 20 years and the evolution of cardiovascular disease studied in relation to their blood pressure.[143] Also, the large collection of data in the Build and Pressure Study of the Chicago Society of Actuaries showed that at any level of diastolic pressure cardiovascular mortality increases in proportion to the associated systolic pressure.[144]

ESSENTIAL HYPERTENSION

The diagnosis of essential hypertension is made by exclusion. After a thorough search for a primary cause, approximately 90–95% of hypertensive individuals are left with the label essential hypertension. The cause is probably multifactorial.

It has long been recognized that essential hypertension tends to occur in families. Observations on identical twins with hypertension suggest that this is due to genetic rather than environmental influences: although they have lived apart for many years similar elevations in blood pressure are generally found in both.[145] In 1967, Pickering,[146] on the basis of population studies, proposed that the inherited influence on arterial pressure was polygenetic: no data have been collected since which contradict this concept. His proposal was supported by the discovery of rat strains with polygenetically inherited primary hypertension.[147] Although the polygenetic predisposition to essential hypertension is now widely accepted, little progress has been made in understanding the mechanism of the hereditary influence at the molecular level.

Certain environmental factors may aggravate and sometimes perhaps even precipitate hypertension if the individual is genetically predisposed. One such factor is the amount of salt eaten in the diet. Although controversial, there is a considerable amount of direct and indirect evidence to suggest that excessive intake of sodium can be associated with an increase in blood pressure.[148] The mechanism for this is unclear. Some experiments indicate that patients with essential, but not secondary, hypertension have a genetically determined defect in cell membrane transport in blood cells which leads to an increase in intracellular sodium. The same defect can be found in normotensive relatives of hypertensive subjects. It is postulated that if this electrolyte transport defect also affects arterial smooth muscle cells it could cause vasoconstriction and produce hypertension.[149] Others claim that there is an inherited defect in the renal excretion of sodium which leads to an increase in a hypothetical circulating natriuretic hormone. This hormone is thought to affect electrolyte transport in cells elsewhere in the body and this might lead to changes in arterioles favouring increased sensitivity to vasoconstrictive stimuli and cause essential hypertension.[150]

There is also a strong correlation between a low dietary intake of calcium and high blood pressure. The reason for this is not known. Some evidence suggests that there is an abnormality of calcium metabolism either within cells or across their membranes in essential hypertension.[151] At present, although it seems clear that there is an abnormal relationship between arterial pressure and electrolytes in patients with essential hypertension, there is disagreement about many of the individual findings and no widely accepted explanation for the agreed observations.[152]

Other environmental factors, particularly those operating through the mind, may also play a part in the genesis of high blood pressure, but they are even more difficult to evaluate.

Essential hypertension may be determined early in life. Some longitudinal studies of arterial pressure have indicated that those whose pressure is at the upper end of the normal range as young adults may become the hypertensives of the future; in general, however, early measures of pressure are not good predictors of future risk. Those who become hypertensive usually show an elevation of pressure beyond the normal range between the ages of 30 and 50 years. This is in contrast to the secondary forms of hypertension, which may appear even during childhood.

Essential hypertension, as indicated by a systolic blood pressure of 140 mmHg or higher or by a diastolic pressure of 90 mmHg or higher, has been discovered in 13–23% of most surveyed populations; some groups of primitive rural people, for example, in Africa and in the Amazon, however, do not develop hypertension, nor does their blood pressure rise with age. Essential hypertension is commoner in women than in men; the sex preponderance is limited to the older age group, in which the prognosis is better. Those who are obese are likelier to develop high blood pressure than those who are lean. Blacks in the USA and other developed countries and in urban communities in less well developed countries are affected twice as frequently as whites.[153]

Benign phase of essential hypertension

Clinical features

The benign phase of essential hypertension is usually symptomless, except sometimes for dyspnoea, until the pressure becomes very high. Signs and symptoms are then related to failure of the heart, narrowing of the coronary arteries and damage to the cerebral circulation. The raised blood pressure is often detected when the patient is seen by a a doctor about some other matter. There may be changes in the fundus of the eyes, usually hypertensive retinopathy and arteriosclerosis; these do not include papilloedema. The urine may be normal, or slight proteinuria may be found. The presence of marked proteinuria should rouse suspicion that the hypertension is not essential but secondary to some primary systemic or glomerular disease. Renal function tests are usually normal at first; as the disease progresses the renal perfusion, main tubular excretory capacity and glomerular filtration rate become lowered.

Renin levels in the blood are low or normal. The incidence of low-renin hypertension increases with age and is commonest in women and blacks. In the sixth decade 37% of patients with benign phase essential hypertension have low blood levels of renin.[154]

Renal changes

The general term *benign nephrosclerosis* is frequently used to encompass all the various renal changes that are encountered in the benign phase of hypertension.

Gross appearance of the kidneys The kidneys may appear normal, particularly if the hypertension is of short duration. Sometimes they are reduced in size and the subcapsular surface is finely granular (Fig. 9.34). Any reduction affects both kidneys equally, is moderate and is more often noted in cases reported from the USA than in those from Europe; it is rare for either kidney to weigh less than 100 g. If there is much atherosclerosis there may also be some coarser scars. On the cut surface there is thinning of the cortex of those kidneys that are smaller than normal and because of the loss of renal mass there is an apparent increase in the amount of fat in the hilum. The arcuate arteries are prominent and appear thick walled.

Light microscopy A variable number of glomeruli show wrinkling and thickening of the capillary basement membrane. In some, this process is accompanied by collapse and shrinkage of the tuft, loss of tuft cellularity, obliteration of the capillary lumen and progressive accumulation of collagen on the inner aspect of Bowman's capsule. These changes are the result of ischaemia and are identical to those that occur in ageing (see

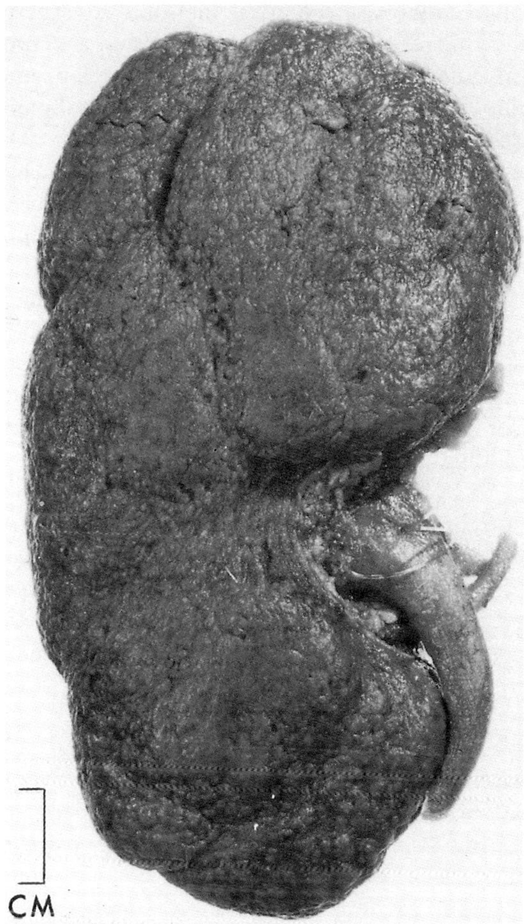

Fig. 9.34 Kidney in long-standing benign phase of hypertension showing the finely granular subcapsular surface. The few coarser scars are caused by concomitant atherosclerosis. There is incidental persistence of traces of fetal lobation.

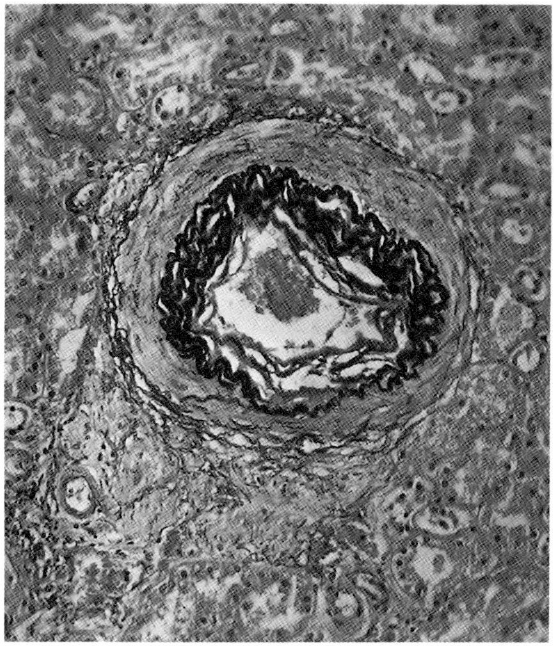

Fig. 9.35 Benign phase of hypertension. Interlobular artery with reduplication of the internal elastic lamina and fibrous thickening of the intima.
Elastic-Van Gieson × 140

p. 25). Continuation of the process leads to shrinkage and global sclerosis of glomeruli. These glomerular changes are focal and even in small kidneys many glomeruli are normal. The shrunken glomeruli may eventually disappear leaving only arteriolae rectae verae, which are channels that open when the glomerular capillary bed is obliterated, joining the afferent and efferent arterioles.

The tubules are atrophic in the depressions between the macroscopic granules. The granules are formed of hypertrophic and dilated tubules. The atrophic tubules have a thickened basement membrane and are usually related to ischaemic glomeruli. Homogeneous eosinophilic casts are sometimes seen in the tubules.

The intima of the interlobular arteries is thickened by fibrous tissue and there is *reduplication of the internal elastic lamina*, with the presence of multiple, roughly concentric, layers of elastic fibres (Fig. 9.35). The media is usually normal. The wall of some of the afferent arterioles may be thickened and largely replaced by a homogeneous material that stains with eosin and periodic acid-Schiff and may contain very fine droplets of lipid. This material is referred to as *hyalin* and the process of alteration in the arteriolar walls is *hyalinization* or *hyalinosis*. It characterizes the condition of *arteriolosclerosis* and occurs focally along the length of the afferent arterioles (Fig. 9.36). It is not pathognomonic of the benign phase of hypertension: it may occur in patients with normal blood pressure as part of the ageing process (see p. 25); it is particularly marked in diabetes mellitus. The efferent arterioles may be involved, but rarely, and not to the degree that is observed in diabetes (see p. 338). The arcuate and larger arteries may be normal but if there is generalized atherosclerosis they may show fibrous intimal

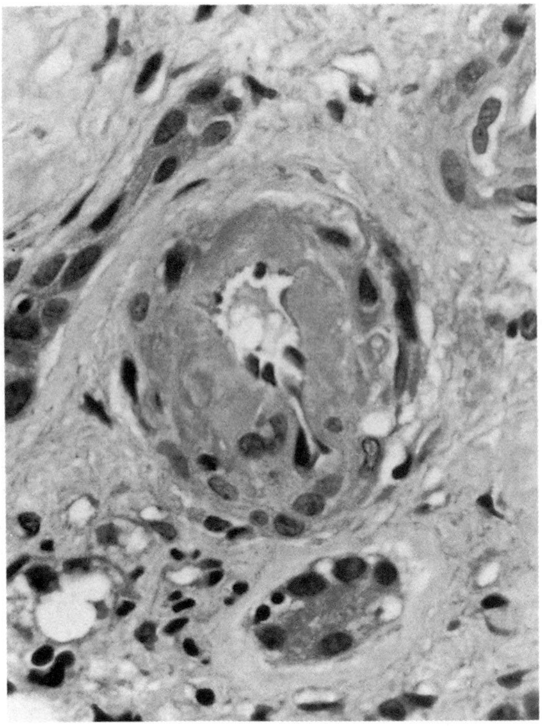

Fig. 9.36 Benign phase of hypertension. Renal arteriole showing hyaline thickening of the wall and reduction of the lumen.
Haematoxylin-eosin × 400

thickening, fraying and splitting of the internal elastic lamina and, sometimes, an increase in the thickness of the media.

The juxtaglomerular apparatus is usually normal in size. The granularity of its cells is normal or decreased.

There is usually some focal fibrosis in the areas of tubular atrophy. Groups of chronic inflammatory cells may also be present, particularly in relation to sclerotic glomeruli.

The renal pelvis is usually normal, in contrast to the changes that affect it in cases of chronic pyelonephritis (see p. 440).

Electron microscopy The thickened intima of those interlobular arteries that show elastic reduplication consists of smooth muscle cells, myointimal cells and fine collagen fibrils. Basement membrane and bundles of elastic fibrils separate the intimal cells. Lipofuscin is common in the smooth muscle and myointimal cells.[155]

The hyaline in the arteriolar walls consists of uniformly very finely granular, moderately electron-dense material that often includes small, osmiophilic droplets of fat and membrane-bound vesicles (Fig. 9.37). The collections of hyaline are predominantly intimal and subendothelial but small deposits are also commonly seen between the smooth muscle cells of the media. Sometimes most of the vessel wall consists of this material.[156]

The wrinkled and collapsed capillary basement membrane of the ischaemic glomeruli is often thickened by 50% or more. The collagen fibrils in the fibrous tissue that accumulates on the inner side of Bowman's capsule show typical periodicity.[157]

Immunofluorescence/immunoperoxidase microscopy The hyalinized arterioles contain granular C3 in their walls. This may be accompanied by IgM. The mesangium also often contains small amounts of granular IgM and C3.[158]

Changes in other organs

Heart The heart responds to the sustained pressure overload in hypertension by gradually increasing its muscle mass. After many years of hypertension it is common for the heart to weigh about 500 g; the greater part of the increase is in the left ventricle. The increase in the weight of the heart and in the thickness of the wall of the left ventricle correlates well with the systemic blood pressure.[159]

Brain High blood pressure is detrimental to the brain. It exerts its effect directly, by accelerating cerebral atherosclerosis and by initiating a series of pathological changes in small arteries and arterioles, or indirectly, by causing cardiac failure, which results in a lowering of cerebral performance.

The relative frequency and severity of atherosclerosis of the intracranial arteries are increased in patients with hypertension.[160] Atherosclerosis also appears in vessels of a calibre smaller than those that generally are affected among normotensive people. These changes predispose to cerebral infarction.

Hyalinization and fibrinoid necrosis ('lipohyalinosis') followed by microaneurysm formation

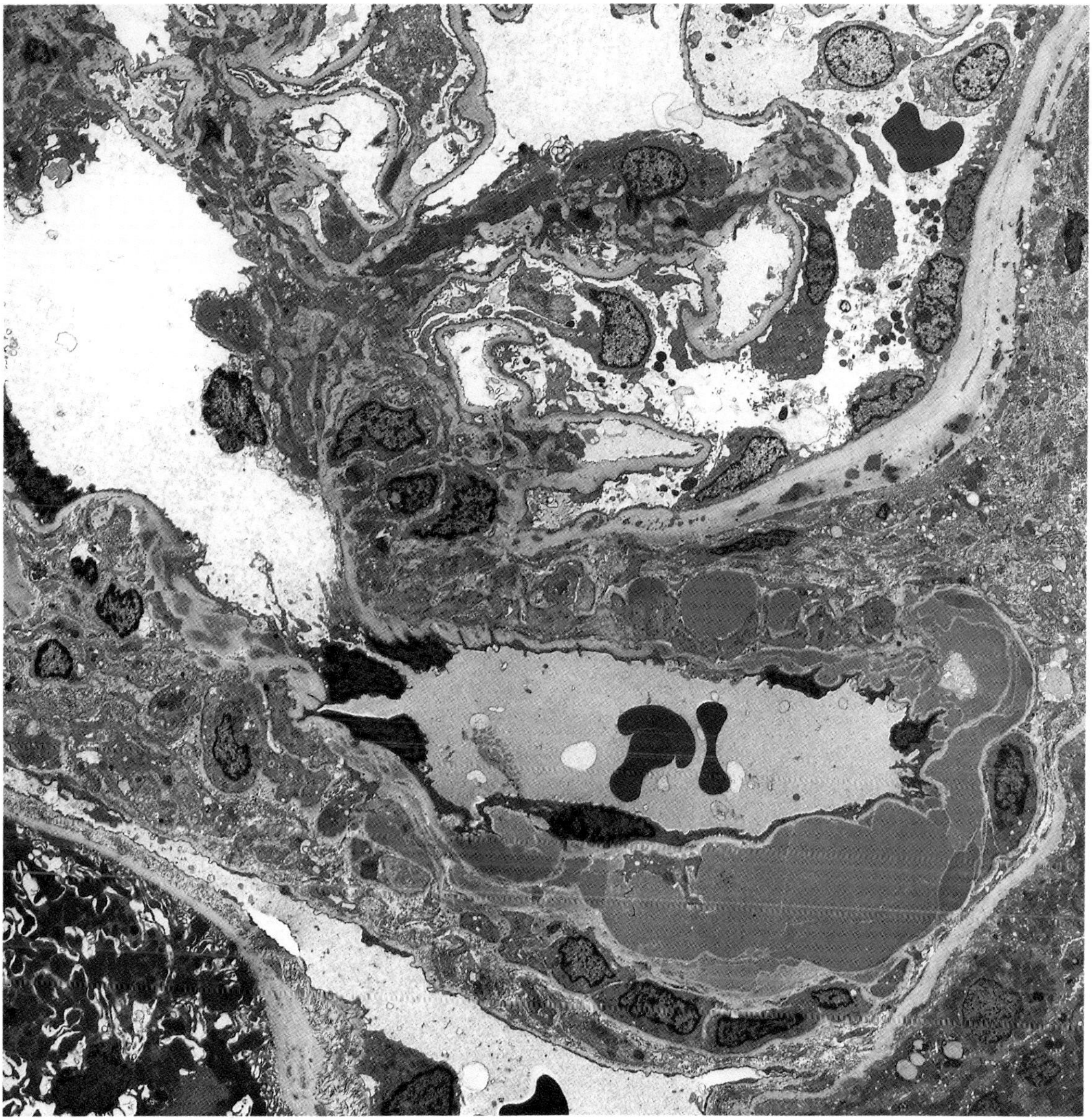

Fig. 9.37 Benign phase of hypertension. Electron micrograph of afferent arteriole at point where it enters glomerulus. The vessel wall contains collections of homogeneous very finely granular hyaline. ×2000

are found in the small arteries and arterioles in the putamen, thalamus, pons, cerebellum and cerebral subcortex.[161] An affected vessel may rupture, causing intracerebral haemorrhage, or segmental arterial occlusion may cause small infarcts that, as they resolve, leave lacunae. The severity of the damage inflicted on these vessels by sustained benign phase hypertension may be related to the fact that the cerebral arteries have relatively thin walls and are the least muscular arteries in the body.

Hypertension has a contributory role in the development and eventual rupture of 'berry' aneurysms at the site of congenital deficiency of the structure of the cerebral arterial vasculature, particularly in the circle of Willis and its branches.

Other viscera Hyalinization of the walls of arterioles is seen commonly in the pancreas, less frequently in the adrenals and the liver and rarely in other organs. Hyaline arteriolosclerosis is common in the spleen, but this is also true of normotensive individuals.

The eyes show the changes of arteriosclerotic and hypertensive retinopathy.

Differential diagnosis

The commonest problem is to differentiate the changes that occur in the kidneys with *increasing age* (see p. 25) from those due to raised blood pressure. The distinction is purely quantitative and impossible to make without knowing the patient's age; even with this knowledge it may be difficult because of the wide differences in the effects of the ageing process on the arteries and arterioles in normotensive individuals.

Arteriolar hyalinization is also a feature of the kidneys in *diabetes mellitus* (see p. 338) but in this disease it is much more severe than in the benign phase of hypertension and the efferent arteriole is invariably involved; in benign nephrosclerosis hyalinization of the efferent arteriolar wall is unusual and rarely pronounced.

Prognosis

The results of the prospective study in Framingham, Massachusetts, USA, showed that the mortality of individuals who had an arterial pressure over 140/90 mmHg on at least three occasions was more than double the mortality in those whose arterial pressure was below that level.[162] A similar increase in risk has been calculated from life insurance data. A claim that hypertensive patients with low levels of circulating renin have a lower morbidity has not been substantiated.

The excess mortality associated with benign phase hypertension is chiefly due to cardiac and other circulatory disease and to cerebral haemorrhage. In particular coronary atherosclerosis and congestive cardiac failure are more common in the hypertensive. The risk of morbidity or death at any level of arterial pressure is accentuated by the presence of other adverse factors such as a raised serum cholesterol, cigarette smoking and diabetes mellitus.

Treatment with antihypertensive drugs reduces the morbidity to one-third of that of the untreated over 5 years. The greatest benefit is to patients with diastolic pressures of 110 mmHg or higher.[163]

Malignant phase of hypertension

Clinical features

The malignant phase of essential hypertension usually follows a period of the benign phase, the mean duration of which is about 8 years.[164] A few patients appear to be in the malignant phase from the beginning of the illness. This phase usually presents between the ages of 35 and 40 years; black patients may develop malignant phase hypertension in their late twenties. Men are affected more often than women.[165] The initial symptoms are commonly acute headache, weight loss and impairment of vision. Occasionally, the patient presents with anuria or with hypertensive encephalopathy. The diastolic blood pressure is usually above 130 mmHg, but this is by no means invariable; in one series 12% had a blood pressure below 180/120 mmHg.[166] The main feature that distinguishes the malignant phase of essential hypertension from the benign phase is the presence of bilateral papilloedema, accompanied by retinal haemorrhages and exudates.

The urine usually contains protein and red cells. The proteinuria is great enough in some patients to produce a nephrotic syndrome; the haematuria may be gross.[165] Renal function rapidly deteriorates during the course of the illness. Left ventricular hypertrophy is frequently observed on the electrocardiogram and cardiac arrhythmias are seen in about a third of the patients.[166] There may be a microangiopathic haemolytic anaemia and a secondary haemolytic uraemic syndrome (see p. 281).[167]

Approximately 75% of patients with malignant hypertension have an increase in plasma renin activity and, consequently, have raised plasma angiotensin II, and aldosterone levels.[166] The oversecretion of aldosterone is accompanied by hypokalaemia.

If untreated the majority of patients in the malignant phase of essential hypertension die in uraemia within a year of the onset of the symptoms.

Renal changes

The combination of changes that occur in the kidneys in the malignant phase of hypertension is often referred to as *malignant nephrosclerosis*.

Gross appearance of the kidneys The size of the kidneys varies greatly from case to case and depends upon the occurrence and duration of a pre-existing benign phase of hypertension. The subcapsular surface of those kidneys that are of normal size is smooth; that of the shrunken ones is finely granular. Petechial haemorrhages are usually present. The cut surface of the cortex is mottled red and yellow.

Light microscopy The most important change is *fibrinoid necrosis* of some of the arterioles (Figs 9.38, 9.39). The wall of the affected part of the vessels is replaced by eosinophilic granular material that gives the staining reactions of fibrin. Red blood cells are often seen in the necrotic tissue and there may be small periarteriolar haemorrhages. The arteriolar lumen is frequently reduced and it may be obliterated by superimposed thrombus. Usually there is minimal or no associated inflammation; rarely neutrophil granulocytes and mononuclear cells are present in and around the wall: the term *necrotizing arteriolitis* is sometimes used to describe this change (Fig. 9.40). Later, varying degrees of fibrosis, recanalization and repair occur in affected arterioles.

The interlobular arteries are drastically narrowed or obliterated by marked intimal thickening in the form of concentric layers of elongated cells in a basophilic matrix that stains for mucin (Figs 9.41, 9.42); sometimes there are relatively

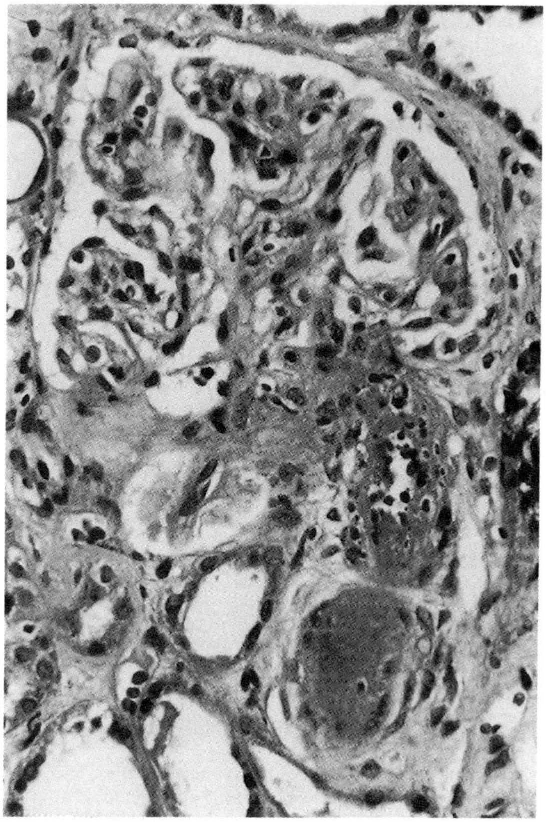

Fig. 9.39 Malignant phase of hypertension. There is necrosis of the afferent arteriole; associated inflammation is minimal.
Haematoxylin-eosin × 280

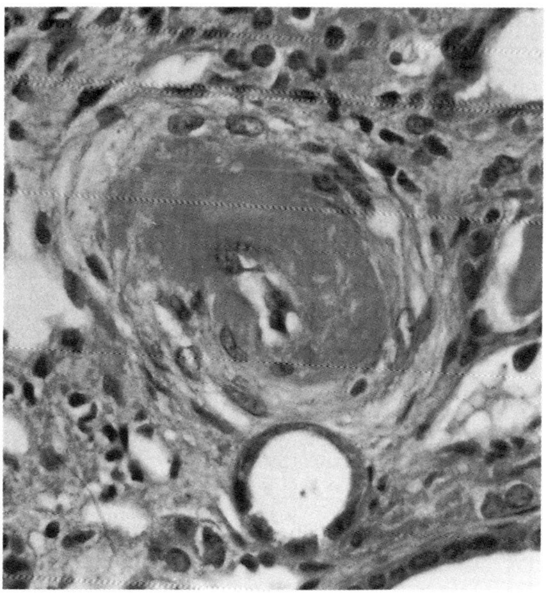

Fig. 9.38 Malignant phase of hypertension. The arteriole shows fibrinoid necrosis of its wall.
Haematoxylin-eosin × 200

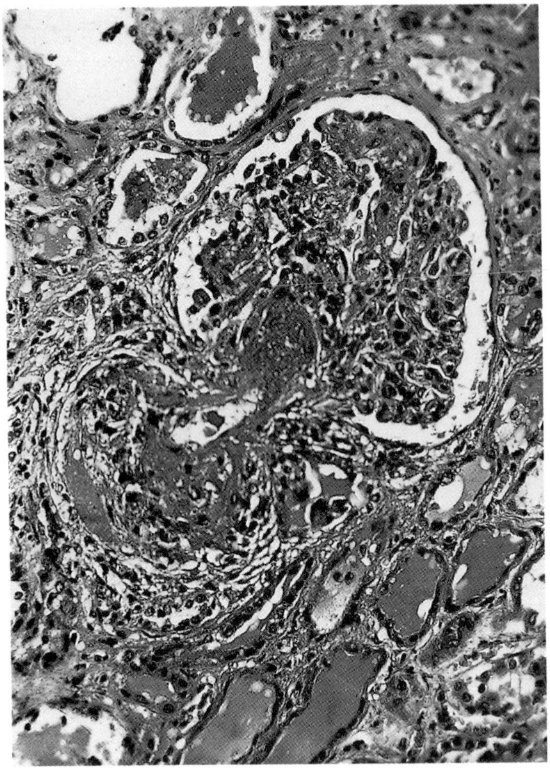

Fig. 9.40 Malignant phase of hypertension. There is necrosis of the afferent arteriole and axial part of the glomerulus. Neutrophil granulocytes and mononuclear cells are present in and around the vessel wall (necrotizing arteriolitis). This degree of associated inflammation is rare in malignant hypertension.
Haematoxylin-eosin × 240

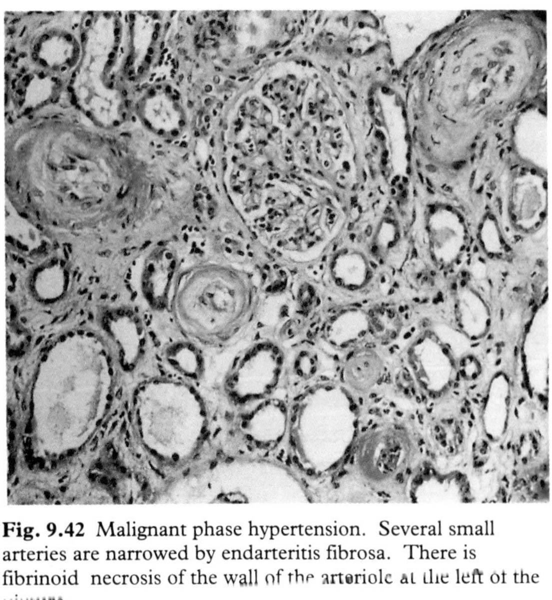

Fig. 9.42 Malignant phase hypertension. Several small arteries are narrowed by endarteritis fibrosa. There is fibrinoid necrosis of the wall of the arteriole at the left of the picture.
Haematoxylin-eosin × 150

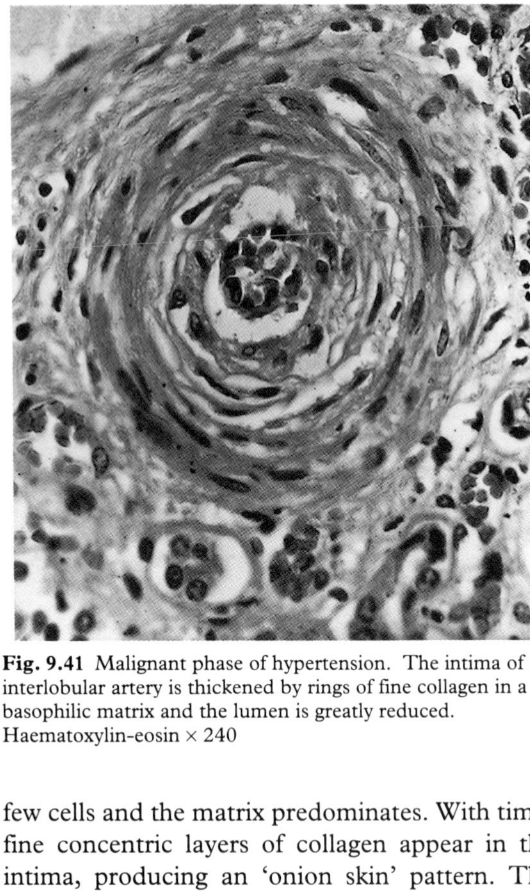

Fig. 9.41 Malignant phase of hypertension. The intima of an interlobular artery is thickened by rings of fine collagen in a basophilic matrix and the lumen is greatly reduced.
Haematoxylin-eosin × 240

few cells and the matrix predominates. With time, fine concentric layers of collagen appear in the intima, producing an 'onion skin' pattern. The terms *endarteritis fibrosa* and *productive endarteritis* have been used to describe these obliterative changes in the interlobular arteries. The amount of collagen is greatest in the kidneys of patients who have been treated with antihypertensive drugs. Small amounts of lipid are occasionally present in the thickened intima. The media is thinner than normal.

The arcuate and larger arteries often appear normal; sometimes there is fibrous intimal thickening and reduplication of their internal elastic lamina. Fibrinoid necrosis is not seen.

Up to 30% of the glomeruli show segmental fibrinoid necrosis of the tuft, usually in continuity with a necrotic afferent arteriole (Fig. 9.40). There is often increased cellularity of part of the tuft, including the presence of neutrophil granulocytes and some proliferation of the parietal epithelial cells in relation to the foci of necrosis. Epithelial crescents may be present, but seldom in large numbers. Lipid and hyaline droplets are common in the visceral epithelial cells and, to a smaller extent, in the parietal epithelial cells. Glomerular necrosis is much less widespread in the kidneys of patients treated with antihypertensive drugs: focal and segmental glomerular scars may be present in those cases and may represent old, healed, necrotic lesions.

In addition, there are often some glomeruli that show ischaemic wrinkling of the capillary walls and some that are sclerotic. These are commonest in shrunken kidneys and are probably an effect of a preceding phase of benign hypertension. In most cases at least half the glomeruli are normal. The juxtaglomerular apparatus is enlarged and the granularity of its cells is increased.[168] These changes are probably related to increased blood levels of renin and angiotensin that occur in the malignant phase of hypertension.

Atrophy and disappearance of groups of tubules are pronounced features of this disease. The atrophic tubules may contain homogeneous eosinophilic casts and red cell casts. Occasionally there are tiny cortical infarcts. Scattered collections of chronic inflammatory cells and some neutrophil granulocytes may be present in the interstitium.

These changes may be superimposed upon those of the benign phase of hypertension in patients whose acute illness was preceded by a period of slowly rising blood pressure.

Electron microscopy[169–171] The walls of arterioles affected by fibrinoid necrosis contain collections of granular, electron-dense material, fibrillar material with a periodicity characteristic of fibrin or fibrinogen, red cells and red cell fragments (Fig. 9.43). Many of the muscle cells of the media are necrotic. Mural or obstructive thrombi, formed of fibrin and platelets, are commonly present.

The thickened intima in the vessels that show endarteritis fibrosa consists of a loose laminar arrangement of basement membrane material, smooth muscle cells and myointimal cells. The electron-lucent spaces between the concentric basement membrane lamellae have a uniform floccular pattern. Collagen fibrils and elastic fibrils are also present but are only prominent in older lesions.

In the glomeruli the focal necrotic lesions are characterized by plugging of the capillaries by platelets, fibrin and necrotic debris. There is rupture of the capillary basement membrane, with extravasation of red cells and neutrophil granulocytes into the mesangium and Bowman's space and deposition there of fibrin.

Immunofluorescence/immunoperoxidase microscopy Fibrinogen is usually present in the walls of necrotic arterioles, in the necrotic foci in glomeruli and in the thickened intima of interlobular arteries. It is often accompanied by IgM and complement components, particularly C3. Other immunoglobulins are less commonly found.

Other organ changes

Fibrinoid necrosis of the arterioles occurs, in order of descending frequency, in the pancreas, adrenals, gastrointestinal tract, brain, eyes, heart and liver. It may also be seen in the spleen but in that organ is difficult to separate from the normal ageing changes. Arteriolar fibrinoid necrosis is not found in the vessels of muscles and skin. In the intestines the arteriolar lesions may cause small foci of haemorrhagic necrosis. The eyes show the changes of hypertensive retinopathy.

The heart is enlarged, mainly by left ventricular hypertrophy. The adrenals are almost always larger than normal.

Differential diagnosis

The morphological lesions produced by the malignant phase of hypertension may be indistinguishable from those seen in *systemic sclerosis* (see p. 243) and the *haemolytic uraemic syndrome* (see p. 283). Clinically there is usually no difficulty in excluding systemic sclerosis, but it can be hard to distinguish the changes of malignant phase hypertension from those of the haemolytic uraemic syndrome. If there are widespread subendothelial electron-lucent deposits in the glomeruli then the haemolytic uraemic syndrome is the more likely diagnosis.

In those rare cases of malignant phase hypertension with necrotizing arteriolar lesions polyarteritis may need to be considered. *Classical polyarteritis* (see p. 268) can usually be excluded

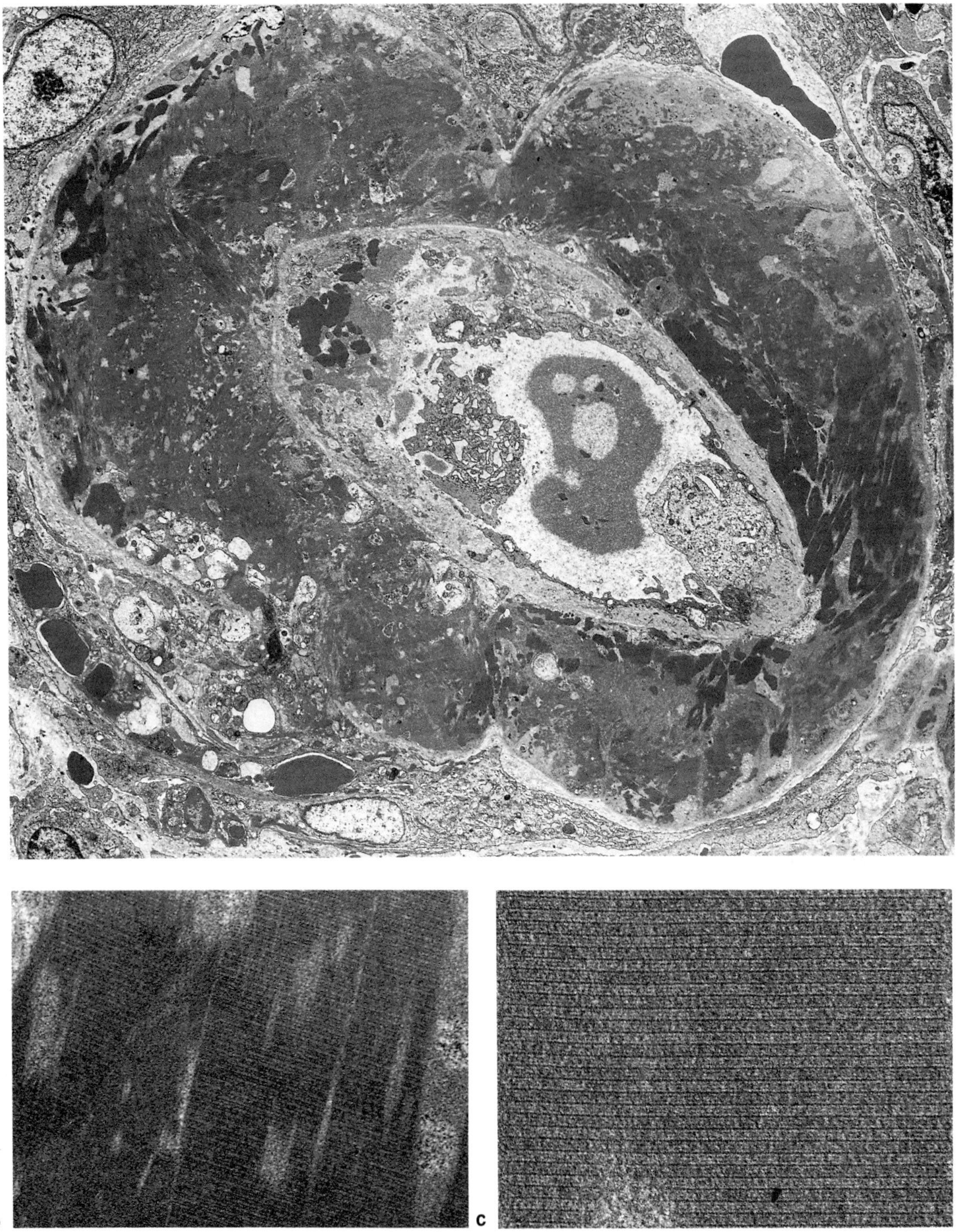

a b c

Fig. 9.43 Malignant phase hypertension. (**a**) Electron micrograph of arteriole affected by fibrinoid necrosis. Many of the muscle cells of the media are necrotic and the wall contains collections of electron-dense material. (**b**) Much of the electron-dense material is fibrillar. (**c**) The fibrils have a periodicity characteristic of fibrin or fibrinogen.
(**a**) × 2460; (**b**) × 25 620; (**c**) × 79 500

because in this condition necrosis is found in the arcuate and larger arteries which are not affected by necrosis in the malignant phase of hypertension. *Microscopic polyarteritis* (see p. 273) may be more difficult to distinguish but in the majority of patients with this condition the glomerular lesions are the only evidence of vasculitis within the kidney. In the 20% who have an arteriolitis or arteritis or both, the presence of autoantibodies to antigens in the cytoplasm of neutrophil granulocytes should be sought in the patient's circulation (see p. 272). Such antibodies are present in microscopic polyarteritis, Wegener's granulomatosis and the Churg–Strauss syndrome; they are absent in malignant nephrosclerosis that is not secondary to one of those conditions.

The arteries and arterioles in *radiation nephritis* (see p. 477) also develop changes indistinguishable from those of malignant phase hypertension but in most instances the clinical history should allow differentiation.

Renal transplantation

Patients whose kidneys are destroyed by malignant phase hypertensive nephrosclerosis sometimes undergo renal transplantation after a variable period on dialysis. The initiation of dialysis removes the retention of sodium and water and in many patients the level of blood pressure falls. In some patients, however, raised renin levels persist or rise further, aggravating the hypertension; when the elevated blood pressure cannot be controlled medically, bilateral nephrectomy, which removes the source of renin, often brings about easier control. The successful transplantation of a normal kidney that can handle sodium and water and is not ischaemic restores and maintains normal blood pressure and induces reversal of the cardiac and retinal complications of hypertension in approximately 75% of patients.[172] It has been suggested that those who receive a kidney from a donor with a family history of essential hypertension are more likely to remain hypertensive after transplantation;[173] this is difficult to prove because there are many other factors that can cause hypertension in the patient with a renal transplant (see p. 662).

Prognosis

In the absence of treatment only 25–30% of patients survive more than 1 year.[165,166] The emergency intensive use of antihypertensive drugs to lower the arterial pressure as rapidly as possible without further impairing blood perfusion to vital organs has greatly improved the outlook for these patients. Four year survival rates of 50% have been recorded.[174] If the patient is in renal failure the problem is much greater. Effective control of the blood pressure may lead to a transitory decline in function followed by a rise in glomerular filtration rate; if the renal failure continues to progress dialysis may be necessary to tide the patient over and allow time to see whether reduction of the blood pressure is going to improve perfusion of the kidneys and ultimately renal function.[175]

Pathogenesis

The rapidly rising blood pressure of the malignant phase of hypertension causes focal but widespread spasm of the walls of the arterioles and small arteries.[176] The segments of intense constriction alternate with segments that are dilated. In the overdistended segments the permeability of the wall is increased and insudation of plasma proteins, particularly fibrinogen, occurs.[177,178] The infiltrating plasma compresses and destroys adjacent smooth muscle cells. The alterations produced in the vessel wall are those referred to as fibrinoid necrosis when they are seen in tissue sections examined by light microscopy. Whether the raised levels of circulating angiotensin II that occur in patients in the malignant phase of essential hypertension play any direct part in producing this increased permeability is unknown. In addition to producing arterial constriction angiotensin II increases the permeability of vascular walls by causing the endothelial cells to contract, which opens the endothelial junctions. Present evidence indicates that the degree of increased permeability in the dilated segments is related to the mean arterial pressure and not to the amount of circulating angiotensin II.

Endarteritis fibrosa is probably the result of organization of mural thrombi that form in consequence of endothelial damage.[179]

SECONDARY HYPERTENSION

High blood pressure in either the benign or the malignant phase may in 5–10% of cases occur as a manifestation of a recognized disease. In such cases it is described as secondary hypertension. Most of the conditions that may lead to secondary hypertension are effects or side-effects of therapeutic drugs, diseases of the kidneys or urinary tract, adrenal disorders, coarctation of the aorta, complications of pregnancy or diseases of the central nervous system.

Despite the rarity of secondary hypertension, it is important to search for an underlying condition because some can be reversed by treatment, sparing the patient from a lifetime of taking antihypertensive drugs. Equally important, the underlying disease may need treatment in its own right, e.g. obstructive uropathy, analgesic kidney damage or diabetes mellitus.

The lesions produced in the kidney in secondary hypertension depend on the gradiant of the rise in blood pressure and are the same as those previously described under the benign and malignant phases of essential hypertension (see p. 306 and 311).

Hypertension secondary to administration of drugs

The oral contraceptive pill and hypertension

Hypertension caused by oral contraceptive pills is one of the commoner forms of secondary hypertension. In one series it accounted for 4% of all cases of hypertension.[180] Benign phase hypertension has been reported to occur in 2–5% of white women taking combined oestrogen-progestogen preparations for a period of 5 years. The rise in pressure occurred in most cases within 2 years.[181] Malignant phase hypertension is rare. Hypertension seldom occurs in women taking 'minipills' which contain only progestogen. The mechanism by which oral contraceptives increase blood pressure is unknown. Withdrawal of the drug usually corrects the pressure within 3 months. The effect of oral contraceptive pills on the kidneys is discussed further on page 524.

Corticosteroids and hypertension

Routine treatment with prednisolone in doses of 10–15 mg/day in adults probably does not contribute in a major way to hypertension. Higher doses, used for example in the first few days after renal transplantation or during rejection (see p. 662), can cause hypertension. The mechanisms are not yet established but probably include sensitization of arterioles to other circulating vasoconstrictor agents and a mineralocorticoid effect.[182]

Cyclosporin-associated hypertension

Doses of cyclosporin currently used in the treatment of recipients of renal, liver, heart, heart-lung and bone marrow allografts, are associated with a progressive and relentless increase in the frequency of hypertension.[183,184] Similarly, cyclosporin-related hypertension occurs in non-transplant patients treated for various immunological diseases.[185] In one series after liver transplantation the incidence of hypertension progressively increased from 15% at 3 months to 64% at 4 years in patients maintained on cyclosporin.

It is not known precisely how cyclosporin causes hypertension. A long-continued vasoconstriction seems likely,[186] but the hypertension does not appear to be directly related to activation of the renin–angiotensin–aldosterone system. In the first year, the vasoconstriction and hypertension are reversible when cyclosporin is discontinued;[186] after this they become progressively more difficult to counter as irreversible ischaemic changes appear in the kidney.

Cyclosporin nephrotoxicity is discussed further on page 520.

Other drugs associated with hypertension

Liquorice, eaten regularly in large quantities, may cause hypertension. The explanation is that liquorice contains glycyrrhetinic acid which suppresses both plasma renin activity and plasma aldosterone. The hypertension is accompanied by hypokalaemic alkalosis; both effects are reversed within a few weeks of stopping the liquorice intake. *Carbenoxolone sodium*, which is a disodium succinate of glycyrrhetinic acid given for peptic ulcer, produces the same features. Hypertension may also complicate the use of *monoamine oxidase inhibitors, sympathomimetics* and the prolonged application of *mineralocorticoid ointment* to the skin.

Hypertension secondary to diseases of the kidneys and urinary tract

Renal vascular disease and renal artery stenosis

Approximately 3% of all cases of hypertension are caused by renal vascular disease.[180] The most common of these conditions is an *atheromatous lesion* compromising the origin of one or both renal arteries (see p. 294). Because the renal arterial lesion is only one aspect of a generalized disease the prognosis for this group of patients is poor, whether they are treated medically or by renovascular surgery. *Dysplasias of renal arteries* are much less frequent causes of hypertension. The most usual form is medial fibroplasia with aneurysms (see p. 296). This disorder occurs most often in young women. The response to reconstructive surgery or balloon angioplasty is generally very good and the long-term prognosis is much better than for atheromatous renal vascular disease.

Classical polyarteritis (see p. 267), *Takayasu's arteritis* (see p. 280), *giant cell arteritis* (see p. 280), *neurofibromatosis* (see p. 111), *aneurysms of the renal artery* (see p. 299), *embolism of the renal artery* (see p. 301), *arteriovenous fistulae* and *trauma to the renal artery* may all cause hypertension. *Distortion and narrowing of the renal arterial supply by a mass*, such as a tumour or cyst, may also rarely induce hypertension.

The indications for investigating the possibility of renal vascular disease as the cause of hypertension include the occurrence of hypertension in patients under the age of 30 years, hypertension in the malignant phase, and the rare combination of severe hypertension with hyponatraemia, hypokalaemia, polyuria, polydipsia and weight loss, suggesting activation of the renin–aldosterone system. Other clinical pointers are drug-resistant hypertension and sudden hypertension following trauma which might have involved the renal areas.[187]

Chronic renal disease

Approximately 2% of all cases of hypertension are caused by chronic renal disease.[180] The renal conditions likeliest to be complicated by hypertension are *glomerulonephritis* (see p. 126), *chronic pyelonephritis* (including reflux nephropathy; see p. 439) and *polycystic disease* (see p. 61). Less frequent causes are the renal lesions of diabetes mellitus (see p. 329), systemic lupus erythematosus (see p. 225), systemic sclerosis (see p. 242), the haemolytic uraemic syndrome (see p. 281), thrombotic thrombocytopenic purpura (see p. 288), amyloidosis (see p. 344), obstruction of the urinary tract (see p. 467), radiation nephritis (see p. 477), analgesic nephropathy (see p. 458) and cortical necrosis (see p. 303), but almost any chronic renal condition may be responsible. Only some of the patients with these disorders develop hypertension. The mechanisms by which the blood pressure is caused to rise are not known.

In a few cases the underlying condition can be successfully treated and the blood pressure returned to normal. In the majority the raised blood pressure can usually be controlled by ultrafiltration haemodialysis and sodium restriction; this suggests that excess sodium and water play a major role in these cases, increased cardiac output rather than increased total peripheral resistance causing the hypertension.

Acute glomerulonephritis

In the acute stage of diffuse endocapillary proliferative glomerulonephritis (see p. 142) hypertension usually is transient and stays in the benign phase but may occasionally enter the malignant phase. Hypertension that occurs in the acute nephritic exacerbations of diffuse mesangiocapillary glomerulonephritis (see p. 164) tends to be persistent. The rise in the blood pressure in acute glomerulonephritis is probably on the basis of sodium and water retention, perhaps with inappropriately high renin activity in the plasma, but the evidence is incomplete.

Hypertension secondary to renin-secreting tumours

Juxtaglomerular cell tumours (see p. 605) produce excess renin which causes hypertension that tends to be severe, although malignant hypertension is uncommon. The tumour is usually small and easily missed on angiography. The blood pressure returns to normal when the tumour is removed. Renin may also be secreted by nephroblastomas (see p. 587) and renal adenocarcinomas (see p. 569) and result in hypertension.

Very rarely hypertension is due to renin production by carcinomas of extrarenal tissues such as pancreas, lung, liver or Fallopian tube.

Hypertension secondary to diseases of the adrenal glands

Recognized diseases of the adrenals are responsible for less than 1% of cases of hypertension.[188]

Primary aldosteronism (Conn's syndrome)

Primary aldosteronism is a useful designation for a rare group of primary or apparently primary diseases of the adrenals that are characterized by excessive and relatively autonomous production of the mineralocorticoid aldosterone. It is associated with three types of adrenal lesion: adrenal cortical adenoma in about 58%, nodular hyperplasia of the adrenal cortex in about 40% and carcinoma in 2%. Primary aldosteronism accounts for approximately 0.4% of all cases of hypertension.[188] The hypertension may be severe but malignant hypertension is uncommon. The excess secretion of aldosterone probably causes retention of sodium in the distal portion of the renal tubules. The total volume of body water, including the volume of extracellular fluid and of plasma, is expanded, causing hypertension and suppression of renin release. Potassium is exchanged, and lost in the urine, resulting in hypokalaemia and a metabolic acidosis.

When an adrenal cortical adenoma is responsible its surgical removal results in cure of the hypertension in 50–60% of cases. In most cases of nodular hyperplasia of the adrenal cortex treatment with spironolactone improves control of arterial pressure; in a small minority of patients, treatment with a glucocorticoid reverses the hypertension and accompanying hypokalaemia and hyperaldosteronism.

Cushing's syndrome[189]

Cushing's syndrome results from overproduction of cortisol as an accompaniment either of ACTH-induced adrenal cortical hyperplasia or of an adrenal cortical tumour. Hypertension occurs in about 85% of patients with the syndrome; in a few cases it may be severe. The mechanisms by which cortisol increases the arterial pressure are still uncertain. In most cases the blood pressure falls after adrenalectomy or pituitary surgery but if the hypertension has been present for a long time it may persist in spite of such treatment.

Hypertension secondary to phaeochromocytoma[190]

The phaeochromocytoma is a neoplasm of the chromaffin cells of the adrenal medulla or, rarely, of chromaffin tissue elsewhere in the body. It occurs with equal frequency in both sexes and may be found at any time in life but is most commonly diagnosed between the ages of 20 and 50 years. Some 10% of adrenal phaeochromocytomas are malignant. The tumour cells elaborate catecholamines; noradrenaline usually predominates, but adrenaline and dopamine may be present in large amounts. The release of these substances into the blood in abnormal amounts is commonly episodic, resulting in paroxsysmal attacks of headache, sweating, palpitation, pallor and hypertension. In about 50% of adults with the disease the hypertension is sustained, although episodic acute rises in pressure are common. If a major product of the tumour is adrenaline the diastolic pressure may remain normal or low even though the systolic pressure is raised. Paroxsysms occur spontaneously; they may also be provoked by exercise and a variety of other factors.

The definitive diagnosis of phaeochromocytoma depends upon a biochemical demonstration of overproduction of catecholamines. Assays of noradrenaline and adrenaline (or of their metabolites normetadrenaline, metadrenaline and vanillylmandelic acid) in 24-hour urine samples or the radioenzymic or high performance liquid chromatography assay of noradrenaline and adrenaline in plasma are used.

Surgical removal of the tumour is curative in approximately 75% of cases; in the others there is either no substantial fall in the blood pressure or hypertension recurs. Failure to respond is sometimes because removal of the tumours has been incomplete but more often it is probably because of persisting hypertensive vascular changes in the kidneys.

Hypertension secondary to inborn errors of corticosteroid synthesis and metabolism

11-β-Hydroxysteroid dehydrogenase deficiency This rare disorder leads to hypertension and hypokalaemia, but with suppression of both aldosterone and renin. The hypertension is aggravated by treatment with hydrocortisone.

Congenital adrenal hyperplasia Among the various conditions associated with adrenal hyperplasia *11-β-hydroxylase deficiency* and *17-α-hydroxylase deficiency* cause hypertension and hypokalaemia. In both conditions renin activity in plasma is suppressed by an overproduction of deoxycorticosterone because of biochemical defects in normal steroid synthesis.

Hypertension secondary to excess endogenous production of deoxycorticosterone and corticosterone

Occasional cases have been recorded of hypertension and hypokalaemia caused by isolated overproduction of deoxycorticosterone. The same syndrome may rarely result from a carcinoma of the adrenal cortex producing an excess of corticosterone.

Coarctation of the aorta[191]

In coarctation of the aorta the blood pressure is reduced in the upper part of the body and normal, low or slightly raised in the lower part. The condition is usually diagnosed in children but it may present later in life with hypertension. The diagnosis is confirmed by radiological examination, if necessary including aortography, or computerized tomographic scanning. After surgical excision of the narrowed segment of aorta the blood pressure usually decreases but is rarely restored to normal levels.

Hypertension complicating pregnancy[192]

Pre-eclamptic toxaemia

In this condition secondary hypertension develops at about the 30th to the 36th week of pregnancy (see p. 554). There is usually a dramatic recovery within a short time of the delivery of the child although in a few cases the blood pressure remains elevated.

In about 30% of women who have had pre-eclampsia the blood pressure rises some years later. It is still not clear whether this is the result of the pre-eclamptic toxaemia or whether pre-eclampsia no more than hastens the onset of essential hypertension in women who otherwise would have acquired it at a later date.

Idiopathic postpartum acute renal failure

This disease is sometimes accompanied by severe hypertension (see p. 565). The fact that hypertension is not invariably present suggests that it is the consequence of the renal lesions rather than their cause.

Hypertension complicating diseases of the central nervous system

The systemic arterial blood pressure rises in cases of increased intracranial pressure. This is presumably a compensatory response to the increasing resistance to the flow of blood through the brain.

Thrombosis of the basilar artery may lead to sudden development of hypertension: it is debatable whether this is compensatory or due to direct disturbance of centres rendered relatively ischaemic by the circulatory disturbance resulting from the thrombosis. There is little evidence, however, that primary organic changes in the central nervous system produce persistent high blood pressure.

Cases of tetanus and poliomyelitis may be complicated by hypertension.

Other causes of secondary hypertension

Alcohol addiction, acute lead poisoning and acute intermittent porphyria can all give rise to secondary hypertension. The hypertension that occurs in acute lead poisoning is due to blunting of β-adrenoceptor-mediated functions with consequent vasoconstriction.[193]

BEHÇET'S DISEASE

Although Behçet's original definition of the disease that bears his name was confined to three features – uveitis with oral and genital ulceration[194] – it is now recognized that many other organs may be involved[195] and that the pathological hallmark of the disease is a leucocytoclastic vasculitis involving primarily the veins, venules and capillaries.

Behçet's disease is most common in Japan where it affects 1 in 10 000 people. Its incidence is also high in countries bordering the Mediterranean and in the Middle East: Italy, Greece, Turkey, Israel, Egypt, Algeria, Tunisia, Lebanon, Syria, Jordan and Saudi Arabia. In Britain the prevalence is approximately 1 in 170 000 people and in the USA about 1 in 800 000.

The disorder may develop at any time; most commonly the onset is between the ages of 20 and 30 years. Male predominance is reported in most series of cases.

Approximately a third of patients with Behçet's disease have proteinuria, haematuria or both; these urinary changes may be intermittent.[196] In at least seven cases a *diffuse crescentic glomerulonephritis* has been reported;[197] in two other patients there was a *focal necrotizing glomerulonephritis* but the percentage of glomeruli with crescents is not given. Three of the seven kidneys with diffuse crescentic glomerulonephritis showed granules of IgG in the glomeruli with subepithelial electron-dense deposits in the one case that was examined by electron microscopy; in four no deposits were shown by immunofluorescence or electron microscopy. Two of the nine patients died and six of the seven survivors developed chronic renal failure; only one had normal renal function 6 months after the onset of the glomerulonephritis. At least seven cases of *IgA nephropathy* have also been described in Japan,[198] but IgA nephropathy is common in that country (see p. 157). Other renal complications that have been reported in Behçet's disease include amyloidosis of AA type, and tubulointerstitial nephritis.

Glomerulonephritis in Behçet's disease seems to be too frequent to be coincidental. Its pathogenesis is not known, but it is probably one of the rarer vasculitic manifestations of the disease. The cause of Behçet's disease is unknown. There is a significant association with HLA-B51 and a viral aetiology has often been claimed, but attempts to isolate a responsible virus from patients have failed.

CONGENITAL HEART DISEASE (POLYCYTHAEMIC NEPHROPATHY)

Approximately 40% of children with cyanotic congenital heart disease have glomerular enlargement (*glomerulomegaly*);[199] in 5% the mesangium is expanded and hypercellular.[200] The renal changes are particularly common in those with transposition of the great vessels.[200] Similar glomerular alterations occasionally occur in patients with idiopathic pulmonary hypertension, chronic cor pulmonale, cardiac fibroelastosis and rheumatic mitral stenosis; they are also found in cystic fibrosis associated with hypoxia (see page 117) and in children living at high altitude.[201]

There are few clinical manifestations; mild proteinuria with or without haematuria has been described most frequently. The natural history of the renal changes is not known because there are no longitudinal studies.

The glomeruli are up to twice their usual diameter[202] but the kidneys are normal in weight because the tubules are not increased in size.[199] In a few studies electron microscopy has shown either diffuse or focal segmental thickening of the glomerular capillary basement membranes in addition to an increase in the amount of mesangial matrix and in the number of mesangial cells. Immunofluorescence microscopy has revealed IgM in the mesangium of some kidneys.[203]

The cause of the renal changes is not known. The one feature common to most of the cases is polycythaemia and there is a positive relationship between the severity of this condition and the glomerular size.[199] Moreover, very similar glomerular changes can be produced in rats by making them polycythaemic.[201]

Because of this association with polycythaemia it has been proposed that all these renal alterations should be grouped together under the term *'polycythaemic nephropathy'*.[201] How polycythaemia might induce glomerulomegaly and mesangial cell proliferation is not clear: a mechanism involving glomerular hyperfiltration and hyperperfusion has been suggested.[201]

Glomerulomegaly also occurs in patients who are enormously fat; it is sometimes accompanied by proteinuria and polycythaemia.[201,204]

REFERENCES

Classical polyarteritis

1. Chen KTK. Renal limited polyarteritis nodosa. Hum Pathol 1987; 18: 1074–1075
2. Rose GA. The natural history of polyarteritis. Br Med J 1957; 2: 1148–1152.
3. Frohnert PP, Sheps SG. Long term follow-up study of polyarteritis nodosa. Am J Med 1967; 43: 8–14.
4. Leib ES, Restivo C, Paulus HE. Immunosuppressive and corticosteroid therapy of polyarteritis nodosa. Am J Med 1979; 67: 941–947.
5. Hind CRK, Savage CO, Winearls CG, Pepys MB. Objective monitoring of disease activity in polyarteritis by measurement of serum C reactive protein concentration. Br Med J 1984; 288: 1027–1030.
6. Gocke DJ, Hsu K, Morgan C, Bombardieri S, Lockshin M, Christian CL. Association between polyarteritis and Australian antigen. Lancet 1970; 2: 1149–1153.
7. Savage COS, Winearls CG, Jones S, Marshall PD, Lockwood CM. Prospective study of radioimmunoassay for antibodies against neutrophil cytoplasm in diagnosis of systemic vasculitis. Lancet 1987; 1: 1389–1393.
8. D'Agati V, Chandler P, Nash M, Mancilla-Jimenez R. Idiopathic microscopic polyarteritis nodosa. ultrastructural observations on the renal vascular and glomerular lesions. Am J Kidney Dis 1986; 7: 95–110.
9. Ralston DE, Kvale WF. The renal lesions of periarteritis nodosa. Proc Mayo Clin 1949; 24: 18–27.
10. Sergent JS, Lockshin MD, Christian CL, Gocke DJ. Vasculitis with hepatitis B antigenaemia: long-term observations in nine patients. Medicine (Baltimore) 1976; 55: 1–18.
11. Montalbert C, Carvallo A, Broumand D, Noble D, Anstine LA, Currier CB. Successful renal transplantation in polyarteritis nodosa. Clin Nephrol 1980; 14: 206–209.
12. Adu D, Howie AJ, Scott DGI, Bacon PA, McGonigle RJS, Michael J. Polyarteritis and the kidney. Q J Med 1987; 62: 221–237.
13. Christian CL, Sergent JS. Vasculitis syndrome. clinical and experimental models. Am J Med 1976; 61: 385–392.
14. Serra A, Cameron JS, Turner DR et al Vasculitis affecting the kidney: presentation, histopathology and long–term outcome. Q J Med 1984; 53: 181–207.
15. Michalak T. Immune complexes of hepatitis B surface antigen in the pathogenesis of polyarteritis nodosa. A study of seven necropsy cases. Am J Pathol 1978; 90: 619–632.
16. Drueke T, Barbanel C, Jungers P et al. Hepatitis B antigen-associated periarteritis nodosa in patients undergoing long-term hemodialysis. Am J Med 1980; 68: 86–90.

Microscopic polyarteritis

17. Davson J, Ball J, Platt R. The kidney in periarteritis nodosa. Q J Med 1948; 17: 175–202.
18. Croker BP, Lee T, Gunnells JC. Clinical and pathologic features of polyarteritis nodosa and its renal-limited variant: primary crescentic and necrotizing glomerulonephritis. Hum Pathol 1987; 18: 38–44.
19. Savage COS, Winearls CG, Evans DJ, Rees AJ, Lockwood CM. Microscopic polyarteritis: presentation, pathology and prognosis. Q J Med 1985; 56: 467–483.
20. Feehally J, Wheeler DC, Walls J, Jones S, Lockwood CM, Savage COS. A case of microscopic polyarteritis associated with antineutrophil cytoplasmic antibodies. Clin Nephrol 1987; 27: 214–215.
21. Venning MC, Arfeen S, Bird AG. Antibodies to neutrophil cytoplasmic antigen in systemic vasculitis. Lancet 1987; 2: 850 (letter).
22. Wainwright J, Davson J. The renal appearances in the microscopic form of periarteritis nodosa. J Pathol Bacteriol 1950; 62: 189–196.
23. Cameron JS. Effect of the recipient's disease on the results of transplantation (other than diabetes mellitus). Kidney Int 1983; 23: suppl 14, S24–33.
24. Lockwood CM, Bakes D, Jones S, Whitaker KB, Moss DW, Savage COS. Association of alkaline phosphatase with an autoantigen recognised by circulating anti-neutrophil antibodies in systemic vasculitis. Lancet 1987; 2: 716–720.
25. Fauci AS, Haynes BF, Katz P. The spectrum of

vasculitis. Clinical, pathologic, immunologic and therapeutic considerations. Ann Intern Med 1978; 89: 660–676.

Wegener's granulomatosis

26. Wegener F. Über generalisierte septische Gefässerkrankungen. Verh Dtsch Pathol Ges 1936; 29: 202–210.
27. Fauci AS, Haynes BF, Katz P, Wolff SM. Wegener's granulomatosis: prospective clinical and therapeutic experience with 85 patients for 21 years. Ann Intern Med 1983; 98: 76–85.
28. Pinching AJ, Lockwood CM, Pusell BA et al. Wegener's granulomatosis: observations on 18 patients with severe renal disease. Q J Med 1983; 52: 435–460.
29. Elkon KB, Sutherland DC, Rees AJ, Hughes GRV, Batchelor JR. HLA-antigen frequencies in systemic vasculitis: increase in HLA-DR2 in Wegener's granulomatosis. Arthritis Rheum 1983; 26: 102–105.
30. Lüdemann J, Gross WL. Autoantibodies against cytoplasmic structures of neutrophil granulocytes in Wegener's granulomatosis. Clin Exp Immunol 1987; 69: 350–357.
31. Weiss MA, Crissman JD. Renal biopsy findings in Wegener's granulomatosis: segmental necrotizing glomerulonephritis with glomerular thrombosis. Hum Pathol 1984; 15: 943–956.
31a. Katzenstein A, Carrington CB, Liebow AA. Lymphomatoid granulomatosis. A clinico-pathologic study of 152 cases. Cancer 1979; 43: 360–373.
32. Curtis JJ, Diethelm AG, Herrera GA, Crowell WT, Whelchel JD. Recurrence of Wegener's granulomatosis in a cadaver renal allograft. Transplantation 1983; 36: 452–454.
33. Steinman TI, Jaffe BF, Monaco AP, Wolff SM, Fauci AS. Recurrence of Wegener's granulomatosis after kidney transplantation. Successful reintroduction of remission with cyclophosphamide. Am J Med 1980; 68: 458–460.
34. Abbott F, Jones S, Lockwood CM, Rees AJ. Autoantibodies to glomerular antigens in patients with Wegener's granulomatosis. Nephrol Dial Transplant 1989; 4: 1–8.
35. Jennette JC, Falk RJ. Antineutrophil cytoplasmic autoantibodies and associated diseases: a review. Am J Kidney Dis 1990; 15: 517–529.
36. Jenne DE, Tschopp J, Lüdemann J, Utecht B, Gross WL. Wegener's autoantigen decoded. Nature 1990; 346: 520.
37. Lüdemann J, Utecht B, Gross WL. Anti-neutrophil cytoplasm antibodies in Wegener's granulomatosis recognize an elastinolytic enzyme. J Exp Med 1990; 170: 357–362.

Churg-Strauss syndrome

38. Churg J, Strauss L. Allergic granulomatosis, allergic angiitis and periarteritis nodosa. Am J Pathol 1951; 27: 277–301.
39. Rose GA, Spencer H. Polyarteritis nodosa. Q J Med 1957; 26: 43–81.
40. Lanham JG, Elkon KB, Pusey CD, Hughes GR. Systemic vasculitis with asthma and eosinophilia: a clinical approach to the Churg–Strauss syndrome. Medicine (Baltimore) 1984; 63: 65–81.
41. Wathen CW, Harrison DJ. Circulating anti-neutrophil antibodies in systemic vasculitis. Lancet 1987; 1: 1037 (letter).
42. Lockwood CM. Reply to correspondence on anti-neutrophil-cytoplasm antibodies in Wegener's granulomatosis. Lancet 1987; 1: 1489–1490.
43. Clutterbuck EJ, Evans DJ, Pusey CD. Renal involvement in Churg–Strauss syndrome. Nephrol Dial Transplant 1990; 5: 161–167.
44. Chumbley LC, Harrison EG, De Remee RA. Allergic granulomatosis and angiitis (Churg–Strauss syndrome). Mayo Clin Proc 1977; 52: 477–484.
45. Phanuphak P, Kohler PF. Onset of polyarteritis nodosa during allergic hyposensitization treatment. Am J Med 1980; 68: 479–485.

Giant cell (temporal) arteritis

46. Elling H, Kristensen IB. Fatal renal failure in polymyalgia rheumatica caused by disseminated giant cell arteritis. Scand J Rheumatol 1980; 9: 206–208.
47. Lie JT. Disseminated visceral giant cell arteritis: histopathologic description and differentiation from other granulomatous vasculitides. Am J Clin Pathol 1978; 69: 299–305.

Takayasu's arteritis

48. Hall S, Barr W, Lie JT, Stanson AW, Kazmier FJ, Hunder GG. Takayasu arteritis. A study of 32 North American patients. Medicine (Baltimore) 1985; 64: 89–99.
49. Wiggelinkhuizen J, Cremin BJ. Takayasu's arteritis and renovascular hypertension in childhood. Pediatrics 1978; 62: 209–217.
50. Weiss RA, Jodorkovsky R, Weiner S et al. Chronic renal failure due to Takayasu's arteritis: recovery of renal function after nine months of dialysis. Clin Nephrol 1982; 17: 104–107.
51. Sinaiko A, Najarian J, Michael AF et al. Renal autotransplantation in the treatment of bilateral renal artery stenosis. Relief of hypertension in an eight year old boy. J Pediatr 1973; 83: 309–314.
52. Yoshimura M, Kida H, Saito Y et al. Peculiar glomerular lesions in Takayasu's arteritis. Clin Nephrol 1985; 24: 120–127.

Haemolytic uraemic syndrome

53. Gasser C, Gautier E, Stech A, Siebermann RE, Oechslin R. Hämolytisch–urämische Syndrome: bilaterale Nierenrindennekrose bei akuten erworbenen hämolytischen Anämien. Schweiz Med Wochenschr 1955; 85: 905–909.
54. Fong JSC, De Chadarevian JP, Kaplan BS. Hemolytic uremic syndrome: current concepts and management. Pediatr Clin North Am 1982; 29: 835–856.
55. Cantrell JE, Phillips TM, Schein PS. Carcinoma associated hemolytic uremic syndrome: a complication of mitomycin C chemotherapy. J Clin Oncol 1985; 3: 723–734.
56. Neild G. The haemolytic uraemic syndrome: a review. Q J Med 1987; 63: 367–376.
57. Sachdev Y, Morley AR, Wiklinson R et al. Addison's disease with renal microangiopathy and renal failure (a new syndrome). Q J Med 1977; 46: 151–162.
58. Loomis LJ, Aronson AJ, Rudinsky R, Spargo BH. Hemolytic uremic syndrome following bone marrow

transplantation: a case report and review of the literature. Am J Kidney Dis 1989; 14: 324–328.
59. Siegler RL. Hemolytic uremic syndrome: clinical observations from the Southwest Pediatric Nephrology Study Group and laboratory findings from the University of Utah Health Sciences Center. In: Murakami K, Kitagawa T, Yabuta K, Sakai T, eds. Recent advances in pediatric nephrology. Oxford: Excerpta Medica, 1987: 581–586.
60. Couser WG, Salant DJ, Adler S, Bernard DB, Stilmant MM. Acute renal failure associated with renal vascular disease, vasculitis, glomerulonephritis and nephrotic syndrome. In: Brenner BM, Lazarus JM, eds. Acute renal failure. Philadelphia: WB Saunders 1983: 339–341.
61. Karmali MA, Petric M, Lim C, Fleming PC, Arbus GS, Lior H. The association between idiopathic haemolytic uraemic syndrome and infection by verotoxin-producing *E. coli.* J Infect Dis 1985; 151: 775–782.
62. Kavi J, Chant I, Maris M, Rose PE. Cytopathic effect of verotoxin on endothelial cells. Lancet 1987; 2: 1035 (letter)
63. Rose PE, Enayat SM, Sunderland R, Short PE, Williams CE, Hill FGH. Abnormalities of factor VIII related protein multimers in the haemolytic uraemic sydrome. Arch Dis Child 1984; 59: 1135– 1140.
64. Drummond KN. Hemolytic uremic syndrome – then and now. N Engl J Med 1985; 312: 116–118.
65. Gianantonio GA, Vitacco M, Mendilaharzu F, Gallo GE, Sojo ET. The hemolytic–uremic syndrome. Nephron 1973; 11: 174–192.
66. De Chadarevian J-P, Kaplan BS. The hemolytic-uremic syndrome of childhood. Perspect Pediatr Pathol 1978; 4: 465–502.
67. Koster F, Levin J, Walker L et al. Hemolytic-uremic syndrome after shigellosis. Relation to endotoxinemia and circulating immune complexes. N Engl J Med 1978; 298: 927–933.
68. Strauss RC, Alexander RW. Post–partum hemolytic uremic syndrome. Obstet Gynecol 1976; 47: 169–173.
69. Clarkson AR, Lawrence JR, Meadows R, Seymour AE. The haemolytic uraemic syndrome in adults. Q J Med 1970; 39: 227– 239.
70. Leung DYM, Moake JL, Havens PL, Kim M, Pober JS. Lytic antiendothelial cell antibodies in haemolytic–uraemic syndrome. Lancet 1988; 2: 183–186.
71. Vitsky BH, Suzuki Y, Strauss L, Churg J. The hemolytic-uremic syndrome. A study of renal pathologic alterations. Am J Pathol 1969; 57: 627–639.
72. Riella MC, George CRP, Hickman RO et al. Renal microangiopathy of the hemolytic-uremic syndrome in childhood. Nephron 1976; 17: 188–203.
73. Morel-Maroger L, Kanfer A, Solez K, Sraer J-D, Richet G. Prognostic importance of vascular lesions in acute renal failure with microangiopathic hemolytic anemia (hemolytic-uremic syndrome): clinicopathologic study in 20 adults. Kidney Int 1979; 15: 548–558.
74. Richardson SE, Karmali MA, Becker LE, Smith CR. The histopathology of the hemolytic uremic syndrome associated with verocytotoxin-producing *Escherichia coli* infection. Hum Pathol 1988; 19: 1102–1108.
75. Habib R, Mathieu H, Royer P. Le syndrome hémolytique et urémique de l'enfant: aspects cliniques et anatomiques dans 27 observations. Nephron 1967; 4: 139–172.
76. Shigematsu H, Dikman SH, Churg J, Grishman E, Duffy JL. Mesangial involvement in hemolytic-uremic syndrome. A light and electron microscopic study. Am J Pathol 1976; 85: 349–362.
77. McCoy RC, Abramowsky CR, Krueger R. The hemolytic uremic syndrome with positive immunofluorescence studies. J Pediatr 1974; 85: 170–174.
78. Gonzalo A, Mampaso F, Gallego N, Bellas C, Sequi J, Ortuno J. Hemolytic uremic syndrome with hypocomplementemia and deposits of IgM and C3 in the involved renal tissues. Clin Nephrol 1981; 16: 193–199.
79. Whittington PF, Friedman AL, Chesney RW. Gastrointestinal disease in the hemolytic–uremic syndrome. Gastroenterology 1979; 76: 728–733
80. Schwartz DL, Becker JM, So HB, Schneider KM. Segmental colonic gangrene: a surgical emergency in the hemolytic–uremic syndrome. Pediatrics 1978; 62: 54–56.
81. Hebert D, Sibley RK, Mauer SM. Recurrence of hemolytic uremic syndrome in renal transplant recipients. Kidney Int 1986; 30: S51–S58.
82. Van den Berg–Wolf MG, Kootte AMN, Weening JJ, Paul LC. Recurrent hemolytic uremic syndrome in a renal transplant recipient and review of the Leiden experience. Transplantation 1988; 45: 248–251.
83. Van Dyck M, Proesmans W, Depraetere M. Hemolytic uremic syndrome in childhood: renal function ten years later. Clin Nephrol 1988; 29: 109–112.
84. Byrnes JJ, Moake JL. Thrombotic thrombocytopenic purpura and the hemolytic-uremic syndrome: evolving concepts of pathogenesis and therapy. Clin Haematol 1986; 15: 413–442.
85. Dungan L, Mai V, Carter A, Carlson JAK, Borczyk A, Karmali M. Outbreaks of gastrointestinal disease – Ontario. Can Dis Wkly Rep 1987; 13: 5–8.
86. Carter AO, Borczyk A, Carlson JAK et al. A severe outbreak of *Escherichia coli* 0157:H7–associated haemorrhagic colitis in a nursing home. N Engl J Med 1987; 317: 1496–1500.
87. Zoja C, Furci L, Ghilardi F, Zilio P, Benigni A, Remuzzi G. Cyclosporine–induced endothelial cell injury. Lab Invest 1986; 55: 455–462.
88. Cattell V. Mitomycin–induced hemolytic uremic kidney. An experimental model in the rat. Am J Pathol 1985; 12: 88–95.
89. Remuzzi G, Medda G, Livio M et al. Prostacyclin generation by cultured endothelial cells in haemolytic uraemic syndrome. Lancet 1980; 1: 656–657.
90. Turi S, Beattie TJ, Belch JJF, Murphy AV. Disturbances of prostacyclin metabolism in children with hemolytic–uremic sydnrome and in first degree relatives. Clin Nephrol 1986; 25: 193–198.

Thrombotic thrombocytopenic purpura

91. Moschcowitz E. An acute febrile pleiochromic anemia with hyaline thrombosis of the terminal arterioles and capillaries: an undescribed disease. Arch Intern Med 1925; 36: 89–93.
92. Ridolfi RL, Bell WR. Thrombotic thrombocytopenic purpura. Report of 25 cases and review of the literature. Medicine (Baltimore) 1981; 60: 413–428.
93. Eknoyan G, Riggs SA. Renal involvement in patients with thrombotic thrombocytopenic purpura. Am J Nephrol 1986; 6: 117–131.

94. Remuzzi G. HUS and TTP: variable expression of a single entity. Kidney Int 1987; 32: 292–308.
95. Symmers WStC. Thrombotic microangiopathic haemolytic anaemia (thrombotic microangiopathy). Br Med J 1952; 2: 897–903.
96. Umlas J. Glomeruloid structures in thrombohemolytic thrombocytopenic purpura, glomerulonephritis and disseminated intravascular coagulation. Hum Pathol 1972; 3: 437–441.
97. Machin SJ. Thrombotic thrombocytopenic purpura. Br J Haematol 1984; 56: 191–197.
98. Wu KK, Hall ER, Rossi EC, Papp AC. Serum prostacyclin binding defects in thrombotic thrombocytopenic purpura. J Clin Invest 1985; 75: 168–174.
99. Lian ECY, Harkness DR, Byrnes JJ, Wallach H, Nunez R. Presence of a platelet aggregating factor in the plasma of patients with thrombotic thrombocytopenic purpura (TTP) and its inhibition by normal plasma. Blood 1979; 53: 333–337.
100. Lian ECY, Mui PTK, Siddiqui FA, Chiu AYY, Chiu LLS. Inhibition of platelet-aggregating activity in thrombotic thrombocytopenic purpura plasma by normal adult immunoglobulin G. J Clin Invest 1984; 73: 548–555.
101. Moake JL, Rudy CK, Troll JH et al. Unusually large plasma factor VIII: von Willebrand factor multimers in chronic relapsing thrombocytopenic purpura. N Engl J Med 1982; 307: 1432–1435.
102. Zimmerman SE, Smith FP, Philips TM, Coffey RJ, Schein PS. Gastric carcinoma and thrombotic thrombocytopenic purpura: association with plasma immune complex concentrations. Br Med J 1982; 284: 1432–1434.

Disseminated intravascular coagulation

103. Bell WR. Disseminated intravascular coagulation. Johns Hopkins Med J 1980; 146: 289–299.
104. Robboy SJ, Major MC, Colman RW, Minna JD. Pathology of disseminated intravascular coagulation (DIC). Hum Pathol 1972; 3: 327–343.
105. Leunissen KML. Intravascular coagulation and kidney donation. Transplantation 1986; 42: 307–308.

Loin pain haematuria syndrome

106. Little PJ, Sloper JS, De Wardener HE. A syndrome of loin pain and haematuria associated with disease of peripheral renal arteries. Q J Med 1967; 36: 253–259.
107. Burden RP, Booth LJ, Ockenden BG, Boyd WN, Higgins PM, Aber GM. Intrarenal vascular changes in adult patients with recurrent haematuria and loin pain – a clinical, histological and angiographic study. Q J Med 1975; 44: 433–447.
108. Fletcher P, Al-Khader AA, Parsons V, Aber GM. The pathology of intrarenal vascular lesions associated with the loin-pain-haematuria syndrome. Nephron 1979; 24: 150–154.
109. Naish PF, Aber GM, Boyd WN. C3 deposition in renal arterioles in the loin pain and haematuria syndrome. Br Med J 1975; 3: 746–751.
110. Hutchison SMW, Doig A, Jenkins A McL. Recurrence of loin pain/haematuria syndrome after renal autotransplantation. Lancet 1987; 2: 1501 1502 (letter).
111. Gazdar AF, Dammin GJ. Neural degeneration and regeneration in human renal transplants. N Engl J Med 1970; 283: 222–224.
112. Aber GM, Higgins PM. The natural history and management of the loin pain/haematuria syndrome. Br J Urol 1982; 54: 613–615.
113. Parbtani A, Cameron JS. Platelet involvement in loin pain/haematuria syndrome. Lancet 1979; 1: 1413 (letter).
114. Siegler RL, Brewer ED, Hammond E. Platelet activation and prostacyclin supporting capacity in the loin pain haematuria syndrome. Am J Kidney Dis 1988; 12: 156–160.
115. Smellie SW, Lambert M, Lavenne E, van Cangh PJ. Factor XII deficiency associated with loin pain/haematuria syndrome. Lancet 1987; 2: 1330 (letter).
116. Jones K, Naish PF, Aber GM. Oestrogen-associated disease of the renal microcirculation. Clin Sci Mol Med 1977; 52: 33–42.

Renal vein entrapment syndrome

117. Buschi AJ, Harrison BB, Brenbridge ANAG, Williamson BRJ, Gentry RR, Cole R. Distended left renal vein: CT/sonographic normal variant. Am J Radiol 1980; 135: 339–342.
118. Wolfish NM, McLaine PN, Martin D. Renal vein entrapment syndrome: frequency and diagnosis. A lesson in conservation. Clin Nephrol 1986; 26: 96–100.

Renal vein thrombosis

119. Arneil GC, MacDonald AM, Murphy AV, Sweet EM. Renal venous thrombosis. Clin Nephrol 1973; 1: 119–131.
120. Belman AB. Renal vein thrombosis in infancy and childhood. A contemporary survey. Clin Pediatr (Phila) 1976; 15: 1033–1044.
121. Llach F, Papper S, Massry SG. The clinical spectrum of renal vein thrombosis: acute and chronic. Am J Med 1980; 69: 819–827.
122. Wagoner RD, Stanson AW, Holley KE, Winter CS. Renal vein thrombosis in idiopathic membranous glomerulopathology and nephrotic syndrome: incidence and significance. Kidney Int 1983; 23: 368–374.
123. Llach F. Hypercoagulability, renal vein thrombosis, and other thrombotic complications of nephrotic syndrome. Kidney Int 1985; 28: 429–439.

Atherosclerosis

124. Glagov S, Rowley DA, Kohut RI. Atherosclerosis of human aorta and its coronary and renal arteries: a consideration of some hemodynamic factors which may be related to the marked differences in atherosclerotic involvement of the coronary and renal arteries. Arch Pathol 1961; 72: 558–571.
125. Gore I, McCombs HL, Lindquist RL. Observations on the fate of cholesterol emboli. J Atheroscler Res 1964; 4: 527–535.
126. Ramirez R, O'Neill WM, Lambert R, Bloomer HA. Cholesterol embolization: a complication of angiography. Arch Intern Med 1978; 138: 1430–1432.
127. Smith MC, Ghose MK, Henry AR. The clinical spectrum of renal cholesterol embolization. Am J Med 1981; 71: 174–180.

128. Williams HH, Wall BM, Cooke CR. Case report: reversible nephrotic range proteinuria and renal failure in atheroembolic renal disease. Am J Med Sci 1990; 229: 58–61.

Dysplasias of the renal arteries

129. Harrison EG, McCormack LJ. Pathologic classification of renal arterial disease in renovascular hypertension. Mayo Clin Proc 1971; 46: 161–167.
130. Weinberger MH. Renovascular hypertension. Introduction: questions, current knowledge and clinical implications. Am J Kidney Dis 1985; 5: A85–A92.
131. Nochy D, Barres D, Camilleri JP, Bariety J, Corvol P, Menard J. Abnormalities of renin containing cells in human glomerular and vascular renal diseases. Kidney Int 1983; 23: 375–379.
132. Graham PC, Stewart HVA, Downie I, Lindop GBM. The distribution of renin-containing cells in kidneys with renal artery stenosis – an immunocytochemical study. Histopathology 1990; 16: 347–355.

Aneurysms of the renal arteries

133. Poutasse EF. Renal artery aneurysms: their natural history and surgery. Trans Am Assoc Genitourin Surg 1965; 57: 55–64.
134. Ratcliff NF. Renal vascular disease: pathology of large blood vessel disease. Am J Kidney Dis 1985; 5: A93–A103.

Renal cortical necrosis

135. Kleinknecht D, Grünfeld J-P, Gomel PC, Moreau J-F, Garcia-Torres R. Diagnostic procedures and long-term prognosis in bilateral renal cortical necrosis. Kidney Int 1973; 4: 390–400.
136. Matlin RA, Gary NE. Acute cortical necrosis. Case report and review of the literature. Am J Med 1974; 56: 110–118.
137. Sheehan HL, Moore HC. Renal cortical necrosis and the kidney of concealed accidental haemorrhage. Oxford: Blackwell, 1952.
138. Deutsch V, Frankel O, Drory Y, Eliahou H, Braf ZF. Bilateral renal cortical necrosis with survival through the acute phase with a note on the value of selective nephroangiography. Am J Med 1971; 150: 828–834.
139. Duff GL, More RH. Bilateral cortical necrosis of the kidneys. Am J Med Sci 1941; 201: 428–450.
140. MacGillivray I. Combined renal and anterior pituitary necrosis. J Obstet Gynaecol Br Comm 1950; 57: 924–930.

Essential hypertension

141. Miall WE, Chinn S. Screening for hypertension: some epidemiological observations. Br Med J 1974; 3: 595–600.
142. Sleight P. Differences between casual and 24hr blood pressures. J Hypertens 1985; 3: suppl 2, S19–23.
143. Kannell WB, Castelli WP, McNamara PM, McKee A, Feinleib M. Role of blood pressure in the development of congestive heart failure. The Framingham Study N Engl J Med 1972; 287: 781–787.
144. Gubner RS. Systolic hypertension: a pathogenetic entity. Significance and therapeutic considerations. Am J Cardiol 1962; 9: 773–776.
145. Thomas CB. Genetic pattern of hypertension in man. In: Onesti G, Kim KE, Moyer JH, eds. Hypertension: mechanisms and management. New York: Grune and Stratton, 1973: 67–73.
146. Pickering GW. The inheritance of arterial pressure. In: Stamler J, Stamler R, Pullman TN, eds. The epidemiology of hypertension. New York: Grune and Stratton, 1967: 18–27.
147. Folkow B. Physiological aspects of primary hypertension. Physiol Rev. 1982; 62: 347–504.
148. MacGregor GA. Sodium is more important than calcium in essential hypertension. Hypertension 1985; 7: 628–637.
149. Semple PF, Lever AF. Glimpses of the mechanisms of hypertension. Br Med J 1986; 293: 901–902.
150. Blaustein MP, Hamlyn JM. Role of natriuretic factor in essential hypertension: an hypothesis. Ann Intern Med 1983; 98: 785–792.
151. Robinson BF. Altered calcium handling as a primary cause of hypertension. J Hypertens 1984; 2: 453–460.
152. Robertson JIS. Salt, volume and hypertension: causation or correlation? Kidney Int 1987; 32: 590–602.
153. Tierney WM, McDonald CJ, Luft FC. Renal disease in hypertensive adults: effect of race and type II diabetes mellitus. Am J Kidney Dis 1989; 13: 485–493.
154. Tuck ML, Williams GH, Cain JP, Sullivan JM, Dluhy RA. Relation of age, diastolic pressure and known duration of hypertension to presence of low renin essential hypertension. Am J Cardiol1973; 32: 637–642.
155. Jones DB. Arterial and glomerular lesions associated with severe hypertension. Light and electron microscopic studies. Lab Invest 1974; 31: 303–313.
156. Biava CG, Dyrda I, Genest J, Bencosme SA. Renal hyaline arteriosclerosis. An electron microscope study. Am J Pathol 1964; 44: 349–363.
157. Thoenes W, Rumpelt HJ. The obsolescent renal glomerulus – collapse, sclerosis, hyalinosis, fibrosis. A light and electron microscopical study on human biopsies. Virchows Arch [A] 1977; 377: 1–15
158. Captopril Collaborative Study Group. Does captopril cause renal damage in hypertensive patients? Lancet 1982; 1: 988–990.
159. Kannell WB, Castelli WP, McNamara PM, McKee A. Feinleib M. Role of blood pressure in the development of congestive heart failure. The Framingham Study. N Engl J Med 1972; 287. 781 787.
160. Baker AB, Resch JA, Loewenson RB. Hypertension and cerebral atherosclerosis. Circulation 1969; 39: 701–710.
161. Rothemund E, Frische M. Klinische-pathologische Studie zur Entstehung der intracerebralen Gefässhyalinose bei Hypertonie. Arch Psychiatr Nervenkr 1973; 217: 195–206.
162. Kannel WB, Wolf PA, Verter J, McNamara PM. Epidemiologic assessment of the role of blood pressure in stroke. The Framingham Study. JAMA 1970; 214: 301–310.
163. Veterans Administration Co-operative Study. Effects of treatment on morbidity in hypertension – results in patients with a diastolic blood pressure averaging 90 through 114 mm Hg. JAMA 1970; 213: 1143–1152.
164. Milliez P, Tcherdakoff P, Samarcq P, Rey LP. The natural course of malignant hypertension. In: Bock KD, Cottier PT, eds. Essential hypertension: an international symposium. Berlin: Springer, 1960; 214.
165. Kincaid-Smith P, McMichael J, Murphy EA. The

clinical course and pathology of hypertension with papilloedema (malignant hypertension). Q J Med 1958; 27: 117–152.
166. Ramos O. Malignant hypertension: the Brazilian experience. Kidney Int 1984; 25: 209–217.
167. Linton AL, Gavras H, Gleadle RI et al. Microangiopathic haemolytic anaemia and the pathogenesis of malignant hypertension. Lancet 1969; 1: 1277–1282.
168. Bohle A, Helmchen U, Grund KE et al. Malignant nephrosclerosis in patients with hemolytic uremic syndrome (primary malignant nephrosclerosis). Curr Top Pathol 1977; 65: 81–113.
169. Jones DB. Arterial and glomerular lesions associated with severe hypertension. Lab Invest 1974; 31: 303–313.
170. Hsu H-C, Churg J. The ultrastructure of mucoid 'onion skin' intimal lesions in malignant nephrosclerosis. Am J Pathol 1980; 99: 67–80.
171. Kashgarian M. Pathology of small blood vessel disease in hypertension. Am J Kidney Dis 1985; 5: A104–110.
172. Curtis JJ, Luke RG, Dustan KP et al. Remission of essential hypertension after renal transplantation. N Engl J Med 1983; 309: 1009–1015.
173. Guidi E, Bianch G, Dallosta V et al. Influence of familial hypertension of the donor on the blood pressure and antihypertensive therapy of kidney graft recipients. Nephron 1982; 30: 318–323.
174. Hood B, Orndahl G, Bjork S. Survival and mortality in malignant (grade IV) and grade III hypertension. Trends in consecutive, actively treated groups. Acta Med Scand 1970; 187: 291–302.
175. Lawton WJ. The short term course of renal function in malignant hypertensives with renal insufficiency. Clin Nephrol 1982; 17: 277–283.
176. Byrom FB. The pathogenesis of hypertensive encephalopathy and its relation to the malignant phase of hypertension. Experimental evidence from the hypertensive rat. Lancet 1954; 2: 201–211.
177. Giese J. The pathogenesis of hypertensive vascular disease. Copenhagen: Munksgaard, 1966.
178. Hill GS, Heptinstall RH. Steroid-induced hypertension in the rat. A microangiographic and histologic study on the pathogenesis of hypertensive vascular and glomerular lesions. Am J Pathol 1968; 52: 1–50.
179. Kincaid-Smith P. Participation of intravascular coagulation in the pathogenesis of glomerular and vascular lesions. Kidney Int 1975; 7: 242–253.

Secondary hypertension

180. Ferguson RK. Cost and yield of the hypertensive evaluation. Experience of a community-based referral clinic. Ann Intern Med 1975; 82: 761–765.
181. Weir RJ, Briggs E, Mack A, Naismith L, Taylor L, Wilson E. Blood pressure in women taking oral contraception. Br Med J 1974; 1: 533–535.
182. Rudnick MR, Bastl CP, Narins RG. Diagnostic approaches to hypertension. Contemp Issues Nephrol (Hypertension) 1981; 8: 270–339.
183. De Plaen JF, Ferrant A, Uten M, Uyttebrouck A, Michaux JL, van Ypersele De Strihou C. Cyclosporine A induced hypertension in bone marrow transplantation. Kidney Int 1985; 28: 394(abst).
184. O'Grady JG, Forbes A, Rolles K, Calne RY, Williams R. An analysis of cyclosporine efficiency and toxicity after liver transplantation. Transplantation 1988; 45: 575–579.
185. Palestine AG, Nussenblatt RB, Chan CC. Side effects of systemic cyclosporine in patients not undergoing transplantation. Am J Med 1984; 77: 652–656.
186. Curtis JJ, Luke RG, Jones P, Dubovsky EV, Whelchel JD, Diethelm AG. Cyclosporine in therapeutic doses increases renal allograft vascular resistance. Lancet 1986; 2: 477–479.
187. Hunt JC, Sheps SG, Harrison EG, Strong CS, Bernatz PE. Renal and renovascular hypertension: a reasoned approach to diagnosis and management. Arch Intern Med 1984; 133: 988–999.
188. Ferris JB, Brown JJ, Fraser R, Lever AF, Robertson JIS. Primary aldosterone excess. Conn's syndrome and similar disorders. In: Robertson JIS, ed. Handbook of hypertension; vol 2: Clinical aspects of secondary hypertension. Amsterdam: Elsevier, 1983: 132–161.
189. Krakoff LR, Elyovich F. Cushing's syndrome and exogenous glucocorticoid hypertension. Clin Endocrinol Metab 1981; 10: 479–488.
190. Manger WM, Gifford RW. Hypertension secondary to phaeochromocytoma. Bull NY Acad Med 1982; 58: 139–158.
191. De Leeuw PW, Birkenhager WH. Coarctation of the aorta. In: Robertson JIS, ed. Handbook of hypertension; vol 2: Clinical aspects of secondary hypertension. Amsterdam: Elsevier, 1983: 1–17.
192. Redman CWG. Hypertension in pregnancy: a case discussion. Kidney Int 1987; 32: 151–160.
193. Bertel O, Buhler FR, Ott J. Lead induced hypertension: blunted beta-adrenoceptor-mediated functions. Br Med J 1978; 1: 551.

Behçet's disease

194. Behçet H. Über rezidivierende, aphthose, durch ein Virus verursachte Geschwüre am Mund, am Auge und an den Genitalien. Dermatol Wochenschr 1937; 36: 1152–1157.
195. International Study Group for Behçet's Disease. Criteria for diagnosis of Behçet's disease. Lancet 1990; 335: 1078–1080.
196. Rosenthal T, Weiss P, Gafni J. Renal involvement in Behçet's syndrome. Arch Intern Med 1978; 138: 1122–1124.
197. Tietjen DP, Moore WJ. Treatment of rapidly progressive glomerulonephritis due to Behçet's syndrome with intravenous cyclophosphamide. Nephron 1990; 55: 69–73.
198. Furukawa T, Hisao O, Furuta S, Shigematsu H. Henoch–Schönlein purpura with nephritis in a patient with Behçet's disease. Am J Kidney Dis 1989; 13: 497–500.

Congenital heart disease

199. Bauer WC. Rosenberg BF. A quantitative study of glomerular enlargement in children with tetralogy of Fallot. A condition of glomerular enlargement without an increase in renal mass. Am J Pathol 1960; 37: 695–712.
200. Spear GS. Glomerular alterations in cyanotic congenital heart disease. Bull Johns Hopkins Hosp 1960; 106: 347–367.

201. Weidner N, Buckalew VM. Polycythemic nephropathy. In: Tisher CC, Brenner, BM, eds. Renal pathology with clinical and functional correlations. Philadelphia: JB Lippincott 1989; 2: 1427–1436.
202. Ingelfinger JR, Kissane JM, Robson AM. Glomerulomegaly in a patient with cyanotic congenital heart disease. Am J Dis Child 1970; 120: 69–71.
203. Burke JR, Glasgow EF, McCredie DA, Powell HR. Nephropathy in cyanotic congenital heart disease. Clin Nephrol 1977; 7: 38–42.
204. Cohen AH. Massive obesity and the kidney: a morphologic and statistical study. Am J Pathol 1975; 81: 117–130.

10

K. A. Porter

The kidneys in metabolic disorders

DIABETES MELLITUS

Diabetes mellitus is a syndrome comprising several disturbances of carbohydrate, fat and protein metabolism. A characteristic feature is permanent impairment of glucose tolerance caused by a defect in the secretion and/or the action of insulin. Liver and tissue use of glucose is lessened and the blood glucose level rises. The hyperglycaemia leads to increased glomerular filtration of glucose; the renal threshold is exceeded and glycosuria occurs.

The disorder may occasionally be secondary to loss of the pancreatic islets through inflammation, surgery, tumours or iron overload (haemochromatosis) or from endocrine disturbances such as Cushing's syndrome, acromegaly or phaeochromocytoma. But usually it is idiopathic.

Idiopathic diabetes mellitus is divided into two variants, *insulin-dependent diabetes mellitus* (IDDM, Type I or juvenile-onset diabetes mellitus) and *non-insulin-dependent diabetes mellitus* (NIDDM, Type II or adult-onset diabetes mellitus).[1]

Ninety per cent of patients who have diabetes have the non-insulin-dependent variant. The lack of insulin is not severe but secretion is deranged and the tissues are unable to respond properly to the hormone. There may be abnormalities of insulin receptors and failure of post-receptor transmission. This form of the disease usually appears in adults over 40 years old. Both genetic and environmental factors seem to be involved in its aetiology; about 60% of the patients are obese. There is no HLA linkage. Non-insulin-dependent diabetes mellitus is most prevalent in rich communities. In Britain it affects approximately 1.8% of people who are over 19 years old.

Ten per cent of patients who have diabetes have the insulin-dependent variant. There is an absolute lack of insulin and these patients require exogenous insulin for their survival. The onset of this variant of the disease is usually in youth, with peaks at 5 years and early adolescence. There are strong associations with HLA-DR3 and -DR4 antigens on chromosome 6 in Caucasians. There is also an association with antibodies directed against pancreatic islet cells. Both genetic and viral factors seem to be involved in the aetiology. In Britain insulin-dependent diabetes mellitus affects approximately 0.2% of individuals aged under 20 years; the prevalence is higher than this in Scandinavia and lower in Asia.[2]

Approximately 10% of all patients with diabetes mellitus die from renal failure[3] and insurance mortality statistics show a 17-fold excess of renal death compared to non-diabetics.[4] The incidence of end-stage renal disease among urban blacks with diabetes mellitus is 3.6 times the rate in whites with this disease. The relative risk for blacks increases with age.[5] The greater susceptibility of blacks to develop hypertension is probably an important reason for this racial difference. Diabetic end-stage renal disease is also more common in Hispanic and American Indian people than in whites.

All forms of diabetes mellitus may be complicated by changes in the kidneys. The proportion of patients with renal lesions is much higher among those with insulin-dependent diabetes mellitus, more than 50% of whom die of renal failure or its consequences if not treated.[3,6] Heredity probably helps to determine susceptibility to diabetic nephropathy.[7] Five renal conditions are encountered: glomerular lesions, vascular lesions, pyelonephritis, papillary necrosis and glycogen and fatty changes in tubular epithelium (Armanni–Ebstein lesion).

Glomerular lesions in diabetes mellitus

The commonest lesion is diabetic glomerulosclerosis.

Diabetic glomerulosclerosis

The morphological changes of diabetic glomerulosclerosis occur in the kidneys of most, if not all, diabetics, usually within a few years of the onset of the disease. The lesions are associated with proteinuria and progressive deterioration in renal function in a proportion of the patients. Diabetic glomerulosclerosis represents the single most important cause of chronic renal failure in adults in the Western world, being responsible for approximately 30% of all new cases of uraemia. Clinical evidence of diabetic glomerulosclerosis is commonest in patients who have had insulin-dependent diabetes mellitus for several years; the incidence after a mean duration of disease of 16 years is 40%.[8] Symptomatic diabetic glomerulosclerosis is less frequent in non-insulin-dependent diabetes mellitus.[9] Once clinically manifest, this complication of diabetes mellitus is at present irreversible, and its progress cannot be arrested. It is often accompanied by diabetic retinopathy, neuropathy and hypertension.

Clinical features Proteinuria is the commonest manifestation of diabetic glomerulosclerosis. Initially it is usually mild and intermittent; the first indication is microalbuminuria which is the excretion of quantities (30–300 mg/24 hours) of albumin insufficient to be demonstrated by reagent strips.[10] After 11–20 years (with great individual variation) the proteinuria becomes continuous and increases in amount, although not usually exceeding 5 g/24 hours. The nephrotic syndrome is uncommon. Microscopic haematuria occasionally occurs but should always arouse suspicions that a glomerular lesion other than diabetic glomerulosclerosis is present. Renal function remains normal for several years, then progressively declines. Radioisotope studies show that the kidneys are frequently increased in size in the early stages of diabetic glomerulosclerosis.[11] Hypertension is common once renal failure develops.

Renal changes

Gross appearance of the kidneys. The kidneys may be enlarged or of normal size and have a smooth subcapsular surface, or they may be shrunken and show subcapsular scarring or granularity. The arteries at the corticomedullary junction are often prominent. There is usually well-marked atherosclerosis of the main renal arteries.

Light microscopy. Three types of abnormality are commonly seen in glomeruli affected by diabetic glomerulosclerosis. These are diffuse glomerulosclerosis, nodular glomerulosclerosis and exudative lesions.

Diffuse glomerulosclerosis is seen in the kidneys of almost all diabetics after a few years of metabolic abnormality. It is characterized by a global and often diffuse increase in the amount of PAS-positive mesangial matrix (Fig.10.1). It is usually accompanied by a diffuse segmental or global thickening of the capillary basement membrane which does not have the refractile appearance that may be seen in diffuse membranous glomerulonephritis. As the mesangium expands, progressive narrowing of the lumen of the capillaries results. Diffuse glomerulosclerosis may occur alone or may be accompanied by nodular glomerulosclerosis. By light microscopy diffuse capillary wall thickening is not seen on its own; there is always some mesangial expansion. The number of mesangial cells may be raised; this is almost always mild (three mesangial cells per mesangial area) and minor compared with the increase in the amount of mesangial matrix.

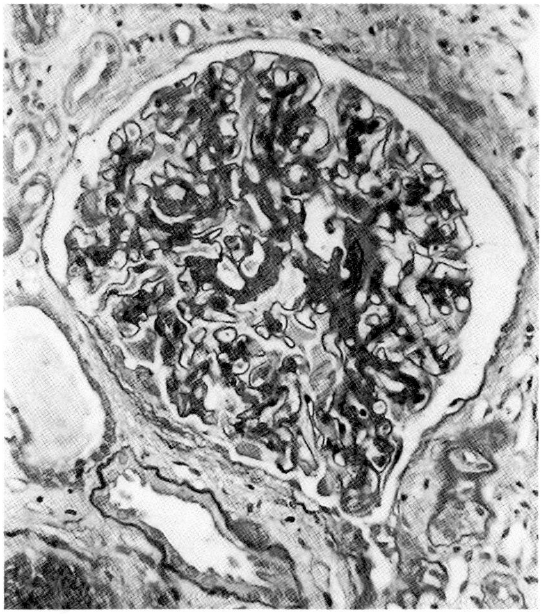

Fig. 10.1 Diabetic glomerulosclerosis – form with diffuse glomerulosclerosis. Glomerulus with global increase in the amount of mesangial matrix. There is also global thickening of the capillary basement membrane. The number of mesangial cells is normal.
Periodic acid-Schiff ×300

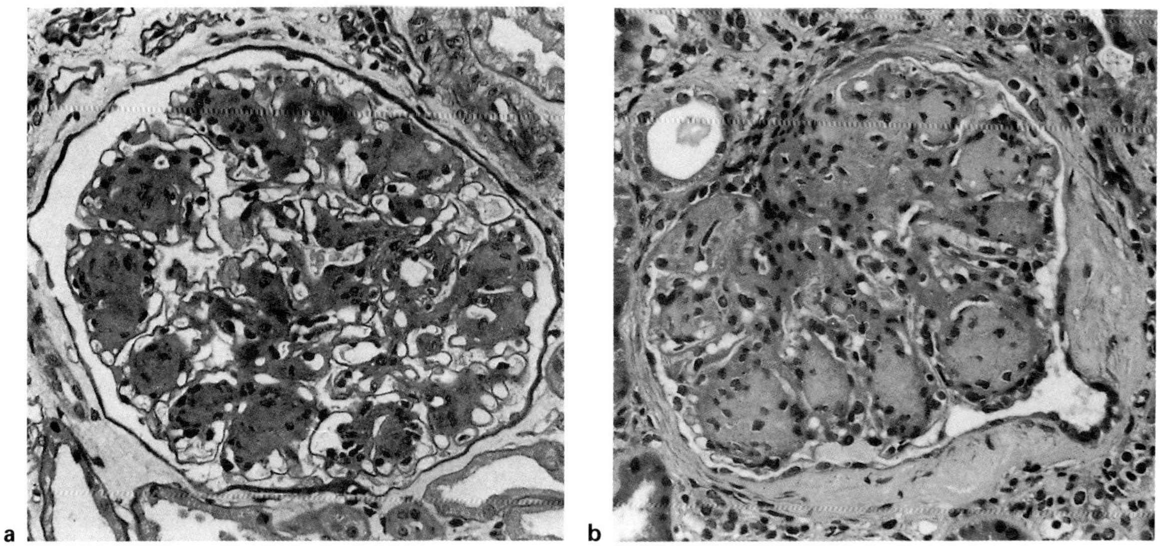

Fig. 10.2 Diabetic glomerulosclerosis – form with nodular glomerulosclerosis (Kimmelstiel–Wilson lesions). Rounded, homogeneous nodules occupy the centre of several lobules in the glomerulus. (**a**) Eariy stage. (**b**) Late stage.
Periodic acid-Schiff: (**a**), (**b**) × 300

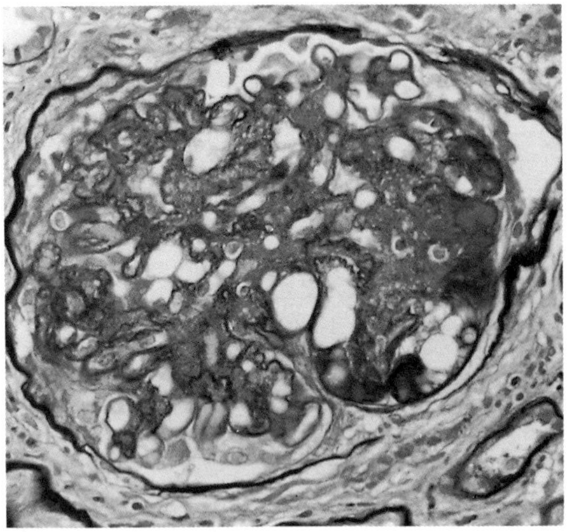

Fig. 10.3 Diabetic glomerulosclerosis – form with exudative lesions. Glomerulus with fibrin caps in capillary walls on right of tuft.
Periodic acid-Schiff × 300

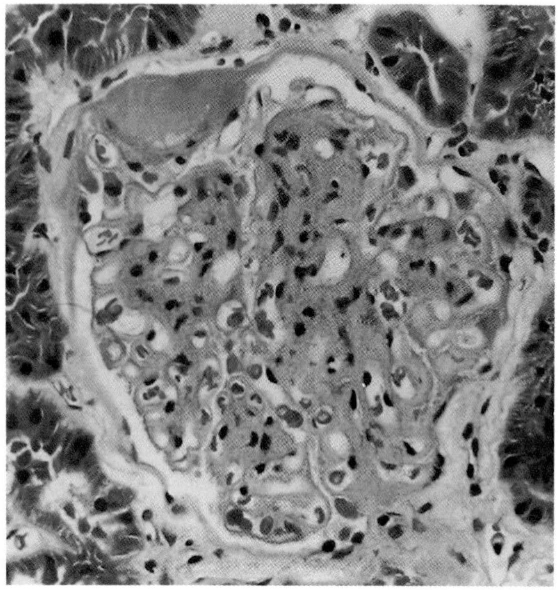

Fig. 10.4 Diabetic glomerulosclerosis – form with exudative lesions. Glomerulus with a 'capsular drop' at 11 o'clock.
Haematoxylin–eosin × 300

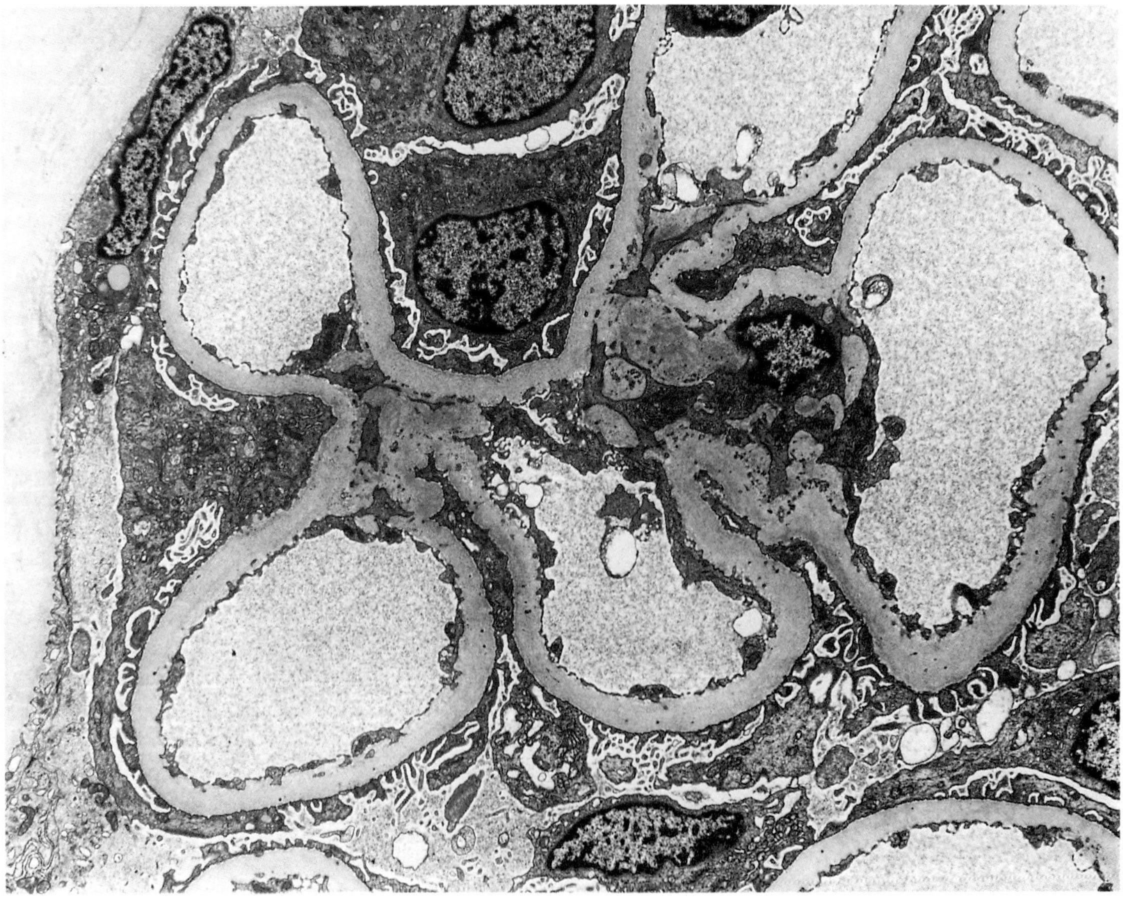

Fig. 10.5 Diabetic glomerulosclerosis. Electron micrograph of part of glomerulus showing thickening of capillary basement membrane.
× 8000

Nodular glomerulosclerosis is present in only about 25% of diabetic kidneys and is invariably accompanied by diffuse glomerulosclerosis. It is the focal lesion that was described first by Kimmelstiel and Wilson in 1936[12] and often bears their names. Rounded, homogeneous, eosinophilic nodules occupy the centre of one or more of the lobules in a variable proportion of the glomeruli (Fig. 10.2). The nodules vary in size. They are usually acellular; silver stains often reveal concentric lamination. The capillaries at the periphery of the nodules are patent and may be dilated, even aneurysmal. Nodular glomerulosclerosis is of diagnostic rather than clinical significance; there is no correlation between its severity and frequency in an individual patient and the degree of functional impairment.

Exudative glomerular lesions, which are also known as insudative lesions, consist of localized accumulations of intensely eosinophilic material in various regions of the glomerulus. They appear as crescentic masses, known as *'fibrin caps'*, lying in the wall of a capillary, usually at the periphery of a lobule (Fig. 10.3), and as small nodules, known as *'capsular drops'*, situated between Bowman's capsule and the parietal epithelium (Fig. 10.4). Lipid globules and foam cells may sometimes be included in both types of exudative lesion.

Electron microscopy Even in cases that appear normal by light microscopy the capillary basement membranes may be thickened and the amount of mesangial matrix slightly increased (Fig. 10.5).[13] As the disease progresses these two changes become more pronounced and either may predominate. The basement membrane may eventually be as much as 10 times thicker than normal.

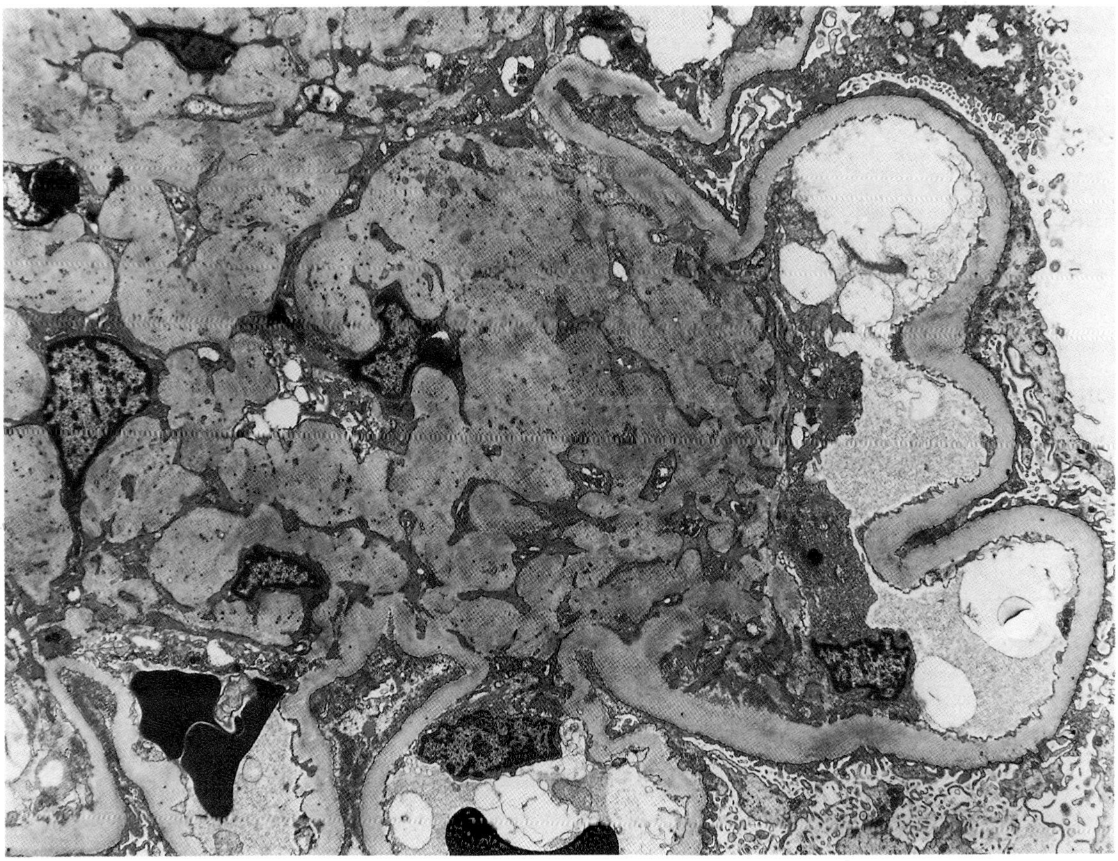

Fig. 10.6 Diabetic glomerulosclerosis. Electron micrograph of part of a glomerulus showing a mesangial nodule composed of matrix.
× 5500

The nodules that sometimes form in the mesangium are composed of matrix that is arranged in either an irregular pattern or in bands (Fig. 10.6). The mesangial cells become elongated and displaced to the periphery of the nodule; later they disappear. Fibrin caps appear as collections of electron-dense finely granular material on the subendothelial aspect of the glomerular capillary basement membranes; they often contain lipid and membranous debris. Capsular drops have a similar composition; they are covered by a thin layer of basement membrane which is continuous with Bowman's capsule (Fig. 10.7).

Immunofluorescence/immunoperoxidase microscopy.[14] A linear distribution of IgG along the basement membranes of the glomerular capillaries, Bowman's capsule and tubules is seen in about half the cases (Fig. 10.8). Similar, but less intense, staining for IgM, fibrin and albumin is less frequent. Staining for C3 is occasionally present but is usually granular. Elution studies show that the IgG has no antibasement-membrane properties. Exudative lesions may contain IgM.

Differential diagnosis Changes resembling diffuse diabetic glomerulosclerosis may be encountered in several forms of mild *mesangial proliferative*

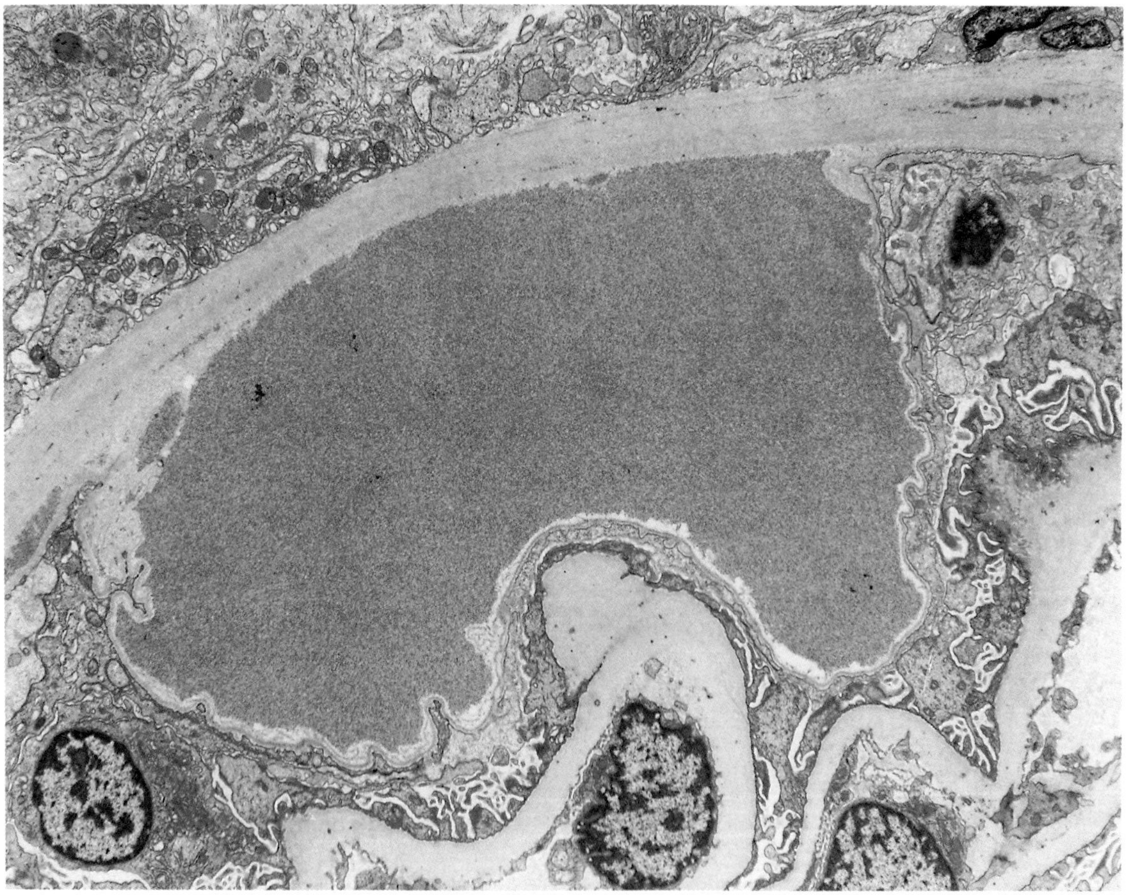

Fig. 10.7 Diabetic glomerulosclerosis – form with exudative lesions. Electron micrograph of part of glomerulus showing capsular drop composed of electron-dense finely granular material. It is covered by a thin layer of basement membrane continuous with Bowman's capsule.
× 8000

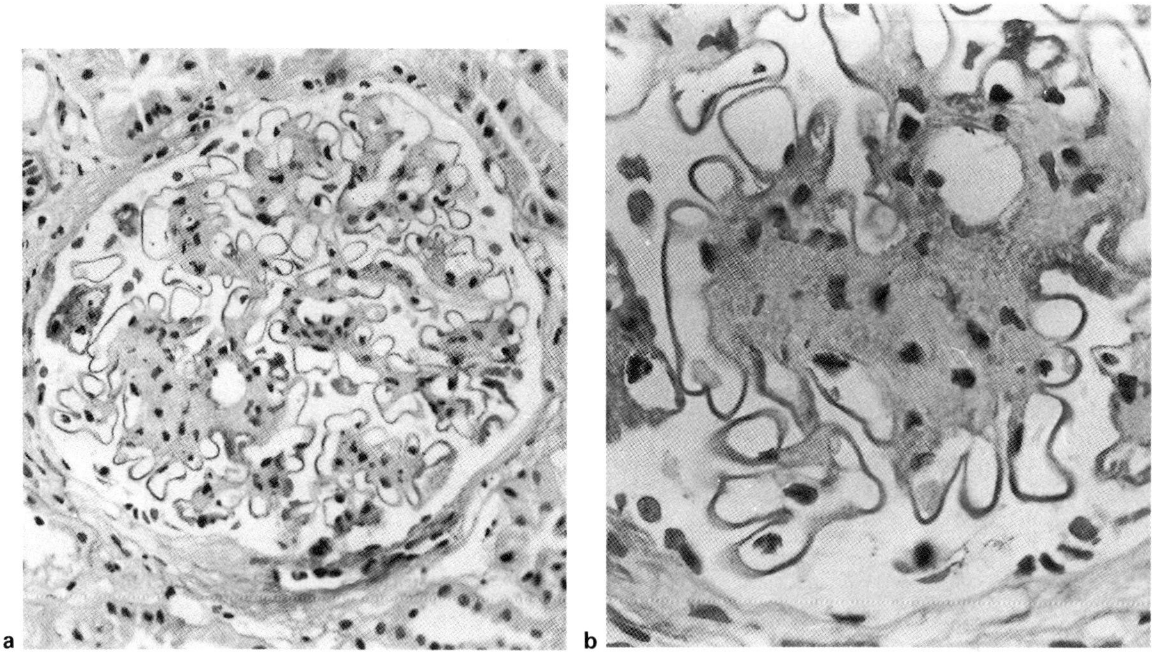

Fig. 10.8 a, b Diabetic glomerulosclerosis. Glomerulus showing linear staining for IgG along the glomerular basement membranes. Immunoperoxidase: (**a**) × 300; (**b**) × 600

glomerulonephritis (see p. 153) in the absence of diabetes. However, none is associated with linear deposition of IgG on the glomerular capillary basement membrane except the glomerulonephritis of *antiglomerular-basement-membrane disease* (see p. 219) and *lupus nephritis* (see p. 228). Even if other features do not make the diagnosis obvious, antiglomerular-basement-membrane glomerulonephritis can be distinguished by the demonstration of antiglomerular-basement-membrane antibodies in the patient's circulation by radioimmunoassay, and lupus glomerulonephritis can be recognized by the demonstration of antibodies to double-stranded DNA in the patient's blood. The problem is greater when the diabetic lesion is not accompanied by linear staining for IgG on the glomerular capillary walls. It is easy to distinguish IgA nephropathy (see p. 159) because of the prominent mesangial deposits of IgA, but the distinction from other forms of mild mesangial proliferative glomerulonephritis may be difficult. The amount of glomerular capillary wall thickening is a help; conditions other than diabetic glomerulosclerosis very rarely show diffuse global thickening of the capillary basement membranes. The diffuseness of the lesion will also usually distinguish diabetic glomerulosclerosis from the essentially focal glomerular changes seen in association with ageing (see p. 25), atherosclerosis (see p. 295) and benign phase hypertension (see p. 306).

Nodular diabetic glomerulosclerosis is almost indistinguishable on light microscopy from *light chain deposition disease* (see p. 363). However, in the latter condition electron microscopy demonstrates a characteristic uniform deposition of electron-dense granular material within the glomerular capillary basement membranes, in the mesangium, in the tubular basement membranes and around blood vessels. This material stains for light chains. Mesangial expansion producing centrilobular nodules also occurs in long-surviving cases of *diffuse mesangiocapillary glomerulonephritis* (see p. 166) and *dense deposit disease* (see p. 180), but the distinctive findings on immunofluorescence or immunoperoxidase microscopy and on electron microscopy should make the differential diagnosis straightforward.

The exudative lesions associated with diabetes

mellitus are completely non-specific and indistinguishable from those that occur in ischaemic and obsolescent glomeruli in a wide range of other renal diseases.

Complications *Glomerulonephritis* may complicate diabetic glomerulosclerosis.[15] Reports have included diffuse endocapillary proliferative glomerulonephritis (see p. 142) diffuse membranous glomerulonephritis (see p. 191) diffuse crescentic glomerulonephritis (see p. 185) and focal segmental glomerulosclerosis (see p. 204) in that order of frequency. The incidence of complicating glomerulonephritis is unknown. There is often a tendency to ascribe all the clinical manifestations of renal dysfunction in diabetic patients to diabetic nephropathy without renal biopsy to exclude the possible presence of complicating glomerulonephritis; even when biopsies are done they are not always examined by electron microscopy and immunofluorescence/immunoperoxidase microscopy. In one series renal biopsies from 18 diabetic patients were reviewed with the individuals' clinical and laboratory findings. Eight (44%) were found to have primary glomerulonephritis in addition to diabetic glomerulosclerosis.[15] Although this almost certainly does not represent the true incidence of complicating glomerulonephritis in diabetics, it is probable that the incidence of this condition has been underestimated.

Diabetic glomerulosclerosis may additionally be complicated by chronic pyelonephritis, papillary necrosis and the vascular and tubular changes that are also associated with diabetes mellitus. Arteriolar hyalinization is particularly common.

Occasionally glomerular lesions from systemic diseases such as systemic lupus erythematosus, amyloidosis and sarcoidosis have been reported.[16,17]

Renal transplantation As present treatment cannot halt the progression of diabetic glomerulosclerosis, dialysis or renal transplantation are eventually needed. Patient and graft survival rates at 2 years post-transplantation in insulin dependent diabetes mellitus are 89% and 83%, comparable to those seen in non-diabetic renal allograft recipients.[18] These are the figures achieved by a group at the University of Minnesota who have the most experience in treating diabetes in end-stage renal failure. They include some related live donor grafts, but the results for the cadaveric grafts are also similar to those in non-diabetics. Other centres are now beginning to obtain similar results. During the next 8 years after transplantation the mortality among the diabetic recipients is considerably higher than in non-diabetics. Myocardial infarction is the commonest cause of death.[19]

Diabetic glomerulosclerosis eventually affects the majority of renal allografts in diabetics but the evolution of the lesions follows a similar time-course to that in the patient's own kidneys (see p. 670). There is usually no significant change during the first 2 years after transplantation. Beyond this time almost all begin to show thickening of the glomerular capillary basement membranes and mesangial expansion.[20] These changes are not seen in non-diabetic patients or in those diabetic patients who are given a simultaneous pancreatic and renal allograft. The slowness and mildness of the diabetic glomerulosclerosis is such that an adverse effect on renal function is not seen for several years and graft failure does not occur for 10–20 years. Nodular glomerulosclerosis rarely occurs in renal allografts; there is a high incidence of hyalinization in afferent and efferent arterioles. Neither change is closely related to functional deterioration of the kidney.

Prognosis Forty-two per cent of the patients with insulin-dependent diabetes mellitus die within 35 years after diagnosis.[21] Many die of renal failure but cardiovascular complications are also an important cause of morbidity and mortality because most of these patients are hypertensive and have hyperlipidaemia and generalized atherosclerosis.[22] Another 42% survive more than 40 years even though they have diffuse diabetic glomerulosclerosis with or without nodules.[23] The single most important prognostic factor is whether a patient develops persistent proteinuria greater than 0.3 g/litre, a level detectable by dipstick. If he or she does, there follows a relentless decline in renal function, albeit at a variable rate, and 50% of such patients reach end-stage renal failure within 7 years.[8] Diabetic patients with proteinuria have a relative mortality 80 times that in the background population for men and 110 times for women; the relative mortality for diabetics without proteinuria is about double that in the general population.[21] Susceptibility to develop proteinuria and eventual renal failure appears to be selective. There is evidence that diabetic glomerulosclerosis is caused by hyperglycaemia but progression to proteinuria and renal failure seems to depend upon some other trigger. Current evidence suggests that this may be hypertension and that a genetic predisposition to high blood pressure may determine susceptibility to diabetic renal failure.[24] Microalbuminuria can be used to predict which patients will progress to clinical proteinuria and renal failure but non-diabetic renal or systemic disease must first be excluded. The exact level of urinary albumin excretion which discriminates between those patients who will progress and those who will not, varies from 15 μg/min to 70 μg/min in different centres. This variability is probably largely due to differences in sampling procedures.[25]

Eythrocyte sodium–lithium countertransport, which is elevated in patients with essential hypertension and in normotensive people from families with a history of hypertension, is also elevated in white patients with insulin dependent diabetes mellitus and nephropathy. As the elevation occurs before there is microalbuminuria, it is suggested that it may be the earliest predictor of which patients with diabetes are going to develop glomerulosclerosis.[26] In blacks the rate of red-cell sodium–lithium countertransport may not be a marker for diabetic renal disease.

In cases of diabetic glomerulosclerosis who develop a complicating glomerulonephritis the prognosis may be adversely affected.

Pathogenesis Very soon after the onset of insulin-dependent diabetes mellitus there is glomerular hyperfiltration, and renal hypertrophy occurs which particularly affects the glomeruli.[27] The rise in single nephron glomerular filtration rate is caused by dilatation of the afferent and efferent arterioles which exposes the glomeruli to systemic blood pressure.[28] What initiates these changes leading to hyperfiltration is not known. They are probably stimulated by one or more of the features of the diabetic state such as extracellular fluid volume expansion due to hyperglycaemia, increased growth hormone and glucagon secretion or altered levels of, or vascular responsiveness to, vasoactive hormones.[29] Of these factors, hyperglycaemia seems likely to be the most important; the others may act as modulatory influences. Glomerular hyperfiltration and hypertrophy are not features of non-insulin-dependent diabetes mellitus.[30]

For the first year or two after the diagnosis of diabetes mellitus the thickness of the glomerular capillary basement membranes and the amount of mesangial matrix remain normal.[13] The same is true of normal kidneys transplanted into patients with insulin-dependent diabetes mellitus.[20] Then the mesangium begins to expand and the basement membrane to thicken. The mesangial expansion could be the result of the glomerular hyperfiltration: the increased transglomerular flow of plasma that occurs in this situation can, in experimental animals, stimulate the mesangial cells to produce more matrix, resulting in mesangial sclerosis.[30] Why nodules should sometimes be formed in the mesangium is not known; the cause of the basement membrane thickening is also obscure.

In those patients who progress to renal failure the onset of hypertension, which in itself leads to high glomerular filtration rates and renal plasma flows, may magnify the glomerular hyperfiltration and hyperperfusion, leading to increased mesangial sclerosis and progressive obsolescence of glomeruli.

The basis for the increased urinary protein excretion in some of the patients who have diabetic glomerulosclerosis is incompletely understood. Whether it can be attributed simply to alterations in glomerular haemodynamics or whether some metabolic effect on the permeability of the glomerular barrier to macromolecules is also involved is at present unknown. Some studies indicate that the charge sites in the glomerular capillary wall (see p. 10), especially those along the lamina rara externa, are diminished and that the severity of this diminution is related to the magnitude of the patient's proteinuria.[31] It is likely that this loss of anionic charge is due to loss of heparin sulphate proteoglycan in the glomerular basement membrane.[32] The local secretion of sialoproteins could be critically influenced by the metabolic changes that exist in the diabetic patient.

Non-diabetic glomerular lesions in diabetic patients

Diabetic patients with proteinuria are generally presumed to have diabetic glomerulosclerosis, usually without biopsy confirmation; but non-diabetic lesions may give rise to proteinuria in diabetic patients. This may happen in the early period after the onset of diabetes mellitus before diabetic glomerulosclerosis has appeared, but more often it complicates the latter.

The prevalence of non-diabetic renal disease in diabetic patients is not known. A wide spectrum of such renal lesions can occur in these patients. These include various forms of glomerulonephritis which have already been described and discussed under complications of diabetic glomerulosclerosis (see p. 336); sometimes they occur before the latter has appeared.[15,17] Steroid-responsive nephrotic syndrome has frequently been reported in diabetes; all cases have been characterized by obliteration of epithelial foot processes without basement membrane or mesangial changes, and by prompt remission of the nephrotic syndrome after treatment with corticosteroids. This is a unique clinical feature because the nephrotic syndrome associated with diabetic glomerulosclerosis does not respond to steroids. Lupus nephritis, sarcoid nephropathy, amyloidosis and chlorpropamide-associated nephropathy have also been recorded in patients with diabetes.[17]

The non-diabetic renal disease may be clinically obvious or present merely as a urinary abnormality. Clues to the possible presence of non-diabetic renal disease are the onset of significant proteinuria earlier than expected in the course of diabetes mellitus, haematuria in the absence of urinary tract infection or urological disorder and deterioration of renal function sooner or faster than anticipated.

The discovery of a non-diabetic renal lesion in a patient with diabetes mellitus may alter the treatment and affect the prognosis.

Vascular lesions of the kidneys in diabetes mellitus

Changes in the blood vessels of the kidneys are very commonly present in diabetic patients.

Arterioles

There is marked hyaline thickening of the walls of the arterioles: this characteristically affects the efferent arterioles as well as the afferent arterioles (Fig. 10.9). By electron microscopy the subendothelial collections of hyalin do not differ from those seen in the benign phase of hypertension (see p. 308). Immunofluorescence or immunoperoxidase microscopy shows that they contain IgM and C3 and sometimes other immunoglobulins and albumin.

Arteriolar hyalinization is not peculiar to diabetes mellitus. It is seen also as part of the ageing process and in patients with benign phase hypertension; however, it occurs far more extensively and at a much earlier age in diabetics, even in the absence of hypertension. The presence of severe arteriolar hyalinization should always raise the suspicion of diabetes mellitus and when both afferent and efferent arterioles are affected it becomes almost diagnostic.[29]

Kidneys with arteriolar hyalinization often show

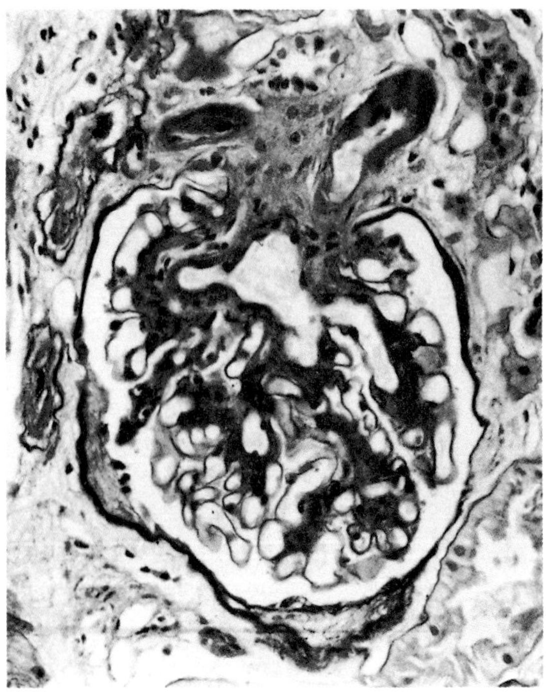

Fig. 10.9 Diabetic vascular lesion. There is marked hyalinization of the walls of the afferent and efferent arterioles.
Periodic acid-Schiff × 425

enlargement of the juxtaglomerular apparatus. There is a linear correlation between mean juxtaglomerular apparatus size and severity of hyalinization of the afferent arteriole.[34]

Arteries

Arteries of all sizes, from the main renal artery downwards, develop atherosclerotic changes (see p. 295). The intimal thickening and elastic changes are more severe and extensive and occur earlier than would be expected in normal or even hypertensive individuals. Atherosclerotic arterial narrowing is an important factor in hastening the onset of renal failure.[35]

Tubular lesions in diabetes mellitus

Diffuse thickening of the basement membrane of tubules undergoing atrophy is common and more marked than is usual in simple ischaemia. Glycogen vacuoles in the cytoplasm of the epithelial cells that line the pars recta of the proximal convoluted tubules (Armanni–Ebstein lesion)[36] are rarely seen now. They occur in uncontrolled hyperglycaemia.

Other renal conditions associated with diabetes mellitus

Papillary necrosis

Renal papillary necrosis (see p. 473) is particularly frequent among diabetics, in whom it is generally a terminal event. It is more likely to occur in women. Both kidneys are usually affected. Ulceration of the necrotic papillae occurs much less frequently than in analgesic abuse. It has been suggested that the kidney with advanced diabetic lesions is more susceptible to papillary necrosis because the circulation to the papillae is impaired by atherosclerotic and hyaline changes. The precipitating factor is often acute pyelonephritis[37] which by producing interstitial oedema may further compromise the papillary blood supply.

Pyelonephritis

It is difficult to assess the frequency of acute and chronic pyelonephritis as complications of diabetes. Quantitative bacteriological examination of the urine indicates that, with the exception of pregnant or older women, urinary infection is not more frequent in patients who are diabetic than in those who are not.[38] Chemotaxis, phagocytosis and the ability of neutrophil granulocytes to kill bacteria are all impaired in hyperglycaemic, poorly controlled diabetes. Infection of the kidneys tends to be a late event in the course of diabetes and the incidence of acute pyelonephritis in diabetic patients at autopsy is raised.[37] The pyelonephritis is often secondary to incomplete bladder emptying due to autonomic neuropathy. Claims for an excessive incidence of infective renal scarring, however, are not convincing. The morphological appearances are described on pages 434 and 440.

The kidneys in secondary diabetes mellitus

Both the nodular and the diffuse form of glomerulosclerosis may be found in patients with haemochromatosis and other forms of secondary diabetes mellitus.[39] Exudative and vascular lesions also occur.

GOUT

Gout is the term used to describe a group of metabolic diseases characterized by hyperuricaemia associated with deposition of crystals of monosodium urate monohydrate in the tissues. The clinical manifestations include acute arthritis, tenosynovitis, bursitis or cellulitis, and chronic deforming arthritis accompanied by periarticular and subcutaneous urate deposits (tophi). Renal and urinary uric acid calculi, urinary abnormalities such as mild proteinuria, and hypertension are common. Renal failure, which was once frequent, is now rare.

Uric acid excreted in the urine is derived from both endogenous purine production and exogenous dietary purines. The uric acid in the plasma passes freely through the glomerular filtration barrier; it is then extensively reabsorbed in the first part of the proximal tubules, secreted back into the proximal tubule and then partly reabsorbed in the proximal and distal tubules. This widely distributed process of secretion and absorption is probably to prevent an extremely high concentration of urate within any one part of the tubule.[40] Hyperuricaemia may result from decreased uric acid excretion or increased uric acid production.[41]

Decreased uric acid excretion In 75–90% of patients with gout, hyperuricaemia occurs because the kidney is unable to excrete the normal uric acid load presented to it. The reason for this under-excretion is often unknown. It may, however, result from a variety of factors that affect renal blood flow and the secretion and reabsorption of uric acid. Examples are: drug administration (e.g. diuretics, cyclosporin and low dose salicylates); lead nephropathy (see p. 503); increased levels of organic acids (e.g. lactic acidosis after over-ingestion of alcohol; ketoacidosis in uncontrolled diabetes mellitus); chronic beryllium poisoning (see p. 508); hypertension (see p. 304); myx-oedema; Bartter's syndrome (see p. 96); Down's syndrome; sarcoidosis (see p. 258); hyperpara-thyroidism (see p. 544), and sickle cell anaemia (see p. 106). Decreased uric acid excretion may also occur because of reduction in functional renal mass brought about by any chronic renal disease, or by a fall in glomerular filtration secondary to plasma volume depletion or nephrogenic diabetes insipidus.

Increased uric acid production Overproduction of uric acid is found in 10–25% of patients with gout. In many of these patients the reason for the increased synthesis of purines is unknown, but in approximately 40% of these overproducers hyperuricaemia results from increased turnover of preformed purines. This occurs whenever there is an increase in the rate of proliferation of cells; it is particularly associated with myeloid and lymphoid proliferative disorders. Hyperuricaemia is common, for example, in polycythaemia rubra vera and chronic granulocytic leukaemia; it also occurs in myeloid metaplasia, acute leukaemia and multiple myeloma. In a few overproducers hyperuricaemia is the result of a specific, inherited defect of a purine enzyme such as a deficiency of hypoxanthine-guanine phosphoribosyltransferase or overactivity of phosphoribosyl-alpha-1-pyrophosphate synthetase. All are X-linked disorders. Hypoxanthine-guanine phosphoribosyltransferase deficiency is associated with the Lesch–Nyhan syndrome (see p. 106). Increased synthesis of purines also occurs in glucose-6-phosphatase deficiency type I glycogen storage disease (see p. 103).

Clinical features

The majority of people with raised levels of monosodium urate in their blood remain asymptomatic throughout life. When gout occurs it is eight time more common in men than in women. It usually presents in men between the ages of 30 and 60 years and in women after the menopause. The first indication is commonly an acute arthritis of the metatarsophalangeal joint of the great toe but sometimes it is an attack of renal colic. Eventually 10% of patients with gout experience renal colic from the passage of calculi down the ureter.

Rarely, acute renal failure may occur from sudden precipitation of crystals of uric acid in the collecting ducts of the kidneys and the ureters; this is most likely to happen when a dehydrated, acidotic patient with leukaemia or lymphoma is treated with cytotoxic drugs. Acute renal failure can be averted by ensuring a large volume of alkaline urine by means of high fluid intake and sodium bicarbonate, and by giving allopurinol to prevent a sudden rise in uric acid.[42]

Mild intermittent proteinuria occurs in about a third of patients with gout. Renal function usually remains normal in young patients unless there is some associated disease (such as glomerulonephritis, pyelonephritis or amyloidosis), or unless hypertension is either present initially or develops later.[43] In patients over the age of 50 years, hypertension, atherosclerotic cardiac disease and cerebrovascular disease are often present, or appear during the course of gout, and are associated with a decrease in renal function. Approximately 8–10% of patients with gout eventually develop chronic renal failure.

An exception to the generalization that patients with uncomplicated gout do not usually develop renal insufficiency is the small group of young patients with a family history of gout which is often of unknown origin but which, in a few instances, is due to a defect in one or more of the enzymes associated with purine synthesis (see p. 106). These patients develop rapidly progressive renal disease in the absence of hypertension and despite treatment with allopurinol that lowers the plasma uric acid.[42]

Renal changes in non-familial gout

There are three principal manifestations of gout in the kidneys: intratubular deposits of uric acid, interstitial deposits of urate, and uric acid calculi. They may be present singly or in various combinations. In addition, pyelonephritis (see p. 440), hypertensive nephrosclerosis (see p. 306), atherosclerotic changes (see p. 295) and the effects of ageing (see p. 25) are also often present.

Intratubular deposits of uric acid [44]

This lesion is found particularly in patients suddenly producing an excess of uric acid because of increased turnover of preformed nucleic acids and hence of purines.

Gross appearance of the kidneys. The collecting ducts full of uric acid can be seen as linear strands in the papillae. Similar yellow material may be present in the renal pelvis and ureters.

Light microscopy. The collecting tubules are distended with uric acid which often appears as amorphous or granular eosinophilic masses or multiple small spherical laminated crystals (Fig. 10.10). In some collecting tubules urate deposits appear as slender birefringent elongated crystals; these are seen best in material that has been fixed in alcohol and stained in such a way as to avoid contact with aqueous solutions. Some of the deposits are surrounded by a palisade of macrophages and multinucleate giant cells, but this is generally a minor feature. The tubules proximal to the obstructed collecting ducts may be dilated. Sometimes the interstitium is oedematous.

a

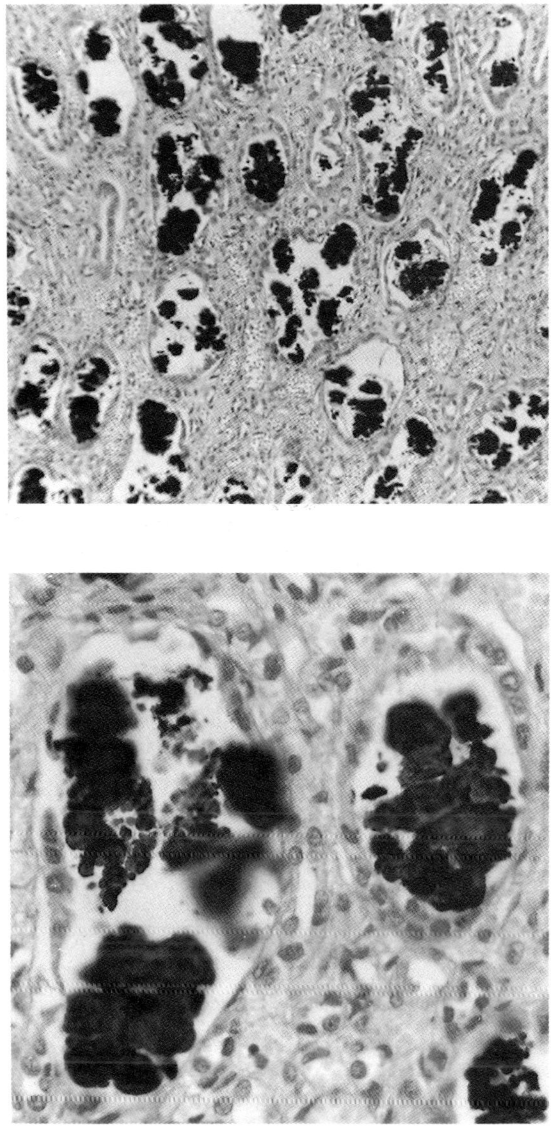

b

Fig. 10.10 a, b Gout. Intratubular deposits of uric acid during treatment of chronic granulocytic leukaemia. Haematoxylin-eosin
(**a**) × 100; (**b**) × 300

Interstitial deposits of urate

This lesion occurs particularly in patients with chronic gout. It used to be very common but since treatment with allopurinol has reduced blood levels of uric acid the once familiar interstitial deposits of urate are seen much less frequently.

Light microscopy The interstitial tissue of the medulla contains crystals of monosodium urate monohydrate surrounded by multinucleate giant cells and mononuclear cells. The crystals are long and slender, disposed in sheaves and arranged radially (Fig. 10.11). In frozen sections or in alcohol-fixed material they are birefringent; in paraffin sections of tissue fixed in formol saline

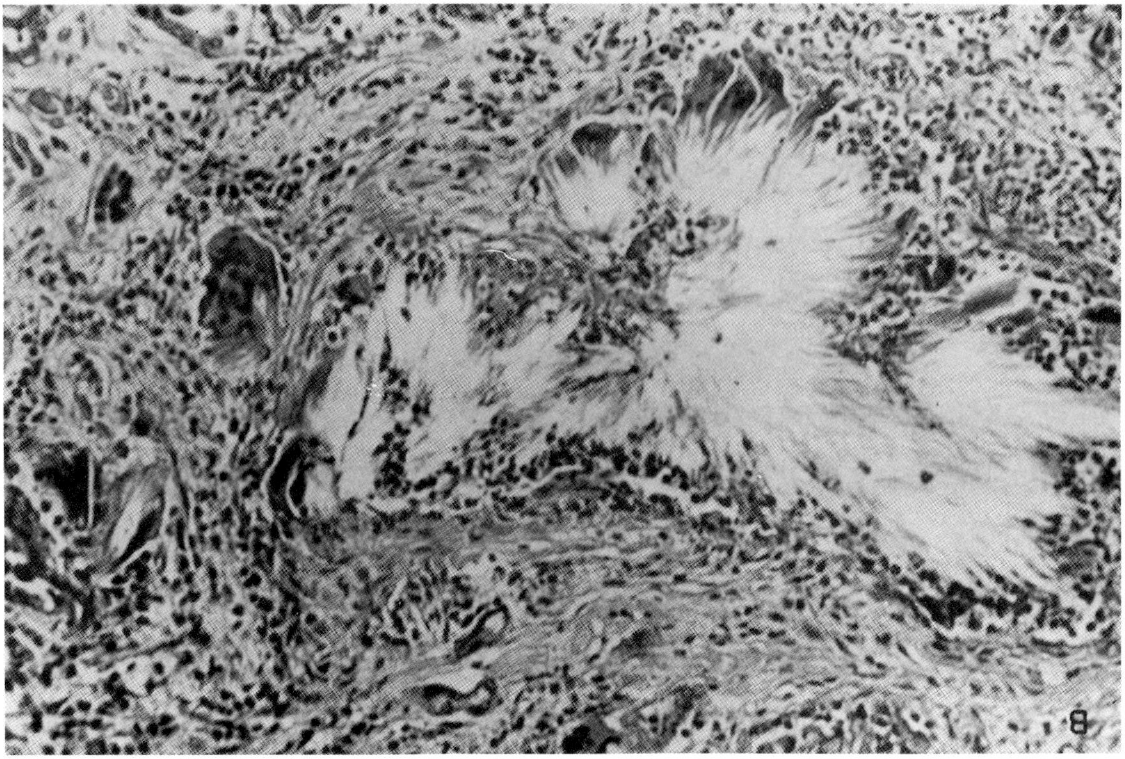

Fig. 10.11 Gout. Interstital deposits of urate. Collection of crystals surrounded by giant cells and macrophages. Haematoxylin-eosin × 250
Reproduced by permission from: Allen AC. The kidney. London: Churchill, 1952 (Fig. 153B)

many of the crystals will have dissolved but they usually leave a characteristically shaped mould. Urate deposits are also present in some of the collecting tubules; the tubular epithelium and the basement membrane about the casts may be focally destroyed. The crystals that are found in the interstitium of the medulla are probably formed within the tubules and continue to grow outside the latter after degeneration of the epithelium and basement membrane. Large crystalline deposits, such as the tophi that occur in the subcutaneous tissues, are rare in the kidneys. Crystal formation seldom takes place in the renal cortex.

As well as the crystalline deposits, various glomerular, tubular and interstitial changes are commonly found. These are of ischaemic or obstructive origin. Changes in blood vessels are frequent and take the form of non-specific thickening of the intima of arteries.

Uric acid calculi [41]

Uric acid calculi (see p. 540) are common, occurring in 15–20% of patients with gout compared to 0.1% in controls. The incidence is particularly high in X-linked familial gout due to enzyme defects (see p. 541). Familial autosomal dominant hyperuricaemic nephropathy is not associated with stones. Pure uric acid calculi are radiolucent but they can generally be distinguished on ultrasonography. They form in acid urine: ensuring that the urine pH stays above 6.0 will usually prevent the development of pure uric acid stones. Uric acid calculi are particularly likely to follow overproduction of uric acid from increased turnover of nucleic acids during treatment of chronic granulocytic leukaemia or lymphoma, or excretion of large quantities of uric acid at the start of treatment of a patient with a uricosuric drug such as probenicid. Mixed uric acid–calcium oxalate stones and calcium oxalate–phosphate stones also occur more frequently than in controls. Possibly uric acid crystals or monosodium urate crystals act as a nidus for calcium stones. Uric acid calculi may cause hydronephrosis and predispose to pyelonephritis.

Renal changes in familial gout[45]

In familial gout there is focal or diffuse interstitial fibrosis, usually with chronic inflammatory cells and tubular atrophy. The presence of urate crystals in the interstitium is not generally a feature. Focal glomerulosclerosis of both segmental and global type occurs in some cases in the absence of hypertension.

Differential diagnosis

Uric acid crystals in the collecting tubules may be seen in any patient who either produces an excess of uric acid or whose kidneys are incapable of excreting a normal uric acid load; the intratubular crystals, however, may not be accompanied by tissue deposits of urate and clinical evidence of gout. A common example is the accumulation of uric acid crystals that occurs in the terminal collecting tubules in some newborn children. These casts are often called '*uric acid infarcts*' because the collecting ducts distended with uric acid form yellow, well-defined wedges located in the papillae of the renal medulla: these lesions superficially resemble infarcts. No renal dysfunction has been attributed to the uric acid casts found in the newborn.

Intratubular deposits of uric acid, producing acute renal failure occasionally occur after multiple epileptic convulsions. The uric acid is thought to come from inosinic acid released during violent protracted ischaemic muscle contraction and from nucleic acids liberated by muscle cell injury.

Complications

Diffuse membranous glomerulonephritis

Diffuse membranous glomerulonephritis producing proteinuria of 1–2 g a day has been recorded in a few patients.[46] It has been suggested that the tubular damage following uric acid deposition releases tubular antigens into the circulation which stimulate autoantibody formation and the production or deposition of immune complexes in the glomerular capillary walls. Evidence has been claimed of human tubular antigen in the subepithelial deposits in one case.[46] The glomerulonephritis progressed to end-stage renal failure in one patient despite treatment with allopurinol; the fate of the other cases in the series is not recorded.[46]

Prognosis

Progression to serious renal insufficiency is uncommon in the majority of patients with typical gout that is being treated with allopurinol. In those patients who do develop renal insufficiency, the renal failure is almost always due to a coexisting condition such as hypertension, hyperlipidaemia or diabetes mellitus.[42]

Patients with typical gout have an incidence of renal insufficiency that is no higher than that of patients of comparable ages and similar degrees of hypertension, diabetes, primary renal disease and urinary obstruction. The minority of patients who have familial gout are the exception. They commonly develop renal failure over a few to several years (see p. 340).

Acute renal failure from intratubular uric acid deposits (acute uric acid nephropathy) is preventable, but cases still occasionally occur. When they do occur prompt haemodialysis to remove the bulk of the excess uric acid load is usually needed.[47] Provided a diuresis can be achieved, the outlook for recovery of renal function is good.

Pathogenesis

In most patients with gout who develop renal failure this is due to nephrosclerosis from chronic hypertension (see p. 306); it is not due to damage induced by chronic hyperuricaemia. The X-linked familial cases are due to purine overproduction (see p. 541). The rare autosomal dominant familial cases probably have a tubular defect in uric acid excretion; hyperuricaemia is only an indication of that fault. Renal failure in acute uric acid nephropathy is the result of mechanical blockage of the collecting ducts.

In some cases of chronic gout an additional confounding factor is present. That factor is lead.[42] In the past this heavy metal has been responsible for several epidemics of gout, often with renal failure, as a result of contamination of port wine by bottles made of lead-containing glass. An example is gout in eighteenth-century England.[48] It continues to be a problem in the South Eastern United States where home-brewed whisky ('moonshine') becomes contaminated with lead from soldered truck radiators used as stills.[49] Lead nephropathy is considered on page 503.

AMYLOIDOSIS

Amyloidosis is a disorder of protein metabolism characterized by extracellular deposits of an abnormal protein that is insoluble in physiological fluids.[50,51] The deposits may be localized or systemic. They can be specifically identified in tissues by their characteristic property of binding Congo red dye; the amyloid stains pinkish orange and then displays a pathognomonic green birefringence when the stained sections are viewed in polarized light. The ultrastructure of almost all forms of amyloid is the same: a feltwork of unbranched fibrils that measure 7.5–10 nm in diameter and are of variable length (Fig. 10.12). Associated with the protein fibrils there are usually non-fibrillar sulphated glycosaminoglycans and a glycoprotein of the pentraxin family known as *amyloid P component*. The exception to these generalizations is the amyloid that is found in the cerebral cortex of old people and particularly in Alzheimer's disease; this intraneuronal amyloid consists of paired helical filaments and lacks amyloid P component.[51]

The fibrils are polymers of small proteins. The protein subunits in the fibrils differ according to the underlying disorder that has caused the amyloid to form. These differences form the basis for the biochemical classification of amyloidosis which recognizes four major forms of systemic amyloid: *AA amyloid* in which the fibrils contain amyloid A (AA) protein, *AL amyloid* in which the fibrils contain immunoglobulin light chain molecules of kappa or lambda type or their amino-terminal fragments, *prealbumin* (now known as *transthyretin*) *amyloid* and *beta$_2$-microglobulin amyloid.* Other protein subunits exist, such as gelsolin, apolipoprotein A-1, cystatin C and beta protein, but the majority of these are uncommon and found mostly in localized amyloidosis.

AA amyloid is most commonly laid down systemically as a secondary response to an underlying chronic inflammatory disorder; it is also found in familial Mediterranean fever (see p. 110) and in association with certain malignant tumours, in particular Hodgkin's disease and renal adenocarcinoma.[52] ***AL amyloid*** is associated with plasma cell and B lymphocyte dyscrasias such as multiple myeloma and monoclonal gammopathy and the isolated nodular deposits of amyloid that are sometimes found in skin, lung or urogenital tract. ***Transthyretin (prealbumin) amyloid*** is found in the predominantly neuropathic and cardio-myopathic forms of hereditary amyloidosis (see p. 109) and in senile systemic amyloidosis (formerly called senile cardiac amyloidosis). ***Beta$_2$-microglobulin amyloid*** is found in association with chronic haemodialysis (see p. 40).

The kidneys may be affected in any of the systemic forms of amyloidosis. They are involved in 76–92% of cases of AA amyloidosis,[53] in about 35% of patients with AL amyloidosis[54] and sometimes in transthyretin amyloidosis.[55] Renal involvement in beta$_2$-microglobulin amyloidosis is at present rare because in this form of the disease amyloid is initially laid down in bones, joints and tendons, and in the carpal tunnel. As deposition continues other tissues, including the kidneys, may become involved, but the frequency with which renal involvement occurs is not yet known.

Clinical features

The frequency of renal amyloidosis varies in different parts of the world and within populations. Countries where leprosy, tuberculosis and chronic suppurative infections remain common have a much greater incidence of AA amyloidosis than is found in those lands where these conditions are

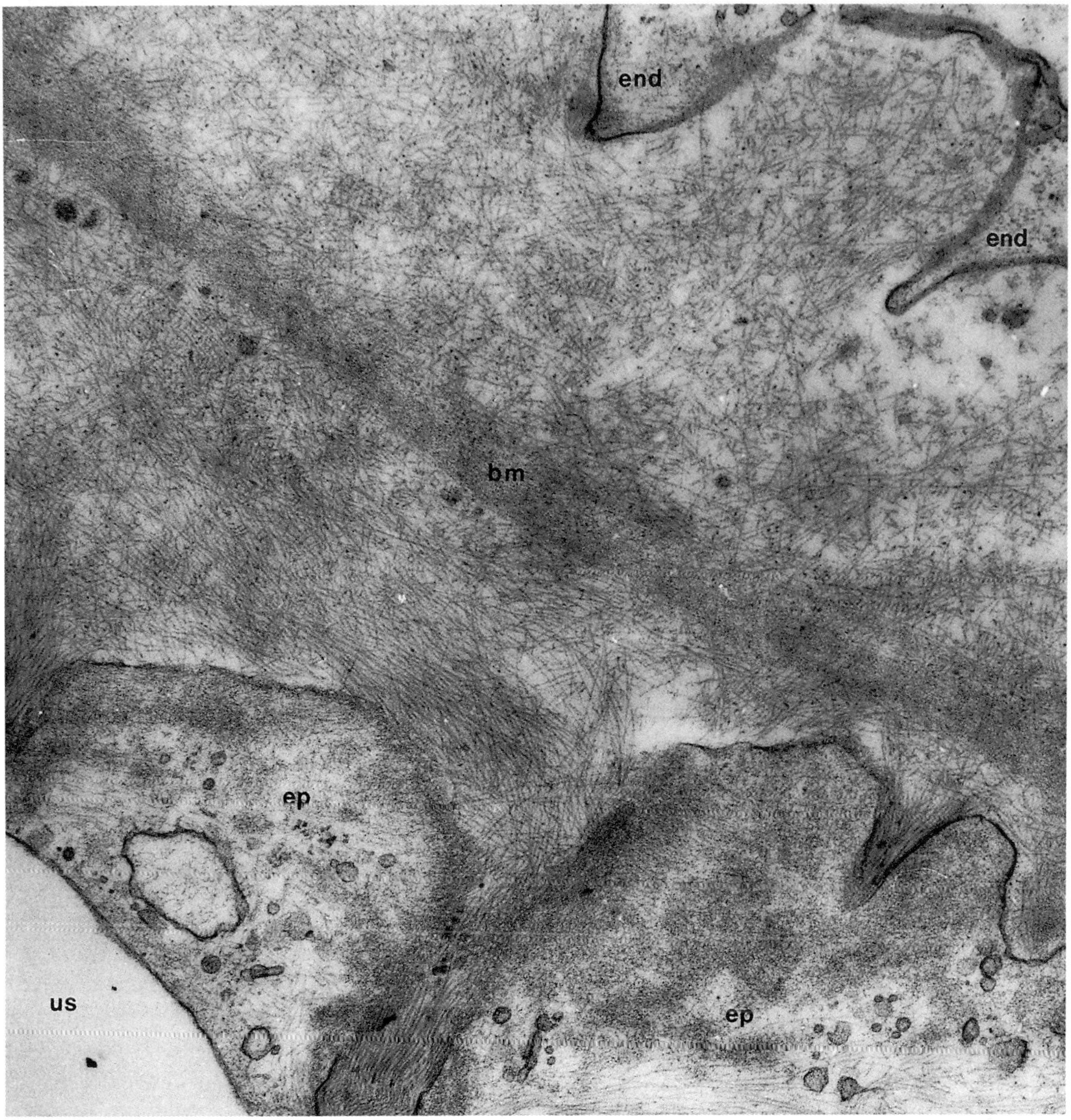

Fig. 10.12 Amyloidosis. Electron micrograph of part of the wall of a glomerular capillary. The subendothelial space, basement membrane and subepithelial space are infiltrated by a meshwork of amyloid fibrils. end, endothelium; bm, basement membrane; ep, retracted foot processes of visceral epithelial cells; us, urinary space.
× 50 000

rare. Some of the hereditary forms of transthyretin amyloidosis, although very rare in most countries, are common within local ethnic groups that carry the appropriate gene (see p. 109).

The mean age at diagnosis is between 20 and 40 years for the hereditary forms of transthyretin amyloidosis, between 45 and 50 years for AA amyloidosis, between 55 and 60 years for AL amyloidosis and 65 and 70 years for senile systemic transthyretin amyloidosis. Renal amyloidosis is rare in children but when it occurs it is usually AA in type and related to chronic infection or familial Mediterranean fever. Males tend to be affected more than females.

In Western Europe and the USA the conditions that most frequently predispose to AA amyloidosis are the chronic rheumatic diseases such as rheumatoid arthritis, juvenile chronic arthritis and ankylosing spondylitis, and other chronic inflammatory states such as Reiter's syndrome, dermatomyositis and Crohn's disease. Local infections such as the chronic urinary tract infections of paraplegic patients, chronically infected burns and the chronic skin infections of heroin addicts who inject the drugs subcutaneously (see p. 511) are other well-recognized causes of amyloidosis.

Proteinuria is the usual presenting sign. It may be a chance finding at routine physical examination or it may occur during the course of one of the diseases known to be associated with amyloidosis. In approximately 50–70% of cases the proteinuria is severe and associated with the nephrotic syndrome.[56] Microscopic haematuria may be found but is unusual. As the condition advances chronic renal failure develops. If renal vein thrombosis supervenes there may be acute renal failure. Hypertension is less frequent than in many other types of chronic renal failure. Many patients suffer from postural hypotension, perhaps because of infiltration of the autonomic ganglia by amyloid.[53] Occasionally patients develop nephrogenic diabetes insipidus or other tubular syndromes secondary to preferential deposition of amyloid around the collecting ducts in the medulla.[57,58] The deposits of amyloid can be localized by scintigraphy after intravenous injection of ^{123}I-labelled purified human serum amyloid P component.[59] The basis of this test is the fact that the polyanionic amyloid fibrils bind relatively large amounts of serum amyloid P components, whereas only very small quantities become attached to normal tissues.

Serology

In AA amyloidosis the concentration in the serum of the precursor protein, an acute-phase reactant called serum amyloid A protein (SAA), is greatly increased. Patients with AL amyloidosis have immunoglobulin light chains, or fragments of such chains, particularly the amino-terminal segments, in the serum. In transthyretin amyloidosis the total circulating transthyretin is lower than normal in patients with the different forms of rare familial amyloid polyneuropathy; also the transthyretin is composed of a mixture of normal and variant molecules.[50] Beta$_2$-microglobulin amyloidosis is associated with raised levels of beta$_2$-microglobulin in the serum (see p. 40).

Renal changes

Gross appearances of the kidneys

Both kidneys are usually enlarged. The subcapsular surface is smooth, and the cut surface pale and firm. When a thin slice is treated with Lugol's aqueous iodine solution the glomeruli appear as deep brown dots in those cases in which they are predominantly involved.

Light microscopy

In typical cases of AA amyloidosis the deposits in the kidneys are mainly in the glomeruli. Deposition is initially focal and segmental in the mesangium, producing palely eosinophilic, PAS-negative masses of varying size (Fig. 10.13). Glomerular tuft cellularity is normal. Mesangial deposition is followed by spread to the capillary wall; this may be accompanied by focal and segmental, irregular, subepithelial spikes, which are visible if silver methenamine is used to stain the capillary basement membrane.[60] As the disease advances more glomeruli become involved: the amyloid deposits enlarge, narrowing and finally obliterating the capillary lumens (Fig. 10.14). Eventually entire glomerular tufts become replaced by amyloid.

Occasionally small crescents occur and very rarely giant cells have been reported in relation to the amyloid deposits, the most striking examples being in cases of familial amyloidosis of the Ostertag variety.[61]

Similar changes are seen in about 50% of cases of AL amyloidosis, but the remainder may show much less or even no glomerular involvement. The same is true of transthyretin amyloidosis in senile systemic amyloidosis[55] and in some of the hereditary forms of amyloidosis.[62] The walls of the arterioles and interlobular arteries are often per-

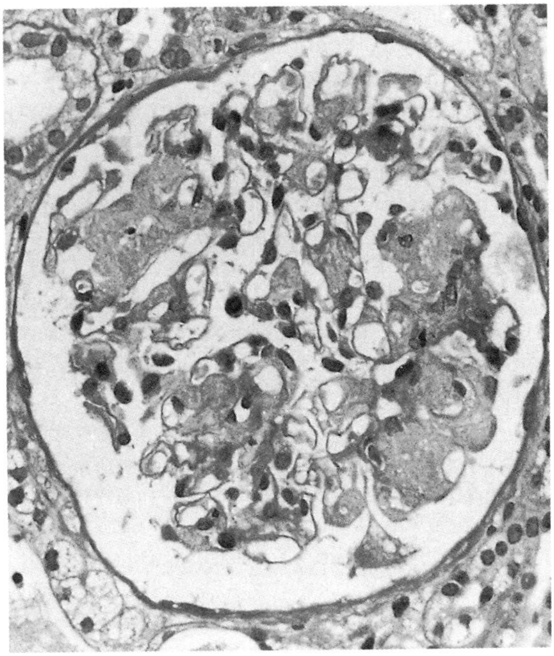

Fig. 10.13 Amyloidosis. Glomerulus showing irregular mesangial deposits of amyloid that are unstained by the periodic acid-Schiff method.
Periodic acid- Schiff × 390

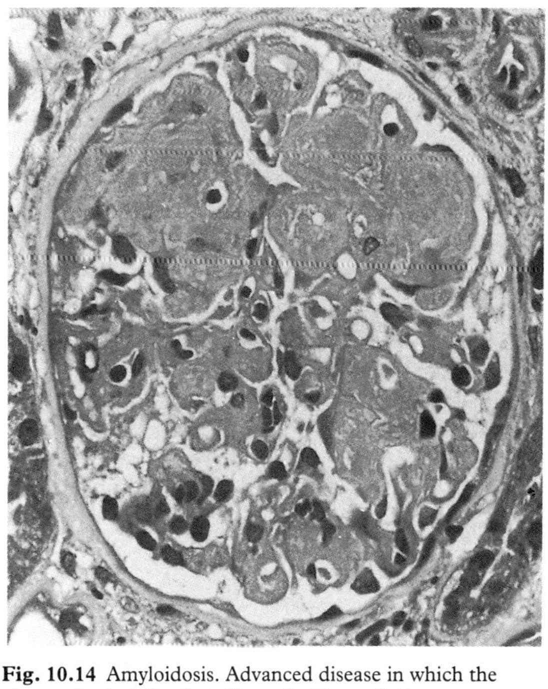

Fig. 10.14 Amyloidosis. Advanced disease in which the glomerulus is diffusely infiltrated with amyloid.
Haematoxylin-eosin × 350

meated by amyloid. In AL amyloidosis and some forms of transthyretin amyloidosis these vessels may be the only structures in the kidney that are affected. The venae rectae may also be involved.

Amyloid may infiltrate the basement membranes of the tubules, particularly the distal tubules and loops of Henle. Occasionally these deposits predominate and also involve the basement membranes of the collecting ducts; in such cases glomerular and vascular deposits, other than in the vasa recta, are inconspicuous.[57] In all patients the tubules atrophy and disappear as the amyloid deposits become more extensive.

The interstitium is sometimes the site of deposits. This usually occurs in the inner medulla but masses of AA amyloid have been recorded in the superficial cortex in patients with chronic paraplegia.[63]

Histochemistry

Detection of amyloid The production of green birefringence by polarized light in Congo red-stained sections is the single most reliable specific method of diagnosis by light microscopy. For this technique to be successful 6–8 μm thick sections should be used; amyloid will often fail to stain in the usual thin sections. In addition appropriate positive and negative controls need to be used. Methyl violet, which stains amyloid a metachromatic pink against a blue background, and thioflavine T, which induces deposits of amyloid to fluoresce under ultraviolet light, are sensitive but not absolutely specific methods.

With all these techniques small amounts of amyloid may be missed because each method requires a critical amount of amyloid to react with the reagent before a positive result can be produced.

Immunohistochemical staining with antibody to amyloid P component also provides additional evidence that deposits are amyloid.

Identification of amyloid fibril type AA amyloid can be distinguished from AL and most other forms of amyloid by incubating Congo red-stained sections with potassium permanganate. This treatment removes the Congo red stain and the green birefringence from AA amyloid; AL and transthyretin amyloid are resistant to permanganate and retain the stain.[64] However, this is not a completely definitive test on its own because the Ostertag type of familial amyloidosis and beta$_2$-immunoglobulin amyloidosis both have permanganate-sensitive fibrils that are not AA in type.[65]

Specific antisera to different amyloid fibril proteins can be used to stain amyloid deposits in tissue sections. Potent anti-AA serum is commercially available and will specifically stain AA deposits (Fig. 10.15).[66] Antisera to transthyretin are easily obtainable but only some transthyretin deposits are stained by them; senile systemic amyloidosis in particular is usually unstained. AL amyloid presents special problems; the subunits are predominantly derived from the variable region of the light chain and therefore usually lack the common characteristic isotopic epitopes of lambda and kappa chains. It is often necessary to use individual anti-idiotypic antisera raised against the patient's own monoclonal protein to obtain positive staining.[67]

Electron microscopy

The amyloid deposits are composed of a meshwork of fine unbranched fibrils, 7.5–10 nm in diameter and 30–1000 nm in length, embedded in a matrix (Fig. 10.12).[68] The fibrils are unimpeded by any natural barrier: they spread in continuity through all structures. Where they penetrate the glomerular capillary basement membrane the fibrils are commonly arranged in parallel arrays perpendicular to the membrane, forming tufts of amyloid fibrils that extend into the urinary space (Fig. 10.16). These bunches of protruding amyloid fibrils give the spicular appearance on light microscopy of silver methenamine preparations that was mentioned earlier.[60] Spicules occur most commonly in AL amyloidosis.[69] What it is that stains with silver is not clear: perhaps it is basement membrane material between the fibrils, or it may be that the parallel arrangement of the fibrils in some unknown manner increases their affinity for silver.

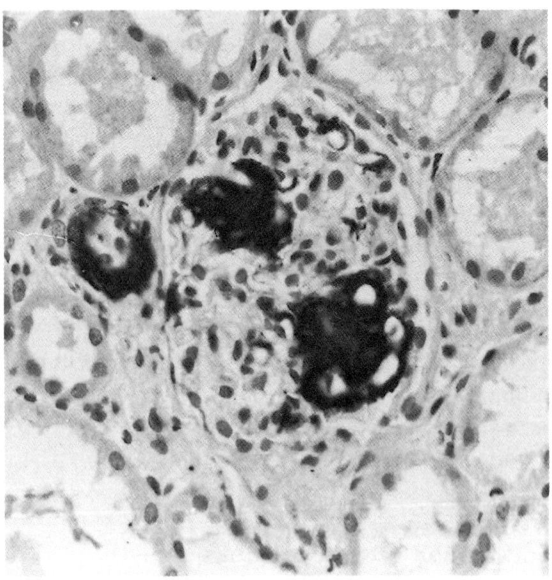

Fig. 10.15 Amyloidosis. Glomerulus stained with an antibody to solubulized AA amyloid fibrils. There are deposits of amyloid in the glomerular mesangium and capillary walls, and in the afferent arteriolar wall. Positively stained fibrils extend out from the capillary walls into Bowman's space.
Immunoperoxidase × 300

Immunofluorescence/immunoperoxidase microscopy

Non-specific mild homogeneous staining of the deposits for IgM, C3 and C1q is often seen and sometimes faint staining for other immunoglobulins or complement components. Amyloid is autofluorescent in ultraviolet light.

Differential diagnosis

Mesangial nodules of amyloid may sometimes resemble those of *diabetic glomerulosclerosis*. Diffuse infiltration of the capillary basement membrane by amyloid may produce an appearance that resembles *diffuse membranous glomerulonephritis*; even the subepithelial spikes on silver staining may be present (see p. 192). Occasionally arteriolar deposits may be misinterpreted as *hyalin*. However, most of these initial difficulties disappear when Congo red staining is done and all can be resolved by the ultrastructural demonstration of amyloid fibrils. The differentiation of amyloid fibrils from other forms of fibril is discussed on page 351.

Renal transplantation

By the time kidneys affected by amyloidosis have progressed to end-stage failure, many of the patients have multiple problems from amyloid deposits elsewhere in the body and from the

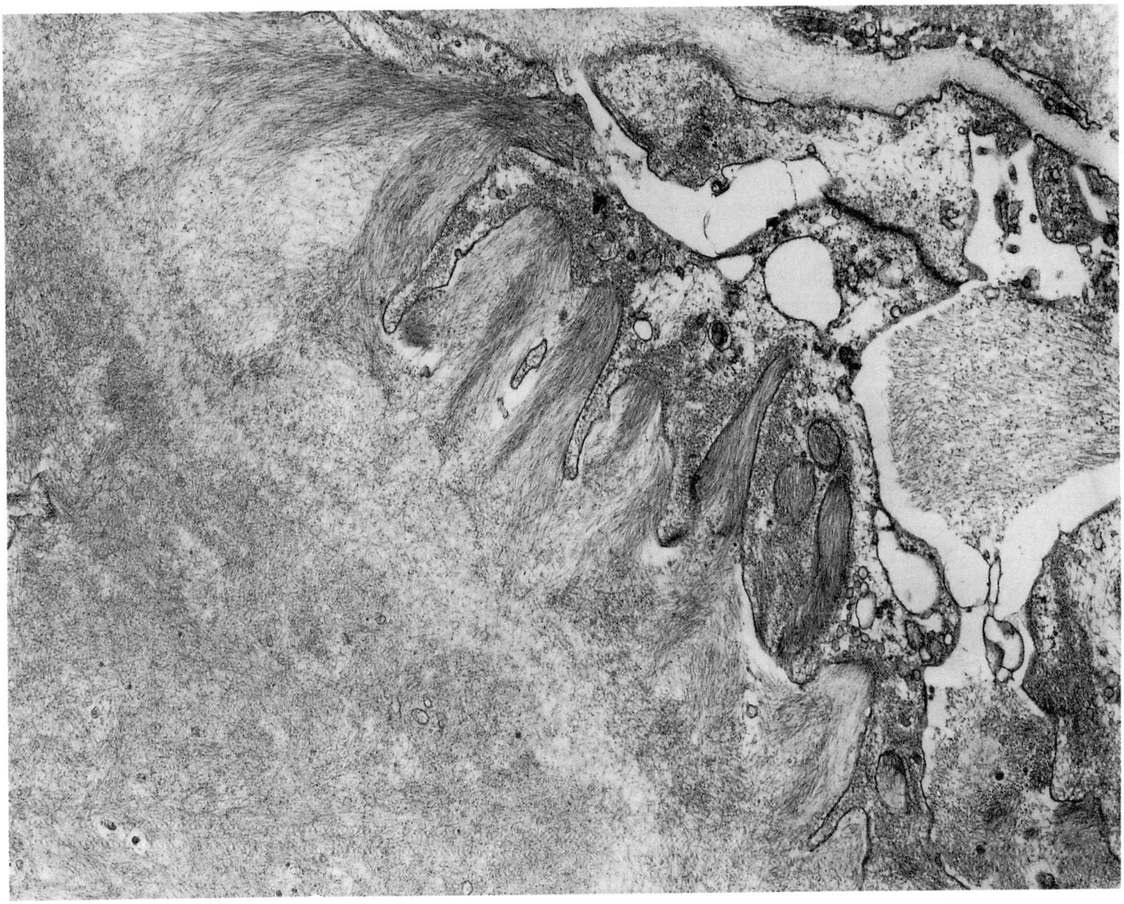

Fig. 10.16 Amyloidosis. Electron micrograph of part of a glomerular capillary basement membrane which is permeated by amyloid fibrils. In the upper and right part of the picture bunches of fibrils have formed spicules that protrude from the epithelial side of the basement membrane into Bowman's space. They are covered by visceral epithelium in which the foot processes are effaced.
× 20 250

underlying disease, and are unsuitable for renal transplantation. Those patients who are given a renal transplant have a lower survival rate than graft recipients who do not have amyloidosis. In one series of 45 patients who received a cadaveric graft the 3-year survival was 51%.[70]

Amyloid develops in the graft in about 20–30% of cases; it does not usually become apparent until 11 months to 3 years after transplantation. Although the amount of amyloid in the kidney and the degree of proteinuria progressively increase these are rarely the main problems; patients are more likely to die from infection following treatment of rejection episodes or from cardiovascular complications related to widespread amyloidosis (see p. 670).

Prognosis

Although there is no specific treatment for any form of amyloidosis, there is evidence that in renal amyloidosis proteinuria may diminish and renal function improve when it is possible to remove or suppress the underlying condition. This has occurred, for example, after a chronic infection causing AA amyloidosis has either been cured by antimicrobial drugs or has been resected,[56] or a chronic rheumatic disease has been treated vigorously.[71] It has also been recorded after successful cytotoxic therapy in AL amyloidosis.[72,73] But only very rarely has convincing evidence of significant reduction in the quantity of amyloid in the kidneys been reported and in none of these has there been complete disappearance of the deposits.[74–76] Amyloid fibrils on the subepithelial side of the glomerular capillary basement membranes become covered by new basement membrane giving the capillary wall a double contour on light microscopy. In one case fibrils, although greatly reduced in quantity, were still present 5½ years after the patient had recovered from infected burns.[74] With $beta_2$-microglobulin amyloidosis it is not yet known whether lowering the circulating $beta_2$-microglobulin concentration by renal transplantation or by using specific absorbents to deplete $beta_2$-microglobulin selectively during dialysis, will lead to resolution of existing amyloid deposits.

If the underlying cause cannot be eliminated the mean duration of life after diagnosis is 14.7 months but there is great variation and patients may survive for 8 or more years.[53] The usual course is of progressive renal failure which may suddenly accelerate if renal vein thrombosis supervenes: this complication occurred in nearly 40% of patients with familial Mediterranean fever in one series.[77]

The development of AA amyloidosis in familial Mediterranean fever can be prevented by long-term treatment with colchicine (see p. 110).[78]

Pathogenesis[50,51,79]

Despite our greatly increased knowledge of the composition, the molecular structure and the properties of many of the constituent elements of amyloid, we still know little about the mechanisms of amyloid fibril formation, deposition and persistence.

The initial event is something which either stimulates overproduction or impairs clearance of an autologous precursor. For example, in the case of AA amyloidosis the production of serum amyloid A protein, one of the acute-phase reactants, is increased greater than 1000-fold by chronic inflammation because the macrophages produce interleukin-1 which induces the hepatic parenchymal cells to synthesize and release large amounts of serum amyloid A protein.

The autologous precursor, which is a protein, is released either into the circulation (e.g. serum amyloid A protein, monoclonal immunoglobulin light chains, transthyretin and $beta_2$-microglobulin) or locally within some part of an organ (e.g. monoclonal immunoglobulin light chains produced by local collections of plasma cells) and is abnormal, either in its structure or in its concentration or in both. In most instances the precursor is then proteolytically cleaved by cells of the mononuclear phagocyte system (in the case of the kidney probably cells in the mesangium) to give a lower molecular weight fragment. As a result of cleavage, the fragment is thought to acquire a tendency to aggregate with other fragments and to interact with precursors of other substances found in amyloid, leading to polymerization and fibril formation.

The persistence of amyloid fibrils in the tissues once they have been laid down has been thought to be due to the presence in the fibrils of extensive antiparallel beta-pleated sheet formation, with segments of polypeptide chains lying side by side at nearly maximal extension. A formation like this is found in silk fibroin, which is particularly resistant to degradation. Recent evidence, however, indicates that the fibrils are not composed solely of beta-pleated sheets but consist of globular subunits, each of which contains some beta-pleated sheets:[80] this suggests that the fibrils are not therefore inherently non-biodegradable.

Variant

Localized amyloidosis

Occasionally isolated deposits of amyloid occur in the renal pelvis without any evidence of deposits elsewhere except sometimes in the ureter.[66,81] They may cause flank pain, gross haematuria, urinary tract infection and rarely hydronephrosis.

The amyloid in those isolated deposits that have been analysed histochemically has been AL in type and composed of lambda light chains.[66] The deposits are surrounded by a dense mononuclear cell infiltrate containing many plasma cells. In some cases the plasma cells have been shown to contain lambda light chains, suggesting that the precursor of the amyloid fibrils was formed locally.[66]

FIBRILLARY GLOMERULOPATHY[82]

In recent years a number of cases have been reported in which the mesangium in many glomeruli is diffusely expanded by material containing microfibrils 10–20 nm in diameter and of variable length. The fibrils show no periodicity, are not arranged in paired bundles and do not stain with Congo red, thioflavine T or other amyloid stains. They often extend into segments of the glomerular capillary basement membranes. In some cases there is slight mesangial proliferation; a few have also shown some extracapillary proliferation. Immunofluorescence/immunoperoxidase microscopy demonstrates diffuse mesangial deposits of IgG, C3 and both kappa and lambda light chains. There may also be lesser staining for other immunoglobulins and complement components.

Clinically, proteinuria is the presenting feature; most patients also have microscopic haematuria and some develop hypertension and impaired renal function. The mean age is 45 years with a range of 25–64 years. The condition is slightly more common in males. There is usually no apparent associated disease; but sometimes fibrillary glomerulopathy occurs during the course of hyperthyroidism, diabetes mellitus, carcinoma of the lung, gastric ulcer, cellulitis, rheumatoid arthritis and cholelithiasis. Proteinuria often becomes severe enough for the nephrotic syndrome to develop. Serology reveals the absence of cryoglobulinaemia and paraproteinaemia.

The fibrils differ from amyloid by being larger in diameter (10–20 nm compared to 7.5–10 nm in amyloid), lacking cross-periodicity, and failing to stain with Congo red. They are smaller than the 20–49 nm diameter fibrils that occur in immunotactoid glomerulopathy and cryoglobulinaemia, and in contrast to some cases of the latter do not appear in bundles composed of two cylinders. Occasionally microfibrils 9–14 nm in diameter have been described in light chain deposition disease (see p. 364), but these fibrils contain only one light chain whereas in fibrillary glomerulopathy the fibrils stain equally intensely for both kappa and lambda light chains as well as gamma and alpha heavy chains and complement components.

Approximately half the patients have progressive deterioration of renal function over a period of 2–8 years. The origin of the fibrils is not known.

CRYOGLOBULINAEMIA

Cryoglobulinaemia is an infrequent disorder characterized by the persistent presence in the blood of proteins that reversibily separate as a gel, or even as crystals, when the plasma is cooled. For diagnosis the blood must be kept at 37°C between collection and analysis. The abnormal protein is usually but not always an immunoglobulin; it may be a paraprotein. The higher the concentration of cryoprotein in the blood, the higher is the temperature at which precipitation occurs.

Cryoglobulins may consist of a single immunoglobulin and are then called *monoclonal cryoglobulins*, the most frequent being IgG or IgM. More often they are composed of two or more immunoglobulins belonging to different classes and are called *mixed cryoglobulins*. Most are IgM – IgG immune complexes: IgM is the antibody and can be either monoclonal or polyclonal; IgG is the antigen and is polyclonal.[83] The IgM acts as a rheumatoid factor against the IgG.

Cryoglobulinaemia may be *secondary* to some underlying disease. If no associated condition can be detected then the term *essential cryoglobulinaemia* is used. Essential cryoglobulinaemia accounts for between a third and a half of all cases of cryoglobulinaemia.

Monoclonal cryoglobulinaemia (type I cryoglobulinaemia) is found in patients with multiple myeloma, Waldenström's macroglobulinaemia or monoclonal gammopathy of undetermined significance and accounts for approximately a quarter of cases of cryoglobulinaemia.

Mixed cryoglobulinaemia in which the IgM is monoclonal (type II cryogloblinaemia) may be secondary to a lymphoproliferative disorder: the letter may be neoplastic, such as a B-lymphocyte neoplasm, chronic lymphocytic leukaemia, diffuse lymphoma, multiple myeloma or Waldenström's macroglobulinaemia, or non-neoplastic, as in Sjøgren's syndrome. Type II cryoglobulinaemia accounts for about a quarter of cases of cryoglobulinaemia.

Mixed cryoglobulinaemia in which both immunoglobulin components are polyclonal (type III cryoglobulinaemia) may be secondary to various autoimmune conditions, such as systemic lupus erythematosus, polyarteritis, Henoch–Schönlein purpura and Sjøgren's syndrome, or to infectious diseases such as diffuse endocapillary proliferative glomerulonephritis, bacterial endocarditis, syphilis, leprosy, hepatitis B virus infection, infectious mononucleosis, malaria, schistosomiasis and coccidioidomycosis. Type III cryoglobulinaemia accounts for about half the cases of cryoglobulinaemia.[83,84]

The kidneys are affected in 35–60% of patients with type II cryoglobulinaemia and uncommonly in patients with types I and III cryoglobulinaemia.[83,84]

Clinical features

The mean age of onset in mixed cryoglobulinaemia is about 50 years, but signs and symptoms can occur as early as the third decade. Men are more likely to develop renal complications than women even though more women have mixed cryoglobulinaemia. Occasionally the disease is familial. Mixed cryoglobulinaemia is encountered in most countries but the majority of cases have been reported from the Mediterranean countries and from the city of New York. In patients with cryoglobulinaemia the underlying disease may only become obvious some years after the detection of cryoglobulins in the blood. Patients typically have episodic purpura, which usually begins in the legs and is often dependent and palpable. This is often associated with arthralgia, and may be accompanied by weakness, peripheral neuropathy and hepatic involvement. Raynaud's phenomenon is frequent.[83,84]

Renal involvement usually presents as proteinuria which is sometimes associated with microscopic haematuria and hypertension. About a fifth of the patients have a nephrotic syndrome when first seen; a further fifth have an acute nephritic syndrome. A few cases rapidly progress to extreme oliguria. Tubular acidosis is sometimes a feature.

Serology

Hypocomplementaemia is characteristic. In patients with renal disease the levels of C4 are very low, and C1q, Cls and C3 depressed. The CH50 level is normal. A cryoglobulin is present in the blood and there is strongly positive rheumatoid factor activity.[84]

Renal changes[84–87]

Light microscopy

In acute cases of type II mixed cryoglobulinaemia the glomeruli are enlarged with diffuse endocapillary proliferation; there is diffuse intracapillary infiltration by macrophages and focal and segmental infiltration by neutrophil granulocytes. Numerous large amorphous masses, often described as '*thrombi*', partly or completely occlude some of the capillary lumens in many of the glomeruli (Fig. 10.17). The intracapillary masses stain strongly with eosin, are PAS-positive and are negative for Congo red and fibrin. Smaller subendothelial collections of similar material are often discernible. Occasional cellular crescents are sometimes present. The arterioles contain similar occlusive masses and in approximately a third of the patients may show focal necrosis of their walls with or without any associated perivascular infiltrating cells. Patchy mononuclear cell infiltration of the interstitium is often present, consisting of macrophages and T lymphocytes, mainly of the CD8 subset. Serial renal biopsies have shown that the endocapillary proliferation and the intracapillary and subendothelial homogeneous eosinophilic masses disappear within a few weeks.[86,88,89]

A more chronic clinical course in type II mixed cryoglobulinaemia is most frequently associated with a diffuse mesangiocapillary glomerulonephritis, but focal segmental endocapillary proliferation, sometimes with crescents, also occurs. Even membranous glomerulonephritis has been described.[83,90] Intracapillary masses are infrequent but segmental subendothelial deposits may produce 'wire loops' (see p. 229). As the disease progresses increasing numbers of glomeruli become sclerotic and any crescents undergo fibrosis. Necrosis of arteriolar walls and interstitial fibrosis with mononulear cell infiltration may be present.[86,88]

Glomerular lesions are occasionally seen in monoclonal (type 1) cryoglobulinaemia and in

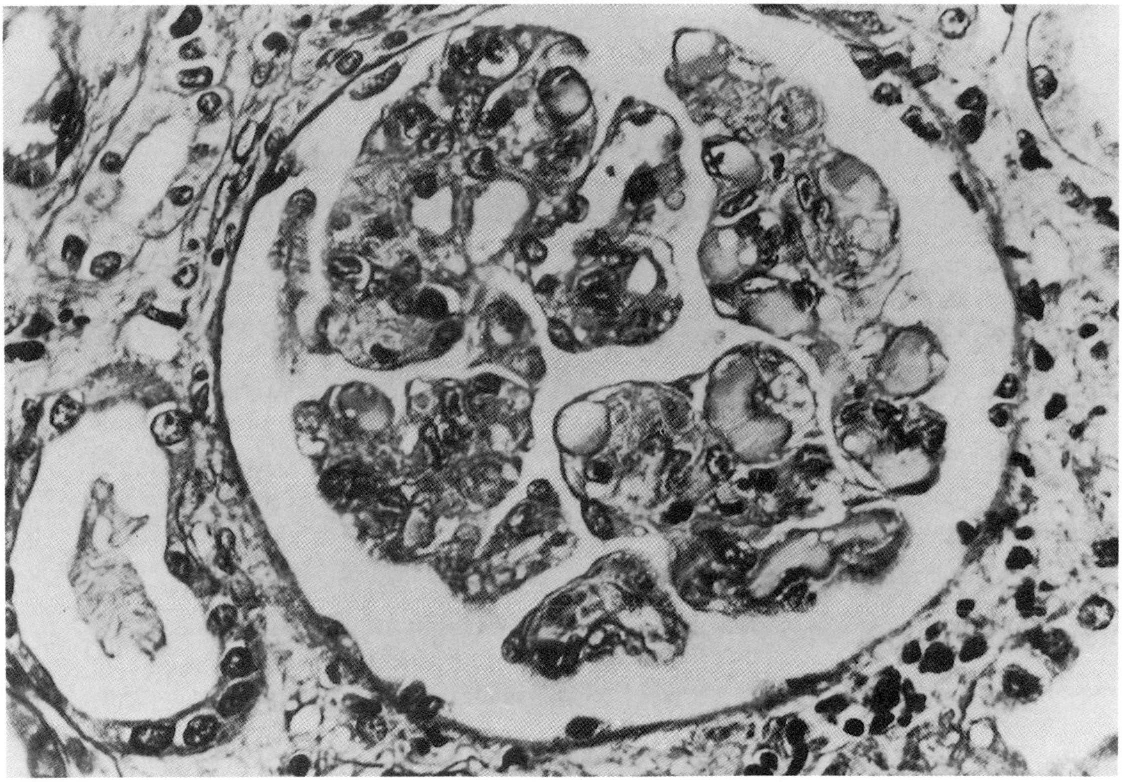

Fig. 10.17 Type II essential mixed cryoglobulinaemia. Acute disease. The glomerulus shows endocapillary proliferation and several of the capillary lumens contain large collections of homogeneous eosinophilic material.
Haematoxylin-eosin × 250
Reproduced by permission from: Verroust P, Morel-Maroger L, Preud'homme JL. Springer Semin Immunopathol 1982; 5: 333 (Fig. 10)

type III mixed cryoglobulinaemia.[83,89,90] They closely resemble those encountered in type II cryoglobulinaemia; the only difference is that in acute type III cryoglobulinaemia intracapillary amorphous masses are not found.[83] Intracapillary amorphous masses seem to be related to the presence of monoclonal immunoglobulin in the cryoglobulin.

Electron microscopy

In mixed cryoglobulinaemia electron-dense deposits are present in the mesangium, on the subendothelial aspects of the glomerular capillary basement membranes and occasionally within the basement membranes and extending on to the subepithelial side of the membranes. Many of the amorphous masses in the capillary lumens are large subendothelial deposits; some appear to be free in the lumen. Under high resolution, in some, but not all, cases, these deposits contain microfibrils or cylinders which are paired. In type II mixed cryoglobulinaemia each fibril measures 20–30 nm in diameter and a bundle of two fibrils is 60–70 nm in diameter. On cross section they appear as annular bodies with a light centre (Fig. 10.18).[91,92] The swollen cytoplasm of the endothelial and mesangial cells may contain crystals of various shapes and electron-lucent needle-shaped spaces.[89]

The deposits in monoclonal IgG cryoglobulinaemia also contain fibrils; they may be straight and arranged in bundles 80 nm in diameter and up to 1 μm in length,[91] or they may be curved and arranged in a fingerprint-like array (Fig. 10.19).[93] The individual fibril diameter is 20–30 nm. Monoclonal IgM cryoglobulins are either amorphous or have only a vaguely fibrillar appearance.

Electron microscopy confirms that monocytes

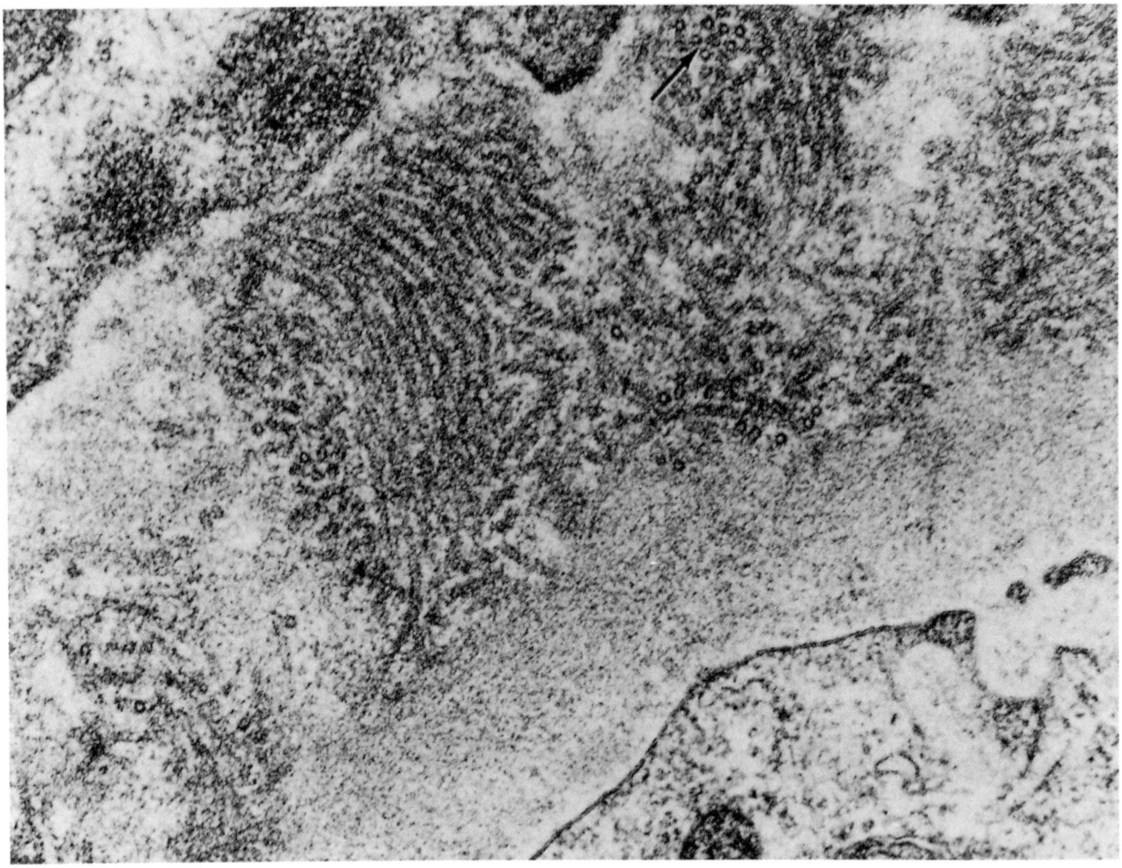

Fig. 10.18 Type II essential mixed cryoglobulinaemia. Acute disease. Electron micrograph of part of a deposit on the subendothelial aspect of the glomerular capillary basement membrane. The deposit contains fibrils which appear annular when cut transversely.
× 48 000
Reproduced by permission from: Spargo BH, Seymour AE, Ordonez NG. Renal biopsy pathology with diagnostic therapeutic implications. New York: John Wiley, 1980 (Fig. 20.1)

in the glomerular capillary lumens are mainly responsible for the intracapillary proliferation in the acute stages. Mesangial cell proliferation and increases in mesangial matrix also occur.[87]

Immunofluorescence/immunoperoxidase microscopy

In mixed cryoglobulinaemia the subendothelial and mesangial fibrillar deposits contain IgG, IgM, C3, C1q and C4, producing a granular pattern in the capillary walls and in the mesangium. Any intraluminal homogeneous masses stain similarly. If the arterioles show focal necroses their walls stain for IgG, IgM and complement.[84,86]

In monoclonal cryoglobulinaemia a particular cryoglobulin may be present either alone or with complement components.[90]

Changes in Other Organs

Fibrillar deposits occur in blood vessels of the skin,[83,94] vasa nervorum, endoneural spaces[95] and Kupffer cells[96] of patients with purpura, peripheral neuropathy and hepatic signs and symptoms. Necrotizing vascular lesions may affect other organs such as the lungs or the gut.

Differential diagnosis

By light microscopy the acute glomerular lesions

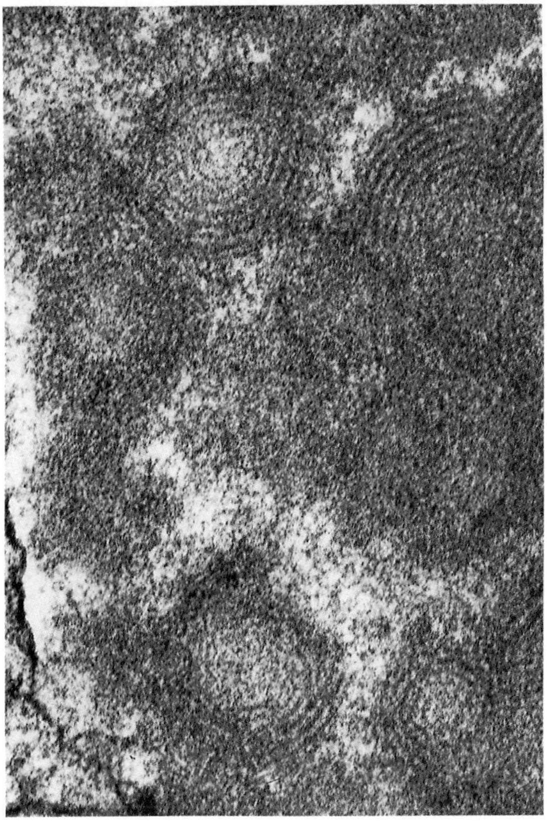

Fig. 10.19 Type 1 monoclonal IgG kappa cryoglobulinaemia. High resolution electron micrograph of part of deposit on subendothelial aspect of glomerular capillary wall. The curved bundles of fibrils resemble finger prints.
× 90 000

may resemble *diffuse endocapillary proliferative glomerulonephritis*. In many cases, however, there are intracapillary amorphous masses which should immediately make one think of cryoglobulinaemia and take a serum sample for confirmation. Similar intraluminal masses are seen in *Waldenström's macroglobulinaemia* but they are unaccompanied by hypercellularity of the glomerular tufts, which is a feature of cryoglobulinaemia and they only contain IgM and a single light chain. In cases of cryoglobulinaemia without intracapillary masses smaller subendothelial deposits can often be seen and electron microscopy will distinguish these from the subepithelial humps that are usually found in diffuse endocapillary proliferative glomerulonephritis (see p. 147). Electron microscopy may also reveal the characteristic 20–30 nm diameter fibrils.

Chronic cases frequently resemble *mesangiocapillary glomerulonephritis* by light microscopy. Electron microscopy may resolve the problem by revealing characteristic fibrils in the subendothelial deposits; if there are no fibrils, differentiation may depend upon the presence or not of a cryoglobulin in the blood. When a cryoglobulin is demonstrated its concentration and the presence or absence of monoclonal components and the presence of extrarenal symptoms, should distinguish between cryoglobulinaemia and primary glomerulonephritis.

The renal lesions of cryoglobulinaemia and *lupus nephritis* may be indistinguishable on morphological grounds, but the associated clinical and laboratory findings usually enable a distinction to be made.

Renal transplantation

There is little known about transplantation in cryoglobulinaemia. The few reports that there have been indicate that persistent cryoglobulinaemia after transplantation does not lead to any obvious lesions in the graft or deterioration in function in the first few months.[97]

Prognosis

The clinical course and prognosis vary widely according to the degree of renal involvement, the type of extrarenal lesions and the presence of an underlying disease, but in one series 65% of patients were alive 10 years after the onset of the disease and still had normal renal function. Cerebral or cardiovascular incident, infections, chronic renal failure, liver failure and neoplasia accounted for most of the deaths in that order of frequency.[98] Occasionally the disease seems to resolve spontaneously. The presence of vasculitis in the renal biopsy is thought to be associated with a worse prognosis.

There is no specific treatment for essential cryoglobulinaemia; methyl prednisolone and plasma exchange are sometimes associated with improvement of renal function.[84]

Pathogenesis

The aetiology and pathogenesis of cryoglobulin

formation, precipitation and tissue damage in essential mixed cryoglobulinaemia remain unclear. There is probably a proliferative disorder of B-lymphocytes[99] with the production of monoclonal IgM kappa with rheumatoid factor activity which binds polyclonal IgG to form a cold-insoluble immune complex.[100] Some evidence suggests that the IgG is bound to some unidentified antigen, probably a viral antigen, so that the monoclonal IgM acts as an anti-immune-complex antibody.

Deposition of the serum cryoglobulins in the glomeruli probably causes the glomerulonephritic lesions, but by what mechanism is not known.[101] The evidence supporting this hypothesis is all indirect and based on three observations: the immunoglobulin classes that characterize the cryoglobulins are nearly always present in the renal deposits; the cryoprecipitates have the same fibrillar ultrastructure as is seen in many of the subendothelial and mesangial deposits; and the IgM found in glomerular deposits has the same cross-reactive idiotype as is present on the IgM rheumatoid factor in the circulating cryoglobulin.[101]

IMMUNOTACTOID GLOMERULOPATHY

Immunotactoid glomerulopathy is a term coined to describe kidneys which contain highly organized tubular structures in areas of immunoglobulin deposition in the glomeruli of patients with no evident systemic disease.[102]

Clinical features

Both sexes are affected in roughly equal numbers. Patients present with proteinuria, microscopic haematuria and hypertension. Proteinuria is almost always the reason for renal biopsy. The patients have no clinical or laboratory evidence of systemic lupus erythematosus or paraproteinaemia. Levels of cryoglobulin and C3 and C4 components of complement are normal. The ANA is negative.

Renal changes

Light microscopy

The mesangium is often globally expanded in the majority of glomeruli; there may also be a mild increase in the number of mesangial cells. The glomerular capillary basement membranes are usually irregularly thickened and prominent subendothelial deposits and intracapillary hyaline thrombi have been described. Stains for amyloid are negative.

Electron microscopy

In most patients there are prominent electron-dense deposits in the mesangium and capillary walls; capillary wall deposits are often subepithelial, subendothelial and intramembranous. The deposits contain microtubules which are usually straight and unbranched, 22–49 nm in diameter and of variable length. They are arranged in a tightly packed feltwork and in some instances form paracrystalline arrays.[102]

Immunofluorescence/immunoperoxidase microscopy

There are coarse granular deposits of IgG and C3 in the glomerular capillary walls and mesangium; IgM and C1q are also sometimes present.[102]

Differential diagnosis

The microtubules differ from amyloid by being larger in diameter (22–49 nm compared with 7.5–10 nm in amyloid), lacking cross-periodicity and failing to stain with Congo red. They are also larger then the 10–20 nm diameter fibrils found in fibrillary glomerulopathy (see p. 351). They closely resemble the microtubules that occur in cryoglobulinaemia, but serum cryoglobulins are not detected.

Prognosis

In a few patients who have been followed up from 22 to 94 months approximately half develop severe hypertension and progressive deterioration of renal function; most require dialysis within 4 years. The others had persistent proteinuria but stable renal function.[102]

Aetiology and pathogenesis

The aetiology and pathogenesis are unknown. One possibility is that the glomerulopathy represents a very early or exclusively renal expression of a monoclonal gammopathy of undetermined significance (see p. 367), in which the aberrant plasma cell clone is not recognized. A case reported recently could be an example of immunotactoid glomerulopathy in which the abnormal plasma cell clone was detected. The patient had an IgG kappa monoclonal gammopathy of undetermined significance and a glomerulonephritis with microtubular deposits of the type found in immunotactoid glomerulopathy.[103] However, light chain deposits are not normally arranged in tubules; when they are they tend to be 9–14 nm in diameter. Another possibility is that the condition is a variant of lupus nephritis; a case has been reported in which deposits of the immunotactoid type were mixed with fingerprint deposits in a patient with mixed connective tissue disease.[104]

PARAPROTEINAEMIA

Paraproteins are immunoglobulins or light chains or heavy chains of immunoglobulins that are either abnormally constituted or present in increased amounts in the blood or urine. They differ from normal polyclonal immunoglobulin in that they are of restricted electrophoretic mobility and of a single heavy and light chain class, e.g. IgG kappa, IgM lambda. They are the result of monoclonal proliferation of B lymphocytes or plasma cells and can be detected as a homogeneous protein band on electrophoresis. The production of paraproteins is often accompanied by secretion of an excess of free immunoglobulin light chains or their fragments.

In some patients the monoclonal proliferation is clinically benign; in other instances it is progressive and autonomous. Patients who have a monoclonal proliferation are often referred to as having a 'paraproteinaemia'. Other terms sometimes used as synonyms are 'plasma cell dyscrasia', 'dysproteinaemia' and 'monoclonal gammopathy'.

Benign paraproteinaemia may be found in approximately 3% of healthy people over the age of 70 years. It also occurs in patients suffering from a wide range of non-lymphoproliferative disorders.

The most important progressive paraproteinaemia is multiple myeloma; others are Waldenström's macroglobulinaemia, the paraproteinaemias that are occasionally associated with lymphomas and chronic lymphocytic leukaemia, light chain deposition disease and the rare heavy chain diseases.

Renal lesions commonly occur in progressive paraproteinaemias; they are very rare in benign paraproteinaemia.

MULTIPLE MYELOMA

Multiple myeloma (myelomatosis) is a malignant disease of plasma cells, but the original mutation and much of the subsequent cell proliferation probably occur at an earlier stage in the maturation sequence of B lymphocytes.[105]

The paraprotein secreted is most commonly IgG (55–60%). IgA production is less common (20–25%), IgD occurs in about 1% and the secretion of IgM or IgE is even less frequent. Very rarely a patient with multiple myeloma produces two paraproteins. In most cases the monoclonal immunoglobulin is accompanied by the secretion of an excess of light chains, but in 20% of patients with multiple myeloma the plasma cells secrete no whole immunoglobulin molecules, only kappa or lambda light chains. Sometimes the paraprotein acts as a cryoglobulin.

Renal lesions are very common. In one autopsy series, the kidneys were abnormal in 88% of patients.[106] The frequency of renal involvement is directly related to the incidence of light chain excretion; it is most common in light chain and IgD myeloma and least frequent in IgG myeloma.[107]

Clinical features

Multiple myeloma is the commonest paraproteinaemia. Its frequency is approximately five new cases per 100 000 of the population and in Britain it accounts for 35 deaths per million of the population each year. Most patients present after the age of 50 years and the peak incidence is in those aged 60–70 years; it is slightly more common in men.[108] The initial symptoms are often weight loss and fatigue but this is frequently followed by bone pain, vertebral collapse or pathological fracture.

Approximately 50% of patients become uraemic during the course of their disease and renal failure may be a presenting feature.[109] Proteinuria is common: in patients with myeloma cast nephropathy (see below) there are almost always copious free light chains in the urine, often as the only component; in patients with light chain deposition (see p. 362) or with large and diffuse amyloid deposits, light chains are scanty or absent.[110]

Renal changes

There are three broad groups of renal lesions specifically related to multiple myeloma: *myeloma cast nephropathy, amyloid deposition* and *light chain deposition.* There is a tendency for cast nephropathy to occur independently of the other two lesions; this seems to be related to differences in the isoelectric point of the light chain and the extent to which the light chains are polymerized. These two factors probably determine whether the light chains will readily pass through the glomerular filtration barrier or be deposited in the glomeruli.[111] Light chains that have a lower isoelectric point and an increased molecular radius because they are polymerized, are less likely to enter the urine and cause cast nephropathy.

Infiltration of the kidney by neoplastic myeloma cells occurs but is unusual.[112] Occasionally *crystalline inclusions* are present in the glomerular epithelial cells and, to a lesser extent, in the mesangial and endothelial cells.[113] Crystals may also occur in tubular and interstitial cells. The crystals are composed of immunoglobulin light chain protein.[114]

In addition to these specific lesions pyelonephritis (see p. 440), nephrocalcinosis (see p. 544) and urate deposition (see p. 341) are also often present.

Myeloma cast nephropathy (Bence Jones cast nephropathy)

Myeloma cast nephropathy is seen in approximately half the patients with renal involvement.[112] The most striking change is the presence in the distal convoluted tubules and collecting ducts of refractile casts which are usually strongly eosinophilic and PAS positive (Fig. 10.20). The casts, which consist primarily of monoclonal immunoglobulin light chains (and sometimes contain amyloid if amyloid is present elsewhere in the kidneys), often appear laminate with fractures in various places; occasionally they contain rhomboid

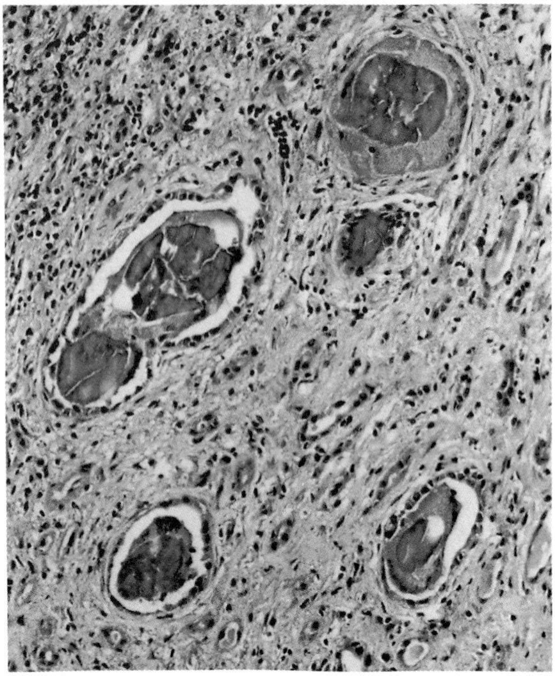

Fig. 10.20 Multiple myeloma – myeloma cast nephropathy. There are fractured tubular casts surrounded by macrophages and multinucleate giant cells.
Haematoxylin–eosin × 250

or needle-shaped crystals composed of light chains. The casts excite a foreign body reaction around their periphery and are characteristically surrounded by multinucleate giant cells (Fig. 10.19). The giant cells originate from macrophages.[115] Myeloma casts are not specific for multiple myeloma; they occur in Waldenström's macroglobulinaemia and occasionally in other conditions.

As the myeloma casts increase in size by progressive lamellar accretions, the tubules dilate and their lining epithelium flattens. Eventually the tubular basement membrane may rupture with extrusion of cast material into the interstitium; this provokes an acute or chronic inflammatory cell reaction in the interstitium. In the infiltrate there are plasma cells but it is usually easy to distinguish this mixed inflammatory infiltration from the rare invasion of the kidneys by a diffuse mass of neoplastic plasma cells.

Severe myeloma cast nephropathy is commonly accompanied by a mild increase in the number of glomerular mesangial cells and in the amount of mesangial matrix caused by light chain deposition in the mesangium and capillary basement membranes. Approximately 25% of patients with cast nephropathy will also have scanty amyloid deposition in the walls of the arterioles and interlobular arteries.

Amyloid deposition[110]

Amyloidosis occurs in approximately 7% of patients with multiple myeloma.[111] It is AL in type (see p. 344) and derived from lambda more commonly than from kappa light chains. In most cases the deposits are scanty and confined to the blood vessel wall, interstitium and tubular basement membranes. They are almost always accompanied by severe myeloma cast nephropathy.

Occasionally amyloid is present throughout the kidneys with prominent glomerular deposits, particularly in the mesangium. Myeloma cast nephropathy is slight or absent in these patients.[110]

Light chain deposition (light chain nephropathy)

The incidence of light chain deposition in multiple myeloma is difficult to assess, but is probably in the region of 20%.[112] Light chain deposition in the glomeruli and tubules produces mesangial expansion which sometimes progresses to nodule formation, and thickening of the glomerular capillary and tubular basement membranes. Light chains are also sometimes deposited in the walls of arterioles and interlobular arteries. Electron microscopy shows characteristic dense linear deposits of granular material in the basement membranes and immunofluorescence/immunoperoxidase microscopy demonstrates either kappa or lambda light chain protein in the glomerular mesangium and along the capillary and tubular basement membranes. These changes are described more fully on page 363.

Changes in other organs

In addition to the infiltrative lesions of multiple myeloma, patients with light chain nephropathy will have light chain deposition in many other organs, including the liver, heart, skin and nervous system. Similarly those patients who develop amyloid in their kidneys will almost always have deposits of this material elsewhere.

Differential diagnosis

Myeloma casts, with their characteristic coating of macrophage-like and multinucleate cells, strongly suggest a diagnosis of paraproteinaemia, although not necessarily multiple myeloma: they also occur in *Waldenström's macroglobulinaemia*, for example. Myeloma casts are not pathognomonic for paraproteinaemia; they are extremely rarely found in other conditions.

Light chain deposition is not unique to multiple myeloma. It is found in various other paraproteinaemias and in some patients who have no evidence of an immunoproliferative disorder. On light microscopy the nodular glomerulosclerosis of light chain nephropathy can resemble *nodular diabetic glomerulosclerosis, renal amyloid* and *diffuse mesangiocapillary glomerulonephritis*. But there are differences. In diffuse mesangiocapillary glomerulonephritis there is extensive mesangial interposition which is absent in light chain nephropathy; in diabetes there is often hyalinization of afferent and efferent arteriolar walls; and in amyloid the nodules stain positively with Congo red dye. With electron microscopy and immunochemistry the difference is clear: only in light chain nephropathy is there the characteristic linear deposition of light chains along the capillary and tubular basement membranes. In *dense deposit disease* there are linear electron-dense deposits along the glomerular and tubular basement membranes that are similar to those seen in light chain nephropathy. However, in dense deposit disease the glomerular electron-dense material lies within the lamina densa of the glomerular basement membrane and not in the lamina rara interna as in light chain nephropathy.

Complications

Acute tubular necrosis may occasionally occur and is one of the more unusual causes of acute renal failure in patients with multiple myeloma. Sometimes it follows treatment with nephrotoxic non-steroidal anti-inflammatory drugs given to relieve musculoskeletal pain, or various potentially nephrotoxic antibiotics given because of infection.

Acute tubular necrosis is usually superimposed on myeloma cast nephropathy or light chain nephropathy but it may occur as an isolated finding.[116]

Renal transplantation

Several renal allografts have been performed and almost all have continued to function well.[117] Light chains may deposit in the graft.[118]

Prognosis

The outlook for all patients with multiple myeloma who have clinical evidence of renal disease is worse than for those who have no apparent involvement of the kidneys. In one series, if the serum creatinine was over 265 μmol/l, median survival was only 1 year 8 months compared with over 2 years 6 months for the other patients.[119] Acute renal failure is associated with a particularly poor prognosis; it occurs in 7–9% of patients with multiple myeloma.[116,120] By eliminating factors predisposing to renal failure, such as dehydration, infection, radiodiagnostic contrast studies and hypercalcaemia, the prognosis can be improved in approximately half the patient who have lesions in their kidneys. The remainder eventually require regular dialysis. Almost all patients, however, die either within 3 years from the cardiovascular or respiratory complications of multiple myeloma or from the direct effects of the tumour; most succumb much sooner.[119]

Pathogenesis

The pathogenesis of myeloma cast nephropathy is incompletely understood. Free light chains are normally removed from the circulation by filtration through the glomeruli. Most are then catabolized in the proximal tubular cells; only a few appear in the urine. In multiple myeloma the number of free light chains or fragments of light chains that pass through the glomerular filtration barrier is often greatly increased and some evidence suggests that the tubular cells become overloaded, which exhausts their lysosomal enzymes. Tubular reabsorption of light chains then falls and large numbers of light chains pass on to the distal tubules. In the distal tubules the light chains are concentrated and in the presence of Tamm–Horsfall protein (see p. 22) and an acid environment, they precipitate to give casts.

However, not all patients with light chain proteinaemia develop tubular casts so other factors are also probably important, in particular the individual characteristics of different light chains. These characteristics include the isoelectric point, glycosylation and amino acid sequence, but the important factor or factors have not yet been defined.

The pathogenesis of light chain nephropathy is also far from clear and is discussed on page 366.

The formation of amyloid is discussed on page 350. In multiple myeloma the focal AL amyloid deposits are derived from either kappa or lambda light chains whereas the diffuse amyloid deposits are almost always of lambda chain origin.

WALDENSTRÖM'S MACROGLOBULINAEMIA

In 1944 Waldenström described two patients who had large amounts of a high molecular weight globulin in their plasma, anaemia, a bleeding tendency and infiltration of their bone marrow by lymphoid cells.[121] Subsequently it has been shown that the high molecular weight globulin is a monoclonal IgM paraprotein which is made by a malignant clone of transformed immature B lymphocytes. The IgM molecule contains a single light chain type; excess free light chains are only occasionally produced by the malignant cells. Sometimes the paraprotein acts as a cryoglobulin.

Waldenström's macroglobulinaemia is an uncommon disease that affects mainly elderly men. In one Australian survey there were 0.5 new cases per 100 000 population per year.[122] The incidence of renal complications is low compared with that in multiple myeloma, probably because of the relative infrequency of free light chains in the plasma.

Clinical features

Proteinuria occurs in approximately one-third of patients with renal lesions;[123] very occasionally it is severe enough to produce the nephrotic syndrome. The urine may contain free light chains, but monoclonal IgM is seldom present. Chronic renal insufficiency is unusual; acute renal failure is rare.

Renal changes

Several types of renal lesion may be encountered.

Glomerular intracapillary amorphous deposits

The characteristic lesion of Waldenström's macroglobulinaemia is the presence in the glomerular capillary lumens of large, amorphous, PAS-positive deposits, often described as *'thrombi'* (Fig. 10.21). The number of deposits is extremely variable.[123] In several cases similar intraluminal deposits have been seen in the arterioles. By immunofluorescence/immunoperoxidase microscopy the deposits stain only for IgM and for the light chain type present in the paraprotein. Glomerular tuft cellularity is normal.

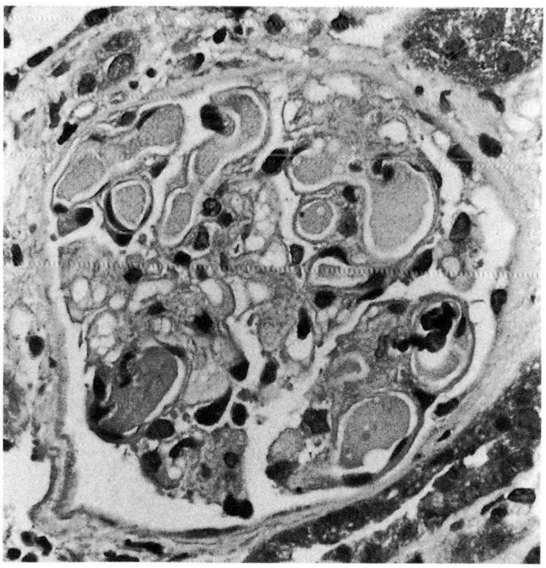

Fig. 10.21 Waldenström's macroglobulinaemia. Several glomerular capillary lumens are occluded by amorphous deposits. Tuft cellularity is normal.
Masson trichrome × 400
Reproduced by permission from: Morel–Maroger L, Basch A, Danon F, Verroust P, Richet G. N Engl J Med 1970; 283: 123 (Fig. 1)

In the few cases in which the paraprotein acts as a cryoglobulin the glomeruli usually show the endocapillary proliferative changes associated with cryoglobulinaemia (see p. 352). Immunofluorescence/immunoperoxidase microscopy reveals complement, in addition to IgM, if the cryoglobulin is type I, and complement and IgG if the cryoglobulin is type II.

Only patients with superadded cryoglobulinaemia are likely to develop renal insufficiency.

Amyloid deposition

Amyloidosis occurs in approximately 5% of patients with Waldenström's macroglobulinaemia;[124] it is usually AL in type (see p. 344). Renal deposits are generally scanty and focal; occasionally they are extensive and diffuse.[127]

Light chain nephropathy

Deposition of light chains may occur in Waldenström's macroglobulinaemia; very few cases have been reported.[126,127] In one of the patients the light chains were confined to the tubular basement membranes.[127]

Infiltration of the kidney by neoplastic lymphoid cells

Invasion of the interstitium by neoplastic lymphocytes similar to those found in the bone marrow is commonly seen (Fig. 10.22); occasionally it is sufficiently marked to cause acute renal failure or massive renal enlargement.[123,125,128] The infiltrate may be cortical but is often more evident in the medulla and may be confined to that region.[129] The lymphoid cells compress the tubules but rarely cause any clinical signs or symptoms. Dutcher bodies (large PAS-positive intranuclear inclusions)[130] may be seen in some of the infiltrating cells; their presence should lead to the suspicion of Waldenström's macroglobulinaemia.

Cast nephropathy

Casts resembling those seen in multiple myeloma (see p. 358) occasionally occur, but they are much less frequent and the multinucleate giant cell response is much less prominent.

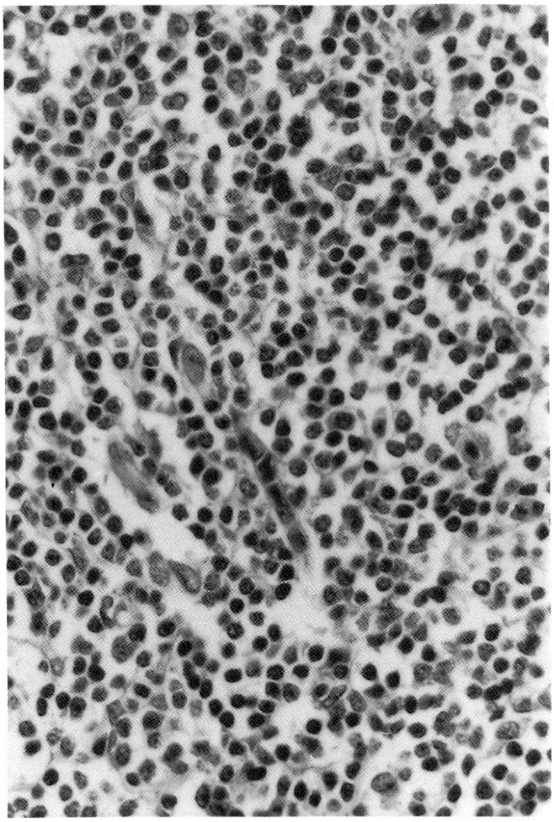

Fig. 10.22 Waldenström's macroglobulinaemia. The interstitium is infiltrated by many lymphocytes and some plasma cells.
Haematoxylin and eosin × 350

Differential diagnosis

Some cases of Waldenström's macroglobulinaemia have the lesions of *cryoglobulinaemia* (see p. 352) because the monoclonal IgM is acting as a type I or II cryoglobulin. The character of the cells infiltrating the interstitium is the only renal morphological feature that may suggest Waldenström's macroglobulinaemia as the cause of the cryoglobulinaemic changes. In those patients in whom the paraprotein is not acting as a cryoglobulin the finding that the glomerular intracapillary amorphous deposits only stain for IgM and a single light chain is a feature that distinguishes Waldenström's macroglobulinaemia from cryoglobulinaemia.

Prognosis

The course of the disease is very variable. Some patients remain asymptomatic for many years; in others progression necessitates chemotherapy which can keep patients in fair health for some years. Death results from intercurrent infection, haemorrhage or thrombosis but rarely renal failure.

Pathogenesis

The pathogenesis of the glomerular intracapillary amorphous deposits is uncertain. It has been suggested that they result from local formation by the monoclonal IgM molecules of complexes with each other or with other serum proteins, a process favoured by the increased protein concentration brought about by ultrafiltration through the glomerular capillary bed.[86] The pathogenesis of the amyloid deposits that may occur is discussed on page 350 and of the light chain nephropathy on page 366.

LIGHT CHAIN DEPOSITION DISEASE

Light chain deposition disease, first described in 1976,[131] is characterized by the accumulation of monoclonal light chains in many organs, including the kidneys, liver, heart, skin and nervous system.[131–133] The light chains may be either kappa or lambda but are usually kappa. In the kidneys they are deposited in the glomerular and tubular basement membranes and in the mesangium (light chain nephropathy); in other organs the deposits are predominantly perivascular.[131] Approximately two-thirds of patients with light chain deposition disease have multiple myeloma (see p. 357) or some other lymphoplasmacytic proliferative disease such as Waldenström's macroglobulinaemia (see p. 360) or lymphoma. Renal involvement is a constant feature of light chain deposition disease; it is the major manifestation in most patients.

Clinical features

Proteinuria or renal insufficiency are the most common presenting manifestation.[132] Exceptionally the early signs and symptoms may be related to involvement of the liver and heart or both.[133,134] The degree of proteinuria varies greatly; sometimes it is sufficiently severe to produce the nephrotic syndrome. In about half the patients with proteinuria the protein in the urine is predominantly light chain. Microscopic haematuria may occur and moderate hypertension is frequent. Characteristically renal failure is common and appears early.[132]

Renal changes

Light microscopy

In approximately 50% of cases the glomeruli are enlarged, with accentuated lobulation of the tuft and nodular expansion of the mesangium by intensely PAS-positive material (Fig. 10.23).[112,132–135] The nodules are not diffuse, are usually of variable size and rarely affect all the lobules. In those cases without nodules there is usually focal or diffuse mesangial expansion. The glomerular capillary walls are often moderately thickened by similar material; sometimes there are small segments of mesangial cell interposition with reduplication of the basement membranes.[112] Mesangial cell proliferation is slight or absent.

The tubules often show some atrophy and their basement membranes are mildly to moderately thickened on the outer side by PAS-positive material (Fig. 10.24); sometimes the thickening is refractile and ribbon like.[132] The deposits are predominantly in the distal tubules and loops of Henle. Congo red staining of the deposits for amyloid is negative.

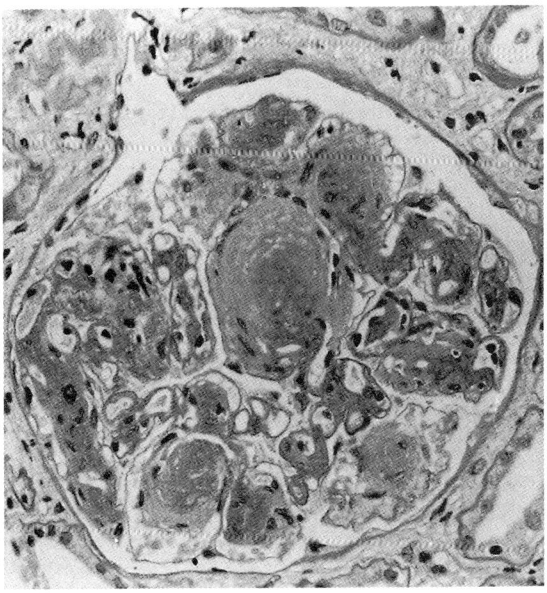

Fig. 10.23 Light chain deposition disease. Glomerulus showing prominent tuft lobulation and mesangial nodules. Periodic acid-Schiff × 250

Electron microscopy

The glomerular capillary basement membranes contain a continuous linear band of finely granular electron-dense material which replaces the lamina rare interna (Fig. 10.25).[112,134,135] A band of similar material is present along the outer side of the tubular basement membranes. Occasionally there are linear deposits in the arterioles and small arteries on the outer side of the media, on the basement membranes of the peritubular capillaries and in the interstitium.[112] In the expanded mesangium, including the nodules, there are finely granular electron-dense deposits which are often poorly demarcated from the greatly increased amounts

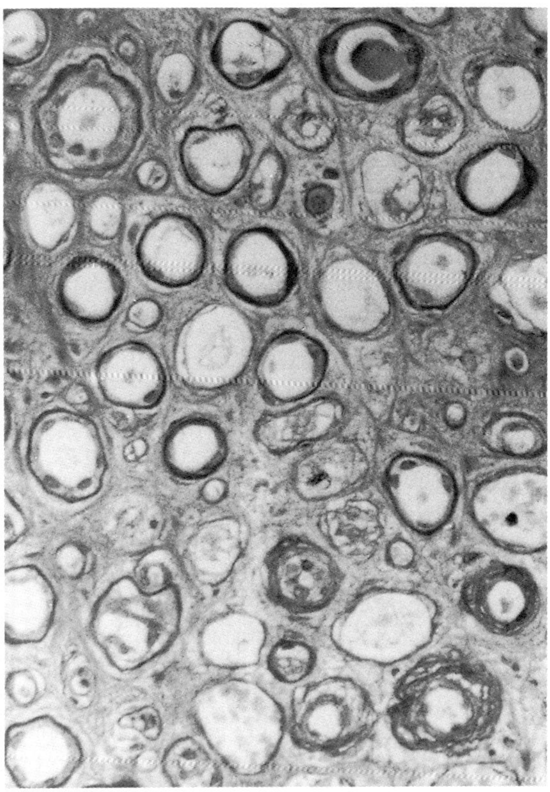

Fig. 10.24 Light chain deposition disease. The tubular basement membranes are thickened and laminated. Periodic acid-Schiff × 300

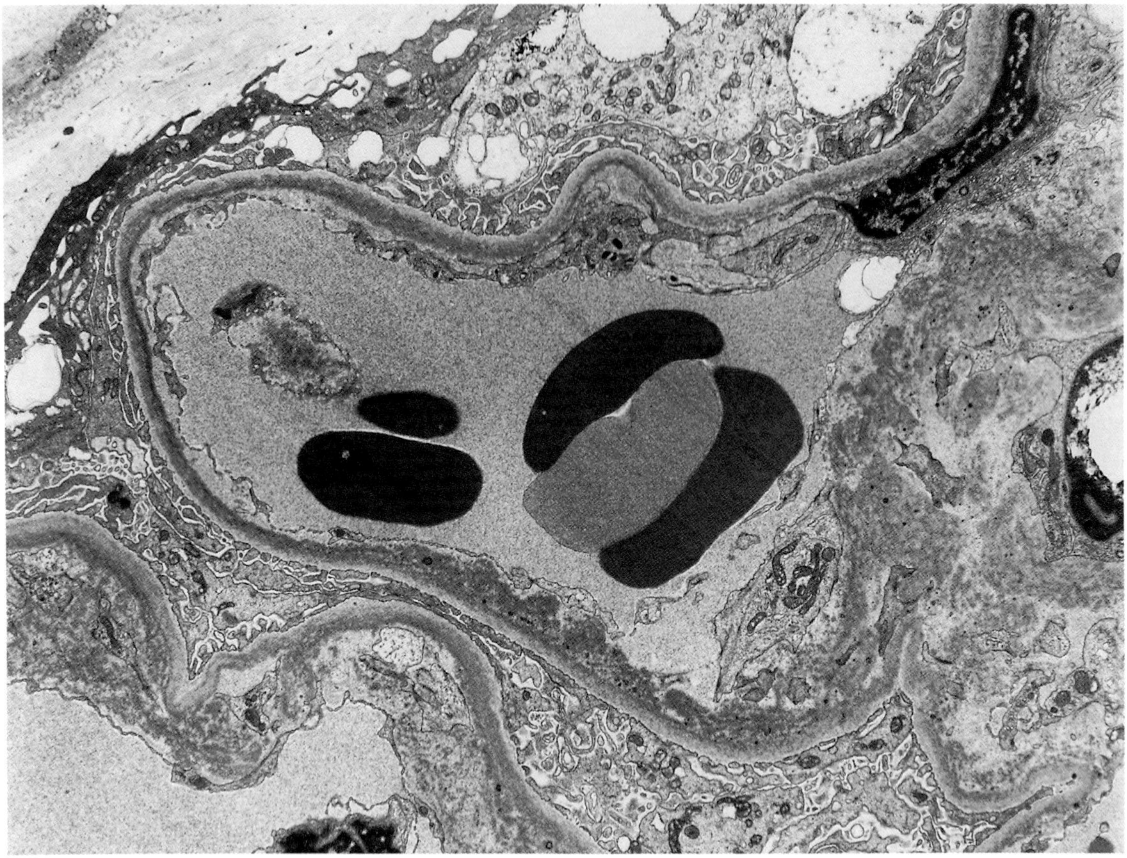

Fig. 10.25 Light chain deposition disease. Electron micrograph of part of a glomerular capillary loop showing a linear band of finely granular electron-dense material replacing the lamina rara interna of the basement membranes.
× 8000

of matrix.(Fig. 10.26). Sometimes small areas of the light chain deposit contain criss-crossing fibrils 9–14 nm in diameter (Fig. 10.27).[136]

Immunofluorescence/immunoperoxidase microscopy

There is granular staining of the mesangium and linear staining along the glomerular and tubular basement membranes exclusively or predominantly for either kappa or lambda light chain protein (Figs 10.28, 10.29).[112,132,134,135,137] In the published cases kappa light chain deposits have been observed four times as frequently as lambda chain. The presence of light chain protein in the deposits may sometimes be difficult to demonstrate, but unless the deposits can be shown to consist exclusively or predominantly of light chain proteins a firm diagnosis of light chain deposition disease cannot be made. The finding of the characteristic deposit on electron microscopy makes the diagnosis very probable but not definite.

Changes in other organs

Deposits of light chain proteins are found in many organs other than the kidney.[138] They are usually perivascular although they are also present on the basement membranes of muscle bundles and the choroid plexuses.[131,132]

Differential diagnosis

The differential diagnosis of light chain deposition disease is discussed on page 359.

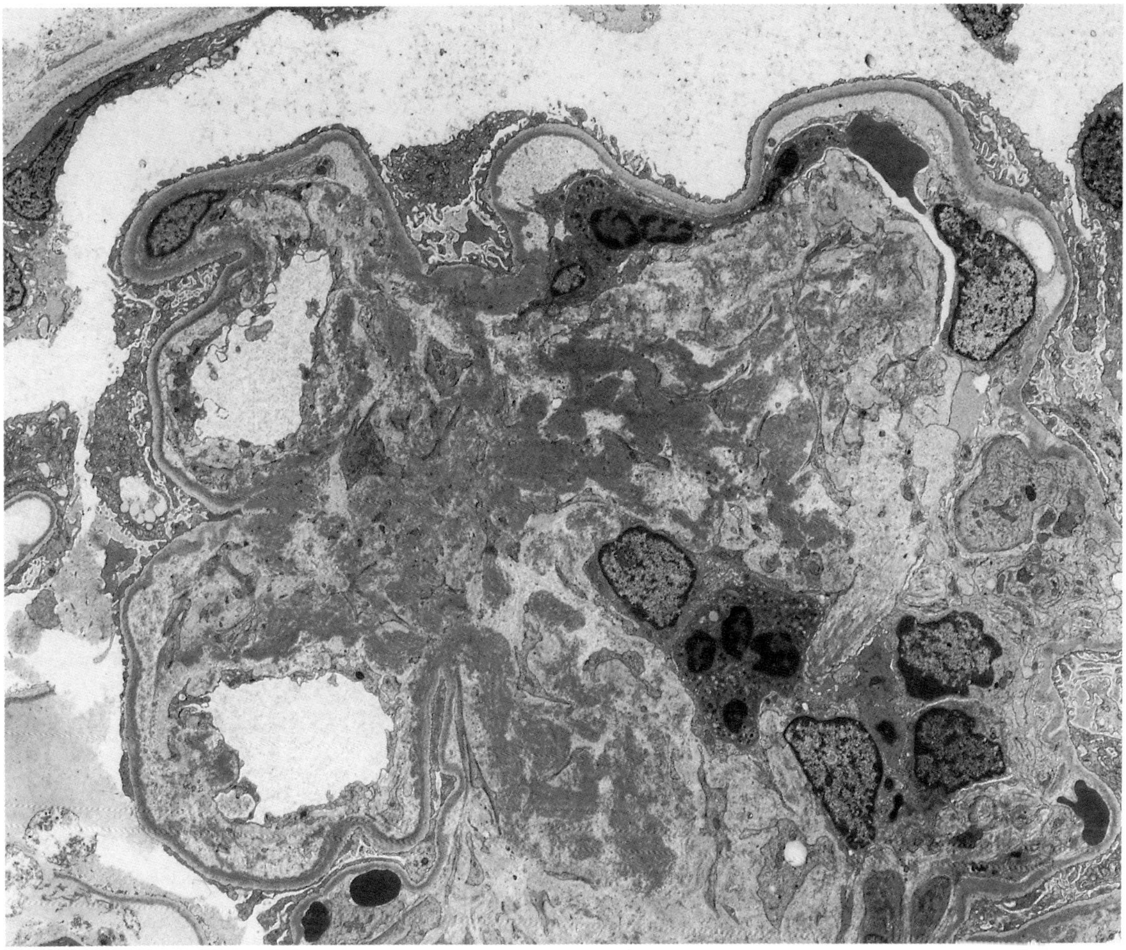

Fig. 10.26 Light chain deposition disease. Electron micrograph of a lobule of a glomerulus. The expanded mesangium contains abundant irregular electron-dense deposits. A linear band of electron-dense material is present in the lamina rara interna of the capillary basement membranes.
× 4550

Complications

Occasionally cellular crescents may be present in up to 50% of the glomeruli. This is associated with haematuria and rapidly progressive deterioration in renal function.[139]

Renal transplantation

Transplantation of a kidney with good subsequent function has been reported in several cases.[117] Commonly over the years light chains gradually deposit in the graft,[118,140] but usually this is unimportant; it is other complications of the underlying lymphoid or plasmacytic proliferative disease that so often lead to death of the patient. Occasionally renal function deteriorates rapidly.[141]

Prognosis

The renal function of patients who do not receive chemotherapy or corticosteroids quickly declines. In one series all needed dialysis within 2–23 months of presentation.[132] Renal failure occurs with equal frequency in patients with slight or heavy proteinuria.

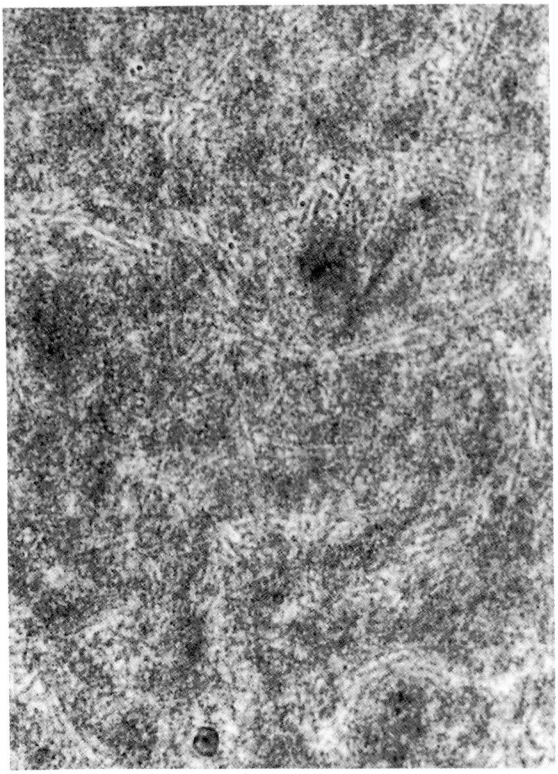

Fig. 10.27 Light chain deposition disease. Electron micrograph of part of a mesangial deposit which contains criss-crossing fibrils 9–14 nm in diameter. × 60 000

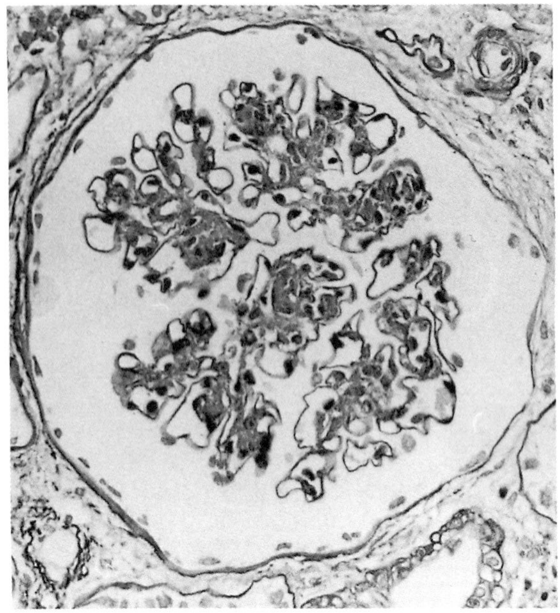

Fig. 10.28 Light chain deposition disease. Granular staining of the mesangium and linear staining along the glomerular capillary basement membranes for kappa light chains. Immunoperoxidase × 250

Early treatment with chemotherapy delays the progression to renal failure. In one series of six patients (five with multiple myeloma and one without any obvious lymphoproliferative disease), five either retained stable renal function or improved over a period of 21–42 months; one needed haemodialysis at 48 months.[132]

Pathogenesis

The pathogenesis of light chain nephropathy is only partly understood. One hypothesis, supported by various pieces of indirect evidence, is that when light chains are highly polymerized to form tetramers they are too big to pass through the glomerular capillary wall; some remain trapped in the region of the lamina rara interna while the remainder leave the glomerulus by the efferent arteriole. In the peritubular capillaries they pass into the interstitium and become deposited on the outer aspect of the tubular basement membranes.[112] It also seems likely that the isoelectric point of the light chains plays a role because a low isoelectric point reduces light chain filtration through the negatively charged glomerular capillary basement membranes.[142]

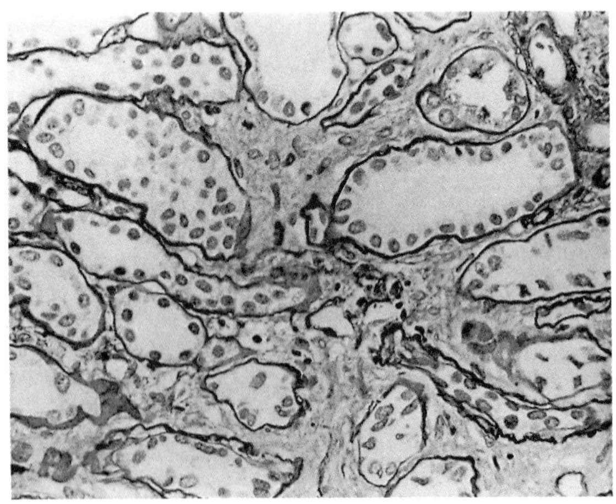

Fig. 10,29 Light chain deposition disease. Linear staining of thickened tubular basement membrane for kappa light chains. Immunoperoxidase × 250

Why the polymerized light chains adhere preferentially to basement membranes in the kidneys is not known. It may be related to electric charge, differences in the amino acid sequence in the variable region of the light chain proteins, or to glycosylation. Certainly patients with light chain deposition disease appear to produce abnormal light chains which become glycosylated before being deposited in the kidneys and other organs.[132]

Variants

In some cases all the deposits of kappa light chains assume a fibrillar structure that resembles amyloid: however, the fibrils are not stained by Congo red.[136,143]

MONOCLONAL GAMMOPATHY OF UNDETERMINED SIGNIFICANCE (BENIGN MONOCLONAL GAMMOPATHY) [144,145]

This phrase is used to describe the presence in the serum of a monoclonal immunoglobulin, in the absence of definite evidence of multiple myeloma or other plasma cell or lymphoproliferative disorder. Monoclonal gammopathy of undetermined significance is due to proliferation of a clone of antibody-secreting plasma cells but to an extent less than in multiple myeloma. Over half the cases do not show progression, even on prolonged follow-up; approximately a quarter develop multiple myeloma or some other lymphoproliferative disorder after many years. The others show a progressive rise in the level of the paraprotein or the appearances of light chains in the urine.

Renal changes

Diffuse deposition of *AL amyloid* is the most frequent renal lesion (see p. 344); *light chain nephropathy* (see p. 362) or the renal lesions associated with *cryoglobulinaemia* (see p. 351) also may occur.

HEAVY CHAIN DISEASES[145,146]

The heavy chain diseases are rare paraproteinaemias in which the malignant cells secrete a heavy chain, or part of a heavy chain, rather than a complete immunoglobulin molecule. The heavy chain may be gamma, mu or alpha. The most frequent is alpha-chain disease. These diseases do not directly cause renal lesions. Amyloidosis occasionally occurs in mu heavy chain disease because there is some additional light chain secretion in these patients. The light and heavy chains do not assemble, however, to form complete IgM molecules. The amyloid deposits sometimes involve the kidneys. Interstitial infiltration by lymphocytes and plasma cells has been recorded.[146]

REFERENCES

Diabetes mellitus

1. Bennett PH. The diagnosis of diabetes: new international classification and diagnostic criteria. Annu Rev Med 1983; 34: 295–309.
2. LaPorte RE, Cruickshanks KJ. Incidence and risk factors for insulin-dependent diabetes. In: National Diabetes Data Group. Diabetes in America, publication no 85–1468, vol 3. Betheseda: NIH, 1985; 1–12.
3. Marble A. The future of the child with diabetes. J Am Diet Assoc 1957; 33: 569–574.
4. Knowles HC. Magnitude of the renal failure problem in diabetic patients. Kidney Int 1974; 6: S2–S7.
5. Stephens GW, Gillaspy JA, Clyne D, Mejia A, Pollak VE. Racial differences in the incidence of end-stage renal disease in types I and II diabetes mellitus. Am J Kidney Dis 1990; 15: 562–567.
6. Goldstein HH. Discussion: the problem of end-stage diabetic nephropathy. Kidney Int 1974; 6: S21–S26.
7. Seaquist ER, Goetz FG, Rich S, Barbosa J. Familial clustering of diabetic kidney disease. Evidence for genetic susceptibility to diabetic nephropathy. N Engl J Med 1989; 320: 1161–1165.
8. Andersen AR, Sandahl-Christiansen J, Andersen JK, Kreiner S, Deckert T. Diabetic nephropathy in type 1 (insulin-dependent) diabetes: an epidemiological study. Diabetologia 1983; 25: 496–501.
9. Takazakura E, Nakamoto Y, Hayakawa H, et al. Onset and progression of diabetic glomerulosclerosis: a prospective study based on renal biopsies. Diabetes 1975; 24: 1–9.
10. Viberti GC, Hill RD, Jarrett RJ, Argyropoulos A, Mahmud U, Keen H. Microalbuminuria as a predictor of clinical nephropathy in insulin-dependent diabetes mellitus. Lancet 1982; 1: 1430–1432.
11. Khan CB, Raman PG, Zic Z. Kidney size in diabetes mellitus. Diabetes 1974; 23: 788–792.
12. Kimmelstiel P, Wilson C. Intercapillary lesions in the glomeruli of the kidney. Am J Pathol 1936; 12: 83–98.
13. Østerby R. Early phases in the development of diabetic glomerulopathy. Acta Med Scand [Suppl] 1974; 574: 3–82

14. Ainsworth SK, Pilia PA, Hirsch HZ, Williams AV, Hennigar GR. Immunopathology of diabetic nephropathy: antibody deposition and antigenic alterations. Diab Nephropath 1983; 2: 4–8.
15. Yum M, Maxwell DR, Hamburger R, Kleit SA. Primary glomerulonephritis complicating diabetic nephropathy: report of seven cases and a review of the literature. Hum Pathol 1984; 15: 921–927.
16. Wass JAH, Watkins PJ, Dische FE, Parsons V. Renal failure, glomerular disease and diabetes mellitus. Nephron 1978; 21: 289–296.
17. Kasinath BS, Mujais SK, Spargo BH, Katz AI. Non-diabetic renal disease in patients with diabetes mellitus. Am J Med 1983; 75: 613–617.
18. Sutherland DER, Fryd DS, Strand M, Ascher N, Simmons RL, Najarian JS. Results of renal transplantation in diabetics at the University of Minnesota since 1979, including a comparison of outcome in diabetic and nondiabetic recipients randomized to cyclosporine versus azathioprine for immunosuppression. Transplant Proc 1984; 16: 629–632.
19. Bentley FR, Sutherland DER, Mauer SM, et al. The status of diabetic renal allograft recipients who survive for 10 or more years after transplantation. Transplant Proc 1985; 17: 1573–1576.
20. Bohman S-O, Wilczek H, Tyden G, et al. Recurrent diabetic nephropathy in renal allografts placed in diabetic patients and protective effect of simultaneous pancreatic transplantation. Transplant Proc 1987; 19: 2290–2293.
21. Borch-Johnsen K, Nissen H, Henriksen E, et al. The natural history of insulin dependent diabetes mellitus in Denmark: 1. Long-term survival with and without late complications. Diab Med 1987; 4: 201–210.
22. Watkins PJ. Diabetic nephropathy – prevalence, complications and treatment. Diab Med 1985; 2: 7–12.
23. Thomsen OF, Andersen AR, Christiansen JS, Deckert T. Renal changes in long term type 1 (insulin dependent) diabetic patients with and without clinical nephropathy: a light microscopic, morphometric study of autopsy material. Diabetologia 1984; 26: 361–365.
24. Krolewski AS, Canessa M, Warram JH, et al. Predisposition to hypertension and susceptibility to renal disease in insulin-dependent diabetes mellitus. N Engl J Med 1988; 318: 140–145.
25. Mogensen CE. Microalbuminuria as a predictor of clinical diabetic nephropathy. Kidney Int 1987; 31: 673–689.
26. Carr S, Mbanya J-C, Thomas T, et al. Increase in glomerular filtration rate in patients with insulin-dependent diabetes and elevated erythrocyte sodium-lithium countertransport. N Engl J Med 1990; 322: 500–505.
27. Morgensen CE, Andersen MJ. Increased kidney size and glomerular filtration rate in early juvenile diabetes. Diabetes 1973; 22: 706–712.
28. Hostetter TH, Troy JL, Brenner BM. Glomerular hemodynamics in experimental diabetes. Kidney Int 1981; 19: 410–415.
29. Hostetter TH, Rennke HG, Brenner BM. The case for intrarenal hypertension in the initiation and progression of diabetic and other glomerulopathies. Am J Med 1982; 72: 375–380.
30. Schmitz A, Nyengaard JR, Bendtsen TF. Glomerular volume in Type 2 (noninsulin-dependent) diabetes estimated by a direct and unbiased stereologic method. Lab Invest 1990; 62: 108–113.
31. Vernier RL, Sisson-Ross S, Mauer SM. Cytochemical studies of the anionic charges in the kidney in type 1 diabetes mellitus. Diab Nephropath 1986; 5: 15–18.
32. Deckert T, Feldt-Rasmussen B, Djurup R, Deckert M. Glomerular size and charge selectivity in insulin-dependent diabetes mellitus. Kidney Int 1988; 33: 100–106.
33. Bell ET. Renal vascular disease in diabetes mellitus. Diabetes 1953; 2: 376–389.
34. Bader H, Meyer DS. The size of the juxtaglomerular apparatus in diabetic glomerulosclerosis and its correlation with arteriosclerosis and arterial hypertension: a morphometric light microscopic study on human renal biopsies. Clin Nephrol 1977; 8: 308–311.
35. Hall GFM. The significance of atheroma of the renal arteries in Kimmelstiel–Wilson's syndrome. J Pathol Bacteriol 1952; 64: 103–120.
36. Ritchie S, Waugh D. The pathology of Armanni–Ebstein diabetic nephropathy. Am J Pathol 1957; 33: 1035–1057.
37. Edmondson HA, Martin HE, Evans N. Necrosis of renal papillae and acute pyelonephritis in diabetes mellitus. Arch Intern Med 1947; 79: 148–175.
38. Vejlsgaard R. Studies on urinary infection in diabetics: 1. Bacteriuria in patients with diabetes mellitus and in control subjects. Acta Med Scand 1966; 179: 173–182.
39. Ireland JT, Patnaik BK, Duncan LJP. Glomerular ultrastructure in secondary diabetics and normal subjects. Diabetes 1967; 16: 628–635.

Gout

40. Diamond HS, Paolino JS. Evidence for a postsecretory reabsorptive site for uric acid in man. J Clin Invest 1973; 52: 1491–1499.
41. Boss GR, Seegmiller JE. Hyperuricemia and gout. Classification, complications and managements. N Engl J Med 1979; 300: 1459–1468.
42. Beck LH. Requiem for gouty nephropathy. Kidney Int 1986; 30: 280–287.
43. Yu T, Berger L, Dorph DJ, Smith H. Renal function in gout. V. Factors influencing the renal hemodynamics. Am J Med 1979; 67: 766–771.
44. Kanwar YS, Manaligod JR. Leukemic urate nephropathy. Arch Pathol 1975; 99: 467–472.
45. Leumann EP, Wegmann W. Familial nephropathy with hyperuricemia and gout. Nephron 1983; 34: 51–57.
46. Yokoyama H, Kida H, Asamato T, Abe T, Koshino Y, Hattori N. Gouty kidney associated with membranous nephropathy: participation of renal tubular epithelial antigen. Nephron 1986; 44: 361–364.
47. Kellstrand CM, Campbell DC, von Hartitzsch B, Buselmeier TJ. Hyperuricemic acute renal failure. Arch Intern Med 1974; 133: 349–359.
48. Ball GV. Two epidemics of gout. Bull Hist Med 1971; 45: 401–408.
49. Ball GV, Morgan JM. Chronic lead ingestion and gout. South Med J 1968; 61: 21–24.

Amyloidosis

50. Cohen AS, Connors LH. The pathogenesis and biochemistry of amyloidosis. J Pathol 1987; 151: 1–10.

51. Pepys MB. Amyloidosis: some recent developments. Q J Med 1988; 67: 283–298.
52. Hind CRK, Tennent GA, Evans DJ, Pepys MB. Demonstration of amyloid A (AA) protein and amyloid P component (AP) in deposits of systemic amyloidosis associated with renal adenocarcinoma. J Pathol 1983; 139: 159–166.
53. Kyle RA, Bayrd ED. Amyloidosis. A review of 236 cases. Medicine (Baltimore) 1975; 54: 271–299.
54. Brandt K, Cathcart ES, Cohen AS. A clinical analysis of the course and prognosis of forty-two patients with amyloidosis. Am J Med 1968; 44: 955–969.
55. Pitkanen P, Westermark P, Cornwall GG. Senile systemic amyloidosis. Am J Pathol 1984; 117: 391–399.
56. Triger DR, Joekes AM. Renal amyloidosis. A fourteen year follow-up. Q J Med 1973; 165: 15–40.
57. Carone FA, Epstein FH. Nephrogenic diabetes insipidus caused by amyloid disease: evidence in man of the role of the collecting ducts in concentrating urine. Am J Med 1960; 29: 539–544.
58. Luke RG, Allison ME, Davidson JF, et al. Hyperkalemia and renal tubular acidosis due to renal amyloidosis. Ann Intern Med 1969; 70: 1211–1217.
59. Hawkins PN, Lavender JP, Pepys MB. Evaluation of systemic amyloidosis by scintigraphy with ^{123}I-labelled serum amyloid P component. N Engl J Med 1990; 323: 508–513.
60. Ansell ID, Joekes AM. Spicular arrangement of amyloid in renal biopsy. J Clin Pathol 1972; 25: 1056–1062.
61. Weiss SW, Page DL. Amyloid nephropathy of Ostertag with special reference to renal glomerular giant cells. Am J Pathol 1973; 72: 447– 460.
62. Heller H, Missmahl HP, Sohar E, Gafni J. Amyloidosis: its differentiation into perireticulin and pericollagen types. J Pathol Bacteriol 1964; 88: 15–34.
63. Tribe CR, Silver JR. Renal failure in paraplegia. London: Pitman, 1969: 54.
64. Wright JR, Calkins E, Humphreys RL. Potassium permanganate reaction in amyloidosis. A histologic method to assist in differentiating forms of this disease. Lab Invest 1977; 36: 274– 281.
65. Lanham JG, Meltzer ML, De Beer FC, Hughes GRV, Pepys MB. Familial amyloidosis of Ostertag. Q J Med 1982; 51: 25–32.
66. Feiner HD. Pathology of dysproteinemia: light chain amyloidosis, non-amyloid immunoglobulin deposition disease, cryoglobulinemia syndromes, and macroglobulinemia of Waldenström. Hum Pathol 1988; 19: 1255–1272.
67. Fujihara S, Glenner GG. Primary localized amyloidosis of the genitourinary tract: immunohistochemical study on eleven cases. Lab Invest 1981; 44: 55–60.
68. Shirahama T, Cohen AS. High resolution electron microscopic analysis of the amyloid fibril. J Cell Biol 1967; 33: 679–708.
69. Silver MM, Hearn SA, Walton JC, Lines LA, Walley VM. Immunogold quantitation of immunoglobulin light chains in renal amyloidosis and kappa light chain nephropathy. Am J Pathol 1990; 136: 997–1007.
70. Pasternack A, Ahonen J, Kuhlback B. Renal transplantation in 45 patients with amyloidosis. Transplantation 1986; 42: 598 601.
71. Bergllund K, Keller C, Thysell H. Alkylating cytostatic treatment in renal amyloidosis secondary to rheumatic disease. Ann Rheum Dis 1987; 46: 757–762.
72. Bradstock K, Clancy R, Uther J, et al. The successful treatment of primary amyloidosis with intermittent chemotherapy. Aust NZ J Med 1978; 8: 176–179.
73. Cohen AS, Rubinow A, Anderson JJ, et al. Survival of patients with primary (AL) amyloidosis. Colchicine-treated cases from 1976 to 1983 compared with cases seen in previous years (1961 to 1973). Am J Med 1987; 83: 1182–1190.
74. Dikman SH, Kahn T, Gribetz D, Churg J. Resolution of renal amyloidosis. Am J Med 1977; 63: 430–433.
75. Van Gise H, Helmchen U, Mikeler E, et al. Correlations between the morphological and clinical findings in a patient recovering from secondary generalized amyloidosis with renal involvement. Virchows Arch [A] 1978; 379: 119–126
76. Falck H, Törnroth T, Skrifvars B, Wegelius O. Resolution of renal amyloidosis secondary to rheumatoid arthritis. Acta Med Scand 1979; 205: 651–656.
77. Reuben A, Hirsch M, Berlyn GM. Renal vein thrombosis as the major cause of renal failure in familial Mediterranean fever. Q J Med 1977; 44: 243–258.
78. Zemer D, Pras M, Sohar E, Modan M, Cabili S, Gafni J. Colchicine in the prevention and treatment of the amyloidosis of familial Mediterranean fever. N Engl J Med 1986; 314: 1001–1005.
79. Castano EM, Frangione B. Biology of disease. Human amyloidosis, Alzheimer disease and related disorders. Lab Invest 1988; 58: 122– 132.
80. Turnell W, Sarra R, Baum JO, et al. X-ray scattering and diffraction by wet gels of AA amyloid fibrils. Mol Biol Med 1986; 3: 409–424.
81. Gelbard M, Johnson S. Primary amyloidosis of renal pelvis and renal cortical adenoma. Urology 1980; 15: 614–617.

Fibrillary glomerulopathy

82. Alpers CE, Rennke HG, Hopper J, Biava CG. Fibrillary glomerulonephritis: an entity with unusual immunofluorescence features. Kidney Int 1987; 31: 781–789.

Cryoglobulinaemia

83. Brouet J-C, Clauvel J-P, Danon F, Klein M, Seligmann M. Biologic and clinical significance of cryoglobulins. A report of 86 cases. Am J Med 1974; 57: 775–788.
84. Cordonnier DJ, Renversez JC, Viatel P, Dechelette E. The kidney in mixed cryoglobulinemias. Springer Semin Immunopathol 1987; 9: 395– 145.
85. Gorevic PD, Kassab HJ, Levo Y, et al. Mixed cryoglobulinemia: clinical aspects and long-term follow up of 40 patients. Am J Med 1980; 69: 287–308.
86. Verroust P, Morel-Maroger L, Preud'homme J-L. Renal lesions in dysproteinemias. Springer Semin Immunopathol 1982; 5: 333–356.
87. D'Amico G, Colasanti G, Ferrario F, Sinico RA. Renal involvement in essential mixed cryglobulinemia. Kidney Int 1989; 35: 1004–1014.
88. Morel-Maroger L, Verroust P. Glomerular lesions in dysproteinemias. Kidney Int 1974; 5: 249–252.
89. Ben-Bassat M, Boner G, Rosenfeld J, et al. The clinicopathologic features of cryoglobulinemic nephropathy. Am J Clin Pathol 1983; 79: 147–156.
90. Abasthi PS, Erickson DG, Williams RC, Tung KSK. Benign monoclonal gammaglobulinemia and glomerulonephritis. Am J Med 1977; 62: 324–329.

91. Feiner H, Gallo G. Ultrastructure in glomerulonephritis associated with cryoglobulinemia: a report of six cases and review of the literature. Am J Pathol 1977; 88: 145–162.
92. Faraggiana T, Parolini C, Previato G, Lupo A. Light and electron microscopic findings in five cases of cryoglobulinemic glomerulonephritis. Virchows Archiv [A] 1979; 384: 29–44.
93. Ogihara T, Saruta T, Saito I, et al. Finger print deposits of the kidney in pure monoclonal IgG kappa cryoglobulinemia. Clin Nephrol 1979; 12: 186–190.
94. Feiner H. Relationship of tissue deposits of cryoglobulin to clinical features of mixed cryoglobulinemia. Hum Pathol 1983; 14: 710–715.
95. Vallat JM, Desproges-Gottenron R, Leboutet MJ, Loubet A, Gualde N, Treves R. Cryoglobulinemic nephropathy: a pathological study. Ann Neurol 1979; 8: 179–185.
96. Zarski JP, Rougier D, Aubert H, et al. Association cryoglobuline et maladie hépatique: frequence, nature et caractères immunocliniques de la cryoglobulinémie. Gastroenterol Clin Biol 1984; 8: 845–850.
97. Andrejak M, Bariety J, Bedrossian J, et al. Cryoglobulinemia in renal transplant recipients. Transplantation 1978; 26: 446–447.
98. Tarantino A, Montagnino G, Baldassari A, et al. Prognostic factors in essential mixed cryoglobulinemia nephropathy. In: Ponticelli C, Minetti L, D'amico G, eds. Antiglobulins, cryoglobulins and glomerulonephritis. Dordrecht: Martinus Nijhoff, 1986: 219.
99. Perl A, Gorevic PD, Ryan DH, Condemi JJ, Ruszkowski RJ, Abraham GN. Clonal B cell expansions in patients with essential mixed cryoglobulinaemia. Clin Exp Immunol 1989; 76: 54–60.
100. Ono M, Winearls CG, Amos N, et al. Monoclonal antibodies to restricted and cross reactive idiotypes on monoclonal rheumatoid factors and their recognition of idiotype-positive cells. Eur J Immunol 1987; 17: 343–349.
101. Sinico RA, Winearls CG, Sabadini E, Fornasieri A, Castiglione A, D'Amico G. Identification of glomerular immune deposits in cryoglobulinemia glomerulonephritis. Kidney Int 1988; 34: 109–116.

Immunotactoid glomerulopathy

102. Korbet SM, Schwartz MM, Rosenberg BF, Sibley RK, Lewis EJ. Immunotactoid glomerulopathy. Medicine (Baltimore) 1985; 64: 228–243.
103. Rollino C, Coppo R, Mazzucco G, et al. Monoclonal gammopathy and glomerulonephritis with organized microtubular deposits. Am J Kidney Dis 1990; 15: 276–280.
104. Lai FM-M, Lai KN, Li EK, Sung JY, Tam JSL. Immunotactoid glomerulopathy. Virchows Archiv [A] 1989; 415: 181–186.

Multiple myeloma

105. Buchsbaum RJ, Schwartz RS. Cellular origins of hematologic neoplasms. N Engl J Med 1990; 322: 694–696.
106. Kapadia SB. Multiple myeloma: a clinicopathologic study of 62 consecutively autopsied cases. Medicine (Baltimore) 1980; 59: 380–392.
107. Pruzanski W. Clinical manifestations of multiple myeloma: relation to class and type of M component. Can Med Assoc J 1976; 114: 896–897.
108. Kyle RA. Multiple myeloma: review of 869 cases. Mayo Clin Proc 1975; 50: 29–40.
109. Johnson WJ, Kyle RA, Dahlberg PJ. Dialysis in the treatment of multiple myeloma. Mayo Clin Proc 1980; 55: 65–72.
110. Hill GS, Morel-Maroger L, Mery JP, Brouet JC, Mignon F. Renal lesions in multiple myeloma: their relationship to the relative electrophoretic mobility of urinary free light chains. Am J Kidney Dis 1983; 3: 423–438.
111. Pasquali S, Zucchelli P, Casanova S et al. Renal histological lesions and clinical syndromes in multiple myeloma. Clin Nephrol 1987; 27: 222–228.
112. Pirani CL, Silva F, D'Agati V, Chander P, Striker LMM. Renal lesions in plasma cell dyscrasias: ultrastructural observations. Am J Kidney Dis 1987; 10: 208–221.
113. Carstens PHB, Woo D. Crystalline glomerular inclusions in multiple myeloma. Am J Kidney Dis 1989; 14: 56–60.
114. Truong LD, Mawad J, Cagle P, Mattioli C. Cytoplasmic crystals in multiple myeloma-associated Fanconi's syndrome. Arch Pathol Lab Med 1989; 113: 781–785.
115. Alpers CE, Magil AB, Gown AM. Macrophage origin of the multinucleated cells of myeloma cast nephropathy. Am J Clin Pathol 1989; 92: 662–665.
116. Cohen DJ, Sherman WH, Osserman EF, Appel GB. Acute renal failure in patients with multiple myeloma. Am J Med 1984; 76: 247–256.
117. Briefel GR, Spees EK, Humphrey RL, Hill GS, Saral R, Zachary JB. Renal transplantation in a patient with multiple myeloma and light chain nephropathy. Surgery 1983; 93: 579–584.
118. Case records of the Massachusetts General Hospital (Case 1–1981). N Engl J Med 1981; 304: 33–43.
119. Rota S, Mougenot B, Baudouin B, et al. Multiple myeloma and severe renal failure: a clinicopathologic study of outcome and prognosis in 34 patients. Medicine (Baltimore) 1987; 66: 126–137.
120. De Fronzo RA, Humphrey RL, Wright JR, Cooke CR. Acute renal failure in multiple myeloma. Medicine (Baltimore) 1975; 54: 209–223.

Waldenström macroglubulinaemia

121. Waldenström JG. Incipient myelomatosis or 'essential' hyperglobulinaemia with fibrinogenopenia – a new syndrome. Acta Med Scand 1944; 117: 216–247.
122. Lowenthal RM, Sawyer PJ, Lickiss JN, Harlow RW, Kirov SM, Woods GM. Immunological types of lymphoproliferative disorders in a cohort: a 4-year study. Aust NZ J Med 1982; 12: 258–262.
123. Morel-Maroger L, Basch A, Danon F, Verroust P, Richet G. Pathology of the kidney in Waldenström's macroglobulinemia. Study of sixteen cases. N Engl J Med 1970; 283: 123–129.
124. MacKenzie MR, Fundenberg HH. Macroglobulinemia: an analysis of forty patients. Blood 1972; 39: 874–889.
125. Verroust P, Mery JPL, Morel-Maroger L, Clauvel JP, Richet G. Glomerular lesions in monoclonal gammopathies and mixed essential cryoglobulinaemias IgG–IgM. Adv Nephrol 1971; 1: 161–194.

126. Preud'homme J-L, Morel-Maroger L, Brouet JC, et al. Synthesis of abnormal immunoglobulins in lymphoplasmacytic disorder with light chain deposition. Am J Med 1980; 69: 703–710.
127. Noël LH, Droz D, Ganeval D, Grünfeld J-P. Renal granular monoclonal light chain deposits: morphological aspects in 11 cases. Clin Nephrol 1984; 21: 263–269.
128. Grossman ME, Bia MJ, Goldwein MI, Hill G, Goldberg M. Giant kidneys in Waldenström's macroglobulinemia. Arch Intern Med 1977; 137: 1613–1616
129. Lindström FD, Hed J, Enestrom S. Renal pathology of Waldenström's macroglobulinaemia with monoclonal antiglomerular antibodies and nephrotic syndrome. Clin Exp Immunol 1980; 41: 196–204.
130. Dutcher TF, Fahey JL. The histopathology of the macroglobulinemia of Waldenström. J Natl Cancer Inst 1959; 22: 887–917.

Light chain deposition disease

131. Randall RE, Williamson WC, Mullinax F, Tung MY, Still WJS. Manifestations of systemic light chain deposition. Am J Med 1976; 60: 293–299.
132. Ganeval D, Noël L-H, Preud'homme J-L, Droz D, Grünfeld J-P. Light chain deposition disease: its relation with AL-type amyloidosis. Kidney Int 1984; 26: 1–9.
133. Fang LST. Light-chain nephropathy. Kidney Int 1985; 27: 582–592.
134. Noël LH, Droz D, Ganeval D, Grünfeld J-P. Renal granular monoclonal light chain deposits: morphological aspects in 11 cases. Clin Nephrol 1984; 21: 263–269.
135. Kubo Y, Morita T, Koda Y, Hirasawa Y. Two types of glomerular lesion in non-amyloid immunoglobulin deposition disease: a case report of IgD-λ myeloma. Clin Nephrol 1990; 33: 259–263.
136. Alpers CE, Hopper J, Biava CG. Light chain glomerulopathy with amyloid-like deposits. Hum Pathol 1984; 15: 444–448.
137. Bradley JR, Thiru S, Evans DB. Light chains and the kidney. J Clin Pathol 1987; 40: 53–60.
138. Bedossa P, Fabre M, Paraf F, Martin E, Lemaigre G. Light chain deposition disease with liver dysfunction. Hum Pathol 1988; 19: 1008–1014.
139. Gerlag P, Koene R, Berden J. Renal transplantation in light chain nephropathy: case report and review of the literature. Clin Nephrol 1986; 25: 101–104.
140. Cadnapaphornchai P, Sillix D. Recurrence of monoclonal gammopathy-related glomerulonephritis in renal allograft. Clin Nephrol 1989; 31: 156–159.
141. Lapenas DJ, Drewry SJ, Luke RL, Leeber DA. Crescentic light-chain glomerulopathy. Report of a case. Arch Pathol Lab Med 1983; 107: 319–323.
142. Baylis C, Falconer-Smith J, Ross BD. The renal handling of human immunoglobulin light chain (IgLC) in the Munich–Wistar rat. Kidney Int 1982; 21: 242 (abstr).
143. Kobayashi Y, Fujii K, Kurokawa A, Kamiyama M, Miyazawa H. Glomerulonephropathy with amyloid-stain-negative microfibrillar glomerular deposits. Nephron 1988; 48: 33–39.

Benign monoclonal gammopathy

144. Mallick NP, Dosa S, Acheson EJ, et al. Detection, significance and treatment of paraprotein in patients presenting with 'idiopathic' proteinuria without myeloma. Q J Med 1978; 47: 145–175.
145. Wickramasinghe SN. Blood and bone marrow. In: Symmers W St C, ed. Systemic pathology, vol 2, 3rd edn. London: Churchill Livingstone, 1986.

Heavy chain disease

146. Fermand J-P, Brouet J-C, Danon F, Seligmann M. Gamma heavy chain 'disease': heterogeneity of the clinicopathologic features. Report of 16 cases and review of the literature. Medicine (Baltimore) 1989; 68: 321–335.

11

K. A. Porter

The kidneys in systemic infections

BACTERIAL INFECTIONS

Various non-specific deep-seated bacterial infections, especially those that are associated with bacteriaemia, may cause a range of renal lesions. This occurs particularly in patients with bacterial endocarditis, infected ventriculoatrial shunts, visceral abscesses, pneumonia, osteomyelitis and septicaemia.

These systemic infections should be distinguished from the various localized bacterial infections of more superfical sites that may also lead to renal lesions. Prime examples are localized infections of the throat or skin by nephritogenic strains of haemolytic streptococci that may lead to diffuse endocapillary proliferative glomerulonephritis (see p. 142).

Certain specific bacterial diseases may also affect the kidneys. Examples are tuberculosis, leprosy, syphilis, leptospirosis and brucellosis.

BACTERIAL ENDOCARDITIS

Bacterial endocarditis continues to be one of the most serious of all infections. It is caused by colonization of the heart valves by any of a variety of organisms. Before colonization the valves may be congenitally malformed, damaged by previous disease or normal. Prosthetic valves are also attacked. The routes of infection, the nature of the causative organisms and the clinical manifestations of the disease have altered greatly over the years as a result of the introduction of antibiotic therapy and prophylaxis, the dramatic fall in the incidence of rheumatic fever in many countries, and the increase in drug addiction and cardiac surgery.[1]

Clinically, bacterial endocarditis has been traditionally divided into acute and subacute forms. Although the distinction is far from absolute, there is an advantage in retaining it because of the very different modes of presentation at the two ends of the disease spectrum.

Both forms of the disease may be complicated by two types of renal lesion – infarcts and glomerulonephritis – which may occur either singly or in various combinations. In addition, in treated cases there may be a tubulointerstitial nephritis caused by an antibiotic.

Subacute bacterial endocarditis

Subacute bacterial endocarditis is usually caused by *Streptococcus viridans, Streptococcus faecalis,* non-enterococcal group D streptococci or true enterococcus species.[2] Occasionally it is caused by *Staphylococcus albus*[3] or some unusual organism, such as *Cardiobacterium hominis, Propionibacterium acnes, Neisseria gonorrhoeae, Proteus mirabilis*[4] and *Actinobacillus actinomycetemcomitans.*[5] In approximately 20% of the infections the organisms are believed to gain access to the circulation from the mouth and in 15% from the colon; in 60% the portal of entry to the blood stream cannot be identified.[2] It is an insidious disease and the patient has often been ill for several weeks before seeking help. There is frequently a known pre-existing heart valve abnormality. The mean age of the patients is just over 50 years. Males outnumber females 2 : 1. Untreated, the duration of the disease often exceeds 6 months.

Clinical features

Microscopic haematuria and moderate proteinuria are the usual signs of renal involvement.[1] Gross haematuria and occasionally sudden pain in the flank may occur if there is renal infarction. Hypertension and oedema are rare. Renal functional impairment is uncommon; when present it is usually caused by diffuse proliferative glomerulonephritis.

Serology

Serum complement levels are depressed in almost all patients with diffuse glomerulonephritis and in approximately 60% of those with focal glomerulonephritis. The degree of complement depression correlates directly with the severity of renal impairment. There is usually evidence of activation of the classical complement pathway, i.e. low levels of C3, Clq and C4. Immune complexes are present in the serum of most patients; high levels are associated with glomerulonephritis.[6] Mixed cryoglobulins are also very commonly present.

Renal changes

Infarcts Macroscopically visible, sterile infarcts, recent or healed (see p. 301), are found in the kidneys at necropsy in over half the cases.[7]

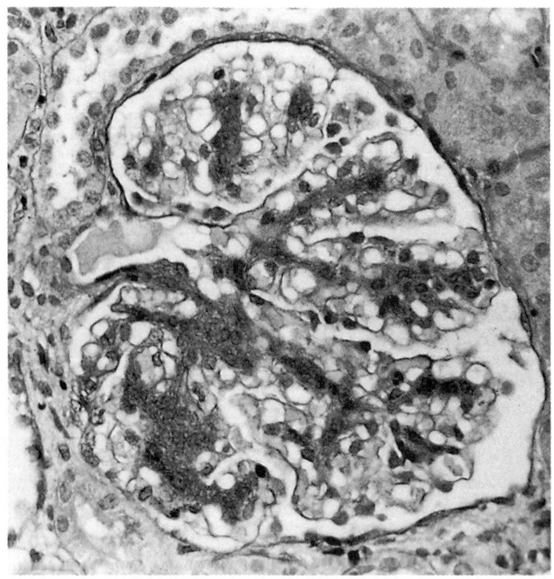

Fig. 11.1 Subacute bacterial endocarditis. Diffuse mesangial proliferative glomerulonephritis. The glomerulus shows segmental accentuation of the proliferation.
Periodic acid-Schiff × 300

Diffuse proliferative glomerulonephritis In addition to infarcts, a diffuse, global or segmental proliferative glomerulonephritis is often seen in cases of subacute bacterial endocarditis. The incidence at necropsy before the advent of antibiotics was about 65%; the incidence subsequent to that time is less clear but is probably approximately 14%.[1]

Light microscopy. The diffuse glomerulonephritis is usually mesangial proliferative in type; segmental accentuation of the mesangial proliferation is common (see p. 153; Fig. 11.1); less frequently it is an endocapillary proliferative glomerulonephritis (see p. 142), sometimes with crescents.[8]

Electron microscopy. Electron-dense deposits are commonly seen in the mesangium and on the subendothelial side of the glomerular capillary basement membrane (Fig.11.2).[8–11] Subepithelial deposits are not usually present. Sometimes no deposits can be detected.[1,11]

Immunofluorescence/immunoperoxidase microscopy. Granular deposits of IgG and C3 are usually present on the glomerular capillary basement membranes or in the mesangium or in both these situations.[8–11] Sometimes there are also deposits of IgM, IgA, Clq and C4.

Focal glomerulonephritis A focal and segmental glomerulonephritis is present in approximately 8% of the cases.[1] In the preantibiotic era

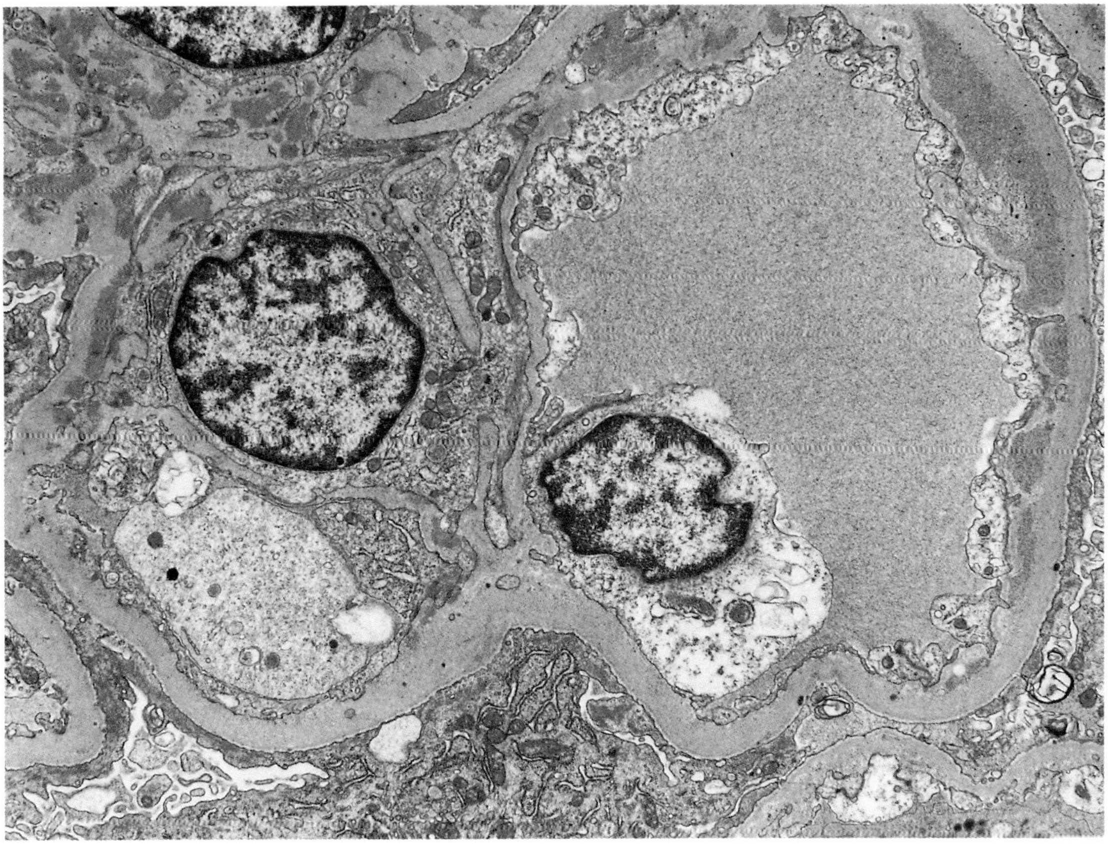

Fig. 11.2 Subacute bacterial endocarditis. Electron micrograph of a glomerular capillary loop showing subendothelial and mesangial electron-dense deposits.
× 9700

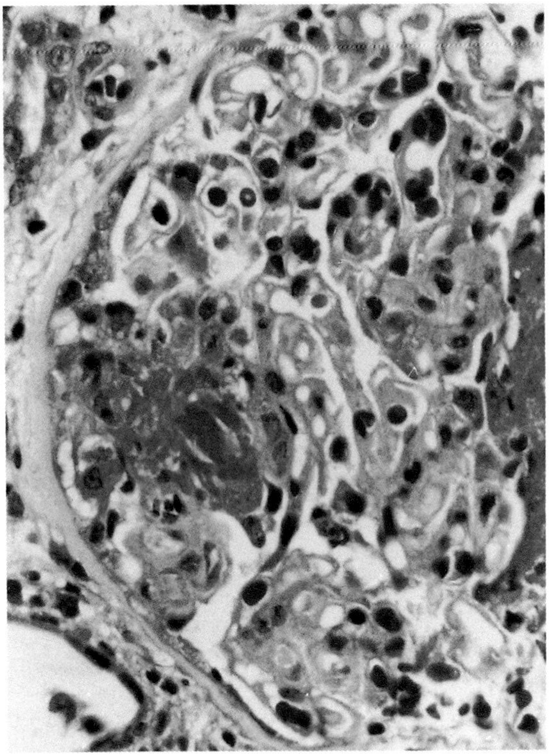

Fig. 11.3 Subacute bacterial endocarditis. Focal glomerulonephritis. Part of a glomerulus showing segmental necrosis.
Haematoxylin-eosin × 500

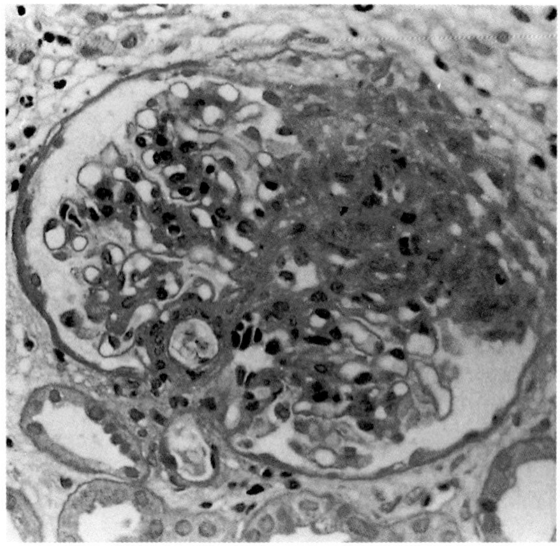

Fig. 11.4 Subacute bacterial endocarditis. Focal glomerulonephritis. A glomerulus showing segmental sclerosis.
Periodic acid-Schiff × 300

the incidence was much higher, the lesion being recorded in about half the cases.[5]

Gross appearance of the kidneys. The subcapsular surface of the kidneys is often speckled with petechial haemorrhages: the designation 'flea bitten' is traditionally applied to this appearance.

Light microscopy. The acute lesion takes the form of a segmental focus of fibrinoid necrosis or intracapillary thrombosis (Fig. 11.3); organisms are not demonstrable. Usually fewer than 15% of the glomeruli bear these lesions. Adjacent to the focus there is generally a segmental increase in the number of mesangial cells. There may be a few crescents.

In cases of longer duration, foci of segmental sclerosis are found (Fig. 11.4); these are thought to represent healed foci of necrosis.

Immunofluorescence/immunoperoxidase microscopy. Diffuse deposits of immunoglobulins and complement are usually present in the glomeruli even though light microscopy reveals only focal lesions. The deposits are granular, predominantly mesangial and mainly composed of IgG, IgM, Clq, C3 and C4. Fibrinogen is usually found only in the focal and segmental lesions that are visible by light microscopy. As the lesions age the immunoglobulins disappear leaving mostly C3 and Clq.

Electron microscopy. Electron-dense deposits are found in the mesangium of most glomeruli and sometimes on the subendothelial aspect of the capillary basement membranes.

Coexistent diffuse and focal proliferative glomerulonephritis In some cases there is mild diffuse global proliferative glomerulonephritis and focal segmental glomerulonephritis.[1,8] The foci of necrosis are usually much less common in these combined forms of glomerulonephritis than in focal glomerulonephritis when it occurs alone.

Tubulointerstitial disease caused by drugs
Occasionally, antibiotics such as penicillin, ampicillin or methicillin, which are used to treat patients with subacute bacterial endocarditis, produce an acute hypersensitivity tubulointerstitial injury (see p. 454).

Differential diagnosis

There is nothing distinctive about the sterile infarcts that occur in subacute bacterial endocarditis.

The diffuse proliferative glomerulonephritis seen in subacute bacterial endocarditis may be indistinguishable morphologically from the *mesangial proliferative glomerulonephritis that occurs in resolving endocapillary proliferative glomerulonephritis* (see p. 150), although subepithelial electron-dense deposits can usually be found in the latter condition. Other forms of *diffuse mesangial proliferative glomerulonephritis* (see p. 153) usually lack subendothelial electron-dense deposits which are common in the diffuse proliferative glomerulonephritis that occurs in subacute bacterial endocarditis. The absence of IgA in the mesangium will distinguish the lesion in subacute bacterial endocarditis from *IgA nephropathy* (see p. 157).

The focal segmental glomerulonephritis that may be found in subacute bacterial endocarditis is often indistinguishable on light microscopy from the focal lesions that occur in a number of other systemic diseases (see p. 211). Immunofluorescence/immunoperoxidase microscopy may help in the distinction; for example, the lesion in *antiglomerular basement membrane disease* (see p. 217) can be distinguished because of the linear deposition of IgG on the capillary basement membranes and the lesions in *Henoch–Schönlein purpura* (see p. 252) and *IgA nephropathy* (see p. 157) can be distinguished by the mesangial deposits of IgA that are characteristic of them. Electron microscopy will often detect an underlying *hereditary nephritis* (see p. 73). To exclude *systemic lupus erythematosus* (see p. 225), *microscopic polyarteritis* (see p. 272) and *Wegener's granulomatosis* (see p. 275), it may be necessary to resort to serological tests. Subepithelial electron-dense deposits are usually present in *resolving endocapillary proliferative glomerulonephritis* (see p. 150) and not in the focal glomerulonephritis that accompanies subacute bacterial endocarditis. The lesions of *idiopathic focal glomerulonephritis* (see p. 211) usually lack deposits of immunoglobulins and complement.

The healed lesions of focal glomerulonephritis occurring in subacute bacterial endocarditis are usually distinguishable from *focal segmental sclerosis* (see p. 204) by the common absence of hyalinosis in the sclerotic foci of the former.

Prognosis

With effective antibiotic therapy patients with diffuse glomerulonephritis usually recover renal function within a few weeks. Immune complexes disappear from the circulation and serum complement levels return to normal. Occasionally microscopic haematuria or proteinuria may persist for months or even years after the bacteria have been eradicated. Recovery is less frequent and death more likely in patients who present with renal failure. Focal glomerulonephritis also usually resolves with control of infection; progression to renal insufficiency is rare.

The glomerulonephritic lesions disappear with clinical recovery; the only residual change after diffuse glomerulonephritis is some expansion of the mesangium and after focal glomerulonephritis is segmental or global scarring of some glomeruli.

Pathogenesis

The *diffuse proliferative glomerulonephritis* that occurs in subacute bacterial endocarditis is caused by immune complexes. Patients with subacute bacterial endocarditis develop high titres of specific opsonic, agglutinating and complement-fixing antibodies to the infecting organisms.[12] As bacterial antigen is continually being released, antigen–antibody complexes either form in the circulation, subsequently lodging in the glomerular filter, or form in the kidneys themselves as the result of circulating antibody reacting with antigen already fixed in the glomerular basement membranes (see p. 128). Bacterial antigen and antibody that specifically reacted with bacteria from the patients' blood have been identified in renal tissue.[13,14] The immune complexes initiate a mesangial proliferative response (see p. 130).

The *focal glomerulonephritis* probably arises by a similar mechanism; that it results from microscopic emboli from the vegetations can be excluded in patients with right-sided endocarditis and it seems unlikely that this mechanism operates in those with lesions on the left.

The *infarcts* result from obstruction of arcuate and interlobular arteries by emboli composed of fragments of the vegetations on the endocardium.

Acute bacterial endocarditis

The organisms causing acute bacterial endocarditis often differ from those responsible for the subacute disease. *Staphylococcus aureus* is the causative agent in approximately 50% of patients; *Streptococcus viridans* is implicated in only about 35%.[15] Other bacteria associated with the acute disease are *Staphylococcus epidermidis*, pneumococci, gonococci, β-haemolytic streptococci and coliforms. Drug addicts are particularly likely to develop this form of bacterial endocarditis (see p. 510). The disease also occurs as a complication of heart surgery, especially in patients receiving prosthetic valves. Acute endocarditis usually begins abruptly and the duration of symptoms prior to presentation is usually brief. In over half the patients acute endocarditis develops in previously normal hearts. The patients are characteristically young. It is a rapidly progressive disease, which if untreated leads to death within days or weeks in 50–60% of patients.

Clinical features

Patients usually present with signs and symptoms of septicaemia. As in the subacute form of the disease microscopic haematuria and proteinuria are the common signs of renal involvement.[1] Renal insufficiency may develop quickly and progress rapidly; it is usually less frequent in those with focal glomerulonephritis.

Serology

The findings are the same as in subacute bacterial endocarditis (see p. 374).

Renal changes

Infarcts Renal infarcts are frequent and, in contrast to those in subacute bacterial endocarditis, are usually infected.

Diffuse proliferative glomerulonephritis A diffuse global or segmental proliferative glomerulonephritis is found at autopsy in approximately 14% of cases of acute bacterial endocarditis.[1]

Light microscopy. In contrast to subacute bacterial endocarditis the diffuse glomerulonephritis in the acute disease is usually of the endocapillary proliferative type (Fig. 11.5),[8,16] sometimes with crescents (see p. 145); only occasionally is the pattern mesangial proliferative.

Electron microscopy. Discrete subepithelial deposits on the glomerular capillary basement membranes are a striking feature (Fig. 11.6);[17,18] they do not differ from those seen in diffuse endocapillary proliferative glomerulonephritis due to other causes. Deposits within the capillary basement membranes (intramembranous deposits) also occur.

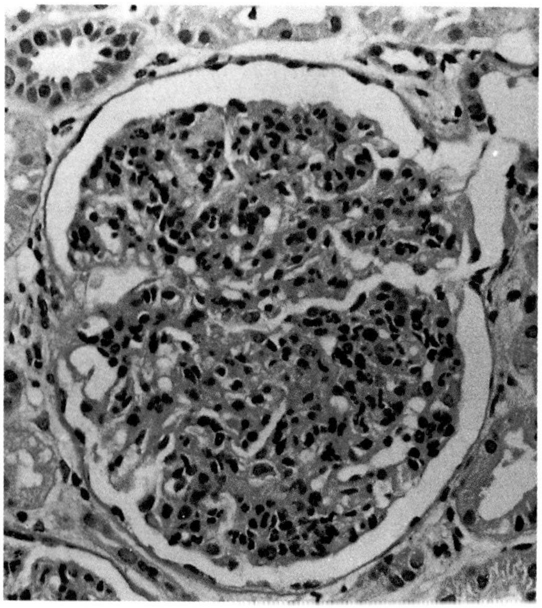

Fig. 11.5 Acute bacterial endocarditis. Diffuse endocapillary proliferative glomerulonephritis.
Periodic acid-Schiff × 340

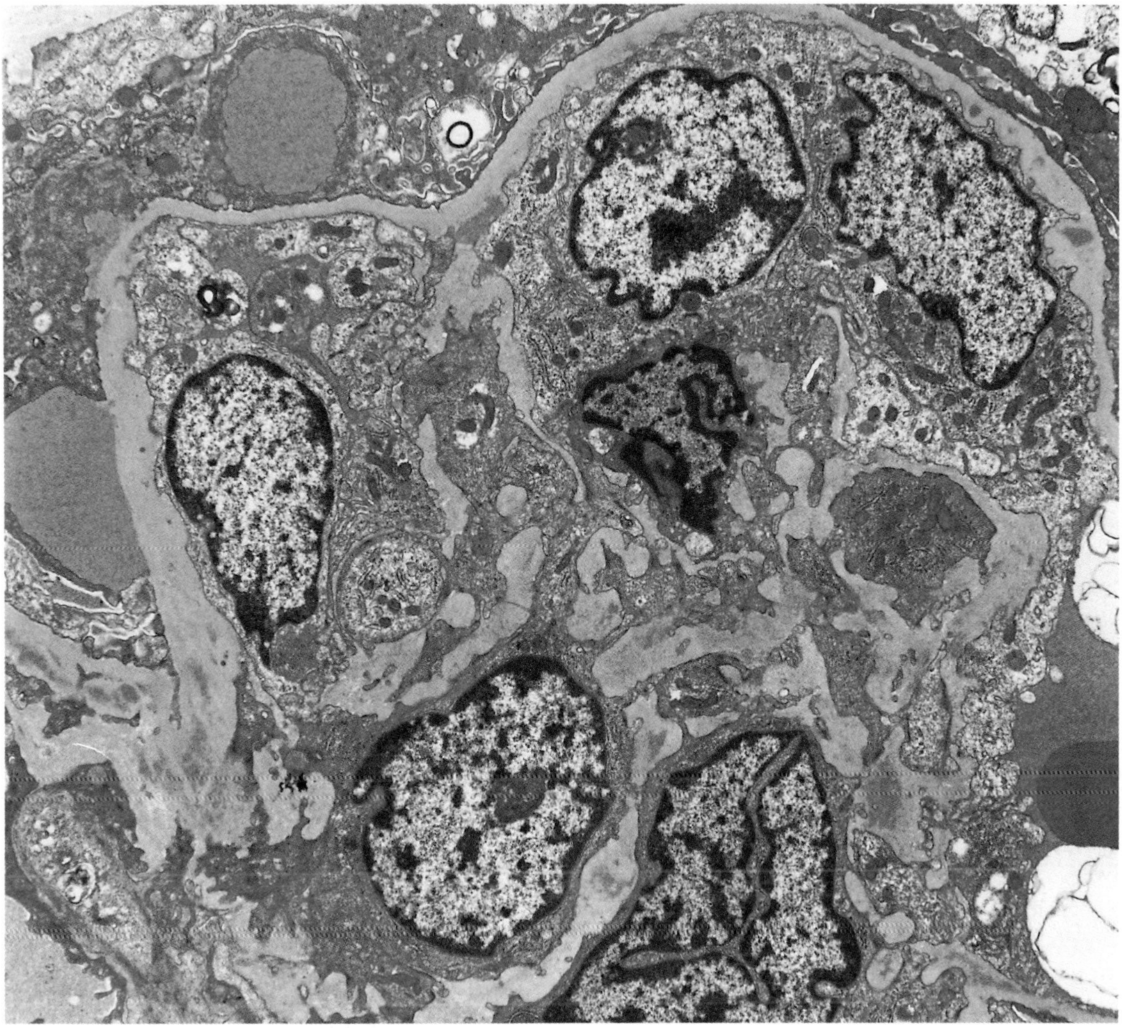

Fig. 11.6 Acute bacterial endocarditis. Electron micrograph of a glomerular capillary loop showing two subepithelial humps. The lumen is occluded by macrophages and mesangial cells.
× 9600

Immunofluorescence/immunoperoxidase microscopy. Granular deposits of IgG and C3, or C3 alone, are common on the glomerular capillary basement membranes and in the mesangium.[18]

Focal glomerulonephritis Focal and segmental glomerulonephritis is present in approximately 10% of the cases at autopsy.[1]

Light microscopy. The findings do not differ from those in subacute bacterial endocarditis (see p. 375).

Immunofluorescence/immunoperoxidase microscopy. Granular deposits of IgG and C3, or C3 alone, are present in the glomerular capillary walls in addition to the mesangium.

Electron microscopy. Scattered subepithelial electron-dense deposits are found on the glomerular capillary basement membranes and in the mesangium. Sometimes subendothelial deposits are also present.

Tubulointerstitial lesions Acute tubular necrosis (see p. 491) is common, probably because shock is frequent in patients with acute bacterial endocarditis.[19] Rarely an acute hypersensitivity tubulointerstitial injury is caused by an antibiotic used in treatment (see p. 454).

Differential diagnosis

The diffuse proliferative glomerulonephritis that occurs in acute bacterial endocarditis may be indistinguishable from the *endocapillary proliferative glomerulonephritis* that occurs in post-streptococcal glomerulonephritis and other conditions (see p. 142).

The focal segmental glomerulonephritis of acute bacterial endocarditis may be indistinguishable on light microscopy from the focal lesions that occur in several systemic diseases. Immunofluorescence/immunoperoxidase microscopy and electron microscopy may help in the distinction (see p. 211).

Prognosis

Many patients die from the non-renal aspects of the disease; if the septicaemia responds to antibiotics the renal failure is reversible. Usually the diffuse endocapillary proliferative glomerulonephritic lesions eventually resolve completely after successful treatment; the focal segmental lesions are often followed by segmental glomerular scars. Depending upon the degree of residual damage there may be some permanent impairment of renal function.

Pathogenesis

The morphological findings, together with the depression of serum complement, strongly suggest that the glomerulonephritis is caused by immune complexes. Supporting this interpretation is the demonstration of *Staphylococcus aureus* antigen in the glomeruli.[17,18] The complexes may be deposited in the kidney from the circulation or may be formed in situ on the glomerular capillary basement membranes (see p. 128). Not all cases of glomerulonephritis in acute endocarditis have an immune complex basis; some may be the direct consequence of complement activation by bacterial cell wall antigens.[20]

VISCERAL SEPSIS

Visceral infections other than bacterial endocarditis (see p. 373) or ventriculoatrial shunt infections (see p. 381) may occasionally be associated with glomerulonephritis.[21,22] Abscesses in the lungs, abdomen and pelvis have been implicated, as have instances of osteomyelitis, mediastinitis, infected skin wounds and infected vascular grafts.[23] A wide variety of Gram-positive, Gram-negative and anaerobic bacteria may be responsible. In the cases reported the duration of visceral sepsis has ranged from weeks to 3 years.

Clinical features

Usually the patient feels ill and has fever and loss of weight. Haematuria is universal and often gross. Oliguria or anuria occurs abruptly in about half the patients. Proteinuria exceeding 2 g per day is common in those patients without oliguria and is sometimes accompanied by the nephrotic syndrome. Hypertension is often present.[21]

Serology

Cryoglobulins and immune complexes are frequently present in the circulation. Levels of serum complement are usually normal; those with hypocomplementaemia usually have associated endocarditis.[22]

Renal changes

Light microscopy

The glomerular lesions are invariably proliferative but the exact pattern varies. Most commonly patients have either a *diffuse mesangiocapillary glomerulonephritis*[18,21,23,24] or a *diffuse endocapillary proliferative glomerulonephritis*.[21,23] Both these patterns may be complicated by variable numbers of crescents of different ages. Pure *diffuse crescentic glomerulonephritis* also occurs.[21] Crescent formation is usually only found when infection has been present for longer than 2 months.

Immunofluorescence/immunoperoxidase microscopy

Diffuse granular deposits of C3 are present on the glomerular capillary walls and in the mesangium of all cases. In those kidneys showing a mesangiocapillary glomerulonephritis the complement is usually accompanied by coarse granular deposits of IgG and IgM; in the others immunoglobulin deposition is inconstant.

Electron microscopy

Electron microscopy has been performed on only a few of these cases. Electron-dense deposits have been recorded in the mesangium and less frequently on the subendothelial and subepithelial aspects of the glomerular capillary basement membranes. Some of the subepithelial deposits have had the appearance of humps (see p. 147).[23]

Prognosis

Clinical recovery and resolution of the renal morphological changes are possible, regardless of the type of glomerulonephritis, if the infection is quickly and completely eradicated. To control infection in a vascular prosthesis early removal of the graft is essential in addition to antibiotic therapy. If the infection is not controlled the early mortality is very high.[23]

Pathogenesis

As in bacterial endocarditis (see p. 373) complexes of bacterial antigen and its specific antibody might form or become trapped in the glomeruli and give rise to mesangial cell proliferation. This possibility is supported by the demonstration of bacterial capsular antigen and antibodies specific to that antigen in the glomeruli of patients with klebsiella pneumonia and glomerulonephritis.[24]

INFECTED VENTRICULOATRIAL SHUNT

The surgical relief of hydrocephalus in the past consisted of the shunting of cerebrospinal fluid from one lateral ventricle into the circulating blood through a catheter inserted into the jugular vein, the vena cava and the atrium. One of the complications of this procedure was colonization of the tubing and valves with microorganisms which sometimes produced a persistent low-grade bacteriaemia. In one series reported in 1975, 27% of hydrocephalic patients who had a ventriculoatrial shunt inserted became infected. Of these 4% developed glomerulonephritis; all were patients with longstanding infections that had not been treated effectively.[25]

'Shunt nephritis' was first described in 1965.[26] Since then, over 100 cases have been reported.[27] In 75% the responsible organism was *Staphylococcus epidermidis*, but other organisms such as diphtheroids, *Staphylococcus aureus, Bacillus subtilis, Serratia* species and *Listeria monocytogenes* have also been reported.[28]

Currently, ventriculoperitoneal shunts are used for the relief of hydrocephalus. The risk of the patient developing glomerulonephritis with this type of shunt is very small; only one case has so far been reported.[29]

Clinical features

Most cases have occurred in children with an equal incidence in males and females. The interval between insertion of the shunt and the onset of glomerulonephritis has varied between 3 weeks and 14 years with a mean of 4½ years.[28]

Fever is the invariable indication of shunt infection and systemic sepsis. The development of glomerulonephritis is almost always heralded by haematuria which is usually microscopic but may be gross. It is often accompanied by proteinuria; in one-quarter of the patients this is of sufficient degree to give a nephrotic syndrome. Impairment of renal function is common.[28]

Serology

Immune complexes and cryoglobulins are present

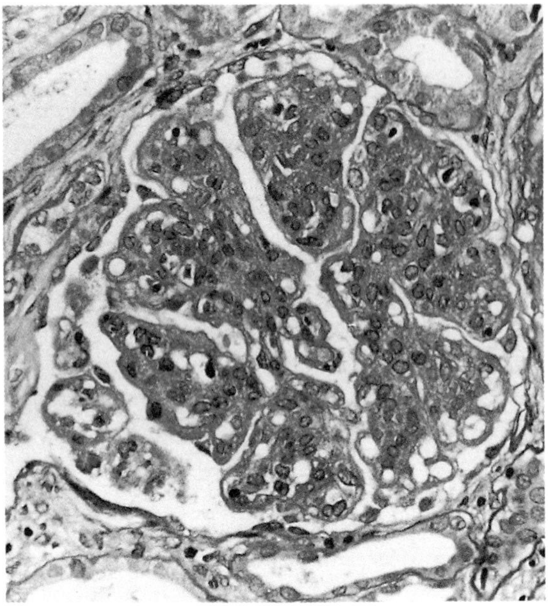

Fig. 11.7 Shunt nephritis. The glomerulus shows a mesangiocapillary pattern of glomerulonephritis. Periodic acid-Schiff × 350

in the circulation. Serum C3 and C4 levels are depressed, indicating activation of complement by the classical pathway.[28]

Renal changes

Light microscopy

In the majority of cases there is a *diffuse mesangiocapillary glomerulonephritis type I* (Fig. 11.7), with or without occasional crescents (see p. 164).[28] A diffuse or focal mesangial proliferative glomerulonephritis or endocapillary proliferative glomerulonephritis has also been occasionally described;[28] rarely these proliferative patterns

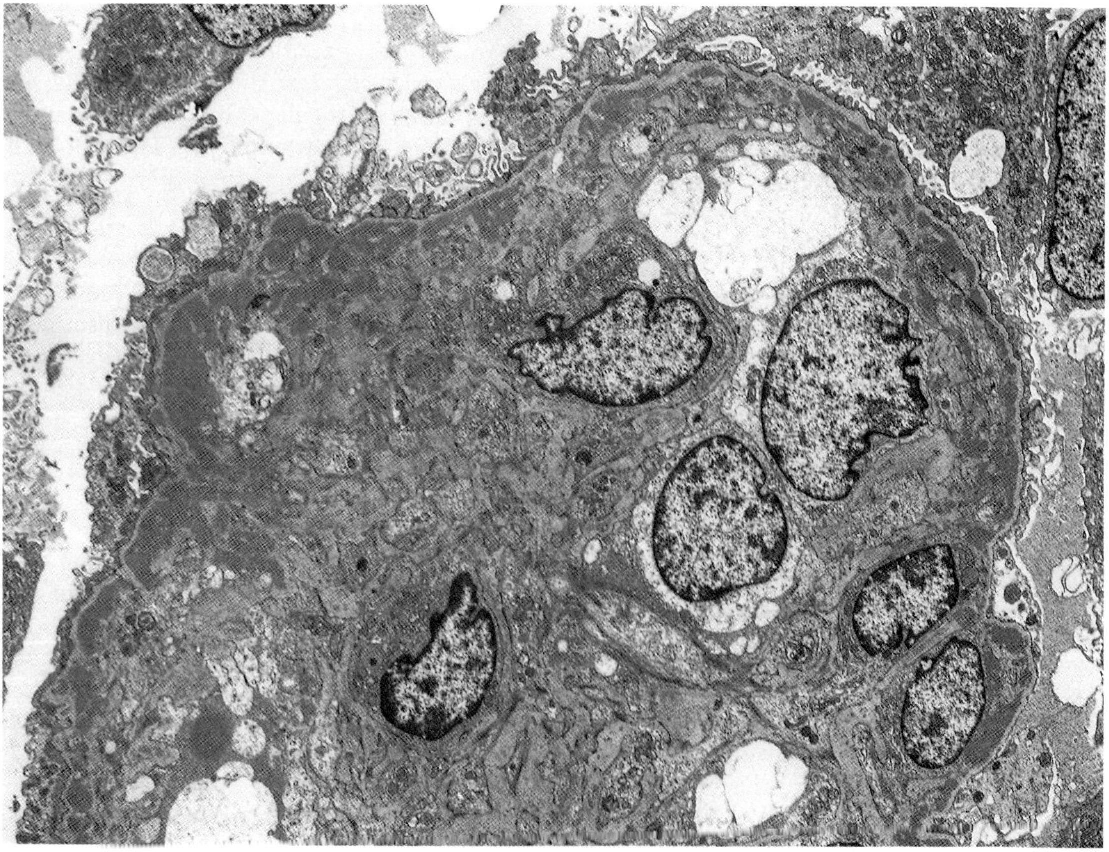

Fig. 11.8 Shunt nephritis. Electron micrograph of part of a glomerulus showing mesangial expansion, increased numbers of mesangial cells, mesangial cell interposition and electron-dense deposits in the mesangium and on the subendothelial aspect of the capillary basement membranes.
× 8000

have been complicated by a diffuse crescentic glomerulonephritis.[27]

Electron microscopy

There are usually subendothelial and mesangial electron-dense deposits in the glomeruli (Fig. 11.8). The number of mesangial cells is increased and in most cases mesangial cell interposition (see p. 167) is present. Sometimes the endothelial cells in the glomerular capillaries are swollen and neutrophil granulocytes and monocytes are present in the capillary lumens, but subepithelial deposits or humps have not been reported.

Immunofluorescence/immunoperoxidase microscopy

Granular deposits of predominantly IgM and C3 are commonly found along the glomerular capillary walls (particularly in the peripheral capillary loops) and in the mesangium (Fig. 11.9); IgG is also often present in the same sites. IgA and other complement components are only infrequently detected.[28]

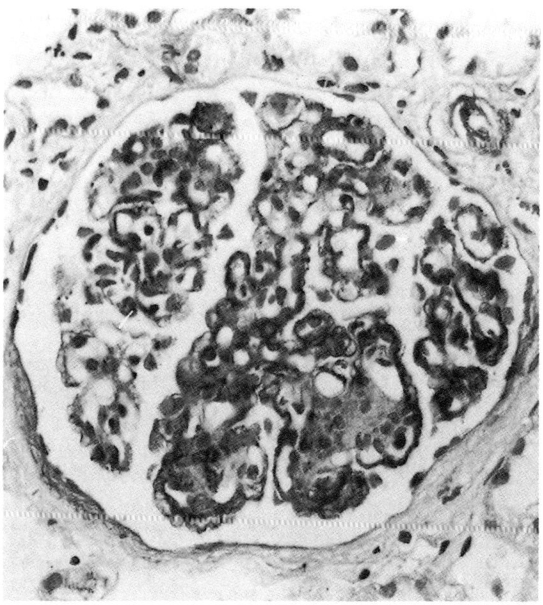

Fig. 11.9 Shunt nephritis. Granules of IgM are present in the walls of the peripheral capillary loops of the glomerulus and in the mesangium.
Immunoperoxidase × 350

Prognosis

To achieve eradication of infection and clinical remission it is usually necessary to remove the shunt as well as give the appropriate antibiotic therapy. Successful treatment of the infection is followed by subsidence of the glomerulonephritis in approximately two-thirds of the patients. The serum complement returns to normal levels and the titres of antibody to bacterial antigen, serum cryoglobulin levels and levels of circulating immune complexes all drop. Renal biopsies performed 2.5–10 months after treatment often disclose only normal glomeruli.[30] However, complete resolution is not always achieved and mild mesangial proliferative glomerulonephritis may persist for years after elimination of the infection;[31] in cases with crescentic glomerulonephritis sclerosis of glomeruli and persistent subendothelial deposits may occur and are associated with proteinuria, microscopic haematuria, hypertension and renal impairment.[30] A few patients progress to end-stage renal disease.[28]

Pathogenesis

'Shunt nephritis' is probably mediated by immune complexes (see p. 128). This hypothesis is supported by the demonstration of bacterial antigen in the glomerular deposits[31,32] and the fact that eradication of the infecting organism results in subsidence of immune complex formation and repair of the glomerular damage.[30,33]

TUBERCULOSIS

Renal tuberculosis is now rare in developed countries. In lands where tuberculosis has not been brought under control and remains rife in all its forms, tuberculosis of the kidneys and urinary tract is as important and frequent a clinical problem as formally it was in, for instance, Western Europe. Also, the decline has not been uniform throughout the populations of developed countries, owing to the immigration of people from countries in which tuberculosis is still prevalent.

The remarkable fall in the frequency of tuberculosis in countries like Britain and the USA, particularly since the introduction of drugs effective against the disease, has tended to lessen clinical awareness of this infection as a cause of urinary symptoms. One consequence is seen in the greater frequency with which renal tuberculosis is mistaken clinically for other diseases.

Renal tuberculosis occurs in two circumstances: most frequently as a late manifestation of an earlier clinical or subclinical infection of the lung or gut, and rarely as part of the widespread infection, disseminated through the vascular system and involving many parts of the body, that characterizes miliary tuberculosis.

Caseous and ulcerative renal tuberculosis

The incidence of caseous and ulcerative renal tuberculosis is greater in men than in women. The disease usually develops between the ages of 20 and 50 years. In approximately one-quarter of cases there is a past history of tuberculosis, usually of the lung; in an additional 25% of patients changes compatible with old pulmonary tuberculosis can be found on chest radiographs.[34] In the remaining cases the disease is apparently confined to the kidneys. Most commonly there is a lapse of 16–25 years between the onset of primary tuberculous infection and the diagnosis of renal involvement; with reactivation pulmonary tuberculosis the lapse is usually about 4–8 years. Of patients infected with tuberculosis less than 0.5% will develop manifestations of renal disease.[35]

Clinical features

Approximately 25% of patients have no constitutional symptoms of tuberculosis or symptoms referable to the urinary tract. The remainder present with symptoms suggesting urinary tract inflammation – dysuria, flank pain, haematuria, nocturia and pyuria. Fewer than 20% of patients will have fever, weight loss, night sweats and anorexia.[34] The urine is almost always abnormal, with pyuria, haematuria or both; culture usually fails to reveal conventional bacterial pathogens. Although there are other causes of 'sterile' pyuria (e.g. *Chlamydia trachomatis* or a fungus), tuberculosis must be excluded in any patient with this finding. *Mycobacterium tuberculosis* is usually demonstrated in the urine, but as bacilluria is often intermittent repeated cultures may be necessary before this is achieved. The tuberculin test will be positive in all patients with renal tuberculosis who are not receiving systemic steroids or who have not been rendered anergic by some condition such as advanced cancer.

Excretion pyelography is the standard diagnostic imaging technique; it will be negative in the earliest stage of renal involvement but with the evolution of cavitation filling defects will appear. Nephrotomograms are particularly helpful. Occasionally sonography may be necessary to confirm the nature of the lesion. Computed tomography does not surpass the sensitivity of conventional pyelography.

Renal changes

Gross appearance of the kidney The tuberculous lesion usually begins in the medulla, near the apex of a pyramid; the papilla then gradually becomes replaced by caseous material. The process spreads to the mucosa of the pelvis and upper part of the ureter and maybe also to adjacent pyramids. The kidney thus comes to contain several soft, caseating foci, 0.5–2.0 cm in diameter, with ragged margins. The mucosal surface of the pelvis is studded with small tubercles and the wall of the ureter is thickened (see p. 687). The caseous masses continue to enlarge and the flow of urine may be obstructed. This may lead to *tuberculous pyonephrosis*, in which part or all of the parenchyma is reduced to a thin shell enclosing a large, caseous mass that fills the greatly dilated calyces and pelvis (Fig. 11.10). The term pyonephrosis is a misnomer when applied to this condition, for there is no pus, except in the rare instance of secondary infection by pyogenic bacteria. In some cases extreme calcification eventually occurs.

Although renal tuberculosis results from haematogenous spread of the infection, clinically evident disease is usually unilateral. At autopsy evidence of involvement of both kidneys is found in 75% of patients, but the infection is usually much more extensive on one side than the other.

Light microscopy Typical caseating granulomas are present (Fig. 11.11). They vary greatly in size, from lesions contained within a single glom-

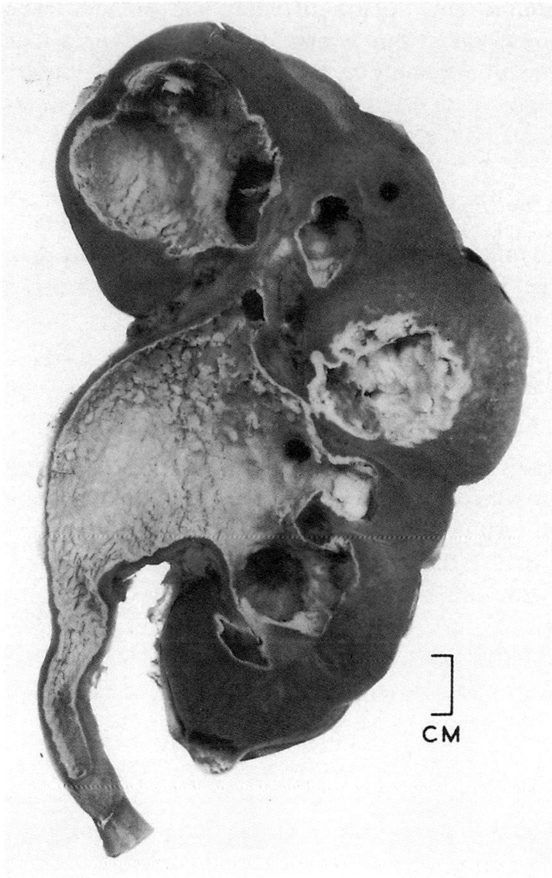

Fig. 11.10 Tuberculous pyonephrosis. In addition to the tuberculous excavation of the substance of the kidney there is extensive tuberculosis of the pelvis and ureter.
Reproduced by permission of the Curator, Gordon Museum, Guy's Hospital, London, UK.

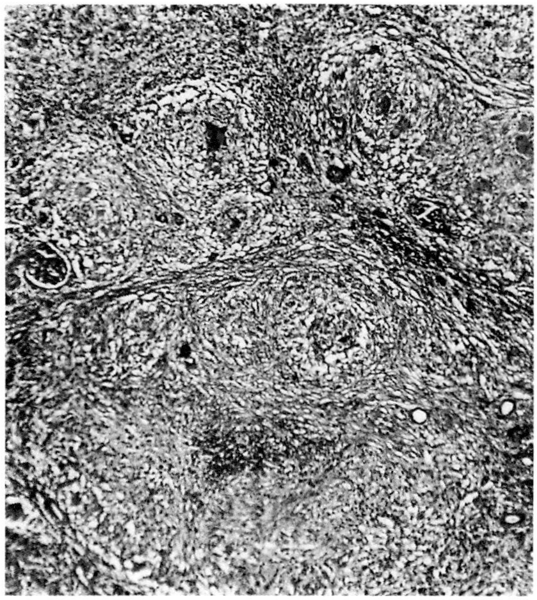

Fig. 11.11 Renal tuberculosis. The cortex contains several granulomas; the one in the lower part of the photograph shows central caseation.
Haematoxylin-eosin × 80

erulus to large caseous lesions. The number of detectable acid-fast bacilli varies greatly. Most granulomas are found initially as segmental lesions in some of the glomeruli, often with accompanying lesions in the loop of Henle or in the collecting ducts. As the disease progresses the lesions in the collecting ducts enlarge, forming a caseous mass which then extends to the papilla.

Changes in other organs

As large numbers of *Mycobacterium tuberculosis* enter the urine from the renal lesions the ureters and the bladder often become infected (see p. 687 and 712).

In men genital infection is also sometimes found in association with renal tuberculosis. Epididymitis, with or without orchitis, is the most common manifestation. Occasionally the genital disease is recognized first and then leads to the recognition of the renal disease. Tuberculous prostatitis also occurs.

Differential diagnosis

Granulomas occur in sarcoidosis (see p. 258), *brucellosis* (see p. 391), *leprosy* (see p. 387), some *fungal infections* (see p. 405), *granulomatous interstitial nephritis* (see p. 454), *Wegener's granulomatosis* (see p. 275) and *xanthogranulomatous pyelonephritis* (see p. 447). These are all non-caseating lesions and most can easily be differentiated from tuberculosis. However, ultimately the demonstration of *Mycobacterium tuberculosis* is the only certain way of being sure of the diagnosis.

Complications

There are three major complications of renal tuberculosis: secondary infection with conventional bacteria, nephrolithiasis and hypertension. *Secondary infection* has been reported in 12–50% of patients with urinary tract tuberculosis.[36] *Nephrolithiasis* (see p. 531) occurs in 7–18% and often causes renal colic.[37] *Hypertension* (see p. 306) affects less than 5% and may not be more common than in the general population.

Prognosis

Without treatment the 5-year survival of patients with renal tuberculosis was 15–42%. With modern chemotherapy and surgery to relieve any obstructions to urinary flow no one should die of urinary tract tuberculosis. The degree of residual impairment will depend upon the amount of irreversible renal destruction that exists before treatment is started.

Pathogenesis

Limited haematogenous dissemination due to low-grade bacteriaemia at the time of the primary (usually pulmonary) infection is common. Since immunity to the mycobacteria is evolving or is already established at this time, small granulomas rapidly form at the metastatic foci. In the kidneys these granulomas are found in the glomeruli. The bacteria within the granulomas may remain viable and may then lie dormant for decades. Only if the host's defences are lowered in some way does bacillary proliferation recur, and lead to rupture of the glomerular capillaries and delivery of organisms into the tubule. Entrapment of mycobacterium-infected macrophages and debris occurs within the loop of Henle and here an expanding granulomatous lesion develops. Caseation, with discharge into the calyceal system leaving a cavity, and papillary necrosis follow. It is not understood why clinically significant disease is usually unilateral.

Miliary tuberculosis

Systemic miliary tuberculosis ensues when a tuberculous lesion erodes the wall of a vessel and highly infected caseous material gains access to the blood stream, leading to an intense bacteriaemia. Granulomas may then result in almost any organ, including the kidneys. The initial site from which dissemination occurs is most commonly in the chest. It may be either a primary or reactivated pulmonary lesion or an associated lymphadenitis.

Clinical features

In miliary tuberculosis the systemic features of the illness dominate. The renal involvement is asymptomatic.

Renal changes

Gross appearance of the kidneys The surfaces of both kidneys are diffusely speckled with uniform yellowish-white foci, each about 1 mm in diameter. The lesions are called miliary because they are roughly the size of millet seed. They are scattered throughout the renal substance but are particularly numerous in the cortex.

Light microscopy The miliary foci are each composed of several coalescent granulomas with central caseation.

Prognosis

The outcome of the illness will depend entirely upon the speed with which specific antibacterial treatment is started. Without treatment the presence of tuberculous meningitis will lead to death. The renal lesions do not affect the prognosis.

ATYPICAL MYCOBACTERIAL INFECTIONS

Atypical mycobacteria are widespread in soil, water, animal excreta and plants. Many are saprophytic or have a very low pathogenicity. The prevalence of infection by these organisms is increasing in Europe and the USA; those affected usually have reduced immunity.

Renal involvement by atypical mycobacteria is rare and usually part of a life-threatening disseminated infection. *Mycobacterium kansasii* has produced miliary granulomatous lesions in the kidneys,[38] and patients with human immunodeficiency virus (HIV) infection and the acquired immune deficiency syndrome (AIDS) may develop bacteriaemias, principally by *Mycobacterium avium-intracellulare*, that result in miliary renal lesions (see p. 398).[39]

Some species of atypical mycobacteria respond only poorly or not at all to antibacterial drugs.

LEPROSY

A wide variety of renal lesions have been described in patients suffering from leprosy. These include amyloidosis, tubulointerstitial nephritis, pyelonephritis, acute tubular necrosis, glomerulonephritis and the glomerular lesions of cryoglobulinaemia. Some of these conditions will be considered briefly.

Amyloidosis

Chronic renal failure resulting from amyloidosis is the leading cause of death in leprosy.[40] The amyloid is AA in type (see p. 344).

Tubulointerstitial nephritis

Chronic tubulointerstitial nephritis has been observed at autopsy in some patients with lepromatous or non-lepromatous leprosy.[41] In one biopsy series the incidence was 22%.[42] The lesions occur particularly in those with advanced disease of long duration. It has been suggested that the lesion may be caused by the prolonged chemotherapy employed in leprosy.

Very rarely granulomas occur in the interstitium; they are characterized by lipid-laden macrophages (lepra cells) and a few giant cells, surrounded by a mantle of lymphocytes. Large numbers of *Mycobacterium leprae* are often present in the cytoplasm of the macrophages and giant cells.

Glomerulonephritis

The incidence of glomerulonephritis in leprosy is difficult to assess. In two renal biopsy series in which patients were selected without regard to clinical evidence of renal disease, glomerulonephritis was found in 37% in one and in 6% in the other.[43,44] In autopsy studies glomerulonephritis has been reported to be more common in leprosy patients than in the general population[45] and was cited as an important complication by Hansen.[46]

Clinical features

Patients may present with an acute nephritic syndrome, a nephrotic syndrome, an asymptomatic proteinuria or haematuria. Hypertension is uncommon. Only rarely is there progression to end-stage renal failure. Cryoglobulinaemia, circulating immune complexes and reduced levels of serum C3 are common.

Renal changes

In most series the two most common morphological patterns of glomerulonephritis observed in leprosy are the *mesangial proliferative* type (see p. 153) and the *diffuse endocapillary proliferative* type (see p. 142);[47–49] in one study of 54 biopsies *diffuse membranous glomerulonephritis* (see p. 191) was the commonest type.[42] A few cases of focal proliferative, diffuse sclerosing, crescentic and mesangiocapillary glomerulonephritis have also been reported.[42,47]

Prognosis

The effect of glomerulonephritis on the prognosis for patients with leprosy is not clear. Uraemia due to chronic glomerulonephritis has been reported in the past as a major cause of death in lepromatous leprosy but episodes with proteinuria, microscopic haematuria, cell casts and oedema suggestive of glomerulonephritis frequently do not lead to end-stage renal failure. Glomerulonephritis may be a mild, self-limited complication in many instances.[47,50]

Pathogenesis

The morphology suggests that the glomerulonephritis is mediated by immune complexes, either circulating or formed in situ. However, there is no other evidence to support or refute this hypothesis.

Some of the cases of diffuse endocapillary glomerulonephritis and mesangial proliferative glomerulonephritis may be poststreptococcal (see p. 143) because the skin lesions in leprosy frequently become secondarily infected with streptococci.

Cryoglobulinaemia

The glomerular lesions of Type III cryoglobulinaemia are sometimes found (see p. 352).[51]

SYPHILIS

Syphilis remains a persistent problem in both developed and undeveloped countries. The dramatic and profound decline in the incidence of new cases of both acquired and congenital syphilis in Britain, the USA and Europe following the advent of penicillin and the end of World War II has been followed in recent years by a slight resurgence of the acquired disease. Congenital syphilis remains extremely rare. However, in some undeveloped countries many cases of syphilis are not treated and congenital syphilis still occurs.

Renal disease is a well-recognized rare complication of syphilis. In the secondary form of syphilis the prevalence is approximately 0.3%;[52] in congenital syphilis the prevalence is probably higher.[53] The most common lesion described is *glomerulonephritis. Tubulointerstitial nephritis, renal gummas* and *amyloid* are still occasionally seen, mostly in countries where there are many cases of untreated syphilis.

Glomerulonephritis

Glomerulonephritis may complicate congenital or acquired secondary syphilis.

Clinical features

Renal involvement generally presents as proteinuria which may be severe enough to produce the nephrotic syndrome. In congenital syphilis the nephrotic syndrome usually occurs in the first 3 weeks after birth. Microscopic haematuria also is often present; rarely, the first manifestation is an acute nephritic syndrome. Renal function is either normal or only modestly impaired.

Serology

Circulating immune complexes are almost always present; cryoglobulins have also been found.[54] In congenital syphilis the serum levels of C3 and C4 are often depressed, indicating activation of complement by the classical pathway;[53] in acquired syphilis the serum complement is usually normal.[54]

Renal changes

The most common form of glomerulonephritis described is *diffuse membranous* (Figs 11.12–11.14; see p. 191).[54–56] Less frequently, *diffuse mesangial proliferative glomerulonephritis* (see p. 153) and *diffuse endocapillary proliferative glomerulonephritis* (see p. 142) are encountered. Rarely, diffuse crescentic glomerulonephritis (see p. 185)[57] or minimal change disease (see p. 135)[58] has been reported.

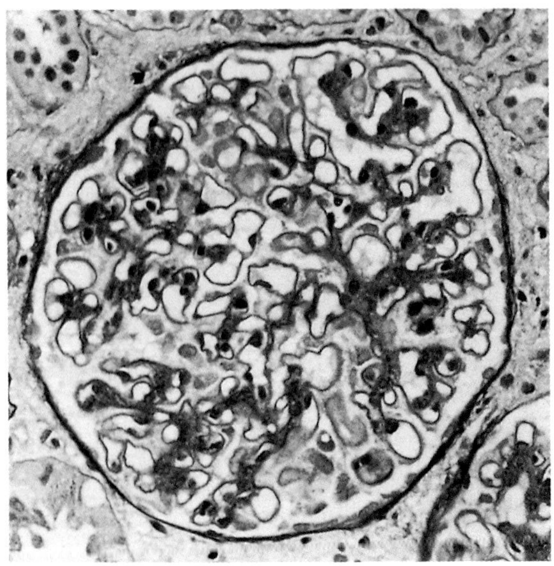

Fig. 11.12 Membranous glomerulonephritis in syphilis. The capillary basement membranes are slightly thickened. Periodic acid-Schiff × 350

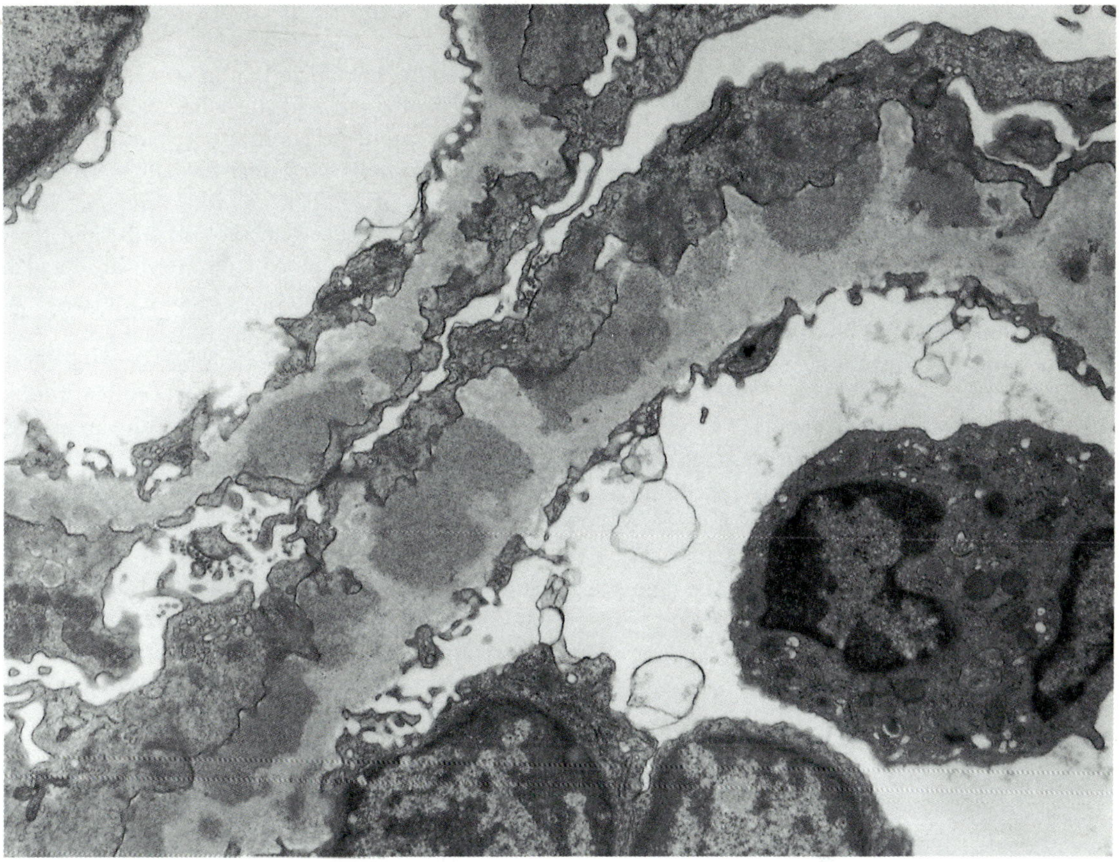

Fig. 11.13 Membranous glomerulonephritis in syphilis. Electron micrograph of part of a glomerulus showing subepithelial electron-dense deposits
× 3 000

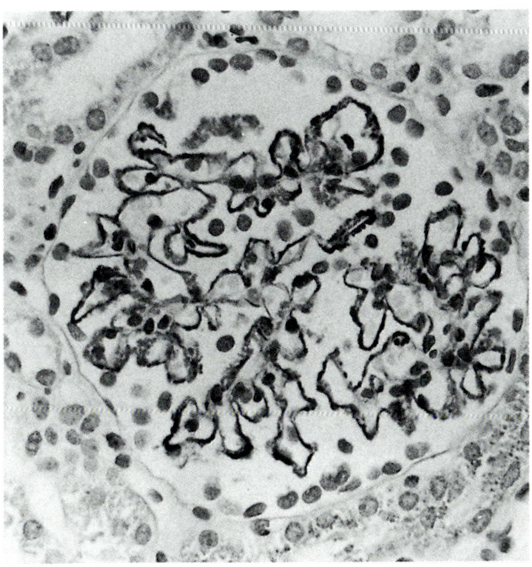

Prognosis

Although spontaneous resolution of the glomerulonephritis associated with syphilis may occur,[59] treatment with appropriate antibiotics usually results in rapid and complete resolution of the urinary abnormalities; permanent impairment of renal function is uncommon[53–58]

Pathogenesis.

The morphological findings suggest an immune-complex-mediated renal injury (see p. 128).

Fig. 11.14 Membranous glomerulonephritis in syphilis. Glomerulus showing granular deposits of IgG on the capillary walls.
Immunoperoxidase × 350

Elution of immune complexes from normal capillary basement membranes and identification of anti-treponemal antibody and treponemal antigen in the eluate support this concept.[54,55,57]

Tubulointerstitial nephritis

In stillborn fetuses from syphilitic mothers there is usually a tubulointerstitial nephritis. Large numbers of spirochaetes are present in the interstitium, tubular cells and tubular lumens; they are demonstrable by Levaditi's silver impregnation method, which renders them thick and black against a yellowish background.

In the tertiary stage tubular damage and focal infiltration of the interstitium by predominantly plasma cells was found in 6.5% of a series of 200 untreated cases in 1932; spirochaetes were not demonstrated in these kidneys.[60] Since then there have been no further reports of this lesion.

Gummas

Gummas have occasionally been found in the kidneys in late cases.

LEPTOSPIROSIS

Leptospirosis is an infectious disease caused by members of the *Leptospira interrogens* complex. These are animal pathogens that only accidentally infect man. There are 26 different serogroups of this organism in the complex including *L. icterohaemorrhagiae, L. canicola, L. hardjo, L. pomona, L. bataviae* and *L. hebdomadis*. The organisms infect many wild and domestic animals; the hosts develop interstitial nephritis and persistently shed leptospirae in their urine. Rodents, especially rats, are the most important reservoir of infection. Contact with contaminated animals, water, soil or sewage or exposure to infected aerosols may transmit the infection to humans.

About one-third of the reported cases of leptospirosis occur in high risk occupations, e.g. farming, abattoir work, sewer maintenance, trout farming and veterinary medicine. Other cases occur in those participating in water-related sports, or exposed in other ways to infected material.

Clinically recognized attacks of leptospirosis are rare in Britain and the USA. Subclinical episodes are more frequent; for example, 10% of Britain's 65 000 dairy farmers show serological evidence of past infection with *L. hardjo*.[61] In less developed countries clinical and subclinal leptospirosis is much more common; in Thailand and in Singapore, leptospirosis is the most important single cause of acute renal failure.[62,63]

All the various pathogenic serogroups of the *L. interrogens* complex can cause either mild or severe disease. The kidneys are invariably involved and renal failure may occur.

Clinical features[64,65]

Patients usually present with fever, myalgia and conjunctival suffusion. There may also be nausea, vomiting, purpura and signs of meningeal irritation. Approximately 10% present as Weil's disease, a severe illness with jaundice and involvement of various organs. Involvement of the kidneys in large series has occurred in approximately 50% of patients;[64] it is indicated by acute oliguric or non-oliguric renal failure. Rarely the haemolytic uraemic syndrome occurs.[66] Of the 43 reported cases of *L. interrogens* infection in Britain in 1982, 11 had renal failure: eight of these were among the 23 patients infected with *L. icterohaemorrhagiae* and three were among the 20 patients with *L. hebdomadis* or *L. canicola* infection.[67]

Serology

The diagnosis is confirmed by a rise in antibody levels. The serogroup of the infecting strain is determined by microscopic agglutination. The serum C3 may be low initially, presumably due to complement activation by the alternative pathway.

Renal changes

Gross appearance of the kidneys

The kidneys are enlarged and pale. There may be haemorrhages on the subcapsular and cut surfaces.

Light microscopy

Biopsies taken during the second and fourth weeks of the disease show a *tubulointerstitial nephritis* (Fig. 11.15).[68,69] There is patchy interstitial oedema and peritubular infiltration of macrophages, lymphocytes and plasma cells. Leptospiral antigen can sometimes be detected within some of the infiltrating mononuclear cells.[70] *Tubular necrosis* is also usually present, often with evidence of epithelial regeneration. The glomeruli may show mild *mesangial proliferation*. In one patient infected with *L. pomona* the glomeruli contained in addition neutrophil granulocytes and there were subepithelial, intramembranous and mesangial electron-dense deposits and granules of C3 and Clq in the glomerular capillary walls.[69] Rarely there may be the changes of the *haemolytic uraemic syndrome* (see p. 281).

a

b

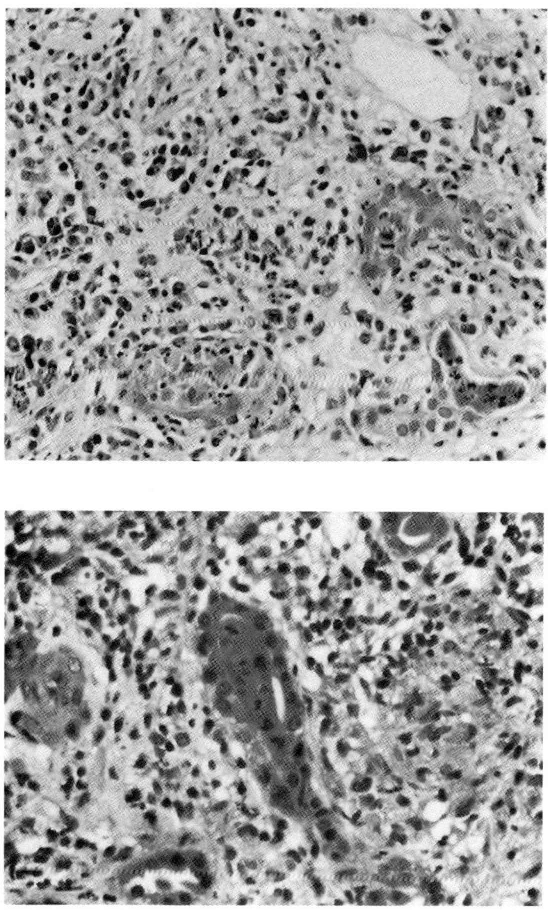

Fig. 11.15 Leptospirosis (*L. icterohaemorrhagiae*). There is an interstitial nephritis with marked cellular infiltration, predominantly mononuclear. (**a**) Some of the tubules show epithelial necrosis. (**b**) A tubule contains a pigment cast. Haematoxylin-eosin: (**a**) × 230; (**b**) × 300

Differential diagnosis

The morphological changes in the kidneys in leptospirosis are non-specific. Their cause must be distinguished from other causes of acute interstitial nephritis by serological studies during the second week of the illness onwards. In the first 10 days isolation of leptospires from the blood or cerebrospinal fluid should be attempted.

Prognosis

Most patients with mild disease recover. The mortality is high in those who are severely ill and require intensive management; as many as 50% of severely jaundiced patients over the age of 50 years may die.[64] However, dialysis has improved the diagnosis and the long term follow-up of patients who developed renal failure shows good recovery of renal function. Penicillin or tetracycline needs to be given within a few days of the onset of the disease if treatment is to have any effect on its natural history; a Jarisch–Herxheimer reaction may occur when penicillin is given at this time.

Pathogenesis

Leptospires gain access to the kidneys by the blood stream within a few hours of infection. Experimental work in hamsters indicates that they initially cause glomerular injury, then migrate to the interstitium and tubules via the peritubular capillaries. It is suggested that the tubulointerstitial changes in leptospirosis result from this spirochaetal migration.[70]

BRUCELLOSIS

Infections in domestic animals by four species of *Brucella* can be transmitted to humans. Invasion occurs through skin abrasions, the gastrointestinal or respiratory mucosa or the conjunctiva. *Br. melitensis* is acquired mainly from goats' milk or fresh cheese, *Br. abortus* from drinking raw cows' milk and *Br. suis* from direct contact with infected blood and tissue of pigs in slaughter houses, on farms and in veterinary practice. Only a few examples of *Br. canis* infection have been reported. Despite eradication programmes brucellosis is still found in many temperate and tropical countries.

Renal involvement is rare, although up to 50% of patients shed the organism in the urine at some point during the course of the disease.

Clinical features

The kidneys may be affected in three circumstances.[71] The first is during the acute stage of brucellosis when there may be proteinuria, haematuria, and signs of a urinary infection or the abrupt onset of a nephritic syndrome. The second is in association with brucella endocarditis, when pain in the back or abdomen may occur together with proteinuria and haematuria. The third is during the chronic stage of the disease when dysuria, haematuria, nocturia and pyuria may occur and the radiological findings may suggest renal tuberculosis or a renal adenocarcinoma. The diagnosis will usually depend upon demonstration of specific agglutinins or complement fixation tests.

Renal changes

Gross appearance of the kidneys

In the acute stage of the disease the kidneys are usually enlarged; in brucella endocarditis there may also be abundant petechiae on the subcapsular and cut surfaces. In the chronic stage of the disease the gross appearances often are indistinguishable from those in caseous and ulcerative renal tuberculosis (see p. 384).[72]

Light microscopy

In acute brucellosis there is usually a non-specific *diffuse tubulointerstitial nephritis* (see p. 432); this may be accompanied by a *focal proliferative glomerulonephritis* (see p. 211).[71] If there is a brucella endocarditis the *proliferative glomerulonephritic lesions* associated with this complication may be present (see p. 375). Granulomatous lesions are not usually found. Stains for organisms are negative. One case has been reported of acute tubular necrosis following rhabdomyolysis which was thought to have been caused by this organism.[73] Another patient had an acute endocapillary proliferative glomerulonephritis with subepithelial humps.[74]

Chronic cases are usually characterized by *focal caseating granulomas* indistinguishable from chronic caseous and ulcerative tuberculosis (see p. 384). Stains usually fail to reveal bacteria. Cultures are frequently positive if plenty of tissue can be taken from multiple sites in the kidney.[72]

Prognosis

Prolonged treatment with rifampicin (rifampin) and deoxycycline usually leads eventually to full recovery even though convalescence may be slow and relapse may occur. Focal proliferative glomerulonephritic lesions may heal to give segmental or global scarring with some impairment of renal function. Progression to chronic renal failure is rare.

LEGIONNAIRES' DISEASE

A mild transient proteinuria, microscopic haematuria and elevation of the serum creatinine level are fairly frequent in Legionnaires' disease; acute renal failure is rare.

Renal changes

Patients with renal failure have either a non-specific *acute tubulointerstitial nephritis* (see p. 432)[75,76] or *acute tubular necrosis* (see p. 491). The organism has been demonstrated in the renal tissue in only one published case of interstitial nephritis;[77] it was found in renal cortical abscesses in a patient with Legionnaires' disease and obstructive nephropathy due to carcinoma of the bladder.[78]

Prognosis

Recovery of function and return of the urinary findings to normal are usual, but may be slow. Approximately 33% of the patients die.[79]

TYPHOID FEVER

Mild proteinuria, sometimes with a few red and white cells, is common in typhoid. Renal biopsies from three such patients showed a mild *focal mesangial proliferative glomerulonephritis* with granules of IgM, salmonella Vi antigen and complement in the mesangium and capillary walls.[80]

Rarely, there is an acute nephritic syndrome with similar morphological changes.[81] Patients occasionally develop gross haematuria and this has been associated with IgA nephropathy in Thailand.[82]

Acute pyelonephritis may also occur and dehydration, if not managed correctly, may lead to *acute tubular necrosis.*

OTHER SYSTEMIC BACTERIAL INFECTIONS

Salmonellosis

In severe systemic infections with salmonellae other than *Salmonella typhi*, acute tubular necrosis (see p. 491) and, less frequently, cortical microabscesses may occur in the kidneys.

Shigellosis

Shigella dysenteriae sometimes causes the haemolytic uraemic syndrome and produces renal changes (see p. 281).

Cholera

Tubular vacuoles occur in cases with potassium loss. A few patients develop acute tubular necrosis (see p. 491); rarely there is cortical necrosis (see p. 303).

Acute bacterial pyelonephritis

The kidney may be infected during the course of septicaemia (see p. 432). There is often an associated obstructive uropathy.

VIRAL INFECTIONS

HEPATITIS B VIRUS INFECTION

The hepatitis B virus consists of a central core or nucleocapsid and an outer coat or envelope. The contents of the nucleocapsid include DNA, a DNA polymerase and hepatitis B core antigen (HBcAg). The envelope consists of proteins, carbohydrates and lipids and carries the hepatitis B surface antigen (HBsAg). When complete viruses are present in the blood, an additional soluble antigen released by disruption of the capsid, the hepatitis B e antigen (HBcAg), is generally detected in the serum. Hepatitis D virus (delta agent) is often found in association with hepatitis B virus; it is a defective transmissible virus which requires multiplication of hepatitis B virus for its own replication.

Asymptomatic people with no evidence of liver damage and patients with symptomatic or asymptomatic chronic liver disease may become carriers of the virus for long periods; they can be detected by the presence of HBsAg in their blood. The prevalence of HBsAg antigenaemia varies greatly throughout the world, ranging from 0.1% in northern and western Europe, Britain, the USA, Canada, Australia and New Zealand to 24% in some populations in South East Asia, China, Japan, and central and southern Africa.[83]

Three main forms of renal disease may be associated with hepatitis B virus: glomerulonephritis, the lesions of cryoglobulinaemia and necrotizing vasculitis.

Glomerulonephritis

In those parts of the world where hepatitis B infection is particularly prevalent, the frequency of hepatitis B antigenaemia is greater among patients with certain forms of glomerulonephritis than in the rest of the population. Most reports have emphasized the strikingly high percentage of children with membranous glomerulonephritis who are HBsAg carriers. In two recent studies, both from areas where infection with hepatitis B virus is rife, the incidence of antigenaemia in such children was 94%[84] in one and 80% in the other.[85] The carrier rate is also raised, but much less dramatically, in adults with membranous glomerulonephritis and in patients with mesangiocapillary glomerulonephritis (type 1).[84,85] There have been occasional observations of a significantly higher prevalence of HBsAg in the blood of patients with mesangial proliferative glomerulonephritis and IgA nephropathy.[84]

The association between HBs antigenaemia and membranous glomerulonephritis also occurs in countries with a low prevalence rate of hepatitis B infection but is much less frequent. In the hospitals in the Southwest Pediatric Nephrology Study Group, based in Texas, USA, approximately 20% of cases of membranous glomerulonephritis newly diagnosed between 1979 and 1984 had an associated HBs antigenaemia; the affected children were predominantly black.[86]

There is evidence from areas in which there are high rates of HBs antigenaemia, that many of the children acquire the hepatitis virus by vertical transmission from their mothers, who are carriers.[87] But even in these populations horizontal transmission may be present in some cases and is probably important in membranous glomerulonephritis in adults and in populations with a low carrier rate.[86]

Few of these patients manifest any clinical evidence of liver disease, although elevated levels of aspartate transaminase and alanine transaminase in the serum are common and liver biopsies often show chronic persistent or active hepatitis.[86,88]

Clinical features

Membranous glomerulonephritis associated with hepatitis B virus is most common in young children but occurs at all ages, with a marked male predominance; mesangiocapillary glomerulonephritis occurs predominantly in adult males. Most patients present with the nephrotic syndrome and the remainder have asymptomatic proteinuria. Microscopic haematuria is detected in most patients; gross haematuria is rare. Hypertension occurs in about half the patients with mesangiocapillary glomerulonephritis and renal impairment occurs in about 20%; both occur only occasionally in membranous glomerulonephritis.[84]

Serology

Approximately a third of the patients have reduced serum levels of C3 and/or C4.[85] By definition all patients have HBsAg in their serum and almost 80% also have HBeAg. Antibody to core antigen (HBcAb) is almost always present, antibody to e antigen (HBeAb) is present in about 25% of cases of membranous glomerulonephritis and in fewer of those with mesangiocapillary glomerulonephritis, but antibody to surface antigen (HBsAb) is absent in children with membranous glomerulonephritis and infrequent in adults with membranous glomerulonephritis or patients with mesangiocapillary glomerulonephritis.[85] Antibody to delta antigen is absent. Circulating immune complexes are common.[88]

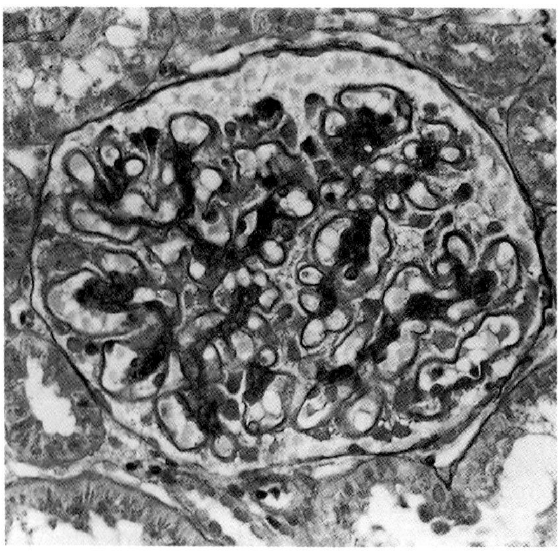

Fig 11.16 Hepatitis-B-associated membranous glomerulonephritis. There is segmental mesangial cell proliferation in addition to global basement membrane thickening.
Periodic acid-Schiff × 350

Renal changes

Membranous glomerulonephritis Most commonly there is a diffuse membranous glomerulonephritis (Fig. 11.16).[89] This differs from the idiopathic lesion (see p. 192) in that approximately half the cases show mild to moderate focal and segmental mesangial cell proliferation (3–4 mesangial cells/mesangial area) with or without increase in the amount of mesangial matrix. The mesangium almost always contains electron-dense deposits (Fig. 11.17)[90] and in approximately a quarter to a third of the kidneys there are small subendothelial and/or intramembranous deposits.[85] Minor degrees of segmental mesangial cell interposition are often present. Tubuloreticular bodies (see p. 232) are present in glomerular and peritubular capillary endothelial cells in up to 25% of the kidneys.[85] Deposits of IgM, IgA, Clq and C4 are more common in hepatitis-B-virus-associated membranous glomerulonephritis than in the idiopathic disease. Occasionally the IgA deposits are prominent in both the capillary walls and mesangium.[91] Spherical particles (Dane particles) have been observed by electron microscopy in the mesangium in a few patients; although not complete viruses their structure has suggested to some that they may be derived from the nucleocapsid.[89,92]

Mesangiocapillary glomerulonephritis Less frequently there is either a focal or diffuse mesan-

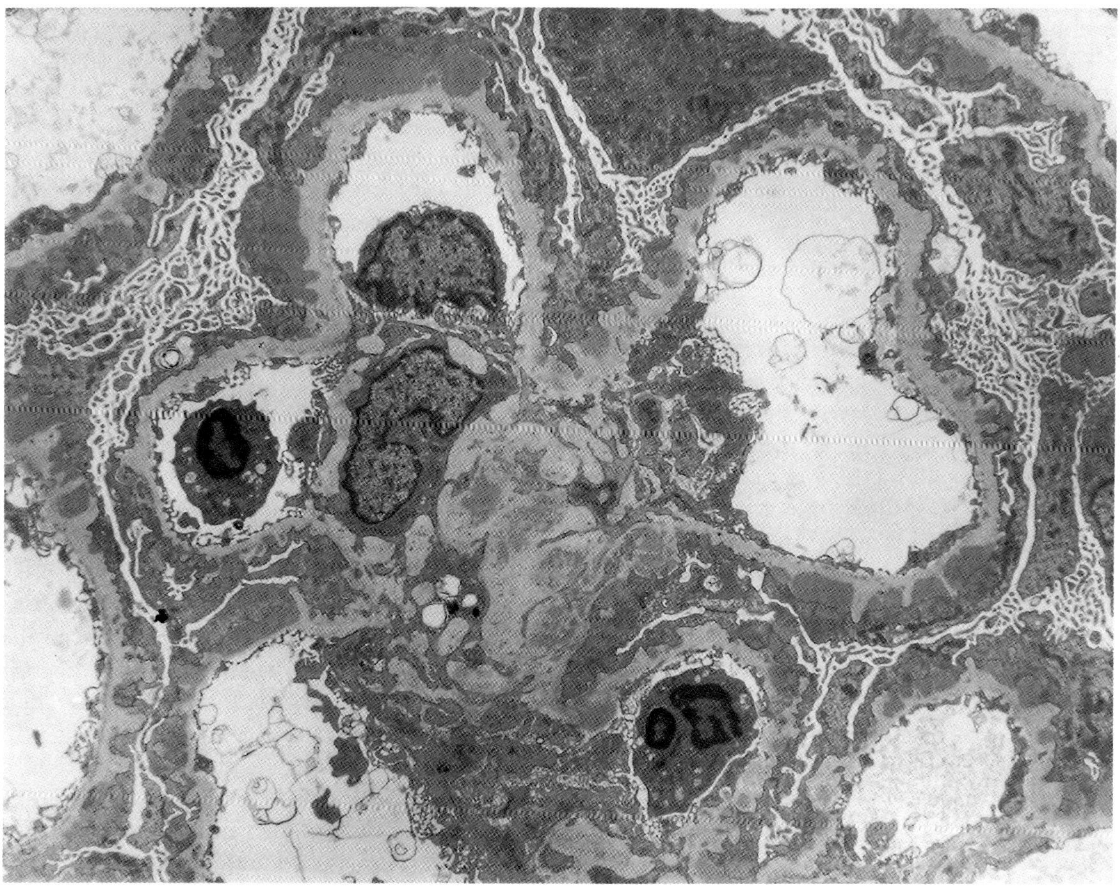

Fig. 11.17 Hepatitis-B-associated membranous glomerulonephritis. Electron micrograph of part of a glomerulus. Mesangial electron-dense deposits are present in addition to those on the subepithelial aspect of the capillary basement membrane. × 8000

giocapillary glomerulonephritis type 1. This does not differ greatly from the idiopathic form (see p. 166) but glomerular deposits of C3 are less frequent, being present in only about 54% of cases, and IgM deposits are more common, being present in almost all the cases. Tubuloreticular bodies are found in the endothelium of approximately 15% of cases.[85]

Mesangial proliferative glomerulonephritis Mesangial proliferative glomerulonephritis associated with hepatitis B virus does not seem to differ from the idiopathic disease (see p. 155). There is usually only slight staining for immunoglobulins. Small discrete electron dense deposits are commonly present in the mesangium.[84]

IgA nephropathy IgA nephropathy associated with HBs antigenaemia is not morphologically distinguishable from the idiopathic lesion (see p. 159).

Combined IgA nephropathy and membranous glomerulonephritis In a few cases biopsies have revealed features of both IgA nephropathy and membranous glomerulonephritis.[92]

Differential diagnosis

Morphologically it is sometimes possible to distinguish membranous glomerulonephritis associated with hepatitis B virus from the *idiopathic disease* by the presence of mesangial electron-dense deposits and by the other criteria discussed earlier, but it is usually impossible to exclude other secondary forms of membranous glomerulonephritis such as *lupus nephritis class V* (see p. 230). To attempt to make the distinction, serological findings, clinical features and other factors have to be taken into account. Hepatitis-B-virus-associated mesangiocapillary glomerulonephritis, mesangial proliferative glomerulonephritis and IgA nephropathy are indistinguishable morphologically from the idiopathic diseases.

Prognosis

In children the nephrotic syndrome usually disappears within approximately 2 years of onset, either spontaneously or following treatment with steroids or interferon.[93–96] Proteinuria may persist but is usually slight. Progressive renal failure and relapse are rare. Remission may be associated with loss of HBeAg from the patient's serum and the appearance of HBeAb, but persistence of HBe antigenaemia is more usual. Most patients who fully recover clinically from their glomerulonephritis remain persistent HBsAg carriers.

Pathogenesis

The likelihood is that the membranous, mesangiocapillary and probably the mesangial proliferative forms of glomerulonephritis that occur in association with hepatitis B infection are due to the accumulation of immune complexes in the glomeruli. However, we have no detailed knowledge of the mechanisms or antigens involved.

The complexes are probably derived either from the circulation or by *in situ* deposition (see p. 128). The evidence concerning the identity of the antigen in the immune complexes is conflicting. HBsAg was detected in the glomerular deposits very frequently in the past but in recent years many investigators have been unable to confirm this observation.[84,85] A possible explanation of this discrepancy is that the glomerular deposits often contain IgM with antiglobulin activity which binds the Fc part of the anti-HBsAg antibody used in the tests and gives a false-positive staining.[97] Investigators using polyclonal antibodies have often found HBeAg and occasionally HBcAg in the deposits. When monoclonal antibodies are used HBe antigen has been demonstrated most consistently, although HBsAg continues to be detected occasionally.[98] When $F(ab^1)_2$ fragments of monoclonal antibodies are employed, only staining for HBe antigen has been reported in the glomerular deposits (Fig. 11.18).[85,99,100] Delta antigen has not been detected in those kidneys.

The isolated cases in which resolution of proteinuria has occurred in cases of hepatitis-B-virus-associated glomerulonephritis following treatment with interferon[95,101] are not strong presumptive evidence for a causal connection between hepatitis B virus antigens and glomerulonephritis because both the glomerulo-

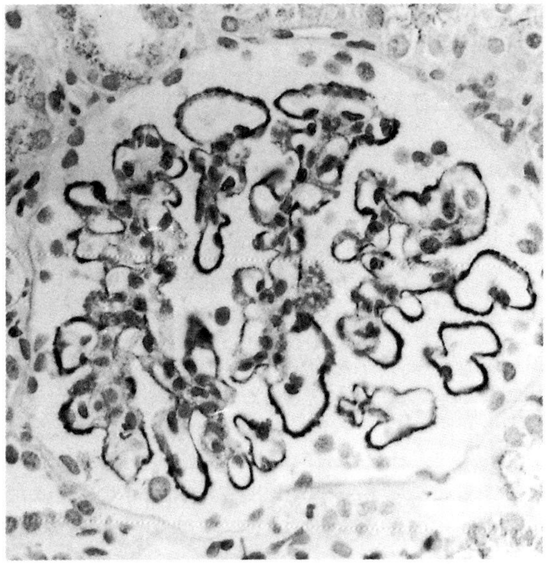

Fig. 11.18 Hepatitis-B-associated membranous glomerulonephritis. Glomerulus showing granular deposits of HBe antigen on capillary walls using a $F(ab^1)_2$ fragment of a monoclonal antibody to HBe.
Immunoperoxidase × 350

nephritis and the hepatitis B viral infection are known to sometimes resolve[96] and this may have occurred in these cases.

The causative role of hepatitis B virus in the pathogenesis of the membranous, mesangio-capillary and probably the mesangial proliferative forms of glomerulonephritis associated with this infection remains probable but uncertain and the identification of HBeAg as the putative antigen is still speculative.[102] Confirmation of the claim that antibodies to HBeAg can be eluted from the glomerulonephritic kidneys would strengthen the case considerably.[103]

The association of IgA nephropathy (see p. 159) and HBs antigenaemia may be due to the viral hepatic lesions leading to IgA deposition in the kidneys in the same way as occurs in cirrhosis (see p. 513). Another suggestion is that HBsAg may be playing a pathogenetic role.[104]

Cryoglobulinaemia

Hepatitis B antigenaemia is sometimes associated with type III cryoglobulinaemia (see p. 352). A high incidence of the virus in these cases compared with the general population has been reported,[105] although this experience has not been without exception. It seems probable that the hepatitis B virus is the primary aetiological factor in a small number of these patients.

The incidence of renal involvement in hepatitis-B-virus-associated type III cryoglobulinaemia is not known; in one selected series of 30 cases it was 50%,[105] but this is almost certainly an unusually high figure. In type III cryoglobulinaemia from all causes, 12% have evidence of renal disease.[106]

The clinical features do not differ from those of other cases of type III cryoglobulinaemia (see p. 352).

The commonest renal change is a glomerulonephritis. Its morphological type is variable: instances of diffuse endocapillary proliferative, mesangial proliferative, focal proliferative with segmental necrosis and membranous glomerulonephritis have been reported.[107] Intracapillary amorphous masses may be present (see p. 352). Segmental subendothelial electron-dense deposits may produce 'wire loops' (see p. 352). There are also mesangial deposits. In some cases these deposits contain paired microfibrils or cylinders (see p. 353). The deposits contain IgG, IgM, C3, Clq and C4, producing a granular pattern in the capillary walls and mesangium. As the disease progresses increasing numbers of glomeruli become sclerotic. Necrotizing vasculitis is occasionally present in cases with an acute course. The interstitium is often focally infiltrated by mononuclear cells; there may be patchy fibrosis.

Information about the prognosis is scanty and incomplete but it is probably similar to that for type III cryoglobulinaemia as a whole, with approximately 75% alive 10 years after the onset of signs and symptoms of renal involvement. Approximately 15% develop acute or chronic renal failure.[108] There is a high prevalence of hypertension among the survivors.

Polyarteritis

Persistent hepatitis B antigenaemia is sometimes associated with polyarteritis, particularly classical polyarteritis (see p. 267). In 1974 it was reported that HBsAg had been found in the sera of 55%

of a series of patients with polyarteritis.[109] The incidence of antigenaemia in subsequent studies has been much lower – in the region of 5%,[110,111] and in a longitudinal investigation of haemodialysed patients who were chronic carriers of HBsAg, polyarteritis developed in 1.2% whereas no cases occurred among similarly dialysed patients who were not carriers.[112] There is also some evidence that the incidence of polyarteritis is higher in populations with many hepatitis B carriers. A study of Eskimos living in south-west Alaska, where the prevalence of hepatitis B infection in some villages is as high as 73%, showed that the apparent incidence of polyarteritis was 150 cases per million which is approximately 75 times the estimated incidence in Michigan, where the prevalence of hepatitis B infection is low.[113]

In some patients HBsAg has been demonstrated in circulating immune complexes and in the vascular lesions[114] but the simultaneous presence of antibodies to HBsAg has not been shown in vessel walls. There is a lack of firm evidence that the circulating immune complexes are implicated in the pathogenesis of the vascular lesions.

The renal vessels are very commonly involved in hepatitis-B-virus-associated classical polyarteritis and the glomerular capillaries in hepatitis-B-associated microscopic polyarteritis. The morphological changes do not differ from those seen in other cases of polyarteritis (see p. 267).

HUMAN IMMUNODEFICIENCY VIRUS INFECTION

Increasing numbers of people throughout the world are becoming infected with the human immunodeficiency virus (HIV); it is believed that most of those infected will eventually develop the acquired immune deficiency syndrome (AIDS).[115] Among the patients with AIDS admitted to hospital there is a high incidence of renal disease. For example, of 182 patients with AIDS treated during the period 1984–88 at a hospital serving the South Bronx region of New York City, USA, 46% were found to have proteinuria, 15% had acute renal failure and 1% were on haemodialysis;[116] in Miami, USA, during the period 1982–87 an average of 6% per year of new patients with AIDS was referred for a nephrological opinion on admission.[117]

The commonest renal lesions associated with infection by HIV type 1 (HIV-1) are focal segmental glomerulosclerosis, glomerulonephritis, acute tubular necrosis and interstitial nephritis.[118] The haemolytic uraemic syndrome (see p. 281) and nephrocalcinosis (see p. 544) may also occur.

Focal segmental glomerulosclerosis

Focal segmental glomerulosclerosis is the most frequent glomerular lesion encountered in patients with HIV infection whose kidneys are either biopsied or examined at autopsy.[116,117,119,120,121] It is much more prevalent in blacks and hispanics than in whites and it is severest in blacks.[122,123]

Clinical features

HIV-associated focal segmental glomerulosclerosis is manifested clinically by proteinuria which is almost always greater than 2 g/24 hours and is often sufficient to cause the nephrotic syndrome. The blood pressure remains normal. Some degree of renal insufficiency is common; it often rapidly worsens. Ultrasonography shows the kidneys to be normal in size or enlarged.

Renal changes

The lesions are in general the same as those in idiopathic focal segmental glomerulosclerosis (Fig. 11.19; see p. 205). The main difference is that in the form of the disease associated with HIV infection there are abundant *tubuloreticular inclusions*[124,125] (see p. 232) in the endothelial cells of the glomerular capillaries (Fig. 11.20) and, less frequently, of peritubular capillaries and of arterioles and arteries. Occasionally tubuloreticular inclusions are also present in the cytoplasm of mesangial cells, interstitial cells and lymphocytes.[126] Other ultrastructural changes such as *cylindrical confronting cisternae* (concentrically arranged cisternae with electron-dense material interposed between the inner lamellae, Fig. 11.21),[125,126] particles resembling viruses and intranuclear inclusions are also sometimes present.[116,126] Another, less specific, difference

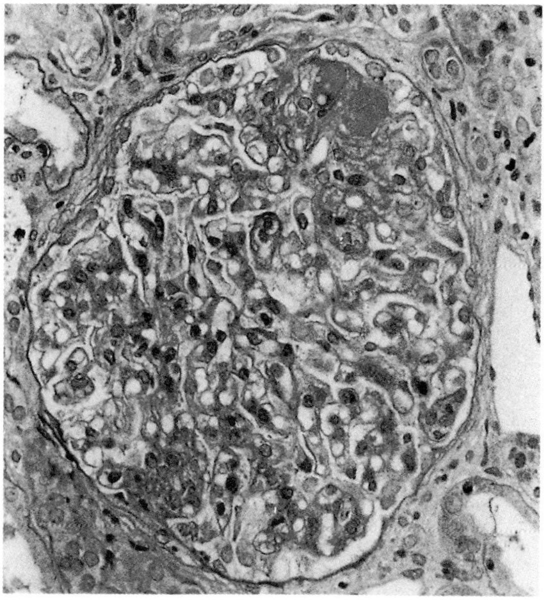

from idiopathic focal segmental glomerulosclerosis is that in the AIDS-associated type the tubular damage is often remarkably severe.

Differential diagnosis

The only feature distinguishing HIV-associated focal segmental glomerulosclerosis from most other forms of focal segmental glomerulosclerosis (see p. 205) is the abundance of tubuloreticular and virus-like inclusions in the endothelial cells. Tubuloreticular inclusions occur in tiny numbers in a variety of diseases but the only other condition in which they are at all common is lupus nephritis (see p. 232).

Fig. 11.19 Human immunodeficiency virus infection. Glomerulus showing segmental sclerosis.
Periodic acid-Schiff × 410

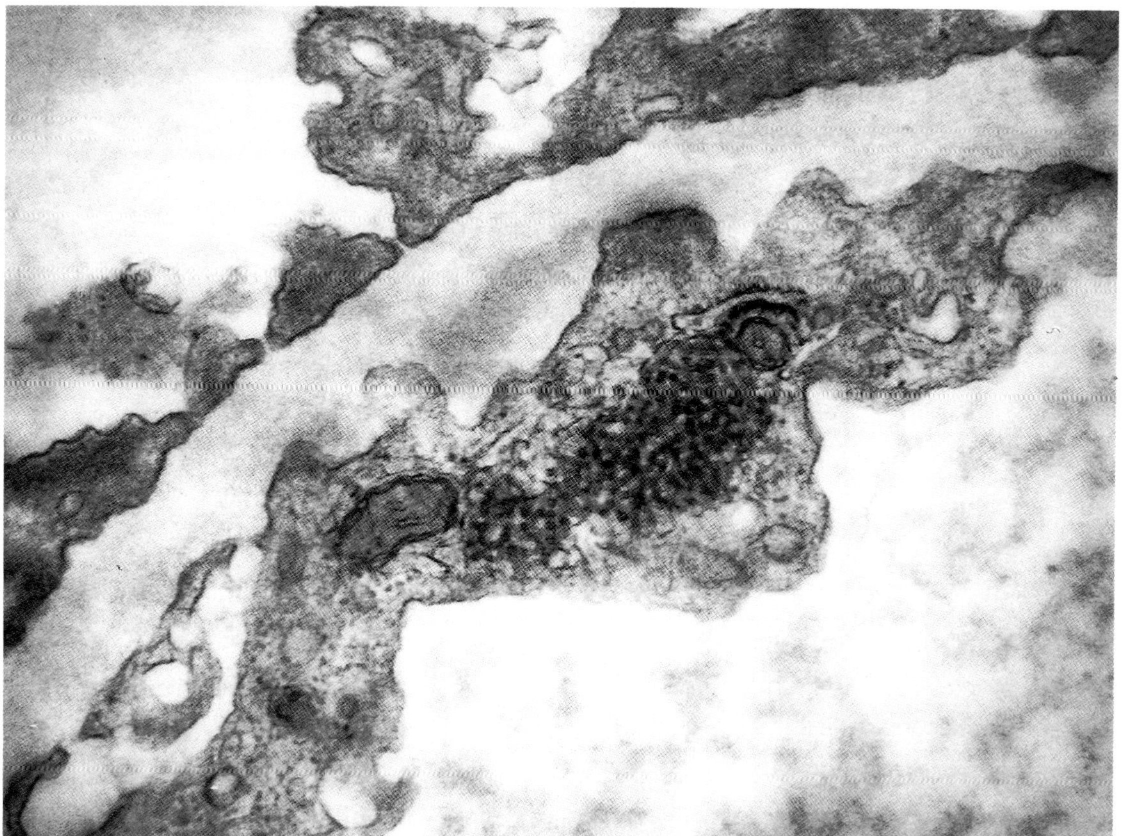

Fig. 11.20 Human immunodeficiency virus infection. Electron micrograph of glomerular capillary endothelial cell. There are tubuloreticular inclusions in the cytoplasm.
x 50 800

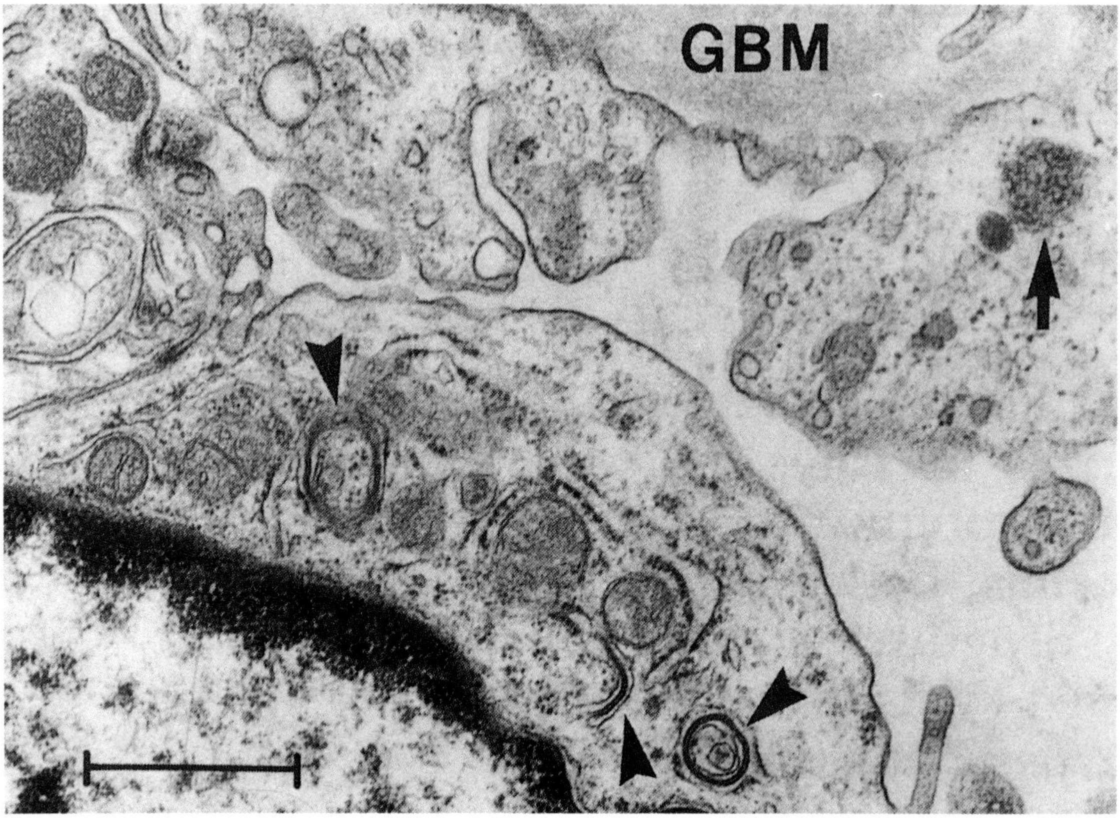

Fig. 11.21 Human immunodeficiency virus infection. Electron micrograph of glomerular capillary endothelial cell. There are cylindrical confronting cisternae in the cytoplasm (arrowheads) and a tubuloreticular inclusion (arrow). GBM, glomerular capillary basement membrane.
× 20 000
Reproduced by permission from: Chander P, Agarwall A, Soni A, Kim K, Tresser G. Hum Pathol 1988;19:1060 (Fig. 1).

Lupus-associated focal segmental glomerulosclerosis is rare and can usually be excluded on the serological findings and on the presence of frequent mesangial and subendothelial immune deposits which are not a feature of HIV-associated focal segmental glomerulosclerosis (see p. 228).

Prognosis

HIV-associated focal segmental glomerulosclerosis is progressive but the rate of progression is variable. In one series approximately 3% rapidly advanced to end stage renal failure within 7 weeks to 8 months after focal segmental glomerulosclerosis was recognized;[116] in another series approximately 82% reached this stage within 8–16 weeks.[120] These patients do badly on haemodialysis.

Pathogenesis

The pathogenesis is unknown. As certain epitopes on the CD4 molecule are the receptors for the envelope glycoprotein of the human immunodeficiency virus and as infection by the latter occurs in cells that express this molecule, it has been suggested that the virus may directly invade the glomerular mesangial cells which also express CD4.[127] However, HIV antigens have not generally been demonstrated in the kidneys, and viral cultures from renal tissue and reverse transcriptase activity have been negative.[116] The exception is a claim to have shown proviral HIV

DNA in tubular and glomerular epithelial cells in renal tissue from HIV-1-infected patients.[128]

Glomerulonephritis

Diffuse mesangial proliferative glomerulonephritis

Diffuse mesangial proliferative glomerulonephritis (see p. 153) occurs in about 8% of patients with AIDS.[123] Mesangial electron-dense deposits are commonly present.

Other forms of glomerulonephritis

Rarely, other forms of glomerulonephritis occur. Patients with minimal change disease, membranous glomerulonephritis, mesangiocapillary glomerulonephritis type III and focal proliferative glomerulonephritis have been recorded.

Acute tubular necrosis

Infections are a prominent feature of AIDS; some are accompanied by episodes of hypotension, hypoxia and dehydration which may lead to acute tubular necrosis. Nephrotoxic drugs used in the treatment of patients with AIDS and radiocontrast agents may also occasionally cause acute tubular necrosis.[129] The morphological changes do not differ from those seen in acute tubular necrosis occurring in other conditions (see p. 491). The prognosis is poor: acute renal failure in patients already critically ill often results in death.

Interstitial nephritis

Patients with AIDS receive many drugs and some of these may cause an allergic interstitial nephritis (see p. 454). Examples of such drugs are trimethoprim, sulphamethoxazole, amphotericin and pentamidine.

Other lesions[121]

A variety of infectious agents may be encountered singly or in combination in the kidneys of patients with AIDS; these include atypical mycobacteria (see p. 386), candida (see p. 405), cryptococcus (see p. 411), nocardia (see p. 415), histoplasma (see p. 412), aspergillus (see p. 408) and cytomegalovirus (see p. 402). The organisms may or may not excite an inflammatory response.

Focal tubular and interstitial calcification may occur; this is usually related to amphotericin toxicity.

Rarely, Kaposi's sarcoma or lymphomas are found in the kidneys. A renal adenocarcinoma has been recorded in one patient.[115]

HANTAVIRUS INFECTION

The genus *Hantavirus*, a subgroup of the Bunyaviridae family, contains several spherical RNA viruses. They are present in healthy rodent and insectivore carriers throughout Europe, Asia and North and South America.[130] The viruses are transmitted to man by excretions and aerosols and are responsible for a large group of endemic, epidemic and sporadic human diseases, collectively known as *haemorrhagic fever with renal syndrome*.[131] Hantavirus can also be transmitted by laboratory rats. Outbreaks of Hantavirus disease have occurred in several countries in laboratory staff handling rats that were subsequently found to be infected. The four major serotypes of Hantavirus are the Hantaan virus, the Seoul virus, the Puumala virus and the Prospect Hill virus.

Hantaan and Seoul virus infections

The Hantaan and Seoul viruses cause epidemic disease in Asia (Korea, Japan, China and eastern parts of the USSR). Epidemic haemorrhagic fever with renal syndrome due to the Hantaan virus attracted great attention during the Korean war and is still a major health problem, particularly in China where 103 778 cases were admitted to hospital in 1985.[130] The Hantaan virus is usually responsible for rural epidemics; urban epidemics are more frequently caused by the Seoul virus.

The disease caused by the Hantaan virus in particular is often severe and is characterized by widespread haemorrhages, shock and renal failure; the mortality rate is about 5%.

The kidneys in the severe cases show acute

tubular necrosis (see p. 491) and focal haemorrhages.[132] In the mild and moderate cases there is an acute tubulointerstitial nephritis similar to that which occurs after infection with the Puumala virus.

Puumala virus infection

The Puumala virus is found predominantly in Europe and causes a milder disease. This form of haemorrhagic disease with renal syndrome, which is usually sporadic and rarely epidemic, has long been recognized in Scandinavia and eastern Europe but it has in recent years been increasingly observed in Belgium, France, The Netherlands and southern Europe.[133,134] The disease occurs predominantly in young men working in agriculture and forestry; it is most common in January and June, times of the year when the density of the rodent population is highest. The incubation period is usually 12–20 days.

The onset of the disease is characterized by an influenza-like syndrome. After 4–14 days intense loin pain develops which is often accompanied by transient acute renal failure, severe proteinuria and microscopic haematuria. Some patients have, in addition, conjunctival haemorrhage, signs of meningeal irritation and thrombocytopenia. Dialysis is only occasionally needed and the serum creatinine returns to normal 2–6 weeks after the attack. Less than 1% of patients die.[133] The diagnosis is confirmed by the demonstration of rising titres of antibodies to the virus, commencing at about 8 days and reaching a peak at about 3 weeks.

The kidneys are enlarged and show an acute tubulointerstitial nephritis (see p. 438).[133,135] The interstitium is diffusely oedematous and there is a marked, patchy, predominantly mononuclear cellular infiltration affecting particularly the medulla, the superficial cortex and the corticomedullary junction (Fig. 11.22). There are also scattered small foci of interstitial haemorrhages, the peritubular capillaries are congested and there is patchy tubular damage and loss. In a few cases there has been a mild mesangial proliferative glomerulonephritis; in one series this was accompanied by scanty focal and segmental intramembranous and subepithelial deposits of immunoglobulins and C3.[136]

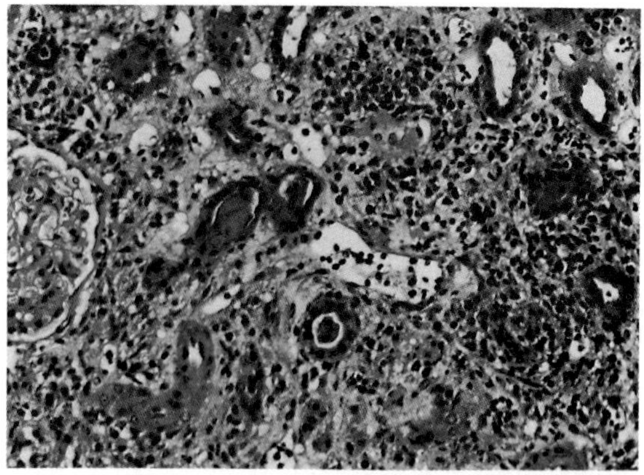

Fig. 11.22 Hantavirus (Puumala serotype) infection. There is interstitial oedema and mononuclear cell infiltration with some tubular loss but normal glomeruli. Haematoxylin-eosin × 250

Prospect Hill virus infection

The Prospect Hill virus occurs in meadow voles in the USA but has not yet been incriminated in human disease.

Pathogenesis

It is not known how the various serotypes of Hantavirus damage the kidney. One hypothesis is that the haemorrhage and oedema are due to a direct viral attack on the vascular endothelial cells and that the interstitial cellular infiltration is the result of an immune response to the organism by the host. So far there has been little evidence to support this proposal. The only claim to have identified viral nucleocapsid-like particles has been in Puumala virus infection and the particles were in the epithelium of the distal tubules not the endothelium.[137]

CYTOMEGALOVIRUS (CMV) INFECTION

The majority of cytomegalovirus (CMV) infections go unnoticed and the normal carrier state is asymptomatic. However, immunosuppression is associated with an increased frequency of clinical disease. Babies in utero, renal transplant recipients and people infected with HIV seem particularly vulnerable.

Renal lesions in congenital CMV disease

Fetal infections are usually the result of a primary maternal CMV infection; a small number are the result of reactivation of infection in a previously immune mother. Infection is most often transplacental, but may be acquired at the time of delivery through contact with an infected birth canal. The incidence of congenital CMV disease has been estimated as 0.4–2.3% of all live births. Renal lesions are common in these cases but produce no clinical symptoms or signs.

Macroscopically the kidneys appear normal. Microscopically there is infection predominantly of the epithelial cells of the distal convoluted tubules and rarely the endothelial cells of the glomeruli.[138] The cells are randomly involved. They are greatly swollen and contain prominent large intranuclear basophilic inclusions that are usually separated from the nuclear membrane by a clear halo (Fig. 11.23). There are often also small basophilic inclusions in the cytoplasm of the infected cells. Electron microscopy shows that the nuclear inclusions contain developing viruses; the intracytoplasmic inclusions contain viral particles arranged in a crystalloid pattern (Fig. 11.24). An interstitial nephritis is common, with focal infiltration of the interstitium by mononuclear cells, with or without small numbers of neutrophil granulocytes. The mononuclear cells are mostly cytotoxic and suppressor CD8+ T lymphocytes and monocytes or natural killer cells.[139] Rarely there is a glomerulonephritis; focal segmental and global necrotizing lesions with and without crescents[140] and various forms of proliferative glomerulonephritis[141] have been recorded.

There is speculation that the interstitial and glomerular lesions are caused by the cytopathic effects of CMV or by CMV/anti-CMV immune complexes but the evidence is equivocal.[142–144]

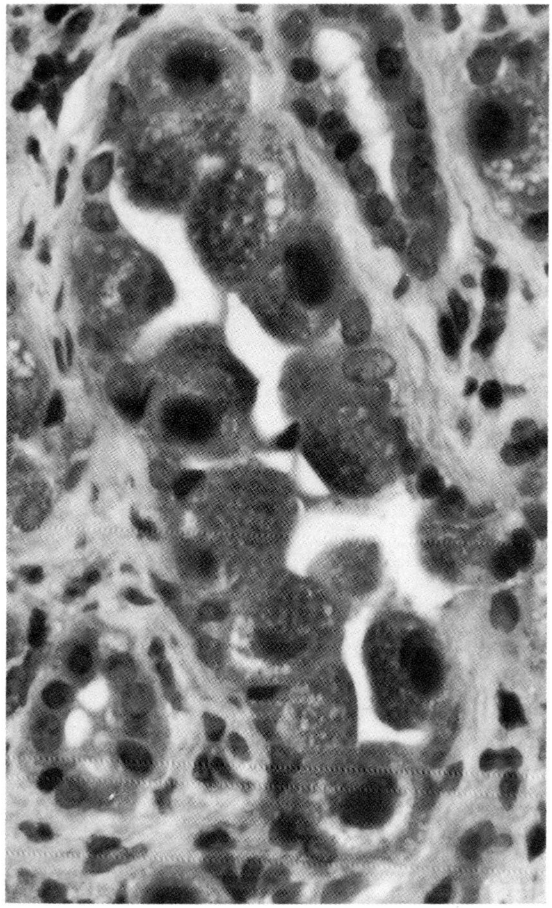

Fig. 11.23 Cytomegalovirus infection. Swollen tubular epithelial cells contain intranuclear inclusions. Haematoxylin-eosin × 900

Lesions in renal allografts

It has been suggested that CMV infection can cause a specific glomerulopathy in renal allografts, and also that it may be associated with an increased incidence of graft rejection. These suggestions are discussed on pages 637, 641 and 653.

Lesions in people infected with HIV

CMV infection occurs frequently in patients infected with HIV. In one series of 50 patients with AIDS who were autopsied 12% had definite CMV inclusions and in another 28% CMV was suspected. CMV infection is often associated with a tubulointerstitial nephritis (see p. 641).[145]

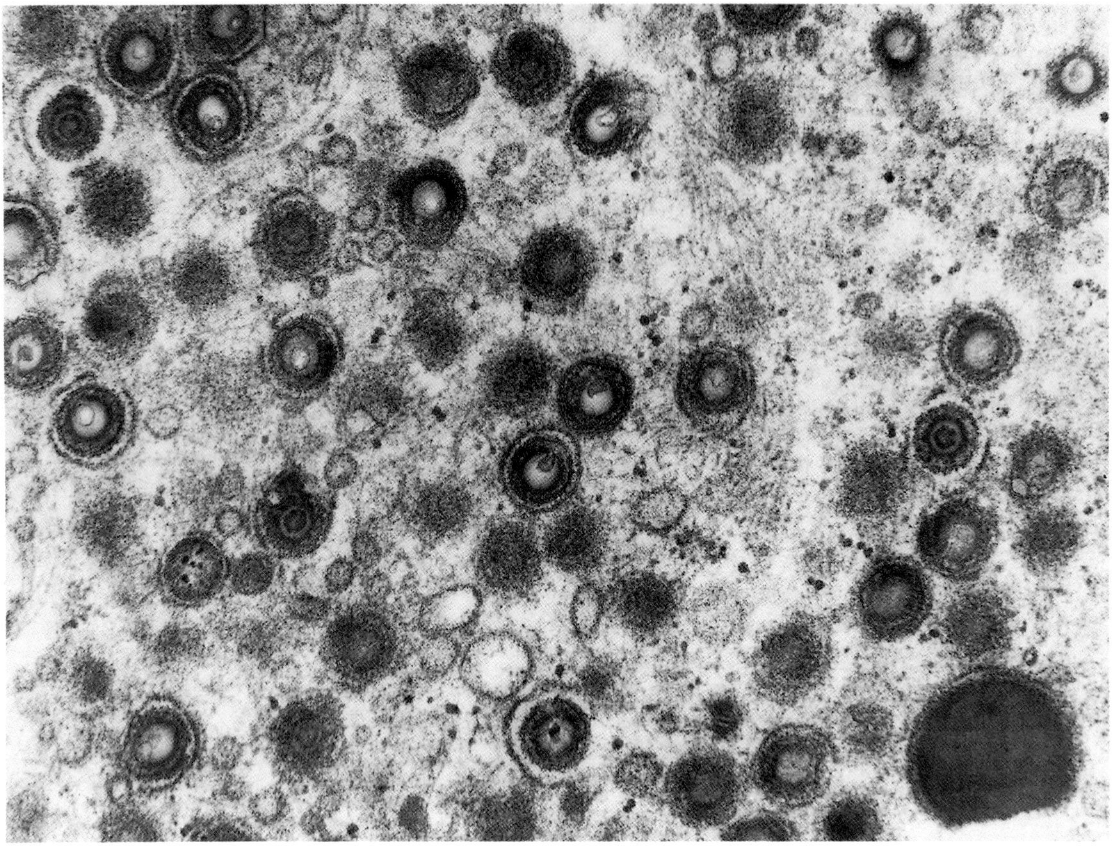

Fig. 11.24 Cytomegalovirus infection. Electron micrograph of tubular epithelial cell showing virions in intracytoplasmic inclusions.
× 80 000

EPSTEIN–BARR (EB) VIRUS INFECTION

In developing countries evidence of infection with Epstein–Barr (EB) virus is present in almost all children by the age of 3 years; acute symptomatic disease is rare. In countries with a higher standard of hygiene infection is delayed until adolescence or early adulthood and causes infectious mononucleosis.

Evidence of renal involvement in infectious mononucleosis is fairly common, with a reported incidence of 5–15% in several large series; it is usually limited to proteinuria and microscopic haematuria but occasionally patients develop gross haematuria, an acute nephritic syndrome or a nephrotic syndrome. Renal failure is a very rare event.[146] The prognosis is excellent, complete resolution being the rule. Only one patient has been recorded as progressing to chronic renal failure.

The usual renal lesion is an acute tubulo-interstitial nephritis (see p. 438) with focal or diffuse mononuclear cell infiltration and marked oedema of the interstitium and scattered foci of tubular damage (Fig. 11.25). The majority of the infiltrating cells are CD8+ suppressor and cytotoxic T lymphocytes.[147] Infrequently there is a mesangial proliferative glomerulonephritis (see p. 153).

The role of the EB virus in the production of these renal lesions is unknown.

OTHER SYSTEMIC VIRAL INFECTIONS

A few cases of glomerulonephritis have been reported following infection with varicella,[148] Coxsackie B,[149] mumps,[150] measles,[151] ECHO 9,[152] Ross river,[153] and dengue haemorrhagic fever

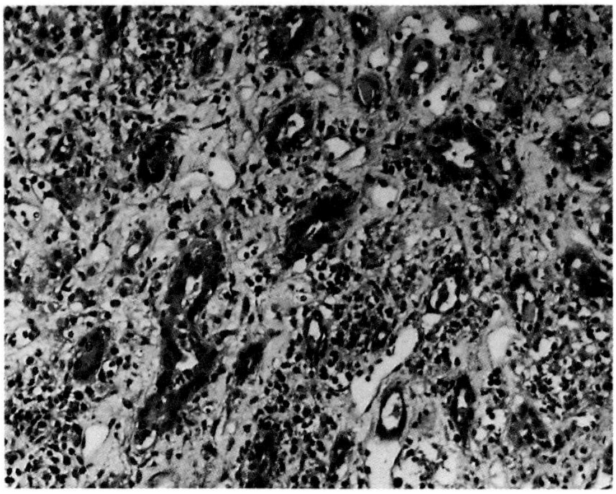

Fig. 11.25 Epstein–Barr virus infection. There is interstitial oedema with mononuclear cell infiltration and a few foci of tubular damage.
Haematoxylin-eosin × 300

viruses;[154] in some of these viral antigens were identified in the glomeruli.

BK polyomavirus has been associated with a chronic tubulointerstitial nephritis.[155]

FUNGAL AND FILAMENTOUS BACTERIAL INFECTIONS

Systemic fungal infections are a major clinical and epidemiological problem; they have assumed particular importance since the introduction of broad spectrum antibiotics, immunosuppressive therapy and the treatment of malignant tumours with cytotoxic drugs, and following the advent of human immunodeficiency virus (HIV) infection.

The kidneys are often involved in systemic mycoses and the possibility that more than one mycotic infection is present in any given case must not be overlooked. Coexistent opportunistic mycoses are common and may be associated with opportunistic bacterial, viral or protozoal infections or even with metazoal infestations.[156]

CANDIDOSIS (CANDIDIASIS)

Candidosis is a primary or secondary opportunistic mucocutaneous or systemic mycotic infection caused by a yeast of the genus *Candida.* It occurs worldwide and is the commonest fungal infection of the kidney.

Candida species are normal commensals of humans and are found on the mucosal surfaces of the mouth, upper respiratory tract, digestive tract and vagina. *Candida albicans* is the species responsible in the majority of cases of renal candidosis; much less frequently *C. tropicalis, C. krusei* and *C. parapsilosis* are the infecting fungi.

Almost all renal candida infections are blood borne and the result of systemic candidosis. They occur when factors are present that impair host resistance and permit invasion of the blood stream by the organism. Such factors include: breaks in the normal skin and mucosal barriers, e.g. burns and gastrointestinal or urological surgery; direct introduction of candida into the blood stream through contaminated intravenous lines, catheters, peritoneal dialysis and cardiac surgery, or the use of contaminated intravenous needles by drug addicts; a lack of granulocytes (the most important line of defence against candida once mucosal penetration has occurred), the result of cytotoxic chemotherapy or in acute leukaemia; defective granulocyte function caused by corticosteroid therapy or inherited disease; local overgrowth and mucosal colonization by candida promoted by broad-spectrum antibiotic therapy; acquired immune deficiency syndrome (AIDS) and other cell-mediated immunodeficiencies; diabetes mellitus; prematurity; and parenteral hyperalimentation.

On rare occasions the candida invades the kidney without evident concomitant invasion of the blood stream. These cases are referred to as primary renal candidosis and are probably the result of ascending infection resulting from vaginal or faecal contamination of the urinary tract. Primary renal candidosis tends to occur in women, in patients with obstruction to the urinary outflow and in those with renal transplants (see p. 662).

Renal candidosis may also develop in the course of candida endocarditis. *C. albicans* is one of the main causes of prosthetic valve infections, very likely gaining entry at the time of heart surgery. Candida endocarditis also occurs in patients with leukaemia and in drug addicts and in such cases is often due to *C. parapsilosis.* Renal infarcts and glomerulonephritis may complicate these forms of fungal endocarditis in the same way as they do bacterial endocarditis (see p. 378).

Dense deposit disease (see p. 179) has been reported in one patient with the candida endocrinopathy syndrome.[157] *C. albicans* antigenic material was detected in the glomeruli. The glomerulonephritis resolved following prolonged antifungal treatment.

Clinical features[158]

Renal involvement in systemic candidosis is often accompanied by a chronic low grade or spiking fever, hypotension, declining renal function, microscopic haematuria, pyuria, proteinuria and flank pain. Renal or ureteric colic can result from the passage of balls of fungus in the urine. The fungal masses may obstruct the ureter and if bilateral or in a transplant can then cause anuria. In neonates the renal signs and symptoms are often particularly marked. Sometimes the renal infection is asymptomatic, the only signs and symptoms being those of a disseminated mycosis, or even non-specific, such as prolonged fever.

Primary renal candidosis is most commonly manifested by the accumulation of fungal material in the renal pelvis producing the various features mentioned above. Clinical indications of renal papillary necrosis (see p. 473) may be present.

Laboratory diagnosis of renal candidosis is very difficult because species of candida are part of the normal human microflora and a positive urine culture is often diagnostically inconclusive. However, recovery of the fungus from the urine together with a positive blood culture is very suggestive of disseminated candidosis and involvement of the kidneys; but blood cultures are positive in only 40–50% of the patients and making the diagnosis is often difficult. No reliable serological diagnostic test is currently available. The only conclusive evidence of renal candidosis is histological demonstration of parenchymal invasion.

Renal changes

In most autopsy series of patients with systemic candidosis, the kidneys are the most frequent site of metastatic candida infection; renal involvement is present in approximately 80% of cases.[159,160]

Gross appearance of the kidneys

There may be multiple white nodules within the cortex and medulla of both kidneys in systemic candidosis; necrosis of the tips of the papillae may also be present. Often there are no grossly recognizable lesions.[159]

Accumulations of white or brown semisolid material in the renal pelvis are more likely in primary renal candidosis although they are occasionally seen in systemic candidosis.[161] The material may be so tightly packed that a pelvicalyceal 'cast' is produced.[162] Obstruction may result in hydronephrosis. Papillary necrosis confined to the distal one-third of the pyramid also occurs in primary renal candidosis.[163]

If there is candida endocarditis petechial haemorrhages or infarcts may be present, as in bacterial endocarditis (see p. 378).

Light microscopy

There may be multiple microabscesses, often involving the glomeruli, with a surrounding neutrophil granulocyte infiltration (Fig. 11.26).

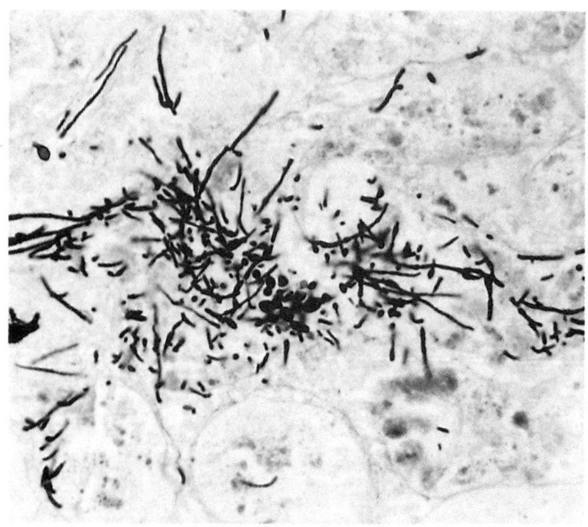

Fig. 11.26 Candidosis. Focus of necrosis containing a mixture of spherical and oval blastoconidia (spores) and pseudohyphae of *Candida albicans*.
Grocott's methenamine silver × 100

In patients with granulocytopenia there are scattered small foci of necrosis and haemorrhage with little or no inflammatory response. Granulomatous inflammation is occasionally seen in those cases which have been treated with antifungal chemotherapy.

The fungi are weakly basophilic and may be difficult to see in sections stained with haematoxylin and eosin; they are readily demonstrated with periodic acid-Schiff or Grocott's methenamine silver stains. They occur as a mixture of spherical to ovoid, non-encapsulated blastoconidia (spores), 2–6μm in diameter, pseudohyphae produced by the budding of greatly elongated yeasts, and occasional true hyphae (Fig. 11.27). The hyphae are septate filaments, measure from 3–5μm in diameter and are not constricted at their point of origin from the yeast surface; the pseudohyphae are constricted at the origin of each elongated yeast and resemble a string of linked sausages.

Mycotic emboli may occur in glomerular and peritubular capillaries. Compact, radiating microcolonies of candida are found in the interstitium and tubules. Hyphae and pseudohyphae often invade arteriolar and arterial walls. The white or brown semisolid material in the pelvis consists of masses of proliferating candida mycelium containing haphazardly arranged hyphae, pseudohyphae and blastoconidia, forming the so-called 'fungus balls'. Necrotic papillae contain masses of fungal elements.

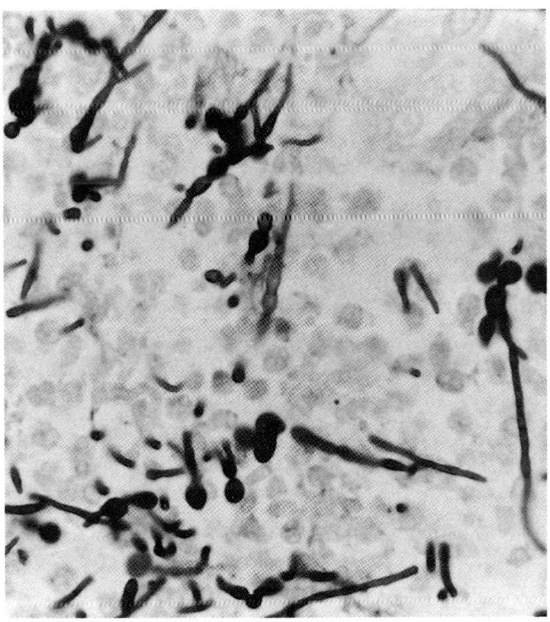

Fig. 11.27 Candidosis. Spherical and oval blastoconidia and narrow frequently constricted pseudohyphae of *Candida albicans* in renal abscess.
Grocott's methenamine silver × 450

Cases with candida endocarditis may show in addition glomerular lesions similar to those encountered in bacterial endocarditis (see p. 378).

Immunofluorescence/immunoperoxidase microscopy

Specific conjugated antibody is available for identifying a fungus in tissue sections as a candida;[164] there are no antisera that will determine the particular species of candida in a section.

Differential diagnosis

The various species of candida can easily be distinguished from most other fungi in sections of the kidney if both yeast-like cells, 2–6μm in diameter, and pseudohyphae and hyphae are present. *Sporothrix schenckii, Blastomyces dermatitidis, Cryptococcus neoformans* and *Histoplasma capsulatum* are yeast-like in tissue but rarely produce filamentous forms. *Torulopsis glabrata* is yeast-like and never produces mycelial elements. Conversely, mycelial pathogens belonging to the genera *Aspergillus, Fusarium* and *Pseudallescheria* do not produce yeast forms in tissues: the only species that produces both yeast-like cells and mycelia is *Trichosporon* and the yeast forms of this fungus are larger and more pleomorphic then those of *Candida* and often accompanied by rectangular arthroconidia.

It is imperative to submit fresh tissue for cultural confirmation of the histological diagnosis and for identification of the species by the organism's patterns of carbohydrate fermentation and assimilation.[165]

Prognosis

Disseminated candidosis is normally progressive and fatal unless treated. Even with intensive treatment with appropriate antifungal drugs the mortality remains high. Survival depends on early diagnosis and treatment, and the control or reversal of the underlying factors that have permitted fungal invasion. Intravenous lines and catheters can often be removed but it is frequently very difficult to reverse conditions such as granulocytopenia.

Primary renal candidosis often responds well to appropriate antifungal treatment if the source of the candida and any predisposing factors such as urinary tract obstruction can be eliminated. Any obstructing fungal masses will have to be removed mechanically if treatment is to succeed.

Untreated candida endocarditis is uniformly fatal. The relapse rate is high even after antifungal therapy.

Pathogenesis

In disseminated candidosis the fungus gains access to the kidneys through the blood. Studies in animals have shown that as the blastoconidia circulate through the renal vasculature they attach themselves to the glomerular and peritubular capillary endothelium by surface fibrils and penetrate through the vessel walls into the renal parenchyma and tubules by germination or the formation of pseudohyphae.[166] This is followed by a neutrophil granulocyte response and the production of microabscesses. If the patient is granulocytopenic focal necrosis of tubules and interstitium may be due to the release of enzymes by the fungus; phospholipase, acid hydrolases and glucosidase have been demonstrated at the tips of the germ tubes put out by germinating blastoconidia.[166] After entering the tubules aggregates of fungal blastoconidia, hyphae and pseudohyphae are excreted into the collecting system and either attach to the papillae, become trapped in the renal pelvis or are excreted in the urine.[167]

Pathogenic candida species are also able to adhere to and gain a foothold on epithelial surfaces.[168] This may explain how they colonize and infect the lower urinary tract in primary renal candidosis. Their passage into the kidney probably depends upon vesicoureteric and intrarenal reflux, as in other forms of pyelonephritis (see p. 436).

ASPERGILLOSIS

Aspergillus species are second only to candida as agents of opportunistic fungal infections in immunosuppressed and debilitated hosts. They are ubiquitous within the environment and their conidia (asexual spores) are constantly present in the air. Although there are hundreds of species only a few cause human disease. The commonest pathogenic species is *A. fumigatus* but *A. flavus*, *A. niger* and *A. glaucus* are sometimes involved.

The aspergilli cause several different diseases; of these invasive necrotizing pneumonia is becoming increasingly common and is often accompanied by widespread haematogenous dissemination with involvement of the kidneys.[169] The factors predisposing to disseminated aspergillosis are similar to those that lead to disseminated candidosis (see p. 405). Sometimes an ascending aspergillosis involves the bladder, ureters and kidneys.[170] Isolated primary renal infection, producing an aspergillus fungal ball ('aspergilloma') or papillary necrosis, is rare.[171–173] Crescentic glomerulonephritis (see p. 185) has been recorded in one patient with aspergillosis; *A. fumigatus* antigens were identified in the subendothelial and mesangial immune deposits.[174]

Clinical features

In disseminated aspergillosis respiratory symptoms predominate; involvement of the kidney is usually asymptomatic. There is microscopic haematuria, pyuria and proteinuria in 60–80% of patients. Diagnosis is very difficult. Urine cultures for aspergillus are positive in 25% of the cases; blood cultures are almost always negative and serological tests are unreliable.[169] Biopsy offers the best chance of establishing the diagnosis.

Ascending panurothelial aspergillosis generally presents with the usual signs and symptoms of a urinary tract infection (see p. 434).[170]

Isolated renal infections occur mostly in patients with diabetes mellitus. Flank pain, renal and ureteral colic, dysuria, haematuria and pyuria may be produced. Balls of fungus are sometimes passed in the urine. If obstructive uropathy occurs there may be renal insufficiency.[171–173]

The case of crescentic glomerulonephritis mentioned above was associated with progressive deterioration of renal function.[174]

Renal changes

Disseminated aspergillosis

Approximately 40% of patients who die of disseminated aspergillosis have multiple cortical and medullary abscesses, 1–3 mm in diameter (Fig. 11.28).[169] Infection is usually bilateral but may occasionally be unilateral.[175] Hyphal invasion of arteries and veins is a major feature resulting in thrombosis which leads to infarction and often to papillary necrosis. Unlike in candidosis, large areas of tissue destruction are common. Septate branching hyphae are found within the abscesses and infarcts and in glomerular capillary loops and Bowman's space. The hyphae have a characteristic appearance: they are 3–6 µm wide, uniform, and regularly septate and they have parallel contours. Branches arise at acute angles and the branching is progressive and dichotomous (Fig. 11.29). Living hyphae are basophilic and although visible in haematoxylin and eosin-stained sections are better demonstrated with periodic acid-Schiff or Grocott's methenamine silver stains. The fungus provokes a neutrophil granulocytic response; in patients with granulocytopenia aspergillus is found in areas of necrosis and haemorrhage with minimal mononuclear cell infiltration. In treated cases a chronic granulomatous inflammatory reaction with giant cells may occur.[174]

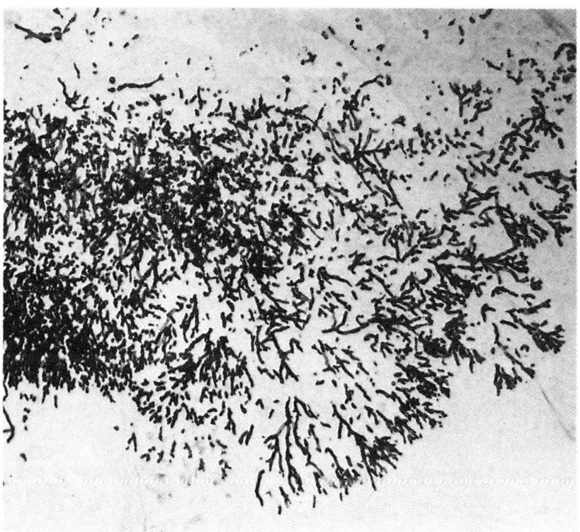

Fig. 11.28 Aspergillosis. Part of a fungal abscess in renal cortex showing typical radial growth pattern. Grocott's methenamine silver × 150

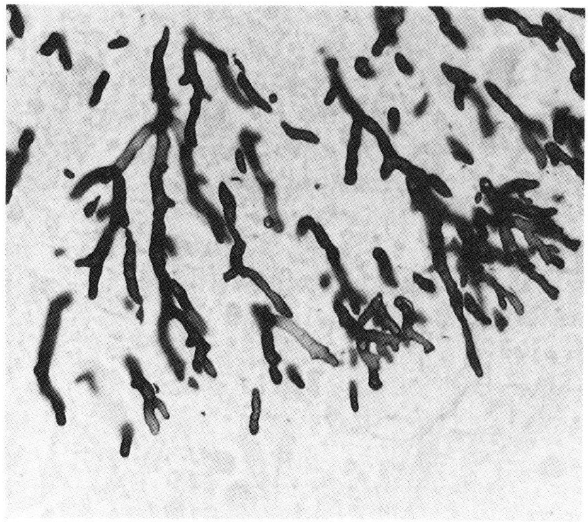

Fig. 11.29 Aspergillosis. Septate branching hyphae in renal abscess. The branching is progressive and dichotomous. Grocott's methenamine silver × 480

Ascending urothelial aspergillosis

The renal pelvis and ureter become almost occluded by debris, fungus and granulation tissue. The bladder is also involved (see p. 713). There is renal papillary necrosis and streaks of fungal inflammation extend into the medulla and cortex.[170]

Isolated renal aspergillosis

Semisolid white or brown masses of mycelium (fungus balls) are present in the renal pelvis and calyces. Fungal material may also be present in the ureter but the bladder is free from infection. The masses consist of tangled hyphae mixed with fibrin and cell debris. There may be hydronephrosis. There is usually no parenchymal or vascular invasion by the fungus.

Differential diagnosis

Aspergillus is easily distinguished histopathologically from candida and trichosporon because the two latter fungi have not only hyphae but also yeast-like cells. However, pathogenic fungi in the genera *Fusarium* and *Pseudallescheria* form branched septate hyphae which may be indistinguishable from those of aspergillus in tissue. For this reason specific conjugated antibody should be applied to the section to positively identify the fungus as aspergillus.[176] Culture of fresh tissue is required in order to determine the species.

Prognosis

More than 70% of patients with disseminated aspergillosis die of the infection. The reason for this poor outlook is that survival is very dependent upon early diagnosis and the reversibility or remission of the underlying disease, conditions that are difficult to satisfy.

The forms of the disease that are confined to the urinary tract usually respond well to a combination of systemic and local antifungal chemotherapy together with surgical treatment if there is obstruction.

MUCORMYCOSIS (ZYGOMYCOSIS)

The term mucormycosis includes all mycotic diseases caused by fungi in the order Mucorales, class Zygomycetes. The Zygomycetes occur worldwide in soil and decaying organic material; the sporadic occurrence of mucormycosis is related mainly to host susceptibility. Disease in humans is caused most commonly by *Rhizopus* species, particularly *R. oryzae*.

Although mucormycosis is the third most common opportunistic mycosis among patients with one or more of the predisposing factors listed under candidosis (see p. 405), disseminated disease is uncommon. The kidneys are involved in approximately 50% of patients who die from disseminated mucormycosis;[177] very rarely, the mycosis is limited solely to one or both kidneys.[178] Mucormycosis only exceptionally occurs in apparently normal people.

Clinical features

Patients usually have persistent fever and those with disseminated disease may have signs and symptoms referable to the primary site of infection. The renal mycosis may be asymptomatic, but often there is flank pain, dysuria and gross haematuria as the result of infarction; pyuria and microscopic haematuria are usual and there may be renal insufficiency.[178,179] Radiology and angiography frequently reveal filling defects, avascular areas and obstruction to arteries.

Renal changes

Thrombosis of various sized branches of the renal artery and sometimes of the main vessel itself is found in almost all cases.[177,178] The thromboses may be unilateral or bilateral and are associated with infarcts of different sizes. Papillary necrosis is also common.

Microscopically, hyphae are scattered throughout the infarcts (Fig. 11.30) and are present within the walls of blood vessels and in thrombi.[175,178,180] They are also present in tubules, glomeruli and partly occluded blood vessels. The infarcts and collections of hyphae are surrounded by a prominent neutrophil granulocyte infiltrate together with mononuclear cells and multinucleate giant cells.

The branching hyphae are broad (10–25 μm in width), ribbon-like, thin-walled, irregular in diameter and usually appear devoid of septa (although rare true septa may be seen after prolonged searching). Care is needed to avoid mistaking artefactual folds in the hyphae for septa. Staining with haematoxylin and eosin demonstrates the hyphae adequately. Occasionally thick-walled, densely stained, spherical chlamydoconidia are found.[181]

Differential diagnosis

The hyphae of *Aspergillus* species can be distinguished from those of the zygomycetes of mucormycosis because they are regularly septate, have an orderly, progressive, dichotomous pattern of branching and are narrower. Specific conjugated antisera are available that enable the

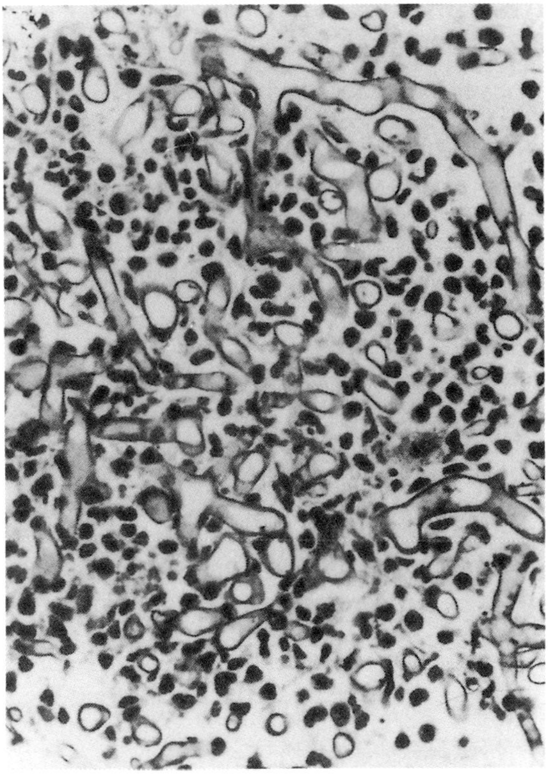

Fig. 11.30 Mucormycosis. Broad, pleomorphic, thin-walled, irregularly branching hyphae adjacent to an infarct. The hyphae lack septa and when cut across appear oval or round. There is a cellular infiltrate.
Grocott's methenamine silver/haematoxylin-eosin × 300
Reproduced by permission from: Chandler FW, Watts JC. in: Dail DH, Hammar SP (eds) Pulmonary pathology. New York: Springer, 1988; 189 (Fig. 8.36A)

Rhizopus group of Zygomycetes to be identified with certainty in deparaffinized sections by direct immunofluorescence.

Prognosis

Disseminated. mucormycosis is almost always fatal because the diagnosis is difficult to establish, the underlying disease is so often uncontrollable and the effectiveness of antifungal drugs is limited by poor penetration into infarcted tissue.

Disease confined to the kidney has been successfully treated by nephrectomy and amphotericin.[182]

CRYPTOCOCCOSIS

Cryptococcosis is a systemic infection caused by a yeast-like organism, *Cryptococcus neoformans*. The fungus is a ubiquitous saprophyte of soil, especially soil contaminated with pigeon or other bird droppings. Although *C. neoformans* is particularly pathogenic, few people develop clinically apparent disease after contact with the yeast. Of those who become ill most have defective cellular immunity or one of the severe underlying diseases listed on page 405. The disease appears to be more prevalent in the USA and Australia than in Africa, Asia and Europe. The organism almost always gains entry to the body through the lungs and from there may spread via the blood stream to affect the brain and meninges. The kidneys are also commonly involved; in an autopsy series the kidneys were infected in 47%.[183]

Clinical features

Renal involvement is usually asymptomatic but there may be pyuria, haematuria and occasionally renal insufficiency. Cryptococci are present in the urine in approximately 40% of patients.[183] The latex agglutination test for capsular polysaccharide antigen is the best method for serological diagnosis.

Renal changes

Gross appearance of the kidneys

There may be scattered small abscesses in the cortex and medulla, with or without papillary necrosis.[184] Often the kidneys appear normal.

Light microscopy

In approximately a quarter of the cases there is extensive focal necrosis of the renal parenchyma producing cyst-like spaces containing numerous organisms. In the other cases cryptococci fill and distend glomerular capillary loops (Fig. 11.31). The organisms are also seen in tubular lumens.

In sections stained with haematoxylin and eosin cryptococci appear as pleomorphic, lightly

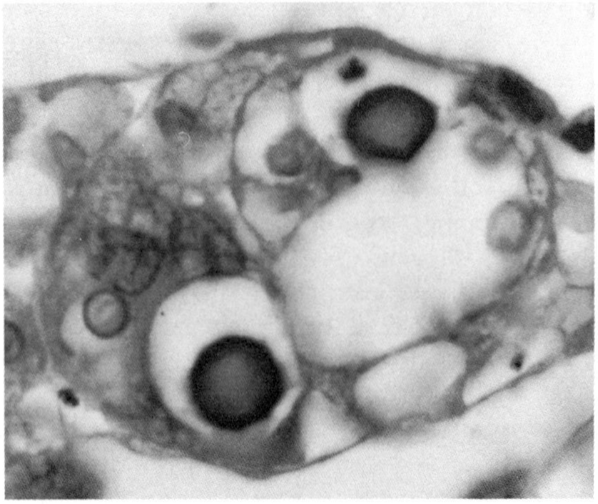

Fig. 11.31 Cryptococcosis. Two cryptococci in interstitium. The eosinophilic fungi are surrounded by wide clear spaces that represent their unstained capsules. Haematoxylin-eosin × 600

eosinophilic, yeast-like cells 2–20 μm in diameter, surrounded by wide clear spaces that represent their unstained capsules. When the capsules are typical they stain with mucin stains such as mucicarmine; the stained capsule often has a spinous appearance because of irregular shrinkage during processing. The capsules are poorly developed in some strains of *C. neoformans*; attention has been drawn to the occurrence of these capsule-deficient cryptococci in some patients with acquired immune deficiency syndrome (AIDS) but they also occur under other circumstances.[185] The organisms are easily demonstrated by either periodic acid-Schiff or Grocott's silver methenamine stains.

There is often a minimal inflammatory response with scattered mononuclear cells. Occasionally an intense granulomatous reaction has been described.[175,183]

Immunofluorescence/immunoperoxidase microscopy

The identity of the organism can be confirmed in deparaffinized sections by direct immunofluorescence using a specific antibody directed against the capsular polysaccharide of *C. neoformans*.[186]

Differential diagnosis

Cryptococcus species are the only pathogenic fungi that produce mucinous capsular material; a positive capsular stain is therefore diagnostic. Capsule-deficient strains can be easily confused with *Histoplasma capsulatum* var. *capsulatum*: direct immunofluorescence can be used to make the distinction. The histological diagnosis should be confirmed by isolating and identifying *C. neoformans* in culture.

Prognosis

In most cases of disseminated infection with renal involvement the course is fulminant and is almost always fatal unless promptly treated with a combination of appropriate antifungal drugs. Even with treatment the prognosis in such cases is poor; next to candidosis, cryptococcosis is the most frequent cause of mycotic deaths in the USA.

Pathogenesis

Cryptococci in the blood lodge within glomeruli. Sometimes this is followed by tissue destruction which allows the fungus to enter the tubules and descend to the papillae.[184] The inflammatory response is often minimal because of defects in the patient's cell-mediated immunity.

OTHER SYSTEMIC FUNGAL INFECTIONS

Histoplasmosis

Histoplasmosis occurs in many parts of the world. It is usually a self-limiting infection and it is highly endemic in the Mississippi and Ohio River valleys in the USA, and in Guatemala, Mexico, Peru and Venezuela. Indigenous histoplasmosis is rare in Europe. Haematogenous dissemination of *Histoplasma capsulatum* var. *capsulatum* from a primary pulmonary focus occurs in approximately 5% of patients with this disease. The immunocompromised, with defective cell-mediated immunity, are particularly at risk of developing generalized infection: histoplasmosis is a major opportunistic infection in patients with the acquired immune deficiency syndrome (AIDS) residing in endemic areas.[187] The disseminated disease is the third most common cause of mycotic deaths in the USA, after candidosis and cryptococcosis. The frequency of involvement of the kidneys at autopsy in these cases has been reported as 11–40%.[188] The renal disease is usually clinically inapparent.

Microscopically there are often small groups of yeast-laden macrophages in glomerular capillary lumens. Less frequently there are granulomas with or without central necrosis and giant cells. In about 10% of cases sheets of macrophages filled with histoplasmas replace the normal renal parenchyma. In some immunodeficient patients the kidneys contain huge numbers of organisms with little or no host response.

The yeast-like cells of *H. capsulatum* var. *capsulatum* are uniform, spherical or oval, 2–4 μm in diameter, have single buds, and are often clustered within macrophages (Fig. 11.32). In sections stained with haematoxylin and eosin the basophilic cytoplasm is retracted from the cell wall creating a false impression of an unstained capsule. Periodic acid-Schiff and Grocott's silver methenamine stains do not give this effect.

The organism has to be differentiated in tissue sections from capsule-deficient cells of *Cryptococcus neoformans*, microforms of *Blastomyces dermatitidis* and yeast forms of *Torulopsis glabrata*: usually a few of the cryptococci will have some mucin-staining capsular material; *B. dermatitidis* cells are multinucleate, have thick double-contoured walls and bud by a broad base; and *Torulopsis* stains entirely with haematoxylin and eosin and does not have a halo. When these differentiating features are equivocal, direct immunofluorescence on a deparaffinized section, using a conjugate directed against *H. capsulatum* cell wall antigen, should be used to confirm the diagnosis.[186] An immunoperoxidase method for use on sections has also been described.[189] Culture will be needed to establish the variety of the particular *Histoplasma capsulatum*.

Without treatment the disseminated disease is almost always fatal. Treatment with amphotericin is reliably effective and the prognosis is greatly improved;[188] in one series the mortality in the treated group was only 7% one year after the onset of the disease.[190]

Blastomycosis

Blastomycosis is endemic in the central and south-eastern parts of the USA; it also occurs

a 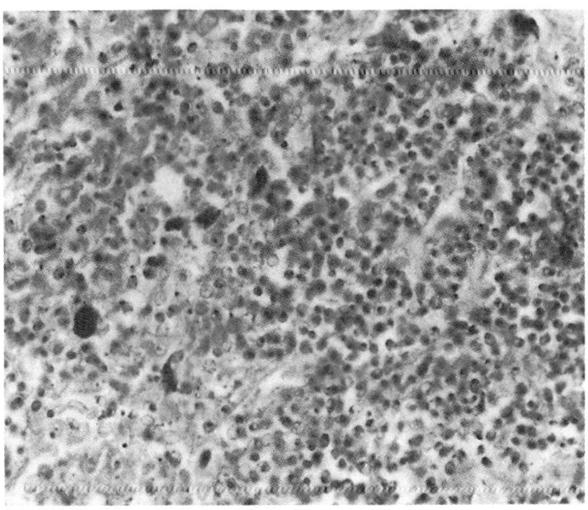 b 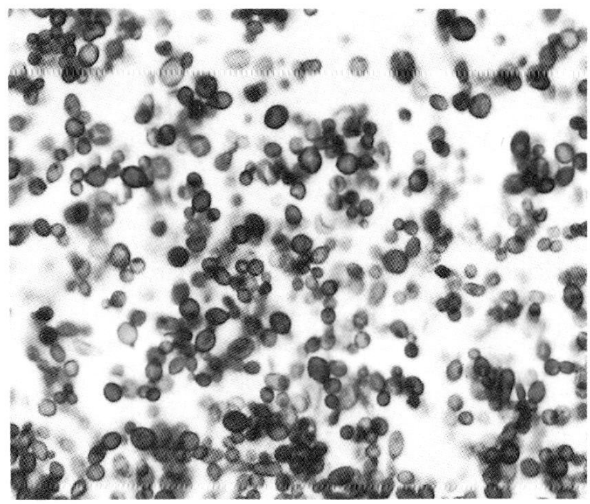

Fig. 11.32 a, b Histoplasmosis. In this immunodeficient patient the renal interstitium contains huge numbers of yeast-like cells of *H.capsulatum* with no host response.
(**a**) Periodic acid-Schiff × 500; (**b**) Grocott's methenamine silver × 760

in eastern Canada, Central America, Africa and the Middle East. *Blastomyces dermatitidis* may disseminate from a primary pulmonary infection via the blood stream to other organs, including the kidneys; this happens most commonly in patients who are immunosuppressed. The disseminated disease is the fifth most common cause of mycotic death in the USA. The kidneys are involved at autopsy in about a quarter of the cases.[191] Renal disease is usually asymptomatic, but there may be flank pain, renal insufficiency and perinephric abscesses with discharging sinuses.

Microscopically, there is usually a granulomatous inflammation with or without giant cells and necrosis and areas of suppuration. The changes may resemble those seen in chronic active tuberculosis (see p. 384). *B. dermatitidis* is present in both the suppurative and the granulomatous areas.

The yeast-like cells are spherical or oval, 8–15 μm in diameter and multinucleate; they have thick, refractile walls with double contours and single, broad-based buds (Fig. 11.33). Occasionally the cells are very small (2–4 μm).

The broad-based attachment of buds to their parent cells is diagnostic and distinguishes the microforms of *B. dermatitidis* from *H. capsulatum* var. *capsulatum*. If in doubt, direct immunofluorescence using a specific conjugate directed against polysaccharide antigens in the wall of the fungus will identify *B. dermatitidis* in deparaffinized tissue sections.[186]

Patients with disseminated disease have a poor prognosis; even with antifungal therapy the outlook is not good.

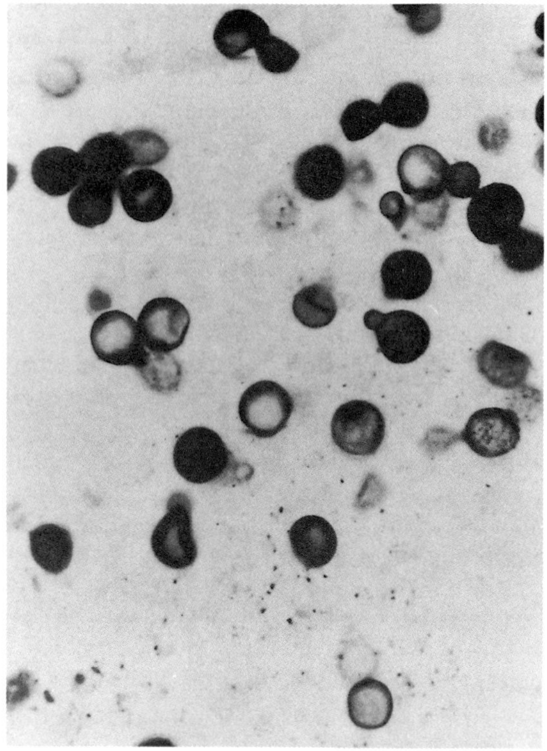

Fig. 11.33 Blastomycosis. Spherical cells of *Blastomyces dermatitidis* in area of suppurative and granulomatous inflammation. The broad-based attachment of buds to their parent cells is diagnostic.
Grocott's methenamine silver × 780
Reproduced by permission from: Chandler FW, Watts JC. in: Dail DH, Hammar SP (eds) Pulmonary pathology. New York: Springer, 1988: 189 (Fig. 8.12B)

Coccidioidomycosis

Coccidioidomycosis is endemic in the southwestern parts of the USA, Mexico, Guatemala, Honduras, Nicaragua, Venezuela, Argentina, Colombia, Bolivia and Paraguay. A few patients develop disseminated disease from a primary pulmonary infection; blacks, males, pregnant women, infants, the elderly and the immunosuppressed are most susceptible. It is the fourth most common cause of mycotic deaths in the USA. The kidneys are involved in approximately one-third of patients who die of disseminated coccidioidomycosis.

The renal lesions consist of miliary granulomas or abscesses scattered throughout the cortex and medulla. Microscopically the granulomas occur in the interstitium and show central necrosis or suppuration. *Coccidioides immitis* is present within the granulomas. The fungus is readily seen in haematoxylin-and-eosin-stained sections but its morphology is clearer with Grocott's silver methenamine stain. In the kidney *C. immitis* exists in the form of spherules that replicate by endosporulation. Mature spherules are 30–100 μm in diameter with refractile walls 1–2 μm thick. They contain uninucleate endospores 2–5 μm in diameter; these are released following rupture of the spherule. The released endospores then enlarge to become spherules.

Endosporulating mature spherules are diagnostic. Immature spherules are less specific; the diagnosis can be confirmed by immunofluorescence on deparaffinized sections using specific conjugates to the fungal cell wall antigens. The labelled antibodies are not widely available and only constantly stain immature spherules and endospores; the walls of mature spherules often fail to react with the conjugate.[192]

The mortality is high with disseminated coccidioidomycosis even when the patients are treated with antifungal drugs.

Paracoccidioidomycosis

Paracoccidioidomycosis is a chronic infection, usually of the lungs, caused by the fungus *Paracoccidioides brasiliensis*. It is endemic in South America, particularly the tropical and subtropical regions of Brazil, Colombia and Venezuela, where it is the most important mycosis.[193] Dissemination occurs eventually in about 60% of patients; the frequency of renal involvement at autopsy is approximately 15%.[194,195] The disease occurs almost exclusively in men over the age of 30 years, many of whom have occupational contact with soil or vegetation. Renal involvement is asymptomatic.

Miliary granulomas with central suppurative necrosis are distributed throughout the cortex and medulla. The yeast-like cells of *P. brasiliensis* are best stained with Grocott's silver methenamine. They vary greatly in size, and are found within the cytoplasm of macrophages and giant cells and lying free at the periphery of areas of necrosis. Non budding and single budding cells usually predominate.

Confusion with *Histoplasma capsulatum* var. *capsulatum* and other yeast-like fungi in most cases can only be resolved by direct immunofluorescence on deparaffinized sections using a specific antibody.

Torulopsosis

Torulopsosis is a rare opportunistic infection caused by a small yeast-like fungus, *Torulopsis (Candida) glabrata*. The organism is part of the normal microflora of the oropharynx, gastrointestinal tract, skin, urethra and vagina of humans. It also occurs as a saprophyte. Predisposing factors are those listed for candidosis (see p. 405); poorly controlled diabetes mellitus is often present. Because of its very low virulence it is rarely of clinical importance; about half the infections caused by *T. glabrata* are self-limiting, clinically inapparent fungaemias and fungurias, often superimposed on bacterial sepsis. Very occasionally it causes life-threatening renal damage.

Renal changes

The kidneys are involved in approximately 50% of patients with disseminated torulopsosis. In most cases, scattered yeast-like cells 2–5 µm in diameter are seen in glomerular capillary loops, Bowman's spaces and, occasionally, tubules. There is usually no apparent tissue reaction or damage. In the uncommon severe infections there may be an acute pyelonephritis with miliary abscesses and papillary necrosis.[196,197] In contrast to candidosis, fungus balls do not occur because *T. glabrata* does not produce hyphae or pseudohyphae in tissue.

Differential diagnosis

T. glabrata may resemble *Histoplasma capsulatum*, especially when the fungal cells are clustered within macrophages. The differentiation can be made by direct immunofluorescence on tissue sections using specific antibodies. Culture of fresh tissue can also be used to identify the organisms.

Prognosis

The occasional severe renal and disseminated infections are treated with amphotericin. The response largely depends upon the reversibility or otherwise of the underlying predisposing factors.

FILAMENTOUS BACTERIAL INFECTIONS

Nocardiosis

Infection with Actinomycetales of the family *Nocardiaceae* may produce an acute, progressive pneumonia in immunocompromised patients.[198] The organism most commonly involved is *Nocardia asteroides*. Blood spread may occur and can involve almost any organ; renal lesions, however, are rare.

Infection of the kidneys presents clinically in the same way as any other bacterial pyelonephritis (see p. 434). The kidneys typically contain multiple microabscesses. Sometimes there are larger abscesses with sinuses.[199,200] The organisms are diffusely distributed in the inflammatory exudate where they appear as tangled, slender (1 μm in diameter), branched and beaded filaments. They do not stain with haematoxylin and eosin or periodic acid-Schiff and are best demonstrated by Grocott's methenamine silver, extending the staining time to 90 minutes.[201] Although nocardiae are Gram positive, they may be difficult to detect among darkly staining fibrin fibrils. They are also weakly acid fast but will not stain with the standard Ziehl–Neelsen procedure – a modified method such as Fite–Faraco, in which an aqueous solution of a weak acid is used for decolorization, is necessary for success: the results are still inferior to those obtained with methenamine silver.[202]

Specific fluorescent antibody conjugates are not available for identifying the species of nocardia. The organism must be identified by culture of fresh tissue.

Early diagnosis and intensive treatment with anti-nocardial drugs are necessary for recovery from systemic nocardiosis.[203]

Actinomycosis

Actinomycosis is a chronic suppurative infection caused by endogenous Actinomycetales of the family Actinomycetaceae; it does not occur preferentially in immunocompromised patients. The organism most usually seen in humans is *Actinomyces israelii*, a common commensal of the mouth and throat. From a primary focus in the abdomen, infection occasionally spreads locally to a kidney;[204] very rarely the kidneys are involved without evidence of such extension.[205]

Renal lesions may be localized, producing abscesses, sinuses and extensive scarring, or diffuse, producing a suppurative and necrotizing pyelonephritis. Abscesses contain 'sulphur granules', which are clusters of organisms embedded in an amorphous matrix and surrounded by eosinophilic, refractile, club-shaped projections (Splendore–Hoeppli reaction).

Morphologically the Actinomycetaceae closely resemble the Nocardiaceae and cannot reliably be distinguished from them by their staining properties. However, specific fluorescent antibody conjugates are available for identifying *A. israelii* and a few other members of the Actinomycetaceae in deparaffinized sections. If immunofluorescence is negative then culture of fresh tissue is essential to determine the nature of the infection. Sulphur granules are not found in nocardiosis but can occur in botryomycosis.[202] Botryomycosis (see p. 446) can be excluded by demonstrating the actinomycetaceal filaments after staining with methenamine silver.

Large doses of penicillin over a period of many weeks are curative in the majority of patients.

PROTOZOAL INFECTIONS

MALARIA

Malaria, the most important parasitic disease of humans, is caused by a protozoon of the genus *Plasmodium*. Four species of the parasite have humans as their natural vertebrate host. Of these *P. falciparum* and *P. malariae* are associated with clinically significant renal disorders; renal changes in *P. vivax* and *P. ovale* infections are rare and when they occur are mild and non-specific. Renal lesions have not been recorded in the very rare zoonotic infections of patients with primate malarias.

Falciparum malaria

P. falciparum is widely prevalent in many tropical areas of the world, particularly in the highly endemic areas of Africa, New Guinea and Haiti. Imported cases (returning travellers and immigrants) are seen in countries where malaria is not a problem; more than 2000 cases each year of all forms of malaria are reported in Britain with 5–10 deaths. Falciparum malaria produces an acute and potentially fatal illness which may be complicated by acute tubular necrosis (see

p. 491) and a transient mesangial proliferative glomerulonephritis (see p. 153).

Acute tubular necrosis

Acute renal failure occurs in fewer than 1% of cases of falciparum malaria,[206] but it is still one of the commoner complications of the disease. It is found only in those patients who have acute intravascular haemolysis either because of a heavy parasitic infection or because of a congenital deficiency of glucose-6-phosphate dehydrogenase (G6PD) making them susceptible to the antimalarial drugs primaquine and quinine. The renal failure is often accompanied by jaundice.

Damage to the tubules varies in severity.[207] Haemoglobin and sometimes haemosiderin granules are present in the proximal tubular cells; haemoglobin casts are common in the lumens of distal tubules and collecting ducts. These changes are most pronounced in blackwater fever.[208] In severe infections the peritubular capillaries and veins are distended by parasitized erythrocytes, macrophages laden with malarial pigment (haematin), lymphocytes and plasma cells; also there may be fibrin thrombi.

Glomerulonephritis

Mild proteinuria (less than 1 g/24 hours), which disappears in a few weeks, is common. There is usually no oedema or hypertension and renal function is normal. A decrease in serum C3 may occur during the acute phase of the disease. *P. falciparum* antigens, antibodies to these antigens, and immune complexes have all been detected in the circulation.[207]

The commonest renal lesion is a mild mesangial proliferative glomerulonephritis (see p. 153). In addition the glomerular capillaries, particularly in autopsy specimens, often have in their lumens monocytes and macrophages containing malarial pigment; parasitized red cells are rare.[207] Mesangial and capillary wall deposits of IgM and C3 are common. Malarial antigen has been demonstrated in the glomeruli by direct immunofluorescence.[207]

This appears to be an immune-complex-mediated glomerulonephritis, the complexes being either formed in situ or filtered from the circulation. Clinically the disease is mild and transient, the proteinuria and immunological abnormalities disappearing within 4–6 weeks following antimalarial treatment.[207,209]

Quartan malaria

Plasmodium malariae is widespread but often overlooked in tropical Africa, parts of the Indian subcontinent, Burma, Sri Lanka, Malaysia and Indonesia. Although the acute symptoms may be severe the mortality is very low. Patients with *P. malariae* infection do not have a phase in which a proportion of the parasites enter the liver and lie dormant for months or years before starting to divide. There are therefore no late relapses due to parasites emerging from the liver. Nevertheless the infection is chronic and undetected parasitaemia may persist for decades causing recrudescences over very long periods.

Quartan malaria may be associated with a glomerulonephritis which is often progressive.

Clinical features

Some patients with quartan malaria have proteinuria and the nephrotic syndrome.[210] The proteinuria is not selective (see p. 136). Microscopic haematuria is often present.

The frequency with which these signs of a renal disorder occur in people infected with *P. malariae* is not known. However, in certain tropical areas where *P. malariae* is common, the incidence of quartan malaria is much higher in children referred to hospital with the nephrotic syndrome than in comparable groups of non-nephrotic sick children seen in the same hospital and unselected children examined in their villages. For example, in one study in Ibadan, Nigeria, 28% of nephrotic children were infected with *P. malariae* alone and a further 60% had a mixed infection with *P. malariae* and *P. falciparum.* The comparable figures for the control groups were 6% and 15–18%.[211]

In quartan malaria the nephrotic syndrome is found most commonly in children. Studies in

Uganda showed that the average age of patients at the onset of the syndrome was 8 years, which coincided with the peak of *P. malariae* infection in the population.[212] The sex incidence is equal.

Renal function and blood pressure are usually normal in the early stages of the disease; in the later stages renal failure with hypertension is common.[210]

Serology

Antibody to *P. malariae* is present.[212] Soluble antigens of *P. malariae* cannot be detected in the circulation by direct techniques; they have been demonstrated, however, by indirect sensitive radioisotope tracer methods.[213] Serum complement (C3) is usually within the normal range.[214] The presence of serum complexes has been inferred from the detection of immunoconglutinins.[214]

Renal changes

A variety of changes have been detected in renal biopsies from patients with quartan malaria and the nephrotic syndrome.

Thirty-nine such biopsies from Ugandans, examined by light microscopy alone, all showed a proliferative glomerulonephritis which was either diffuse or focal; an unstated proportion of these appeared to be mesangiocapillary glomerulonephritis.[215]

A study of biopsies from 45 Nigerian children revealed a different picture; in this later investigation the material was also examined by electron microscopy and immunofluorescence microscopy. Eighty-four per cent of the kidneys had basically normal glomerular tuft cellularity, thickening of the glomerular capillary walls with double contouring, and increased amounts of mesangial matrix. Lacunae containing electron-dense particles were observed in the basement membranes. In some patients the process was focal and segmental; in others the majority of the glomeruli were involved, the lesions were global, and there were also focal glomerulosclerosis, tubular atrophy and interstitial cellular infiltration. There were coarse or fine granular deposits of IgG, IgM and C3, particularly in the glomerular capillary walls. Because this combination of changes did not match any of the generally recognized morphological patterns of glomerulonephritis (see p. 132), the term 'quartan malarial nephropathy' was coined. *P. malariae* antigen was demonstrated in the glomeruli of approximately a quarter of the patients using immunofluoresence and an anti-*P.-malariae* serum. Malarial antigen was not found in the glomeruli of patients with disease of long duration.[216]

In a third study of 13 nephrotic Nigerian children infected with *P. malariae* the glomeruli in the biopsies were said to show variable endothelial cell proliferation, patchy basement membrane thickening and splitting, and an increase in the amount of mesangial matrix (Fig. 11.34). Granules of immunoglobulin and complement were present along the glomerular capillary walls (Fig. 11.35). The emphasis, however, was laid on the presence of electron-dense deposits on the glomerular capillary basement membranes (Fig. 11.36).[217] Patients with mild symptoms and short duration of the disease had only a few subepithelial deposits; patients with progressive disease had massive thickening of the glomerular capillary basement membranes with many large intramembranous deposits as in stage IV membranous glomerulonephritis (see p. 197).[218]

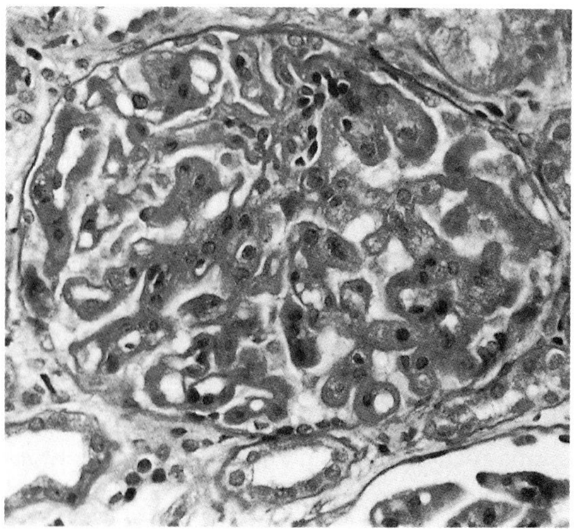

Fig. 11.34 Quartan malaria. The glomerular capillary walls are thickened and have double contours. The amount of mesangial matrix is increased; the number of mesangial cells is slightly raised.
Periodic acid-Schiff × 250

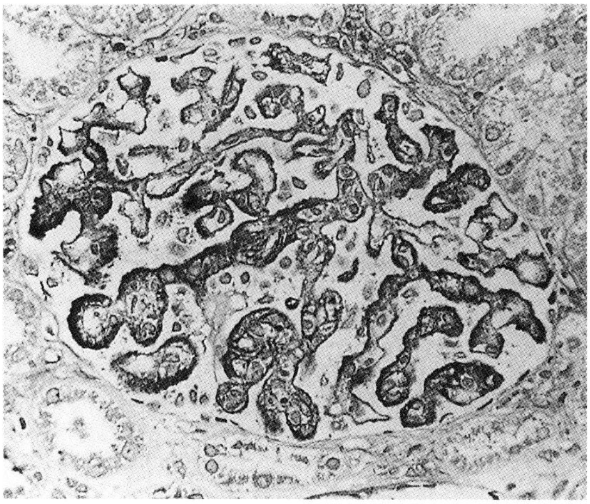

Fig. 11.35 Quartan malaria. Granular deposits of IgG mainly along glomerular capillary walls.
Immunoperoxidase × 250

Subendothelial deposits were found in those specimens with fine granular deposits of immunoglobulin and complement.[213] This investigation, in addition to detecting *P. malariae* antigen in the glomerular capillary walls, also showed that antibodies eluted from renal specimens were directed against *P. malariae*.[218,219]

In the fourth and most recent study quartan malarial nephropathy was defined as variable degrees of focal and segmental glomerulitis, capillary wall thickening and accumulation of PAS positive material in the mesangium. With increased severity the lesion becomes diffuse, with progressive glomerular sclerosis. There is little or no endothelial cell proliferation.[220] Using this histological definition it was decided that 20 of 100 children presenting with the nephrotic syn-

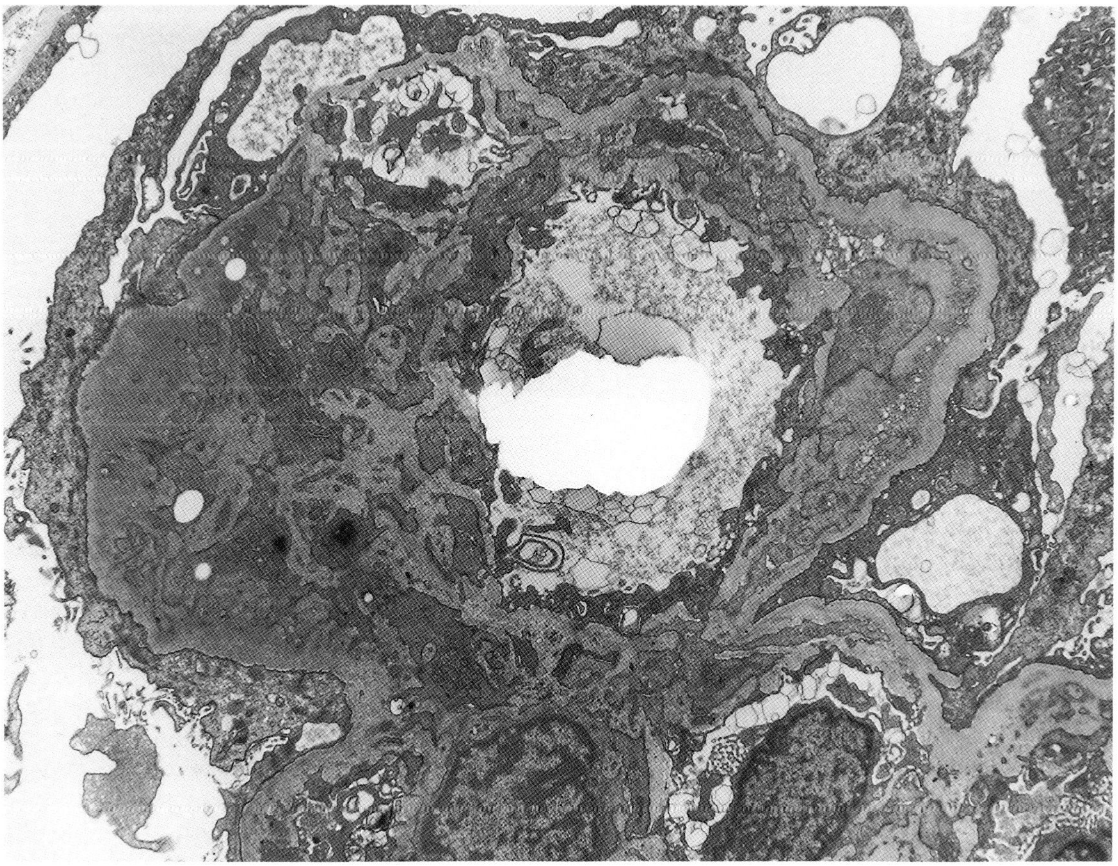

Fig. 11.36 Quartan malaria. Electron micrograph of part of glomerular capillary wall. The basement membrane is thickened and there are subendothelial and intramembranous electron-dense deposits. There is also some mesangial cell interposition.
× 8000

drome in Northern Nigeria had quartan malarial nephropathy; eight of these patients had evidence of *P. malariae* on peripheral blood smears. Of the other 80 children 25 had mesangiocapillary glomerulonephritis, 19 proliferative glomerulonephritis, nine minimal change disease and 19 various other lesions. Twenty three of the 80 children had evidence of *P. malariae* in peripheral blood smears (29%, compared to the 40% of those diagnosed on histological grounds as having quartan malarial nephropathy). *P. malariae* antigen, however, was detected by immunofluorescence in 11 of 15 cases that were diagnosed histologically as quartan malaria compared with eight of 55 patients with other histological diagnoses.[220]

Differential diagnosis

The various glomerular lesions are not specific. Similar patterns have been observed at different stages after other infections and in renal biopsies from children with the nephrotic syndrome who live in the tropics but have no evidence of infection with *P. malariae*.[221]

Prognosis

In most patients renal function slowly deteriorates and hypertension supervenes or worsens. Some patients lose their oedema but continue to have symptomless proteinuria. Remission, either stable or transient, is rare. Antimalarial treatment fails to improve the symptoms or prognosis; the response to steroids is poor.[211,219]

Pathogenesis

The association between *P. malariae* infection and renal disease is not proof of cause and effect. The high incidence of the nephrotic syndrome in areas where quartan malaria is common and its virtual disappearance after a malaria eradication campaign in Guyana are strong circumstantial evidence, and indeed the most convincing evidence, for an aetiological role of *P. malariae*.[222] However, it is worth remembering that a similar decline in tuberculosis and some other diseases was also observed. The finding of *P. malariae* antigen in the glomerular lesions is not such strong direct evidence as it first appears, for two reasons. First, in all the studies the best control is lacking, that is, labelled serum that has been specifically adsorbed with *P. malariae* antigen. Second, the majority of the investigations were performed with the same serum from a patient with post-transfusion malaria.[217] That serum has now been used up, and reliable replacements have been difficult to find. The problem has always been to obtain a serum that would react only with *P. malariae* antigens. It may be hoped that DNA probes specific for *P. malariae* will soon become available and enable the veracity of the finding of malarial antigen in the glomeruli to be determined. The possibility that antibody to *P. malariae* antigens in eluates is serum antibody trapped in the renal tissue needs to be excluded.

If the presence in the glomeruli of *P. malariae* antigens and antibody to those antigens is confirmed this would suggest that the renal changes are a form of immune complex glomerulonephritis, the complexes probably being formed in situ.

VISCERAL LEISHMANIASIS

Chronic infection with the protozoon *Leishmania donovani* is associated with mild proteinuria, microscopic haematuria and pyuria in about 50% of patients. Renal function is sometimes impaired in severe cases.

Histological examination of the kidneys has shown diffuse interstitial nephritis (see p. 439) and mild mesangial proliferative glomerulonephritis (see p. 153). In one series of seven patients examined at autopsy a mild to moderate diffuse interstitial nephritis with mononuclear cell infiltration was present in all the kidneys; there was mild focal and segmental proliferative glomerulonephritis in five of the cases.[223] There are granular deposits of immunoglobulins and complement but leishmania antigen or antibody to that antigen has not been detected. Renal amyloidosis may also occur in leishmaniasis.

The signs of renal involvement improve after effective treatment of the leishmaniasis.

There is no evidence at present to indicate

whether any of these renal lesions are caused either by the parasitic invasion or by the host's response to that infection.

TOXOPLASMOSIS

In disseminated infection with *Toxoplasma gondii* there is sometimes renal involvement. Usually there is mild proteinuria; occasionally patients present with a nephritic syndrome. The nephrotic syndrome very rarely occurs in infants with congenital toxoplasmosis; such cases should be distinguished from congenital nephrotic syndrome of Finnish type (see p. 82).[224]

In cases with the nephritic syndrome there may be a diffuse endocapillary proliferative glomerulonephritis (see p. 145) with granular deposits of immunoglobulin, complement and toxoplasma antigen.[225] Other cases that have been biopsied have shown a focal interstitial nephritis. Cyst forms of the toxoplasma have been seen in the glomeruli of a few patients.

Some of the renal lesions may have been mediated through immune complexes that were either formed in situ with planted *T. gondii* antigen (see p. 128) or filtered from the circulation.[226]

METAZOAL INFESTATIONS

SCHISTOSOMIASIS

Schistosomiasis, an infestation by trematodes (flukes) of any species of the genus *Schistosoma*, affects approximately 10% of the world's population. It is spreading geographically and increasing in prevalence. Renal disease associated with this parasitic infestation may take the form of obstructive uropathy, glomerulonephritis or, rarely, amyloidosis.

Obstructive uropathy

In *S. haematobium* infestations eggs are deposited in the urinary bladder and ureters (see pp. 713–715). Obstruction to the urinary flow and vesicoureteric and intrarenal reflux may be caused. The outcome may be hydronephrosis (see p. 468); sometimes secondary infection, which is common, leads to acute pyelonephritis or pyonephrosis (see p. 472). These complications can result in renal failure and death. This progression is frequent in Egypt and Central Africa but occurs less often in South Africa.[227] In young patients, hydronephrosis is usually reversible with schistosomicidal treatment.

Glomerulonephritis

Clinically apparent glomerulonephritis has been consistently described only in the hepatosplenic form of schistosomiasis caused by *S. mansoni*. Its true prevalence in *S. mansoni* infestation is not known; it has been demonstrated at autopsy in 12% of those with hepatosplenic schistosomiasis admitted to hospitals in endemic areas[228] but these patients are a selected group because hepatosplenic schistosomiasis occurs in only 2–5% of patients infected with *S. mansoni* and not all patients with this form of the disease are admitted to hospital.

Clinical features

Glomerulonephritis particularly affects young adults, usually males, who come from an endemic area. They have hepatomegaly and splenomegaly. The majority present with proteinuria which is usually sufficiently severe to produce the nephrotic syndrome; there is often hypertension and in a few this is the initial sign of the disease. Most of the patients have microscopic haematuria.[229,230]

Serology

The serum level of the third component of complement (C3) may be reduced but is often normal; no correlation has been found between activity of the disease and complement level.[231] Circulating immune complexes are common.[232]

Renal changes

Diffuse mesangiocapillary glomerulonephritis (see

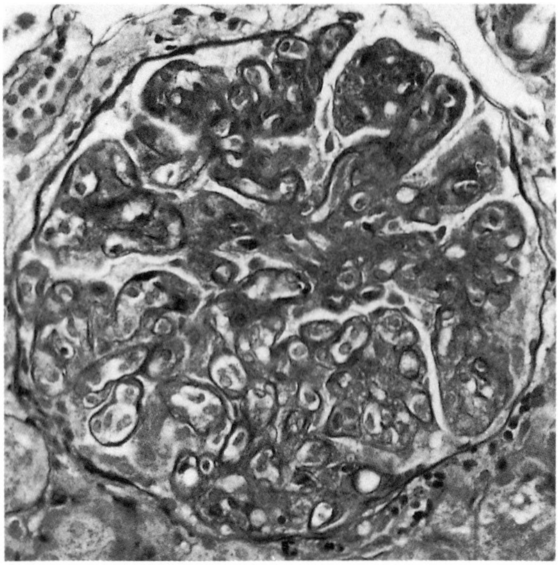

Fig. 11.37 Schistosomiasis. Glomerulus showing the changes of mesangiocapillary glomerulonephritis from a patient with hepatosplenic form of *Schistosoma mansoni* infestation.
Periodic acid-Schiff × 200

p. 116) is the most frequent glomerular lesion associated with renal signs and symptoms resulting from *S. mansoni* infestation (Fig. 11.37).[229,230] The second most common change observed in biopsy material is *focal segmental glomerulosclerosis* (see p. 205), often with diffuse or focal proliferative glomerulonephritis (see pp. 153, 211).[229,232] Other types of glomerulonephritis are sometimes seen.[228,233]

Differential diagnosis

The diffuse mesangiocapillary glomerulonephritis associated with *S. mansoni* infection does not differ morphologically from that due to many other causes and from the idiopathic type I lesion (see p. 166). The distinction largely depends upon the exclusion of other possible associated conditions; identification of schistosomal antigen in glomeruli should be attempted.[230]

Renal transplantation

Very little is known about the outcome of renal transplantation in treated *S. mansoni* schistosomiasis. Mesangiocapillary glomerulonephritis developed in one renal allograft 3 years after transplantation;[234] this might have been the disease recurring in the transplant, but there is no proof. A few other grafts have functioned normally.

A transitory glomerulonephritis has been reported in a patient with *S. mansoni* hepatosplenic schistosomiasis who, 6 months after renal transplantation, was treated with the schistosomicidal drug niridazole. Three weeks after the treatment there was slight proteinuria, a rise in serum creatinine and hypocomplementaemia. A biopsy of the renal allograft revealed that the mesangium was expanded and contained *S. mansoni* antigen, immunoglobulins and complement.[235] Renal function recovered and the proteinuria disappeared spontaneously within 4 days without change in the patient's maintenance immunosuppression.

Prognosis

The clinical course of the renal lesion is progressive and similar to that of idiopathic mesangiocapillary glomerulonephritis (see p. 165). It is not influenced by antiparasitic or immunosuppressive treatment.[230]

Pathogenesis

Schistosomal antigens from different morphological stages of *S. mansoni* have been demonstrated in the glomeruli of animals[236] and human patients[233] with this disease and schistosomal specific antibodies have been eluted from their kidneys.[233] The major antigen in the glomerular lesions is a polysaccharide with a molecular weight of 10 000 Da which occurs in the intestinal lining of adult worms;[237] it is continuously synthesized and then eliminated by regurgitation into the circulation of the host.[238]

This evidence strongly suggests that the renal lesions in schistosomiasis are caused by immune complexes composed of schistosomal antigens and of antibodies produced against those antigens. Whether the complexes are formed in situ or come from the circulation is not clear.

The probable reason why schistosomiasis-associated glomerulonephritis is usually restricted to patients with portal hypertension is that in these patients the collateral circulation allows schistosomal antigens entering the portal system, and any immune complexes formed in the portal circulation, to bypass the hepatic Kupffer cells, which would normally phagocytose and denature them, and reach the systemic circulation and the kidneys.

Amyloid

Renal amyloidosis has been reported in children from Central, East and West Africa infested with *S. mansoni*;[239,240] it has not been found in Brazilian and Egyptian patients.

FILARIASIS

The kidneys are sometimes involved in filariasis caused by nematodes of the superfamily Filarioidea. The commonest lesion is a glomerulonephritis which may produce either a nephritic or a nephrotic syndrome.

Infections with *Wuchereria bancrofti* and *Brugia malayi* have been associated with *diffuse endocapillary proliferative* and *mesangial proliferative glomerulonephritis*. In *Loa loa* infestations *membranous glomerulonephritis* (see p. 191) is more common and in *Onchocerca volvulus* infestations mesangial proliferative and mesangiocapillary are the commonest forms of glomerulonephritis. Filarial antigen has been demonstrated in association with the accompanying granular deposits of immunoglobulins and complement in the patients infested by *O. volvulus*.[241]

Microfilariae are sometimes seen in the glomeruli accompanied by eosinophil and neutrophil granulocytes. Interstitial nephritis has also been described; occasionally this is granulomatous. Renal amyloidosis has occurred after prolonged infestation by *Brugia pahangi* and *Dirofilaria immitis*.

The evidence suggests that in some cases of *O. volvulus* infestation the glomerulonephritis may be induced by immune complexes in which the antigen is filarial.[241] Soluble filarial antigens and antibodies to these antigens are present in the circulation of most patients.[242]

ECHINOCOCCOSIS (HYDATID DISEASE)

Echinococcosis is an infestation caused by cestodes of the genus *Echinococcus*. Of the species known to be capable of infesting humans *E. granulosus* is the most important. *E. granulosus* is found throughout the world and is endemic in sheep and cattle rearing areas in Australia, New Zealand, Argentina, Brazil, Chile, Uruguay, Peru, the western United States of America, some eastern European countries, Sardinia, Cyprus, the Middle East, East Africa, northern India and Pakistan.[243]

When humans become the intermediary hosts the invasive embryo tape worms form cysts (hydatid cysts) in the liver and many other organs. The kidneys are involved in approximately 4% of cases of echinococcosis.[243]

Renal hydatid cysts

The cysts are usually single and unilocular, and vary from a few centimetres in diameter to a huge mass occupying the entire kidney.[244,245] They are lined by a 1 mm thick translucent white laminated membrane and filled with watery fluid that often contains pale, finely granular material (hydatid sand). On the inner side of the membrane there is a germinal layer and within fertile cysts there are distinctive brood capsules and developing larval scolices.

Renal hydatid ctysts often have long periods of silent growth. The main clinical manifestations are caused by mechanical pressure at the site of the enlarging cyst; haematuria and proteinuria may also occur. Pain sometimes results as the cyst expands. Occasionally the cyst ruptures into the peritoneum giving peritonitis.[244,245]

Glomerulonephritis

A case of *diffuse membranous glomerulonephritis* associated with intrahepatic echinococcosis has been reported.[246] *E. granulosus* antigen was demonstrated along the glomerular capillary basement membranes by indirect immunofluorescence and antibodies to the antigen were eluted from the renal tissue. The serum contained antibodies to *E. granulosus*, both free and in immune complexes.

In another report five patients with echinococcosis were treated with mebendazole, a drug that is now little used. Subsequently four developed *diffuse mesangial proliferative glomerulonephritis* and the fifth *diffuse mesangiocapillary glomerulonephritis type I*.[247] As mebendazole causes necrosis of the hydatid cyst wall, these glomerular changes may have resulted from immune complexes formed in the kidneys following release of echinococcal antigens.

REFERENCES

Bacterial infections

1. Neugarten J, Gallo GR, Baldwin DS. Glomerulonephritis in bacterial endocarditis. Am J Kidney Dis 1984; 3: 371–379.
2. Bayliss R, Clarke C, Oakley CM, Somerville W, Whitfield AGW, Young SEJ. The microbiology and pathogenesis of infective endocarditis. Br Heart J 1983; 50: 513–519.
3. Geraci JE, Hanson KC, Giuliani ER. Endocarditis caused by coagulase-negative staphylococci. Mayo Clin Proc 1968; 43: 420–434.
4. Bayliss R, Clarke C, Oakley CM, Somerville W, Whitfield AGW, Young SEJ. The bowel, the genito-urinary tract and infective endocarditis. Br Heart J 1984; 51: 339–345.
5. Shah GM, Winer RL. Glomerulonephritis associated with endocarditis caused by *Actinobacillus actinomycetemcomitans*. Am J Kidney Dis 1981; 1: 113–115.
6. Kauffman RH, Thompson J, Valentijn RM, Daha MR, van Es LA. The clinical implications and the pathogenetic significance of circulating immune complexes in infective endocarditis. Am J Med 1981; 71: 17–25.
7. Heptinstall RH. Pathology of the kidney, 3rd edn. Boston: Little, Brown and Co, 1983; 2: 583.
8. Gutman RA, Striker GE, Gilliland BC, Cutler RE. The immune complex glomerulonephritis of bacterial endocarditis. Medicine (Baltimore) 1972; 51: 1–24.
9. Ebright JR, Komorowski R. Gonococcal endocarditis associated with immune complex glomerulonephritis. Am J Med 1980; 68: 793–796.
10. Porter GA, Bennett WM, Wilson JW. Renal consequences of valvular heart disease. Am J Cardiol 1975; 35: 886–897.
11. Boulton-Jones JM, Sissons JGP, Evans DJ, Peters DK. Renal lesions of subacute infective endocarditis. Br Med J 1974; 2: 11–14.
12. Laxdal T, Messner RP, Williams RC, Quie PG. Opsonic, agglutinating, and complement-fixing antibodies in patients with subacute bacterial endocarditis. J Lab Clin Med 1968; 71: 638–653.
13. Levy RL, Hong R. The immune nature of subacute bacterial endocarditis (SBE) nephritis. Am J Med 1973; 54: 645–652.
14. Perez GO, Rothfield N, Williams RC. Immune-complex nephritis in bacterial endocarditis. Arch Intern Med 1976; 136: 334–336.
15. Kaplan EL, Rich H, Gersony W, Manning J. A collaborative study of infective endocarditis in the 1970's. Emphasis on infections in patients who have undergone cardiovascular surgery. Circulation (New York) 1979; 59: 327–335.
16. Tu WH, Shearn MA, Lee JC. Acute diffuse glomerulonephritis in acute staphylococcal endocarditis. Ann Intern Med 1969; 71: 335–341.
17. Yum MN, Wheat LJ, Maxwell D, Edwards JL. Immunofluorescent localization of *Staphylococcus aureus* antigen in acute bacterial endocarditis nephritis. Am J Clin Pathol 1978; 70: 832–835.
18. Pertschuk LP, Woda BA, Vulentin JC, Brigati DJ, Soriano CB, Nicastri AD. Glomerulonephritis due to *Staphylococcus aureus* antigen. Am J Clin Pathol 1976; 65: 301–307.
19. Beaufils M, Gilbert C, Morel-Maroger L et al. Glomerulonephritis in severe bacterial infections with and without endocarditis. Adv Nephrol 1978; 7: 217–234.
20. Craddock CF, Richards NP, Powell RJ, Morgan AG. Novel C3 nephritic factor activity in the glomerulonephritis of staphylococcal endocarditis. Q J Med 1987; 65: 895–898.
21. Beaufils M, Morel-Maroger L, Sraer JD, Kanfer A, Kourilsky O, Richet G. Acute renal failure of glomerular origin during visceral abscesses. N Engl J Med 1976; 295: 185–189.
22. Beaufils M. Glomerular disease complicating abdominal sepsis. Kidney Int 1981; 19: 609–618.
23. Coleman M, Burnett J, Barratt LJ, Dupont P. Glomerulonephritis associated with chronic bacterial infection of a dacron arterial prosthesis. Clin Nephrol 1983; 20: 315–320.
24. Forrest JW Jr, John F, Mills LR et al. Immune complex glomerulonephritis associated with *Klebsiella pneumoniae* infection. Clin Nephrol 1977; 7: 76–80.
25. Schoenbaum SC, Gardner P, Shillito J. Infections of cerebrospinal fluid shunts: epidemiology, clinical manifestations and therapy. J Infect Dis 1975; 131: 543–552.
26. Black JA, Challacombe DN, Ockenden BG. Nephrotic syndrome associated with bacteraemia after shunt operations for hydrocephalus. Lancet 1965; 2: 921–924.
27. Wakabayashi Y, Kobayashi Y, Shigematsu H. Shunt nephritis: histological dynamics following removal of the shunt. Case report and review of the literature. Nephron 1985; 40: 111–117.

28. Arze RS, Rashid H, Morley R, Ward MK, Kerr DNS. Shunt nephritis: report of two cases and review of the literature. Clin Nephrol 1983; 19: 48–53.
29. Noe HN, Roy S. Shunt nephritis. J Urol 1981; 125: 731–733.
30. Wegmann W, Leumann EP. Glomerulonephritis associated with infected ventriculoatrial shunt. Clinical and morphological findings. Virchows Arch [A] 1973; 359: 185–200.
31. O'Regan S, Makker SP. Shunt nephritis: demonstration of diphtheroid antigen in glomeruli. Am J Med Sci 1979; 278: 161–165.
32. Groeneveld ABJ, Nommensen FE, Mullink H, Ooms ECM, Bode WA. Shunt nephritis associated with *Propionibacterium acnes* with demonstration of the antigen in the glomeruli. Nephron 1982; 32: 365–369.
33. Zunin C, Castellani A, Olivetti G, Marini G, Gabriele PW. Membranoproliferative glomerulonephritis associated with infective ventriculo-atrial shunt: report of two cases recovered after removal of the shunt. Pathologia 1977; 69: 297–305.
34. Simon HB, Weinstein AJ, Pasternak MS, Swartz MN, Kunz LJ. Genitourinary tuberculosis. Clinical features in a general hospital population. Am J Med 1977; 63: 410–420.
35. Alvarez S, McCabe WR. Extrapulmonary tuberculosis revisited: a review of experience at Boston City Hospital and other hospitals. Medicine (Baltimore) 1984; 63: 25–55.
36. Cinman AC. Genitourinary tuberculosis. Urology 1982; 20: 353–358.
37. Christensen WI. Genitourinary tuberculosis: review of 102 cases. Medicine (Baltimore) 1974; 53: 377–390.
38. Listwan WJ, Roth DA, Tsung SH, Rose HD. Disseminated *Mycobacterium kansasii* infection with pancytopenia and interstitial replication. Ann Intern Med 1975; 83: 70–73.
39. Elliott JL, Hoppes WL, Platt MS, Thomas JG, Patel IP, Gansei A. The acquired immunodeficiency syndrome and *Mycobacterium avium-intracellulare* bacteremia in a patient with hemophilia. Ann Intern Med 1983; 98: 290–293.
40. Williams RC, Cathcart EC, Calkins E. Secondary amyloidosis in lepromatous leprosy. Possible relationships of diet and environment. Ann Intern Med 1965; 62: 1000–1007.
41. Desikan KV, Job CK. A review of postmortem findings in 37 cases of leprosy. Int J Lepr 1968; 36: 32–44.
42. Grover S, Bobhate SK, Chaubey BS. Renal abnormality in leprosy. Lepr India 1983; 55: 286–291.
43. Johny KV, Karat AMA, Rao PS, Date A. Glomerulonephritis in leprosy – a percutaneous renal biopsy study. Lepr Rev 1975; 46: 29–37.
44. Gupta JC, Diwakar R, Singh S, Gupta DK, Panda PK. A histopathologic study of renal biopsies in fifty cases of leprosy. Int J Lepr 1977; 45: 167–170.
45. Kean BH, Childress ME. A summary of 103 autopsies on leprosy patients on the Isthmus of Panama. Int J Lepr 1942; 10: 51–59.
46. Hansen AG, Looft C. Die Lepra vom clinischen und pathologisch-anatomischen Standpunkte. Translated by Walder N. Bristol: John Wright, 1895.
47. Ng WL, Scollard DM, Hua A. Glomerulonephritis in leprosy. Am J Clin Pathol 1981; 76: 321–329.
48. Gupta SC, Bajaj AK, Govil DC, Sinha SN, Kumar R. A study of percutaneous renal biopsy in lepromatous leprosy. Lepr India 1981; 53: 179–186.
49. Ponce P, Ramos A, Ferreira ML, Pinto G, Lacerda MH. Renal involvement in leprosy. Nephrol Dial Transplant 1989; 4: 81–84.
50. Iveson JMI, McDougall AC, Leathem AJ, Harris HJ. Lepromatous leprosy presenting with polyarthritis, myositis, and immune-complex glomerulonephritis. Br Med J 1975; 2: 619–621.
51. Weiner ID, Northcutt AD. Leprosy and glomerulonephritis: case report and review of the literature. Am J Kidney Dis 1989; 13: 424–429.
52. Thomas EW, Schur M. Clinical nephropathies in early syphilis. Arch Intern Med 1946; 78: 679–686.
53. Sanchez-Bayle M, Ecija JL, Estepa R, Cambronero MJ, Martinez MA. Incidence of glomerulonephritis in congenital syphilis. Clin Nephrol 1983; 20: 27–31.
54. Gamble CN, Reardan JB. Immunopathogenesis of syphilitic glomerulonephritis. Elution of antitreponemal antibody from glomerular immune-complex deposits. N Engl J Med 1975; 292: 449–454.
55. O'Regan S, Fong JSC, De Chadarevian J-P, Rishikof JR, Drummond KN. Treponemal antigens in congenital and acquired syphilitic nephritis. Demonstration by immunofluorescence studies. Ann Intern Med 1976; 85: 325–327.
56. Losito A, Bucciarelli E, Massi-Benedetti F, Lato M. Membranous glomerulonephritis in congenital syphilis. Clin Nephrol 1979; 12: 32–37.
57. Walker PD, Deeves EC, Sahba G, Wallin JD, O'Neill WM. Rapidly progressive glomerulonephritis in a patient with syphilis. Identification of antitreponemal antibody and treponemal antigen in renal tissue. Am J Med 1984; 76: 1106–1112.
58. Krane NK, Espenan P, Walker PD, Bergman SM, Wallin JD. Renal disease and syphilis: a report of nephrotic syndrome with minimal change disease. Am J Kidney Dis 1987; 9: 176–179.
59. Sterzel RB, Krause PH, Zobl H, Kuhn K. Acute syphilitic nephrosis: a transient glomerular immunopathy. Clin Nephrol 1974; 2: 164–168.
60. Rich AR. The pathology of nineteen cases of a peculiar and specific form of nephritis associated with acquired syphilis. Bull Johns Hopkins Hosp 1932; 50: 357–382.
61. Hodnett T, Waitkins SA, Platt DW. Prevalence of leptospirosis in dairy farm workers. Israeli J Vet Med 1987; 43: 345–346.
62. Ku G, Lim CH, Pwee HS et al. Review of renal failure. Ann Acad Med Singapore [Suppl] 1975; 4: 115–120.
63. Sitprija V, Benyajati C. Tropical diseases and acute renal failure. Ann Acad Med Singapore [Suppl] 1975; 4: 112–114.
64. Heath CW, Alexander AD, Galton MM. Leptospirosis in the United States, analysis of 483 cases in man 1949–1961. N Engl J Med 1965; 273: 857–864, 915–922.
65. Winearls CG, Chan L, Coghlan JD, Ledingham JGG, Oliver DO. Acute renal failure due to leptospirosis: clinical features and outcome in six cases. Q J Med 1984; 53: 487–495.
66. Hanvanich M, Moollaor P, Suwangool P, Sitprija V. Hemolytic uremic syndrome in *Leptospirosis bataviae.* Nephron 1985; 40: 230– 231.
67. Leptospirosis Reference Laboratory and Communicable Disease Surveillance Centre (Public Health Laboratory

Service). Leptospirosis in man, British Isles, 1982. Br Med J 1983; 287: 1365–1366.
68. Sitprija V, Evans H. The kidney in human leptospirosis. Am J Med 1970; 49: 780–788.
69. Lai KN, Aarons I, Woodroffe AJ, Clarkson AR. Renal lesions in leptospirosis. Aust NZ J Med 1982; 12: 276–279.
70. Sitprija V, Pipatanagul V, Mertowidjojo K, Boonpucknavig V, Boonpucknavig S. Pathogenesis of renal disease in leptospirosis: clinical and experimental studies. Kidney Int 1980; 17: 827–836.
71. Dunea G, Kark RM, Lannigan E, D'Alessio D, Muehrcke RC. Brucella nephritis. Ann Intern Med 1969; 70: 783–790.
72. Kelalis PP, Greene LF, Weed LA. Brucellosis of the urogenital tract: a mimic of tuberculosis. J Urol 1962; 88: 347–353.
73. Wasserheit JN, Dugdale DC, Agosti JM. Rhabdomyolysis and acute renal failure: a new presentation of acute brucellosis. J Infect Dis 1984; 150: 782–783.
74. Doregatti C, Volpi A, Tarelli LT et al. Acute glomerulonephritis in human brucellosis. Nephron 1985; 41: 365–366.
75. Relman AS, McCluskey RT. Case records of the Massachusetts General Hospital. Acute renal failure and hemoptysis in a 44 year old man. N Engl J Med 1978; 298: 1014–1019.
76. Poulter N, Gabriel R, Porter KA et al. Acute interstitial nephritis complicating Legionnaires' disease. Clin Nephrol 1981; 15: 216–220.
77. Weisenburger DD, Helms CM, Renner ED. Sporadic Legionnaires' disease. A pathologic study of 23 fatal cases. Arch Pathol Lab Med 1981; 105: 130–137.
78. Dorman SA, Hardin NJ, Winn WC. Pyelonephritis associated with *Legionella pneumophila*, serogroup 4. Ann Intern Med 1980; 93: 835–837.
79. Fenves AZ. Legionnaires' disease associated with acute renal failure: a report of two cases and review of the literature. Clin Nephrol 1985; 23: 96–100.
80. Sitprija V, Pipatanagul V, Boonpucknavig V, Boonpucknavig S. Glomerulitis in typhoid fever. Ann Intern Med 1974; 81: 210–213.
81. Buka I, Coovadia HM. Typhoid glomerulonephritis. J Clin Pathol 1980; 33: 305–307.
82. Indraprasit S, Boonpucknavig V, Boonpucknavig S. IgA nephropathy associated with enteric fever. Nephron 1985; 40: 219–222.

Viral infections

83. Gust I, Crowe S. The global importance of viral hepatitis. In: Zuckerman AJ, ed. Clinics in tropical medicine and communicable diseases. London: WB Saunders, 1986; 281.
84. Lai KN, Lai FM-M, Chan KW, Chow CB, Tong KL, Vallence-Owen J. The clinicopathologic features of hepatitis B virus-associated glomerulonephritis. Q J Med 1987; 63: 323–333.
85. Lee HS, Choi Y, Yu SH, Koh HI, Kim MJ, Ko KW. A renal biopsy study of hepatitis B virus-associated nephropathy in Korea. Kidney Int 1988; 34: 537–543.
86. Southwest Pediatric Nephrology Study Group. Hepatitis B surface (HBs) antigenemia in North American children with membranous glomerulopathy. J Pediatr 1985; 106: 571–578.
87. Stevens CE, Beasley RP, Tsui J, Lee W-C. Vertical transmission of hepatitis B antigen in Taiwan. N Engl J Med 1975; 292: 771–774.
88. Furose A, Hattori S, Terashima T, Karashima S, Matsuda I. Circulating immune complex in glomerulonephropathy associated with hepatitis B virus infection. Nephron 1982; 31: 212–218.
89. Hsu H-C, Lin G-H, Chang M-H, Chen C-H. Association of hepatitis B surface (HB_s) antigenemia and membranous nephropathy in children in Taiwan. Clin Nephrol 1983; 20: 121–129.
90. Makker SP. Hepatitis B associated membranous glomerulonephritis. Indian J Pediatr 1986; 53: 317–319.
91. Chen A, Ho Y-S, Tu Y-C. Is there a simultaneous involvement of membranous and IgA nephropathy in hepatitis B antigenemia? Hum Pathol 1988; 19: 120–121 (letter).
92. Magil A, Webber D, Chan V. Glomerulonephritis associated with hepatitis B surface antigenemia. Report of a case with features of both membranous and IgA nephropathy. Nephron 1986; 42: 335–339.
93. Wiggelinkhuizen J, Sinclair-Smith C, Stannard LM, Smuts H. Hepatitis B virus associated membranous glomerulonephritis. Arch Dis Child 1983; 58: 488–496.
94. Yoshikawa N, Ito H, Yamada Y et al. Membranous glomerulonephritis associated with hepatitis B antigen in children: a comparison with idiopathic membranous glomerulonephritis. Clin Nephrol 1985; 23: 28–34.
95. Garcia G, Scullard G, Smith C et al. Preliminary observation of hepatitis B-associated membranous glomerulonephritis treated with leukocyte interferon. Hepatology 1985; 5: 317–320.
96. Knecht GL, Chisari FV. Reversibility of hepatitis B virus induced glomerulonephritis and chronic active hepatitis after spontaneous clearance of serum hepatitis B surface antigen. Gastroenterology 1978; 75: 1152–1156.
97. Maggiore Q, Bartolomeo F, L'Abbate A, Misefari V. HBsAg glomerular deposits in glomerulonephritis: fact or artifact? Kidney Int 1981; 19: 579–586.
98. Takeda S-I, Kida H, Katagiri M, Yokoyama H, Abe T, Hattori N. Characteristics of glomerular lesions in hepatitis B virus infection. Am J Kidney Dis 1988; 11: 57–62.
99. Hirose H, Udo K, Kojima M et al. Deposition of hepatitis Be antigen in membranous glomerulonephritis: identification by $F(ab^1)_2$ fragments of monoclonal antibody. Kidney Int 1984; 26: 338–341.
100. Hsu H-C, Wu C-Y, Lin C-Y, Lin G-J, Chen C-H, Huang F-Y. Membranous nephropathy in 52 hepatitis B surface antigen (HBsAg) carrier children in Taiwan. Kidney Int 1989; 36: 1103–1107.
101. Mizushima N, Kanai K, Matsuda H. Improvement of proteinuria in a case of hepatitis B–associated glomerulonephritis after treatment with interferon. Gastroenterology 1987; 92: 524–526.
102. Johnson RJ, Couser WG. Hepatitis B infection and renal disease: clinical, immunopathogenetic and therapeutic considerations. Kidney Int 1990; 37: 663–676.
103. Hattori S, Furuse A, Matsuda I. Presence of HBe antibody in glomerular deposits in membranous glomerulonephritis is associated with hepatitis B virus infection. Am J Nephrol 1988; 8: 384–387.
104. Lai KN, Lai FM-M, Tam JS. IgA nephropathy associated with chronic hepatitis B virus infection in

adults: the pathogenetic role of HBsAg. J Pathol 1989; 157: 321–327.
105. Levo Y, Gorevic PD, Kassab HJ, Zucker-Franklin D, Franklin EC. Association between hepatitis B virus and essential mixed cryoglobulinemia. N Engl J Med 1977; 296: 1501–1504.
106. Brouet J-C, Clauvel J-P, Danon F, Klein M, Seligmann M. Biologic and clinical significance of cryoglobulins. Am J Med 1974; 57: 775–788.
107. Cordonnier DJ, Renversez JC, Vialtel P, Dechelette E. The kidney in mixed cryoglobulinemias. Springer Semin Immunopathol 1987; 9: 395–415.
108. Tarantino A, De Vecchi A, Montagnino G et al. Renal disease in essential mixed cryoglobulinaemia. Long-term follow-up of 44 patients. Q J Med 1981; 50: 1–30.
109. Trepo CG, Zuckerman AJ, Bird RC, Prince AM. The role of circulating hepatitis B antigen/antibody immune complexes in the pathogenesis of vascular and hepatic manifestations in polyarteritis nodosa. J Clin Pathol 1974; 27: 863–868.
110. Conn DL, McDuffie FC, Holley KE, Schroeter AL. Immunologic mechanisms in systemic vasculitis. Mayo Clin Proc 1976; 51: 511–518.
111. D'Agati V, Chandler P, Nash M, Manuilla-Jimenez R. Idiopathic microscopic polyarteritis nodosa: ultrastructural observations on the renal vascular and glomerular lesions. Am J Kidney Dis 1986; 7: 95–110.
112. Drueke T, Barbanel C, Jungers P et al. Hepatitis B antigen-associated periarteritis nodosa in patients undergoing long-term hemodialysis. Am J Med 1980; 63: 86–90.
113. McMahon BJ, Bender TR, Templin DW et al. Vasculitis in Eskimos living in an area hyperendemic for hepatitis B. JAMA 1980; 244: 2180–2182.
114. Michalak T. Immune complexes of hepatitis B surface antigen in the pathogenesis of periarteritis nodosa. A study of seven necropsy cases. Am J Pathol 1978; 90: 619–632.
115. Center for Disease Control (CDC). Revision of the CDC surveillance case definition for acquired immunodeficiency syndrome. MMWR 1987; 36: suppl, 1S–16S.
116. Soni A, Agarwal A, Chander P et al. Evidence for an HIV-related nephropathy: a clinico-pathological study. Clin Nephrol 1989; 31: 12–17.
117. Bourgoignie JJ, Meneses R, Ortiz C, Jaffe D, Pardo V. The clinical spectrum of renal disease associated with human immunodeficiency virus. Am J Kidney Dis 1988; 12: 131–137.
118. Glassock RJ et al. Human immunodeficiency virus (HIV) infection and the kidney. Ann Intern Med 1990; 112: 35–49.
119. Pardo V, Aldana M, Colton RM et al. Glomerular lesions in the acquired immunodeficiency syndrome. Ann Intern Med 1984; 101: 429–434.
120. Rao TKS, Filippone EJ, Nicastri AD et al. Associated focal and segmental glomerulosclerosis in the acquired immunodeficiency syndrome. N Engl J Med 1984; 310: 669–973.
121. Gardenswartz MH, Lerner CW, Seligson GR et al. Renal disease in patients with AIDS: a clinicopathologic study. Clin Nephrol 1984; 21: 197–204.
122. Bourgoignie JL. Renal complications of human immunodeficiency virus type 1. Kidney Int 1990; 37: 1571–1584.
123. Pardo V, Meneses R, Ossa L et al. AIDS-related glomerulopathy: occurrence in specific risk groups. Kidney Int 1987; 31: 1167–1173.
124. D'Agati V, Suh J-I, Carbone L, Cheng J-T, Appel G. Pathology of HIV-associated nephropathy: a detailed morphologic and comparative study. Kidney Int 1989; 35: 1358–1370.
125. Luu J, Bockus D, Remington F, Bean MA, Hammar SP. Tubuloreticular structures and cylindrical confronting cisternae: a review. Hum Pathol 1989; 20: 617–627.
126. Chander P, Agarwal A, Soni A, Kim K, Tresser G. Renal cytomembranous inclusions in idiopathic renal disease as predictive markers for the acquired immunodeficiency syndrome. Hum Pathol 1988; 19: 1060–1064.
127. Karlsson-Parra A, Dimény E, Fellström B, Klareskog L. HIV receptors (CD4 antigen) in normal human glomerular cells. N Engl J Med 1989; 320: 741 (letter).
128. Cohen AH, Sun NC, Shapshak P, Imagawa DT. Demonstration of human immunodeficiency virus in renal epithelium in HIV-associated nephropathy. Modern Pathol 1989; 2: 125–128.
129. Humphreys RH, Schoenfeld PY. Renal complications in patients with the acquired immunodeficiency syndrome (AIDS). Am J Nephrol 1987; 7: 1–7.
130. Lee HW. Hantavirus infection in Asia. In: Davison AM, ed. Nephrology 2: Proceedings of the Xth International Congress of Nephrology. London: Baillière Tindall, 1988: 816–831.
131. Lee HW. Hemorrhagic fever with renal syndrome. History, Hantaan virus and epidemiological features. Scand J Infect Dis [Suppl] 1982; 36: 82–85.
132. Lukes RJ. The pathology of thirty-nine fatal cases of epidemic haemorrhagic fever. Am J Med 1954; 16: 639–650.
133. Ypersele De Strihou C, Méry JP. Hantavirus-related acute nephritis in Western Europe. Expansion of a world-wide zoonosis. Q J Med 1989; 73: 941–950.
134. Osterhaus ADME, Groen J, UytdeHaag FGCM et al. Hantavirus nephropathy in Netherlands. Lancet 1989; 2: 338–339 (letter).
135. Lähdevirta J. Nephropathia epidemica in Finland. A clinical, histological and epidemiological study. Ann Clin Res 1971; 3: suppl 8, 1–154.
136. Jokinen EJ, Lähdevirta J, Collan Y. Nephropathia epidemica: immunohistochemical study of pathogenesis. Clin Nephrol 1978; 9: 1–5.
137. Collan Y, Lähdevirta J. Electron microscopy of nephropathia epidemica. Cell nuclei in kidney biopsies. Acta Pathol Microbiol Scand [A] 1979; 87: 71–77.
138. Fetterman GH, Sherman FE, Fabrizio NS, Studnicki FM. Generalized cytomegalic inclusion disease of the newborn. Arch Pathol 1968; 86: 86–94.
139. Platt JL, Sibley RK, Michael AF. Interstitial nephritis associated with cytomegalovirus infection. Kidney Int 1985; 28: 550–552.
140. Pyanov RP. Changes in the kidneys in infants with cytomegaly. Arkh Patol 1969; 31: 50–53.
141. Beneck D, Greco MA, Feiner HD. Glomerulonephritis in congenital cytomegalic inclusion disease. Hum Pathol 1986; 17: 1054–1059.
142. Sissons JGP. Biology of persistent virus infections affecting the kidney with reference to cytomegalovirus and hepatitis B virus. In: Davison AM, ed. Nephrology 2: Proceedings of the Xth International Congress of Nephrology. London: Baillière Tindall, 1988: 781–789.

143. Battegay EJ, Mihatsch MJ, Mazzucchelli L et al. Cytomegalovirus and kidney. Clin Nephrol 1988; 30: 239–247.
144. Herrera GA, Alexander RW, Cooley CF et al. Cytomegalovirus glomerulopathy: a controversial lesion. Kidney Int 1986; 29: 725–733.
145. Seney FD, Burns DK, Silva FG. Acquired immunodeficiency syndrome and the kidney. Am J Kidney Dis 1990; 16: 1–13.
146. Lee S, Kjellstrand CM. Renal disease in infectious mononucleosis. Clin Nephrol 1978; 9: 236–240.
147. Kopolovic J, Pinkus G, Rosen S. Interstitial nephritis in infectious mononucleosis. Am J Kidney Dis 1988; 12: 76–77.
148. Minkowitz S, Wenk R, Friedman E, Yuceoglu A, Berkovich S. Acute glomerulonephritis associated with varicella infection. Am J Med 1968; 44: 489–492.
149. Burch GE, Colcolough H. Progressive Coxsackie viral pancarditis and nephritis. Ann Intern Med 1969; 71: 963–970.
150. Monteiro GE, Lillicrap CA. Case of mumps nephritis. Br Med J 1967; 4: 721–722.
151. Lin CY, Hsu HC. Measles and acute glomerulonephritis. Pediatrics 1983; 71: 398–401.
152. Yuceoglu AM, Berkovich S, Minkowitz S. Acute glomerulonephritis associated with Echo virus type 9 infection. J Pediatr 1966; 69: 603–609.
153. Fraser JRE, Cunningham AL, Muller HK, Sinclair RA, Standish HG. Glomerulonephritis in the acute phase of Ross River virus disease (epidemic polyarthritis). Clin Nephrol 1988; 29: 149–152.
154. Boonpucknavig V, Bhamarapravati N, Boonpucknavig S, Futrakul P, Tanpaichitr P. Glomerular changes in dengue hemorrhagic fever. Arch Pathol Lab Med 1976; 100: 206–212.
155. Rosen S, Harmon W, Krensky AM et al. Tubulointerstitial nephritis associated with polyomavirus (BK type) infection. N Engl J Med 1983; 308: 1192– 1196.

Fungal and filamentous bacterial infections

156. Symmers WStC. Histopathology of opportunistic fungal infections. In: Chick EW, Balows A, Furcolow ML, eds. Opportunistic fungal infections. Proceedings of the Second International Conference. Springfield, Illinois: Charles C Thomas, 1975: 269–284.
157. Chesney RW, O'Regan S, Guyda HJ, Drummond KN. Candida endocrinopathy syndrome with membranoproliferative glomerulonephritis: demonstration of glomerular candida antigen. Clin Nephrol 1976; 5: 232–238.
158. Dreetz DJ, Fetchick R. Fungal infections of the kidney and urinary tract. In: Schrier RW, Gottschalk CW, eds. Diseases of the kidney, 4th edn. Boston: Little, Brown and Co, 1988; 1: 1015–1047.
159. Parker JC, McCloskey JJ, Knauer KA. Pathobiologic features of human candidiasis. A common deep mycosis of the brain, heart and kidney in the altered host. Am J Clin Pathol 1976; 65: 991–1000.
160. Myerowitz RL, Pazin GJ, Allen CM. Disseminated candidiasis. Changes in incidence, underlying diseases, and pathology. Am J Clin Pathol 1977; 68: 29–38.
161. Aragona F, Glazel GP, Pavanello L, Perale R, Rizzoni C, Pagano F. Upper urinary tract obstruction in children caused by *Candida* fungus balls. Eur Urol 1985; 11: 188–191.
162. Eckstein CW, Kass EJ. Anuria in a newborn secondary to bilateral ureteropelvic fungus balls. J Urol 1982; 127: 109–110.
163. Tomashefski JF, Abramowsky CR. *Candida*-associated renal papillary necrosis. Am J Clin Pathol 1981; 75: 190–194.
164. Humphrey DM, Weiner MH. Candidal antigen detection in pulmonary candidiasis. Am J Med 1983; 74: 630–640.
165. Rippon JW. Medical mycology: the pathogenic fungi and the pathogenic antinomycetes, 2nd edn. Philadelphia: WB Saunders, 1982: 484–531.
166. Barnes JL, Osgood RW, Lee JC, King RD, Stein JH. Host–parasite interactions in the pathogenesis of experimental renal candidiasis. Lab Invest 1983; 49: 460–467.
167. Winblad B. Experimental renal candidiasis in mice and guinea pigs. Acta Pathol Microbiol Scand 1975; 83: 406–414.
168. King RD, Lee JC, Morris AL. Adherence of *Candida albicans* and other *Candida* species to mucosal epithelial cells. Infect Immun 1980; 27: 667–674.
169. Young RC, Bennett JE, Vogel CL, Carbone PP, de Vita VT. Aspergillosis. The spectrum of the disease in 93 patients. Medicine (Baltimore) 1970; 49: 147–173.
170. Flechner SM, McAninch JW. Aspergillosis of the urinary tract: ascending route of infection and evolving patterns of disease. J Urol 1981; 125: 598–601.
171. Comings DE, Turbow BA, Callahan DH, Waldstein SS. Obstructing *Aspergillus* cast of the renal pelvis. Report of a case in a patient having diabetes mellitus and Addison's disease. Arch Intern Med 1962; 110: 255–261.
172. Eisenberg RL, Hedgcock MW, Shanser JD. *Aspergillus* mycetoma of the renal pelvis associated with ureteropelvic junction obstruction. J Urol 1977; 118: 466–467.
173. Salgia P, Mani MK. Renal aspergillosis – case report. Nephron 1985; 40: 376–378.
174. Slater DN, Brown CB, Ward AM et al. Immune complex crescentic glomerulonephritis associated with pulmonary aspergillosis. Histopathology 1983; 7: 957–966.
175. Raghavan R, Date A, Bhaktaviziam A. Fungal and nocardial infections of the kidney. Histopathology 1987; 11: 9–20.
176. El Nageeb S, Hay RJ. Immunoperoxidase staining in the recognition of *Aspergillus* infections. Histopathology 1981; 5: 437–444.
177. Meyer RD, Rosen P, Armstrong D. Phycomycosis complicating leukemia and lymphoma. Ann Intern Med 1972; 77: 871–879.
178. Low AI, Tulloch AGS, England EJ. Phycomycosis of the kidney associated with a transient immune defect and treated with clotrimazole. J Urol 1974; 111: 732–734.
179. Dansky AS, Lynne CM, Politano VA. Disseminated mucormycosis with renal involvement. J Urol 1978; 119: 275–277.
180. Langston C, Roberts DA, Porter GA, Bennett WM. Renal phycomycosis. J Urol 1973; 109: 941–944.

181. Chandler FW, Watts JC, Kaplan W, Hendry AT, McGinnis MR, Ajello L. Zygomycosis. Report of four cases with formation of chlamydoconidia in tissue. Am J Clin Pathol 1985; 84: 99–103.
182. Prout GR, Goddard AR. Renal mucormycosis. Survival after nephrectomy and amphotericin B therapy. N Engl J Med 1960; 263: 1246–1248.
183. Salyer WR, Salyer DC. Involvement of the kidney and prostate in cryptococcosis. J Urol 1973; 109: 695–698.
184. Randall RE, Stacy WK, Toone EC et al. Cryptococcal pyelonephritis. N Engl J Med 1968; 279: 60–65.
185. Bottone EJ, Toma M, Johansson BE, Wormser GP. Capsule-deficient cryptococcus neoformans in AIDS patients. Lancet 1985; 2: 400 (letter).
186. Kaplan W, Kraft DE. Demonstration of pathogenic fungi in formalin-fixed tissues by immunofluorescence. Am J Clin Pathol 1969; 52: 420–432.
187. Wheat LJ, Slama TG, Zeckel ML. Histoplasmosis in the acquired immune deficiency syndrome. Am J Med 1985; 78: 203–210.
188. Goodwin RA, Shapiro JL, Thurman GH, Thurman SS, Des Prez RM. Disseminated histoplasmosis: clinical and pathologic correlations. Medicine (Baltimore) 1980; 59: 1–33.
189. Klatt EC, Cosgrove M, Meyer PR. Rapid diagnosis of disseminated histoplasmosis in tissues. Arch Pathol Lab Med 1986; 110: 1173–1175.
190. Reddy P, Gorelick DF, Brasher CA, Larsh H. Progressive disseminated histoplasmosis as seen in adults. Am J Med 1970; 48: 629–636.
191. Schwarz J, Salfelder K. Blastomycosis. A review of 152 cases. Curr Top Pathol 1977; 65: 165–200.
192. Kaplan W. Direct fluorescent antibody tests for the diagnosis of mycotic diseases. Ann Clin Lab Sci 1973; 3: 25–29.
193. Restrepo A, Robledo M, Giraldo R et al. The gamut of paracoccidioidomycosis. Am J Med 1976; 61: 33–42.
194. Salfelder K, Doehnert G, Doehnert A. Paracoccidioidomycosis: anatomic study with complete autopsies. Virchows Arch [A] 1969; 348: 51–76.
195. Pena CE. Deep mycotic infections in Colombia. A clinicopathologic study of 162 cases. Am J Clin Pathol 1967; 47: 505–520.
196. Kauffman CA, Tan JS. *Torulopsis glabrata* renal infection. Am J Med 1974; 57: 217–224.
197. Vordermark JS, Modarelli RO, Buck AS. *Torulopsis* pyelonephritis associated with papillary necrosis: a case report. J Urol 1980; 123: 96–97.
198. Krick JA, Stinson EB, Remington JS. *Nocardia* infection in heart transplant patients. Ann Intern Med 1975; 82: 18–26.
199. Murray JF, Finegold SM, Froman S, Will DW. The changing spectrum of nocardiosis. Am Rev Respir Dis 1961; 83: 315–330.
200. Parmentier JC, Vanladuyt HW, Prignotj J, Tanghe W. A case of disseminated nocardiosis. Br J Dis Chest 1968; 68: 46–51.
201. Emmons CW, Binford CH, Utz JP, Kwon-Chung KJ. Medical mycology, 3rd edn. Philadelphia: Lea & Febiger, 1977; 111.
202. Robboy SJ, Vickery AL. Tinctorial and morphologic properties distinguishing actinomycosis and nocardiosis. N Engl J Med 1970; 282: 593–596.
203. Frazier AR, Rosenow EC, Roberts GD. Nocardiosis. A review of 25 cases occurring during 24 months. Mayo Clin Proc 1975; 50: 657–663.
204. Ellis LR, Kenny GM, Nellans RD. Urogenital aspects of actinomycosis. J Urol 1979; 122: 132–133.
205. Anhalt M, Scott R. Primary unilateral renal actinomycosis: case report. J Urol 1970; 103: 126–129.

Protozoal infections

206. Sheehy TW, Reba RC. Complications of falciparum malaria and their treatment. Ann Intern Med 1967; 66: 807–809.
207. Boonpucknavig V, Sitprija V. Renal disease in acute *Plasmodium falciparum* infections in man. Kidney Int 1979; 16: 44–52.
208. Rosen S, Hano JE, Inman MM, Gilliland PF, Barry KG. The kidney in blackwater fever. Light and electron microscopic observations. Am J Clin Pathol 1968; 49: 358–370.
209. Sitprija V. Nephropathy in falciparum malaria. Kidney Int 1988; 34: 867–877.
210. Hendrickse RG, Adeniyi A. Quartan malarial nephrotic syndrome in children. Kidney Int 1979; 16: 64–74.
211. Gilles HM, Hendrickse RG. Nephrosis in Nigerian children. Role of *Plasmodium malariae*, and effect of antimalarial treatment. Br Med J 1963; 2: 27–31.
212. Kibukamusoke JW, Hutt MSR, Wilks NE. The nephrotic syndrome in Uganda and its association with quartan malaria. Q J Med 1967; 36: 393–408.
213. Houba V, Lambert PH, Voller A, Soyanwo MAO. Clinical and experimental investigation of immune complexes in malaria. Clin Immunol Immunopathol 1976; 6: 1–12.
214. Soothill JF, Hendrickse RG. Some immunological studies of nephrotic syndrome of Nigerian children. Lancet 1967; 2: 629–632.
215. Kibukamusoke JW, Hutt MSR. Histological features of the nephrotic syndrome associated with quartan malaria. J Clin Pathol 1967; 20: 117–123.
216. Hendrickse RG, Glasgow EF, Adeniyi A, White RHR, Edington GM, Houba V. Quartan malarial nephrotic syndrome. Collaborative clinicopathological study in Nigerian children. Lancet 1972; 1: 1143–1149.
217. Allison AC, Houba V, Hendrickse RG, de Petris S, Edington GM, Adeniya A. Immune complexes in the nephrotic syndrome of African children. Lancet 1969; 1: 1232–1238.
218. Houba V, Lambert PH. Immunological studies on tropical nephropathies. Adv Biosci 1974; 12: 617–629.
219. Houba V. Immunologic aspects of renal lesions associated with malaria. Kidney Int 1979; 16: 3–8.
220. Abdurrahman MB, Aikhionbare HA, Babaoye FA, Sathiakumar N, Narayana PT. Clinicopathological features of childhood nephrotic syndrome in Northern Nigeria. Q J Med 1990; 75: 563–576.
221. Morel-Maroger L, Saimot AG, Sloper JC et al. 'Tropical nephropathy' and 'Tropical extramembranous glomerulonephritis' of unknown aetiology in Senegal. Br Med J 1975; 1: 541–546.
222. Giglioli G. Malaria and renal disease with special reference to British Guiana. II: The effect of malarial eradication on the incidence of renal disease in British Guiana. Ann Trop Med Parisitol 1962; 56: 224–241.
223. Dutra M, Martinelli R, De Carvalho EM, Rodrigues

LE, Brito E, Rocha H. Renal involement in visceral leishmaniasis. Am J Kidney Dis 1985; 6: 22–27.
224. Shahin B, Papadopoulou ZL, Jenis EH. Congenital nephrotic syndrome associated with congenital toxoplasmosis. J Pediatr 1974; 85: 366–370.
225. Ginsburg BE, Wasserman J, Huldt G, Bergstrand A. Case of glomerulonephritis associated with acute toxoplasmosis. Br Med J 1974; 3: 664–665.
226. Couvreur J, Alison F, Boccon-Gibod L, Desmont G, Tournier G. Rein et toxoplasmoses. Ann Pédiatr (Paris) 1984; 31: 847–852.

Metazoal infestations

227. Naude JH. The natural history of ureteric bilharzia. Br J Urol 1984; 56: 599–601.
228. Andrade ZA, Andrade SG, Sadigursky M. Renal changes in patients with hepatosplenic schistosomiasis. Am J Trop Med Hyg 1971; 20: 77–83.
229. Andrade ZA, Rocha H. Schistosomal glomerulopathy. Kidney Int 1979; 16: 23–29.
230. Martinelli R, Noblat ACB, Brito E, Rocha H. *Schistosoma mansoni*-induced mesangiocapillary glomerulonephritis: influence of therapy. Kidney Int 1989; 35: 1227–1233.
231. Bout D, Santaro F, Capron A. Détection des immunocomplexes dans la bilharziose. Med Mal Infect 1975; 12: 631–636.
232. Rocha H, Cruz T, Brito E, Susin M. Renal involvement in patients with hepatosplenic *Schistosomiasis mansoni.* Am J Trop Med Hyg 1976; 25: 108–115.
233. Sobh MA, Moustafa FE, El-Housseini F, Basta MT, Deelder AM, Ghoniem MA. Schistosomal specific nephropathy leading to end-stage renal failure. Kidney Int 1987; 31: 1006–1011.
234. Azevedo LS, De Paula FJ, Ianhez LE, Saldanha LB, Sabbaga E. Renal transplantation and *Schistosomiasis mansoni.* Transplantation 1987; 44: 795–798.
235. Falcão HA, Gould DB. Immune complex nephropathy in schistosomiasis. Ann Intern Med 1975; 83: 148–154.
236. Houba V. Experimental renal disease due to schistosomiasis. Kidney Int 1979; 16: 30–43.
237. Mariearty PL, Brito E. Elution of renal antischistoma antibodies in human *Schistosomiasis mansoni.* Am J Trop Med Hyg 1977; 26: 717–722.
238. Von Lichtenberg F, Bawden MP, Shealey SH. Origin of circulating antigen from the schistosome gut: an immunofluorescent study. Am J Trop Med Hyg 1974; 23: 1088–1091.
239. Omer HO, Wahab SMA. Secondary amyloidosis due to *Schistosoma mansoni* infection. Br Med J 1976; 1: 375–377.
240. Barsoum RS, Bassily S, Soliman MM, Ramzy MF, Milad M, Hassaballa AM. Renal amyloidosis and schistosomiasis. Trans R Soc Trop Med Hyg 1979; 73: 367–374.
241. Ngu JL, Chatelanat F, Leke R, Ndumbe P, Youmbissi J. Nephropathy in Cameroon: evidence for filarial derived immune-complex pathogenesis in some cases. Clin Nephrol 1985; 24: 128–134.
242. Lal RB, Paranjape RS, Briles DE, Nutman TB, Ottesen EA. Circulating parasite antigen(s) in lymphatic filariasis: use of monoclonal antibodies to phosphocholine for immunodiagnosis. J Immunol 1987; 138: 3454–3460.
243. Sparks AK, Connor DH, Neafie RC. Echinococcosis. In: Binford CH, Connor DH eds. Pathology of tropical and extraordinary diseases. Washington: Armed Forces Institute of Pathology, 1976; 2: 530–533.
244. Ferreira AM, Rangel AJR. Hydatid cyst of the kidney: eight cases. Br J Urol 1979; 51: 345–348.
245. Kottasz S, Koranyi E. Echinococcosis of the kidney. Int Urol Nephrol 1984; 16: 199–209.
246. Vialtel P, Cheais F, Desgeorges P, Couderc P, Micouin C, Cordonnier D. Membranous nephropathy associated with hydatid disease. N Engl J Med 1961; 304: 610–611.
247. Kung'u A. Glomerulonephritis following chemotherapy of hydatid disease with mebendazole. East Afr Med J 1982; 59: 404–409.

12

K. A. Porter

Tubulointerstitial disease (interstitial nephritis)

INTRODUCTION

The terms 'tubulointerstitial disease', 'interstitial nephritis' and 'tubulointerstitial nephritis' are frequently used to describe those situations in which the predominant morphological changes occur in the renal interstitium and tubules. The interstitium contains inflammatory cells and is oedematous or fibrotic; there is also usually a variable degree of accompanying tubular necrosis, atrophy or loss.

The traditional classification of tubulointerstitial disease is into acute and chronic forms; these forms are then subdivided into primary and secondary. In primary interstitial disease any glomerular damage appears to be the result of the tubulointerstitial changes; when the term interstitial nephritis is used without any further qualification it is the primary condition that is meant. Commonly, tubulointerstitial disease is not primary but secondary to damage elsewhere.

The main difficulty with this traditional, predominantly histological, classification is that it does not specifically recognize the wide variety of aetiological agents and diverse mechanisms that produce very similar morphological patterns of tubulointerstitial injury. To overcome the problem, the World Health Organization (WHO) Collaborating Centre for the Histological Classification of Renal Diseases proposed a new classification[1] that takes into account aetiological, pathogenetic and clinical features in addition to the histology. The WHO classification (Table 12.1) is used in this chapter.

In approximately a third of the patients with acute tubulointerstitial nephritis and in a smaller number of cases of chronic tubulointerstitial disease no cause can be identified and they do not seem to fit into any of the recognized categories of tubulointerstitial nephritis. The lesions are granulomatous in some of these cases.

Inflammation of the interstitium affects renal function and may lead to renal failure.

TUBULOINTERSTITIAL DISEASE CAUSED BY INFECTION

Infection is an important cause of tubulointerstitial disease. Renal involvement may take four forms:

1. *Acute infectious tubulointerstitial nephritis*, which is brought about by direct invasion of the renal parenchyma by organisms and their subsequent proliferation within the kidney.
2. *Acute tubulointerstitial nephritis associated with systemic infection* but not caused directly by organisms invading the kidneys.
3. *Chronic infectious tubulointerstitial nephritis.*
4. *Specific renal infections* such as tuberculosis and leprosy.

ACUTE INFECTIOUS TUBULOINTERSTITIAL NEPHRITIS

The use of the term 'acute' indicates the rapidity of the onset of this form of tubulointerstitial nephritis rather than the character of the inflammatory reaction. Included under the heading are acute infections by bacteria, fungi and viruses.

Bacterial infections known to cause acute tubulointerstitial nephritis include leptospirosis, brucellosis and Legionnaires' disease. These conditions are described from page 390 onwards. However the commonest renal infection is by one of the particular strains of *Escherichia coli* which produce acute pyelonephritis.

Acute pyelonephritis (acute bacterial tubulointerstitial nephritis)

Acute pyelonephritis is a common non-specific bacterial infection of the kidneys which affects the pelvis, the calyces and the renal parenchyma. It is usually part of a generalized urinary tract infection. Acute pyelonephritis occurs some 10 times more frequently in females than in males, and is particularly often seen in childhood and during pregnancy. Most first attacks of acute pyelonephritis are caused by *Escherichia coli.* There are many serotypes of this organism, but only about 5% are frequent causes of infection of the urinary tract: these 5% of serotypes account for some 75% of such infections. Other organisms that are occasionally responsible, particularly in cases of recurrent pyelonephritis, include species

Table 12.1 Classification of tubulointerstitial diseases (interstitial nephritis)

- **Infection**
  - *Acute infectious tubulointerstitial nephritis*
    - Acute bacterial (acute pyelonephritis)
    - Fungal
    - Viral
  - *Acute tubulointerstitial nephritis associated with systemic infection*
    - Group A streptococcal infection
    - Diphtheria
    - Toxoplasmosis
    - Legionnaires' disease
    - Brucellosis
    - Viral infection
    - Other variants
  - *Chronic infectious tubulointerstitial nephritis (chronic pyelonephritis)*
    - Non-obstructive reflux-associated chronic pyelonephritis
    - Other variants
    - Chronic obstructive pyelonephritis
    - Xanthogranulomatous pyelonephritis
    - Malakoplakia
    - Megalocytic interstitial nephritis
  - *Specific renal infection*
    - Tuberculosis
    - Leprosy
    - Syphilis
    - Epidemic haemorrhagic fever
    - Other variants
- **Drug-induced tubulointerstitial nephritis**
  - *Acute drug-induced tubulotoxic injury*
    - Direct
    - Indirect
  - *Drug-induced hypersensitivity tubulointerstitial nephritis*
  - *Chronic drug-induced tubulointerstitial nephritis*
    - Analgesic nephropathy
    - Lithium nephropathy
    - Other, e.g. chloroethyl-cyclohexyl nitrosourea (lomustine)
- **Tubulointerstitial nephritis associated with immune disorders**
  - *Induced by antibodies reacting with tubular antigens*
    - Antiglomerular-basement-membrane glomerulonephritis or Goodpasture's syndrome
    - Immune complex glomerulonephritis
    - Drugs
    - Idiopathic
    - Renal allografts
  - *Induced by autologous or exogenous antigen–antibody complexes*
    - Systemic lupus erythematosus
    - Mixed cryoglobulinaemia
    - Bacterial immune complex glomerulonephritis
    - Sjøgren's syndrome
    - Hypocomplementaemic glomerulonephritis with vasculitis
    - Renal allografts
  - *Induced by, or associated with, cell-mediated hypersensitivity*
    - Bacterial, viral, or parasitic infection, drugs, chemicals
  - *Induced by immediate (IgE-type) hypersensitivity*
    - Drugs, parasitic infection(?)
- **Obstructive uropathy**
  - Without infection (hydronephrosis)
  - With infection
  - Pyonephrosis
- **Vesicoureteral reflux associated nephropathy (reflux nephropathy)**
- **Tubulointerstitial nephritis associated with papillary necrosis**
  - Diabetes mellitus
  - Obstructive uropathy
  - Analgesic nephropathy
  - Sickle cell disease nephropathy
  - Haemorrhagic necrosis of papillae in the newborn
  - Other variants (e.g. vascular disease, tuberculosis)
- **Heavy metal-induced tubular and tubulointerstitial lesions**
  - Lead nephropathy
  - Mercury nephropathy
  - Cisplatin nephropathy
  - Cadmium nephropathy
  - Nephropathy induced by other heavy metals (gold, silver, copper, iron)
- **Acute tubular injury/necrosis**
  - Toxic
  - Ischaemic
  - Severe crushing injury
  - Abortion
  - Extensive burn injury
  - Shock
  - Septicaemia
  - Other variants
  - Incompatible blood transfusion
  - Myoglobulinuria
- **Tubular and tubulointerstitial nephropathy caused by metabolic disturbances**
  - Hypercalcaemic nephropathy
  - Urate nephropathy
  - Oxalate nephropathy
  - Cystinosis
  - Hypokalaemic nephropathy
  - Vacuolar change (osmotic nephropathy)
  - Glycogen deposition (as in glycogenosis or diabetes mellitus)
  - Fatty changes
  - Hyaline droplet degeneration
  - Bile pigment deposition (bile nephrosis)
  - Copper deposition (Wilson's disease)
  - Iron deposition
- **Hereditary renal tubulointerstitial disorders**
  - Medullary cystic disease (juvenile nephronophthisis)
  - Familial interstitial nephritis of unknown aetiological basis
  - Alport's syndrome
- **Tubulointerstitial nephritis associated with neoplastic disorders**
  - Plasma cell dyscrasias
    - Myeloma kidney
    - Light-chain nephropathy
  - Mixed IgG–IgM cryoglobulinaemia
  - Waldenström's macroglobulinaemia
  - Leukaemic and lymphomatous infiltration
- **Tubulointerstitial lesions in glomerular and vascular diseases**
  - Acute and chronic glomerular diseases
  - Ischaemic atrophy
  - End-stage kidney
- **Miscellaneous disorders**
  - Radiation nephritis
  - Balkan endemic nephropathy
  - Sarcoid granulomatous nephropathy
  - Tubulointerstitial nephritis of unknown aetiological basis (idiopathic)
    - Acute idiopathic tubulointerstitial nephritis
    - Idiopathic granulomatous tubulointerstitial nephritis
    - Chronic idiopathic tubulointerstitial nephritis

Reproduced by permission from: Churg J, Cotran RS, Sinniah R, Sakaguchi H, Sobin LH. Renal disease. Classification and atlas of tubulo-interstitial diseases. New York: Igaku-Shoin, 1985; 2.

of other Enterobacteriaceae (particularly species of *Klebsiella* and *Proteus*), *Streptococcus faecalis*, *Staphylococcus* species and, rarely, *Pseudomonas aeruginosa* and some other bacteria. The organisms are the same as those responsible for cystitis; they are described on page 706. Recurrent attacks of acute pyelonephritis may occur; these are usually reinfections caused by different serotypes of *E. coli*. Bacterial invasion of the kidneys occurs by ascent from the bladder or occasionally by haematogenous spread from other foci.

Acute pyelonephritis is commoner in patients with obstructive lesions of the urinary tract. Any congenital or acquired lesion that causes obstruction and stasis, even of quite short duration, is likely to increase the liability to infection or to exacerbate an infection that is already established. The obstruction may be caused by such conditions as benign or malignant enlargement of the prostate, congenital valve-like folds in the prostatic part of the urethra, calculi, carcinoma of the uterine cervix involving the lower end of one or both ureters, and retroperitoneal fibrosis. Atony of the bladder – for instance, accompanying paraplegia – and vesicoureteric reflux also predispose to acute pyelonephritis. Pregnancy is a cause of urinary obstruction with atonia and dilatation of the ureters. The special risks of introducing infection by catheterization and by the use of indwelling catheters are also well known.

Acute pyelonephritis ranges in severity from a few scattered foci of inflammation or abscess formation to widespread bilateral suppuration.

Clinical features

The onset of acute pyelonephritis is usually abrupt with fever, pain in the loins, dysuria and increased frequency of urination. As the attack develops rigors occur. The urine contains pus cells, casts formed of pus cells, and bacteria, the latter in numbers usually greater than 100 000 per millilitre (see p. 706). The pus cell casts distinguish between cystitis and pyelonephritis; they indicate that inflammation is occurring in the kidney. There is a leucocytosis. Renal function may be temporarily abnormal.

Serology

The level of C3 reactive protein in the serum is raised when the kidney is infected; it is normal if the infection is confined to the lower urinary tract.[2] There is a rapid IgM antibody response following a first attack of acute pyelonephritis; this is followed by a fall to normal levels after 2–3 months. If recurrent attacks occur IgG antibodies appear.

Renal changes

Gross appearance of the kidneys In severe cases of acute pyelonephritis both kidneys are often involved. They are enlarged. Small, yellow abscesses, each with a hyperaemic rim, may be seen on the subcapsular surface (Fig. 12.1). When the kidneys are cut the abscesses are present in both cortex and medulla, but principally in the cortex. They appear round or wedge shaped, the apex pointing to the medulla. The medulla is usually patterned with radial, yellow streaks of suppuration. The mucosa of the pelvis is thickened and congested, and often coated with purulent exudate. If there is an obstruction to the outflow of urine the calyces are widened and the pelvis and ureter dilated.

Light microscopy Where there are abscesses there is extensive destruction of tubules, the proximal convoluted segment being particularly involved. The interstitium locally is densely packed with neutrophil granulocytes and there is surrounding oedema. The cellular infiltrate also includes some lymphocytes, plasma cells, macrophages and, occasionally, eosinophils. The collecting tubules and ducts of Bellini draining the infected areas are filled with neutrophil granulocytes; this exudate acounts for the yellow streaks seen with the naked eye. Microorganisms may sometimes be seen in appropriately stained sections. The glomeruli are usually normal. Between the abscesses there are large areas of normal parenchyma. The blood vessels of the pelvis and calyces are dilated and engorged, and the mucosa is infiltrated with neutrophil granulocytes.

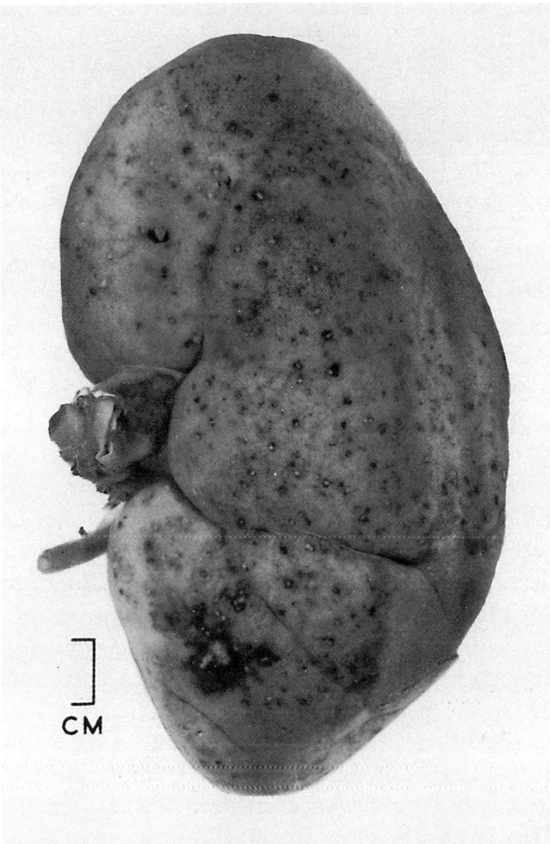

Fig. 12.1 Acute pyelonephritis. The kidney is enlarged. There are small abscesses, each with a hyperaemic rim, on the subcapsular surface.

Complications

Papillary necrosis may complicate severe acute pyelonephritis. It is particularly common in diabetes mellitus; 25% of diabetic patients with acute pyelonephritis develop papillary necrosis (see p. 473).[3]

Occasionally in severe acute pyelonephritis the suppurative lesions may develop into a multilocular abscess, or a honeycombed cluster of small abscesses, which are referred to as a ***renal carbuncle***. Carbuncles are usually unilateral; rarely they rupture through the capsule to produce a perinephric abscess.

Pyonephrosis (see p. 472) may occur when there is severe obstruction to the outflow of urine. Purulent exudate fills the dilated renal pelvis, calyces and ureter. The kidney is sometimes eventually converted into a bag of pus.

Emphysematous pyelonephritis (see p. 438) is a rare complication most often seen in elderly women with diabetes mellitus. The acute pyelonephritis is associated with necrosis of the renal parenchyma and gas formation produced by fermentation of the dead tissue by the urinary pathogen, usually *E. coli*.

Prognosis

Primary non-obstructive acute pyelonephritis In primary non-obstructive acute pyelonephritis appropriate antibiotic treatment is usually curative, but if the infection is not controlled the papilla is gradually destroyed by the inflammatory process and as the scar contracts the calyx becomes club shaped. The small cortical abscesses may spread in the affected lobes of the kidney but eventually heal with the formation of a depressed scar. A recent report suggests that as many as one-third of kidneys affected by primary non-obstructive acute pyelonephritis progress to cortical scars.[4]

Acute pyelonephritis tends to recur; in one series recurrence of infection was found in 33 cases out of 93.[5] In school children 90% of the recurrences are infections with a different serological type of *E. coli* or with a different species of organism. Recurrence occurs within 1 year of treatment in half the cases.[6]

Acute pyelonephritis associated with obstruction When there is obstruction, both failure to eradicate the infection and recurrence are more frequent, and progressive renal damage occurs.[7]

Pathogenesis

Theoretically, organisms may reach the kidneys by the blood stream, or by ascending the lumen of the ureters, or by lymphatic spread from the intestines or from the lower parts of the urinary tract. There is no evidence to support the concept of lymphatic spread. In contrast, there is plenty of evidence that under very special circumstances the kidneys can be attacked by blood-borne bacteria. In the human, for example, the kidneys may become infected in the course of a blood stream infection by *Staphylococcus aureus*; in animals, species of *Pseudomonas* may infect normal kidneys with unobstructed urinary outflow. However, *E. coli*, the organism that is most commonly found in the urine of patients experiencing a first attack of acute pyelonephritis, does not produce lesions in normal kidneys when injected intravenously into animals: renal infection will occur in the course of such experiments only if the ureter has previously been partly obstructed[8] or if the renal vein has been constricted.[9] These experimental findings are mirrored by the observations in man, for escherichial bacteriaemia seems to be the source of renal infection only in those people who have some obstructive lesion of the urinary tract. It seems probable, therefore, that blood-borne infection accounts for only a small proportion of cases of acute pyelonephritis.

The ascending route, by the ureter from the bladder, is now accepted as the way in which the kidneys are most commonly infected. Infection of the urine in the bladder is frequent, and often asymptomatic, occurring at some time during school life in 5% of girls and in 0.03% of boys (see p. 707).[10] The bacteria that cause spontaneous infection of the urinary tract come from the patient's faeces; the representation of serotypes of the escherichia in infections of the bladder is in proportion to their prevalence in faeces (see p. 705).[11] These organisms commonly soil the vulva and occasionally establish themselves in the vaginal introitus, in the outer part of the urethra and on the area immediately around the urethral orifice.[12] At the end of urination, closure of the urethra, which takes place from before backwards, results in the return to the bladder of a minute quantity of urine that has been contaminated by bacteria in the urethra. The shortness of the female urethra probably accounts for the greater frequency of such contamination of the bladder in girls and women than in boys and men. The use of catheters or other instruments increases the chances of transferring infection from the urethra to the bladder.[13]

Ascent of organisms from the bladder to the kidneys is aided by vesicoureteric reflux (see p. 685). In a normal person the vesicoureteric valve mechanism is competent and prevents reflux of urine into the ureters during urination (see p. 685).[14] In individuals with primary or secondary vesicoureteric reflux and an infected bladder, contaminated urine is forced up the ureter from the bladder to the pelvis and calyces.[15] Experiments have shown that once the organisms are in the pelvis they may reach the parenchyma of the kidney either through the tubules or by direct invasion of the interstitium.[16] Their entry is greatly facilitated by the phenomenon of *intrarenal or calicotubular reflux*, by which, during urination, urine flows back up the ducts of Bellini at the tips of one or more of the papillae and then spreads outwards along the collecting tubules. Intrarenal reflux occurs in only the compound papillae which constitute 12% of the total papillae in the kidney; 80% of the compound papillae are situated in the upper pole (see p. 4). The compound papillae (Fig.12.2) are the result of fusion of two or three

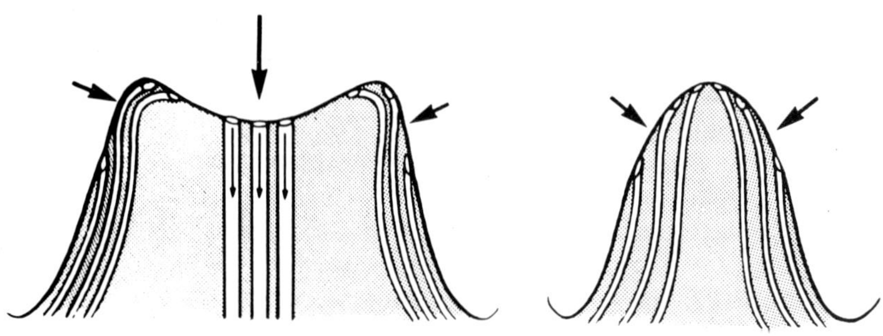

Fig. 12.2 Diagram of compound papilla (left) and simple papilla (right). The orifices of the ducts of Bellini are gaping in the compound papilla and slit-like in the simple papilla.
Reproduced by permission from: Ransley PG. Urol Res 1977; 5: 61 (Fig. 10)

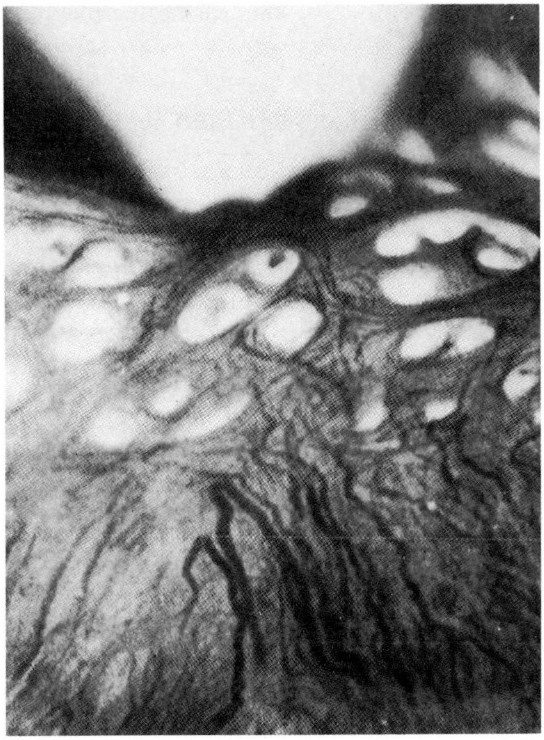

Fig. 12.3 Human compound papilla with prominent gaping openings of ducts of Bellini.
× 25
Reproduced by permission from: Ransley PG, Risdon RA. Urol Res 1975; 3: 111(Fig. 1)

pyramids; the area cribrosa covering them is flattened or concave and the orifices of the ducts of Bellini are round or oval (Fig.12.3). It seems probable that when the pressure within the renal pelvis rises, the slit-like orifices of the single papillae close and prevent entry of urine, while the gaping mouths of the ducts of Bellini in the compound papillae fail to close and allow the urine to enter.[17] Intrarenal reflux is commonest in children with severe grades of vesicoureteric reflux (Fig.12.4).[18]

The types of *E. coli* that cause the first attack of acute pyelonephritis possess a wide range of properties that probably assist them to invade the kidneys. These include a short generation time in urine and the ability to resist the bactericidal effect of serum, produce haemolysin and attach to the epithelial cells of the urinary tract. The capacity to firmly adhere to the epithelium by means of an adhesin appears to be of major importance.

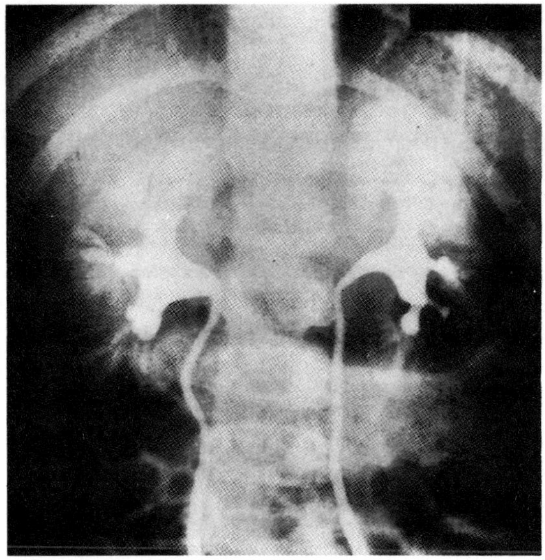

Fig. 12.4 Micturating cystogram in a child. There is extensive reflux throughout the upper third of both kidneys and in scattered small segments in the right middle and lower zones and at the left lower pole.
Reproduced by permission of the late Dr John Hodson formerly of Department of Radiology, Memorial University of Newfoundland.

The adhesin is associated with certain types of fimbriae or pili (long rigid protein structures, 6–7 nm in diameter, which extend for considerable distances from the surface of the bacterium like spokes radiating from the hub of a wheel).[19] For example, in P-fimbriated strains of *E. coli* the adhesin, which is a small peptide confined to the tip of the fimbriae, recognizes and specifically binds to a receptor structure, α-galactosyl-1,4-β-galactose, which is present on the cell membrane of human urinary tract epithelium. This receptor disaccharide sequence is related to the blood group P antigen system on membrane glycolipids. Other fimbriated strains of *E. coli* bind to a selected glycoprotein oligosaccharide rich in mannose residues, or to Dr^a blood group antigen. Since bacteria can each carry between 10 and 20 adhesin-tipped fimbriae, they are well equipped to probe the urinary tract epithelium for receptor molecules.[19] Yet other strains have adhesive properties unrelated to the presence of fimbriae.[20,21] Clinical studies and experiments in mice and primates indicate that P-fimbrae are probably essential if a strain of *E. coli* is to produce pyelonephritis in a woman with an anatomically normal urinary tract.[19] Women with recurrent urinary tract infections have fewer soluble adhesin-receptor compounds in their mucosal secretions (i.e. they are non-secretors) and their uroepithelium does not express A, B and H blood group oligosaccharides. The lack of receptor compounds in their secretions means that the adhesin on the invading bacterium is not blocked before attaching to an epithelial receptor; the failure to express blood group substances means that the less prominent adhesin-receptor oligosaccharides are not covered by the A, B and H oligosaccharides and are more readily accessible.[22] Once attached to the epithelium, the bacteria produce a covering polysaccharide capsule termed the glycocalyx which is resistant to antibiotics and host defences.[20]

This understanding of the properties of the strains of *E. coli* that cause acute pyelonephritis has encouraged attempts to prepare a vaccine against pyelonephritis based upon stimulating immunity to a combination of adhesin, K polysaccharide and modified haemolysin antigen.

The normal bacterial flora of the urogenital tract has the ability to inhibit the growth of *E. coli* and competitively exclude its attachment to the urinary epithelium. Preliminary studies suggest that this property can be exploited and urinary tract infections prevented in humans by intravaginal implantation of carefully selected strains of lactobacilli.[23]

Women of blood groups AB and B who are non-secretors of blood group substances have been shown to be particularly susceptible to urinary tract infections because, as explained earlier, the adhesin receptors on their uroepithelium are not obscured by blood group oligosaccharides.[22]

The arrival of bacteria in the renal tubules and interstitium is followed by an intense acute inflammatory reaction that results in destruction of tissue. Experimental evidence suggests that the acute inflammatory response soon changes to a lymphocytic one[16] and that specific antibody is formed against the organisms involved, both by lymphoid cells in the kidney itself and by those in the lymphoid tissues elsewhere.[24] Antibody to the *E. coli* P fimbriae is synthesized locally in the kidney. Perhaps this antibody prevents further bacterial adherence to the kidney and limits the attack of pyelonephritis.[25] In most cases the organisms are killed and healing follows.

Acute fungal tubulointerstitial nephritis

Fungal infection of the urinary tract is rare; it is most commonly seen in patients whose immune system is in some way compromised. In most cases the kidneys are involved by blood-borne spread from an extrarenal focus of infection. The fungi most commonly responsible are yeasts of the genus *Candida*; other species only rarely invade the kidney. An acute tubulointerstitial nephritis may be induced with clinical findings indistinguishable from those of acute bacterial pyelonephritis. The diagnosis of acute fungal tubulointerstitial nephritis is made by demonstrating the fungi with the Gomori (Grocott) methenamine silver stain. Fungal infections of the kidney are discussed on pages 405–415.

Acute viral tubulointerstitial nephritis

An acute interstitial nephritis can be caused by viruses belonging to the Hantavirus genus[1] in the course of haemorrhagic fever with renal syndrome. Severe tubulointerstitial nephritis has also been associated with BK-type polyomavirus infection.[26] Viral infections of the kidney are discussed on pages 393–404.

Emphysematous pyelonephritis[27,28]

Rarely acute pyelonephritis will progress to renal necrosis with gas formation. This condition is called emphysematous pyelonephritis. The necrotic tissue has been infected by gas-forming urinary pathogens, particularly *Escherichia coli. Clostridium welchii* plays no part in this disease. Urine and blood cultures often reveal the responsible organisms.

Clinical features

Emphysematous pyelonephritis is commonest in elderly women with diabetes mellitus, persistent urinary infection and renal vascular disease. There is usually obstruction to urinary outflow. The presenting signs and symptoms are those of acute pyelonephritis with severe systemic effects (see p. 434). The gas can be demonstrated on plain abdominal X-ray and by the use of tomography.

Renal changes

The disease is usually unilateral; bilateral involvement is rare. There is severe acute pyelonephritis (see p. 434) with areas of necrosis of the kidney in half the patients, and multiple cortical abscesses in about a third. Obstructive chronic pyelonephritis (see p. 444) may also be present. Papillary necrosis (see p. 473) and intrarenal arterial and venous thrombi are each present in approximately 20% of the patients. In about a fifth of the patients the entire kidney appears necrotic.

Prognosis

Emphysematous pyelonephritis is a potentially fatal condition. Massive antibiotic treatment together with correction of fluid and electrolyte balance and of any hyperglycaemia is essential but alone is still associated with a mortality of over 70%. It must be combined with immediate nephrectomy. Combined medical and surgical treatment results in a survival rate of approximately 90%.

Pathogenesis

E. coli is the causative organism in 70% of cases. Less commonly *Klebsiella pneumoniae, Aerobacter aerogenes* or *Proteus mirabilis* is responsible. Even *Candida albicans* has been implicated.[29] These organisms use the necrotic renal tissue as a substrate for the production of hydrogen and carbon dioxide.

ACUTE TUBULOINTERSTITIAL NEPHRITIS ASSOCIATED WITH SYSTEMIC INFECTION

Occasionally cases are reported in which acute interstitial nephritis is associated with systemic infection but cannot be readily ascribed to invasion of the kidneys by an organism or to drugs given to treat the infection. It was, of course, the changes in the kidneys of just such cases associated with diphtherial and streptococcal infections that caused William Councilman to introduce the term 'acute interstitial nephritis' in 1898.[30] A wide range of organisms can cause the associated systemic infection.[31]

The tubulointerstitial changes in these cases closely resemble the lesions seen in acute drug-induced hypersensitivity tubulointerstitial nephritis (see p. 454).

The mechanisms involved in the pathogenesis of this form of acute tubulointerstitial nephritis are unknown, but a hypersensitivity reaction is suspected.

CHRONIC PYELONEPHRITIS (CHRONIC INFECTIOUS TUBULOINTERSTITIAL NEPHRITIS)

Chronic pyelonephritis is the late stage of bacterial infection of the kidney. It is the cause of renal failure in up to 25% of children and young adults requiring dialysis or renal transplantation.[32] In most cases of chronic pyelonephritis there is an obvious obstruction of the urinary tract – *obstructive chronic pyelonephritis*. The small proportion of cases in which there is little or no evident obstruction – *non-obstructive chronic pyelonephritis* – is almost always associated with vesicoureteric reflux.

Non-obstructive chronic pyelonephritis (reflux nephropathy)

This is a relatively uncommon disease. In the absence of urinary tract obstruction it is usual for acute pyelonephritis to heal completely. In some cases, however, there is persistence of a significant degree of bacteriuria or recurrence of infection; very rarely there is progressive renal deterioration, ending in uraemia and, if dialysis or renal transplantation is not undertaken, death. In a large necropsy study the incidence of non-obstructive chronic pyelonephritis was found to be only 0.23%; the patient's death had been associated with renal failure in less than half of these cases.[33]

However, non-obstructive chronic pyelonephritis is found in 12–20% of children investigated for persistent urinary infection.

Vesicoureteric reflux is present in the majority of children with non-obstructive chronic pyelonephritis. In one important study of 400 children under the age of 13 years, 86% of those with chronic non-obstructive pyelonephritis also had reflux.[34] In contrast, only about 37% of adults with non-obstructive chronic pyelonephritis have reflux.[35] It is known that in children vesicoureteric reflux tends to cease spontaneously after some years;[36] this might account for its absence in many adults and some children with non-obstructive chronic pyelonephritis. Even in the absence of vesicoureteric reflux virulent bacteria may be able to reach the kidney if ureteral peristalsis is paralysed by the effect of the organism's endotoxins.[37]

Because non-obstructive chronic pyelonephritis is so often associated with vesicoureteric reflux, the alternative term *reflux nephropathy* is now frequently used. If this is done it should be remembered that present evidence indicates that vesicoureteric reflux on its own will not cause non-obstructive chronic pyelonephritis. It has to be combined with urinary infection if renal scarring is to occur. Only in animals with bladder neck obstruction has vesicoureteric reflux with sterile urine been shown to cause renal damage (see p. 472).

Non-obstructive chronic pyelonephritis affects females more often than males and may be found at any age. It is in childhood that scar formation is observed radiologically, usually before the age of 6 years.[38] The formation of new scars is rarely observed in adults except in cases in which there is very severe vesicoureteric reflux.

Clinical features

Non-obstructive chronic pyelonephritis produces no direct symptoms. The only physical abnormalities are those attributable to renal insufficiency (see p. 127) or high blood pressure (see p. 306). Approximately 25% of patients will have had symptoms suggestive of a urinary tract disorder at some time in the past.

Proteinuria is variable in amount and usually not heavy except in patients with malignant hypertension or in those with focal segmental glomerulosclerosis (see p. 204). In the latter patients the proteinuria may be sufficiently great to cause a nephrotic syndrome. Bacteriuria is usually, but not always, present. Excretion of leucocytes in the urine can generally be provoked by the intravenous administration of a pyrogen,[39] but this result is not pathognomonic of chronic pyelonephritis.

Radiological examination is the most helpful aid to diagnosis. An intravenous pyelogram (urogram) shows localized narrowing of the renal substance, with distortion, blunting or loss of the related papilla.[40] Vesicoureteric reflux is detected by micturating cystourography (voiding cystourethrography).[14]

Renal changes

Gross appearance of the kidneys The affected kidney is reduced in size. When the disease is bilateral, which is slightly more common, the two kidneys are characteristically involved unequally (Fig. 12.5). The reduction in size may be very marked, particularly when the disease is unilateral. The capsule is adherent and the subcapsular surface is deformed by a variable number of coarse, rather flattened scars, most commonly situated at the poles of the kidneys. Between the scars the surface of the kidneys may be smooth or finely granular. Each scar lies immediately over a dilated and deformed calyx, the renal parenchyma in the affected area being reduced to a few millimetres. The relation of the scars of non-obstructive chronic pyelonephritis to dilated calyces distinguishes them from vascular scars[41] and accounts for their characteristic pyelographic appearance.[40] In keeping with the radiological findings, the papillae in the scarred areas are retracted, distorted and blunted. Occasionally, the pyramid adjacent to the scar has completely disappeared. Some scars are so extensive that they must represent destruction of tissue amounting to most of a renal pole. The epithelium of the pelvis is thickened and granular.

Light microscopy

Changes in the pyelonephritic areas. In the scars the damage to the tubules is often disproportion-

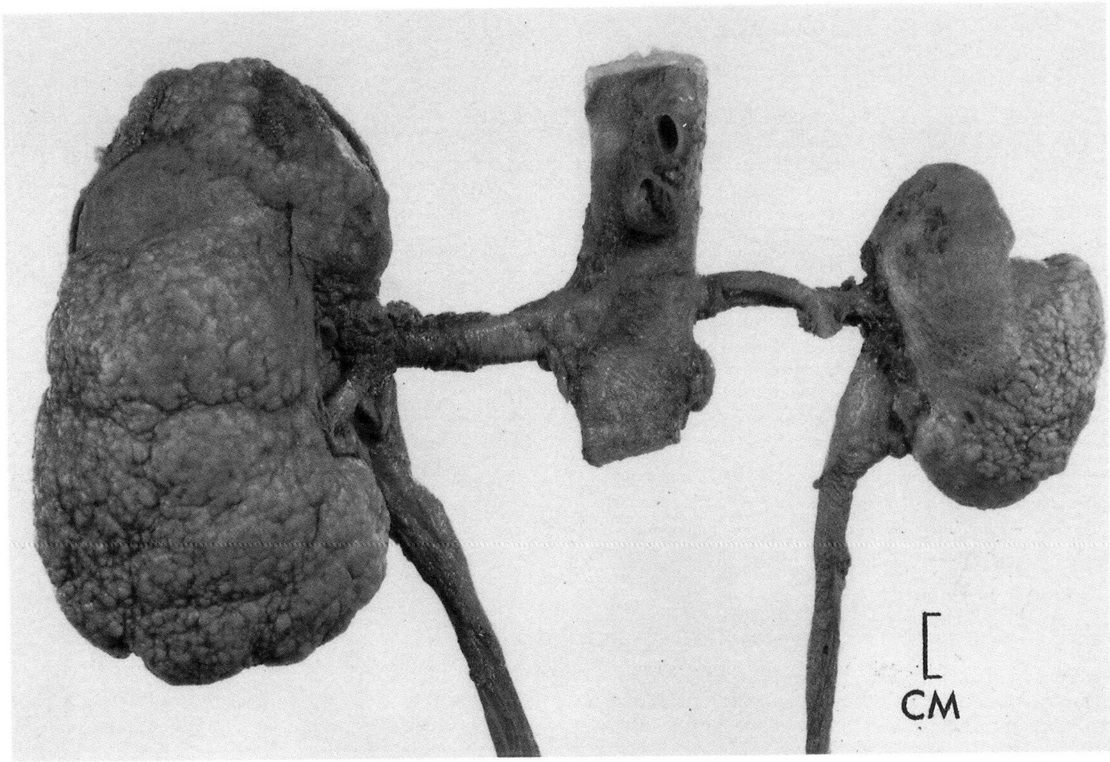

Fig. 12.5 Bilateral non-obstructive chronic pyelonephritis. Characteristically, one kidney is more affected than the other. There is an area of gross scarring of the parenchyma at the upper pole of the more severely damaged (smaller) kidney. The granularity of both kidneys is a feature sometimes seen in chronic pyelonephritis

ately greater than that to glomeruli. Many of the tubules are completely destroyed and have disappeared. The surviving tubules are atrophic and lined by flattened epithelium; they contain homo geneous eosinophilic casts (Fig. 12.6). Often large areas of the histological sections are filled with such tubules; this may give a picture that has been likened to that of thyroid tissue. Many of the atrophic tubules consist of blind, sequestered segments.[42] Neutrophil granulocytes may be present in the lumen of some of the tubules. Occasionally casts composed of basophilic granular material, nuclear debris and cholesterol clefts, are found.

The glomeruli may show few changes. Frequently, however, collagen is laid down, either external or internal to Bowman's capsule; when external to the capsule the process is referred to as *periglomerular fibrosis* (Fig. 12.7). Less commonly, focal segmental glomerulosclerosis and hyalinosis and fibrin caps are found. In some pyelonephritic areas the glomeruli are obsolete and converted into small, acellular, eosinophilic spheres. Occasionally some of the glomeruli show segmental mesangial cell proliferation and an increase in the amount of mesangial matrix. Because of the destruction of tubules the glomeruli lie much closer to one another than is normal (Fig.12.6).

Interstitial fibrosis is common. Often the interstitium is densely infiltrated with lymphocytes and plasma cells, and sometimes with eosinophils also; occasionally there are lymphoid follicles. Cellular infiltration is least in cases of dense fibrosis and obsolescence and loss of glomeruli. Tamm–Horsfall protein may be present in the interstitium; there may be a surrounding mononuclear cellular reaction.

In many instances there is fibrous intimal thickening of the arterioles and arteries (Fig. 12.8).

The papilla is usually indistinguishable as a histological anatomical feature. The dilated calyx

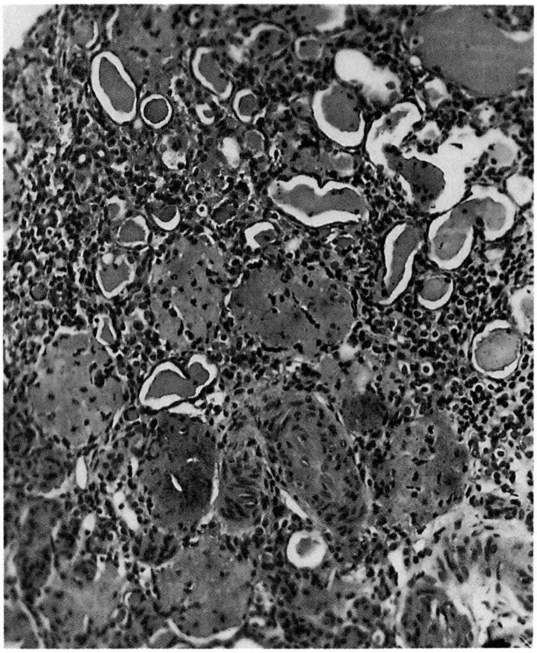

Fig. 12.6 Non-obstructive chronic pyelonephritis. Scar containing small obsolete glomeruli, atrophic tubules with homogeneous eosinophilic casts and an interstitial accumulation of lymphocytes. Haematoxylin-eosin × 160

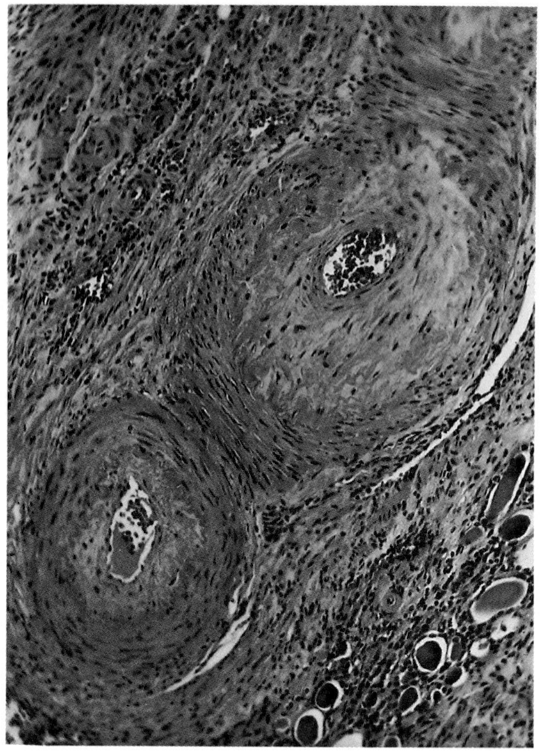

Fig. 12.8 Non-obstructive chronic pyelonephritis. The arteries show marked fibrous intimal thickening. Van Gieson-elastic × 100

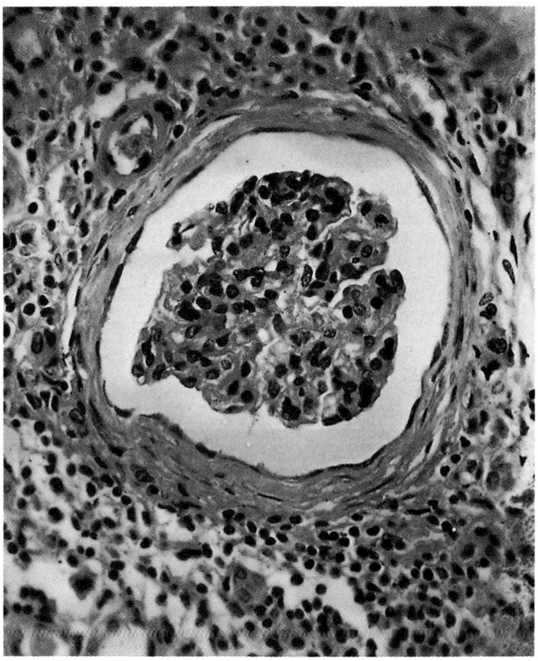

Fig. 12.7 Non-obstructive chronic pyelonephritis. Periglomerular fibrosis. Haematoxylin-eosin × 320

is lined by thickened epithelium, beneath which are large numbers of chronic inflammatory cells. Lymphoid follicles may be present. Neutrophil granulocytes are often numerous if there is active infection.

The cortical and medullary changes are non-specific. Only when they are combined with pelvi-calyceal deformation, and there is in addition evidence of bacterial infection, is it permissible for the diagnosis of non-obstructive chronic pyelonephritis to be made.

Changes in the unscarred areas. Initially in the unscarred areas of the kidney there are usually no changes unless there is high blood pressure or the patient is elderly, when the lesions discussed on pages 25 and 306 may be present. Later, focal segmental glomerulosclerosis (see p. 205) may occur. Similar changes occasionally develop in the opposite uninvolved kidney in patients with severe unilateral non-obstructive chronic pyelonephritis with reflux.

Electron microscopy Any glomerular changes are usually of the type seen in ischaemia (see p. 308). Electron-dense deposits are rarely found either in the mesangium or on the glomerular capillary basement membranes. The exception is when there is focal segmental glomerulosclerosis and hyalinosis; the lesions in these cases are the same as those discussed on page 207.

Immunofluorescence/immunoperoxidase microscopy Usually immunoglobulins and complement are not present in the kidneys of uncomplicated non-obstructive chronic pyelonephritis. If there is secondary hypertension there may be C3 in arteriolar and arterial walls; if focal segmental glomerulosclerosis and hyalinosis are present the glomerular lesions often contain IgM and complement.[43]

Differential diagnosis

Many chronic tubulointerstitial diseases can produce changes in the renal parenchyma that are identical to those seen in non-obstructive chronic pyelonephritis. Common examples are *ischaemia* of various types, *obstruction to the urinary outflow tract, drug reactions* and *analgesic abuse*, but there are numerous others. For this reason non-obstructive chronic pyelonephritis cannot be diagnosed on a renal biopsy. A firm diagnosis depends upon examination of the renal pelvis, calyces and papillae. In practice information on these structures is usually provided by the radiologist rather than the histopathologist. At times even the radiologist cannot separate non-obstructive chronic pyelonephritis from obstructive chronic pyelonephritis due to a stone which has temporarily lodged in an upper pole calyx and then been passed down the ureter.

Complications

The main complications are hypertension and focal segmental glomerulosclerosis.

Hypertension. Approximately 50% of adults with non-obstructive chronic pyelonephritis associated with vesicoureteric reflux develop a raised blood pressure.[44] It is also frequent in children, in whom it is often of the malignant type.[45] In both children and adults hypertension is most common when the chronic pyelonephritis is bilateral. The factor initiating hypertension in the cases with bilateral chronic pyelonephritis is probably hypervolaemia; in some of the unilateral forms of the disease, the renin–angiotensin system is responsible, triggered by ischaemia of the parenchyma.[45]

Focal segmental glomerulosclerosis. Focal segmental glomerulosclerosis commonly complicates non-obstructive chronic pyelonephritis, particularly in patients with bilateral disease. Its frequency in various series has varied from 28%[46] to 78%[47]. It is associated with progressive renal disease and the lesions are most advanced and widespread in patients with renal failure. It is also associated with proteinuria and approximately 60% of patients with focal segmental glomerulosclerosis excrete in excess of 1 g of protein per 24 hours and 25% excrete more than 3 g per 24 hours.[46]

Renal transplantation

Renal transplantation is widely used for the treatment of end-stage non-obstructive chronic pyelonephritis. The results are good and there is nothing to indicate in long-term follow-up studies that the chronic pyelonephritis in the patient's own kidneys affects either patient or graft survival. Pyelonephritis is no more frequent in the transplant in patients whose own disease was non-obstructive chronic pyelonephritis than in control groups. The secondary focal segmental glomerulosclerosis that is so commonly present in late non-obstructive chronic pyelonephritis almost certainly does not recur in the transplanted kidney. In the one case in which focal segmental glomerulosclerosis was found after transplantation severe chronic rejection was present and this was thought to be the cause.[43]

Prognosis

There is a scarcity of reliable data on which to

assess prognosis. In one series of 217 adults with non-obstructive chronic pyelonephritis, 75% were alive 15 years after diagnosis.[48] The prognosis was significantly worse for males, only about 45% of whom were alive at 10 years. Proteinuria seemed to be the feature which provided the best guide to prognosis; onset of heavy proteinuria was soon followed by impaired renal function. The renal lesion associated with the proteinuria was focal segmental glomerulosclerosis.

Progression to end-stage renal failure usually only occurs when there is evidence of bilateral scarring on radiological assessment; occasionally it happens despite apparent unilateral disease. In some young girls who develop end-stage renal failure there is a history of inadequate treatment of recurrent episodes of acute pyelonephritis. Failure to control hypertension will worsen the prognosis.

Patients found to have renal scarring at the time the first episode of acute pyelonephritis is recognized can probably be prevented from developing further renal scarring by keeping them free of infection. The effect of surgical correction of vesicoureteric reflux on subsequent scarring is uncertain. Both forms of treatment are the subject of an international study.[49]

Pathogenesis

The initial events in the development of chronic non-obstructive pyelonephritis are probably the same as those that lead to acute pyelonephritis, but in man there is still a paucity of convincing clinical observations on the development and progression of the renal damage. The assumption is that recurrent or continued bladder infection, in the presence of vesicoureteric and intrarenal reflux, repeatedly delivers bacteria into the collecting tubules and that the inflammation in the kidney becomes chronic. Gross progressive scarring of the calyces and of the renal parenchyma results. The scars develop predominantly at the poles of the kidneys because those are the papillary areas that are particularly affected by intrarenal reflux.

Most evidence suggests that the renal scarring in chronic non-obstructive pyelonephritis occurs mainly in infancy and early childhood and that further focal scarring of the kidney is rare in adult life.[14,38] The loss of renal tissue in the scars is followed by compensatory enlargement of the remaining nephrons.[49] In the case of bilateral scarring the nephron loss may be sufficient to result in chronic hyperfiltration in the residual glomeruli and development of focal segmental sclerosis and hyalinosis (see p. 26). This would explain why some patients develop proteinuria and undergo progressive functional deterioration independently of vesicoureteric reflux, urinary infection or hypertension. The finding of correlates between glomerular hypertrophy, focal segmental sclerosis and proteinuria in patients with chronic non-obstructive pyelonephritis is consistent with this proposal.[50] It is more difficult to accept this explanation for the decline in function in those patients in whom the disease apparently involves only one kidney. In experimental rats five-sixths of the renal mass has to be removed before glomerular hypertrophy is followed by proteinuria and focal segmental sclerosis.[51] However, unilateral renal agenesis does appear to predispose children to the development of focal segmental glomerulosclerosis and renal failure in early adult life (see p. 55).[52]

Obstructive chronic pyelonephritis

Chronic pyelonephritis associated with obstruction of the urinary tract is a commoner condition than non-obstructive chronic pyelonephritis. In the necropsy study referred to under non-obstructive chronic pyelonephritis (see p. 439) the incidence of chronic pyelonephritis associated with obstruction was 1.41%.[33]

There are many causes of urinary obstruction (see pp. 468–469); they include benign senile hyperplasia of the prostate, renal calculi, carcinoma of the cervix with involvement of the lower end of the ureter, and congenital valves in the prostatic urethra. Obstruction also occurs in pregnancy. Paralysis of the bladder in its effects has much in common with organic obstruction and chronic pyelonephritis is a major cause of death in cases of paraplegia.[53]

When acute pyelonephritis is associated with obstruction to urine outflow it tends to recur and to progress. Repeated catheterization is a factor in many of these cases. Continuing renal obstruction, ending in uraemia and death, is more frequently a feature than in non-obstructive chronic pyelonephritis.

The sex incidence of obstructive chronic pyelonephritis is about equal. Many of the men have prostatic enlargement. Most of the deaths from renal infection occur after the age of 70 years.

Clinical features

Sixty to seventy per cent of the patients give a definite history of acute urinary infection and symptoms referable to the lower parts of the urinary tract.[54] There may be high blood pressure. Evidence of renal failure is present in late cases. Bacteriuria is a frequent accompaniment, and neutrophil granulocytes are often present in the urinary sediment. Radiological examination shows dilatation of the ureteric pelvis and calyces, localized blunting of the renal papillae, and narrowing of the renal parenchyma.

Renal changes

The pathological changes in the kidney are a combination of those due to obstruction (see p. 469) and those due to infection (see p. 440).

Gross appearance of the kidneys The affected kidney may be enlarged, normal in size or smaller than normal; it is often segmentally scarred. Between the scars the subcapsular surface is frequently granular. The renal pelvis and calyces are usually diffusely dilated and the thickness of the renal parenchyma is uniformly reduced. The scars are coarse but they are shallower and less prominent than in non-obstructive chronic pyelonephritis. The renal pelvic epithelium may be thickened and finely granular.

Light microscopy Changes attributable to obstruction alone (see p. 469), such as marked interstitial fibrosis, tubular dilatation, and sclerosis and crowding together of glomeruli, are usually present. Superimposed on these there will be the lesions described under non-obstructive chronic pyelonephritis (see p. 440), including focal or diffuse scarring. Lymphoid follicles and collections of Tamm–Horsfall protein are often prominent in the interstitium.

Differential diagnosis

The distinction between uninfected obstruction and obstructive chronic pyelonephritis may be difficult, but in the latter condition there are characteristically discrete parenchymal scars of varying size.

Complications

Pyonephrosis (see p. 472) or *papillary necrosis* (see p. 473) may complicate obstructive chronic pyelonephritis. *Xanthogranulomatous pyelonephritis* (see p. 447) is a rare complication; it is most likely to occur when obstruction is due to renal calculi.

Prognosis

Bacteriuria can rarely be eradicated in the presence of urinary tract obstruction; recurrent infections and attacks of acute pyelonephritis occur with increased frequency. In addition, the obstruction in itself causes progressive parenchymal damage. As a result uraemia and death occur more frequently in obstructive than in non-obstructive chronic pyelonephritis.

The prognosis in a particular case will depend upon the underlying cause of the obstruction, its duration and degree, and the feasibility of relieving that obstruction by surgical or other means. When it is possible to remove the obstruction surgically, renal function usually ceases to decline and often improves, at least in the short term. However, in some patients with bilateral disease and much scarring deterioration of function may progress despite adequate relief of obstruction. This is particularly likely to happen in children in whom the obstruction to urine outflow is often accompanied by dysplasia or some other renal maldevelopment.[55] In these patients focal segmental glomerulosclerosis occurs.

Pathogenesis

When obstruction occurs at the bladder outlet or below, urine remains in the bladder after micturition. Once the residual urine becomes infected the organisms persist and are very difficult to eliminate by treatment with antibiotics. As the degree of obstruction increases urine flow is slowed, ureteric peristalsis becomes ineffective and the ascent of bacteria to the renal pelvis is assisted. High degrees of back pressure caused by obstruction lead to incompetence of the papillary valves and intrarenal reflux, allowing the infected urine to reach the renal parenchyma.[56] Blood-borne infection of the kidney is also facilitated by urinary tract obstruction. Intravenous injection of *Escherichia coli* in animals with one ureter tied leads to renal infection in the obstructed kidney but not in the other.[8] How obstruction promotes blood-borne infection is unknown; slowing of the renal circulation is probably important.

Patients with obstruction are more likely to be catheterized, which provides a potential source of bacteria. Also obstruction, sufficiently severe that the ureter becomes incompetent and allows transmission of voiding pressure to occur continuously, causes renal damage even in the absence of infection (see p. 472).[57] If hypertension occurs this will be an additional factor producing ischaemic focal renal scarring (see p. 306).

Once extensive damage has been inflicted on the kidneys by these combined mechanisms the destruction may become progressive even if the obstruction and infection are relieved; this happens because focal segmental glomerulosclerosis develops in the surviving renal tissue. Why this occurs is not clear, but the results of animal experiments suggest that glomerular hyperfiltration may be the factor that damages the glomeruli and leads to their sclerosis (see p. 206).

Botryomycosis [58,59]

Botryomycosis is a term applied to chronic progressive bacterial infections in which the pus contains characteristic granules composed of bacteria. The granules superficially resemble those that occur in an actinomycotic lesion. Indurated inflammatory masses and abscesses with draining sinuses are produced. The condition is uncommon and may involve many tissues and organs including the kidney; sometimes the infection starts in the kidney and is largely confined to that organ and the perinephric tissues.

There has usually been a severe, persistent and refractory urinary infection. This condition is most frequently caused by *Staphylococcus aureus*, but many common bacteria such as streptococci, *Escherichia coli* and *Pseudomonas aeruginosa* may be responsible. The organism can usually be cultured from the urine and sometimes from the blood.

In most patients treatment with antibiotics alone is insufficient; surgical drainage or excision or both are also required. Of the cases reported, nearly 50% died.[59]

Renal changes

The kidneys are enlarged and numerous abscesses are visible on the subcapsular and cut surfaces. Sometimes there is a perinephric abscess continuous with one of the intrarenal lesions. The abscesses are surrounded by granulation and fibrous tissue. In the pus at the centre of each are colonies of bacteria surrounded by eosinophilic homogeneous material which may have club-like extensions (Fig. 12.9). There is a superficial resemblance to mycetoma or actinomycosis but Gomori's silver

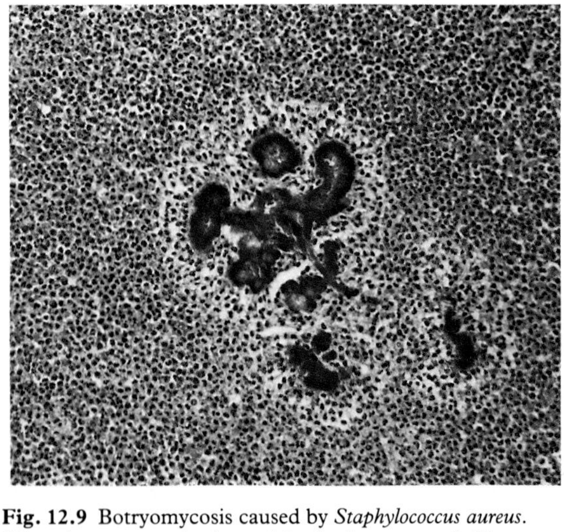

Fig. 12.9 Botryomycosis caused by *Staphylococcus aureus*. Microabscess contains bacterial colonies surrounded by eosinophilic homogeneous material. Haematoxylin-eosin × 95

methenamine stain fails to demonstrate any filaments, hyphae or spores. Giemsa and tissue Gram stains, such as the Brown–Hopps method, reveal bacteria in and adjacent to the mass.

Pathogenesis

Why the organisms form granules in some patients is not clear. Among the many suggested mechanisms one is that the lesion represents a balance between the virulence of the infecting organism and the defences of the host, allowing a state of symbiosis to occur.[59]

Xanthogranulomatous pyelonephritis

Xanthogranulomatous pyelonephritis is an uncommon form of chronic infectious tubulo-interstitial nephritis: the incidence in Sheffield, UK, has been estimated at 1.4 cases per 100 000 population per annum.[60] It is characterized by the accumulation in the kidney of lipid-laden foamy macrophages in sufficient numbers to produce yellow areas visible to the naked eye. There may be one or more localized intrarenal masses, an abscess cavity containing stones, or a diffuse replacement of most of the kidney by firm yellow tissue. Unlike chronic pyelonephritis the condition may spread into the perinephric tissues. It is usually unilateral and results in a non-functioning kidney. It almost always develops as a complication of prolonged, frequently low-grade, suppuration in a kidney in which the flow of urine is obstructed, usually by calculous disease.

The most common infecting organisms are *Escherichia coli* and *Proteus mirabilis*; other bacteria such as *Streptococcus faecalis* and *Pseudomonas aeruginosa* are occasionally cultured.[61]

Clinical features

Xanthogranulomatous pyelonephritis affects patients of all ages, but it is commonest in the age group 50–70 years and rare in childhood. Females predominate, with a ratio in one large series as high as 5 : 1.[60] Most patients present with fever, pain in one loin, malaise and weight loss; in about 40% there are symptoms of a urinary tract infection. Patients often have tenderness and a poorly defined mass in one loin. The urine contains protein and pus cells; haematuria is rare. Anaemia, a raised erythrocyte sedimentation rate and a neutrophil granulocytosis are common. Liver dysfunction is frequent.[61]

Conventional radiography reveals a stone in the urinary tract of about 80% of patients; in most this is a staghorn calculus. The affected kidney is sometimes enlarged and the outline ill defined. Intravenous urography often demonstrates a non-functioning kidney. Ultrasonography and computerized tomography show dilatation of the calyces and parenchymal cavitation.

Renal changes

Gross appearance of the kidney[60,61] The kidney is usually enlarged, the capsule is thickened and there are often adhesions to the adjacent tissues. On section the pelvis is characteristically dilated, filled with thick yellow fluid and contains a staghorn calculus and necrotic debris. Less frequently, smaller calculi or other causes of obstruction may be encountered such as congenital pyeloureteric stenosis, carcinoma of the renal pelvis, ureter or bladder, and schistosomiasis. The papillae are lost and the expanded calyces are lined by a friable yellowish layer, giving an appearance resembling that of renal tuberculosis. The narrowed parenchyma contains yellow nodules, some of which are centrally softened to form abscesses (Fig. 12.10). In most cases the whole of one kidney is affected but in about one-third there is a solitary focus of xanthogranulomatous pyelonephritis with a background of generalized acute or chronic obstructive pyelonephritis.

Light microscopy In the yellow areas there is a diffuse infiltrate consisting of large numbers of macrophages which have a cytoplasm that is vacuolated (foamy) and also contains PAS-positive, diastase-resistant, granules (Fig. 12.11). The cytoplasm is vacuolated because it contains large amounts of neutral fat and cholesterol esters which stain positively with oil red O. There are also variable but much smaller numbers of neutrophil granulocytes, plasma cells, lympho-

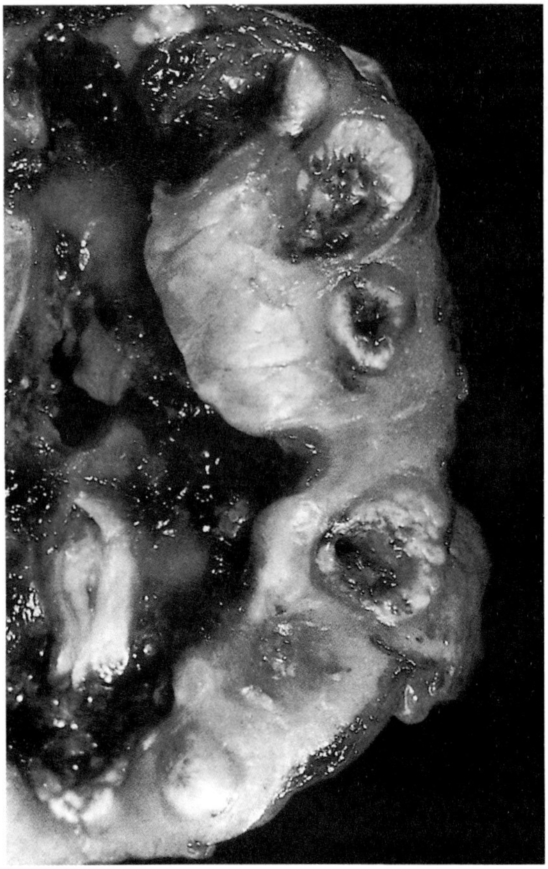

Fig. 12.10 Xanthogranulomatous pyelonephritis. Extensive hydronephrosis and parenchymal destruction by abscess cavities and yellow nodules.
Reproduced by permission from Churg J, Cotran RS, Sinniah R, Sakaguchi H, Sobin LHC, eds. Renal disease. Classification and atlas of tubulo-interstitial disease. New York, Igaku-Shoin, 1985; 39 (Fig. 4.2)

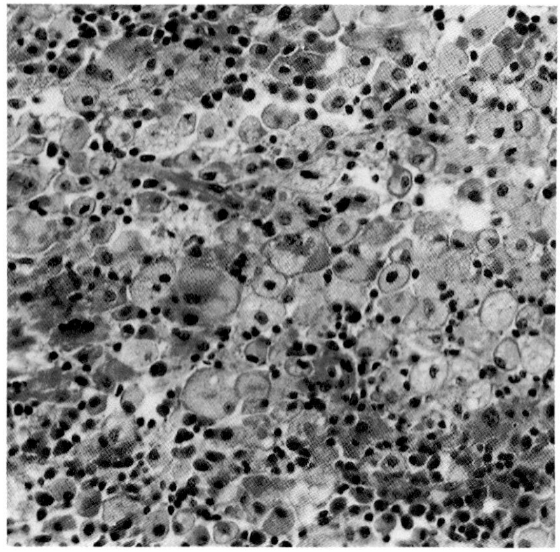

Fig. 12.11 Xanthogranulomatous pyelonephritis. There are sheets of 'foamy' macrophages and numerous plasma cells in the interstitium.
Haematoxylin-eosin × 800

cytes and multinucleate foreign body giant cells. Gram-negative bacilli may be demonstrated in the areas of cellular infiltration in sections stained by the Dieterle method.[62] Variable amounts of haemosiderin are nearly always present in the lesions; it is both within macrophages and in the extracellular tissues.[63] Focal necrosis and calcification are common and cholesterol clefts occur. At the edge of the yellow tissue are fibroblasts and collagen. In a minority of cases there may be palisading granulomas; in such cases tuberculosis must be excluded.[60]

The cortex away from the yellowish masses usually shows the changes of obstructive chronic or acute pyelonephritis (see pp. 434 and 445). Recanalized, organized thrombi are found in the large veins in about 20% of cases.

Electron microscopy The cytoplasm of the infiltrating macrophages contains numerous lipid droplets and variable numbers of phagolysosomes. Bacteria are often present in the exudate and within neutrophil granulocytes; they are only occasionally seen in macrophages.[62]

Immunofluorescence/immunoperoxidase microscopy Many of the infiltrating plasma cells contain IgA or IgG; only a few contain IgM;[61] there are no glomerular or other deposits of immunoglobulins or complement components.

Differential diagnosis

In small needle biopsy samples the distinction from *renal cell carcinoma* may be difficult; staining the cells with a monoclonal antibody that is specific for macrophages will solve the problem (see p. 452). *Malakoplakia* may appear similar to xanthogranulomatous pyelonephritis but the macrophages in malakoplakia contain Michaelis–Gutmann bodies, which are diagnostic (see p. 450).

Megalocytic interstitial nephritis may be indistinguishable from xanthogranulomatous pyelonephritis by light microscopy; electron microscopy in one case revealed rod-shaped electron-lucent crystalline material in the macrophages which may be distinctive (see p. 453). Occasionally in a biopsy the presence of giant cells and granulomas might indicate that tuberculosis should be excluded.

Complications

Xanthogranulomatous pyelonephritis may spread in any direction. It often extends into the perinephric tissues producing a *perinephric abscess*; *fistulae* occasionally form and affect the small or large bowel or extend to the skin in the loin.[64]

Prognosis

Xanthogranulomatous pyelonephritis progressively destroys the kidney, eventually leading to cessation of function. When the condition is unilateral (as it is in practically all cases) nephrectomy is curative. Systemic signs and symptoms disappear and liver function returns to normal.[61] Prolonged antibiotic therapy is unsuccessful. Conservative surgical treatment leads to fistula formation.

Pathogenesis

The pathogenesis is not known. A possible explanation is that in the course of an acute pyelonephritis in an obstructed kidney the pelviureteric epithelium becomes ulcerated and inflammation extends into the pelvicalyceal fat. Fat necrosis is followed by release of lipid which accumulates in the obstructed pelvis and is then phagocytosed by macrophages. Experimental production of the lesion in rats by permanent ligature of one ureter and intravenous administration of a suspension of *E. coli* supports this explanation.[65]

Malakoplakia

Malakoplakia is an uncommon chronic granulomatous inflammation characterized by dense collections of large macrophages (von Hansemann cells) whose cytoplasm contains haematoxyphil inclusions (Michaelis–Gutmann bodies). It may occur in several parts of the body, but its most frequent location is in the urinary bladder (see p. 711). Renal involvement is rare.

Clinical features[66]

Renal malakoplakia affects women far more frequently than men. It can occur at any age but the peak incidence is in the fifth decade. Patients present with pain in the flank, fever and rigors and often give a history of recurrent urinary tract infections. The urine contains protein, white blood cells and red cells. Occasionally macrophages with Michaelis–Gutmann bodies can be recognized in bladder washings. Bilateral disease may cause renal failure.

In most cases *Escherichia coli* is isolated from the urine; occasionally other bacterial species, including *Proteus vulgaris*, *Aerobacter aerogenes* and *Klebsiella pneumoniae* have been implicated.

Renal changes

Gross appearance of the kidneys Solitary or multiple yellowish-brown nodules, ranging in size from 1 to 20 mm in diameter, occur in one or both kidneys; they are often visible on the subcapsular as well as on the cut surfaces. The multifocal form is more common, occurring in 75% of cases; in approximately half these the renal involvement is bilateral. The lesions are well demarcated, often contain foci of suppuration and haemorrhage and may show central necrosis; isolated nodules may be mistaken for neoplasms. They are predominantly cortical in distribution; occasionally the medulla is affected and a necrotizing papillitis may be produced. The kidneys may be enlarged because they contain many nodules; they may be hydronephrotic because malakoplakia around the ureteric orifices or the urethra has caused obstruction (see p. 712).

Light microscopy The nodules are composed of closely packed large macrophages (von Hansemann cells) with small, dark, frequently eccentric nuclei (Fig.12.12). The abundant cytoplasm contains many eosinophilic, PAS-positive,

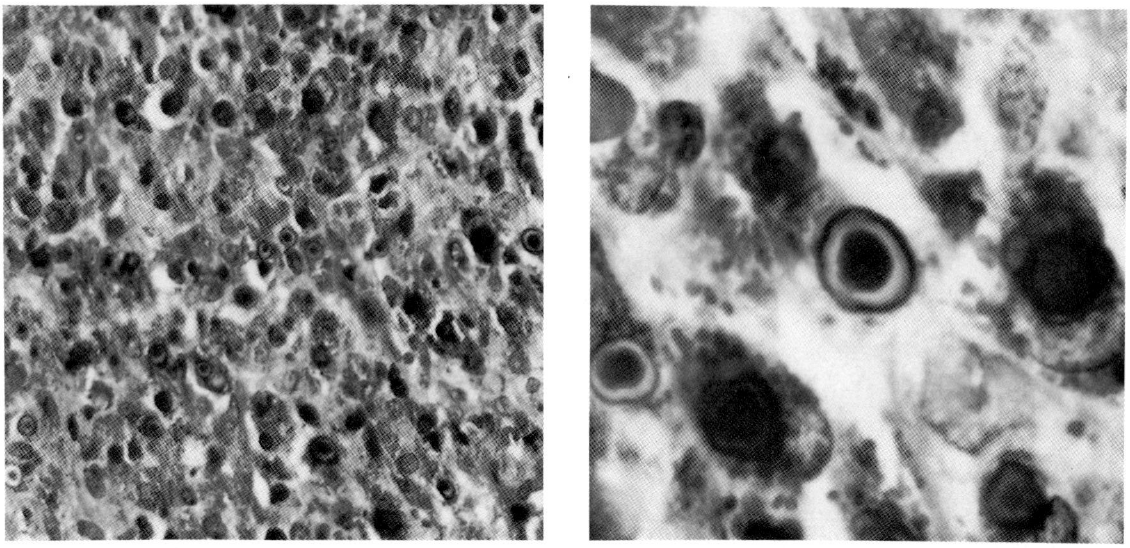

a b

Fig. 12.12 Malakoplakia. (**a**) There are sheets of macrophages (von Hansemann cells) with abundant, granular cytoplasm and small, dark, often eccentric, nuclei.Scattered Michaelis–Gutmann bodies can just be seen. There are also some infiltrating acute and chronic inflammatory cells. (**b**) Two Michaelis–Gutmann bodies with characteristic 'owl's eye' appearance. Periodic acid-Schiff: (**a**) × 150; (**b**) × 650

granules. The cytoplasm also contains characteristic deeply haematoxyphil homogeneous or laminated inclusions, 4–10 μm in diameter; similar structures are also found lying outside cells. These intracellular and extracellular bodies are named after Michaelis and Gutmann, who reported the first cases of malakoplakia.[67] Michaelis–Gutmann bodies stain positively for calcium (Fig.12.13) and iron, and are visible in unstained preparations as strongly refractile spheres. They also stain positively with the periodic acid-Schiff technique (with and without diastase). Michaelis–Gutmann bodies may be difficult to see in haematoxylin and eosin-stained sections; special stains and electron microscopy may be needed to demonstrate them. Gram-negative bacteria may be found in some of the macrophages.

Frequently the nodules also contain a few neutrophil granulocytes, lymphocytes and plasma cells. Vascular granulation tissue, collagen and abscesses may be present in some cases.

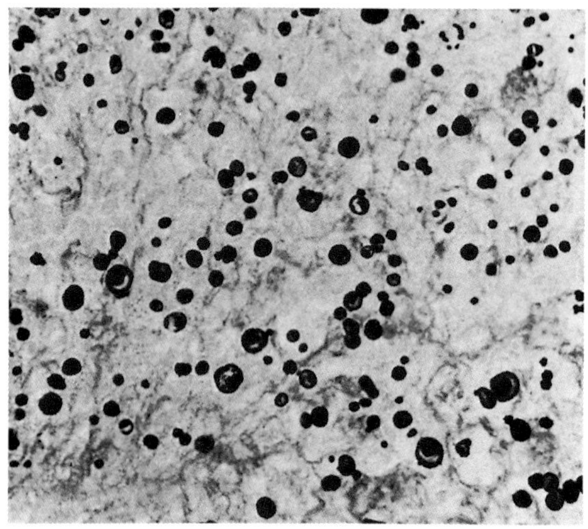

Fig. 12.13 Malakoplakia. Numerous Michaelis–Gutmann bodies staining positively for calcium. They vary greatly in size. A few are laminated.
Von Kossa × 300

Electron microscopy [68] The von Hansemann macrophages contain numerous phagolysosomes of various sizes (Fig.12.14), these structures account for the PAS-positive granularity of the cytoplasm. Bacilli have occasionally been detected within phagolysosomes in von Hansemann macrophages. Some of the larger phagolysosomes show central calcification. Typical Michaelis–Gutmann bodies are larger and have a central core

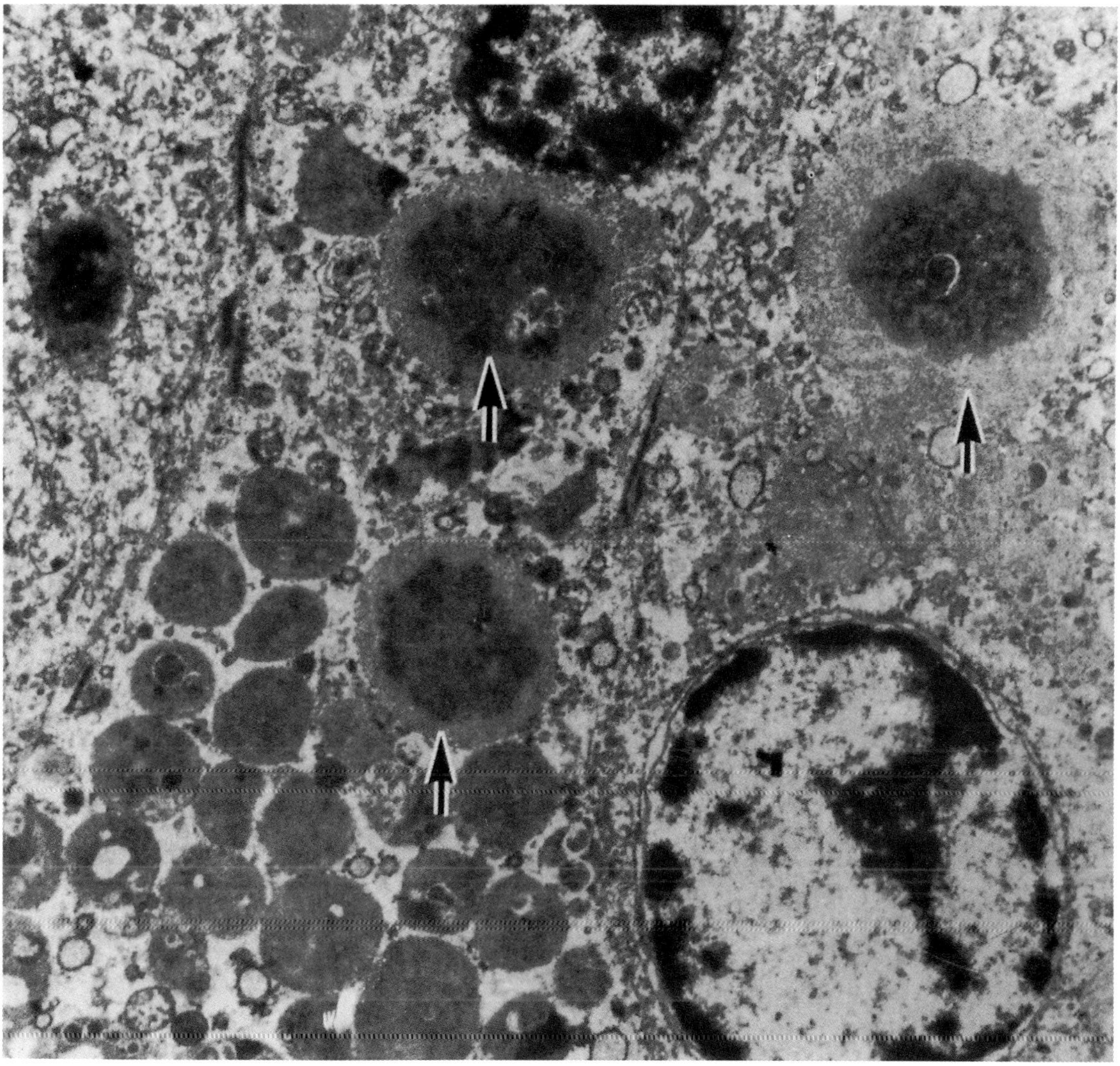

Fig. 12.14 Malakoplakia. Electron micrograph of von Hansemann macrophage. The cytoplasm contains numerous phagolysosomes; those arrowed show central calcification.
× 12 000
Reproduced by permission from: McClure J, Cameron CHS, Garrett R. J Pathol 1981; 134: 13 (Fig. 1)

of electron-dense fibrillar material surrounded by multiple concentric laminae of calcium hydroxyapatite crystals (Fig. 12.15).

Changes in other organs

Accompanying the renal nodules there are frequently malakoplakic changes at other sites, most commonly the urinary bladder, ureter and retroperitoneum (see p. 711).[66]

Differential diagnosis

The importance of recognizing renal malakoplakia lies in not confusing it in a biopsy with *renal adenocarcinoma, histoplasmosis* or *cryptococcosis.* Accurate diagnosis involves an awareness of the condition and the use of special stains to demonstrate the pathognomonic Michaelis–Gutmann bodies. In aspiration biopsies von Hansemann macrophages can be rapidly distinguished from

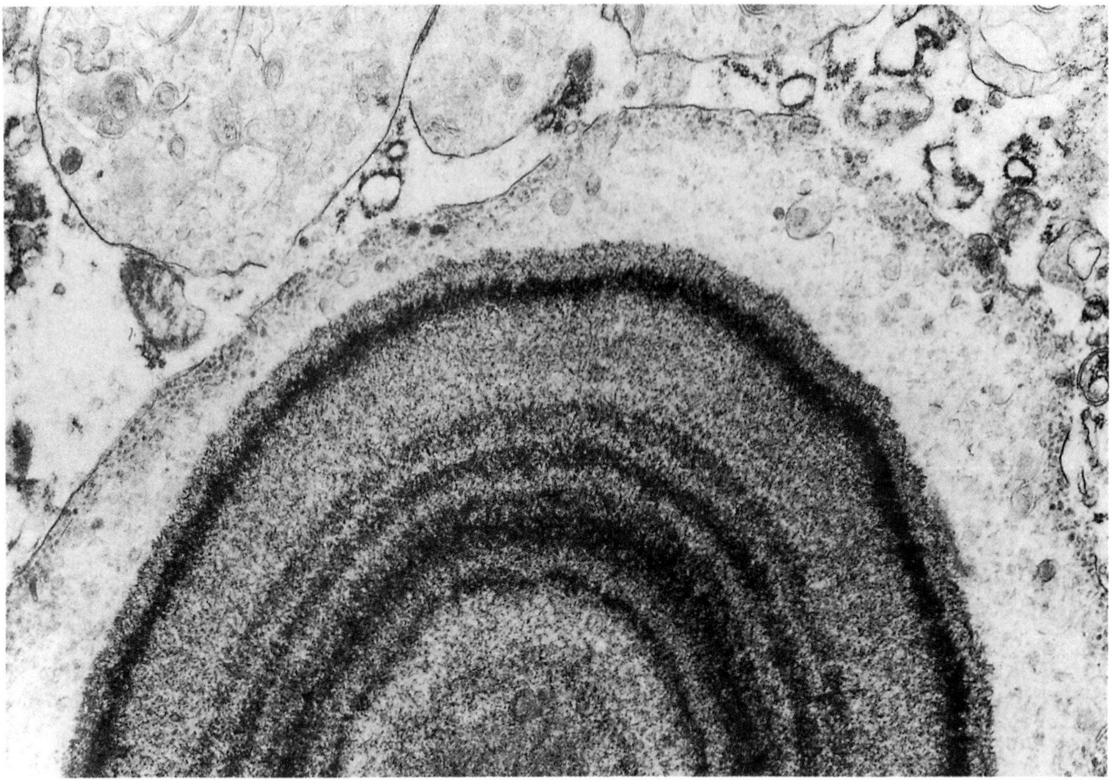

Fig. 12.15 Malakoplakia. Electron micrograph of a Michaelis–Gutmann body showing the concentric lamination of the calcium hydroxyapatite crystals.
× 27 000
Reproduced by permission from: Kelly DR, Murad TM. Am J Clin Pathol 1981; 75: 333 (Fig. 12 lower)

renal adenocarcinoma cells by either staining for alpha-l-antitrypsin or by using a monoclonal antibody specific for macrophages; in common with other macrophages von Hansemann cells stain positively while renal adenocarcinoma cells do not.

Prognosis

Renal failure may occur when kidneys are extensively damaged either by ureteric obstruction or by bilateral replacement of the parenchyma by malakoplakic nodules. Recovery has followed intensive treatment with antibiotics.

Pathogenesis

The pathogenesis of malakoplakia is unknown. It has been suggested that there is infection with an unusual strain of bacteria. Another proposal is that the abnormal reaction is caused by a defect in lysosomal activity following normal phagocytosis of bacteria. A third explanation is that the patient has an immunological abnormality which affects the intracellular killing of bacteria. There is little strong support for any of these theories. Even simple overload by the presentation of a large quantity of bacterial antigen for phagocytosis has been proposed; certainly malakoplakia can be produced experimentally by delivering a large bolus of highly concentrated bacterial cell wall derivative into the rat kidney.[69]

Megalocytic interstitial nephritis

Megalocytic interstitial nephritis was described in 1945.[70] It is an extremely rare disease affecting

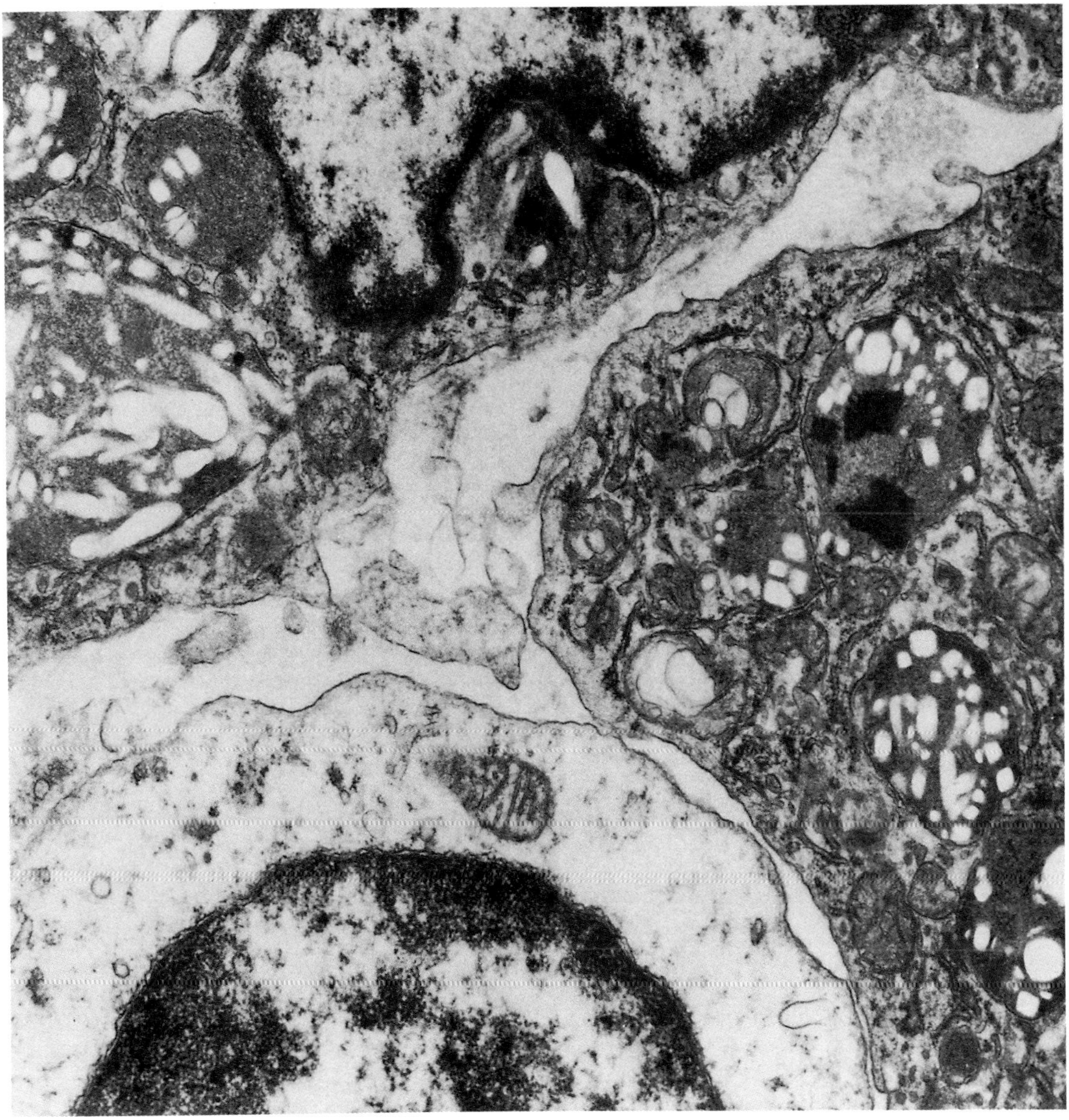

Fig. 12.16 Megalocytic interstitial nephritis. Electron micrograph of macrophages showing phagolysosomes containing electronlucent crystalloids.
× 27 000
Reproduced by permission from: Kelly DR, Murad TM. Am J Clin Pathol 1981; 75: 333 (Fig. 5)

primarily the renal cortex in an otherwise normal kidney.[71] There are discrete or confluent yellow foci composed of macrophages containing many PAS-positive cytoplasmic granules; the cells closely resemble those in malakoplakia but lack Michaelis–Gutmann bodies and contain more cytoplasmic lipid inclusions. It was the presence of these large polyhedral macrophages that led Zollinger in 1945 to use the term 'megalocytic' in describing this form of interstitial nephritis.[70] Electron microscopy of the macrophages reveals abundant cytoplasmic phagolysosomes, several of which contain electron-lucent crystalloids (Fig. 12.16). It has been suggested that the crystalloid bodies are specific.[72] The condition is probably a variant of malakoplakia.[73]

SPECIFIC RENAL INFECTIONS

Many other infectious agents can induce tubulo-interstitial disease. Some of these produce distinctive morphological patterns or are caused by organisms that can be readily identified. Examples are tuberculosis, syphilis, brucellosis, coccidioidomycosis and nocardiosis. These are discussed in Chapter 11 (see p. 383).

TUBULOINTERSTITIAL DISEASE CAUSED BY DRUGS

Drug-induced tubulointerstitial nephritis may be either acute or chronic.

ACUTE DRUG-INDUCED TUBULOINTERSTITIAL NEPHRITIS

Acute drug-induced tubulointerstitial injury is uncommon.[74] In some cases it seems to result from direct toxicity, in others from a hypersensitivity (allergic) reaction.

The evidence that hypersensitivity is involved is usually largely clinical. It consists of the frequent presence of a rash and eosinophilia; the fact that acute drug-induced tubulointerstitial nephritis occurs in only a minority of patients taking normal doses of the drug; that the disease recurs on re-exposure to the drug; and that the nephritis responds to corticosteriod therapy. In most instances the immune mechanisms involved have been difficult to define and proof that the renal lesions are the result of a hypersensitivity is usually lacking.

Direct acute drug-induced tubulointerstitial nephritis

Direct acute drug-induced tubulointerstitial injury may be caused by a variety of agents such as heavy metals (see p. 475), lithium (see p. 463), aminoglycosides (see p. 517) and urates (see p. 475).[75] The morphological changes produced are considered under the individual agents.

Drug-induced acute hypersensitivity tubulointerstitial injury

Many drugs can cause acute hypersensitivity injury. Those most often implicated are methicillin, sulphonamides, rifampicin (rifampin), frusemide (furosemide), thiazides, phenytoin, glafenine, phenindione, allopurinol, cimetidine, fenoprofen and mefenamic acid. Others are listed in Table 12.2.[74] Tubulointerstitial injury occurs in only a few of the patients taking any of these drugs and appears not to be dose related.

Patients usually have a fever, arthralgia is common and there may be a maculopapular rash and acute renal failure. There is microscopic haematuria, pyuria and proteinuria; gross haematuria, red cell casts and the nephrotic syndrome are sometimes found. Eosinophilia occurs in the peripheral blood of approximately half the patients, particularly in methicillin-related cases. Hyperchloraemic acidosis and impaired ability to concentrate urine are common. The latter may persist for many months after the acute episode in those patients who regain renal function. Intravenous urography frequently reveals enlarged kidneys.

Penicillins

Many cases of methicillin-associated tubulointerstitial nephritis have been recorded;[76] with the introduction of other agents for the treatment of resistant staphyloccocal infections this antibiotic is now little used. Acute tubulointerstitial nephritis occasionally occurs with other penicillins that are still in use (Table 12.2). Males are affected more frequently than females and all ages are at risk. The interval between exposure to the particular penicillin and the onset of symptoms is 5–21 days.[77]

Light microscopy[76] The interstitium is oedematous and infiltrated by a variable number of mononuclear cells and eosinophils (Fig. 12.17). The infiltrate is characteristically focal, particularly prominent at the corticomedullary junction

Table 12.2. Drugs associated with acute tubulointerstitial nephritis

Antimicrobial drugs	Non-steroidal anti-inflammatory drugs	Other drugs
METHICILLIN*	FENOPROFEN	PHENYTOIN
Penicillin G	MEFENAMIC ACID (MEFENAMATE)	GLAFENINE†
Ampicillin	Naproxen	PHENINDIONE
Amoxycillin	Ibuprofen	ALLOPURINOL
Carbenicillin	Ketoprofen	CIMETIDINE
Oxacillin*	Indomethacin	Sulphinpyrazone
Nafcillin	Tolmetin	Carbamazepine
Cephalothin*	Zomepirac	Clofibrate*
Cephalexin	Phenylbutazone*	Azathioprine
Cephradine	Aspirin	Phenobarbitone
Cefoxitin	Diflunisal	Methyldopa
Cefotaxime	Piroxicam	Gold and bismuth salts
RIFAMPICIN (RIFAMPIN)		Diazepam
SULPHONAMIDES	Diuretics	Penicillamine
Co-trimoxazole	FRUSEMIDE (FUROSEMIDE)	Interferon
Polymyxin B	THIAZIDES	Phenacetin
Kanamycin	Triamterene	Phenazone (antipyrine)*
Gentamicin		Carbimazole
Colistin		
Ethambuton		
Chloramphenicol		
Tetracyclines		
Vancomycin		
Erythromycin		

Drugs reported with any frequency are shown in capitals.
* No longer in regular use.
† Not in use in Britain or the USA
Reproduced by permission from: Cameron JS, Q J Med 1988; 66: 97

and often surrounds tubules. The mononuclear cells are mostly lymphocytes with some macrophages and plasma cells. The macrophages may appear as epithelioid cells and sometimes they form granulomas.[78,79] A few of the infiltrating cells may be in mitosis. The eosinophils tend to be concentrated in small foci and may form microabscesses.[77] Neutrophil granulocytes are rare. The majority of the mononuclear cells are T lymphocytes; in the few biopsies analysed those expressing the CD4 molecule outnumber those with the CD8 molecule.[80]

Characteristically the tubules are focally invaded by lymphocytes (tubulitis) but may show a range of lesions from focal necrosis with regeneration to patchy atrophy or dilatation. Extensive necrosis of the epithelium is rare. In most cases there is enhanced expression of HLA class II antigens on the tubular epithelium.[81] In some patients the distal tubules appear to be more severely affected.

The glomeruli are usually normal; occasionally there is mild mesangial hypercellularity. Blood vessels are usually normal but a mild arteriolitis has been seen in a few cases.[77]

Electron microscopy The tubules show focal loss of their brush borders, occasional necrotic epithelial cells and infiltration of lymphocytes between epithelial cells.[77] Immune deposits are not usually found either in glomeruli or on tubular basement membranes.

Immunofluorescence/immunoperoxidase microscopy In a few patients there is linear staining of the tubular basement membrane for IgG with or without C3 (Fig.12.18). Most kidneys are negative or show only trace amounts of a variety of immunoglobulins or complement components.

Differential diagnosis It may be difficult on morphological grounds to distinguish acute drug-induced hypersensitivity tubulointerstitial nephri-

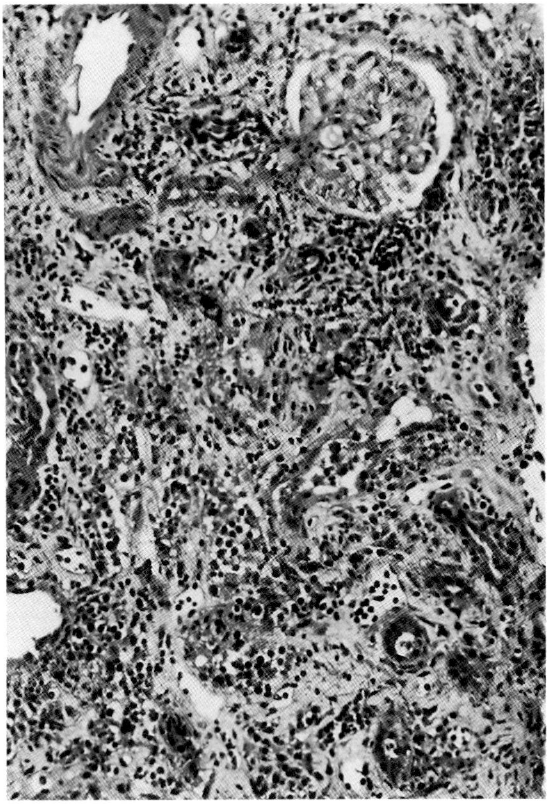

Fig. 12.17 Drug-induced acute hypersensitivity tubulointerstitial nephritis due to methicillin. There is prominent interstitial mononuclear cell infiltration and oedema.
Haematoxylin-eosin × 180

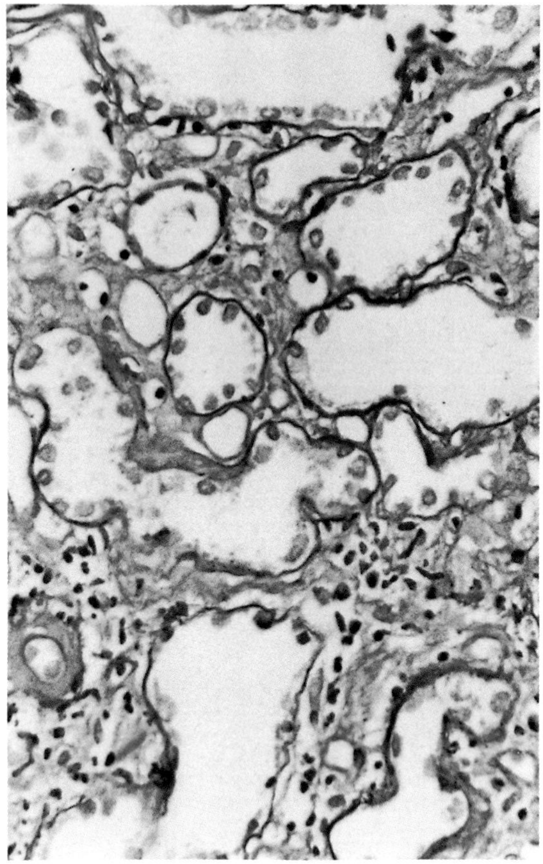

Fig. 12.18 Drug-induced acute hypersensitivity tubulointerstitial nephritis due to methicillin. There is linear staining for IgG along tubular basement membranes.
Immunoperoxidase × 230

tis from acute ischaemic or nephrotoxic injury unless the interstitial infiltrate of mononuclear cells and eosinophils is intense. The morphological and phenotypic pattern of cellular infiltration is also insufficiently specific to permit distinction between acute hypersensitivity tubulointerstitial nephritis induced by one of the penicillins and acute hypersensitivity tubulointerstitial nephritis caused by some other drug.[80]

Prognosis Once the drug is withdrawn most patients eventually recover full renal function; in only a few is there permanent damage. The outcome is worst in patients with oliguric renal failure and those with diffuse interstitial infiltrates.[74] Treatment with prednisolone seems to hasten recovery.[77] Rechallenge with the drug leads to recrudescence.

Pathogenesis In a few patients with methicillin-induced tubulointerstitial nephritis the serum has contained antibody directed against dimethoxyphenylpenicilloyl, the major haptenic antigen determinant of methicillin. Additionally in those cases the hapten has been demonstrated in a linear pattern on the tubular basement membranes.[82] Based on these observations it has been proposed that methicillin, when bound to the tubular basement membrane as a hapten–protein conjugate, stimulates the production of antibodies capable of reacting with normal tubular basement membranes. As a consequence of antibody deposition the tubules are damaged and this induces an acute interstitial reaction. Laboratory experiments support this hypothesis: animals actively immunized with tubular basement membrane antigens may develop severe tubulointerstitial nephritis.[83] However, in all the animal models the injury is determined at least in part by a cell-mediated second phase.

In the majority of patients with tubulointerstitial nephritis induced by one of the penicillins, antitubular basement membrane antibodies are not detectable and the pathogenesis of the nephritis remains unknown.

Rifampicin (rifampin)

Intermittent treatment with the antituberculous drug rifampicin is occasionally associated with acute tubulointerstitial nephritis. About 60 cases have been reported in the 17 years since the first report. Patients range in age from 20 to 66 years with an almost equal number of affected men and women. The interval between the commencement of treatment with the drug and the onset of symptoms ranges from 3 to 12 months. There is no correlation between the single or cumulative dose of rifampicin and the development of tubulointerstitial nephritis. Patients develop an influenza-like syndrome consisting of fever, nausea, malaise, chills, headache and lumbar pain, quickly followed by oliguria and sometimes anuria.[84] Antibodies to rifampicin have sometimes been detected in the circulation.

Renal changes The histological changes are usually similar to those seen in acute tubulointerstitial nephritis induced by penicillin although in some patients there has been more marked proximal tubular injury and less interstitial infiltrate.[85] Occasionally glomerular immune complex disease has also been present.

Pathogenesis The pathogenesis is unclear. Although most of the evidence points to a hypersensitivity mechanism there is a close correlation between the presence of anti-rifampicin antibodies and the tubulointerstitial nephritis. An acute immune complex pathogenesis has been suggested but the immunofluorescence results are against this explanation.[86]

Prognosis Most patients make a good recovery after withdrawal of the drug; a few are left with interstitial nephritis.

Non-steroidal anti-inflammatory drugs

Non-steroidal anti-inflammatory drugs are widely used in the management of musculoskeletal disorders. Large numbers of mainly older individuals are taking these drugs, which are available without prescription in many countries.[74] The incidence of complicating tubulointerstitial nephritis is unknown; the number of reported cases is small when compared with the large number of patients treated with non-steroidal anti-inflammatory drugs.[87] Although many different compounds in this groups have been associated with acute tubulointerstitial nephritis (Table 12.2), propionic acid derivatives are implicated in 64%, fenoprofen alone accounting for 52% of the reported cases.[87]

An interesting clinical feature of tubulointerstitial nephritis induced by non-steroidal anti-inflammatory drugs is the concurrent presence of protein within the nephrotic range in most of the patients. The interval between exposure to the drug and the onset of symptoms ranges from a few days up to 36 months and averages 5 months. A rash and eosinophilia occur in only 25% of the cases; renal failure severe enough to require temporary dialysis occurs in about a third.

Renal changes The renal histology in general resembles that seen in penicillin-induced tubulointerstitial nephritis, although eosinophils are usually sparse or absent. When a nephrotic syndrome accompanies acute tubulointerstitial nephritis the otherwise normal glomeruli show retraction and obliteration of epithelial foot processes. Immunofluorescent staining for immunoglobulins and complement is usually negative.[88]

Prognosis Withdrawal of the drug usually leads to recovery but in about 10% of the cases there is residual renal insufficiency and interstitial fibrosis.[89]

Pathogenesis Most cases are probably due to a cell-mediated immune response. This is suggested by the prolonged drug exposure, as well as by the predominance in the interstitial infiltrate of CD8-positive T lymphocytes.[90]

Other drugs[74,75]

Many other drugs have been implicated as causing acute interstitial nephritis (Table 12.2). *Phenindione*, an anticoagulant now little used, in the past caused about 30 cases. *Thiazides* and *frusemide (furosemide)*, used as diuretics, have been linked with about 20 cases. Several instances of tubulointerstitial nephritis have been reported in patients with hyperuricaemia treated with *allopurinol*; the nephritis in these cases is often characterized by granulomas in the interstitium. *Cimetidine*, used in the treatment of peptic ulceration, has been the cause of several cases. *Glafenine*, an analgesic drug commonly used in Europe, although not in Britain and the USA, is thought to have caused a number of cases of acute tubulointerstitial nephritis. *Phenytoin*, used extensively for the treatment of seizures and of cardiac arrhythmias, has been incriminated in several reports. *Sulphonamides* are thought to have caused some cases of acute tubulointerstitial nephritis.

The other drugs listed in Table 12.2 have been associated with very few cases.

CHRONIC DRUG-INDUCED TUBULOINTERSTITIAL NEPHRITIS

Analgesic nephropathy

The association between chronic tubulointerstitial nephritis and the excessive use of analgesic drugs was first described in 1953.[91] Since then many cases have been reported, particularly from Australia, Switzerland and Scandinavian countries. The incidence of analgesic nephropathy is closely related to the prevalence of regular, usually daily, consumption of analgesics.[92-94] In England, Wales and the northern and eastern parts of the USA the percentage of the population habitually taking analgesics is low, and analgesic nephropathy is uncommon, accounting for 1–3% of patients in end-stage renal failure.[95] In contrast to this in localized areas of Australia, Denmark, Sweden, Finland and Switzerland 17–31% of the population are habitual consumers[93] and analgesic nephropathy accounts for up to 20% of dialysis cases.[95] The prevalence is highest in areas where caffeine-containing mixed analgesic powders are available without prescription and are widely advertised. The powders are often taken for their stimulant and mood-altering effects rather than as analgesics. The prevalence is also high where free headache powders are given to employees in factories. Women are more prone to this habit and the ratio of females to males with analgesic nephropathy is approximately 4 : 1. Affected women are often middle aged and have a history of social problems or psychological disorders. Some of the patients who develop nephropathy take analgesics because they suffer from a chronic and disabling painful condition, such as rheumatoid arthritis. However, severe renal failure is rare in patients with rheumatoid arthritis; when present the patient has usually been ingesting large quantities of compound analgesics rather than aspirin alone.

The magnitude of the risk of developing chronic renal failure after ingestion of large amounts of analgesics cannot be calculated with any precision from the published studies. The risk appears to be in the order of six times higher in those who daily consume 1.25 g or more of analgesics.[92]

The primary lesion in analgesic nephropathy is usually renal papillary necrosis (see p. 473). Obstruction of tubules in the necrotic papillae then causes secondary interstitial changes in the cortex.

Clinical features[96]

The patients present with a variety of complaints. These include nocturia, renal colic, haematuria and symptoms of urinary infection. All patients show reduced urinary concentrating capacity; persistent pyuria, renal insufficiency and hypertension are common. Proteinuria occurs in about a third of the patients. Impaired urinary acidification and clinical gout are seen in approximately

20%. Occasionally, separated papillae produce ureteric obstruction and acute renal failure. Fragments of papillae may be found in the urine. Radiology may demonstrate medullary or papillary cavities or the presence of rings of calcification around necrotic papillae.[97] As many patients deny habitual use of analgesics, testing the urine for metabolites of phenacetin and aspirin can be helpful in making a diagnosis.

Sometimes the disease is recognized in the course of investigating dyspepsia or anaemia.

Renal changes

Gross appearance of the kidneys[98,99] In the early stages of the disease, the kidneys are normal in size with smooth subcapsular surfaces. Yellow streaks radiate into the pyramids from the tips of the papillae (Fig. 12.19). Usually almost all the pyramids in both kidneys are affected. The outer medulla and cortex appear normal. The mucosa of the renal pelvis and ureter may show a brownish discolouration.[100]

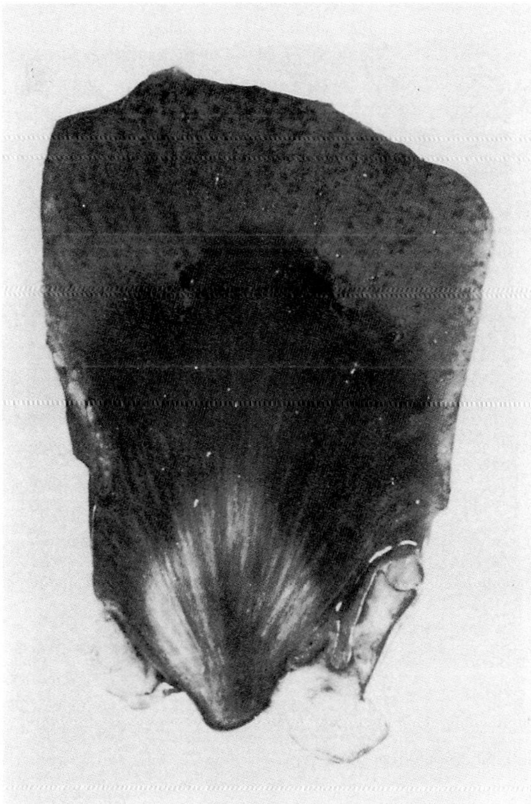

Fig. 12.19 Analgesic nephropathy. Early stage. Part of a kidney showing pale streaks radiating from the tip of a papilla. *Reproduced by permission from: Burry A. Kidney Int 1978; 13: 34 (Fig. 1a)*

Later the kidneys are usually smaller than normal. The subcapsular surface is pale and often coarsely granular. Varying numbers of papillae are either necrotic or have been shed. The necrotic parts are yellow or brown, of variable shape and usually confined to the apical region of the papillae. They are fairly sharply demarcated from the adjoining renal substance, sometimes by a congested zone (Fig. 12.20). There are ragged cavities where papillae have sloughed. Incomplete detachment may leave a small dark fragment attached to the papillary stump. Typically there is extensive cortical thinning; the cortex in the columns of Bertin usually survives, however, producing narrow bars or ridges.

Light microscopy[98,99] In the early stages changes within the kidneys are confined to the papillae and inner medulla. There is patchy necrosis of interstitial cells and of the cells lining Henle's loops and capillaries. The basement membranes of Henle's loops and the capillary basement membranes are markedly thickened. The interstitial matrix is swollen (Fig. 12.21). These changes extend in columns from the papillae and alternate with spared areas. There is little or no cellular infiltrate. Thickening of the basement membranes also occurs in the capillaries lying directly beneath the epithelium in the pelvic, ureteric and bladder mucosa.[101]

As the disease advances the tissues at the tip of the papillae become necrotic, only collecting ducts and occasional vasa recta being spared (Fig. 12.22). Later papillary necrosis becomes total. Small or large necrotic fragments are shed and the raw area may become lined by epithelium. Calcium may be deposited in the outer part of the necrotic zone. In the outer medulla a band of fibrous tissue may be laid down.

Only when this stage is reached are changes found in the cortex. They are at first focal but tend to become diffuse later. Oedema and sparse mononuclear cell infiltration around medullary rays progress to tubular atrophy and interstitial

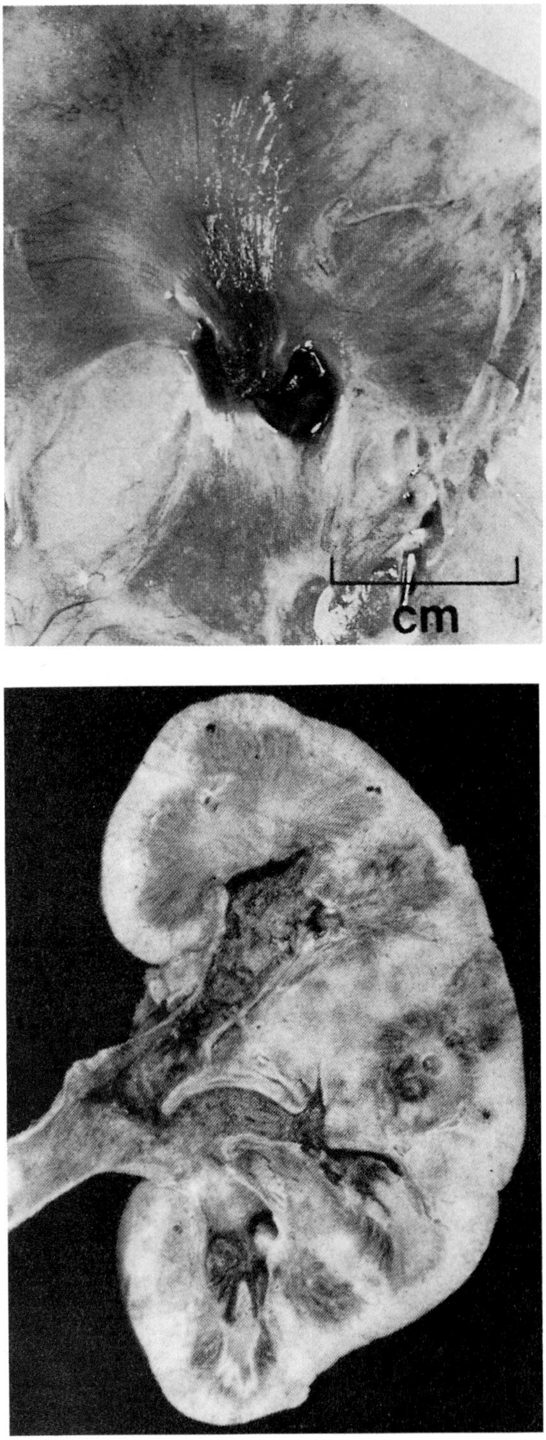

a

b

Fig. 12.20 Analgesic nephropathy. Papillary necrosis. (**a**) Part of kidney showing dark necrotic papilla about to be shed. (**b**) Bisected kidney. Several of the necrotic papillae have become separated and shed, leaving ragged cavities.
(**a**) *Photograph provided by Dr JG Jackson, Charing Cross Hospital Medical School, London, UK*

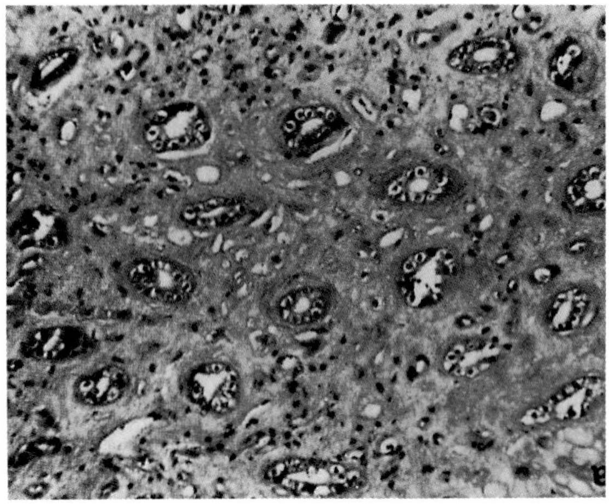

Fig. 12.21 Analgesic nephropathy. Early stage. Necrosis of capillaries, ascending limbs of Henle's loops and interstitial cells. Intact collecting ducts run through the area of necrosis. Haematoxylin-eosin × 90
Reproduced by permission from: Burry A. Kidney Int 1978; 13: 34 (Fig. 2a)

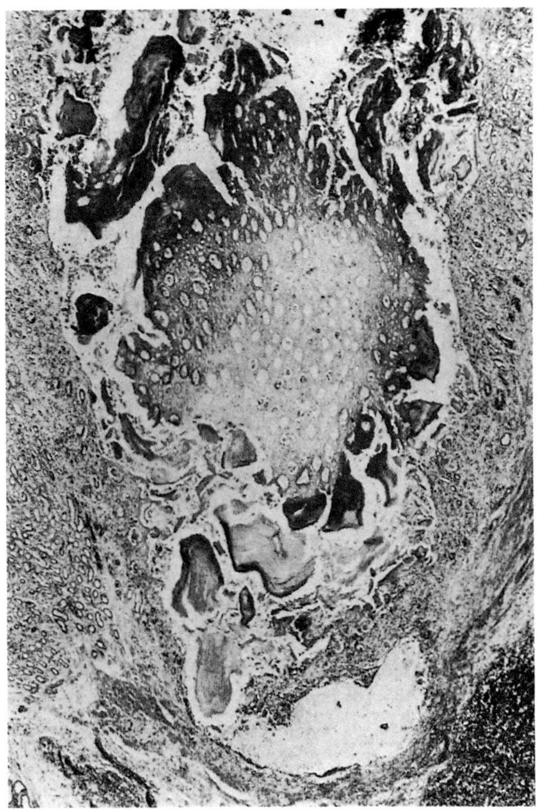

Fig. 12.22 Analgesic nephropathy. Papillary necrosis. The necrotic papilla illustrated in Figure 12.20a has become almost separated from the surrounding tissue. This lesion was responsible for a characteristic ring shadow in the pyelograph. Haematoxylin-eosin × 20
Photograph provided by W. St C. Symmers

fibrosis. The glomeruli become crowded because of the tubular atrophy, but they remain intact for a long time; eventually periglomerular and intracapsular fibrosis and focal segmental glomerulosclerosis and hyalinosis appear. The arcuate and interlobular arteries usually show intimal thickening.

Electron microscopy[99] The earliest lesion is thickening of the basement membranes of the loop of Henle and of the capillaries in the inner medullary zone. This is followed by stratification of the membranes into thin concentric lamellae between which cell debris and lipids accumulate. Lipids are also deposited in the surrounding interstitial ground substance. The lumen of the affected tubules and capillaries becomes narrowed and there is necrosis of some of the epithelial and endothelial cells. The interstitial cells lose their processes and their cytoplasm becomes vacuolated.

The basement membrane changes in the renal pelvis and ureter are similar to those seen in the papillae and inner medulla.[101]

Changes in other organs

Thickening of the walls of capillaries in the submucosa of the ureter[100] and bladder[102] has already been mentioned. This vascular change is thought to be specific for analgesic abuse.[101]

Peptic ulceration is present in about a third of patients taking analgesic mixtures which include aspirin. *Anaemia* may occur because of renal failure, haemolysis and gastrointestinal blood loss. *Premature atheroma* is said to be common and leads to myocardial infarction, renal artery stenosis and intermittent claudication.

Differential diagnosis

Renal papillary necrosis occurs in a number of other conditions (see p. 473). In the form associated with *non-steroidal anti-inflammatory drugs* the papillae are not pigmented and separation of necrotic papillae occurs rarely. In *diabetes mellitus* there is usually evidence of severe acute pyelonephritis, the necrotic papillae most commonly remain attached and between the necrotic tissue and the surrounding parenchyma there is usually a broad zone of neutrophil granulocytes. In renal papillary necrosis complicating *sickle cell disease* the papillae are not pigmented but otherwise the changes very closely resemble those of analgesic nephropathy. In the remaining conditions in which renal papillary necrosis occurs the lesions resemble those seen in diabetes mellitus and the necrotic papillae are demarcated from the adjacent healthy kidney by a cream-coloured band of granulocytes.

The presence of thickening of the walls of capillaries in the submucosa of the renal pelvis, ureter and bladder strongly suggests that the disease underlying the renal papillary necrosis is either diabetes mellitus or analgesic abuse.

Complications

Transitional cell tumours Transitional cell tumours of the renal pelvis, ureter and bladder are more common in analgesic abusers.[103,104] Approximately 8% of patients with analgesic nephropathy in Sweden and Switzerland develop uroepithelial tumours.[99,105] It is estimated that in some areas of Switzerland transitional cell tumours occur 77 times more frequently in the renal pelvis, 89 times more frequently in the ureter and seven times more frequently in the bladder in analgesic abusers than in non-abusers.[106] The tumours are more common in women, in contrast to the usual 2 : 1 ratio of males to females with uroepithelial tumours not associated with analgesic abuse. The mean induction time for these renal pelvic transitional cell carcinomas has been calculated to be 22 years (see also p. 720).[107]

Morphologically the neoplasms do not differ from other transitional cell tumours of the urinary tract. They are, however, reputed to have a worse prognosis; the major factor contributing to this is the coexisting chronic nephropathy.[108] They are frequently multiple and there is often an accompanying extensive uroepithelial dysplasia, with focal carcinoma *in situ*; both features suggest a diffuse alteration of the transitional epithelium throughout the urinary tract.

Renal cell carcinoma (renal adenocarcinoma) Regular consumption of analgesic mixtures appears to double the risk of developing a renal cell carcinoma.[109,110]

Other renal complications Ureteric obstruction by separated papillae may lead to hydronephrosis or pyonephrosis. Calculous disease may also occur.

Renal transplantation

If analgesic abuse ceases, renal transplantation for end-stage renal failure is uncomplicated and the outlook is good. Unfortunately some patients surreptitiously return to excessive consumption of analgesics and if unchecked this may lead to papillary necrosis in the renal transplant. To avert this problem it may be necessary periodically to test the urine of these patients for metabolites of phenacetin and aspirin.

Prognosis

After excessive intake of analgesics has been stopped most patients survive for many years with impaired but stable renal function. A few patients with severe renal dysfunction progress to end-stage renal failure despite cessation of analgesic abuse. Any deaths are usually from complications such as myocardial infarction and uroepithelial transitional cell carcinoma.[111]

Pathogenesis

Analgesic nephropathy The bulk of the evidence suggests that analgesic mixtures, rather than any one agent, cause the renal damage in patients. Most of the mixed compounds contain two or more of the following substances: aspirin, phenazone (antipyrine), amidopyrine (aminopyrine), paracetamol (acetaminophen), codeine, caffeine or non-steroidal anti-inflammatory drugs. Before 1975 phenacetin (acetophenetidin) was common in these mixtures but this is no longer the case. The renal damage is very probably caused by combined chronic toxicity of the ingredients of the mixed compounds. Feeding rodents with any of the compound analgesics that are associated with clinical analgesic nephropathy leads to papillary necrosis and chronic interstitial nephritis.[96] Single analgesics usually produce papillary necrosis in fewer animals.

The mechanism of this toxicity is far from clear. One possible explanation is that there is interference with the blood supply to the papillae and in one study of experimental analgesic nephropathy a reduction in medullary blood flow was demonstrated.[112] Aspirin and other non-steroidal anti-inflammatory agents inhibit renal prostaglandin synthesis and thus have the potential to induce papillary ischaemia. Another possible explanation is that one or more of the chemicals in the analgesic compound directly damage the cells of the renal papillae. After ingestion both paracetamol and aspirin are concentrated in the renal papillae where they may cause oxidative damage.[113] These two possible mechanisms are not mutually exclusive and may work in combination. Other factors may also be important. For example, dehydration, which markedly increases the concentration of both paracetamol and aspirin in the renal medulla, may increase the toxicity of some analgesics.[113]

Uroepithelial and renal parenchymal neoplasms Epidemiological surveys indicate that it is the regular consumption of analgesics containing phenacetin rather than of those containing no phenacetin that confers an increased risk of cancer of the renal pelvis,[114] ureter,[115] bladder[114] and renal parenchyma[116] Experiments in rodents have also implicated phenacetin[117] and possibly paracetamol,[118] but not other analgesics, in the production of uroepithelial tumours. The carcinogenic effect of phenacetin is thought to result from the potent alkylating action of the N-O-sulphate and N-O-glucuronide conjugates of N-hydroxyphenacetin.[119]

Lithium nephropathy

Lithium is an effective and widely used agent in the long-term management of manic depressive psychosis and endogenous depression. Its prolonged administration is associated in about half the patients with an impairment of urinary concentrating ability; in approximately 20% there is polyuria (an output of more than 3 litres in 24 hours), which is primarily due to nephrogenic diabetes insipidus.[120] In most cases the renal functional abnormalities abate when the drug is discontinued; in a few they persist and there is a chronic interstitial nephritis.[121,122]

Renal changes

Within days of commencing lithium treatment glycogen begins to accumulate in the epithelial cells of the distal tubules and collecting ducts (Fig. 12.23). The cells become swollen and their cytoplasm vacuolated; this lesion appears to be specific to lithium therapy.[123] Later, features of non-specific focal tubulointerstitial nephritis are found in some patients. Areas of interstitial fibrosis and tubular atrophy are accompanied by mild infiltration by mononuclear cells. There is tubular dilatation and microcyst formation which is often more pronounced than in control biopsies from psychiatric patients not treated with lithium. The interstitial fibrosis extends into the medulla, where it is more diffuse.[124] Sometimes there is also segmental and global sclerosis of glomeruli. Casts containing Tamm–Horsfall protein are frequent in the distal tubules and collecting ducts. The extent of tubular atrophy and interstitial fibrosis is related to the duration of lithium therapy; the number of atrophic tubules corresponds with impairment in concentrating ability.

Electron microscopy confirms the presence of glycogen in the epithelial cells of the distal tubules and collecting ducts. Immunofluorescence/immunoperoxidase microscopy is usually negative[123]

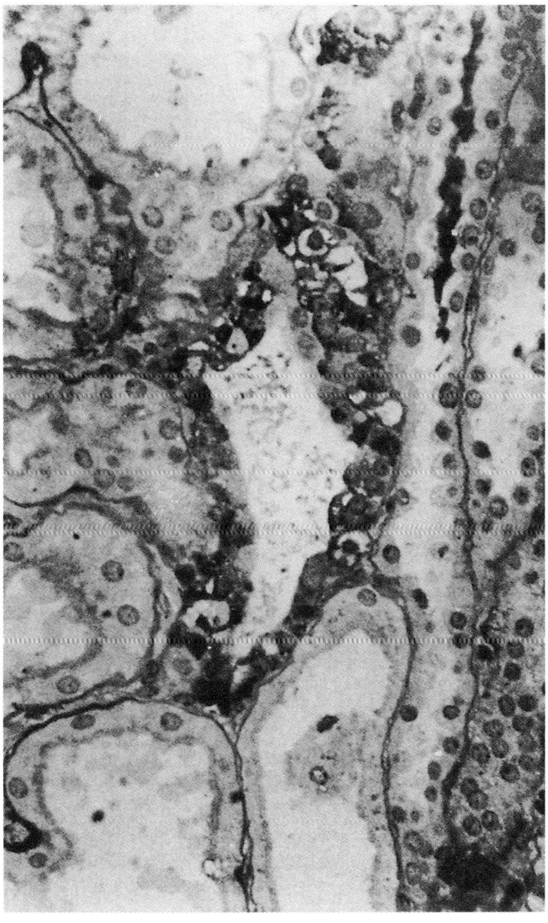

Fig. 12.23 Lithium nephropathy. The cytoplasm of the cells lining a cortical collecting duct shows vacuolation and PAS-positive granules. This lesion is thought to occur only in patients being treated with lithium
Periodic acid-Schiff × 400
Reproduced by permission from: Walker RG, Bennett WM, Davies BM, Kincaid-Smith P. Kidney Int 1982; 21: suppl, 11, S13 (Fig. 5)

Differential diagnosis

Although the presence of prominent tubular dilatation and microcysts is suggestive, only the presence of glycogen and vacuolation of the distal tubular and collecting duct epithelium distinguishes the tubulointerstitial nephropathy of lithium therapy from that induced by many other conditions.

Prognosis

The accumulation of glycogen in the distal tubules and collecting ducts is reversible. The chronic tubulointerstitial changes are probably not reversible; they may lead to a persistent defect in concentrating ability and the potential risk of dehydration.[120] Glomerular filtration rate is only rarely reduced; when this happens it is probably related to factors other than lithium, such as the common use of other psychotropic drugs.

Pathogenesis

Lithium accumulates within the cells of the collecting tubules, interfering with cyclic adenosine 3',5'-monophosphate (cAMP) formation and inhibiting antidiuretic-hormone-mediated water reabsorption. The vacuolation and glycogen accumulation in the epithelial cells of the collecting tubule may represent a response to intracellular accumulation of lithium.[120] In rabbits this reversible lesion can be produced by chronic lithium administration; later it is accompanied by a progressive irreversible focal interstitial nephritis.[125]

Whether the focal tubulointerstitial nephritis in humans is also caused by lithium is unknown. It probably is, but doubt remains because some psychiatric patients who are not being treated with lithium develop very similar changes;[122,126] these may be caused by other psychotropic agents, analgesic abuse and hypertension.

TUBULOINTERSTITIAL NEPHRITIS ASSOCIATED WITH IMMUNE DISORDERS

Tubulointerstitial nephritis may occur in immune complex disorders, in the presence of cell-mediated or immediate hypersensitivity, or associated with antibodies reacting with tubular antigens.

TUBULOINTERSTITIAL NEPHRITIS ASSOCIATED WITH IMMUNE COMPLEX DISORDERS

Immune complex-mediated nephritis is characterized by granular immune deposits along tubular basement membranes and in the interstitium. It is often found in systemic lupus erythematosus and occasionally in Sjøgren's syndrome and mixed cryoglobulinaemia; it may also occur with certain forms of glomerulonephritis. A few cases have been recorded in cutaneous vasculitis and bacterial endocarditis. Immune complex tubulointerstitial nephritis is occasionally found in renal allografts (see p. 660). The antigens involved are usually unidentified.

Systemic lupus erythematosus (see p. 225)

Tubulointerstitial nephritis associated with local deposits of immunoglobulin or complement is common only in systemic lupus erythematosus. Immune deposits are found in 30–60% of patients.[127,128] The frequency of tubulointerstitial disease correlates with the activity of the glomerular lesions and, to a lesser extent, with the severity of the lupus nephritis as reflected in its World Health Organization (WHO) classification. The prevalence of tubulointerstitial nephritis increases progressively from 14% in WHO class IIa to 50% in class IV; it is unusual in the membranous form of lupus nephritis (class V), affecting only 7% of these patients.[128]

The immune deposits usually contain IgG associated with C1q, C3 or both; C4, IgM and IgA are also often present (Fig. 12.24). Staining for Clq is frequently intense. The deposits appear coarsely or finely granular and are predominantly seen along the basement membrane of all parts of the tubules; they also occur in the walls of peritubular capillaries and larger vessels and in the interstitium.[127] By electron microscopy discrete electron-dense deposits may be found at all these

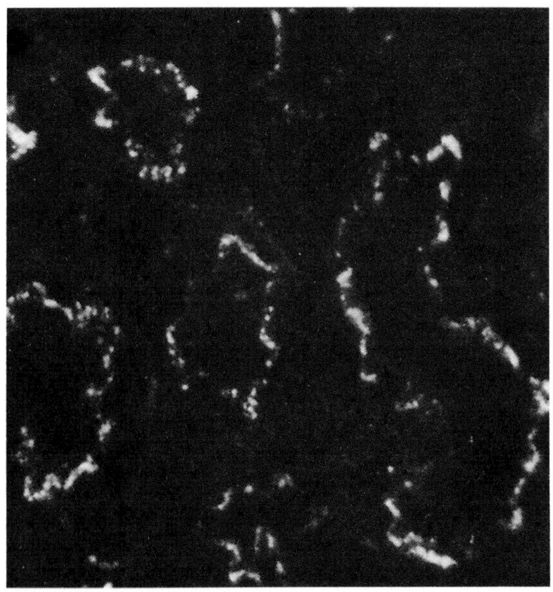

Fig. 12.24 Tubulointerstitial disease associated with systemic lupus erythematosus. Granular deposits of C3 are present along the tubular basement membranes. Immunofluorescence × 240
Reproduced by permission from: Park MH, D'Agati V, Appel GB, Pirani CL. Nephron 1986; 44: 309 (Fig. 1)

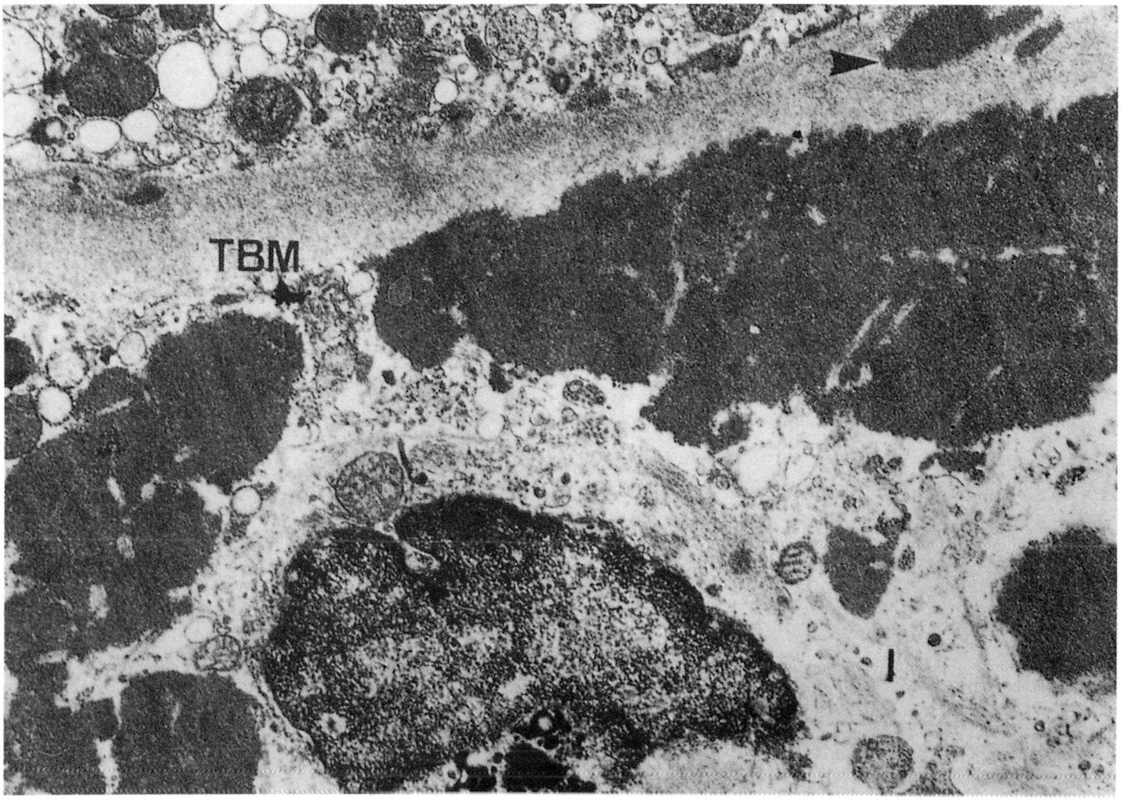

Fig. 12.25 Tubulointerstitial disease associated with systemic lupus erythematosus. Part of tubule and adjacent interstitium. There are large electron-dense deposits on the outer aspect of the tubular basement membrane (TBM). A small deposit is also present within the tubular basement membrane (arrowhead). I, interstitium.
× 12 000
Reproduced by permission from: Park MH, D'Agati V, Appel GB, Pirani CL. Nephron 1986; 44: 309. (Fig. 5)

sites; on the tubules they are usually located on the outer surface of the basement membranes (Fig. 12.25). Immune deposits in tubulointerstitial nephritis are usually more easily detected by immunofluorescence/immunoperoxidase microscopy than by electron microscopy. Very rarely, there are linear deposits on the tubular basement membranes (see p. 467).

The interstitial cellular infiltrate is composed predominantly of T lymphocytes with or without plasma cells and neutrophil granulocytes. Within the T lymphocyte population there is great variability in the relative number of CD4-positive and CD8-positive subsets, but in the majority of patients the ratio of T4 to T8 positive cells is less than one.[129] Interstitial fibrosis, thickening and duplication of tubular basement membranes and tubular damage are frequent. The severity of tubulointerstitial damage correlates poorly or not at all with the presence of immune deposits,[128,130] but it correlates well with the degree of renal insufficiency and is an accurate prognostic indicator of progressive deterioration of renal function.[128]

Why tubulointerstitial deposits are common in systemic lupus erythematosus is not known. One possibility is that the mononuclear phagocytic system, which is the usual mechanism for the removal of circulating immune complexes, is saturated by high levels of complexes. As a result the complexes overflow, reach the peritubular capillaries and pass through their wall into the interstitium.[131] Another possibility is that tubulointerstitial immune complexes are formed locally following the release of DNA or other intracellular antigens from tubular cells.[131] There is no direct evidence concerning the way in which tubulointerstitial deposits mediate renal injury; the frequent presence of complement components suggests a pathogenetic role for the complement system. Local cell-mediated mechanisms are also probably involved.[129]

Sjøgren's syndrome

Focal tubulointerstitial nephritis occurs in approximately one-third of patients with Sjøgren's syndrome (see p. 248) but the presence of immune complexes has been described in only a few patients.[132,133] It has been suggested that the tubulointerstitial immune deposits may be formed locally; antibodies to renal tubular antigens are detected in the sera of some cases.[132]

Other conditions[134]

Immune complex tubulointerstitial nephritis has also been described in a few patients with mesangiocapillary glomerulonephritis, membranous glomerulonephritis, crescentic glomerulonephritis and shunt-associated glomerulonephritis. In addition, it has been described in mixed cryoglobulinaemia, acute bacterial endocarditis and cutaneous vasculitis.[135] The occurrence of immune complex tubulointerstitial nephritis in renal allografts is described on page 660.

TUBULOINTERSTITIAL NEPHRITIS ASSOCIATED WITH ANTIBODIES REACTING WITH TUBULAR ANTIGENS

Tubulointerstitial disease associated with antitubular-basement-membrane antibodies occurs in several human diseases but is rare. It has also been described in a few renal allografts (see p. 660). Antitubular-basement-membrane antibodies are present in the circulation and can be detected by radioimmunoassay or enzyme-linked immunosorbent assay.[136] In the kidneys there are linear deposits of IgG and C3 along variable numbers of tubular basement membranes (Fig. 12.26).[137] The proximal tubules are most affected. When adequate tissue is available, antitubular-basement-membrane antibodies can be found in eluates of the kidneys. The linear tubular basement membrane staining sometimes

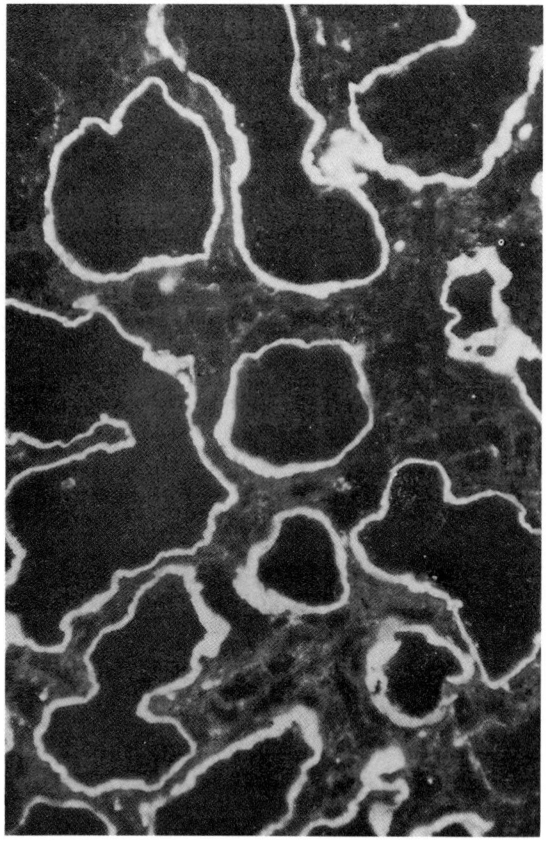

Fig. 12.26 Tubulointerstitial nephritis associated with antitubular-basement-membrane antibodies. There is linear staining of the tubular basement membranes for IgG. Immunofluorescence × 250
Reproduced by permission from: Bergstein J, Litman N. N Engl J Med 1975; 292: 875 (Fig. 2)

diminishes with time; it was scanty in one case after the disease had been present for 2 years.[138] In diabetes mellitus linear basement membrane staining for IgG also occurs, but this is accompanied by staining for albumin and there is no staining for C3, so confusion with antitubular-basement-membrane antibody should not arise (see p. 334). However, proof that linear staining is due to antitubular-basement-membrane antibody must be obtained in each case by demonstrating the antibody in either the serum or in a renal eluate.

Antiglomerular-basement-membrane disease

Tubulointerstitial nephritis associated with antibodies to tubular basement membrane antigens is principally found in cases of antiglomerular-basement-membrane disease (see p. 217), including patients with Goodpasture's syndrome (see p. 224). More than half of all patients with antiglomerular-basement-membrane disease have evidence of antitubular-basement-membrane antibodies.[137] The most prominent renal change is an interstitial mononuclear cell infiltrate.[139] The proximal tubules may show loss of brush borders, atrophy and thickening or rupture of their basement membranes. Electron microscopy demonstrates invasion of the tubules by lymphocytes and gaps in their basement membrane. There are no electron-dense deposits.[139]

The antitubular-basement-membrane antibodies are probably responsible for at least some of the tubulointerstitial nephritis because the tubular and interstitial damage is more severe in patients with diffuse crescentic glomerulonephritis who have these antibodies than in those who have only antibodies directed against glomerular basement membrane.[139] Animal experiments suggest that the antitubular-basement-membrane antibody probably damages the tubules through Fc receptors on macrophages and perhaps by complement fixation. T lymphocytes are essential for their action.[140] Little is known about the nature of the antigens against which human antitubular-basement-membrane antibodies react in antiglomerular-basement-membrane disease. Attempts to induce tubulointerstitial nephritis in animals by the transfer of human serum containing antitubular-basement-membrane antibodies have not been successful.

Other diseases

Antitubular-basement-membrane antibodies and tubulointerstitial nephritis have been found in several children and adults with *membranous glomerulonephritis* (see p. 200).[137,138] Some of these cases seem to be secondary to the use of diuretics in the treatment of the disease; in others the connection is unclear. Familial membranous glomerulonephritis with antitubular-basement-membrane antibodies has also been reported.[141] A few patients with *systemic lupus erythematosus* have had tubulointerstitial nephritis and antitubular-basement-membrane antibodies.[142]

Linear staining for IgG along tubular basement membranes, suggestive of antitubular-basement-membrane antibodies, has been recorded in *nephronophthisis* (see p. 68) and in a few patients with *endocapillary proliferative glomerulonephritis* (see p. 142).

Drug induced tubulointerstitial nephritis

Tubulointerstitial nephritis associated with linear deposits of IgG along tubular basement membranes develops in a small percentage of patients who receive penicillins or phenytoin (see p. 455).

TUBULOINTERSTITIAL NEPHRITIS ASSOCIATED WITH CELL-MEDIATED HYPERSENSITIVITY

Lymphocytic infiltration is present in all forms of tubulointerstitial nephritis but, with one exception, there is no proof that the lymphocytes actually mediate the injury. The exception is acute rejection in allografts (see p. 636). However, persuasive indirect evidence suggests a role for T cells in the pathogenesis of drug-induced interstitial nephritis (see p. 457).

OBSTRUCTIVE UROPATHY

Obstruction to the outflow of urine at any point will increase back pressure and may cause structural changes in the urinary tract. This condition is referred to as *obstructive uropathy*. The type of change will depend upon the severity, site and duration of the obstruction. Back pressure on the kidney will result in dilatation of the pelvis and of the calyces and eventually in parenchymal damage.

The term *hydronephrosis* is used to describe dilatation of the pelvis and calyces; it is usually, but not always, the result of obstructive uropathy. *Obstructive nephropathy* refers to the renal parenchymal damage that ensues from obstruction to the flow of urine. As hydronephrosis often leads to obstructive nephropathy the former term is commonly used to embrace both the pelvicalyceal and renal parenchymal changes. If infection develops in an obstructed kidney, pus may collect in the dilated pelvis. This condition is called *pyonephrosis*.

HYDRONEPHROSIS

Hydronephrosis is common, occurs at all ages and is a frequent cause of renal failure. There is a peak incidence below the age of 1 year and then again in the elderly. In adults aged 20–60 years it is more frequent in women because of pregnancy and carcinoma of the cervix; after the age of 60 years it is commoner in men due to hyperplasia and carcinoma of the prostate. In infants and children the obstruction is commonly congenital. Early recognition of obstructive uropathy is important since correction of the lesion may prevent, halt or reduce deterioration of renal function.

Causes

The commonest cause of hydronephrosis is obstruction. Rarely hydronephrosis may occur for some other reason.

Obstruction The obstruction may be structural or functional. In either case it can be acute, subacute or chronic, bilateral or unilateral, and partial or complete. In infants and children obstruction is almost always partial and chronic.

Structural obstruction. Some of the structural causes of urinary tract obstruction are listed in Table 12.3.

Functional obstruction. This is due to a dynamic abnormality in the urinary tract. Some of the

Table 12.3. Some structural causes of urinary tract obstruction

Infants and children	Adults
Urethra or bladder neck	
Meatal stenosis	Benign hyperplasia of the prostate
Phimosis	Carcinoma of the prostate
Urethral valves	Urethral stricture
Bladder	
Calculus	Calculus
Blood clot	Blood clot
	Carcinoma of the bladder
	Foreign body
Ureter	
Congenital stricture	Pregnancy, uterine prolapse
Ureterocele	Carcinoma of the cervix
Blood clot	Calculus
Retroperitoneal tumour	Carcinoma of ureter
	Blood clot
	Papillary tissue in renal papillary necrosis
	Stricture
	Retroperitoneal tumour
	Retroperitoneal fibrosis
	Abdominal aortic aneurysm
	Surgical ligation
Ureteropelvic junction and renal pelvis	
Congenital stricture	Calculus
Aberrant renal artery	Carcinoma of the pelvis
Blood clot	Blood clot
	Papillary tissue in renal papillary necrosis
	Aberrant renal artery
	Fibrous band
	Ball of fungus

Reproduced by permission from: Wilson DR. Urinary tract obstruction. In: Schrier RW, Gottschalk CW, eds. Diseases of the kidney, vol 1, 4th edn. Boston: Little, Brown, 1988: 716.

Table 12.4. Some functional causes of urinary tract obstruction

Infants and children	Adults
Bladder	
Neurogenic bladder	Neurogenic bladder
Congenital spinal cord defects	Multiple sclerosis
Myelodysplasia	Paraplegia
	Tabes dorsalis
	Diabetes mellitus
	Parkinson's disease
Ureter	
Primary megaureter	Vesicoureteric reflux
Vesicoureteric reflux	Pregnancy
Acute pyelonephritis	Acute pyelonephritis

Reproduced by permission from: Wilson DR. Urinary tract obstruction. In: Schrier RW, Gottschalk CW, eds. Diseases of the kidney, vol 1, 4th edn. Boston: Little, Brown, 1988: 717.

causes of functional obstruction are listed in Table 12.4. In the ureter the dysfunction is usually impaired peristalsis (see p. 684); in the urinary bladder failure of neurogenic control may produce involuntary micturition or a flaccid atonic bladder (see p. 700). These functional changes can cause a significant increase in back pressure and produce hydronephrosis. Certain strains of *Escherichia coli* introduced into the ureter of a monkey will paralyse peristalsis and produce obstruction with increased ureteral perfusion pressure;[143] this form of functional obstruction probably also occurs in some cases of acute pyelonephritis in humans.

Physiological dilatation of the ureters, including the pelvis, may occur in pregnancy (see p. 549). It is commoner on the right side and it may persist for weeks after delivery. Its origin is probably in part structural obstruction by the enlarged uterus, in part functional, but it is far from adequately understood. The importance is that in the minority of cases it may predispose to the development of pyelonephritis.

Non-obstructive causes Rarely hydronephrosis arises from a non-obstructive cause. An example is when there is a high flow of urine, such as in mannitol-induced diuresis. This causes a transitory dilatation of the pelvis and calyces.

Clinical features[144,145]

The clinical features are very variable; patients may present with an acute illness, with chronic or slowly progressive symptoms, or with minimal or no symptoms or signs. The form of presentation will depend upon the cause of the obstruction, whether it is unilateral or bilateral, partial or complete, its duration and on the presence or not of complications such as urinary tract infection.[145] There may be bladder symptoms if there is partial bilateral obstruction; acute renal failure if there is complete bilateral obstruction or complete obstruction of a solitary kidney; chronic renal failure if there is severe partial bilateral obstruction; polyuria if there is chronic partial bilateral obstruction; flank pain or enlarged tender kidney if there is complete or partial unilateral obstruction; and resistant or recurrent urinary tract infections with any obstructive lesion.[145] The initial clinical picture may relate only to the underlying process causing the obstruction.

Chronic obstructive uropathy should be suspected if there is deterioration of renal function associated with proteinuria of less than 2 g/24 hours and only occasional leucocytes and granular casts in the urine. Deterioration of renal function without apparent cause should always raise the possibility of obstruction.[144]

The diagnosis is usually made by intravenous pyelography; if renal function is impaired sonography or computerized axial tomography may provide the answer.

Renal changes

Gross appearance of the kidneys[146] The pelvis and calyces are dilated. With time the pressure of the enclosed fluid gradually obliterates the pyramids and compresses the columns of Bertin

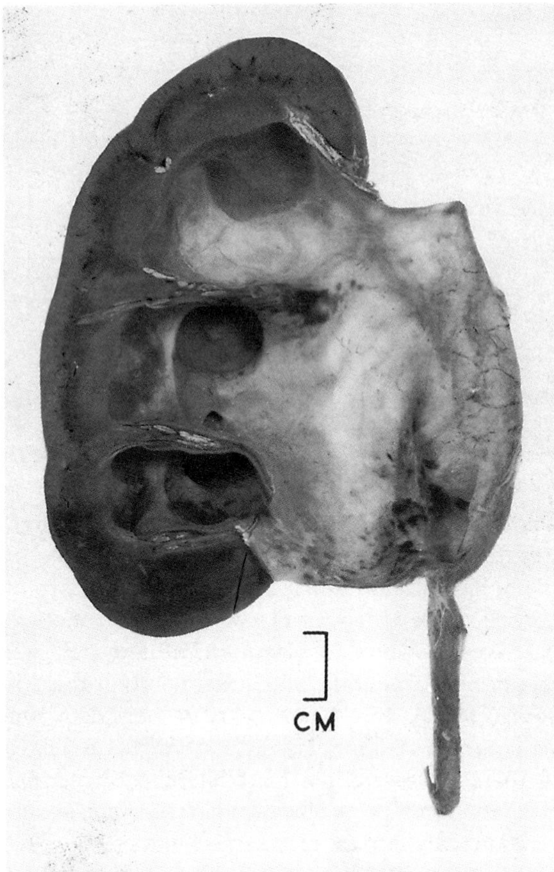

Fig. 12.27 Hydronephrosis caused by obstruction at the pelviureteric junction.
Reproduced by permission of the Curator of the Gordon Museum, Guy's Hospital, London, UK

into thin septa (Fig. 12.27). These papillary and calyceal changes are widespread and not confined to one or two collecting units. The cortex then becomes reduced in thickness and the surface of the kidney becomes bosselated. Eventually the septa disappear and all that remains of the kidney is a thin fibrous pouch filled with fluid. If the condition is unilateral the contralateral kidney undergoes progressive compensatory hypertrophy.

Light microscopy Within 24 hours of the onset of obstruction widespread dilatation of the collecting ducts occurs and the interstitium becomes oedematous, especially in the region of the collecting ducts. A few days later the lining epithelium of the ducts becomes flattened and basophilic and small groups of epithelial cells undergo necrosis. Slight dilatation is found in the distal convoluted tubules but dilatation of the proximal tubules is variable and patchy. Proximal tubules with collapsed lumen are frequent, particularly in slight to moderate hydronephrosis. If the hydronephrosis is severe the proximal tubules lose their microvilli.[147] Over the next few weeks the number of fibroblasts increases in the oedematous interstitium and is followed by laying down of collagen. Collections of Tamm–Horsfall protein often appear in the interstitium. Sometimes the protein can be seen extruding from tubules, in lymphatics or projecting into veins to form polyps.[148] If the obstruction is not relieved the proximal tubules become atrophic, with very thick basement membranes; some of the tubules may contain hyaline casts. The interstitium remains prominent. The glomeruli are little affected initially, an increase in Bowman's space and pericapsular fibrosis being the only changes; with progression of the disease an increasing number become sclerosed. Superimposed on this picture there may be focal areas of inflammatory infiltration in the interstitium relating to episodes of bacterial infection (see p. 434).

Electron microscopy In the proximal tubules there is loss of microvilli, reduction in the number of unfoldings of the basolateral membrane and lateral cellular interdigitations, flattening of the nuclei, and reduction in the number of mitochondria, of the amount of endoplasmic reticulum and of the size of the Golgi complex. All these changes seem to be related in their severity to the degree of tubular atrophy.[147]

Differential diagnosis

The microscopic changes in the cortex in hydronephrosis and obstructive nephropathy are very similar to those seen when the tubules are obstructed in the medulla in *analgesic nephropathy* (see p. 458) or *nephronophthisis medullary cystic disease* (see p. 68). Cortical damage due to slowly progressive ischaemia, as in *renal artery stenosis* (see p. 298), may be distinguished because in this condition there tends to be less interstitial fibrosis and oedema. In ischaemic atrophy the tubules are usually closely apposed, especially in the early stages; in obstructive nephropathy the atrophic tubules are usually separated by abundant interstitial tissue. Hydronephrosis without superimposed infection is characterized by minimal cellular infiltration in the interstitium and can be separated from both obstructive and non-obstructive chronic pyelonephritis by this interstitial difference. However, bouts of infection are so common in hydronephrosis that this distinction is of little practical use in most instances.

Complications

Urinary tract infection Chronic bacteriuria is frequent and difficult to eradicate in patients with obstructive uropathy. As a result acute pyelonephritis and chronic obstructive pyelonephritis are common complications of hydronephrosis. The infection can be blood borne or ascending by the ureter from the bladder. In animal experiments *Escherichia coli* injected intravenously will cause acute infection of the kidney if the ureter has been partially obstructed.[8] Ascending infections are also more common in the presence of obstruction and intrarenal reflux. Infection is particularly frequent if the obstruction is below the level of the bladder, probably mainly because the increased volume of residual urine left after urination provides an excellent medium in which bacteria may multiply.

Acute pyelonephritis may progress to pyonephrosis (see p. 472).

Renal calculi Magnesium ammonium phosphate (struvite) stones are a frequent and serious complication (see p. 538). They occur when there is already infection with bacteria which produce urease and break down urea in the urine to ammonia. The ammonia raises the pH of the urine which causes struvite to precipitate with eventual formation of a renal pelvic staghorn calculus. The resulting obstruction at the ureteropelvic junction frequently causes complete loss of renal function.

Hypertension In bilateral hydronephrosis hypertension may result from fluid retention with extracellular fluid volume expansion. Occasionally, hypertension complicates unilateral hydronephrosis and obstructive nephropathy; this is sometimes renin dependent. In both circumstances the hypertension may improve after relief of the obstruction.

Polycythaemia A few patients with hydronephrosis and obstructive nephropathy develop polycythaemia, presumably as a consequence of increased synthesis and release of erythropoietin.

Prognosis

Recovery of renal function after relief of total obstruction is related to the duration of obstruction. Function is frequently regained after obstruction of less than 3 weeks' duration, and some recovery of function was demonstrated in one patient when the duration of unilateral obstruction was 3 months.[19] The potential for recovery is better in partial than in complete obstruction, and when there is no complicating pyelonephritis. A marked and sometimes prolonged diuresis may follow the relief of obstruction; this is attended by massive losses of sodium and other solutes that can cause severe hypovolaemia if not treated.[150]

Pathogenesis

Atrophy of the renal parenchyma Two main mechanisms have been proposed to explain the atrophy of the renal parenchyma that occurs in sustained hydronephrosis.

Ischaemia. Obstruction to the outflow of urine from the kidneys is followed by a progressive and eventually very marked reduction in renal blood flow.[151] The reasons for this diminution in flow are complex;[152] they probably involve mechanical venous obstruction consequent upon pelvic dilatation and increased pressure,[153] stretching of vessels,[146] intrarenal vasoconstriction [154] and possibly contraction of interstitial myofibroblasts affecting the circulation through the peritubular capillaries.[155] It seems probable that the parenchymal atrophy that occurs in unrelieved hydronephrosis is in part due to the ischaemia that results from this impairment of blood flow. During atrophy some of the renal parenchymal cells shrink and are then phagocytosed and digested by adjacent cells, the process known as apoptosis.[152,156]

Pressure atrophy. Compression of renal tissue by the accumulation of urine in the renal pelvis and tubules may be another important factor.[157] The finding that the renal papillae are flattened and atrophied out of proportion to the cortex is in agreement with this concept.[145] Intrarenal reflux (see p. 436) is common, probably because the increased pelvicalyceal pressure flattens the pliant renal papillae and causes the slit-like openings of the ducts of Bellini to gape. It is suggested that the mechanical effect of this raised pressure in the collecting tubules may also be contributary.

Interstitial oedema The interstitial oedema seems to result partly from fluid being forced under pressure through the tubular walls into the surrounding tissues and by backflow of urine into the parenchyma through ruptures in the pelvic epithelium in the region of the renal fornices (evaginations of the minor calyces which penetrate outward into the renal parenchyma). Dilated tubules also rupture into thin-walled veins, forming tubulovenous anastomoses with extravasation of urine into the veins.[158] Dyes and other markers placed in the obstructed pelvis of a hydronephrotic kidney progressively disappear from the pelvis and appear in the lymph and general circulation.

PYONEPHROSIS

If acute pyelonephritis develops in an obstructed, hydronephrotic kidney, the dilated pelvis and calyces may become filled with pus. The term 'pyonephrosis' is used to describe this appearance. Eventually, in advanced cases, the kidney is sometimes converted into a sac of pus.

TUBULOINTERSTITIAL NEPHRITIS ASSOCIATED WITH VESICOURETERIC REFLUX

Vesicoureteric reflux is the regurgitation of urine through an incompetent vesicoureteric junction (see p. 685). It may be either primary or secondary. In primary vesicoureteric reflux the generally accepted view is that the defect is one of shortness of the submucosal segment of the ureter due to congenital lateral ectopia of the ureteric orifice.[159] Secondary vesicoureteric reflux may be a complication of several conditions, including obstructive uropathy (see p. 467), inflammatory disorders such as tuberculosis (see p. 383) and schistosomiasis (see p. 421) involving the vesicoureteric junction, surgery to the ureteric orifice, irradiation of the bladder, and renal transplantation (see p. 625). Urinary tract infections may temporarily induce reflux.

Whether the kidney is scarred by vesicoureteric reflux seems to depend on whether the urine is infected or sterile.

RENAL DISEASE ARISING FROM VESICOURETERIC REFLUX AND INFECTED URINE

Vesicoureteric reflux associated with infected urine may lead to either acute pyelonephritis (see p. 432) or chronic pyelonephritis (see p. 439). This may happen either in the presence of obstruction or without it. The term *reflux nephropathy* is commonly used to describe non-obstructive chronic pyelonephritis arising in these circumstances (see p. 439).

RENAL DISEASE ARISING FROM VESICOURETERIC REFLUX AND STERILE URINE

Although it is now clear from studies in pigs and monkeys that high grade vesicoureteric reflux of sterile urine at great pressure can lead to focal scarring of the kidney,[57,160] there is still controversy about whether such scarring can be produced in humans without infection. The work in animals has shown that loss of renal function will occur in the presence of sterile urine only if there is bladder neck obstruction of such severity that the ureter becomes incompetent and allows transmission of voiding pressure to occur continuously.[57,160]

The extreme urodynamic conditions required

to produce sterile reflux scarring in animals are rarely encountered in patients. They might operate in some male infants with posterior urethral valves or in some children with a neuropathic bladder.[160] Even in these situations it is difficult to be sure that urinary infection has never occurred; moreover, in patients with urethral valves any scars encountered have to be distinguished from lesions due to dysplastic development.[161]

Sterile reflux in animals with bladder neck obstruction produces a diffuse dilatation of pelvis and calyces with focal scars morphologically similar to those seen in patients with non-obstructive chronic pyelonephritis (see p. 440) but lacking lymphoid follicles in the interstitium.[160,162]

There have been claims that sterile reflux causes widespread renal damage in humans.[163] However, in all these patients it is impossible to be sure that the urine has been constantly sterile. This applies particularly to those who give no history of urinary tract infection and present with renal scarring and end-stage renal failure. Careful follow-up of children with all grades of vesicoureteric reflux has shown no development of scarring in those in whom regular testing of the urine has revealed no evidence of infection.[36] This suggests that if sterile reflux nephropathy occurs it is probably rare.

RENAL SEGMENTAL ATROPHY (ASK-UPMARK KIDNEY)[164]

In renal segmental atrophy one or both kidneys are small and bear deep transverse grooves on the cortical surface. Each groove extends downwards to a dilated calyx from which it is separated by a fibrous plaque. The condition is rare and predominantly affects females. It causes hypertension and this is often discovered in adolescence. Initially the Ask-Upmark kidney was considered a developmental abnormality in which nephrogenesis had been arrested in one or a few adjacent renal lobes after the formation of the juxtamedullary nephrons. However, in 70% of cases the Ask-Upmark kidney is associated with vesicoureteric reflux and this and infection are probably responsible for the condition.[165,166]

TUBULOINTERSTITIAL NEPHRITIS ASSOCIATED WITH PAPILLARY NECROSIS

RENAL PAPILLARY NECROSIS

There are several conditions in which necrosis occurs in the papillary part of the medulla of one or both kidneys. The commonest of these are diabetes mellitus (see below), acute obstructive pyelonephritis (see p. 432) and ingestion of large quantities of compound analgesics (see p. 458) or non-steroidal anti-inflammatory drugs (see p. 474) In some areas of certain countries with a high incidence of renal papillary necrosis, such as Australia, Switzerland and Scandinavia, most cases are associated with analgesic abuse; in countries with a relatively low prevalence of renal papillary necrosis, such as Britain and much of the USA, diabetes mellitus, acute obstructive pyelonephritis and the consumption of non-steroidal anti-inflammatory drugs account for the majority of cases. Renal papillary necrosis is also occasionally encountered in the sickle cell haemoglobinopathies (see p. 106),[167] in renal transplants (see p. 625), in renal vein thrombosis (see p. 293), in Wegener's granulomatosis (see p. 275),[168] in pancreatitis, in candidosis (see p. 406), in aspergillosis (see p. 409), in mucormycosis (see p. 410) and in chronic alcoholism.[169] In infancy and childhood, it may be seen in association with shock, septicaemia, severe dehydration and diarrhoea.[170]

Renal papillary necrosis in analgesic nephropathy

The association between renal papillary necrosis and the excessive use of analgesic drugs is discussed on page 458. The signs and symptoms produced and the morphological changes in the kidneys are described there.

Renal papillary necrosis in diabetes mellitus

Renal papillary necrosis is found in approximately a quarter of diabetic patients who die and are examined at autopsy.[171] The incidence is greater in females. In countries where analgesic abuse is uncommon diabetes mellitus accounts for about

50–60% of the cases of renal papillary necrosis reported in the major series.

Clinical features

The clinical picture is variable but a fulminating course with septicaemia and acute renal failure is more common than in cases of renal papillary necrosis arising in analgesic nephropathy.

Renal changes

Gross appearance of the kidneys The kidneys are more likely to be normal in size when renal papillary necrosis occurs in diabetes mellitus than when it complicates analgesic abuse. The necrosis usually affects the distal two-thirds of the papilla and is frequently surrounded by a cream zone; in analgesic nephropathy the lesion usually lacks a pale zone and often involves only the tip of the papilla. In diabetes mellitus the necrotic papillae usually remain attached; in analgesic nephropathy they frequently separate and are shed. The cortex is usually not thinned. The changes of acute pyelonephritis (see p. 434) are usually evident in the renal parenchyma and pelvis.

Light microscopy Even in the early stages the affected papillae generally exhibit necrosis of all the tissue; it is unusual to find preservation of collecting ducts and vasa recta as often occurs in analgesic nephropathy. The damaged papilla is commonly separated from the adjacent tissues by a broad band of neutrophil granulocytes (the cream zone seen with the naked eye). Because the renal papillary necrosis is so acute in diabetic patients the cortex does not usually show the extensive tubular atrophy and interstitial fibrosis that eventually occurs in analgesic nephropathy. The usual diabetic glomerular and vascular changes are present (see p. 330).

Pathogenesis

The probable importance of the diabetic vascular changes and acute pyelonephritis in precipitating renal papillary necrosis in diabetes mellitus is discussed on page 339.

Renal papillary necrosis in acute pyelonephritis

Acute obstructive pyelonephritis has been reported as the cause of renal papillary necrosis in 15–40% of cases. *Acute non-obstructive pyelonephritis* and *emphysematous pyelonephritis* can also result in papillary necrosis (see pp. 435, 438); usually they are associated with diabetes mellitus.

The clinical features and the renal morphology usually resemble those that occur in diabetes mellitus. With obstruction there will be in addition hydronephrosis or pyonephrosis.

Renal papillary necrosis associated with non-steroidal anti-inflammatory drugs

All non-steroidal anti-inflammatory drugs that have been tested have caused renal papillary necrosis in experimental animals, but there are few reports of this disorder in humans treated with these agents.[172] The evidence from patients with chronic painful arthritis who take these drugs over many years is difficult to interpret. Renal papillary necrosis is found at autopsy in 20–30% of patients with rheumatoid arthritis,[173] whereas screening in arthritis clinics has revealed little evidence of nephrotoxicity[174] and renal papillary necrosis has been infrequently reported as a complication during life.[175] This discrepancy is unexplained.

The fact that non-steroidal anti-inflammatory drugs inhibit prostaglandin synthesis and diminish medullary blood flow suggests that they should predispose to renal papillary necrosis. Only after further use and greater length of exposure to these drugs will we know if this prediction is false.

Clinical features

In most cases the onset has been insidious. Episodes of gross or microscopic haematuria have been early signs in some children.[170]

Renal changes

The papillary lesions resemble those in analgesic nephropathy in being small and multiple but they are not pigmented and the necrotic papillae more often remain attached to the medulla. No distinctive features are shown by light microscopy.

Renal papillary necrosis in sickle cell disease

Various types of papillary abnormality thought to indicate papillary necrosis are seen radiologically in approximately 50% of patients with sickling disorders.[176] The papillary lesions develop slowly and do not usually cause renal failure. The clinical manifestations do not differ from those encountered in renal papillary necrosis in analgesic nephropathy.

Renal changes

The renal changes usually resemble those seen in the form of renal papillary necrosis that occurs in analgesic nephropathy, except that pigmentation is not present.

Pathogenesis

The conditions in the medulla in sickle cell disease that predispose to necrosis of renal papillae are discussed on page 106.

Renal papillary necrosis in other conditions

When renal papillary necrosis occurs in association with *renal vein thrombosis, arteritis* and *renal transplantation* the clinical features and the renal morphology usually resemble those that occur in renal papillary necrosis in diabetes mellitus. In *chronic alcoholism* the lesions may resemble either those of the acute type of renal papillary necrosis that occurs in diabetes or the chronic type that is associated with analgesic abuse; in patients with the latter pattern it is possible that excessive ingestion of analgesics is the reason.

HEAVY METAL-INDUCED TUBULOINTERSTITIAL LESIONS

Chronic exposure to lead (see p. 503), mercury (see p. 505) and cisplatin (see p. 516) will lead to tubulointerstitial disease. The other heavy metals cause predominantly tubular damage. Heavy metal poisoning is discussed in Chapter 13 (see p. 502).

ACUTE TUBULAR NECROSIS

In acute tubular necrosis the injury is predominantly to the tubules. This condition is considered in Chapter 13 (see p. 491).

TUBULOINTERSTITIAL NEPHROPATHY CAUSED BY METABOLIC DISTURBANCES

Hypercalcaemic nephropathy

Hypercalcaemia may initially cause an acute and reversible fall in glomerular filtration rate; if persistent it will eventually lead to the development of nephrocalcinosis with calcium deposits and a tubulointerstitial nephritis (see p. 544).

Urate nephropathy

Deposition of urates in the kidneys is often associated with a tubulointerstitial nephritis. Urate nephropathy is discussed under hyperuricaemia and gout on page 341.

Oxalate nephropathy

In this condition there is deposition of calcium oxalate crystals in the kidney, accompanied by tubulointerstitial damage. Oxalate nephropathy due to primary hyperoxaluria is discussed on page 103. Secondary hyperoxaluria can develop as a consequence of poisoning with ethylene glycol, anaesthesia with methoxyflurane or deficiency of pyridoxine.

Cystinosis

Cystinosis is a rare disorder of metabolism in which there is widespread deposition of cystine crystals in the lysosomes of cells that exhibit phagocytosis and pinocytosis. In the adult form there is no renal involvement, but in the infantile and adolescent forms intracellular cystine accumulation eventually leads to atrophy of the tubules, interstitial fibrosis and focal infiltration by mononuclear cells. These changes are most severe in the infantile form. Cystinosis is discussed on page 93.

Other metabolic disorders

Hypokalaemic nephropathy (see p. 97), glycogen storage disease (see p. 102), iron deposition, copper deposition, bile deposition, hyaline droplet degeneration and fatty change are all predominantly or exclusively tubular disorders.

HEREDITARY TUBULOINTERSTITIAL DISORDERS

NEPHRONOPHTHISIS–MEDULLARY CYSTIC DISEASE COMPLEX

This heterogeneous group of hereditary disorders is considered on page 68. They are diffuse renal diseases typically characterized by variable numbers of tiny medullary cysts, progressive tubular atrophy and interstitial fibrosis. Because medullary cysts do not inevitably occur, it has been suggested that cysts are not essential to either the pathogenesis or the evolution of this complex of diseases and that, as severe tubulointerstitial disease often dominates, these conditions should be regarded as genetically determined tubulo-interstitial conditions.[177]

OTHER HERITABLE SYNDROMES

Jeune's syndrome

This rare autosomal recessive syndrome consists of chondrodysplasia with short-limbed dwarfism and a narrow thoracic cage which produces severe neonatal respiratory distress. The kidneys contain cysts and there is a progressive tubulointerstitial nephritis which gives impaired urinary concentrating ability in those who survive into infancy.[177]

Laurence–Moon–Biedl–Bardet syndrome[178–180]

The rare Laurence–Moon–Biedl–Bardet syndrome is autosomal recessive and is characterized by obesity, mental retardation, polydactyly, retinitis pigmentosa and hypogenitalism. Renal disease occurs in more than 70% of cases and is an important cause of death. There is often a progressive tubulointerstitial nephritis but there are also glomerular lesions and there may be medullary and cortical cysts. The glomerular lesions include accumulation of granular material within the inner third of the capillary basement membrane; it is not known how specific this lesion is and whether it precedes the tubulointerstitial changes.

Alström's syndrome

Alström's syndrome is an extremely rare autosomal recessive condition characterized by blindness, nerve deafness, obesity and diabetes mellitus in adults.[181] It is accompanied by a progressive tubulointerstitial nephropathy with impaired urinary concentrating ability and aminoaciduria. The renal lesions do not seem to be secondary to the diabetes.

TUBULOINTERSTITIAL NEPHRITIS ASSOCIATED WITH NEOPLASTIC DISORDERS

Prominent tubulointerstitial nephritis may be associated with various non-renal neoplastic disorders. Examples are multiple myeloma (see p. 387), Waldenström's macroglobulinaemia (see p. 360), light chain deposition disease (see p. 362) and cryoglobulinaemia (see p. 351).

TUBULOINTERSTITIAL NEPHRITIS IN GLOMERULAR AND VASCULAR DISEASES

GLOMERULAR DISEASES

Tubulointerstitial nephritis is common in many forms of glomerulonephritis. Occasionally it is associated with immune deposits on the tubular basement membranes and in the interstitium (see p. 466).

In the advanced sclerosing stages of any type of chronic glomerulonephritis tubulointerstitial lesions are usually prominent. The tubular atrophy and interstitial fibrosis are probably caused mainly by ischaemia. The mononuclear cellular infiltrate may reflect cell mediated immunity (see p. 130); sometimes it may be evidence of ascending infection.

Tubulointerstitial nephritis is also often present in antiglomerular-basement-membrane disease (see p. 466) and in systemic lupus erythematosus (see p. 464).

VASCULAR DISEASES

Ischaemic lesions, particularly in the superficial cortex, are very common and produce tubulointerstitial changes which can closely resemble those that occur in chronic pyelonephritis (see p. 306); in the past the distinction was not always clearly made, with the result that chronic pyelonephritis was overdiagnosed.

MISCELLANEOUS INSTANCES OF TUBULOINTERSTITIAL DISEASE

RADIATION NEPHRITIS

Impairment of renal function and hypertension may result from inadvertent ionizing irradiation of the kidneys during treatment of malignant tumours; it may also follow total body irradiation in preparation for bone marrow transplantation.[182] It is today uncommon because of improved shielding of the kidney during radiotherapy. The dose of ionizing radiation that is required to produce nephritis is about 23 Gy (2300 rad) over a period of less than 5 weeks.[183] However, when radiotherapy is combined with cytotoxic drugs the kidneys may be damaged by lower doses of radiation. This seems to apply particularly to young children, in whom a dose as low as 15 Gy (1500 rad) has produced radiation nephritis.[184] Now that children with a nephroblastoma or with a bone marrow transplant survive for long periods after treatment (see p. 594), it has become even more important to avoid radiation nephritis.

Clinical features[185–187]

The clinical presentation of radiation injury may be either acute or chronic.

Acute presentation

The term 'acute' refers to the development of hypertension, often malignant, and uraemia approximately 6–12 months after irradiation; when a combination of radiation and chemotherapy is used the onset may be as early as 5 weeks after the treatment.[188] There may also be dependent oedema and effusions. In most cases there is severe anaemia; usually this is normochromic normocytic in type but occasionally it is microangiopathic and associated with a haemolytic uraemic syndrome (see p. 281).[189] The urine contains red cells and granular casts. Proteinuria, usually of less than 2 g/24 hours, is present in most patients. In the latent period before the onset of signs and symptoms the urine is generally normal and the blood urea nitrogen not raised.

Chronic presentation

In the chronic group are patients who first develop clinical manifestations years after their radiation therapy. There is insidious onset of renal insufficiency with mild proteinuria and often polyuria. Some patients lose sodium in their urine or develop hypoaldosteronism with hyperkalaemia and hyperchloraemic metabolic acidosis, but the signs and symptoms are usually no different from those in patients with renal failure from other causes. Hypertension is commonly present but rarely severe; a few patients develop malignant hypertension late in the course of the disease.[186]

Renal changes

Acute radiation nephritis

Gross appearance of the kidneys The kidneys usually appear normal.

Light microscopy The changes are principally in the glomeruli and in the arterioles and small arteries. Most glomeruli show expansion of the mesangium and thickening and duplication of the capillary walls (Fig. 12.28).[189] Sometimes there is focal necrosis of mesangial cells, fibrin thrombi in capillary lumens and swelling of endothelial cells.[182]

Focal fibrinoid necrosis of the walls of arterioles and small interlobular arteries is common (Fig. 12.29);[190] usually there is no cellular infiltration either around or within the walls. The larger

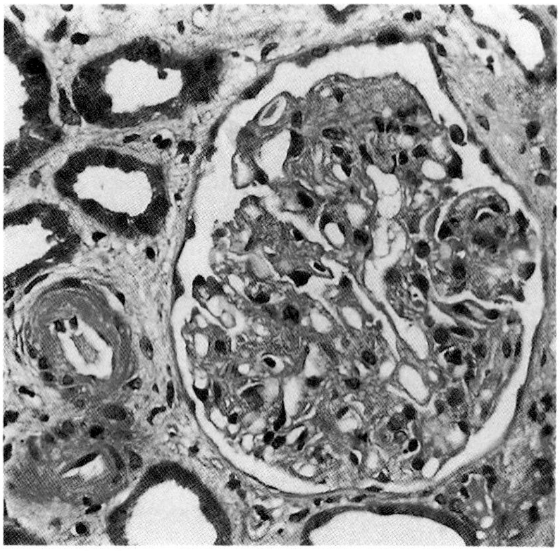

Fig. 12.28 Acute radiation nephritis. Glomerulus showing mesangial expansion and duplication of some of the capillary walls.
Haematoxylin-eosin × 460

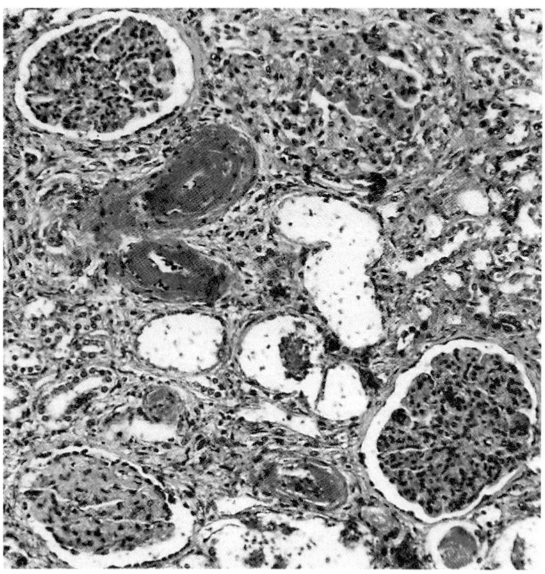

Fig. 12.29 Acute radiation nephritis. There is fibrinoid necrosis of the walls of arterioles.
Haematoxylin-eosin × 155

interlobular arteries often show a marked focal intimal thickening that narrows the lumens of these vessels. Lipid-containing foam cells are common in the thickened intima (Fig. 12.30).[189] Intravascular thrombi may occur. These changes do not extend to the arcuate, interlobar or segmental arteries.

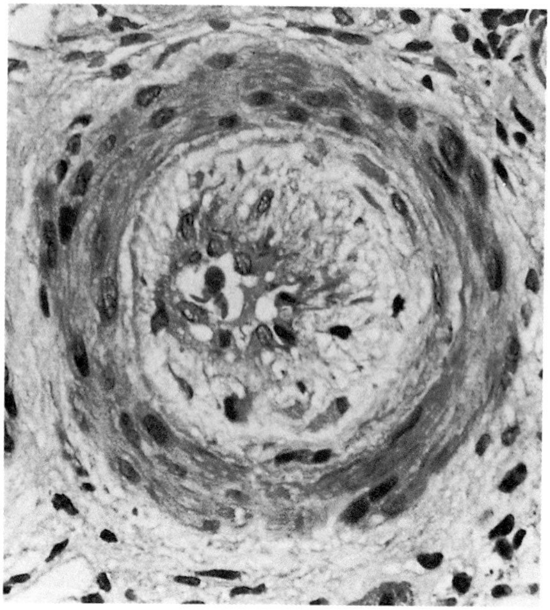

Fig. 12.30 Acute radiation nephritis. The intima of a small interlobular artery is thickened by loose tissue that contains foam cells. The arterial lumen is greatly reduced.
Haematoxylin-eosin × 350

Tubulointerstitial changes may be slight or there may be focal tubular damage and necrosis, affecting particularly the proximal tubules, and interstitial oedema.

Electron microscopy Characteristically in the glomerular capillary walls electron-lucent material accumulates between the basement membrane and the endothelium. This is often accompanied by formation of a new thin basement membrane beneath the displaced endothelium (Fig. 12.31).[189,190] The mesangium may appear expanded.

Immunofluorescence/immunoperoxidase microscopy Immunoglobulin M, complement and sometimes IgG have been found in the glomerular capillary and arteriolar walls of some patients.[182,191] In other cases staining has been negative.[192]

Chronic radiation nephritis

Gross appearance of the kidneys The kidneys are usually shrunken and the thickened cap-

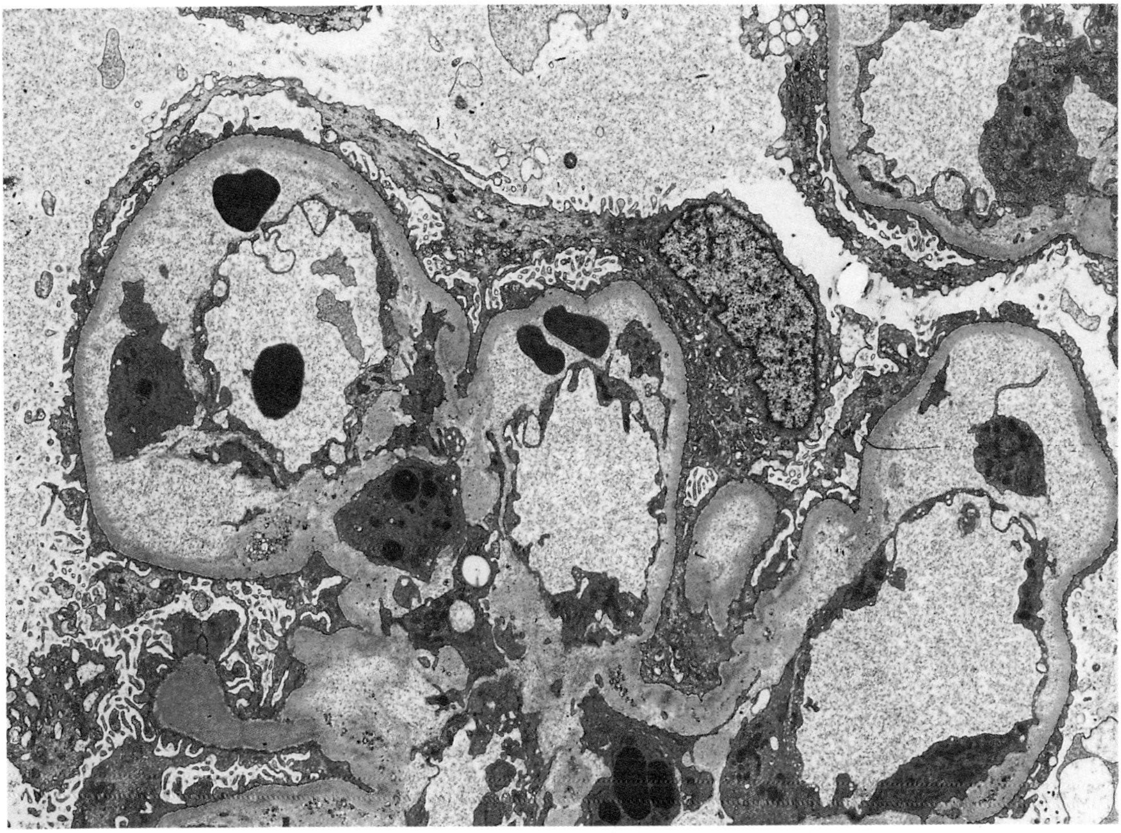

Fig. 12.31 Acute radiation nephritis. Electron micrograph of part of glomerulus showing marked thickening of the capillary wall by accumulation of electron-lucent material between the endothelium and the basement membrane. ×3600

sule is adherent to the surrounding tissues. The subcapsular surface is often granular.

Light microscopy The changes are principally in the tubules and glomeruli. Tubular atrophy is severe and extensive and the tubular basement membranes are thickened (Fig. 12.32). Many of the glomeruli are sclerosed; some may show the changes that are more characteristically encountered in acute radiation nephritis (see above). Focal or diffuse interstitial fibrosis is usual; sometimes there are a small number of infiltrating mononuclear cells. Some degree of narrowing of the larger interlobular arteries by intimal thickening is usually present but it is frequently minor in comparison with the tubular atrophy. The kidneys from patients with malignant hypertension will in addition usually show focal fibrinoid necrosis of arterioles.

Electron microscopy The proximal tubular cells are atrophic, with great reduction in the size of the microvilli. The glomerular capillary basement membranes appear tortuous, wrinkled and collapsed; they may also show subendothelial accumulation of electron-lucent material.

Differential diagnosis

The morphological changes in acute radiation nephritis may be indistinguishable from those seen in *malignant hypertension* (see p. 311), the *haemolytic uraemic syndrome* (see p. 283) and *thrombotic thrombocytopenic purpura* (see p. 289). The distinction between acute radiation nephritis and *progressive systemic sclerosis* (see p. 243) may sometimes be difficult on morphological grounds but widespread subendothelial electron-lucent collections in the glomeruli favour acute

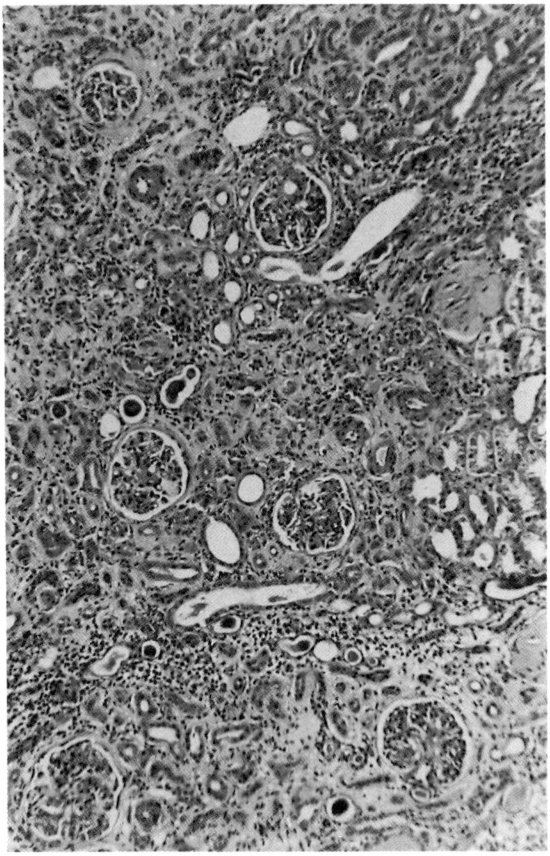

Fig. 12.32 Chronic radiation nephritis. There is widespread tubular atrophy.
Haematoxylin-eosin × 150

radiation nephritis and review of the clinical data should decide the issue. Extensive arteriolar damage sometimes may suggest *polyarteritis* (see p. 273) but the glomerular lesions of acute radiation nephritis, which are not present in polyarteritis, will usually distinguish the two conditions. Chronic radiation nephritis may closely resemble the ischaemic changes that arise in the kidney from *renal artery stenosis* (see p. 298), but characteristic glomerular and interlobular artery changes can usually be found in chronic radiation nephritis.

Complications

There is a risk that radiation-induced tumours may arise but the incidence is low.[193]

Prognosis[187]

The prognosis in acute radiation nephritis is related to the severity of the hypertension. If this can be controlled patients will survive but may be left with some degree of chronic renal failure. Chronic radiation nephritis is compatible with some years of life, depending on the severity of the renal failure.

Pathogenesis[187,194]

The precise way in which ionizing radiation exerts its effect on renal cells is still not known. One possibility is that most of the damage is caused by oxygen-derived free radicals, released from the cell water, which react with the cell membranes, cytoskeletal proteins, DNA and RNA, leading to biochemical changes which cause disordered function or death. DNA is considered to be the most critical target; breaks in the DNA strand have been observed in cells exposed to radiation.[195] Agents such as cysteine and dimethylsulphoxide that directly or indirectly remove free radicals reduce radiation damage.

The acute manifestations of radiation injury to the kidney are probably largely due to vascular damage. The vascular endothelial and smooth muscle cells normally have a very low turnover; after injection of tritiated thymidine (^{3}H-thymidine) the number of endothelial cells that become labelled is less than 1% and their turnover time has been calculated to be between 50 and 1000 days. After irradiation the number of endothelial and smooth muscle cells slowly begins to diminish as cells that die are not replaced; the severity of this process is dose dependent. Attempts at replacement occur but proliferation of the irradiated cells is abnormal and ineffective. Basement membranes become exposed and this leads to activation of the coagulation system with vascular narrowing or occlusion, reduction in blood flow and ischaemic damage to the tissue.

The severe tubular atrophy in chronic radiation nephritis is probably partly due to vascular injury and partly due to progressive loss of tubular cells as a direct consequence of radiation injury. The ability of the irradiated but surviving tubular cells to proliferate effectively is reduced.

BALKAN ENDEMIC NEPHROPATHY

An unusual form of chronic renal disease is prevalent among the inhabitants of a few villages in a small area in the vicinity of the Danube and its tributaries in adjacent parts of Romania, Yugoslavia and Bulgaria. The disease most commonly affects people between the ages of 30 and 60 years. It often occurs in families, progressively more of the members showing evidence of the disease as they age. It is not found among those who have lived for only a short time in the endemic areas; however, people from regions where the condition does not occur are liable to develop it if they live for 15 years or more in villages in which it is prevalent.[196,197] The incidence of the disease within the endemic area is variable, but levels as high as 10% of the population have been claimed for some villages.[198]

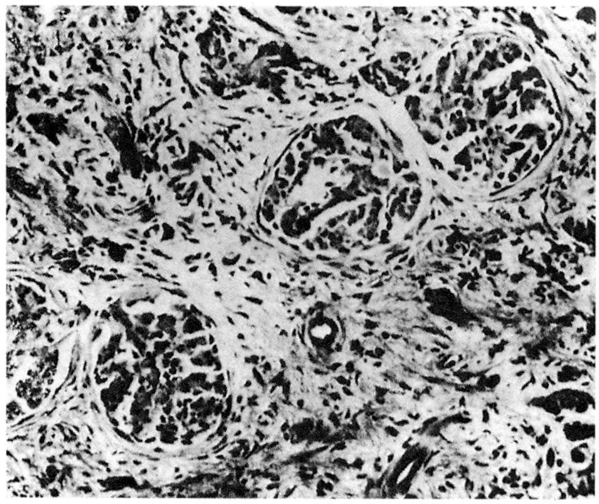

Fig. 12.33 Balkan endemic nephropathy. There is widespread tubular atrophy and loss, dense interstitial fibrosis and relatively unaffected glomeruli. The tubular basement membranes are thickened and distorted (arrows).
Periodic acid-Schiff × 250
Reproduced by permission from: Dammin GJ. Arch Pathol 1972; 93: 372 (Fig. 1)

Clinical features

The onset of the disease is insidious, with weakness, anorexia, lumbar pain and progressive renal failure, usually unaccompanied by salt retention or hypertension. The skin becomes pale and yellow; severe anaemia, which may be normochromic or hypochromic, is usual. Tubular proteinuria, shown by increased excretion in the urine of β_2-microglobulin, is the earliest manifestation of the disease.[196,199] Overt proteinuria, detected by routine tests, is a late feature; it is usually slight. The patients do not develop a nephrotic syndrome.

Renal changes

Gross appearance of the kidneys

At autopsy the kidneys are shrunken and the subcapsular surface is finely granular.[200] Carcinoma of the pelvis or ureter may be present because these neoplasms are unusually frequent among the same population and affect about a third of patients dying from Balkan endemic nephropathy (see pp. 613, 720).[201,202]

Light microscopy[199,203]

In the earlier stages of the disease the tubular cells, particularly those of the lower parts of the proximal convoluted tubules and the loops of Henle, show epithelial degeneration or regeneration. Some tubules are atrophic. There is interstitial oedema and fibrosis but only slight mononuclear cell infiltration. The glomeruli often show focal and segmental thickening of the capillary basement membranes and an increase in the number of mesangial cells and in the amount of mesangial matrix. There may be periglomerular fibrosis.

Later, there is widespread extreme tubular atrophy (Fig. 12.33). The cortical interstitium may become infiltrated by variable numbers of lymphocytes. In one small group of cases some of the renal veins showed muscular hypertrophy with or without obliteration and recanalization of the lumen.[203] There is usually prominent interstitial fibrosis in the inner cortex. Glomerulosclerosis and hyalinosis may be found, particularly in the subcapsular areas. Mild intimal thickening of arteries is frequent.

Electron microscopy

In a few cases subendothelial and intramembranous electron-dense deposits have been reported in the glomerular capillary basement membranes.[204]

These changes have not been seen in other cases.[199]

Immunofluorescence/immunoperoxidase microscopy

There are usually no deposits of immunoglobulin, complement or fibrin.[199] Granular deposits of IgG and C3 in the glomerular capillary walls have only been reported in small numbers of cases, including those with electron-dense deposits at this site.[204,205] Deposits on tubular basement membranes have also been recorded in a few of these patients.[205]

Differential diagnosis

Balkan endemic nephropathy can be differentiated from *non-obstructive chronic pyelonephritis* (see p. 439) by the lack of the calyceal distortion and segmental scarring with dense mononuclear cell infiltration that characterize pyelonephritis. The absence of papillary necrosis and the diffuseness of the change distinguish Balkan endemic nephropathy from *analgesic nephropathy* (see p. 458). Glomerular and vascular changes are usually more pronounced in *lead nephropathy* (see p. 503). *Cadmium poisoning* (see p. 504) is not usually associated with such marked and diffuse tubular atrophy. The morphological changes are very similar to those that occur in *chronic radiation nephritis* (see p. 478) and *obstructive uropathy* (see p. 468).

Prognosis

Survival after symptoms have appeared ranges from a few months to nearly 10 years, with approximately half the patients dying within 2 years. The natural history of the disease is almost certainly much longer than this because many asymptomatic patients are found to have proteinuria in village surveys.[199]

Pathogenesis

The pathogenesis of Balkan endemic nephropathy is not known and the relationship with tumours of the uroepithelium is unexplained.

Because of the geographical clustering all the early attention was focused on possible local environmental factors. Abnormal levels of trace elements such as cadmium, lead, copper, zinc, barium, chromium, fluorine, cobalt and silicon in the soil and water and in tissue from patients with the disease were sought but not detected. Radioactivity in the area was not unusually high. The disease existed before synthetic chemicals came to be used in agriculture. Searches for bacteria such as leptospirae, brucellae and streptococci have not been successful.[199] Claims of a causative role for arboviruses and slow porcine coronaviruses have been made but have not been adequately substantiated.[204] Plant nephrotoxins and fungi, especially *Penicillium verrucosum* var. *cyclopium*, have been suspected as possible causes because some of them have been found to produce lesions in the pars recta and junctional zone of the proximal tubules of experimental animals that closely resemble the changes in patients with Balkan endemic nephropathy.[199]

Recently there has been renewed interest in genetic factors and it has even been claimed that pedigree analysis reveals an autosomal dominant type of inheritance.[206] However, this is contrary to most studies, which still indicate that genetic factors are unlikely to be playing a direct role,[197] although an inherited predisposition to damage by some environmental factor may be an element in the story. Claims that there is a partial lecithin-cholesterol acyltransferase deficiency in patients with this disease have yet to be confirmed.[207]

SARCOID GRANULOMATOUS INTERSTITIAL NEPHRITIS

Granulomatous lesions in the interstitium of the kidneys occur in about 20% of patients with generalized sarcoidosis; in most cases they have little clinical relevance. Occasionally isolated sarcoid granulomatous interstitial nephritis causes acute renal failure. This is discussed on page 259.

INTERSTITIAL NEPHRITIS WITH UVEITIS

In 1975 a syndrome of acute tubulointerstitial nephritis with eosinophils, acute renal failure, anterior uveitis and granulomas in the bone marrow, was described in two patients.[208] Since then approximately 35 similar cases have been reported although in only a few was the bone marrow examined so identity cannot be assumed. The patients are mainly female, usually adolescents but sometimes adults.[209–211]

Clinical features

Presentation is with anorexia, weight loss and ocular symptoms. There is azotaemia, the erythrocyte sedimentation rate is raised and most patients are anaemic. Polyuria, glycosuria, aminoaciduria and mild proteinuria are common. About a quarter of the patients have an eosinophilia. In the adolescents the serum IgG is raised; this has not been described in adults.[212]

Renal changes

Light microscopy

The interstitium is infiltrated by eosinophils, lymphocytes and plasma cells. The number of eosinophils may decrease in the later stages of the disease or after treatment with steroids. A few granulomas were present in the interstitium of one of the first cases described; they have not been mentioned in subsequent cases. The lymphocytes are mostly CD4-positive T cells. There is focal necrosis or atrophy of the proximal convoluted tubules. The glomeruli show minimal mesangial expansion or are normal. The blood vessels are normal.

Immunofluorescence/immunoperoxidase microscopy

No tubulointerstitial or glomerular deposits have been detected.

Other organ changes

Non-caseating granulomas with Langhans giant cells have been found in the bone marrow. These lesions disappear after treatment.

Differential diagnosis

Toxoplasmosis and *infectious mononucleosis* may give a similar picture and should be excluded by appropriate staining of the biopsy in the former and by serology in both. *Sarcoidosis, brucellosis, tuberculosis* and *histoplasmosis* should be considered but are usually easily differentiated.

Prognosis

The renal disease may remit spontaneously or after treatment with steroids. Full recovery seems to occur in children; the outlook for adults is not yet clear.

Pathogenesis

The aetiology and pathogenesis are unknown. There is some evidence that the uveitis may be caused by immune complexes,[213] but on morphological evidence the interstitial nephritis appears to be a T-lymphocyte-mediated reaction.

REFERENCES

Introduction

1. Churg J, Cotran RS, Sinniah R, Sakaguchi H, Sobin LH. Renal disease. Classification and atlas of tubulointerstitial disease. New York: Igaku-Shoin, 1984.

Tubulointerstitial disease caused by infection

2. Hanson LÅ. Prognostic indicators in childhood urinary infections. Kidney Int 1982; 21: 659–667.
3. Robbins SL, Mallory GK, Kinney TD. Necrotizing renal papillitis: a form of acute pyelonephritis. New Engl J Med 1946; 235: 885–893.
4. Meyrier A, Condamin M-C, Fernet M et al. Frequency of development of early cortical scarring in acute primary pyelonephritis. Kidney Int 1989; 35: 696–703.
5. Kunin CM. The natural history of recurrent bacteriuria in school girls. In: Kincaid-Smith P, Fairley KF, eds. Renal infection and renal scarring. Melbourne: Mercedes, 1970; 3–23.
6. Smellie JM. Do urinary tract infections really matter in children? Proc R Soc Med 1972; 65: 513–514.
7. Smellie JM. Childhood urinary infections and their significance. In: Asscher AW, ed. The management of urinary infection. An international symposium. Oxford: Medicine Publishing Foundation, 1980: 29.
8. Brumfitt W, Heptinstall RH. Experimental

pyelonephritis: the influence of temporary and permanent ureteric obstruction on the localization of bacteria. Br J Exp Pathol 1958; 39: 610–617.
9. Brumfitt W, Heptinstall RH. Experimental pyelonephritis: the effect of renal vein constriction on bacterial localisation and multiplication in the rat kidney. Br J Exp Pathol 1959; 40: 145–148.
10. Kunin CM. Emergence of bacteriuria, proteinuria and symptomatic urinary tract infections among a population of school girls followed for 7 years. Pediatrics 1968; 41: 968–976.
11. Gruneberg RN, Leigh DA, Brumfitt W. *Escherichia coli* serotypes in urinary tract infection: studies in domiciliary, antenatal and hospital practice. In: O'Grady F, Brumfitt W, eds. Urinary tract infection. London: Oxford University Press, 1968; 68.
12. Stamey TA, Timothy M, Miller M, Mihara G. Recurrent urinary infections in adult women. The role of introital enterobacteria. Calif Med 1971; 115: 1–19
13. Windberg J, Bollgren I, Källenius G et al. Clinical pyelonephritis and focal renal scarring. A selected review of pathogenesis, prevention and prognosis. Pediatr Clin North Am 1982; 29: 801–814.
14. Hodson CJ, Edwards D. Chronic pyelonephritis and vesicoureteric reflux. Clin Radiol 1960; 11: 219–231.
15. Edwards D. Significance of vesico-ureteric reflux in childhood. In: O'Grady F, Brumfitt W, eds. Urinary tract infection. London: Oxford University Press, 1968: 104–107.
16. Heptinstall RH. Experimental pyelonephritis: bacteriological and morphological studies on the ascending route of infection in the rat. Nephron 1964; 1: 73–92 .
17. Ransley PG, Risdon RA. Renal papillary morphology and intrarenal reflux in the young pig. Urol Res 1975; 3: 105–109.
18. Rolleston GL, Maling TMJ, Hodson CJ. Intrarenal reflux and the scarred kidney. Arch Dis Child 1974; 49: 531–539.
19. Schoolnik GK. How *Escherichia coli* infects the urinary tract. N Engl J Med 1989; 320: 804–805 .
20. Costerton JW, Marrie TJ, Cheng K-T. Phenomena of bacterial adhesion. In: Savage DC, Fletcher M, eds. Bacterial adhesion: mechanisms and physiological significance. New York: Plenum Press, 1985; 3–43 .
21. Rosenstein IJ, Stoll MS, Mizouchi T, Childs RA, Hounsell EF, Feizi T. New type of adhesive specificity revealed by oligosaccharide probes in *Escherichia coli* from patients with urinary tract infection. Lancet 1988; 2: 1327–1330 .
22. Sheinfeld L, Schaeffer AJ, Cordon-Cardo C, Rogatko A, Fair WR. Association of Lewis blood group phenotype with recurrent urinary tract infections in women. N Engl J Med 1989; 320: 773–777.
23. Reid G. Host versus bacterial factors in the pathogenesis of urinary tract infections. In: Davison AM, ed. Nephrology. London: Baillière Tindall,1988; 2: 860–866
24. Miller TE, North JDK. Host response in urinary tract infections. Kidney Int 1974; 5: 179–186 .
25. Smith JW. Microbial and host factors that influence adherence of *Escherichia coli* to kidney epithelium. Am J Kidney Dis 1986; 7: 368–374 .
26. Rosen S, Harmon W, Krensky AM, et al. Tubulo-interstitial nephritis associated with polyoma (BK type) infection. N Engl J Med 1983; 308: 1192–1196 .
27. Michaeli J, Mogle P, Perlberg S, Heiman S, Caine M. Emphysematous pyelonephritis. J Urol 1984; 131: 203–208.
28. Evanoff GV, Thompson CS, Foley R, Weinman EJ. Spectrum of gas within the kidney. Emphysematous pyelonephritis and emphysematous pyelitis. Am J Med 1987; 83: 149–154.
29. Johnson JR, Ireton RC, Lipsky BA. Emphysematous pyelonephritis caused by *Candida albicans*. J Urol 1986; 136: 80–82.
30. Councilman WT. Acute interstitial nephritis. J Exp Med 1898; 3: 393–420 .
31. Cameron JS. Allergic interstitial nephritis: clinical features and pathogenesis. Q J Med 1988; 66: 97–115.
32. Advisory Committee to the Renal Transplant Registry. The twelth report of the Human Renal Transplant Registry. JAMA 1975; 233: 787– 796 .
33. Farmer ER, Heptinstall RH. Chronic non-obstructive pyelonephritis – a reappraisal. In: Kincaid-Smith P, Fairley KF, eds. Renal infection and renal scarring. Melbourne: Mercedes Publishing Services, 1971; 233–236 .
34. Smellie JM, Hodson CJ, Edwards D, Normand ICS. Clinical and radiological features of urinary infection in childhood. Br Med J 1964; 2: 1222–1226 .
35. Arze RS, Ramos JM, Owen IP et al. The natural history of chronic pyelonephritis in the adult. Q J Med 1982; 51: 396–410.
36. Smellie JM, Edwards D, Hunter N, Normand ICS, Prescod N. Vesicoureteric reflux and renal scarring. Kidney Int 1975; 8: S65– S72 .
37. Roberts JA, Suarez GM, Kaack B et al. Experimental pyelonephritis in the monkey. VII. Ascending pyelonephritis in the absence of vesicoureteric reflux. J Urol 1985; 133: 1068–1075.
38. Hodson CJ, Wilson S. Natural history of chronic pyelonephritic scarring. Br Med J 1965; 2: 191–194.
39. Pears MA, Houghton BJ. Response of infected urinary tract to bacterial pyrogen. Lancent 1959; 2: 1167–1172.
40. Hodson CJ. Radiological diagnosis of pyelonephritis. Proc R Soc Med 1959; 52: 669–672 .
41. Smith JF. The diagnosis of the scars of chronic pyelonephritis. J Clin Pathol 1962; 15: 522–526.
42. Shimamura T, Heptinstall RH. Experimental pyelonephritis: nephron dissection of the kidney of experimental chronic pyelonephritis in the rabbit. J Pathol Bacteriol 1963; 85: 421–423.
43. Bhathena DB, Weiss JH, Holland NH et al. Focal and segmental glomerular sclerosis in reflux nephropathy. Am J Med 1980: 68: 886–892.
44. Kincaid-Smith P, Becker G. Reflux nephropathy and chronic atrophic pyelonephritis: a review. J Infect Dis 1978; 138: 774–780.
45. Holland NH, Kotchen T, Bhathena D. Hypertension in children with chronic pyelonephritis. Kidney Int 1975; 8: S243–S251.
46. Cotran RS. Glomerulosclerosis in reflux nephropathy. Kidney Int 1982; 21: 528–534.
47. Kincaid-Smith P. Glomerular lesions in atrophic pyelonephritis (RN). In: Hodson J, Kincaid-Smith P, eds. Reflux nephropathy. New York: Masson. 1979; 268.
48. Kincaid-Smith P, Whitworth JA. The kidney. A clinicopathological study, 2nd edn. Oxford: Blackwell Scientific, 1987; 248.
49. Tamminen-Möbius T. International reflux study in

children. In: Davison AM, ed. Nephrology. Proceedings of the Xth International Congress of Nephrology. 1988; 2: 854–859.
50. El-Khatib MT, Becker GJ, Kincaid-Smith PS. Morphometric aspects of reflux nephropathy. Kidney Int 1987; 32: 261–266.
51. Shimamura T, Morrison AB. A progressive glomerulosclerosis in partial five-sixth nephrectomized rats. Am J Pathol 1975; 79: 95–106.
52. Kiprov DD, Colvin RB, McCluskey RT. Focal and segmental glomerulosclerosis and proteinuria associated with unilateral renal agenesis. Lab Invest 1982; 46: 275–281.
53. Tribe CR. Causes of death in the early and late stages of paraplegia. Paraplegia 1963; 1: 19–47.
54. Kleeman CR, Hewitt WL, Guze LB. Pyelonephritis. Medicine (Baltimore) 1960; 39: 3–116.
55. Warshaw BL, Edelbrock HH, Ettenger RB et al. Progression to end-stage renal disease in children with obstructive uropathy. J Pediatr 1982; 100: 183–187.
56. Roberts JA, Angel JR, Roth JK. The hydrodynamics of pyelorenal reflux. II. The effect of chronic obstructive changes on papillary shape. Invest Urol 1981; 18: 296–301.
57. Mendoza JM, Roberts JA. Effects of sterile high pressure vesicoureteral reflux on the monkey. J Urol 1983; 130: 602–606.
58. Winslow DJ, Chamblin SA. Disseminated visceral botryomycosis. Report on a fatal case probably caused by *Pseudomonas aeruginosa*. Am J Clin Pathol 1960; 33: 43–47.
59. Brunken RC, Lichon-Chao N, van den Broek H. Immunologic abnormalities in botryomycosis. A case report with review of the literature. J Am Acad Dermatol 1983; 9: 428–434.
60. Parsons MA, Harris SC, Longstaff AJ, Grainger RG. Xanthogranulomatous pyelonephritis: a pathological, clinical and aetiological analysis of 87 cases. Diagn Histopathol 1983; 6: 203–219.
61. Antonakopoulos GN, Chapple CR, Newman J et al. Xanthogranulomatous pyelonephritis. A reappraisal and immunohistochemical study. Arch Pathol Lab Med 1988; 112: 275–281.
62. Khaly-Mawad J, Greco MA, Schinella RA. Ultrastructural demonstration of intracellular bacteria in xanthogranulomatous pyelonephritis. Hum Pathol 1982; 13: 41–47.
63. McDonald GSA. Xanthogranulomatous pyelonephritis. J Pathol 1981; 133: 203–213.
64. Tolia BM, Iloreta A, Freed SZ, Fruchtman B, Bennett B, Newman HR. Xanthogranulomatous pyelonephritis. Detailed analysis of 29 cases and a brief discussion of atypical presentations. J Urol 1981; 126: 437–442.
65. Povysil C. Ultrastructure of experimental xanthogranulomatous pyelonephritis. Virchows Arch [B] 1976; 20: 155–167.
66. McClure J. Malakoplakia. J Pathol 1983; 140: 275–330.
67. Michaelis L, Gutmann C. Ueber Einschlüsse in Blasentumoren. Z Klin Med 1902; 47: 208–215.
68. McClure J, Cameron CHS, Garett R. The ultrastructural features of malakoplakia. J Pathol 1981; 134: 13–25.
69. Garrett IR, McClure J. Renal malakoplakia. Experimental production and evidence of a link with interstitial megalocytic nephritis. J Pathol 1982; 136: 111–122.
70. Zollinger HU. Die interstitielle Nephritis. Basel: Karger, 1945.
71. Jander HP, Pujara S, Murad TM. Tumefactive megalocytic interstitial nephritis. Radiology 1978; 129: 635–636.
72. Kelly DR, Murad TM. Megalocytic interstitial nephritis, xanthogranulomatous pyelonephritis and malakoplakia. Am J Clin Pathol 1981; 75: 333–344.
73. Esparza AR, McKay DB, Cronan JJ, Chazan JA. Renal parenchymal malakoplakia. Histologic spectrum and its relationship to megalocytic interstitial nephritis and xanthogranulomatous pyelonephritis. Am J Surg Pathol 1989; 13: 225–236.

Tubulointerstitial disease caused by drugs

74. Cameron JS. Allergic interstitial nephritis: clinical features and pathogenesis. Q J Med 1988; 66: 97–115.
75. Cotran RS, Brenner BM, Stein JH. eds. Tubulointerstitial nephropathies. New York: Churchill Livingstone, 1983.
76. Ditlove J, Weidmann P, Bernstein M, Massry SG. Methicillin nephritis. Medicine (Baltimore) 1977; 56: 483–491.
77. Galpin JE, Shinaberger JH, Stanley TM et al. Acute interstitial nephritis due to methicillin. Am J Med 1978; 65: 756-765.
78. Mayaud C, Kanfer A, Kourilsky O, Sraer JD. Interstitial nephritis after methicillin. N Engl J Med 1975; 292: 1132–1133.
79. Codding CE, Ramseyer L, Allon M, Pitha J, Rodriguez M. Tubulointerstitial nephritis due to vancomycin. Am J Kidney Dis 1989; 14: 512–515.
80. Boucher A, Droz D, Adafer E, Nöel L-H. Characterization of mononuclear cell subsets in renal cellular interstitial infiltrates. Kidney Int 1986; 29: 1043–1049.
81. Cheng H-F, Nolasco F, Cameron JS, Hildreth G, Neild G, Hartley B. HLA-DR display by renal tubular epithelium and phenotype of infiltrate in interstitial nephritis. Nephron Dial Transplant 1989; 4: 205–215 .
82. Border W, Lehman D, Egan J, Sass H, Glode J, Wilson C. Antitubular basement membrane antibodies in methicillin-associated interstitial nephritis. N Engl J Med 1974, 291. 381–384.
83. Brentjens JR, Noble B, Andres GA. Immunologically mediated lesions of kidney tubules and interstitium in laboratory animals and in man. Semin Immunopathol 1982; 5: 357–378.
84. Adler SG, Cohen AH, Border WA. Hypersensitivity phenomenon and the kidney: role of drugs and environmental agents. Am J Kidney Dis 1985; 5: 75–96.
85. Flynn CT, Rainford DJ, Hope E. Acute renal failure and rifampicin: danger of unsuspected intermittent dosage. Br Med J 1974; 2: 482 .
86. Kleinknecht D, Kanfer A, Morel-Maroger L, Méry JP Immunologically mediated drug-induced acute renal failure. Contrib Nephrol 1978; 10: 42–52.
87. Pirson Y, van Ypersele de Strihou C. Renal side effects of nonsteroidal antiinflammatory drugs: clinical relevance. Am J Kidney Dis 1986; 8: 338–344.
88. Bender WL, Whelton A, Beschorner WE, Darwish MO, Hall-Craggs M, Solez K. Interstitial nephritis, proteinuria and renal failure caused by nonsteroidal anti-inflammatory drugs. Immunologic characterization of the inflammatory infiltrate. Am J Med 1984; 76: 1006–1012.

89. Adams DH, Howie AJ, Michael J, McConkey B, Bacon PA, Adu D. Non-steroidal anti-inflammatory drugs and renal failure. Lancet 1986; 1: 57–60.
90. Stachura I, Jayakumar S, Burke E. T and B lymphocyte subsets in fenoprofen nephropathy. Am J Med 1983; 75: 9–16.
91. Spuhler O, Zollinger HU. Die chronisch-interstitielle Nephritis. Z Klin Med 1953; 151: 1–49.
92. Dubach UC, Rosner B, Pfister E. Epidemiologic study of abuse of analgesics containing phenacetin. Renal morbidity and mortality (1968–1979). N Engl J Med 1983; 308: 357–362.
93. Buckalew VM, Schey HM. Renal disease from habitual antipyretic analgesic consumption: an assessment of the epidemiologic evidence. Medicine (Baltimore) 1986; 11: 291–303.
94. Sandler DP, Smith JC, Weinberg CR et al. Analgesic use and chronic renal disease. N Engl J Med 1989; 320: 1238–1243.
95. Wing AJ, Brunner FP, Brynger HOA et al. Comparative review between dialysis and transplantation. In: Drukker W, Parsons FM, Maher JF, eds. Replacement of renal function by dialysis, 2nd edn. The Hague: Martinus Nijhoff, 1983: 850–871.
96. Nanra RS. Renal effects of antipyretic analgesics. Am J Med 1983; 75: 70–81.
97. Lindvall N. Radiological changes of renal papillary necrosis. Kidney Int 1978; 13: 93–106.
98. Burry A. Pathology of analgesic nephropathy: Australian experience. Kidney Int 1978; 13: 34–40.
99. Gloor FJ. Changing concepts in pathogenesis and morphology of analgesic nephropathy as seen in Europe. Kidney Int 1978; 13: 27–33.
100. Mihatsch MJ, Torhorst J, Steinmann E et al. The morphologic diagnosis of analgesic (phenacetin) abuse. Pathol Res Pract 1979; 164: 68–79.
101. Mihatsch MJ, Hofer HO, Gudat F, Knüsli C, Torhorst J, Zollinger HU. Capillary sclerosis of the urinary tract and analgesic nephropathy. Clin Nephrol 1983; 20: 285–301.
102. Hesse VE, van Tonder H, Abrahams C. Analgesic cystitis: an unusual microangiopathy of the bladder. J Urol 1976; 116: 176–177.
103. Hultengren N, Lagergren C, Ljungqvist A. Carcinoma of the renal pelvis in renal papillary necrosis. Acta Chir Scand 1965; 130: 314–320.
104. Piper JM, Tonascia J, Matanoski GM. Heavy phenacetin use and bladder cancer in women aged 20 to 49 years. N Engl J Med 1985; 313: 292–295 .
105. Bengtsson U, Angervall L, Ekman H, Lehman L. Transitional cell tumours of the renal pelvis in analgesic abusers. Scand J Urol Nephrol 1968; 2: 145–150.
106. Mihatsch MJ, Manz T, Knüsli C et al. Phenacitinabusus III. Schweiz Med Wochenschr 1980; 111: 255–264 .
107. Johansson S, Wahlqvist T. Tumours of urinary bladder and ureter associated with abuse of phenacetin-containing analgesics. Acta Pathol Microbiol Scand [A] 1977; 85: 768–774.
108. Johansson S, Angervall L, Bengtsson U, Wahlqvist L. A clinicopathologic and prognostic study of epithelial tumours of the renal pelvis. Cancer 1976; 37: 1376–1383.
109. McCredie M, Stewart JH, Carter JJ, Turner J, Mahoney JF. Phenacetin and papillary necrosis: independent risk factors for renal pelvic cancer. Kidney Int 1986; 30: 81–84.
110. McLaughlin JK, Mandel JS, Blot WJ, Schuman LM, Mehl ES, Fraumeni JF. A population-based case-control study of renal cell carcinoma. J Natl Cancer Inst 1984; 72: 275–284.
111. Kincaid-Smith P, Nanra RS, Fairley KF. Analgesic nephropathy: a recoverable form of chronic renal failure. In: Kincaid-Smith P, Fairley KF, eds. Renal infection and renal scarring. Melbourne: Mercedes, 1971: 385–400
112. Nanra RS, Chirawong P, Kincaid-Smith P. Medullary ischaemia in experimental analgesic nephropathy. The pathogenesis of renal papillary necrosis. Aust NZ J Med 1973; 3: 580–586.
113. Murray TG. Drug-induced chronic tubulo-interstitial renal disease. In: Cotran RS, Brenner BM, Stein JH, eds. Tubulo-interstitial nephropathies. Edinburgh: Churchill Livingstone, 1983: 187–209.
114. McCredie M, Stewart JH, Ford JM. Analgesics and tobacco as risk factors for cancer of the ureter and renal pelvis in men. J Urol 1983; 130: 28–30.
115. McCredie M, Stewart JH, Ford JM, MacLennan RA. Phenacetin-containing analgesics and cancer of the bladder or renal pelvis in women. Br J Urol 1983; 55: 220–224.
116. McCredie M, Ford JM, Stewart JH. Risk factors for cancer of the renal parenchyma. Int J Cancer 1988; 42: 13–16.
117. Isaki H, Yoshi H, Otsuji A et al. Tumours of Sprague–Dawley rats induced by long-term feeding of phenacetin. Gann 1979; 70: 29–36.
118. Flaks B, Flaks A, Shaw APW. Induction by paracetamol of bladder and liver tumours in the rat. Acta Pathol Microbiol Immunol Scand [A] 1985; 93: 367–377.
119. Mulder GJ, Hinson JA, Gillette JR. Generation of reactive metabolites of *N*-hydroxyphenacetin by glucuronidation and sulfation. Biochem Pharmacol 1977; 26: 189–196.
120. Boton R, Gaviria M, Batile DC. Prevalence, pathogenesis, and treatment of renal dysfunction associated with chronic lithium therapy. Am J Kidney Dis 1987; 10: 329–345.
121. Hestbech J, Hansen H, Amdisen A, Olsen S. Chronic renal lesions following long-term treatment with lithium. Kidney Int 1977; 12: 205–213.
122. Jorkasky DK, Amsterdam JD, Oler J et al. Lithium-induced renal disease: a prospective study. Clin Nephrol 1988; 30: 293–302.
123. Walker RG, Dowling JP, Alcorn D, Ryan GB, Kincaid-Smith P. Renal pathology associated with lithium therapy. Pathology 1983; 15: 403–411.
124. Aurell M, Svalander C, Wallin L, Alling C. Renal function and biopsy findings in patients on long-term lithium treatment. Kidney Int 1981; 20: 663–670.
125. Walker RG, Escott M, Birchall J et al. Chronic progressive renal lesions induced by lithium. Kidney Int 1986; 29: 875–881.
126. Walker RG, Bennett WM, Davies BM. Structural and functional aspects of long-term lithium therapy. Kidney Int 1982; 21: 513–519.

Tubulointerstitial nephritis associated with immune disorders

127. Brentjens JR, Sepulveda M, Baliah T et al. Interstitial immune complex nephritis in patients with systemic lupus erythematosus. Kidney Int 1975; 7: 342–350.

128. Park MH, D'Agati VD, Appel GB, Pirani CL. Tubulointerstitial disease in lupus nephritis: relationship to immune deposits, interstitial inflammation, granular changes, renal function, and prognosis. Nephron 1986; 44: 309–319.
129. D'Agati VD, Appel GB, Estes D, Knowles DM, Pirani CL. Monoclonal antibody identification of infiltrating mononuclear leukocytes in lupus nephritis. Kidney Int 1986; 30: 573–581.
130. Magil AB, Tyler M. Tubulointerstitial disease in lupus nephritis. A morphometric study. Histopathology 1984; 8: 81–87.
131. McCluskey RT. Evidence for an immune complex disorder in systemic lupus erythematosus. Am J Kidney Dis 1982; 2: Suppl 1, 119–125.
132. Winer RL, Cohen AH, Sawhney AS, Gorman JT. Sjøgren's syndrome with immune complex tubulointerstitial renal disease. Clin Immunol Immunopathol 1977; 8: 494–503.
133. Cotran RS, Galvanek E. Immunopathology of human tubulointerstitial diseases: localization of immunoglobulins, complement and Tamm-Horsfall protein. Contrib Nephrol 1979; 16: 126 131
134. McCluskey RT. Immunologically mediated tubulo-interstitial nephritis. In: Cotran RS, Brenner BM, Stein JH. ed. Tubulo-interstitial nephropathies. New York: Churchill Livingstone, 1983: 121–149.
135. Nojima Y, Terai C, Takano K, Takehara K, Yamada A, Takaku F. Tubulointerstitial immune complex nephritis in a patient with cutaneous vasculitis. Clin Nephrol 1986; 25: 48–51.
136. Cattran DC. Circulating anti-tubular basement membrane antibody in a variety of human renal diseases. Detection and significance. Nephron 1980; 26: 13–19.
137. Lehman DH, Wilson CB, Dixon FJ. Extraglomerular immunoglobulin deposits in human nephritis. Am J Med 1975; 58: 765–796.
138. Levy M, Gagnadoux MF, Beziau A, Habib R. Membranous glomerulonephritis associated with anti-tubular and anti-alveolar basement membrane antibodies. Clin Nephrol 1978; 10: 158–165.
139. Andres G, Brentjens J, Kohli R et al. Histology of human tubulo-interstitial nephritis associated with antibodies to renal basement membranes. Kidney Int 1978; 13: 480–491.
140. Zakheim B, McCafferty E, Phillips SM, Clayman M, Nielson EG. Murine interstitial nephritis II. The adoptive transfer of disease with immune T lymphocytes produces a phenotypically complex interstitial lesion. J Immunol 1984; 133: 224–239.
141. Freycon MT, Gilly J, Bouvier R, Braye A. Néphrite tubulointerstitielle chronique familiale à anticorps antimembrane basale tubulaire. Pédiatrie 1982; 37: 371–381.
142. Makker SP. Tubular basement membrane antibody induced interstitial nephritis in systemic lupus erythematosus. Am J Med 1980; 69: 949–952.

Obstructive uropathy

143. Roberts JA. Experimental pyelonephritis in the monkey. III. Pathophysiology of ureteral malfunction induced by bacteria. Invest Urol 1975; 13: 117–120.
144. Arruda JAL. Obstructive uropathy. In: Cotran RS, Brenner BM, Stein JH. ed. Tubulo-interstitial nephropathies. New York: Churchill Livingstone, 1983; 243-273.
145. Wilson DR. Urinary tract obstruction. In: Schrier RW, Gottschalk CW, eds. Diseases of the kidney, 4th edn. Boston: Little, Brown, 1988; 1: 715–746.
146. Hinman F. Hydronephrosis. I. The structural changes. Surgery 1955; 17: 816–835.
147. Moller JC, Skriver E, Olsen S, Maunsbach AB. Ultrastructural analysis of human proximal tubules and cortical interstitium in chronic renal disease (hydronephrosis). Virchows Arch [Pathol Anat] 1984; 402: 209–237.
148. Barrie HJ. Herniations into the renal veins with special reference to hydronephrosis. J Pathol Bacteriol 1961; 82: 177–182.
149. Better OS, Arieff AI, Massry SG, Kleeman CR, Maxwell MH. Studies on renal function after relief of complete unilateral ureteral obstruction of 3 months duration in man. Am J Med 1973; 54: 234–240.
150. Witte MH, Short FA, Hollander W. Massive polyuria and natriuresis following relief of urinary tract obstruction. Am J Med 1964; 37: 320–326.
151. Huland H, Leichtweiss H-P, Augustin HJ. Changes in renal hemodynamics in experimental hydronephrosis. Invest Urol 1981; 18: 274–277.
152. Gobe GC, Axelsen RA. Genesis of renal tubular atrophy in experimental hydronephrosis in the rat. Role of apoptosis. Lab Invest 1987; 56: 273–281.
153. Rao NR, Heptinstall RH. Experimental hydronephrosis: a microangiographic study. Invest Urol 1968; 6: 183–204.
154. Arenshorst WJ, Finn WF, Gottschalk CW. Nephron stop-flow pressure response to obstruction for 24 hours in the rat kidney. J Clin Invest 1974; 53: 1497–1500.
155. Nagle RB, Kneiser MR, Bulger RE, Benditt P. Induction of smooth muscle characteristics in renal interstitial fibroblasts during obstructive nephropathy. Lab Invest 1973; 29: 422–427.
156. Kerr JFR, Bishop CJ, Searle J. Apoptosis. Rec Adv Histopathol 1984; 12: 1–15.
157. Wyker AT, Ritter C, Marion DN, Gillenwater JY. Mechanical factors and tissue stresses in chronic hydronephrosis. Invest Urol 1981; 18: 430–436.
158. Bhagavan BS, Wenk RE, Dutta D. Pathways of urinary backflow in obstructive uropathy. Demonstration by pigmented gelatin injection and Tamm-Horsfall uromucoprotein markers. Hum Pathol 1979; 10: 669–683.

Tubulointerstitial nephritis associated with vesicoureteric reflux

159. McGovern JH, Marshall VF, Paquin AJ. Vesicoureteral regurgitation in children. J Urol 1960; 80: 122–149.
160. Ransley PG, Risdon RA, Godley ML. High pressure sterile vesicoureteral reflux and renal scarring: an experimental study in the pig and minipig. Contrib Nephrol 1984; 39: 320–343.
161. Risdon RA. Pyelonephritis and reflux nephropathy. In: Tisher CC, Brenner BM, eds. Renal pathology with clinical and functional correlations. Philadelphia: JB Lippincott, 1989; 1: 777–808.
162. Hodson CJ, Maling TMJ, McManamon PJ, Lewis MG. The pathogenesis of reflux nephropathy (chronic atrophic pyelonephritis). Br J Radiol [Suppl] 1975; 13: 1–26 .

163. Bailey RR. End stage reflux nephropathy. Nephron 1981; 27: 302–306.
164. Ask-Upmark E. Über juvenile maligne Nephrosklerose und ihr Verhältnis zu Störungen in der Nierenentwicklung. Acta Pathol Microbiol Scand 1929; 6: 383–442.
165. Arant BS, Sotelo-Avilia C, Bernstein J. Segmental 'hypoplasia' of the kidney (Ask-Upmark). J Pediatr 1979; 95: 931–939.
166. Shindo S, Bernstein J, Arant BS. Evolution of renal segmental atrophy (Ask-Upmark kidney) in children with vesicoureteric reflux: radiographic and morphologic studies. J Pediatr 1983; 102: 847–854.

Tubulointerstitial nephritis associated with papillary necrosis

167. Harrow BR, Sloane JA, Liebman NC. Roentgenologic demonstration of renal papillary necrosis in sickle cell trait. N Engl J Med 1963; 268: 969–976.
168. Watanabe T, Nagafuchi Y, Yoshikawa Y, Toyoshima H. Renal papillary necrosis associated with Wegener's granulomatosis. Hum Pathol 1983; 14: 551–557.
169. Edmondson HA, Reynolds TB, Jacobson HG. Renal papillary necrosis with special reference to chronic alcoholism. Arch Intern Med 1966; 118: 255–264
170. Watanabe S, Sakaguchi H. Renal papillary necrosis in the newborn – report of three cases with autopsy findings and review of the literature. Acta Pathol Jpn 1969; 19: 419–431
171. Edmondson HA, Martin HE, Evans NG. Necrosis of renal papillae and acute pyelonephritis in diabetes mellitus. Arch Intern Med 1947; 79: 148–175.
172. Garella S, Matarese RA. Renal effects of prostaglandins and clinical adverse effects of nonsteroidal anti-inflammatory agents. Medicine (Baltimore) 1984; 63: 165–181.
173. Nanra RS, Kincaid-Smith P. Renal papillary necrosis in rheumatoid arthritis. Med J Aust 1975; 1: 194–197.
174. Emkey RD, Mills JA. Aspirin and analgesic nephropathy. JAMA 1982; 247: 55–57.
175. Allen RC, Petty RE, Lirenman DS, Malleson PN, Laxer RM. Renal papillary necrosis in children with chronic arthritis. Am J Dis Child 1986; 140: 20–22.
176. Eckert DE, Jonutis AJ, Davidson AJ. The incidence and manifestations of urographic papillary abnormalities in patients with S hemoglobulinopathies. Diagn Radiol 1974; 113: 59–63

Hereditary tubulointerstitial disorders

177. Bernstein J, Gardner KD. Hereditary tubulo-interstitial nephropathies. In: Cotran RS, Brenner BM, Stein JH, eds. Tubulo-interstitial nephropathies. Contemporary issues in nephrology. Edinburgh: Churchill Livingstone, 1983; 10: 335–357.
178. Hurley RM, Dery P, Nogrady MB, Drummond KN. The renal lesion of the Laurence–Moon–Biedl–Bardet syndrome. J Pediatr 1975; 87: 206–209.
179. Price D, Gartner JG, Kaplan BS. Ultrastructural changes in the glomerular basement membrane of patients with Laurence–Moon–Biedl–Bardet syndrome Clin Nephrol 1981; 16: 283–288.
180. Harnett JD, Green JS, Cramer BC, et al. The spectrum of renal disease in Laurence–Moon–Biedl–Bardet syndrome. N Engl J Med 1988; 319: 615–618.
181. Goldstein JL, Fialkow PJ. The Alström syndrome. Report of three cases with further delineation of the clinical, pathophysiological, and genetic aspects of the disorder. Medicine (Baltimore) 1973; 52: 53–71.

Miscellaneous instances of tubulointerstitial disease

182. Bergstein J, Andreoli SP, Provisor AJ, Yum M. Radiation nephritis following total body irradiation and cyclophosphamide in preparation for bone marrow transplantation. Transplantation 1986; 41: 63–66.
183. Kunkler PB, Farr RF, Luxton RW. The limit of renal tolerance of X-rays: an investigation into renal damage occurring following the treatment of tumours of the testis by abdominal baths. Br J Radiol 1952; 25: 190–205.
184. Arneil GC, Emmanuel IC, Flatman GE, Harris F, Young DG, Zachary RB. Nephritis in two children after irradiation and chemotherapy for nephroblastoma. Lancet 1974; 1: 960–963 .
185. Luxton RW. Radiation nephritis. Q J Med 1953; 22: 215–242.
186. Luxton RW. Radiation nephritis: a long-term study of 54 patients. Lancet 1961; 2: 1221–1224 .
187. Krochak RJ, Baker DG. Radiation nephritis. Clinical manifestations and pathophysiologic mechanisms. Urology 1986; 27: 389–393.
188. Churchill DN, Hong K, Gault MH. Radiation nephritis following combined abdominal radiation and chemotherapy (bleomycin-vinblastine). Cancer 1978; 41: 2161–2164.
189. Keane WF, Crosson JT, Staley NA, Anderson WR, Shapiro FL. Radiation-induced renal disease: a clinicopathologic study. Am J Med 1976; 60: 127–137 .
190. Steele BT, Lirenman DS. Acute radiation nephritis and the hemolytic uremic syndrome. Clin Nephrol 1979; 11: 272–274.
191. Jennette JC, Ordonez NG. Radiation nephritis causing nephrotic syndrome. Urology 1983; 22: 631–634.
192. Cogan MG, Arieff AI. Radiation nephritis and intravascular coagulation. Clin Nephrol 1978; 10: 74–78.
193. National Research Council Committee on the Biological Effects of Ionizing Radiations. The effects on populations of exposure to low levels of ionizing radiation. Washington: National Academy Press, 1980; 400–406.
194. Hopewell JW, Campling D, Calvo W, Reinhold HS, Wilkinson JH, Young TK. Vascular irradiation damage: its cellular basis and likely consequences. Br J Cancer 1986; 53: suppl 7,181–191.
195. Maehara Y, Anai H, Kusumoto T, Sakagushi Y, Sugimachi K. Nick translation detection *in situ* of cellular DNA strand break induced by radiation. Am J Pathol 1989; 134: 7–10.
196. Craciun EC, Rosculescu I. On Danubian endemic familial nephropathy (Balkan nephropathy). Some problems. Am J Med 1970; 49: 774–779.
197. Čeovic S, Hrabar A, Radonić M. An etiological approach to Balkan endemic nephropathy based on the investigation of two genetically different populations. Nephron 1985; 40: 175–179.
198. Moroeanu SB. Epidemiological observations on the endemic nephropathy in Rumania. In: Wolstenholme GEW, Knight J, eds. The Balkan nephropathy. Ciba

Foundation Study Group No. 30. London: Churchill, 1967: 4–13.
199. Hall PW, Dammin GJ. Balkan nephropathy. Nephron 1978; 22: 281–300.
200. Hall PW, Dammin GJ, Griggs RC, Fajgelj A, Zimonijic B, Gaon J. Investigation of chronic endemic nephropathy in Yugoslavia – II. Renal pathology. Am J Med 1965; 39: 210–217.
201. Petkovic S, Mutavdzic M, Petronic V, Markovic M. Comparative incidence pattern of urothelium tumours in and beyond endemic nephropathy regions. In: Puchlew A, Dincu IV, Milev B, Doichinov D, eds. Proceedings of the Second International Symposium on Endemic Nephropathy. Sofia: Publishing House of the Bulgarian Academy of Sciences, 1974: 114–116 .
202. Atanassov N, Donovski L, Kumanov H. Tumours of the urinary passages in endemic nephropathy. In: Puchlev A, Dincu IV, Milev B, Doichinov D, eds. Proceedings of the Second International Symposium on Endemic Nephropathy. Sofia: Publishing House of the Bulgarian Academy of Sciences, 1974: 117–123.
203. Mandal AK, Sindjic M, Sommers SC. Kidney pathology in endemic nephropathy. Clin Nephrol 1987; 27: 304–308.
204. Apostolov K, Spasić P, Bojanić N. Evidence of a viral aetiology in endemic (Balkan) nephropathy. Lancet 1975; 2: 1271–1273.
205. Macanović M, Rezaković D, Bašagic E, Brkić N. Endemic (Balkan) nephropathy. Lancet 1976; 1: 541 (letter).
206. Toncheva D, Dimitrov T, Tzoneva M. Cytogenetic studies in Balkan endemic nephropathy. Nephron 1988; 48: 18–21.
207. Pavlović NM, Strahinjić S, Varghese Z et al. Possible role of partial lecithin:cholesterol acyltransferase (LCAT) deficiency in pathogenesis of Balkan endemic nephropathy (BEN). In: Strahinjić S, Stefanovic V, eds Etiology of endemic (Balkan) nephropathy. Niš: University Press 1987: 121–146.
208. Dobrin RS, Vernier RL, Fish AL. Acute eosinophilic intersitial nephritis and renal failure with bone marrow-lymph node granulomas and anterior uveitis: a new syndrome. Am J Med 1975; 59: 325–333.
209. van Haesebrouck P, Carton D, de Bel C, Praet M, Proesmans W. Acute tubulointerstitial nephritis and uveitis syndrome (TINU). Nephron 1985; 40: 418–422.
210. Catalano C, Harris PE, Enia G, Postorino M, Martorano C, Maggiore Q. Acute interstitial nephritis associated with uveitis and primary hypoparathyroidism. Am J Kidney Dis 1989; 14: 317–318.
211. Cacoub P, Deray G, le Hoang P et al. Idiopathic acute interstitial nephritis associated with anterior uveitis in adults. Clin Nephrol 1989; 31: 307–310.
212. Burnier M, Jaeger P, Campiche M, Wauters JP. Idiopathic acute interstitial nephritis and uveitis in the adult. Report of one case and review of the literature. Am J Nephrol 1986; 6: 312–315.
213. van Acker KJ, Buyssens N, Neetens A, Lequesne M, Desmet N. Acute tubulointerstitial nephritis with uveitis. Acta Paediatr Belg 1980; 33: 171–177.

13

K. A. Porter

Acute tubular necrosis and renal lesions caused by poisoning, addiction and therapy

ACUTE TUBULAR NECROSIS

Acute tubular necrosis (ATN) is the name used to describe the tubular damage that is found in the approximately 75% of patients with acute renal failure who have no obvious causative primary glomerular, vascular or interstitial disease and in whom there is no obstruction to the urinary tract. Despite the designation 'necrosis' in the name used for the condition, dead cells are not always demonstrable by light microscopy in ATN, although cell loss can usually be seen; the damage may be apparent only when the tubular epithelium is examined under an electron microscope.

There are many causes of ATN; very loosely these may be divided into two main groups:

1. The *ischaemic causes*, which precipitate an episode of renal hypoxia; this is often associated with hypotension or hypovolaemia or both. Examples are crushing injuries of muscles, septic abortion and burns.
2. The *nephrotoxic causes*, poisonous agents that directly damage the tubules, chiefly the proximal convoluted segments. Examples are chemicals, such as mercury and carbon tetrachloride, and the poisons in some toxic fungi (toadstools, mushrooms).

The morphological changes produced in the tubules by the two groups of agents are initially different; later in the course of the condition they often overlap. ATN produced by causes that act predominantly through ischaemia is often referred to as ischaemic ATN; that due to toxic agents as nephrotoxic ATN.

ISCHAEMIC ACUTE TUBULAR NECROSIS

Although German surgeons in the 1914–18 World War were aware that soldiers suffering from crush injuries often developed acute renal failure,[1] and in the post-war years several reports of acute renal failure following shock or incompatible blood transfusions appeared, it was not until 1941 that attention was really focused on the problem. During the Battle of Britain and for the next 2 years, from 1940 to 1942, London and other major cities were exposed to heavy air raids, and large numbers of people were buried beneath fallen masonry and beams. Many of them later developed acute renal failure from which they died. The publication of two papers in 1941 and 1942 by Bywaters and his colleagues,[2,3] describing some of these patients and the lesions in their kidneys, was followed by a great surge of interest in ischaemic ATN.[4] This interest was one of the factors that helped stimulate investigators to perfect methods of microdissection of renal tubules[5] and renal biopsy[6] which were then applied to the problem in 1950. Fascination with the enigma of ischaemic ATN has still not abated.

Causes of ischaemic acute tubular necrosis

In times of war burns and extensive traumatic injuries, including those involving muscle necrosis, are the commonest causes of the circulatory shock and hypovolaemia that lead to renal tubular ischaemia and ATN. In peace time surgical complications precipitate about half of the cases of ischaemic ATN; traumatic and non-traumatic rhabdomyolysis accounts for about a quarter of all cases; and accidental or suicidal poisoning and reaction to therapeutic drugs together account for roughly 15% of cases; only approximately 5% are associated with obstetrical complications, such as septic abortion and postpartum haemorrhage. A miscellaneous group of conditions is responsible for the remaining small percentage of cases of ATN: it includes acute pancreatitis, dehydration following excessive diarrhoea, vomiting or sweating, septicaemia and peritonitis, haemolysis caused by incompatible blood transfusion, blackwater fever, paroxysmal haemoglobulinuria, and distilled water irrigation during transurethral prostatectomy. Major earthquakes lead to large numbers of cases of ischaemic ATN: following the earthquake in Armenia in 1988 there were at least 600 patients with acute renal failure following crush injuries who required haemodialysis treatment.[7]

Clinical features

The first indication of ATN is when the excretory function of the kidneys begins to fail and the concentrations of creatinine and urea in the blood rise rapidly. This is often accompanied by oliguria but some patients continue to produce more than 500 ml of urine per day. Non-oliguric forms of ATN are now as common or more common than oliguric; they occur most frequently in drug-induced ischaemic ATN.[8] Anuria is rare.

The urine is loaded with granular and cellular casts and with isolated tubular epithelial cells; red cells are infrequent or absent. If the cause of the ATN is haemolysis or myolysis there will also be many pigmented casts. The osmolarity of the urine is close to that of plasma. The urinary sodium concentration is usually greater than 300 mmol/l, indicating the inability of the tubules to reabsorb sodium. There is commonly a mild degree of 'non-selective' proteinuria. There is sometimes a slight rise in blood pressure during this stage. Anaemia is very common and particularly severe in those in whom haemolysis is occurring.

The stage of marked acute renal failure may last from a few days up to several weeks; the average is about 11 days.[9] In the past it was commonly followed by an early diuretic phase in which urine outputs exceeding 2 litres per day sometimes occurred while the glomerular filtration rate remained only a few millilitres per minute. This phase is seldom seen these days, probably because of better control of fluid and electrolyte balance during the period of acute renal failure. Improvement in renal function may occur suddenly or gradually. The glomerular filtration rate increases, proteinuria diminishes and microscopic abnormalities of the urine disappear; tubular functions, such as maximum urine concentration and acidification, recover more slowly. By the end of 3 months most of the excretory function that is going to return has been regained; there is some further slow improvement over the following year.

Renal changes

Gross appearance of the kidneys

The kidneys are enlarged and smooth; the cut surface bulges. The cortex is pale and contrasts with the congested medulla.[3]

Light microscopy

The important changes are in the tubules; the alterations in other structures are variable and non-specific.

Tubules The appearance of the tubules varies depending on the time of biopsy in relation to the onset of renal failure and whether hypertonic solutions have been given intravenously.[10]

In the oliguric phase focal necrosis is usually, but not invariably, found in the tubules, all parts of which may be affected. Necrosis was detectable by light microscopy in 80% of cases in one series.[10] It is relatively rare to see necrotic epithelial cells attached to the tubular basement membrane; patchy gaps where individual cells or clusters of cells have been shed is the usual finding (Fig. 13.1). The focal necrotic lesions are commonest in the distal convoluted segments and infrequent in the proximal segments of the tubules. In approximately 5% of cases the basement membrane of the tubule is focally ruptured (tubulorrhexis): this may cause a reaction in the adjacent interstitial tissue, producing a peritubular granuloma (Fig. 13.2), or it may give rise to a tubulovenous communication.[10]

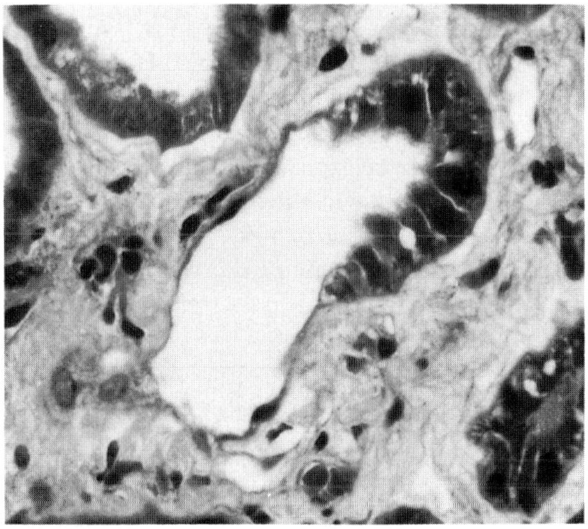

Fig. 13.1 Ischaemic acute tubular necrosis in the oliguric phase. The tubule is dilated and there is a large gap in its lining epithelium where necrotic cells have been shed. The interstitium is oedematous.
Haematoxylin-eosin × 400

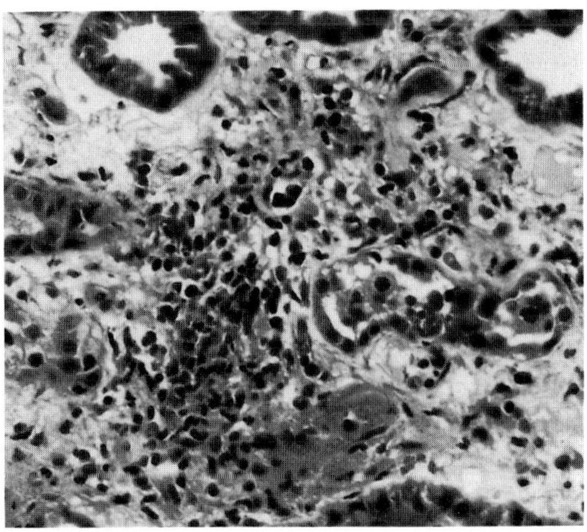

Fig. 13.2 Ischaemic acute tubular necrosis in the oliguric phase. There is a cellular reaction in the interstitium adjacent to a rupture in a tubule.
Haematoxylin-eosin × 300

Many of the distal convoluted and collecting tubules contain casts. Hyaline, granular and pigmented casts in various combinations are seen. The pigmented casts appear brown to brownish-orange in preparations stained with haematoxylin and eosin; they are composed mainly of Tamm–Horsfall protein in conjunction with haemoglobin or myoglobin. The two types of pigmented cast can be distinguished from one another in histological sections by applying peroxidase labelled monoclonal antibodies that are specific for either haemoglobin or myoglobin (Fig. 13.3). Such antibodies are commercially available. Haemoglobin casts are particularly common when ATN follows a transfusion reaction or accompanies blackwater fever or a sickle cell crisis. Myoglobin casts are a prominent feature when the renal damage follows injury to muscle (see p. 509). Desquamated tubular cells often become mixed with the pigment and neutrophil granulocytes may accumulate around some of the casts.

The tubules often appear dilated and lined by flatter epithelial cells than normal (Fig. 13.4). The flattened epithelium shows increased basophilia of

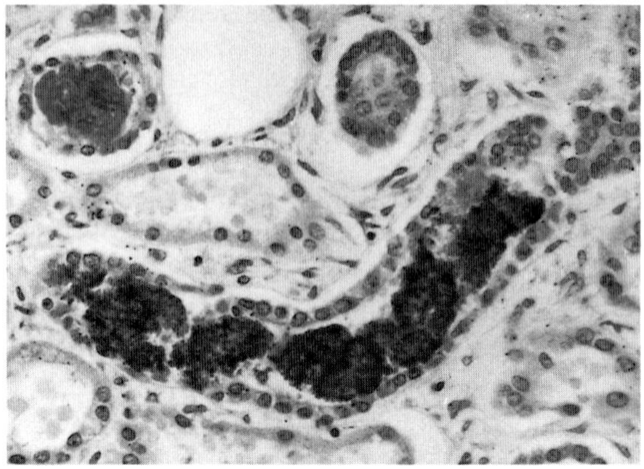

Fig. 13.3 Ischaemic acute tubular necrosis in the oliguric phase. A granular pigmented cast is present in a tubule. It has been stained positively by a monoclonal antibody to haemoglobin.
Immunoperoxidase × 350

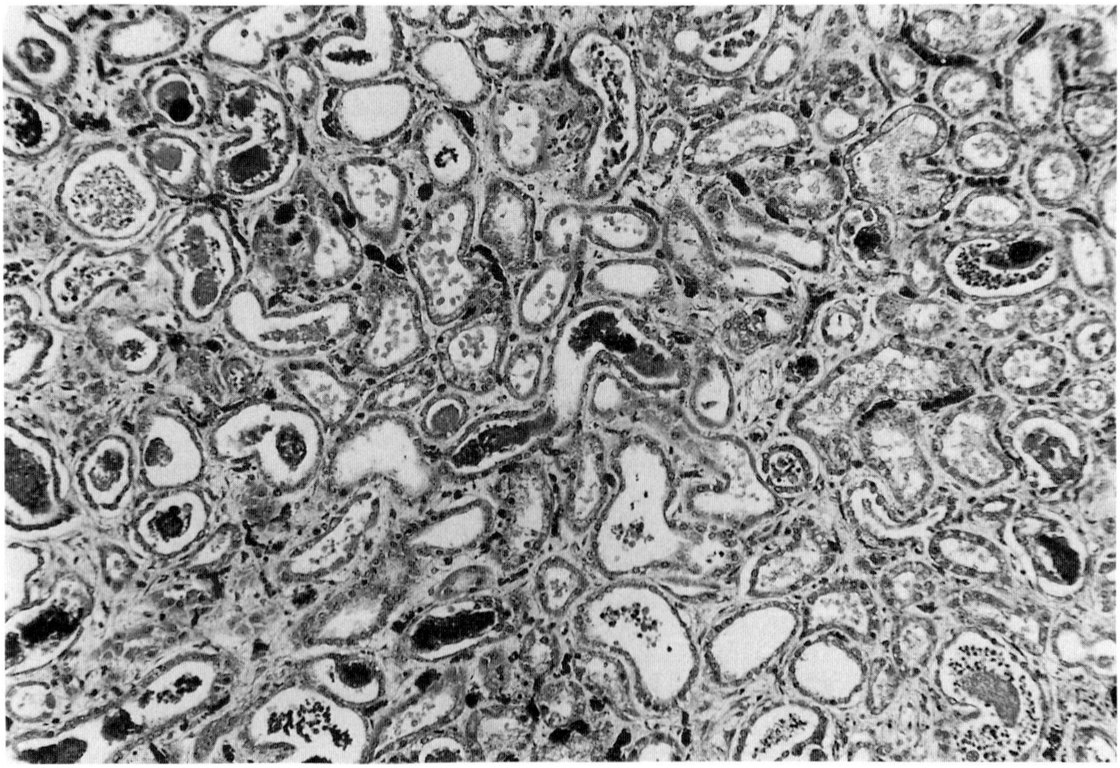

Fig. 13.4 Ischaemic acute tubular necrosis in the oliguric phase. The tubules appear dilated and lined by flatter epithelial cells than normal. There are pigmented granular casts.
Haematoxylin-eosin × 60

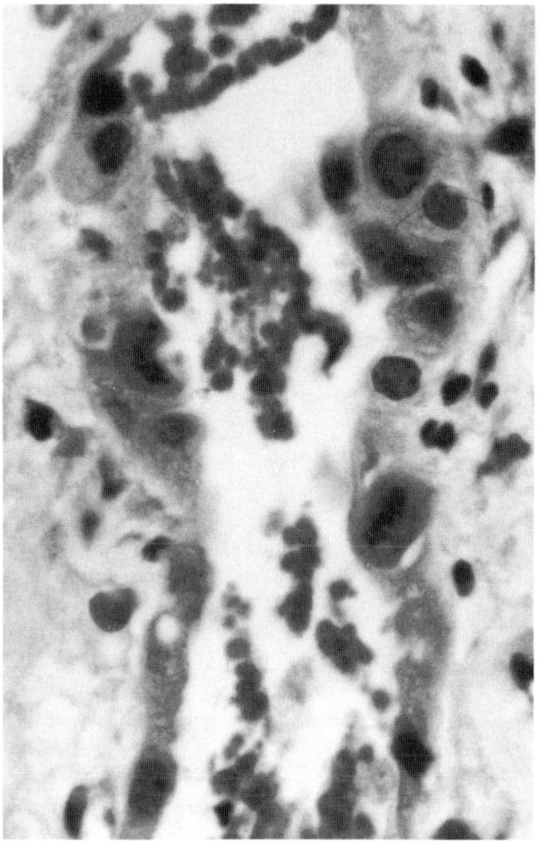

Fig. 13.5 Ischaemic acute tubular necrosis in the oliguric phase. One of the epithelial cells lining the tubule is in mitosis.
Haematoxylin-eosin × 300

its cytoplasm and occasional mitotic figures are present (Fig. 13.5). In some cases the epithelium partly covers the casts in the lumens. These appearances are more marked in the distal convoluted tubules than in the proximal. In the proximal convoluted tubules the PAS-positive brush border is thinned or absent. The alterations in the morphology of the proximal tubules often make it difficult in a biopsy to distinguish proximal from distal tubules.

Most of these epithelial changes are evidence of regeneration. The flattened epithelium is composed of newly formed cells that are replacing those that have been lost. The thinned or absent brush borders in the proximal tubular epithelial cells reflect the initial inability of regenerating proximal tubular cells to form normal microvilli; this has been shown in experimental animals following temporary occlusion of the renal pedicle.[11] There is also the possibility that in the proximal tubules some of the cells with attenuated brush borders were damaged by the ischaemia that followed the event that precipitated acute renal failure. This seems unlikely, however, because in experimental animals the loss of microvilli that occurs after an ischaemic injury is quickly reversed. The brush border is reconstituted within a few hours through a process by which fragments of membrane, previously incorporated into the apical cytoplasm, are recycled to form new microvilli.[12] Also the brush border usually appears intact by transmission electron microscopy in biopsies obtained from patients who have had ischaemic ATN for only a few days.[13]

The cytoplasm of some or many of the proximal tubular epithelial cells may be filled with fine vacuoles. This hydropic change happens if the patient is treated with hypertonic solutions such as dextran or mannitol. It is sometimes referred to as *osmotic nephrosis*; it is reversible and probably has no influence on renal function.

Abundant casts and regeneration of tubules are still present at the start of the diuretic phase but the patchy necrosis and loss of tubular epithelial cells, and the thinning of the brush border of the proximal epithelium, lessen as recovery occurs. All the changes disappear over the next few weeks.

In those cases in which the normal glomerular filtration rate is not regained, occasional collections of tubules with flattened epithelium remain.

Interstitium The interstitium is oedematous and often contains small numbers of lymphocytes, macrophages, plasma cells and neutrophil and eosinophil granulocytes. The cells tend to be clustered around necrotic and ruptured segments of tubules (Fig. 13.2). Severe interstitial oedema in the early stages of ischaemic ATN is frequently followed by interstitial fibrosis.[14]

Glomeruli The glomeruli usually appear normal. In biopsies obtained shortly after recovery, the parietal epithelial cells lining Bowman's capsule are often unduly prominent; this non-specific change may be related to the regeneration of the proximal tubular epithelium that is occurring.[10]

Juxtaglomerular apparatus The juxtaglomerular apparatus frequently appears hyperplastic in biopsies obtained in the recovery phase of ischaemic ATN.[10]

Blood vessels Leucocytes are very commonly found in the vasa recta of the medulla.[15] In the first few days lymphocytes predominate; later they are followed by cells of the myeloid series. Their presence is unexplained; one suggestion is that they indicate intravascular haemopoiesis. A similar accumulation occurs in acute pyelonephritis and leukaemia.

Microdissection studies

Nephron dissection has shown that the lesions in the tubules are patchily scattered throughout its length and are often more severe and extensive than would be anticipated from the appearance in histological sections. They are most common in the pars recta of the proximal convoluted tubule at the corticomedullary junction and in the distal convoluted tubule. Necrotic lesions appear at an early stage in ischaemic ATN. Microdissection remains the only means of accurately assessing tubular obstruction by casts: a single cast in a medullary collecting duct can obstruct hundreds of nephrons and yet not be seen in standard histological sections. Tubular dissection has shown that dilatation may sometimes occur without any evidence of cast formation lower in the nephron. Many of the casts have proved to be as much as 2–3 cm in length.[5,16]

Electron microscopy

Transmission electron microscopy Scattered epithelial cells showing degenerative changes and single dead cells in the process of desquamation and disintegration are frequent (Fig. 13.6).[17,18] Nearly all the tubules are affected to some extent. The necrotic cells often lie adjacent to damaged but intact tubular cells or even to cells with almost normal morphology. Intercellular spaces are also present where necrotic cells have been desquamated, exposing the tubular basement membrane. Both the proximal and distal convoluted tubules exhibit dilatation of their lumens and flattening and simplification of their lining epithelial cells. The cells of the proximal tubules have flatter and shorter microvilli than normal. There are also fewer basal and lateral infoldings of the plasma membrane than normal in both the proximal and distal convoluted tubules. The glomeruli appear normal.

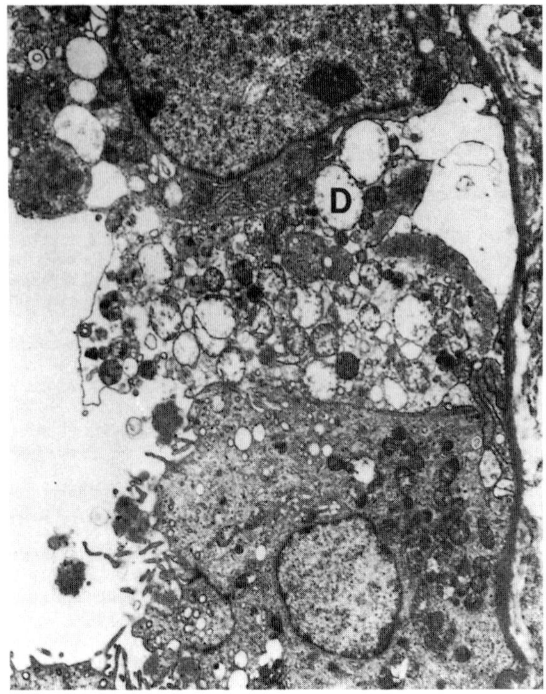

Fig.13.6 Ischaemic acute tubular necrosis in the oliguric phase. Electron micrograph of part of a tubule showing a dead epithelial cell (D) in the process of disintegration. × 3500
Reproduced by permission from: Jones DB. Lab Invest 1982; 46: 254 (Fig. 14)

Scanning electron microscopy Scanning electron microscopy confirms that in the oliguric phase there is a decrease in the number and height of brush border microvilli in the proximal tubules. The extent of these changes varies from one proximal tubule to the next and between individual epithelial cells.[17]

Immunofluorescence/immunoperoxidase microscopy

In most cases immunofluorescence and immunoperoxidase studies for immunoglobulins and complement are negative.

Differential diagnosis

The main distinctions that have to be made are between ischaemic ATN and acute tubulointerstitial nephritis and between idiopathic ischaemic ATN and tubular necrosis complicating some primary renal disease.

Acute tubulointerstitial nephritis

The distinction between acute tubulointerstitial nephritis and ischaemic ATN may at times be very difficult. In most cases the differentiation can be made because a moderate to marked mononuclear cell infiltrate is rare in ischaemic ATN but usual in acute tubulointerstitial nephritis; similarly, the presence of many neutrophil granulocytes or eosinophils is rare in ischaemic ATN but frequent in acute tubulointerstitial nephritis.

Tubular necrosis complicating primary renal disease

When lesions compatible with the diagnosis of ischaemic ATN are found in a biopsy from a patient with acute renal failure it is important to look carefully for evidence of any primary renal disease, such as glomerulonephritis, which could be responsible.

Prognosis

Many patients with ischaemic ATN die during the illness. With the widespread use of dialysis, however, up to 50% of the deaths are due to underlying disease rather than to complications of acute renal failure.[19] The three most important factors deciding the outcome are the severity of the renal failure as judged by urinary output, the severity of the condition that precipitated the attack of ischaemic ATN, and the age of the patient. Non-oliguric patients have consistently lower mortality than oliguric patients. Ischaemic ATN without severe primary disease in young people is associated with a mortality of less than 10%. In obstetric cases the mortality is about 15%. The presence of respiratory, circulatory or hepatic failure, alone or combined, increases the mortality to approximately 70%. The most common cause of death is sepsis, followed, in order, by gastrointestinal haemorrhage and myocardial failure. Mortality increases with age, irrespective of precipitating causes. Survival from ischaemic ATN in elderly patients who have just had surgical operations is low. The great majority of deaths occur within the first week after the onset of acute renal failure.[19]

Of those who survive, approximately 40% regain normal renal function; minor defects in glomerular filtration or tubular function remain for long periods in 50%; 10% are left with permanent impairment of renal function.[20] Very few patients require maintenance dialysis or renal transplantation.

Pathogenesis

The pathogenesis of ischaemic ATN is still unclear. Various animal models exist but the majority differ substantially from ischaemic ATN in humans; the most appropriate is probably that in which the pedicle of one kidney in a rabbit is clamped and the other kidney is removed.[21] Several hypotheses have been proposed on the basis of data obtained from these animal models and from patients with ischaemic ATN;[21,22] they include prolonged renal vasoconstriction, tubular obstruction by casts, leakage of tubular fluid, tubuloglomerular feedback and changes in glomerular permeability. However, no one of these hypotheses by itself will adequately explain all the findings in ischaemic ATN.

Prolonged renal vasoconstriction

In the vascular theory it is proposed that there is intense vasoconstriction of the renal arterioles and arteries which reduces the blood flow to the glomeruli; this results in diminished glomerular filtration and oliguria. Supporting this theory is the fact that the renal blood flow is reduced to 25–50% of normal in patients with ischaemic ATN; this reduction affects particularly the cortex.[23,24] Recovery from post-ischaemic ATN in rodents is preceded by an increase in renal blood flow.[25] The marked rise in plasma renin activity that occurs during the acute renal failure phase of ischaemic ATN in patients, and its subsequent fall in the recovery phase, suggest that angiotensin II might mediate the cortical vasoconstriction.[26]

Tubular obstruction by casts

One of the earlier pathogenetic suggestions was that in ischaemic ATN the casts of necrotic cells and precipitated proteins obstruct the tubules, raising intratubular pressure and thus decreasing the glomerular filtration rate and producing oliguria. The persistent dense nephrogram frequently observed following pyelography in patients with ischaemic ATN suggests that tubular obstruction may be present[27] and micropuncture studies in animal models of ischaemic ATN have shown increased intratubular pressure.[28]

Leakage of tubular fluid

The leakage theory proposes that glomerular filtration continues normally but that the filtrate leaks back into the peritubular circulation via injured tubular cells. There is much circumstantial evidence that leakage of tubular fluid occurs in patients. Foci in which the tubular basement membrane is bared or ruptured occur and these lesions are significantly more prominent in biopsies obtained during the acute renal failure stage of ischaemic ATN than in those obtained shortly after recovery.[10] Studies of the clearance of inulin in patients also suggests that leakage of tubular fluid is occurring.[22] In animal models, the existence of a back leak of tubular fluid has been confirmed using inulin, to which tubular epithelium is normally impermeable. Only 40–60% of inulin injected by a microtechnique into the lumen of a proximal tubule can be recovered from the urine produced by kidneys subjected to ischaemia.[22,29] Restoration of tubular impermeability to inulin coincides with recovery from acute renal failure in ATN.[25]

Leakage of tubular fluid and tubular obstruction are closely related. Increased intratubular pressure brought about by obstruction increases back leak and may lead to tubular rupture. Conversely, if extensive leakage of tubular fluid occurs, intratubular pressure cannot rise to a level that will cause obstructive casts to be expelled.[21]

Tubuloglomerular feedback

The tubuloglomerular feedback hypothesis proposes that the proximal tubular damage due to ischaemic injury results in failure of the normal reabsorption of the filtered sodium chloride, the concentration of this substance therefore rising in the distal tubule. The raised sodium chloride is sensed by the macula densa which responds by inducing the release of renin leading to local generation of angiotensin II. The angiotensin II causes arteriolar constriction, decreased filtration pressure and a fall in glomerular filtration rate.[30] The signal for arteriolar constriction will persist until tubular function is restored. Healing of the damaged epithelium requires from a few days to 2 or more weeks, depending on the severity of the lesion; the period of oliguria reflects this variable time. Until the newly regenerated epithelium completely regains its normal absorptive function, small increases in glomerular filtration rate may result in large increases in urine flow resulting in a period of polyuria and salt loss (the early diuretic phase).[30]

A more recent refinement of this theory is to suggest that even in cases in which proximal tubular damage appears minimal, lesions in the thick ascending limb of Henle's loop may be sufficient to initiate tubuloglomerular feedback. There is evidence that this part of the tubule is especially susceptible to hypoxic injury because of its high energy requirements for ion transport and its location in a region where there is always a precarious balance between oxygen supply and demand.[31]

Altered glomerular permeability

The altered glomerular permeability theory proposes that ATN results from decreased permeability of the glomerular capillary basement membranes. The glomerular ultrafiltration coefficient has been found to be reduced in some animal models of ATN; this reduction has been associated with a decrease in both the diameter and the density of the fenestrae in the glomerular capillary endothelium.[32] It is not known whether comparable alterations occur in the glomeruli of patients with ischaemic ATN because the appropriate measurements have not been made on scanning electron micrographs. It has also been suggested that lowered glomerular ultrafiltration may result from reduction in the surface area of the glomerular capillary basement membranes caused by mesangial cell contraction under the influence of various local stimuli, in particular angiotensin II. This proposal is based on the morphological demonstration that the part of the glomerular basement membrane that overlies the mesangium (the perimesangial glomerular basement membrane) is extensively attached to mesangial cells either directly or through microfibrils.[33] These connections are most prominent at the points (the mesangial angles) where the glomerular basement membrane (pericapillary glomerular basement membrane) leaves the capillary lumen and begins to cover the mesangium. Contraction of the mesangial cells may bring the glomerular basement membrane from opposing mesangial angles closer together, causing increased wrinkling of the perimesangial glomerular basement membrane and diminution of the area of the filtration barrier (see Fig. 1.5b, p. 9).

Summary

A generally acceptable coherent account of the pathogenesis of ischaemic ATN still cannot be given. My own view is that the hypotension produced by the initiating event leads to tubular injury which may range from damage confined to the particularly vulnerable thick ascending limb of Henle's loop to widespread proximal tubular injury. This damage may be made worse by an accompanying excessive, inappropriate and transitory renal vasoconstriction.[34] The tubular damage, acting through a tubuloglomerular feedback mechanism, induces persistent afferent arteriolar constriction which causes acute renal failure. The vasoconstriction continues until the tubular cells regenerate and mature sufficiently to regain their ability to reabsorb sodium chloride and until the composition of the tubular fluid ceases to stimulate the macula densa. It seems to me unlikely that tubular leakage and obstruction, or changes in the glomerular ultrafiltration coefficient, play an essential role in the pathogenesis of ischaemic ATN.

NEPHROTOXIC ACUTE TUBULAR NECROSIS

For a long time it has been known that poisoning with heavy metals and organic solvents may lead to a dose-dependent acute tubular necrosis. In more recent years the range of substances found to be toxic to the renal tubules has been greatly extended.

Causes of nephrotoxic acute tubular necrosis

Ingested nephrotoxic chemicals

The substances in this category are mainly industrial and agricultural chemicals. They include compounds of heavy metals (arsenic, barium chloride, mercuric chloride, uranium and bismuth), herbicides (chlorates, chlorphenoxyacetic acid derivatives, diquat and paraquat), disinfectants (lysol, cresol and phenol) and rat poisons (yellow phosphorus and zinc phosphide).[35]

Inhaled or cutaneously absorbed nephrotoxins

Chemicals in this group often produce nephrotoxic ATN after acute excessive exposure at work. They include carbon tetrachloride, arsine, carbon monoxide, toluene and trichlorethylene.[35]

Nephrotoxic plants and fungi

Toxic fungi may be ingested in the belief that they are edible. Children may eat attractive but poisonous berries, for example those of *Daphne mezereum.* In Africa herbal remedies prepared from nephrotoxic plants are a common cause of ATN.[35]

Nephrotoxic animal venoms

Snake bites are responsible for numerous cases of ATN in rural areas of the tropics, especially in India and South East Asia.[36,37]

Nephrotoxic therapeutic agents

Various antibiotics, such as the aminoglycosides (e.g. gentamicin), cephalosporins and amphotericin, can produce a nephrotoxic ATN. Cisplatin (*cis*-dichlorodiammine platinum II), widely used in the treatment of cancer resistant to other agents, is also nephrotoxic. These and other therapeutic agents that may damage the kidneys are referred to further on pages 514 to 525.

Clinical features

In addition to clinical manifestations due to the local and general effects of the poison (which may, for example, include liver failure), there will be acute renal failure which may or may not be accompanied by oliguria. The course is very similar to that of ischaemic ATN (see p. 492).

Renal changes

Gross appearance of the kidneys

The kidneys are usually moderately enlarged. The cortex is pale and swollen; the medulla is deep red.

Light microscopy

As in ischaemic ATN all the important changes are in the tubules, but, in contrast to ischaemic ATN, the tubular necrosis is almost always obvious and usually affects the great majority of nephrons.

Tubules In the first 2 days after exposure to the toxic agent there is extensive necrosis that usually involves all nephrons uniformly and is often confined to the proximal part of the nephron. Within the proximal tubule some poisons cause maximum damage in only certain segments. For example, mercuric chloride, potassium chlorate and diethylene glycol tend to involve particularly the convoluted and straight parts of the proximal tubules, while uranyl nitrate and dioxane predominantly affect the initial and convoluted parts. The extent of the necrosis is dose dependent. If the patient has been exposed to large doses of the nephrotoxic agent the lesion may extend beyond these localized segments of the proximal tubule. The necrotic cells are often partly desquamated and the tubular lumens are filled with cellular debris (Fig. 13.7). The tubular basement membranes are usually intact. Casts are often present in the collecting ducts. Calcification of necrotic epithelial cells may occur.[21]

Regeneration of the tubular epithelium begins after 3–5 days and is accompanied by gradual clearing of debris from the tubular lumens. By about 10 days after exposure to the toxin, the proximal tubules are dilated and lined by flattened basophilic cells which often show mitosis. Over the next few days the cells become first cuboidal, then columnar, and then gradually develop brush borders.[21]

Interstitium The interstitium is oedematous and often contains scattered small groups of mononuclear cells.

Glomeruli The glomeruli usually appear normal.

Blood vessels Leucocytes are common in the vasa recta of the medulla (see p. 496).

Microdissection studies

Nephrons dissected from cases of nephrotoxic ATN usually have intact tubular basement membranes; all show necrosis of tubular cells. The proximal part of the tubule is generally the most affected.[5]

Electron microscopy

Electron microscopic studies have confirmed the widespread necrosis of epithelial cells in the proximal tubules and the slow acquisition of microvilli by the regenerating epithelium.

Immunofluorescence/immunoperoxidase microscopy

There is usually no staining for immunoglobulins or complement.

Changes in other organs

Changes are usually present in other organs and vary according to the particular poison involved. Lesions in the liver are common.

Differential diagnosis

The uniform extensive necrosis, largely confined

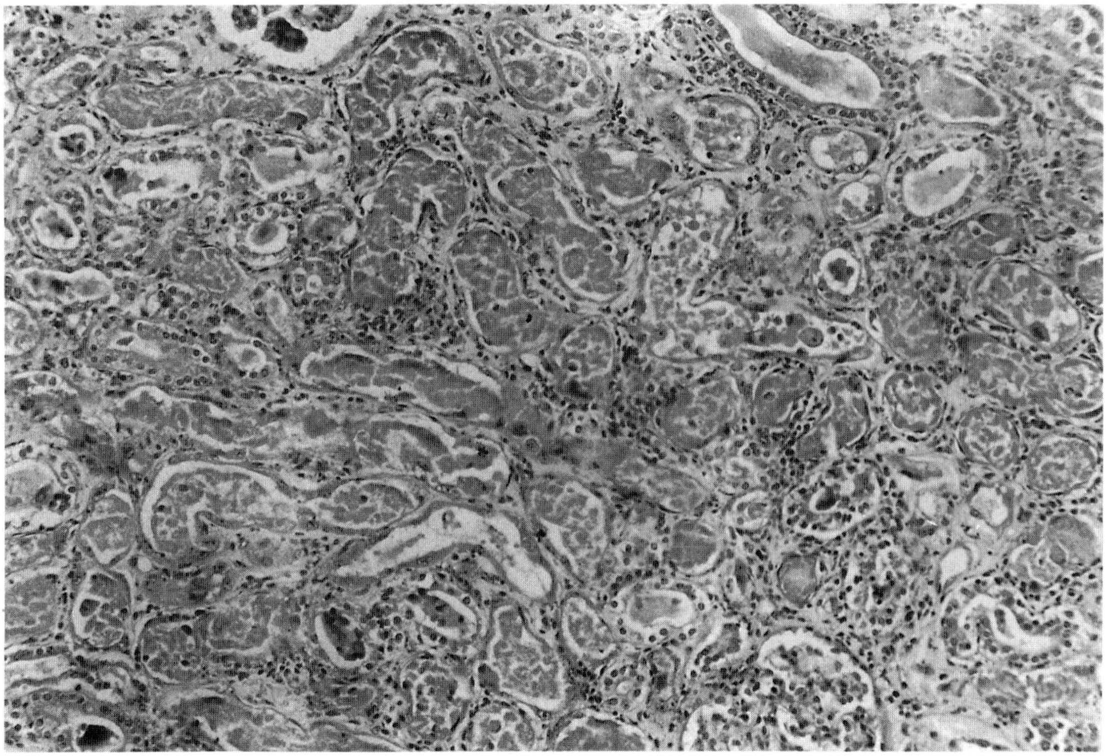

Fig. 13.7 Nephrotoxic acute tubular necrosis. From a woman who died 4 days after taking mercuric chloride by mouth. There is widespread necrosis of the proximal convoluted tubules.
Haematoxylin-eosin × 150

to one part of the tubule, is characteristic and nephrotoxic ATN is unlikely to be confused with acute interstitial nephritis. The greatest difficulty in biopsy specimens is to differentiate this type of ATN from *bilateral cortical necrosis*, particularly from patchy forms of the latter. However, in bilateral cortical necrosis all segments of the tubules and the glomeruli are affected, and microthrombi are common in the arterioles and glomerular capillaries; in nephrotoxic ATN the tubular lesions are confined to one part of the nephron and microthrombi are rare. The preferential location of the necrosis in certain parts of the proximal tubule may on occasion be of some help in deciding which of several possible nephrotoxins caused the renal damage (see also below, 'Pathogenesis').

Prognosis

The course of nephrotoxic ATN is very similar to that of ischaemic ATN. Recovery may occur after dialysis, depending on the dose of toxin and on the severity of the lesions in organs other than the kidneys.

Pathogenesis

In nephrotoxic ATN there is general agreement that the tubular necrosis is brought about primarily by a direct action of the poison on the epithelial cells. The kidneys are particularly likely to be damaged by such agents for three main reasons. Firstly, their disproportionately high blood flow (25% of the resting cardiac output) means that they receive a greater exposure to any blood-borne toxin than most other organs. Secondly, the nephrons concentrate solutes filtered by the glomeruli and may, therefore, be exposed to very high concentrations of any toxic agent. Thirdly, the tubular cells have complicated enzyme systems and transport mechanisms that are probably very vulnerable to noxious substances; also, potential toxins are sometimes actively transported into the tubular cells where they may be metabolized to nephrotoxic substances, or they may simply accumulate until the intracellular concentration reaches a lethal level.[38]

Chloroform is an example of a substance which is taken into proximal tubular cells and then activated by cytochrome P–450 to phosgene which binds irreversibly to protein. This causes damage and death of the proximal tubular cells.[38] Cephaloridine selectively accumulates in the proximal tubules because it is actively transported into these cells.[39] Gentamicin is excreted primarily by glomerular filtration; it then binds specifically to phospholipid receptors on the brush border membranes of the proximal tubular cells. The bound gentamicin is then engulfed by absorptive endocytosis and stored in phagolysosomes. The gentamicin injures the membranes of the lysosomes which leads to the release of damaging enzymes into the cytoplasm and so to death of the proximal tubular cells.[38,39]

How the injury to the proximal tubular cells brings about acute renal failure is not known. The same five hypotheses have been suggested as in ischaemic ATN (see p. 497). There is evidence for and against the importance of each of these theories, but no consensus has been reached on the most likely mechanism. In nephrotoxic ATN intratubular obstruction and perhaps backleak are probably more important than they seem to be in ischaemic ATN.[39]

ACUTE TUBULAR NECROSIS IN RENAL ALLOGRAFTS

Renal allografts often undergo a period of ATN immediately after transplantation. The incidence in different series has been between 14 and 53%.[40] Function may be delayed for varying periods depending upon the severity of the damage. Unless rejection or other complications occur in the oliguric period, ATN in a transplant rarely has any adverse effect on graft or patient survival (see p. 627).[40]

Compared with ATN in non-transplanted (native) kidneys, in grafts there is less flattening of the proximal tubular epithelium, much less damage to the brush border of the tubules, greater numbers of necrotic tubular cells, fewer casts, more birefringent oxalate crystals, and a three-fold increase in the number of mononuclear cells infiltrating the interstitium. Electron microscopy shows only slight reduction in the microvilli of the proximal tubular epithelial cells and preservation of the basolateral infoldings of the plasma membrane.[40]

These differences in the degree and amount of tubular damage in ATN in a graft compared with ATN in a native kidney may be because in transplants there is complete interruption of blood flow and much of the ischaemic injury occurs while the kidney is cold; in ATN in native kidneys the blood flow is reduced but does not stop, and the ischaemic injury occurs when the kidney is at body temperature.[40] The increased amount of mononuclear cell infiltration in the interstitium is almost certainly due to the host's cell-mediated immunological response to the graft; all renal allografts contain considerable numbers of such infiltrating cells in the first few weeks after transplantation, even if there is no evidence of either ATN or rejection (see p. 640).

RENAL DISEASE CAUSED BY POISONING AND OCCUPATIONAL HAZARDS

HEAVY METALS

Four metals with a specific gravity greater than 5 are widely recognized as nephrotoxic following environmental or occupational exposure: lead, cadmium, mercury and arsenic. Gold, platinum and bismuth may also damage the kidneys but usually after their therapeutic use (see p. 514). Other heavy metals such as uranium, chromium, cobalt, copper, antimony and nickel are nephrotoxic after massive accidental absorption, but there is little clinical evidence to suggest that low-dose industrial exposure to these elements leads to renal injury.

Lead nephropathy

Exposure to lead may be occupational or environmental. Examples of occupations where workers may develop lead poisoning are manufacture of paint, paint spraying, plumbing, lead smelting, mining, battery making and burning, making stained glass, welding, glazing pottery, foundry work, brass working, use of oxyacetylene torches by demolition workers to cut through metal covered in lead based paints, and manufacture of pewter. Environmental exposure may occur from drinking water supplied through lead pipes or pipes with lead soldered joints, from paint dust and flakes from older houses where paints based on lead pigments were used, through air and soil pollution from leaded petrol (gasoline), from cooking in leaded pots, through lead-contaminated home-made wines, cider, rum or whisky, and from chewed or burnt newsprint. The lead is absorbed either through the gastrointestinal tract or the lungs into the blood. Inhaled lead is more dangerous because almost all of it is absorbed; by contrast, only about 10% of ingested lead is absorbed. Absorbed lead is excreted via the kidneys, thereby exposing these organs to potential damage. The exposure may be acute or chronic.

Acute lead nephropathy

Patients known to have absorbed an excess of inorganic lead, who display the classic clinical manifestations of acute lead poisoning (abdominal colic, extensor muscle weakness, encephalopathy and anaemia), may develop a proximal tubular reabsorptive defect characterized by aminoaciduria, phosphaturia and glycosuria (Fanconi's syndrome).[41] The defect appears in the presence of blood lead levels usually in excess of 150 μg/dl and is rapidly reversed by the chelation therapy that is used to treat the encephalopathy. Acute lead nephropathy is most commonly seen in childhood lead poisoning. It can be induced experimentally in rats by giving lead in their diet.

Renal changes In both patients and experimental animals, acute lead nephropathy is consistently associated with the appearance of intranuclear inclusions in the tubular cells, particularly of the proximal convoluted tubules and loops of Henle. The inclusions vary in size and shape; they are eosinophilic and PAS positive, and are acid-fast with the Ziehl–Neelsen stain. They stain red with Giemsa (Fig. 13.8).[42] The inclusions consist of a lead–protein complex; they contain about 50 μg of lead per milligram of protein, which is 60–100 times the concentration found in control nuclei.[43] The proximal tubular cells are often flattened and basophilic. Desquamated cells may be found in the urine. The intranuclear inclusions persist for

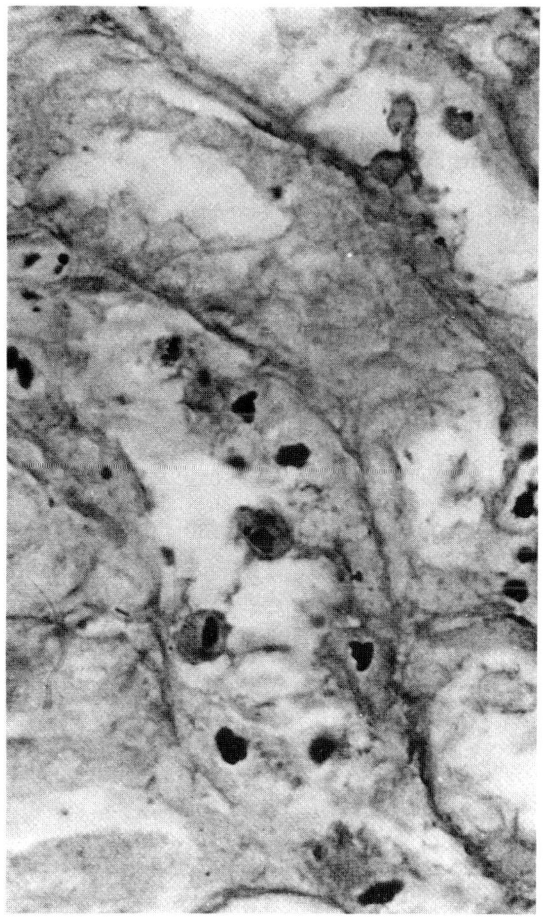

Fig.13.8 Acute lead nephropathy. Several of the tubular cells contain dark intranuclear inclusions. A few of the cells with inclusions are sloughing into the tubular lumen.
Acid permanganate aldehyde-fuchsin × 650
Reproduced by permission from: Landing BH, Nakai H. Am J Clin Pathol 1959;31:499 (Fig. 2)

long periods and in one case they were still present 10 years after the last exposure to lead.[44] Acute poisoning is also associated with morphological and functional defects in the mitochondria.[45]

Acute lead nephropathy is usually considered to be a transient phenomenon with no late sequelae.[46,47] However, the acute lead poisoning that occurred among children in Queensland, Australia, between 1915 and 1935 was associated with a greatly increased mortality in those individuals from renal and vascular causes 10–30 years later. It has been suggested that this was because they developed chronic lead nephropathy.[48,49]

Chronic lead nephropathy

Contraction and granularity of the kidneys were recognized as regular features of chronic lead poisoning during the late nineteenth and early twentieth centuries. Following legislation which defined safe limits of lead exposure in industry, overt chronic lead poisoning largely disappeared.[48] However, a group of physicians in Queensland, Australia, continued to see cases of renal insufficiency occurring many years after childhood acute lead poisoning. The children had originally been acutely ill because they had ingested lead paint from the railings of the house verandas where they played. Clinically, in these patients, hypertension and chronic renal failure preceded death, which was usually due to uraemia. Both direct measurements of bone and the ethylenediaminetetraacetic acid (EDTA) lead-mobilization test showed that these patients had excessive body stores of lead.[47]

Renal changes In most of the Queensland cases the kidneys were small and granular. Microscopically, there was patchy interstitial fibrosis, tubular atrophy and a small number of mononuclear cells infiltrating the interstitium; many of the glomeruli were sclerotic or had disappeared, and the arterioles and arteries showed benign hypertensive changes.[49] Tubular intranuclear inclusions were very rare. A similar chronic tubulointerstitial nephritis has been described in consumers of lead-contaminated home-distilled whisky in the south-eastern USA[50] and also in American industrial workers whose exposure to lead was never severe enough to produce acute symptoms of poisoning.[51] There is no evidence that established symptomatic chronic tubulointerstitial nephritis in patients with excessive amounts of lead in their bodies can be reversed by chelation therapy; in its early presymptomatic stages, however, it may be reversible.[52]

That acute lead nephropathy can evolve into chronic renal disease and that the excessive amounts of lead in the body are the cause of these non-specific renal changes is still not accepted by all nephrologists and pathologists. Some feel that the evidence is circumstantial and not very convincing; they argue that the patients may have hypertensive nephrosclerosis or some other kind of chronic renal disease and that the lead overload is coincidental.[53] However, evolution of acute lead nephropathy to chronic lead nephropathy has been observed in experimental animals.[54]

The same scepticism has been expressed about the suggestion that environmental chronic lead intoxication is responsible for some cases of 'essential' hypertension. The main supporting evidence for this notion comes from an epidemiological survey which showed that in over 9000 Americans, selected to represent the United States population as a whole, raised blood lead concentrations correlated with hypertension.[55] It has also been shown in another survey that 135 hypertensive patients had higher blood lead concentrations than did sex- and age-matched normotensive controls.[56]

Cadmium nephropathy

Cadmium is used in the manufacture of alloys, paints, plastics, glass and electrical equipment, in electroplating and soldering, and in the production of zinc, copper and nickel products.

Absorbed cadmium becomes bound to metallothionein, a cysteine-rich apoprotein. Much of the cadmium–metallothionein complex is initially stored in the liver but about a third is taken up by epithelial cells of the renal proximal tubules, where it is sequestered with a biological half-life of over 15 years. Body stores of cadmium increase steadily with age; when the concentration in the renal cortex reaches approximately 200 μg/g urinary changes occur.[57]

Acute absorption of as little as 10 mg of cadmium as dust or fumes may induce severe gastrointestinal symptoms and fatal pulmonary oedema. Chronic exposure to low doses causes slowly progressive emphysema, anosmia and proximal tubular reabsorption defects. The tubular dysfunction is characterized by aminoaciduria, hypercalciuria, glycosuria, uricosuria, phosphataemia and renal tubular acidosis.[57] The clinical picture of cadmium nephropathy is often dominated by the effects of the calcium loss in the urine. Urinary calculi occur in up to 40% of workers who are exposed in industry to cadmium[58] and osteoporosis, osteomalacia and pseudofractures are present in severe cases. Ureteral colic is a common complaint among cadmium workers.

Renal failure is rare after occupational exposure to cadmium. However, renal failure and kidney stones have been described in Japanese villagers eating rice and vegetables grown in soil heavily contaminated by cadmium emitted from adjacent industrial plants. In Japan, this syndrome has been called itai-itai disease,[59,60] which roughly translated means 'ouch-ouch' disease indicating the severe bone pain suffered by its victims.

Renal changes

A non-specific tubulointerstitial nephritis is found in the kidneys of patients with itai-itai disease and in a few of those from individuals chronically exposed to cadmium in their occupations.[59,61] In some patients much of the damage is secondary to calcium stones.

Chronic interstitial fibrosis and tubular loss have been produced in animals exposed to cadmium,[62] but whether low-level occupational exposure has similar consequences in humans is uncertain. It is also unclear whether cadmium contributes to hypertension.[57]

Mercury

The toxicity of mercury and the type of renal lesion it may produce depend on both its chemical form and its route of absorption. All chemical forms of mercury accumulate in the cells of the proximal tubules; once there the effect of the various mercury compounds varies from inducing necrosis of the proximal cells (mercuric chloride) to producing a diuresis (chlormerodrin). It has been suggested that the variable effect of different mercury compounds on the kidney is due to variability in their transformation to inorganic mercury within the body.[57] Mercury in one or more of its forms may produce acute nephrotoxic tubular necrosis, diffuse membranous glomerulonephritis, or antiglomerular-basement-membrane antibody glomerulonephritis.

Nephrotoxic acute tubular necrosis

ATN may be produced by both inorganic and organic mercury compounds.

Poisoning with mercuric chloride (corrosive sublimate) was once a relatively common cause of ATN. When mercuric chloride was widely available as a disinfectant it was sometimes drunk accidently by children or purposely by people trying to commit suicide; it was also used to induce abortion. Ingestion of as little as 0.5 g of mercuric chloride will produce nephrotoxic ATN. During the first 2 days, while the clinical picture is dominated by gastrointestinal symptoms, chelation therapy with dimercaprol (British anti-Lewisite, BAL) limits renal damage and may be life saving.[63]

Organic mercurial diuretics, which were at one time used for treating the oedema of cardiac failure, occasionally produced ATN similar to that induced by mercuric chloride.[64]

Renal changes There is widespread necrosis of the proximal convoluted tubules and the appearances are those of nephrotoxic ATN (see p. 500). In experimental animals the lesion affects primarily the pars recta of the proximal tubules but extends to more proximal segments after larger doses of mercuric chloride.[65] If the patient does not die from infection, uraemia, haemorrhage or other complications, spontaneous regeneration of the tubular epithelium occurs, with recovery. Restoration of function is sometimes limited by residual tubular atrophy and calcification, and interstitial fibrosis.[57]

Diffuse membranous glomerulonephritis

Proteinuria and often the nephrotic syndrome might occur during the treatment of cardiac failure with organic mercurial diuretics (now no longer used),[66] and are seen today following the external use of mercurial ointments and powders (e.g. the application of ointments which contain ammoniated mercury [aminomercuric chloride] by black women to lighten the colour of their skin,[67] or the use of mercury-containing ointments by patients with psoriasis[68]). These effects are also seen following industrial exposure,[69,70] for example among those making thermometers and barometers, mercury vapour lamps, and explosives (mercury fulminate) and in the felting of hats and furs (mercury nitrate).

Renal changes In all cases in which renal biopsies have been obtained and electron microscopy has been undertaken the histological picture has been that of a diffuse membranous glomerulonephritis (see p. 192). Improvement with loss of proteinuria occurred in most patients when the source of mercury was withdrawn.

Diffuse membranous glomerulonephritis caused by mercury poisoning differs from idiopathic membranous glomerulonephritis in that it is almost always accompanied by proximal tubular damage. The damage may take the form of necrosis or flattening of the epithelium. Mercury can be detected in phagolysosomes in the tubular epithelial cells;[69] it has not been found in the glomerular subepithelial deposits.

Tubular damage caused by the mercury may perhaps release tubular antigen and lead to the formation of antibody. If this happens the antibody will combine with the antigen to form complexes in the glomerular capillary walls as occurs in Heymann's model of membranous glomerulonephritis in the rat (see p. 202).

Antiglomerular-basement-membrane antibody glomerulonephritis

Occasionally, when exposure to mercury leads to proteinuria, the renal lesion is characterized by deposits of antiglomerular-basement-membrane (anti-GBM) antibody in the glomeruli.[70] Anti-GBM antibodies are also induced in animals injected with mercuric chloride.[71] The nature of the reactive antigens within the glomerular basement membrane is unknown; perhaps mercury alters one or more basement membrane constituents and renders them autoimmunogenic.

Arsenic

Arsenical substances are used extensively in industry, agriculture and husbandry. Arsenic trioxide remains an important by-product of copper smelting and arsenic compounds are still used in sheep dips, pesticides and weed killers. Arsenic is also sometimes found as a contaminant in illicitly distilled whisky. Arsenic is known to produce ATN and perhaps patchy cortical necrosis.

Acute tubular necrosis

ATN has been caused by inhalation of arsine (AsH_3), a highly toxic odourless gas, produced when arsenicals react with acid. Almost invariably the result of an industrial accident, exposure to arsine produces haemolysis, haematuria and abdominal pain within a few hours, followed by acute oliguric renal failure and jaundice.[72] The histological picture is of ischaemic ATN with haemoglobin casts. In patients who survive, recovery from the ATN is often incomplete, the kidneys showing residual interstitial fibrosis, tubular atrophy and glomerular sclerosis.[73]

Cortical necrosis

Patchy cortical necrosis has been reported following consumption of contaminated whisky.[74]

Other heavy metals

Acute tubular necrosis of nephrotoxic type due to massive accidental or parenteral absorption of chromium, bismuth, copper and antimony compounds is well recognized. Occupational renal disease as a result of chronic low-dose exposure has not been reported. Uranium workers have a statistically significant increase in mean urinary β_2-microglobulin excretion compared to controls, but as the levels are well within normal limits and there is no reduction in glomerular filtration rate, the clinical significance of this indication of tubular dysfunction is doubtful.[75]

ORGANIC CHEMICALS

Organic chemicals are in use everywhere in industrialized societies. Most will cause acute tubular necrosis in experimental animals if administered intravenously in sufficient quantity. However, relatively few are recognized nephrotoxins in the workplace or the home. The nephrotoxicity of organic chemicals is roughly dose-related: massive exposure leads to ATN and low doses to defects in tubular function and increased susceptibility to other nephrotoxins.[76]

Solvents

Many halogenated hydrocarbons, including chloroform, carbon tetrachloride, trichlorethylene, and ethylene dichloride are highly nephrotoxic. Their use as industrial cleaners and for removing greasy spots from clothing may be followed by ATN if the ventilation is inadequate.[76] Neurological, hepatic, pulmonary and intestinal symptoms dominate initially but acute renal failure may appear within the first week, causing death unless dialysis is provided.

There is some pathological evidence suggesting that solvents may induce immunologically mediated glomerular disease as well as the more clearly defined ATN.

Acute tubular necrosis

Initially in some cases neutral fat appears in the basal part of the cells of the convoluted tubules.[77] A little later degenerative changes with patchy necrosis occur in the same cells, accompanied by tubulorrhexis and protein, red cell or bile casts in the tubular lumens.[78] In some reports the lesions have been less extensive and not confined to the proximal tubules, resembling more closely those seen in ischaemic ATN.[79]

Glomerular disease

On the basis of analysis of case histories it has been claimed that there is an association between inhalation of organic solvents and the appearance of glomerulonephritis, in particular the form associated with anti-GBM antibodies.[80] A suggested explanation for this association is that the solvent may induce a change in the pulmonary alveolar basement membrane, causing formation of anti-basement membrane antibodies, which cross-react with glomerular basement membranes.[80] A case control study, comparing patients with a recent diagnosis of glomerular disease with controls with non-renal diagnoses, failed to corroborate this association.[81] However, speculation continues.[82] No convincing animal model of solvent-induced glomerulonephritis has yet been produced.

Glycols

A variety of glycols are toxic to the kidney. Ethylene glycol nephrotoxicity is the most frequently observed.

Ethylene glycol

Ethylene glycol is a colourless, odourless fluid used as an antifreeze solution in motor vehicle radiators. It has a not unpleasant, bitter sweet flavour and may be ingested as a substitute for alcohol for its intoxicating effects or it may be consumed by mistake as in the cases in the German army in World War II in which it was inadvertently used in the preparation of coffee.[83] The fatal dose is about 100 ml. Death often occurs within 48 hours as a result of damage to the central nervous system; if the patient survives acute renal failure may develop.

Renal changes The striking feature is the presence of masses of birefringent needle-shaped calcium oxalate crystals arranged in sheaves in the tubular lumens.[84,85] Initially the crystals are mainly in the proximal convoluted tubules; from the third day onwards they are also present in large numbers in the distal tubules and collecting ducts. The proximal tubular epithelium may appear normal for the first day or two but later the cells become swollen and contain variable numbers of hydropic vacuoles with pyknosis or loss of the nuclei. Tubular dilatation occurs and focal necroses may appear in the distal parts of the nephron. In severe cases there may be patchy bilateral cortical necrosis.

Although this histological picture is characteristic, the presence of large numbers of oxalate crystals is not specific for ethylene glycol poisoning; they are also found in hyperoxaluria and oxalic acid poisoning (see p. 104). Small numbers of oxalate crystals are commonly found in the kidneys of patients with long-standing chronic renal failure from various causes.

MISCELLANEOUS SUBSTANCES

Silicon

The possibility that inhalation of silicon can cause renal disease was first considered following the observation that in a series of patients with severe silicosis, 40% had renal insufficiency, 20% had proteinuria and 45% showed impaired urine concentration.[86] Since then, in two series, glomerular and tubular lesions have been reported in 51% and 45% of patients who died of advanced pulmonary silicosis.[87,88] In addition to these autopsy studies, there have been at least 11 reports of cases of glomerulonephritis, and a few of polyarteritis, discovered at renal biopsy in workers exposed over long periods to high concentrations of silicon.[89,90] Some population-based epidemiological evidence suggests that the mortality from renal disease is increased in workers exposed to silicon.[91]

Renal changes

Among the glomerular lesions a focal and a diffuse proliferative glomerulonephritis, with subendothelial deposits on the glomerular capillary basement membranes, were the two most common histological patterns. Crescents were present in a few cases; three showed crescentic mesangial IgA nephropathy.[92] Increased numbers of tubuloreticular structures in the endothelial cytoplasm, and a high silicon concentration in the renal tissue compared to normal, were present in approximately half the biopsied cases; in one case silicon crystals were identified in the tubules.[89] However, the silicon content of kidneys in patients with pulmonary silicosis but no renal disease is not known.

In experimental animals silicon is nephrotoxic and this toxicity is dose related. Short-term administration causes mainly degenerative changes in the tubular epithelium; long-term administration leads to a tubulointerstitial nephritis and glomerulosclerosis. Proliferative glomerulonephritis has not been produced.[89]

Conclusion

A causal relationship between silicon inhalation and nephropathy has yet to be established. The association may simply be due to chance. Systematically conducted epidemiological studies could help resolve this question.

Beryllium

The granulomatous pulmonary interstitial fibrosis which may follow occupational exposure to beryllium in the aerospace and electronic industries, in the manufacture of fluorescent lights, and in the mining and extracting of beryllium ores, is often associated with hypercalciuria and, less commonly, hypercalcaemia. The hypercalciuria leads to an increased incidence of *renal stones*;[93] the hypercalcaemia may cause *nephrocalcinosis*. The altered calcium metabolism in berylliosis is probably related to increased sensitivity to vitamin D associated with reduced circulating parathormone levels.

RENAL COMPLICATIONS OF DRUG AND ALCOHOL DEPENDENCE

ADDICTION TO NARCOTIC DRUGS

Renal lesions in people dependent upon narcotic drugs are frequent. Some are the result of the response made by the addict to bacterial, viral or fungal infection acquired because the drug, or the needles used to administer it, were contaminated by these organisms. A few are the result of damage to striated muscles when the addict is unconscious. Occasionally lesions may be induced by direct toxicity of the drug or of adulterating substances added to the drug. Which of these renal complications occur will depend in part upon the route of administration of the narcotic.

Renal complications that may occur in any narcotic drug addict

Ischaemic acute tubular necrosis with myoglobinuria

An overdose of heroin (diamorphine), cocaine or other narcotic drug, self-administered or given by another person, will lead to stupor and collapse; this is often associated with shock. On occasion the weight of the slumped body may then exert prolonged pressure on one or more of the limb muscles which injures the cells allowing myoglobin to escape into the circulation.[94] Sometimes in drug addicts with rhabdomyolysis there is no evidence of external muscle compression; it is postulated in these cases that the muscle damage results from either a toxic or allergic reaction to the drug or an adulterant.[95] In the case of cocaine abuse vasoconstriction causing muscle ischaemia may be a factor.[96] The myoglobin is excreted in the urine and in a patient who is hypotensive, hypoxic, acidotic and dehydrated it predisposes to acute tubular necrosis (ATN). The urine containing myoglobin is often dark brown. The acute renal failure is usually transient and the serum creatinine returns to normal levels within a month.[96] In some cases, however, there is also liver failure; in one series of 13 cocaine abusers in acute renal failure, 11 had severe hepatic dysfunction which was accompanied by disseminated intravascular coagulation in seven of the patients: six of these seven died within 2–15 days.[97]

Renal changes The appearances are those of ischaemic ATN (see p. 493). Pigment casts are prominent and there may be calcification of cell debris in the lumens of the tubules.[95] Myoglobin casts can be differentiated from haemoglobin casts by applying a commercially available specific fluorescein- or peroxidase-labelled antibody to human myoglobin to sections of either fresh frozen or formalin-fixed paraffin-embedded tissue.[98]

Pathogenesis It is generally thought that, in addition to the five mechanisms that might be responsible for any case of ischaemic ATN (see p. 497), in myoglobinuric ATN the myoglobin being excreted by the kidney has a direct toxic effect on the tubular epithelium. It is known that under acid conditions the iron-containing porphyrin ring is split from the myoglobin, producing haematin (ferrihaemate), and some evidence indicates that the haematin damages the proximal tubular epithelial cell membranes, probably by lipid peroxidation, and suppresses transport in the cells. Other evidence suggests that Tamm–Horsfall protein is particularly likely to be precipitated and form casts with myoglobin in acid urine; the tubular obstruction then leads to increased proximal tubular uptake of myoglobin which is itself in some way toxic to the proximal tubular cells.[99]

Renal complications in those injecting drugs intravenously

Heroin available 'on the street' often contains various contaminants. The mixture is dissolved by the addict in water or saliva, usually using some unsterile container, before injection into a vein. The syringe and needle are often unsterile and needles are frequently shared with other addicts. Bacterial and viral infections are therefore common in these patients. Human immunodeficiency virus type 1 (HIV-1) infections may be complicated by nephropathy; hepatitis B virus (HBV) may be associated with glomerulonephritis and necrotizing angiitis; and septicaemia and infective endocarditis can lead to glomerulonephritis, renal infarcts and abscesses. In addition, heroin is associated with a nephropathy which seems to be related to substances adulterating the drug rather than to any accompanying infection.

Nephropathy associated with human immunodeficiency virus type 1 (HIV-1)

Infection with HIV-1 is common in those taking drugs intravenously. Once infected the patient may develop focal segmental glomerulosclerosis (HIV-1 associated nephropathy) and/or any one or more of a wide range of renal lesions, including various forms of glomerulonephritis, ATN, the haemolytic uraemic syndrome, involvement by various infectious agents, and, rarely, Kaposi's sarcoma or a lymphoma involving the kidney (see p. 398).

Renal complications of infection with hepatitis B virus (HBV)

People who take drugs intravenously often become infected with HBV. This infection may produce glomerulonephritis, or the renal lesions of cryoglobulinaemia and necrotizing vasculitis. The most frequent lesion is glomerulonephritis and most commonly this is a diffuse membranous glomerulonephritis or a mesangiocapillary glomerulonephritis type I (see p. 393).

Renal complications of septicaemia and infective endocarditis

There is an increased frequency of infective endocarditis and septicaemia in intravenous drug abusers.[100] Endocarditis is often caused by coagulase-positive *Staphylococcus aureus* affecting normal valves on the right side of the heart. Infective endocarditis may lead to glomerulonephritis (which may be focal or diffuse) and infarction or abscesses in the kidney (see p. 378). Septicaemia may produce glomerulonephritis, ischaemic acute tubular necrosis or abscesses (see p. 432).

Heroin-associated nephropathy

Some heroin addicts, who are not infected with the human immunodeficiency virus (HIV), develop massive proteinuria and rapidly progress to end-stage renal failure. The underlying renal lesion is most commonly a focal segmental glomerulosclerosis which develops into global sclerosis (obsolescence) of most glomeruli. Similar lesions have been found in addicts taking the opiates pentazocine (Fortral, Talwin) and tripelennamine (Pyribenzamine) intravenously.[101] The incidence of heroin-associated nephropathy amongst addicts is not known, but in the Buffalo area of New York State in the USA the prevalence of this nephropathy in 1980 was 10% among patients with end-stage renal disease who were 18–45 years of age.[102]

Clinical features Heroin-associated nephropathy occurs 45 times more commonly in black drug addicts than in white and is most frequent in men aged 18–40 years. The patients usually present with the nephrotic syndrome, but proteinuria may be detected incidentally. Renal insufficiency is often present and may be advanced when the patient is first seen. Hypertension is frequent.[103]

Renal changes The great majority of patients show a spectrum of lesions ranging from focal to diffuse segmental or global glomerulosclerosis according to the stage of the disease.[103–105] Occasionally there is minimal change disease or focal mesangiocapillary glomerulonephritis.[104] Electron microscopical studies reveal the same changes as are seen in idiopathic or secondary focal segmental glomerulosclerosis associated with other conditions. Immunofluorescent or immunoperoxidase studies have shown either IgM and C3 in the sclerotic lesions or non-specific fine linear deposits of IgG along the capillary basement membranes.[103]

Differential diagnosis The glomerulosclerotic lesions of heroin-associated nephropathy are non-specific and are often indistinguishable from those seen in *idiopathic* or *secondary focal segmental glomerulosclerosis*. If they occur in an HIV-positive patient they cannot be distinguished from HIV-associated focal segmental glomerulosclerosis because the only distinctive feature of this latter condition – the large number of tubuloreticular structures and cylindrical confronting cisternae in the endothelial cells and leucocytes – is a general feature of HIV-1 infection and is not specific for HIV-1 nephropathy per se.[106,107]

Prognosis Heroin-associated glomerulosclerosis pursues a rapidly progressive course and terminates in end-stage renal failure in 6 months to 4 years.[108] If the patient stops taking heroin the renal failure may stabilize.

Renal transplantation Successful renal transplantation has been carried out in some addicts with heroin-associated nephropathy, but patients often continue to take heroin afterwards.[109] Glomerulosclerosis has been seen in some of the grafts in patients who have failed to overcome their addiction, but convincing evidence that this represents recurrence of heroin-associated nephropathy has yet to be produced.

Pathogenesis The pathogenesis of heroin nephropathy is not known. One possibility is that heroin itself produces the glomerular lesion; against this is the failure to induce the change in experimental animals given pure heroin. Another possibility is that the contaminating substances in the injected heroin are nephrotoxic; the material injected by an addict is often only 3% heroin and 97% adulterants. Supporting this notion is the claim that heroin plus contaminants will produce glomerulosclerosis in rats.[110] There is also some evidence which suggests that there may be a genetic predisposition to the disease; this might explain the great predilection of the lesion for blacks.

Necrotizing angiitis

Rarely, a necrotizing angiitis, indistinguishable from idiopathic classic polyarteritis (see p. 267), occurs in addicts taking drugs parenterally in whom there is no evidence of infection by hepatitis B virus. The kidneys are often involved. Originally this form of arteritis was thought to occur only in patients taking methylamphetamine (methamphetamine),[111] but it has since been seen in association with the use of other hallucinogenic drugs and of heroin. The polyarteritis has a poor prognosis; its progress has occasionally been halted by treatment with cytotoxic drugs.

Renal infarction

Multiple renal infarcts have been described in intravenous cocaine abusers.[112] They have been attributed to cocaine-induced vasospasm leading to arterial thrombosis.

Renal complications in those injecting drugs subcutaneously

Amyloidosis

Amyloidosis is a frequent complication of long-standing drug addiction.[113,114] It occurs mostly in people who inject drugs subcutaneously ('skin poppers') because they so commonly have extensive chronic suppurating skin infections;[113,114] it is rare in addicts who inject only into their veins ('mainliners').[114] The incidence of amyloidosis in addicts with widespread chronic infections of the skin in one series was 26%.[113] It occurs particularly in those with a long history of drug addiction. The mean duration of drug taking in one series was 16 years, and the mean age of the patients 40 years.

The amyloid is AA in type and it is often found in the kidneys.[113] The distribution does not differ from that seen in amyloidosis complicating various chronic infections in non-addicts (see p. 346).

The patient develops marked proteinuria, often accompanied by the nephrotic syndrome. The blood pressure is usually normal or low. In most centres amyloidosis is the second most common reason for the nephrotic syndrome in drug addicts, the usual cause being focal segmental glomerulosclerosis (heroin-associated nephropathy). In a few centres amyloidosis has become the most frequent cause because patients are surviving longer, exhausting suitable intravenous sites, and consequently changing to injecting their drugs subcutaneously.[115]

Progress to end-stage renal disease usually occurs within months of amyloidosis being recognized. Treatment of the skin infections may induce remissions.

Amyloidosis can be very largely prevented if rigorous attempts are made to avoid skin infections and if any that occur are treated promptly and effectively.

Renal complications in those sniffing solvents

Acute tubular necrosis

Inhalation of the fumes of toluene or toluene-containing compounds is a favourite of glue and paint 'sniffers' who deliberately breathe in sufficient of the solvent to induce intoxication. Benzoic and hippuric acid metabolites of this aromatic hydrocarbon are excreted by the kidneys and undergo transient intracellular storage in the proximal tubular epithelial cells.[76]

Neurological symptoms usually dominate the clinical picture immediately after inhalation, but muscle weakness and rhabdomyolysis may occur in habitual inhalers of toluene. The rhabdomyolysis is not usually related to muscle compression; it is possibly related to the combined effects on muscle of the hypokalaemia and hypophosphataemia that occur after inhalation of toluene. Not all cases show these electrolyte disturbances and a direct toxic effect on skeletal and cardiac muscle has been suggested.

Addicts may develop acute tubular necrosis. In a few this is hypotension-induced ischaemic acute tubular necrosis; in others it is associated with pigment casts and myoglobinuria. Occasionally the ATN is not completely reversible and progressive tubulointerstitial injury has been reported.[116]

Acute tubular necrosis may also occur when other solvents, such as trichlorethylene, are inhaled by addicts.

ALCOHOLISM

Alcoholism may be associated with renal complications. These include acute tubular necrosis (ATN) with myoglobinuria, hepatorenal syndrome, glomerular lesions (in particular IgA nephropathy) and hypertension.

Acute tubular necrosis with myoglobinuria

Ischaemic ATN induced by ethyl alcohol is occasionally seen;[117] it is usually associated with rhabdomyolysis. Often there is a clear history of the patient having lain immobile through a long period while drunk, in such a position that the trunk has produced a continuous pressure on a limb. The capillary occlusion induced by the pressure causes muscle ischaemia and rhabdomyolysis, with pain, swelling or impaired mobility of the affected muscles.[118] Sometimes there are no symptoms or signs of muscle injury in spite of a marked elevation of serum creatine kinase which is also released from injured muscles.[117] There is evidence that chronic alcoholics may be predisposed to rhabdomyolysis and ATN following episodes of acute alcoholic myopathy (affecting type 1 fibres) and after periods of acute medical or surgical stress, as, for example, after haematemesis or acute urinary retention. The muscle damage in these patients may be due to impaired intracellular glycogen metabolism.[119]

The ATN causes acute renal failure: this is often oliguric but may be non-oliguric. The changes in the kidneys[119] do not differ from those seen in cases of ischaemic ATN with myoglobinuria induced by causes other than alcoholism (see p. 509). The prognosis is good. Most patients whose cases have been reported regained full renal function in a relatively short time.[117]

Hepatorenal syndrome

Some patients with alcoholic cirrhosis develop progressive renal failure. It is an example of the hepatorenal syndrome, a term originally introduced to describe acute renal failure occurring after biliary tract surgery,[120] but now usually defined as acute renal failure induced specifically as a result of cirrhosis or some other severe parenchymal liver disease.[121] It occurs in about half the patients dying from alcoholic cirrhosis.

The pathophysiology of acute renal failure in decompensated alcoholic cirrhosis is controversial. Using light microscopy, most observers have found either normal-looking kidneys or inconstant and mild tubular lesions which they felt did not amount to ischaemic ATN.[122] However, an electron microscopic study of kidneys from five patients who died with the hepatorenal syndrome demonstrated focal necrosis and tubulorrhexis consistent with an ischaemic ATN.[123] In jaundiced patients the tubules may contain deposits of bile pigment – a condition at one time referred to as cholaemic nephrosis.

The enigma of the hepatorenal syndrome is that intense renal and cerebral vasoconstriction occurs in the face of generalized vasodilatation. This is in contrast to hypovolaemic or haemorrhagic hypotension in which total peripheral resistance is increased. It may be that some renal vasoconstrictor, present in the blood stream but normally inactivated by the liver, remains active in cases of alcoholic cirrhosis because of inadequacy of the diseased liver. Certainly transplantation of a normal liver to patients suffering from the hepatorenal syndrome may cause the syndrome to reverse and resolve.[124] The prognosis is very poor because of the underlying hepatic dysfunction.

Glomerular disease in cirrhosis

Glomerular disease occurs in more than half the patients with alcoholic cirrhosis of the liver. The most characteristic finding is the presence of IgA in the mesangium.

IgA nephropathy

In 1970 Manigand first described glomerular deposits of predominantly IgA and C3 in biopsy specimens from 75% of 20 patients with alcoholic liver cirrhosis.[125] This finding of an IgA nephropathy has since been amply confirmed.[126] In patients with alcoholic cirrhosis studied at autopsy the incidence of glomerular mesangial deposits of IgA has been in the range 61–66%.[127,128] IgG or IgM or both are also often present, but IgA is the main immunoglobulin; Clq is uncommon.

Renal changes In many, but not all, of the patients the IgA deposits are accompanied by mesangial proliferative changes.[127] The non-proliferative form is characterized by mesangial electron-dense deposits that frequently extend into the subendothelial space; this group is clinically silent. The proliferative form is usually a mesangiocapillary glomerulonephritis type 1; most of these cases are associated with clinical manifestations. Progression from non-proliferative to proliferative glomerulonephritis was observed in two of eight patients whose kidneys were serially biopsied.[129]

Clinical features In general the more severe the proliferative changes in the glomeruli, the more common are proteinuria and microscopic haematuria. Gross haematuria is much less frequent than in primary IgA nephropathy. In a series of 752 consecutive patients with cirrhosis, haematuria and proteinuria were present in 9.2% and the nephrotic syndrome in 1.6%.[130]

Serum levels of IgA are increased in cirrhotics; in one study they were raised in 54% of patients whether there was renal disease or not.[126] In patients with IgA mesangial deposits increased serum levels of IgA are more common, occurring in 91–96% of the patients.[126] Circulating IgA immune complexes are also common. Levels of serum C3 are usually decreased.

Renal insufficiency is infrequent and usually mild; it is most likely to occur in cases of mesangiocapillary glomerulonephritis type I.

Differential diagnosis IgA nephropathy secondary to alcoholic cirrhosis is often morphologically indistinguishable from primary IgA nephropathy. However, in the form associated with cirrhosis there is a greater tendency to mesangial interposition in the glomeruli, producing a mesangiocapillary pattern.[130] Clq is more likely to be present in the mesangium, serum C3 levels are usually lower and the frequency of circulating IgA immune complexes is higher.[131]

Prognosis The overall prognosis is that of the underlying alcoholic cirrhosis; in most cases the IgA nephropathy seems to influence the outcome very little. A few patients with bouts of gross haematuria have developed acute renal failure due to acute tubular necrosis.[132]

Pathogenesis The pathogenesis of IgA nephropathy in association with alcoholic cirrhosis is not established. One suggestion is that the sequestration of circulating IgA polymers and IgA immune complexes, which happens in the normal liver, is defective in alcoholic cirrhosis; as a result, levels of circulating immune complexes and serum IgA rise and may be responsible for the glomerular deposits.[133] Alternatively, it has been speculated that the complexes may be derived from IgA aggregates combining with proteins of the hepatocyte membranes or with Mallory body proteins in the alcohol-damaged liver.[134] The observation that a Mallory-body antigen (JMB2) is sometimes present in association with the mesangial deposits of IgA, in patients with alcoholic cirrhosis, supports the possibility that this antigen may be involved in the pathogenesis of the nephropathy.[135]

Hypertension and Cushingoid syndrome

The association between hypertension and alcohol consumption is well recognized.[136] It has been suggested that this might be related to abnormalities of adrenocortical activity because the hypertension is occasionally accompanied by a rise in hydrocortisone concentrations to such an extent that Cushing's syndrome is mimicked.[137]

ABUSE OF ANALGESIC DRUGS

People who become addicted to analgesics may develop renal disease. The addiction is often to caffeine-containing mixed analgesic powders which are taken for their stimulant and mood-altering effects rather than as analgesics. Most of the mixed compounds contain two or more of the following substances: aspirin, paracetamol (acetaminophen), codeine, phenazone (antipyrine), amidopyrine (aminopyrine), caffeine or non-steroidal anti-inflammatory drugs. Before 1975 phenacetin (acetophenetidin) was common in these mixtures but legislation in several countries and general awareness of the dangers of phenacetin have greatly reduced its use. The prevalence of addiction is highest in those areas where caffeine-containing mixed analgesic powders are available without prescription and are widely advertised. Addiction is also very high where free headache powders are given to employees in industries that involve work that causes either eye-strain or extreme boredom.

Renal changes

Abuse of analgesic drugs primarily causes renal papillary necrosis and transitional cell tumours of the renal pelvis. Other changes are mostly complications of renal papillary necrosis, such as tubulointerstitial nephritis, hydronephrosis or pyonephrosis, and renal calculi; the risk of developing a renal adenocarcinoma is also doubled.

Analgesic nephropathy is discussed in detail on pages 458–462.

RENAL COMPLICATIONS OF THERAPEUTIC AND DIAGNOSTIC AGENTS

Many therapeutic agents, used in normal doses, may be complicated by changes in the kidneys. Some of the more important are various metals, non-steroidal anti-inflammatory agents, antibiotics, sulphonamides, cyclosporin, hydralazine, penicillamine, captopril, the contraceptive pill and ionizing radiation. Diagnostic aids such as iodine-containing radiocontrast agents may also lead to renal damage.

METALS

Gold

Gold is an effective and widely used treatment for active and erosive rheumatoid arthritis that is progressing despite treatment with other agents such as salicylates and non-steroidal anti-inflammatory drugs.[138] The benefits of gold therapy are slow to appear; at least 3–6 months of treatment are necessary before any appreciable effect can be expected, and then to prevent relapse the patient must be kept on a maintenance dose for months or years. With such prolonged treatment renal toxicity occurs quite frequently. All gold preparations at present available for parenteral or oral use have, on occasion, been shown to be nephrotoxic.

Clinical features

Proteinuria develops in 2–10% of patients being treated with gold, with occasional reports of up to 26%;[138,139] in half the patients the onset occurs in the first 6 months of treatment and in 85% by 2 years.[138] The peak incidence is between 4 and 6 months after the start of treatment. The severity and duration of the proteinuria are not related to the total amount of gold received, to the duration of treatment, or to the peak or mean gold levels in the blood. In approximately one third of patients the proteinuria is sufficiently severe to cause the nephrotic syndrome.[138] The proteinuria gradually reduces after gold treatment is stopped and usually disappears within 2 years; rarely it has persisted for as long as 3¼ years.[138]

Occasionally gold nephrotoxicity may present as microscopic haematuria with or without proteinuria. There is usually no deterioration in the glomerular filtration rate.

Renal changes

Membranous glomerulonephritis Membranous glomerulonephritis is the renal lesion most commonly associated with gold treatment (see p. 191).[140–143] It occurs in approximately 70% of patients with proteinuria. The subepithelial deposits are often smaller than those generally observed in idiopathic membranous glomerulonephritis and they are usually at stage I or II. In 30–50% of biopsies the deposits are segmental; some capillary loops may appear normal. The number of mesangial cells and the amount of mesangial matrix may be increased.[143] Gold is often detectable in the proximal tubular epithelial cells, and occasionally within glomerular visceral epithelial cells, mesangial cells and endothelial cells;[140,141] it has not been identified in the subepithelial deposits. The gold appears as electron-dense, finely beaded, curvilinear particles contained within intracytoplasmic membrane-bound lysosomes (Fig. 13.9).

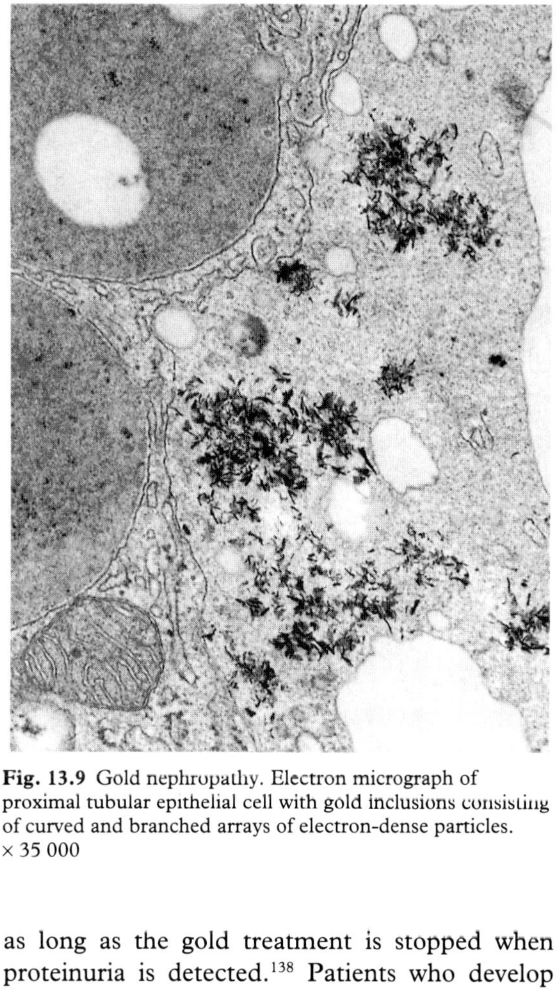

Fig. 13.9 Gold nephropathy. Electron micrograph of proximal tubular epithelial cell with gold inclusions consisting of curved and branched arrays of electron-dense particles. × 35 000

Minimal change lesions Minimal change lesions occur in approximately 10% of patients with proteinuria during gold treatment. There is extensive obliteration of epithelial foot processes without other significant glomerular, tubular or interstitial abnormalities.[143]

Other renal lesions In the remaining 20% of patients about half show a mild *mesangial proliferative glomerulonephritis* with or without electron-dense deposits in the mesangium.[144,143] Most of the other patients have a *tubulointerstitial nephritis* with foci of tubular cell damage, interstitial mononuclear cell infiltration, tubular atrophy and interstitial fibrosis. A few cases with glomerular subendothelial and mesangial electron-dense deposits have been described.[140]

Prognosis

The long-term prognosis is almost always good as long as the gold treatment is stopped when proteinuria is detected.[138] Patients who develop proteinuria with gold treatment have an increased (17–83%) chance of developing proteinuria if they are subsequently given penicillamine.[138]

Pathogenesis

The injection of gold in therapeutic doses into rodents induces a membranous glomerulonephritis. As gold has not been demonstrated in the glomerular subepithelial immune deposits in man or experimental animals, it is very unlikely that the metal is acting as a hapten or inducing immunogenic gold protein conjugates.[138] The most likely explanation for the membranous glomerulonephritis is that the gold, which is a potent nephrotoxin, damages the brush borders of the proximal tubules with the consequent release of autoantigen. The autoantigen induces antibodies which combine with the antigen to form immune complexes on the glomerular capillary basement membrane, as in Heymann's model of membranous glomerulonephritisin rats (see p. 202)

There is also a genetic predisposition in some individuals who develop membranous glomerulonephritis during gold treatment; the predisposition is associated with HLA-DR3, the allele that also favours idiopathic membranous glomerulonephritis. Fifty per cent of DR3-positive individuals treated with gold develop membranous glomerulonephritis.[145]

Platinum – cisplatin

Cisplatin (*cis*-dichlorodiammine platinum 11) is an inhibitor of DNA synthesis which is widely used in the treatment of solid tumours that are resistant to other forms of therapy. It is nephrotoxic and even at very low doses it may cause acute renal failure, especially after its repeated administration. Approximately one-third of patients receiving a single course of cisplatin 2 mg/kg body weight develop acute renal failure.[146] This is reversible but a gradual irreversible decline in glomerular filtration rate may occur with successive courses of cisplatin. Commonly cisplatin nephropathy causes defective magnesium reabsorption. The resulting very low blood levels of magnesium may be life-threatening.

Renal changes

The kidneys accumulate platinum and retain it to a greater degree than other organs; they are the predominant route of excretion for cisplatin. The primary site of renal damage is the tubule; a *nephrotoxic acute tubular necrosis* is produced. Autopsy studies in patients suggest that the distal tubules and collecting ducts are most affected,[147] but in animal studies the pars recta of the proximal tubules is the initial site of cell damage.[148]

Lithium

Prolonged administration of lithium is common in the management of patients with manic depressive psychosis and endogenous depression. Such treatment is commonly associated with impairment of urinary concentrating ability and a *chronic interstitial nephritis*. Lithium nephropathy is described in detail on page 462.

A few patients develop a nephrotic syndrome with renal changes indistinguishable morphologically from *minimal change disease* (see p. 135). Recovery occurs in 2–12 weeks following discontinuation of the lithium; patients relapse within 5 weeks if lithium treatment is reinstated.[149] The pathogenesis is unknown; a direct action of lithium on the glomerular epithelial cells or an indirect effect on lymphocytes has been suggested.

NON-STEROIDAL ANTI-INFLAMMATORY DRUGS

Non-steroidal anti-inflammatory drugs are chemically diverse but they all act as analgesic and anti-inflammatory agents and they all inhibit prostaglandin synthesis. The group includes salicylates (e.g. aspirin), propionic acid derivatives (e.g. fenoprofen, ibuprofen and naproxen), indole derivatives (e.g. indomethacin, tolmetin, sulindac and zomepirac), anthranilic acid derivatives (e.g. mefenamic acid and meclofe-namate), pyraxolene derivatives (e.g. phenylbutazone and oxyphenbutazone) and oxicam derivatives (e.g. piroxicam). Their use is occasionally associated with acute renal failure; this complication usually occurs only in elderly patients who have low cardiac output, the nephrotic syndrome, cirrhosis or pre-existing renal dysfunction.[150] Three main patterns of acute renal failure may occur: transient renal dysfunction with no morphological changes, acute tubular necrosis (ATN), and acute interstitial nephritis. Non-steroidal anti-inflammatory drugs may also give rise to the nephrotic syndrome: this may be accompanied by acute renal failure or occur on its own. Long-term use of these drugs may cause papillary necrosis.

Transient renal dsyfunction with no morphological changes

The renal dysfunction is usually mild; there is often oliguria but the urine appears normal. Urinary sodium is usually low. Morphologically the kidneys usually appear normal. When the drug is withdrawn renal function returns to baseline level within 5 days. This syndrome is thought to be due to intense renal vasoconstriction due to inhibition of renal prostaglandin by the drug.

Acute tubular necrosis

Oliguric or non-oliguric acute renal failure occurs within days or weeks of starting on the drug. There is sometimes severe hyperkalaemia, there is mild proteinuria, the urine contains granular casts, and urinary sodium is usually raised. Recovery is gradual after withdrawal of the drug; occasionally the patient is left with permanent renal impairment.

Renal changes

The renal changes are those of ischaemic ATN (see p. 493).[151] The ATN is probably caused by the intense renal vasoconstriction that follows inhibition of renal prostaglandin by the drug; the non-steroidal anti-inflammatory agent may also directly damage the tubular epithelium.

Acute tubulointerstitial nephritis

Acute tubulointerstitial nephritis due to non-steroidal anti-inflammatory drugs is discussed on pages 457–458.

Nephrotic syndrome

When acute renal failure is accompanied by the nephrotic syndrome the kidneys usually show an acute tubulointerstitial nephritis with the additional feature that electron microscopy demonstrates moderate to severe effacement of the foot processes of the epithelial cells.[152] The nephrotic syndrome without acute renal failure has been reported with sulindac, tolmetin and zomepirac; the renal changes were those of minimal change disease.[153]

Papillary necrosis

Papillary necrosis has been reported in association with long-term use of aspirin, indomethacin, phenylbutazone, ibuprofen and fenoprofen.[154,155] The pathological features are described on page 474. The lesions differ slightly from those in classic analgesic nephropathy in that they are not pigmented, necrosis tends to affect all papillae, and the majority of necrotic papillae are not shed but remain attached to the medulla. Because the necrotic papillae remain attached, radiological confirmation of the diagnosis is difficult; cavities within the necrotic tissue can sometimes be demonstrated.

ANTIBIOTICS

Some antibiotics occasionally give rise to renal complications. Of those most often involved, several (e.g. methicillin) are now prescribed less frequently and others (e.g. cephaloridine) are no longer used.

Penicillins

The penicillins may give rise to an *acute interstitial nephritis*. The changes that occur in the kidneys are described on page 454. With methicillin now used less often, ampicillin and oxacillin are the penicillins most likely to be involved. The penicillins do not cause nephrotoxic acute tubular necrosis (ATN); *ischaemic ATN* occurs very rarely following allergic shock induced by one of the antibiotics in this group.

Aminoglycosides – gentamicin

The majority of aminoglycosides are nephrotoxic. In a prospective study it was found that 11% of cases of acute renal failure acquired in hospital were due to the use of aminoglycosides.[156] These antibiotics are excreted in the urine and part of the filtered load is absorbed by the proximal tubules in which the aminoglycosides are retained with a tissue half-life of several days. Gentamicin is currently the most widely used aminoglycoside. When the aminoglycosides produce renal damage it is usually ATN; less commonly they produce acute tubulointerstitial nephritis.

Acute tubular necrosis

Clinical features As early as 24 hours after a single therapeutic dose of an aminoglycoside the amounts of proximal tubular brush border and lysosomal enzymes in the urine start to increase and then go on rising. Glycosuria, aminoaciduria and tubular proteinuria with beta-microglobulinuria develop. There may also be loss of potassium and magnesium in the urine leading to decreased plasma levels of these cations. Polyuria and nephrogenic diabetes insipidus sometimes occur. In the next few days there is progression to non-oliguric acute renal failure. When the drug is discontinued renal function recovers.

Renal changes In experimental animals the ATN induced by aminoglycosides is nephrotoxic in type and confined almost exclusively to the convoluted and straight segments of the proximal tubules.[157] The earliest change, seen by electron microscopy, is the appearance in the cytoplasm of the tubular cells of large numbers of structures composed of concentric electron-dense lamellae. These so-called *myeloid bodies* (Fig. 13.10) lie within phagolysosomes and may be detected within 48 hours of gentamicin administration; they are a characteristic consequence of the administration of aminoglycosides but they are not specific for these compounds. Myeloid bodies occur in all patients being treated with aminoglycosides, not just in those with acute renal failure. Subsequently, the height and number of the microvilli decrease, the mitochondria swell and the rough endoplasmic reticulum dilates. These

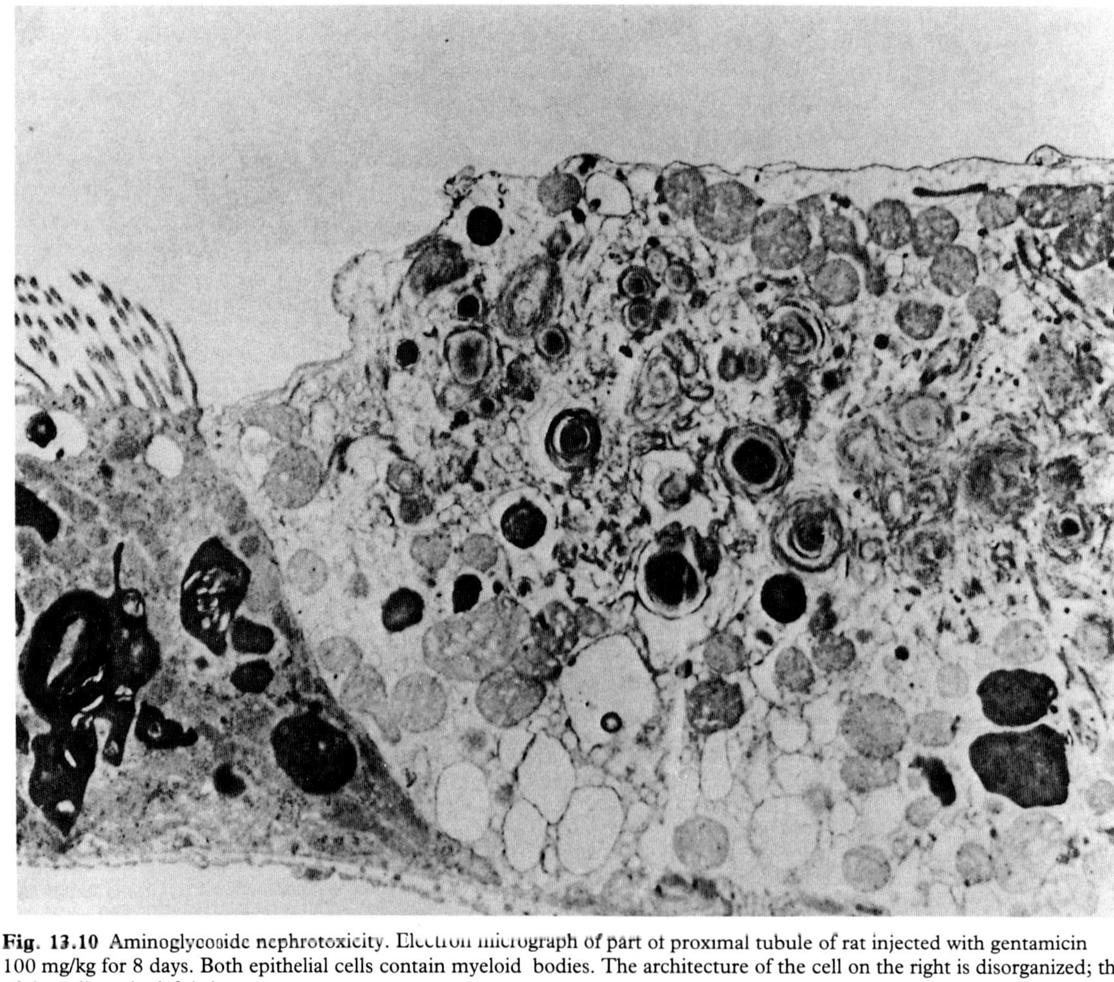

Fig. 13.10 Aminoglycoside nephrotoxicity. Electron micrograph of part of proximal tubule of rat injected with gentamicin 100 mg/kg for 8 days. Both epithelial cells contain myeloid bodies. The architecture of the cell on the right is disorganized; that of the cell on the left is intact.
× 11 250
Reproduced by permission from: Kaloyanides GH, Pastoriza-Munoz E. Kidney Int 1980;18:571 (Fig. 2)

changes progress to necrosis of the proximal tubular cells. The number of cells underlying necrosis depends on the dosage of the drug; the lesions may therefore be focal or diffuse. Signs of regeneration of tubular cells occur early, despite continued treatment with aminoglycosides.

There are few reports on renal biopsies from patients in acute renal failure induced by aminoglycosides. In would appear that, at least in some cases, the lesions resemble more closely those seen in ischaemic ATN (see p. 493), but with two additional features: rather coarse vacuolization of the cytoplasm of the proximal tubules and the presence of myeloid bodies.[158] Administration of an aminoglycoside in combination with a cephalosporin (see below) increases the incidence and severity of ATN in the patients.[157]

Pathogenesis Aminoglycoside in the glomerular filtrate binds to phospholipid receptors on the membranes of the microvilli of the proximal tubular cells. The bound aminoglycoside is then taken into the cells by endocytosis and stored in phagolysosomes. The aminoglycoside injures the lysosomal membrane, releasing damaging enzymes into the cytoplasm which kill the cells.[38,39] How injury to the proximal tubular cells causes acute renal failure is not known. The various hypotheses are described on pages 501–502.

Myeloid bodies are probably collections of incompletely degraded cell membranes; the phospholipid-rich material accumulates in phagolysomes because the aminoglycoside has impaired the activity of one or more lysosomal enzymes.[157]

Acute interstitial nephritis

In some patients gentamicin gives rise to an acute interstitial nephritis. Morphologically this does not differ from that produced by the penicillins (see p. 454).[159] Evidence points to an allergic mechanism in these cases.

Cephalosporins

Cephaloridine, now replaced by other compounds, caused dose-related nephrotoxic ATN affecting predominantly the proximal tubules; it was accompanied by early calcification of the necrotic epithelium. Among the newer cephalosporins, cephalothin, although much less toxic than cephaloridine, may induce either a *nephrotoxic ATN*[160] or an *allergic type of acute interstitial nephritis*[161]. The ATN only develops after very large doses of cephalothin.[160] When cephalothin and gentamicin are used together ischaemic ATN may be produced.[162] There is some evidence that the ATN produced by cephalosporins is at least partly mediated by an inhibitory effect on mitochondrial respiration in the tubular cells.[163]

Amphotericin (amphotericin B)

Nephrotoxic ATN is frequently produced by amphotericin. The necrosis affects both the proximal and distal tubules; calcification of the necrotic cells is often a striking feature.[164] The ATN is usually reversible, but renal function is permanently impaired in 40% of patients who receive more than 5 g of amphotericin.[165]

The cause of the tubular damage is not known. Amphotericin has two actions which might be relevant: one is to bind to steroid-containing membranes, causing their permeability to change; the other is to cause vasoconstriction.

Amphotericin also causes vasopressin-related nephrogenic diabetes insipidus and renal tubular acidosis.

Rifampicin (rifampin)

Rifampicin may cause acute renal failure. This is most commonly associated with an acute tubulointerstitial nephritis, but occasionally ATN is produced.

Acute tubulointerstitial nephritis

The tubulointerstitial nephritis produced by rifampicin is an acute hypersensitivity injury resembling that produced by a number of other drugs. It is discussed on page 457. Rarely, the acute tubulointerstitial nephritis is accompanied by the nephrotic syndrome and effacement of the glomerular epithelial foot processes.[166]

Acute tubular necrosis

Occasionally with low doses there is ischaemic

ATN; with higher doses the tubular changes more closely resemble those of nephrotoxic ATN.[167] The tubular damage may be due to interference with mitochondrial DNA transcription, a known effect of rifampicin.

SULPHONAMIDES

Sulphonamides may produce acute renal failure because of obstruction, acute tubulointerstitial nephritis or ATN.

Obstruction

Acute renal failure due to concretions of sulphonamide crystals in the tubules and in the urinary tract is very rarely seen these days, probably because of the use of more soluble sulphonamides and improvements in clinical management. Sulphapyridine, sulphathiazole and sulphadiazine are most likely to induce this complication. Obstruction is characterized by microscopic or gross haematuria, cystalluria and renal colic.

Acute tubulointerstitial nephritis

Occasional cases of acute tubulointerstitial nephritis have been reported.[168] There are no distinctive morphological features.

Acute tubular necrosis

A few cases of ischaemic ATN occur. Nephrotoxic ATN has not been reported.

CYCLOSPORIN (CYCLOSPORINE A)

Treatment with the immunosuppressive drug cyclosporin is frequently complicated by acute, subacute and chronic nephrotoxicity. The lesions produced by cyclosporin in renal allografts are described on page 661.

Acute nephrotoxicity

Clinical features

Within a few days of starting a daily oral dose of 10 mg/kg of cyclosporin a slight increase in the level of serum creatinine almost always occurs, due to a reduction in the glomerular filtration rate and renal plasma flow. The increase is reversible if the dose of cyclosporin is reduced.[169]

Renal changes

Morphologically, the kidney is often normal at the time the level of serum creatinine starts to rise. Sometimes there is isometric vacuolization of the cells of the straight part of the proximal tubule (Fig. 13.11).[170] The vacuolization is due to dilatation of the smooth and rough endoplasmic reticulum and is identical with osmotic nephrosis; it may be due to a direct toxic effect of the drug on the epithelial cells. Claims that giant mitochondria and microcalcification are commoner in the tubular cells of patients being treated with cyclosporin are controversial.[170] Many hold that their incidence is no greater than in controls.

Pathogenesis

The pathogenesis of acute nephrotoxicity is poorly understood. Present evidence suggests that cyclosporin causes a selective vasoconstriction of the afferent arterioles.[169] How this vasoconstriction is brought about is not clear – it seems to be largely

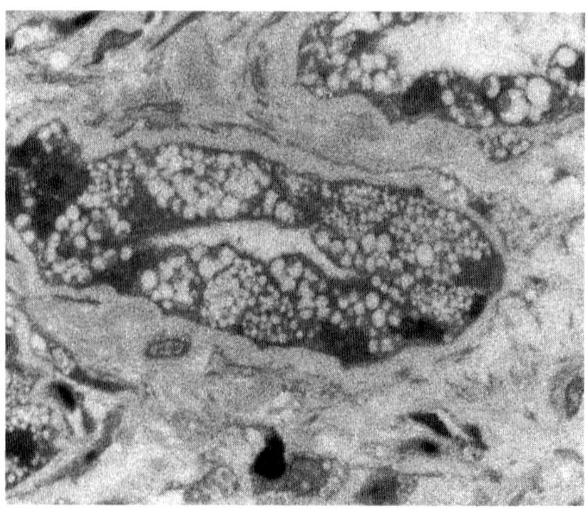

Fig. 13.11 Cyclosporin nephrotoxicity. Isometric vacuolization of cells of straight part of proximal tubule. Epon-embedded tissue, section 0.5 μm thick, azur II × 600

independent of the renin–angiotensin system and of the tubuloglomerular feedback mechanism; atrial natriuretic hormone is normal. A sympathomimetic effect has been suggested because in rats cyclosporin produces catecholamine release and neural stimulation.[169] Another hypothesis is that cyclosporin increases transmembrane calcium ion influx causing exaggerated contractile responses in arteriolar smooth muscle and mesangial cells.[171] A direct cytotoxic effect on endothelial cells and an inhibitory influence on their regeneration has been suggested on the basis of cell-culture studies.[172] The most likely hypothesis, however, is that cyclosporin alters the balance between the vasodilator prostacyclin (PGI_2) and its vasoconstrictor antagonist thromboxane A_2 in the cortex of the kidneys.[169] Of course, endothelial cell damage or inhibition of endothelial cell replication could also result in a decrease in total prostacyclin production.[173]

Prognosis

The fall in glomerular filtration rate is progressive for the first 6 months of treatment leading to at least a 20% reduction in renal function in almost all patients. After this time in many patients there seems to be little further deterioration:[174] in these cases the fall in glomerular filtration rate can be reversed within 2 weeks after cyclosporin is discontinued, even after many months of treatment; renal blood flow also increases.[175]

Subacute and chronic nephrotoxicity

Clinical features

After usually about a year of continuous treatment with cyclosporin, but sometimes much earlier, the elevated renal vascular resistance and the azotaemia cease to be fully reversible in some patients. This evidence of chronic nephrotoxicity appears in about 15% of renal transplant patients treated with cyclosporin.[169]

Continued administration of cyclosporin to patients showing evidence of chronic nephrotoxicity is often followed by the development of hypertension and proteinuria. In one series of liver transplants in patients maintained on cyclosporin, the incidence of hypertension progressively increased from 15.3% at three months to 63.6% at 4 years; the occurrence of hypertension was independent of corticosteroid treatment.[176]

Renal changes

Biopsies of the kidneys in the *subacute* stage of *nephrotoxicity* reveal hyalinization of afferent arteriolar walls with protein deposit replacing necrotic smooth muscle cells (Figs 13.12, 13.13).[170,177] The pericytes also show degenerative changes and some are replaced by hyaline material. Claims that there may be mucoid thickening of the intima are not so well established. Similarly, reports that arteriolar or glomerular fibrin or platelet thrombi are caused by cyclosporin are controversial; they have only been found in patients with transplants and not in patients with autoimmune disease treated with cyclosporin.[170] In transplants thrombi are more likely to be due to rejection (see p. 648).

In *chronic nephrotoxicity* the arteriolar hyaline changes are progressively accompanied by interstitial fibrosis, tubular atrophy and glomerular sclerosis.[170,177] The interstitial fibrosis is focal and often forms streaks or stripes: claims that these are specific are unfounded. Comparable stripes may be seen in other conditions: they correspond

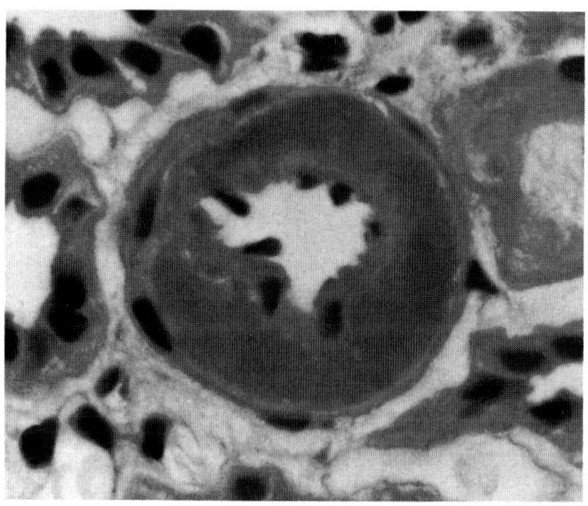

Fig. 13.12 Cyclosporin nephrotoxicity. Hyaline change in wall of afferent arteriole.
Haematoxylin-eosin × 250

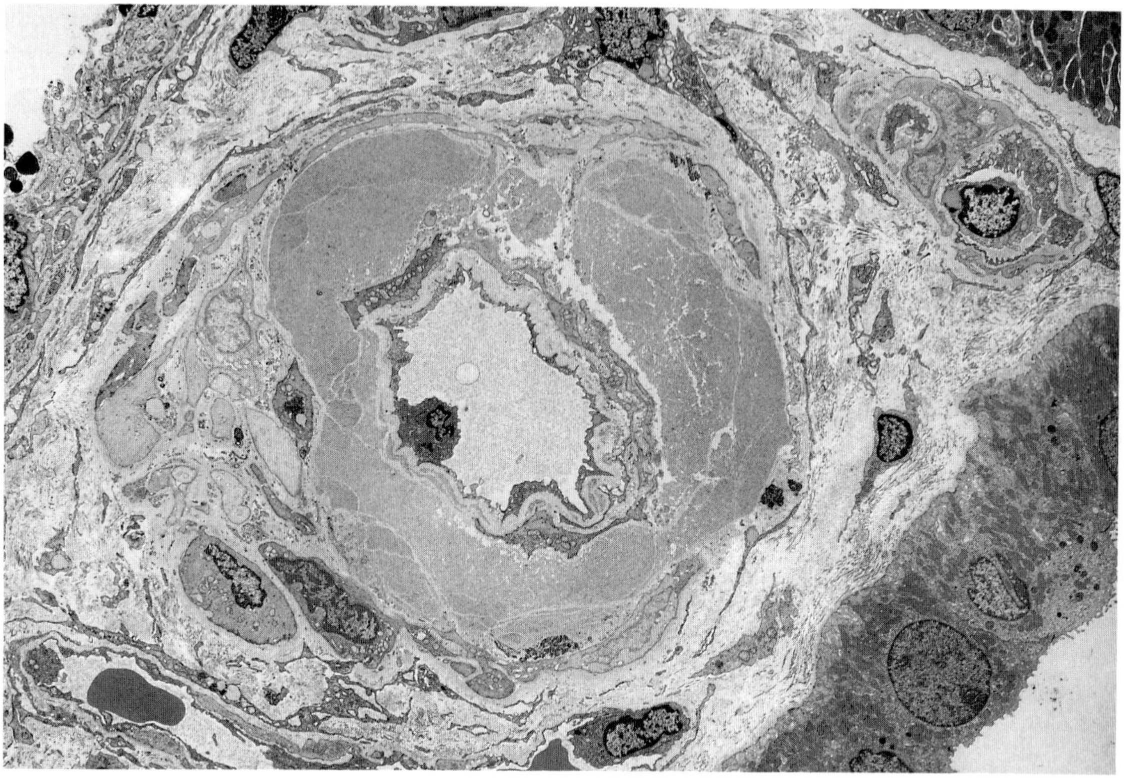

Fig. 13.13 Cyclosporin nephrotoxicity. Electron micrograph of an afferent arteriole. There are subintimal and medial hyaline deposits in its wall. Several degenerated pericytes are partially or completely replaced by hyalin. × 2000

to groups of tubules supplied by narrowed arterioles. The glomerular sclerosis may be global or segmental.

The arteriolar, tubular and interstitial changes are all non-specific. The diagnosis of cyclosporin nephrotoxicity is always one of exclusion.

Prognosis

Chronic cyclosporin nephrotoxicity can progress to end-stage renal disease within 5 years.[178]

Pathogenesis

This is not known. It is generally assumed that sustained afferent arteriolar vasospasm associated with long-term cyclosporin administration leads eventually to degeneration of the smooth muscle in the vessel walls; ultimately the arterioles become obliterated and the glomeruli they supply become sclerosed.[178] When a certain critical number of glomeruli is lost, hyperfiltration in the others triggers progressive focal glomerular sclerosis, even if the cyclosporin has by this time been withdrawn (see p. 26).

HYDRALAZINE

Hydralazine dilates peripheral blood vessels and is commonly used in treating patients with hypertension. Its long-term administration is very often associated with the appearance of anti-nuclear antibodies and, in approximately 7% of the patients, with a syndrome resembling systemic lupus erythematosus (SLE). Of the patients showing the clinical manifestations of SLE 20–50% have lupus nephritis, usually the Class III focal form. This drug-induced SLE is discussed on page 240.

PENICILLAMINE

Penicillamine is an effective, widely prescribed, second-line treatment for rheumatoid arthritis; it is also used to treat hepatolenticular degeneration (Wilson's disease), cystinuria and lead poisoning. Complications are common and include renal damage in 5–30% of patients.[179] The incidence is highest in those with rheumatoid arthritis and cystinuria.

Clinical features

Renal involvement presents as proteinuria of varying severity; the nephrotic syndrome occurs in 16–70% of cases. The peak incidence of proteinuria occurs in the second 6 months of treatment.

Renal changes

Membranous glomerulonephritis

In approximately 90% of patients there is membranous glomerulonephritis. The subepithelial deposits are smaller than those usually observed in idiopathic membranous glomerulonephritis (see p. 191); in addition, they are often segmental.

Other renal lesions

Minimal change nephropathy is occasionally seen and in a few cases electron-dense deposits have been present in the mesangium but not on the capillary basement membranes.[179] Rarely a *proliferative glomerulonephritis* or a *necrotizing arteritis* has been reported; both may be complicated by the formation of *crescents*.[180,181]

Prognosis

When treatment is stopped the proteinuria declines and disappears within 2 years; its median duration in one series of patients was 8 months.[179] The immune deposits resolve as the proteinuria reduces and the basement membrane is gradually restored to a normal appearance. Several years may be required for complete disappearance of all structural abnormalities.

Pathogenesis

Penicillamine is a hapten and may present renal tubular and glomerular basement membrane antigens to the immune system, producing membranous glomerulonephritis and anti-GBM disease, respectively. Penicillamine may also alter polymeric proteins, enhancing the nephritogenic potential of existing rheumatoid immune complexes.[179]

CAPTOPRIL

Captopril is a drug which lowers blood pressure by inhibiting angiotensin-converting enzyme. Occasionally it is associated with membranous glomerulonephritis.

Clinical features

Proteinuria of 3 g/24 hours or more occurs in about 1% of patients treated with this drug for 8 months or longer. If patients with pre-existing renal disease or proteinuria are excluded, the incidence is about 0.5%. Approximately 20% of those with proteinuria develop the nephrotic syndrome. Deterioration in renal function has not been reported.

Renal changes

Some of the nephrotic patients when biopsied show the histological changes of *membranous glomerulonephritis*;[182] the subepithelial deposits are usually small and discrete (stage I). In one reported case a pretreatment biopsy did not show this lesion, whereas a second biopsy after 6 months of captopril therapy revealed membranous glomerulonephritis.[183] Abnormalities within the basement membrane in patients with proteinuria have been attributed to captopril but were probably present before the drug was started.

Prognosis

Discontinuation of the drug usually leads to resolution of the proteinuria; histological lesions may persist for long periods.[184]

Pathogenesis

Although it has been questioned, a causal relationship between captopril and membranous glomerulonephritis probably does exist. Captopril, or one of its metabolites, may act as a hapten and initiate antibody formation. Another possibility is that captopril interferes with the regulation of the immune system, autoantibody formation resulting from abnormalities in lymphocyte function.

Reports of captopril-associated membranous glomerulonephritis have become scarce in recent years; perhaps the risks were higher when the drug was first used and dosages of 450 mg/day or more were common.

CONTRACEPTIVE PILLS

Oral contraceptive pills may contain a combination of oestrogen and progestational compounds (combination-type oral contraceptives); a second type contains only progestogens with no oestrogen component ('minipills'). The use of combination-type oral contraceptives may give rise to hypertension, haemolytic uraemic syndrome and acute renal vein thrombosis, and perhaps to the loin pain haematuria syndrome. 'Minipill' users very rarely develop these complications.[185]

Hypertension

Women taking combination-type oral contraceptive pills may develop hypertension; withdrawal of the compound causes the blood pressure to fall and on its reintroduction the blood pressure rises again.[186] Usually the woman has been taking the contraceptive pill for several months before hypertension occurs. The incidence of hypertension is not known accurately because there have been so few prospective studies; in one study the frequency of a blood pressure over 140/90 mm Hg was about three times greater in women taking oral contraceptives than in age-adjusted controls.[187]

The hypertension induced by oral contraceptives varies in severity: usually it is mild but rarely it may be very severe (malignant hypertension).[188] In most cases the patients have been normotensive prior to starting the oral contraceptive although sometimes there is a history of transient hypertension during pregnancy. Some of the patients with malignant hypertension do not respond to withdrawal of the contraceptive pill, the renal damage being too severe to be reversed.[189]

In recent years the change to combination-type compounds containing relatively low oestrogen doses (low-dose oestrogen oral contraceptives) and to 'minipills' containing no oestrogen, has progressively lowered the risk of women on the contraceptive pill developing hypertension.

The mechanism by which combination-type oral contraceptives increase blood pressure is not known. Various components of the renin–angiotensin system are altered and there is sodium and water retention, but these changes occur to the same degree in women whose blood pressure does not rise as in those in whom it does.

Haemolytic uraemic syndrome

The haemolytic uraemic syndrome may rarely occur in women taking an oral contraceptive; this is particularly likely to happen following a change from a low-dose to a high-dose oestrogen pill.[190]

Acute renal vein thrombosis

Combination-type oral contraceptives occasionally cause renal vein thrombosis.[191] This complication is rare; its exact frequency is not known.

Loin pain haematuria syndrome

In a subset of patients with the loin pain haematuria syndrome (see p. 291) oestrogen-containing oral contraceptives seem to be either the cause of the signs and symptoms or an aggravating factor increasing their severity. Discontinuation of the contraceptive pill results in amelioration of the syndrome in these cases.[192]

RADIOCONTRAST MATERIALS

Radiocontrast materials are an important cause of acute renal failure. The older agents containing soluble iodine were more nephrotoxic than the triiodinated benzoic acid derivatives in current use. In an investigation of 129 consecutive cases of hospital-acquired renal insufficiency, radiocontrast studies were found to be the cause in 12% of the patients.[156] Acute renal failure is more likely to occur if the patient already has chronic renal failure or diabetes mellitus; a combination of the two is especially dangerous. Excessive dehydration is sometimes a contributory factor, especially in patients with multiple myeloma. Angiography seems to present more of a hazard than intravenous urography, computerized tomography or oral cholecystography.

The incidence of acute renal failure induced by radiocontrast materials is not known. Figures vary from 0.15% to 17%, according to whether the patients have normal or abnormal renal function prior to the procedure and according to what arbitrary change in serum creatinine is used to make the diagnosis.[193]

Clinical features

The onset of acute renal failure is usually 12–48 hours after the investigation; it may be non-oliguric or oliguric. The non-oliguric episodes are not always recognized and may only be diagnosed in retrospective studies.

Renal changes

Alterations compatible with *ischaemic acute tubular necrosis* are found, particularly in those who are oliguric.[194] In approximately 20% of the kidneys there is also an intense vacuolization of the proximal tubular cells (*osmotic nephrosis*);[195,196] this change may be diffuse or focal and probably has no adverse effect on renal function because it is present in the same percentage of recipients of radiocontrast material who have not developed acute renal failure.

Prognosis

Approximately 65% of the patients make a complete recovery within 2 weeks; 33% suffer permanent impairment of renal function and a few die.

Pathogenesis

The pathogenesis is not known. A direct nephrotoxic effect of the radiocontrast material on the tubular cells is the most widely held theory. Radiocontrast material is not nephrotoxic in rodents and dogs unless injected intra-arterially. The tri-iodinated agents are hyperosmolar compared with plasma. This accounts for the vacuolization of the epithelial cells in some cases; it may also cause a depression of glomerular filtration rate. The newer non-ionic contrast agents have a much lower osmolality.

IONIZING RADIATION

Radiation nephritis, leading to renal dysfunction and hypertension, may result from inadvertent irradiation of the kidneys during treatment of malignant tumours; it may also follow total body irradiation in preparation for bone marrow transplantation. It is today uncommon because of improved shielding of the kidneys during radiotherapy. Radiation nephritis is discussed on page 477.

REFERENCES

Acute tubular necrosis

1. Hackradt A. Über akute tödliche, vasomotorische Nephrosen nach Verschüttung. München: Wagner, 1917: 43.
2. Bywaters EGL, Beall D. Crush injuries with impairment of renal function. Br Med J 1941; 1: 427–432.
3. Bywaters EGL, Dible JH. The renal lesion in traumatic anuria. J Pathol Bacteriol 1942; 54: 111–120.
4. Lucké B. Lower nephron nephrosis. The renal lesions of the crush syndrome, of burns, transfusions and other conditions affecting the lower segments of the nephrons. Milit Surg 1946; 99: 371–396.
5. Oliver J, MacDowell M, Tracy A. The pathogenesis of acute renal failure associated with traumatic and toxic injury. Renal ischemia, nephrotoxic damage and the ischemuric episode. J Clin Invest 1951; 30: 1307–1439.
6. Iversen P, Brun C. Aspiration biopsy of the kidney. Am J Med 1951; 11: 324–330.
7. Collins AJ. Renal dialysis treatment for victims of the

Armenian earthquake. N Engl J Med 1989; 320: 1291–1292.
8. Dixon BS, Anderson RJ. Nonoliguric acute renal failure. Am J Kidney Dis 1985; 6: 71–80.
9. Loughridge IW, Milne MD, Shackman R, Wootton IDP. Clinical course of uncomplicated acute tubular necrosis. Lancet 1960; 1: 351–355.
10. Solez K, Morel-Maroger L, Sraer J-D. The morphology of 'acute tubular necrosis' in man: analysis of 57 renal biopsies and a comparison with the glycerol model. Medicine (Baltimore) 1979; 58: 362–376.
11. Cuppage FE, Neagoy DR, Tate A. Repair of the nephron following temporary occlusion of the renal pedicle. Lab Invest 1967; 17: 660–670.
12. Venkatachalam MA, Jones DB, Rennke HG, Sandstrom D, Patel Y. Injury and repair of proximal tubule microvilli. Evidence for membrane recycling. J Cell Biol 1977; 75: 220a.
13. Olsen S. Ultrastructure of the renal tubules in acute renal insufficiency. Acta Pathol Microbiol Scand 1967; 71: 203–218.
14. Bohle A, Jahnecke J, Meyer D, Schubert GE. Morphology of acute renal failure. Comparative data from biopsy and autopsy. Kidney Int 1976; 10: S9–16.
15. Solez K, Kramer EC, Heptinstall RH. The pathology of acute renal failure: leukocyte accumulation in the vasa recta. Am J Pathol 1974; 74: 31a.
16. Darmardy EM, Stranack F. Microdissection of the nephron in disease. Br Med Bull 1957; 13: 21–26.
17. Jones DB. Ultrastructure of human acute renal failure. Lab Invest 1982; 46: 254–264.
18. Dunnill MS, Jerrome DW. Renal tubular necrosis due to shock: light and electron-microscope observations. J Pathol 1976; 118: 109–112.
19. Anderson RJ, Schrier RW. Acute tubular necrosis. In: RW Schrier, CW Gottschalk, eds. Diseases of the kidney, 4th edn. Boston: Little, Brown, 1988; 2: 1413–1446.
20. Kennedy AC. Long-term follow-up of renal function after recovery from acute tubular necrosis. In: Andreucci, ed. Acute renal failure. Boston: Nijhoff, 1984: 481–485.
21. Solez K. Pathogenesis of acute renal failure. Int Rev Exp Pathol 1983; 24: 277–333.
22. Myers BD, Moran SM. Hemodynamically mediated acute renal failure. N Engl J Med 1986; 314: 97–105.
23. Hollenberg N, Epstein M, Rosen R, Basch RI, Oken DE, Merrill JP. Acute oliguric renal failure in man: evidence for preferential renal cortical ischemia. Medicine (Baltimore) 1968; 47: 455–474.
24. Oken DE. Hemodynamic basis for human acute renal failure (vasomotor nephropathy). Am J Med 1984; 76: 702–710.
25. Finn WF, Chevalier RL. Recovery from postischemic acute renal failure in the rat. Kidney Int 1979; 16: 113–123.
26. Moran SM, Myers BD. Pathophysiology of protracted acute renal failure in man. J Clin Invest 1985; 76: 1440–1448.
27. Fry IK, Cattell WR. The nephrographic pattern during excretion urography. Br Med Bull 1972; 28: 227–232.
28. Burke TJ, Cronin RE, Duchin KL, Peterson LN, Schrier RW. Ischemia and tubular obstruction in acute renal failure in dogs: role of mannitol in prevention. Am J Physiol 1980; 238: F305–314.
29. Donohoe JF, Venkatachalam MA, Bernard DB, Levinsky NG. Tubular leakage and obstruction after renal ischemia: structural-functional correlations. Kidney Int 1978; 13: 208–222.
30. Thurau K, Boylan JW. Acute renal success. The unexpected logic of oliguria in acute renal failure. Am J Med 1978; 61: 308–315.
31. Brezis M, Rosen S, Silva P, Epstein FH. Renal ischemia: a new perspective. Kidney Int 1984; 26: 375–383.
32. Evan AP, Gattone VH, Luft FC. Glomerular filtration barrier in ischemic and nephrotoxic acute renal failure. In: Solez K, Whelton A, eds. Acute renal failure. New York: Marcel Dekker, 1984; 119–133.
33. Sakai T, Kriz W. The structural relationship between mesangial cells and basement membrane of the renal glomerulus. Anat Embryol (Berl) 1987; 176: 373–388.
34. Ratcliffe PJ, Endre ZH, Tange JD, Ledingham JGG. Ischaemic acute renal failure: why does it occur? Nephron 1989; 52: 1–5.
35. Abuelo JG. Renal failure caused by chemicals, foods, plants, animal venoms, and misuse of drugs. An overview. Arch Intern Med 1990; 150: 505–510.
36. Chugh KS. Snake-bite-induced acute renal failure in India. Kidney Int 1989; 35: 891–907.
37. George A, Varghese TT, Solez K. Viper bite poisoning in India: a review with special reference to renal complications. Renal Fail 1987; 10: 91–99.
38. Hook JB, Smith JH. Biochemical mechanisms of nephrotoxicity. Transplant Proc 1985; 17: suppl 1, 41–50.
39. Humes HD. Aminoglycoside nephrotoxicity. Kidney Int 1988; 33: 900–911.
40. Olsen S, Burdick JF, Keown PA, Wallace AC, Racusen LC, Solez K. Primary acute renal failure ('acute tubular necrosis') in the transplanted kidney: morphology and pathogenesis. Medicine (Baltimore) 1989; 68: 173–187.

Renal disease caused by poisoning and occupational hazards

41. Pueschel SM, Kopito L, Schwachman H. Children with an increased lead burden: a screening and follow-up study. JAMA 1972; 222: 462–466.
42. Landing BH, Nakai H. Histochemical properties of renal lead inclusions and their demonstration in urinary sediment. Am J Clin Pathol 1959; 31: 499–503.
43. Goyer RA. Ascorbic acid and EDTA treatment of lead toxicity in rats. Life 1979; 24: 433–438.
44. Galle P, Morel-Maroger L. Les lésions rénales du saturnisme humain et expérimental. Nephron 1965; 2: 273–286.
45. Goyer RA. The renal tubule in lead poisoning. I. Mitochondrial swelling and aminoaciduria. Lab Invest 1968; 19: 71–77.
46. Chisolm JJ, Harrison HC, Eberlein WR, Harrison HE. Amino-aciduria, hypophosphatemia and rickets in lead poisoning: study of a case. Am J Dis Child 1955; 89: 159–168.
47. Burde B, Choate MS. Does asymptomatic lead exposure in children have any latent sequelae? Pediatrics 1972; 81: 1088–1091.
48. Emmerson BT. Chronic lead nephropathy. Kidney Int 1973; 4: 1–5.

49. Inglis JA, Henderson DA, Emmerson BT. The pathology and pathogenesis of chronic lead nephropathy occurring in Queensland. J Pathol 1978; 124: 65–76.
50. Morgan JM, Hartley MW, Miller RE. Nephropathy in chronic lead poisoning. Arch Intern Med 1966; 118: 17–29.
51. Wedeen RP, Maesaka JK, Weiner B et al. Occupational lead nephropathy. Am J Med 1975; 59: 630–641.
52. Wedeen RP, Mallik DK, Batuman V. Detection and treatment of occupational lead nephropathy. Arch Intern Med 1979; 139: 53–57.
53. Bennett MW. Lead nephropathy. Kidney Int 1985; 28: 212–220.
54. Aviv A, John E, Bernstein J, Goldsmith DI, Spitzer A. Lead intoxication during development: its effect on kidney function and blood pressure. Kidney Int 1980; 17: 430–437.
55. Wedeen RP. Blood lead levels, dietary calcium, and hypertension. Ann Intern Med 1985; 102: 403–404.
56. Beevers DG, Erskine E, Robertson M, et al. Blood lead and hypertension. Lancet 1976; 2: 1–8.
57. Wedeen RP. Heavy metals. In: Schrier RW, Gottschalk CW. eds, Diseases of the kidney, 4th edn. Boston: Little, Brown, 1988; 2: 1359–1376.
58. Scott R, Cunningham C, McLelland A, Fell GS, Fitzgerald-Finch OP, McKellar N. The importance of cadmium as a factor in calcified upper urinary tract stone disease – a prospective 7 year study. Br J Urol 1982; 54: 584–589.
59. Nomiyama K. Recent progress and perspectives in cadmium health effects studies. Sci Total Environ 1980; 14: 199–232.
60. Saito H, Shioji R, Hurukawa Y et al. Chronic cadmium poisoning induced by environmental cadmium pollution. Renal lesions (multiple proximal tubular dysfunctions) identified in residents of cadmium-polluted Hosogoe, Kosaka town, Akita prefecture, Japan. Jpn J Med 1977; 16: 2–13.
61. Kazantzis G. Renal tubular dysfunction and abnormalities of calcium metabolism in cadmium workers. Environ Health Perspect 1979; 28: 155–159.
62. Cherian MG, Goyer RA, Delaquerriere-Richardson L. Cadmium-metallothionein-induced nephropathy. Toxicol Appl Pharmacol 1976; 38: 399–408.
63. Schreiner GE, Maher JF. Toxic nephropathy. Am J Med 1965; 38: 409–449.
64. Freeman RB, Maher JF, Schreiner GF, Mostafi FK. Renal tubular necrosis due to nephrotoxicity of organic mercurial diuretics. Ann Intern Med 1962; 57: 34–43.
65. Biber TUL, Mylle M, Baines AD, Gottschalk CW, Oliver JR, MacDowell MC. A study of micropuncture and microdissection of acute renal damage in rats. Am J Med 1968; 44: 664–705.
66. Mandema E, Arends A, van Zeijst J, Vernier G, van der Henn GK, van der Slikke LB. Mercury and the kidney. Lancet 1963; 1: 1266 (letter).
67. Kibukamusoke JW, Davies DR, Hutt MSR. Membranous nephropathy due to skin-lightening cream. Br Med J 1974; 2: 646-647.
68. Gartner HV. Membranous (peri-, epi-, extramembranous) glomerulonephritis – prototype of an immune complex glomerulonephritis: a clinical morphological study. Veröff Pathol 1980; 113: 1–136.
69. Tubbs RR, Gephardt GN, McMahon JT et al. Membranous glomerulonephritis associated with industrial mercury exposure. Am J Clin Pathol 1982; 77: 409–413.
70. Druet P, Bernard A, Hirsch F et al. Immunologically mediated glomerulonephritis induced by heavy metals. Arch Toxicol 1982; 50: 187–194.
71. Sapin C, Druet E, Druet P. Induction of anti-glomerular basement membrane antibodies in the Brown-Norway rat by mercuric chloride. Clin Exp Immunol 1977; 28: 173–179.
72. Fowler BA, Weissberg JB. Arsine poisoning. N Engl J Med 1974; 291: 1171–1174.
73. Muehrcke RO, Pirani CL. Arsine-induced anuria: a correlative clinicopathological study with electron microscopic observations. Ann Intern Med 1968; 68: 835–866.
74. Gerhardt RE, Crecelius EA, Hudson JB. Moonshine-related arsenic poisoning. Arch Intern Med 1980; 140: 221–213.
75. Thun MJ, Baker DB, Smith AB. Uranium and nephrotoxicity. NIOSH health hazard evaluation report. Canon City, CO: Cotter Corp 1981: HETA 81–055–954.
76. Wedeen RP. Occupational renal disease. Am J Kidney Dis 1984; 3: 241–257.
77. Jennings RB. Fatal fulminant acute carbon tetrachloride poisoning. Arch Pathol 1955; 59: 269–284.
78. Schreiner GE, Maher JF. Toxic nephropathy. Am J Med 1965; 38: 409–449.
79. Woods WW. The changes in the kidneys in carbon tetrachloride poisoning, and their resemblance to those in the 'crush syndrome'. J Pathol Bacteriol 1946; 58: 767–773.
80. Beirne G. Glomerulonephritis associated with hydrocarbon solvents. Environ Res 1980; 23: 422–428.
81. Van der Laan G. Chronic glomerulonephritis and organic solvents. A case control study. Int Arch Occup Environ Health 1980; 47: 1–8.
82. Churchill DN, Fine A, Gault MH. Association between hydrocarbon exposure and glomerulonephritis. An appraisal of the evidence. Nephron 1983; 33: 169–172.
83. Boemke F. Beitrag zur Toxikologie und Pathologie des Athylenglykols (Glysantin). Virchows Arch [A] 1943; 310: 106.
84. Smith DE. Morphologic lesions due to acute and subacute poisoning with antifreeze (ethylene glycol). Arch Pathol 1951; 51: 423–433.
85. Friedman EA, Greenberg JB, Merrill JP, Dammin GJ. Consequences of ethylene glycol poisoning. Report of four cases and review of the literature. Am J Med 1962; 32: 891–902.
86. Saita G, Zavaglia O. La funzionalità renale nei silicotici. Med Lav 1951; 42: 41–48.
87. Kolev T, Doitschinov D, Todorov D. Morphologic alterations in the kidneys by silicosis. Med Lav 1970; 61: 205–210.
88. Slavin RE, Swedo JL, Brandes D, Gonzalez-Vitale JC, Osornio-Vargas A. Extrapulmonary silicosis: a clinical, morphologic and ultrastructural study. Hum Pathol 1985; 16: 393–412.
89. Osorio AM, Thun MJ, Novak RF, van Cura EJ, Avner ED. Silica and glomerulonephritis: case report and review of the literature. Am J Kidney Dis 1987; 9: 224–230.
90. Arnalich F, Lahoz C, Picazo ML et al. Polyarteritis nodosa and necrotizing glomerulonephritis associated

with long-standing silicosis. Nephron 1989; 51: 544–547.
91. Thun MJ, Stayner L, Brown D, Maxweiler R. Mining and deaths from chronic renal failure. Lancet 1982; 2: 606 (letter).
92. Bonnin A, Mousson C, Justrabo E, Tanter Y, Chalopin JM, Rifle G. Silicosis associated with crescentic IgA mesangial nephropathy. Nephron 1987; 47: 229–230.
93. Stoeckle JD, Hardy HL, Weber AL. Chronic beryllium disease. Long-term follow-up of sixty cases and selective review of the literature. Am J Med 1969; 46: 545–561.

Renal complications of drug and alcohol dependence

94. Schreiber SN, Liebowitz MR, Bernstein LH, Srinivasan K. Limb compression and renal impairment (crush syndrome) complicating narcotic overdose. N Engl J Med 1971; 284: 368–369.
95. Schwartzfarb L, Singh G, Marcus D. Heroin-associated rhabdomyolysis with cardiac involvement. Arch Intern Med 1977; 137: 1255–1257.
96. Pogue VA, Nurse HM. Cocaine-associated acute myoglobinuric renal failure. Am J Med 1989; 86: 183–186.
97. Roth D, Alarcón FJ, Fernandez JA, Preston RA, Bourgoignie JJ. Acute rhabdomyolysis associated with cocaine intoxication. N Engl J Med 1988; 319: 673–677.
98. Williams GA, Kent SP. Specific identification of hemoglobin and myoglobin in renal tubular casts by the fluorescent antibody technic on fixed embedded tissues. Am J Clin Pathol 1981; 75: 726–730.
99. Zager RA. Studies of mechanisms and protective maneuvers in myoglobinuric acute renal injury. Lab Invest 1989; 60: 619–629.
100. Craven DE, Rixinger AI, Goularte TA, McCabe WR. Methicillin-resistant *Staphylococcus aureus* bacteremia linked to intravenous drug abusers using a 'shooting gallery'. Am J Med 1986; 80: 770–776.
101. May DC, Helderman JH, Eigenbrodt EH, Silva FG. Chronic sclerosing glomerulopathy (heroin-associated nephropathy) in intravenous T's and blues abusers. Am J Kidney Dis 1986; 8: 404–409.
102. Zielezny MA, Cunningham EE, Venuto RC. The impact of heroin abuse on a regional end-stage disease program. Am J Public Health 1980; 70: 829–831.
103. Cunningham EE, Brentjens JR, Zielezny MA, Andres GA, Venuto RC. Heroin nephropathy. A clinicopathologic and epidemiologic study. Am J Med 1980; 68: 47–53.
104. Grishman E, Churg J, Porush JG. Glomerular morphology in nephrotic heroin addicts. Lab Invest 1976; 35: 415–424.
105. Stachura I. Renal lesions in drug addicts. Pathol Annu 1985; 20: pt 2, 83–89.
106. Chander P, Agarwal A, Soni A, Kim K, Treser G. Renal cytomembranous inclusions in idiopathic renal disease as predictive markers for the acquired immunodeficiency syndrome. Hum Pathol 1988; 19: 1060–1064.
107. D'Agati V, Cheng JI, Carbone L, Cheng JT, Appel G. The pathology of HIV-nephropathy: a detailed morphologic and comparative study. Kidney Int 1989; 35: 1358–1370.
108. Rao TKS, Nicastri AD, Friedman EA. Natural history of heroin-associated nephropathy. N Engl J Med 1974; 290: 19–23.
109. Gordon MJV, White R, Matas AJ et al. Renal transplantation in patients with a history of heroin abuse. Transplantation 1986; 42: 556–557.
110. Moody C, Kaufman R, McGuire D, Grossman M, Khan Y, Lasker N. The role of adulterants in heroin nephropathy. Am J Kidney Dis 1985; 6: A12 (abstr.).
111. Citron BP, Peters RL. Angiitis in drug abusers. N Engl J Med 1971; 284: 112.
112. Wohlman RA. Renal artery thrombosis and embolization associated with intravenous cocaine injection. South Med J 1987; 80: 928–930.
113. Menchel S, Cohen D, Gross E, Frangione B, Galo G. AA protein-related renal amyloidosis in drug addicts. Am J Pathol 1983; 112: 195–119.
114. Neugarten J, Gallo G, Buxbaum J, Katz LA, Rubenstein J, Baldwin DS. Amyloidosis in subcutaneous heroin abusers ('skin poppers' amyloidosis'). Am J Med 1986; 81: 635–640.
115. Dubrow A, Mittman N, Ghali V, Flamenbaum W. The changing spectrum of heroin-associated nephropathy. Am J Kidney Dis 1985; 5: 36–41.
116. Russ G, Clarkson AR, Woodroffe AJ, Seymour AE, Cheng IKP. Renal failure from 'glue sniffing'. Med J Aust 1981; 2: 121–122.
117. Haapanen E, Pellinen TJ, Partanen J. Acute renal failure caused by alcohol-induced rhabdomyolysis. Nephron 1984; 36: 191–193.
118. Owen CA, Mubarak SJ, Hargrens AR, Rutheford L, Garetto LP, Akeson WH. Intramuscular pressures with limb compression. Clarification of the pathogenesis of the drug-induced muscle compartment syndrome. N Engl J Med 1979; 300: 1169–1172.
119. Saltissi D, Parfrey PS, Curtis JR et al. Rhabdomyolysis and acute renal failure in chronic alcoholics with myopathy, unrelated to acute alcohol ingestion. Clin Nephrol 1984; 21: 294–300.
120. Helwig FC, Scutz CB. A liver kidney syndrome. Clinical, pathological and experimental studies. Surg Gynecol Obstet 1932; 55: 570–580.
121. Conn HO. A rational approach to the hepatorenal syndrome. Gastroenterology 1973; 65: 321–340.
122. Papper S. The hepatorenal syndrome. In: Epstein M, ed. The kidney in liver disease, 2nd edn. New York: Elsevier Biomedical, 1983; 87–106.
123. Mandal AK, Lansing M, Fahmy A. Acute tubular necrosis in hepatorenal syndrome: an electron microscopy study. Am J Kidney Dis 1982; 2: 363–374.
124. Iwatsuki S, Popovtzer MM, Corman JL et al. Recovery from 'hepatorenal syndrome' after orthotopic liver transplantation. N Engl J Med 1973; 289: 1155–1159.
125. Manigand G, Morel-Maroger L, Simon J et al. Lésions rénales glomérulaires et cirrhose du foie: note préliminaire sur les lésions histologiques du rein au cours des cirrhoses hépatiques, d'après 20 prélèvements biopsiques. Rev Eur Étud Clin Biol 1970; 15: 989–996.
126. Newell GC. Cirrhotic glomerulonephritis: incidence, morphology, clinical features, and pathogenesis. Am J Kidney Dis 1987; 9: 183–190.
127. Berger J, Yaneva H, Nabarra B. Glomerular changes in patients with cirrhosis of the liver. Adv Nephrol 1977; 7: 3–14.
128. Kawaguchi K, Koike M. Glomerular lesions associated

with liver cirrhosis: an immunohistochemical and clinicalpathologic analysis. Hum Pathol 1986; 17: 1137–1143.
129. Nochy D, Callard P, Bellon B, Bariety J, Druet P. Association of overt glomerulonephritis and liver disease: a study of 34 patients. Clin Nephrol 1976; 6: 422–427.
130. Nakamoto Y, Iida H, Kobayashi K et al. Hepatic glomerulonephritis. Characteristics of hepatic IgA glomerulonephritis as the major part. Virchows Arch [A] 1981; 392: 45–54.
131. Woodroffe AJ, Gormly AA, McKenzie PE et al. Immunologic studies in IgA nephropathy. Kidney Int 1980; 18: 366–374.
132. Praga M, Costa JR, Shandas GJ, Martinez MA, Miranda B, Rodici JL. Acute renal failure in cirrhosis associated with macroscopic hematuria of glomerular origin. Arch Intern Med 1987; 147: 173–174.
133. Gormly AA, Smith PS, Seymour AE, Clarkson AR, Woodroffe AJ. IgA glomerular deposits in experimental cirrhosis. Am J Pathol 1981; 104: 50–54.
134. Swerdlow MA, Chowdhury LN, Horn T. Patterns of IgA deposition in liver tissues in alcoholic liver disease. Am J Clin Pathol 1982; 77: 259–266.
135. Burns J, D'Ardenne AJ, Morton JA, McGee JO'D. Immune complex nephritis in alcoholic cirrhosis: detection of Mallory body antigen in complexes by means of monoclonal antibodies to Mallory bodies. J Clin Pathol 1983; 36: 751–755.
136. Klatsky AL, Friedman GD, Siegelaub AB, Gérard MJ. Alcohol consumption and blood pressure. Kaiser-Permanente multiphasic health examination data. N Engl J Med 1977; 296: 1194–1200.
137. Smals AG, Kloppensborg PW, Njo KT, Knoben JM, Ruland CM. Alcohol-induced Cushingoid syndrome. Br Med J 1976; 2: 1298.

Renal complications of therapeutic and diagnostic agents

138. Hall CL. Gold nephropathy. Nephron 1988; 50: 265–272.
139. Furst D, Levine S, Srenvasan R, Metzgar AL, Bangert R, Paulus HE. A double-blind trial of high versus conventional dosages of gold salts for rheumatoid arthritis. Arch Rheum 1977; 20: 1473–1480.
140. Francis KL, Jenis EH, Jensen GE, Calcagno PL. Gold-associated nephropathy. Arch Pathol Lab Med 1984; 108: 234–238.
141. Ainsworth SK, Swain RP, Watabe N, Brackett NC, Pilia P, Hennigar GR. Gold nephropathy. Ultrastructural, fluorescent, and energy-dispersive X-ray microanalysis study. Arch Pathol Lab Med 1981; 105: 373–378.
142. Tönroth T, Skrifvars B. Gold nephropathy prototype of membranous glomerulonephritis. Am J Pathol 1974; 75: 573–584.
143. Hall CL, Fothergill NJ, Blackwell MM, Harrison PR, MacKenzie JC, MacIver AG. The natural course of gold nephropathy: long term study of 21 patients. Br Med J 1987; 295: 746–748.
144. Helin H, Korpela M, Mustonen J, Pasternack A. Mild mesangial glomerulopathy, a frequent finding in rheumatoid arthritis patients with haematuria or proteinuria. Nephron 1986; 42: 224–230.
145. Kolb H, Toyka KV, Gleichmann E. Histocompatibility antigens and chemical reactivity in autoimmunity. Immunol Today 1987; 8: 3–6.
146. Madias NE, Harrington JT. Platinum nephrotoxicity. Am J Med 1978; 65: 307–314.
147. Tanaka H, Ishikawa E, Teshima S, Shimizu E. Histopathologic study of human cisplatin nephropathy. Toxicol Pathol 1986; 14: 247–257.
148. Safirstein R, Winston J, Goldstein M, Moel D, Dikman S, Guttenplan J. Cisplatin nephrotoxicity. Am J Kidney Dis 1986; 8: 356–367.
149. Alexander F, Martin J. Nephrotic syndrome associated with lithium therapy. Clin Nephrol 1981; 15: 267–271.
150. Blackshear JL, Napier JS, Davidman M, Stillman MT. Renal complications of nonsteroidal anti-inflammatory drugs: identification and monitoring of those at risk. Semin Arthritis Rheum 1985; 14: 163–175.
151. Fong HJ, Cohen AH. Ibuprofen-induced acute renal failure with acute tubular necrosis. Am J Nephrol 1982; 2: 28–37.
152. Wolters J, van Breda Vriesman PJ. Minimal change nephropathy and interstitial nephritis with diclofenac. Neth J Med 1985; 28: 311–314.
153. Feinfeld DA, Olesnicky L, Pirani CL, Appel GB. Nephrotic syndrome associated with use of the nonsteroidal anti-inflammatory drugs. Case report and review of the literature. Nephron 1984; 37: 174–199.
154. Munn E, Lynn KL, Bailey RR. Renal papillary necrosis following regular consumption of non-steroidal anti-inflammatory drugs. NZ Med J 1982; 95: 213–214.
155. Shah GM, Muhalwas KK, Winer RL. Renal papillary necrosis due to ibuprofen. Arthritis Rheum 1981; 24: 1208–1213.
156. Hou SH, Bashinsky DA, Wish JB, Cohen JJ, Harrington JT. Hospital-acquired renal insufficiency. A prospective study. Am J Med 1983; 74: 243–248.
157. Kaloyanides GJ, Pastoriza-Munoz E. Aminoglycoside nephrotoxicity. Kidney Int 1980; 18: 571–582.
158. Houghton DC, Campbell-Boswell MV, Bennett WM, Porter GA, Brooks RE. Myeloid bodies in the renal tubules of humans: relationship to gentamicin therapy. Clin Nephrol 1978; 10: 140–145.
159. Pusey CD, Saltissi D, Bloodworth L, Rainford DJ, Christie JL. Drug associated acute interstitial nephritis: clinical and pathological features and the response to high dose steroid therapy. Q J Med 1983; 52: 194–211.
160. Barrientos A, Bello I, Gutierrez-Millet V. Renal failure and cephalothin. Ann Intern Med 1976; 84: 612.
161. Barza M. The nephrotoxicity of cephalosporins: an overview. J Infect Dis 1978; 137: S60–S73.
162. Kleinknecht D, Ganeval D, Droz D. Acute renal failure after high doses of gentamicin and cephalothin. Lancet 1973; 1: 1129 (letter).
163. Tune BM, Fravert D. Mechanisms of cephalosporin toxicity: a comparison of cephaloridine and cephaloglycin. Kidney Int 1980; 18: 591–599.
164. Wertlake PT, Butler WT, Hill GJ, Utz JP. Nephrotoxic tubular damage and calcium deposition following amphotericin B therapy. Am J Pathol 1963; 43: 449–457.
165. McCurdy DK, Frederic M, Elkinton JR. Renal tubular acidosis due to amphotericin B. N Engl J Med 1968; 278: 124–130.
166. Neugarten J, Gallo GR, Baldwin DS. Rifampin induced

nephrotic syndrome and acute interstitial nephritis. Am J Nephrol 1983; 3: 38–42.

167. Campese VM, Marzullo F, Schena FP, Coratelli P. Acute renal failure during intermittent rifampicin therapy. Nephron 1973; 10: 256–261.
168. Schreiner GE, Maher JF. Toxic nephropathy. Am J Med 1965; 38: 409–449.
169. Kahan BD. Cyclosporine. N Engl J Med 1989; 321: 1725–1738.
170. Mihatsch MJ, Thiel G, Spichtin HP et al. Morphological findings in kidney transplants after treatment with cyclosporine. Transplant Proc 1983; 15: suppl 1, 2821–2835.
171. Goldberg HJ, Wong PY, Cole EH, Levy GA, Skorecki KL. Dissociation between the immunosuppressive activity of cyclosporine derivatives and their effects on intracellular calcium signalling in mesangial cells. Transplantation 1989; 47: 731–733.
172. Zoja C, Furci L, Ghilardi F, Zilio P, Benigni A, Remuzzi G. Cyclosporin-induced endothelial cell injury. Lab Invest 1986; 55: 455–462.
173. Lau DCW, Wong K-L, Hwang WS. Cyclosporine toxicity on cultured rat microvascular endothelial cells. Kidney Int 1989; 35: 604–613.
174. Lewis RM, Janney RP, Golden DL et al. Stability of renal allograft function associated with long-term cyclosporine immunosuppressive therapy – five year follow-up. Transplantation 1989; 47: 266–272.
175. Tegzess AM, Doorenbos BM, Minderhound JM, Donker AJ. Prospective serial renal function studies in patients with nonrenal disease treated with cyclosporine A. Transplant Proc 1988; 20: suppl 2, 390–393.
176. O'Grady JG, Forbes A, Rolles K, Calne RY, Williams R. An analysis of cyclosporine efficacy and toxicity after liver transplantation. Transplantation 1988; 45: 575–579.
177. Myers BD, Sibley R, Newton L et al. The long-term course of cyclosporine-associated chronic nephropathy. Kidney Int 1988; 33: 590–600.
178. Myers BD, Newton L, Boshkos C et al. Chronic injury of human renal microvessels with low-dose cyclosporine therapy. Transplantation 1988; 46: 694–703.
179. Hall CL, Jawad S, Harrison PR et al. Natural course of penicillamine nephropathy: a long term study of 33 patients. Br Med J 1988; 296: 1083–1086.
180. Ntoso KA, Tomaszewski JE, Jimenez SA, Neilson EG. Penicillamine-induced rapidly progressive glomerulonephritis in patients with progressive systemic sclerosis: successful treatment of two patients and a review of the literature. Am J Kidney Dis 1986; 8: 159–163.
181. Banfi G, Imbasciati E, Guerra L, Mihatsch MJ, Ponticelli C. Extracapillary glomerulonephritis with necrotizing vasculitis in D-penicillamine-treated rheumatoid arthritis. Nephron 1983; 33: 56– 60.
182. Textor SC, Gephard TGN, Bravo EL et al. Membranous glomerulopathy associated with captopril therapy. Am J Med 1983; 74: 705–712.
183. Sturgill BC, Shearlock KT. Membranous glomerulopathy and nephrotic syndrome after captopril therapy. JAMA 1983; 250: 2343–2345.
184. Hoorntje SJ, Donker AJ, Prins EJ, Weening JJ. Membranous glomerulopathy in a patient on captopril. Acta Med Scand 1980; 208: 325–329.
185. Hall WD, Douglas MB, Blumenstein BA, Hatcher RA. Blood pressure and oral progestational agents. A prospective study of 119 black women. Am J Obstet Gynecol 1980; 136: 344–348.
186. Laragh JH, Sealey JE, Ledingham JGG, Newton MA. Oral contraceptives: renin, aldosterone, and high blood pressure. JAMA 1967; 201: 918–922.
187. Fisch IR, Frank J. Oral contraceptives and blood pressure. JAMA 1977; 237: 2499–2503.
188. Hodsman GP, Robertson JIS, Semple PF, Mackay A. Malignant hypertension and oral contraception: four cases, with two due to the 30 microgram oestrogen pill. Eur Heart J 1982; 3: 255–259.
189. Zacherle BJ, Richardson JA. Irreversible renal failure secondary to hypertension induced by oral contraceptives. Ann Intern Med 1972; 77: 83–85.
190. Jackson B, Clarkson AR, Seymour AF. The haemolytic-uraemic syndrome and oral contraceptives. Aust NZ J Med 1976; 6: 580–582.
191. Slick GL, Schnetzler DE, Koloyanides GJ. Hypertension, renal vein thrombosis and renal failure occurring in a patient on an oral contraceptive agent. Clin Nephrol 1975; 3: 70–74.
192. Aber GM, Higgins PM. The natural history and management of the loin pain/haematuria syndrome. Br J Urol 1982; 54: 613–615.
193. Cronin RE. Radiocontrast media-induced acute renal failure. In: RW Schrier, CW Gottschalk, eds. Diseases of the kidney, 4th edn. Boston: Little, Brown, 1988; 2: 1301–1317.
194. Van Zee BE, Hoy WE, Talley TE, Jaenike JR. Renal injury associated with intravenous pyelography in non-diabetic and diabetic patients. Ann Intern Med 1978; 89: 51–54.
195. Moreau J-F, Droz D, Sabto J et al. Osmotic nephrosis induced by water soluble triiodinated contrast media in man. Radiology 1975; 115: 329–336.
196. Moreau J-F, Droz D, Noël L-H, Liebowitch J, Jungers P, Michel J-R. Tubular nephrotoxicity of water soluble iodinated contrast media. Invest Radiol 1980; 15: S54–S60.

14

K. A. Porter

Nephrolithiasis and nephrocalcinosis

NEPHROLITHIASIS (RENAL CALCULI)

Calculi may form at any level in the urinary tract, but most arise in the kidneys. Stones formed in the bladder are discussed on page 703; the few that arise in the ureters are described on page 686.

Renal stones are composed of masses of aggregated crystals and a small amount of matrix. The crystals, which are created from precipitated urinary solutes, constitute 95–98% of the total weight of the stone; they are arranged in and between the matrix which extends out in lamellae and radial formations from a central core of the same material.[1] The cut surface of a bisected renal stone is concentrically laminated and a skeleton of matrix can be seen after removal of the crystals.[1] The matrix is mainly mucoprotein and comprises 3–5% of the total weight of the stone.[1]

Calculi are common in the renal pelvis, calyces and collecting ducts of people in industrialized countries; in these lands nephrolithiasis is the third most common disorder of the urinary tract.[2] In underdeveloped countries nephrolithiasis is rare; this is in contrast to the very high incidence of bladder stone disease in children in Third World nations (see p. 703).[2,3] Renal stones were not always common in the countries that are now industrialized: in 1900 they were unusual. In Britain and the USA the incidence of renal calculi has become at least 10 times higher in the past 90 years.[3] This increase may be related to changes in diet (see p. 535).

It is difficult to be sure of the exact frequency of renal stones because patients may have no symptoms, and very few surveys of whole populations have been made; most of the available information is based on hospital admissions and occasional analyses of selected groups of people at autopsy. Estimates of the current annual incidence in Britain and the USA range from 6.87 to 20.8 per 10 000 of the population.[2] From these figures it has been calculated that at least 5% of women and 12% of men living to the age of 70 years experience one bout or more of renal colic caused by the passage of a stone down the ureter.[2] However, even within a particular country regional differences in the incidence of renal stones can be marked. Their high incidence in industrialized countries is thought to be still increasing.[2]

The crystals in a stone in the kidney are commonly mixed, although there is usually a preponderance of crystals from one particular solute. In Britain and much of the rest of Europe, North America, Australasia and South Africa, about 70% of renal stones are composed almost entirely of calcium oxalate in its monohydrate or dihydrate forms, or of calcium oxalate mixed with calcium phosphate in the form of hydroxyapatite. Approximately 15% of calculi consist predominantly of magnesium ammonium phosphate (struvite). Uric acid stones and cystine stones together account for about 10% of calculi.[2] Very rarely, stones are made up of almost pure xanthine, 2,8-dihydroxyadenine, silica, or some chemical foreign to the body.

Little is known about the composition of renal stones in Third World countries, but some evidence suggests that while calcium oxalate and mixed calcium oxalate and phosphate calculi occur in all these countries, uric acid stones are commoner in some parts of the Middle East, India and North Africa than they are in Europe and the USA.[4]

The formation of stones within the kidney is not a specific disease; it is a potential complication of many different disorders.

CALCIUM OXALATE AND MIXED CALCIUM OXALATE AND CALCIUM PHOSPHATE (HYDROXYAPATITE) STONES

Clinical features

Calcium oxalate and mixed calcium oxalate and calcium phosphate stones are found most commonly in men: four of every five patients are males. In both sexes the peak age of onset is between 20 and 30 years, but stones continue to be common up to the age of 50 years. They are uncommon in children.[2]

Many renal stones produce no symptoms for long periods. They generally manifest themselves clinically when they begin to pass down the ureter, producing renal colic, or when they predispose to urinary infection giving dysuria, or when they traumatize the renal pelvis causing haematuria. Anuria due to impaction of stones in both ureters is very rare. The passing of a stone, or radiographic evidence of the calculus, which is very opaque to X-rays, confirms the diagnosis.

Approximately 40% of calcium oxalate or mixed calcium oxalate and phosphate stones are passed spontaneously in the urine; about 10–15% lodge in the bladder.[4] Any stone passed by the patient must be analysed quantitatively. Methods currently available, particularly infrared spectroscopy, allow identification not only of the chemical composition of the calculus but also of its crystalline phases; the changing composition of a stone from its nidus to its surface can help in determining the factors that were involved in its formation.

Renal changes

Calcium oxalate and hydroxyapatite stones may be unilateral or bilateral, solitary or multiple; most commonly they are unilateral and solitary. They are usually either yellow-brown, or dark from altered blood, and hard. Predominantly oxalate calculi may be nodular with small blunt spikes; mixed oxalate and phosphate stones may be fairly smooth. If small, both forms of stones are sometimes triangular in section. The nodular form is sometimes called the mulberry type in Britain or the jackstone type in the USA.

Complications

The complications of calcium oxalate and hydroxyapatite renal calculi are *acute* and *chronic pyelonephritis* (see pp. 432 and 444), *hydronephrosis* (see p. 468) and *obstructive nephropathy* (see p. 467).

Complications may also arise as a result of

treatment of a renal stone by extracorporeal shock wave lithotripsy. This non-invasive method of removing renal stones has become increasingly popular and it is now the commonest technique for removing stones in industrialized countries. Hydraulic shock waves, generated outside the body, are focused on the stone, which they then pulverize.[5] Three main complications may arise. The stone fragments may *obstruct the ureter*; this occurs in 5–15% of cases but is usually not a serious problem. Secondly, about 8% of patients develop *hypertension* or experience an exacerbation of pre-existing hypertension within 1 year of treatment. Thirdly, there is a risk of renal damage. One sequel of injury to the structure of the glomerular basement membrane that has been reported is the onset of *antiglomerular-basement-membrane antibody disease* about 7 months later.[6] Presumably the globular domain NC1 of collagen IV (see p. 218) is disrupted by the shock waves and the Goodpasture antigen, which it contains, is exposed or released. Antiglomerular-basement-membrane antibody disease could then be precipitated in genetically predisposed patients.[6] Other renal lesions that have been reported include alterations in the endothelium and glomerular epithelium, and haemosiderin accumulation in tubule cells.[7]

Prognosis

The prognosis will largely depend upon the underlying condition causing the renal stones. Calcium oxalate and hydroxyapatite stones *per se* rarely lead to renal failure. If at the time of diagnosis there is renal damage due to the calculi then this may cause renal dysfunction and hypertension. The main problem is recurrence unless the causative condition can be treated; the recurrence rate is high, approaching 70% by 10 years after spontaneous passage or surgical removal of a calculus.[7]

Predisposing conditions

The urine is normally supersaturated with respect to calcium oxalate so, in principle, such stones can form in all people. The risk of calculi is increased by conditions that raise the amount of calcium or oxalate in the urine or decrease the volume of urine. Persistent hypercalciuria is present in approximately 70% of patients who form calcium oxalate and mixed calcium oxalate and phosphate renal stones; hyperoxaluria occurs in 5%. In both groups there is sometimes a decrease in the volume of urine due to a fall in the amount of water drunk. The remaining 25% of patients with stones have no known, easily recognized, major predisposing condition.

Other factors that may make nephrolithiasis more likely are lack of the normal diurnal rhythm of the hydrogen ion concentration of the urine, and deficiency of the inhibitors of crystallization that are present in normal urine. The importance of these factors is less well established and is the subject of controversy.

Hypercalciuria

A raised output of calcium in the urine occurs in idiopathic hypercalciuria, primary hyperparathyroidism, medullary sponge kidney, renal tubular acidosis, immobilization in bed for long periods, sarcoidosis, osteolytic metastatic tumours in bone, excessive intake of calcium and the milk-alkali syndrome, treatment with carbonic anhydrase inhibitors, increased protein in the diet, increased carbohydrate in the diet and exposure to beryllium or cadmium.

Patients with idiopathic hypercalciuria, renal tubular acidosis, medullary sponge kidney, increased dietary intake of protein or carbohydrate, and cadmium poisoning have normal levels of serum calcium. Patients with the other conditions in which hypercalciuria occurs have an accompanying hypercalcaemia.

Idiopathic hypercalciuria Idiopathic hypercalciuria is the commonest cause of nephrolithiasis in Europe and North America,[4] occurring in approximately 50% of all patients who form calcium oxalate or calcium oxalate and calcium phosphate stones.[8] The term is used to describe a syndrome in which excessive calcium excretion occurs in the urine but no cause can be found, and in which plasma calcium is consistently normal. Excessive calcium excretion is defined as more than 4 mg of calcium/kg/day in the urine.[8] There is often a mild hyperuricaemia.[4] Idiopathic hypercalciuria is a diagnosis of exclusion.

The syndrome occurs more often in men than women; patients with idiopathic hypercalciuria are usually 30–50 years old when the diagnosis is first made. By definition the metabolic lesion is unknown. It has been suggested that idiopathic hypercalciuria is caused by a primary increase in absorption of calcium by the gut due to either increased production of 1,25-dihydroxy-vitamin D_3 or an intrinsic abnormality of calcium transportation in the intestinal epithelial cells independent of vitamin D.[8] There may also be in some cases a defect in calcium reabsorption by the kidneys due to a fault in the transportation of calcium within the tubular cells.[4,8]

Family studies suggest that idiopathic hypercalciuria may be the expression of a complex, or polygenic, trait resulting from alleles at several loci. Attempts to link hypercalciuria to specific chromosomal gene rearrangements have not been successful.[8]

Primary hyperparathyroidism (see p. 544) This condition is present in approximately 5% of patients with calcium oxalate and phosphate renal stones. The hypercalciuria is principally the result of increased reabsorption of calcium from the intestine brought about by 1,25-dihydroxy-vitamin D_3.[9] Roughly 55% of patients with primary hyperparathyroidism have nephrolithiasis.[9] The stones often contain calcium phosphate; the formation of this salt is favoured by the slightly alkaline urine in this condition.[4]

Medullary sponge kidney (see p. 66) Hypercalciuria occurs in approximately 42% of patients with medullary sponge kidney.[10] The cause of the calcium loss is unknown; it may be due to impaired calcium reabsorption in the terminal part of the nephron.

Medullary sponge kidney is often found in patients with nephrolithiasis but the exact incidence is uncertain; figures of 2.6–21% have been reported. In one large series, medullary sponge kidney was found in 12% of 624 male patients and 19% of 175 female patients with renal stones.[10]

Renal tubular acidosis Renal tubular acidosis (RTA) is a term applied to several conditions in which metabolic acidosis is caused by specific defects in renal tubular hydrogen ion secretion.[11] There are two broad categories of RTA: type 1 (distal RTA or classic RTA) and type 2 (proximal RTA). Nephrolithiasis occurs only in type 1 RTA: this form of RTA is responsible for between 0.3 and 8.0% of calcium oxalate or calcium oxalate and calcium phosphate stones.[11] Patients with type I RTA have three abnormalities that make them particularly prone to develop renal stones: hypercalciuria, a raised urinary pH, and low levels of citrate in the urine. In addition, about 20% of those who form stones have hyperuricosuria.[11]

Type 1 renal tubular acidosis This category of RTA is caused by an inability on the part of the distal tubules to establish adequate hydrogen ion (pH) gradients between the fluid in the tubular lumen and the blood in the peritubular capillaries; the distal tubules may also be unable to secrete hydrogen ion. The majority of the patients with this defect develop calcium oxalate or mixed calcium oxalate and calcium phosphate stones and nephrolithiasis.[11] In one series 77% of patients with type 1 RTA had nephrolithiasis and 52% had nephrocalcinosis.[12] Type 1 RTA may be transmitted as an autosomal dominant inherited disease, or, slightly more commonly, it may occur spontaneously or in association with a systemic disease, such as Sjøgren's syndrome, systemic lupus erythematosus, Wilson's disease (hepatolenticular degeneration), primary biliary cirrhosis, a dysproteinaemia, lymphocytic thyroiditis, or jejunal and ileal bypass or disease.[13]

Patients with type 1 RTA are unable to excrete urine of pH less than 5.4. In addition to urolithiasis they may have muscle weakness and osteomalacia. Patients with inherited type 1 RTA commonly present with renal stones in childhood. The acquired form may present at any age.[13] The diagnosis is established by demonstrating the patient's inability to acidify the urine in the presence of systemic acidosis and in the absence of defects in renal bicarbonate and ammonia metabolism.

Type 2 renal tubular acidosis This category of

RTA is caused by a proximal tubular defect in bicarbonate reabsorption and is not associated with urolithiasis or nephrolithiasis.[13]

Immobilization in bed for long periods Immobilization, particularly in adolescence when active bone growth is present, may be complicated by hypercalciuria and occasionally by stone formation. Prolonged periods of immobilization seem to disrupt the balance between bone reabsorption and formation: osteoclastic activity predominates and calcium is mobilized.[13]

Sarcoidosis (see p. 258) In sarcoidosis there is increased sensitivity to vitamin D; when the disease is active there may be hypercalcaemia, massive hypercalciuria and nephrolithiasis.[13]

Osteolytic metastatic tumours in bone Bone metastases only rarely cause calcium oxalate and mixed calcium and phosphate stones; perhaps there is usually insufficient time for stones to form because hypercalciuria tends to be a late or terminal complication of malignant disorders.[13]

Excessive intake of calcium and the milk-alkali syndrome Excessive intake of calcium only rarely causes hypercalciuria. In the past, patients with peptic ulcers sometimes consumed huge quantities of calcium carbonate and milk: as a result they developed hypercalcaemia, alkalosis and renal impairment (milk-alkali syndrome), and occasionally nephrocalcinosis; hypercalciuria and renal stones were rare.[14]

Carbonic anhydrase inhibitors These drugs are commonly used in glaucoma. They produce various abnormalities of acid-base metabolism in the kidneys, including a type 1 RTA. As a result approximately 10% of patients treated with them will begin to form calcium oxalate and phosphate stones. Some of these patients give a past history of stone formation that has been inactive until treatment with the carbonic anhydrase inhibitor was started.[13]

Increased protein in the diet The increase in the frequency of nephrolithiasis that has occurred in the developed nations of the world closely correlates with economic wealth, increased per capita expenditure on food, and a diet relatively high in animal protein. One explanation of these associations is that the high dietary protein is an important factor contributing to nephrolithiasis.[15]

Supporting this hypothesis are the data on normal people showing that urinary calcium, oxalate and uric acid levels increase immediately following ingestion of a large amount of protein. The acidifying effects of a high protein intake also reduce the amount of citrate in the urine. All these changes would certainly be expected to increase the probability of initiation and growth of stone-forming crystals. It is also known that there is a low incidence of nephrolithiasis in vegetarians in industrialized nations, and reduction in dietary protein lowers the risk of stone formation in patients with hypercalciuria who have a history of recurrent stone formation.[15] During World Wars I and II, as animal protein consumption fell the incidence of nephrolithiasis declined; this is shown very clearly in the figures from autopsies done in one centre in Germany from 1913 to 1958.[16]

However, most patients with recurrent calcium oxalate and/or phosphate stones consume a diet that is similar in composition to that of case controls. Where those who form stones differ is that the linear relationship between dietary protein intake and the amount of calcium excreted in the urine is much stronger in them than in the controls. On the basis of this finding it has been speculated that patients who form stones are more sensitive to the hypercalciuric action of protein and excrete more calcium in their urine for any given increase in dietary protein intake than do control subjects.[15]

Not everyone believes that dietary protein is important in stone formation: some rightly argue that other variables that parallel the intake of dietary protein could be the real cause of stone formation.

Increased carbohydrate in the diet A raised dietary carbohydrate intake has a hypercalciuric effect in both normal people and patients who form renal stones. Hypersensitivity to this effect has been observed not only in stone formers but also in their close relatives.[17] Because insulin has a direct hypercalciuric action on the kidney it has been suggested that in stone formers insulin secretion in response to ingested carbohydrates may be exaggerated.

Exposure to beryllium or cadmium Exposure to beryllium (see p. 508) and cadmium (see p. 504) are the only well recognized industrial hazards associated with hypercalciuria and an increased incidence of nephrolithiasis. Calculi occur in up to 40% of those who are exposed in their work to cadmium (see p. 504).[18] In beryllium workers the incidence is much lower: in one series of 60 patients renal stones occurred in four (7%).[19]

Hyperoxaluria

Hyperoxaluria may be primary, due to overproduction in hereditary disorders of metabolism (primary oxaluria), or secondary, due to intestinal disease (enteric hyperoxaluria) or excessive ingestion of oxalate in the diet. Drinking ethylene glycol also leads to hyperoxaluria because this substance is converted to glycoaldehyde and to glycolate in the liver (see p. 507).[13] The anaesthetic methoxyflurane can also be converted to oxalate and occasional cases of hyperoxaluria and oxalate stones have followed the use of this agent.[20]

Of the approximately 5% of patients with oxalate stones who have hyperoxaluria, this is secondary in about 4% and primary in 1% or less.[13]

Primary hyperoxaluria (see p. 103) This term refers to two autosomal recessive, genetically distinct, inherited enzyme deficiencies (see p. 103). In type I, the commoner form, there is a deficiency of peroxisomal alanine-glyoxylate aminotransferase in the cells of the liver, which leads to increased excretion of oxalic and glycolic acids in the urine. In type II, there is a deficiency of D-glyceric dehydrogenase, which is associated with increased excretion of oxalic and L-glyceric acids.[20] Both are associated with the early onset of recurrent calcium oxalate stones and eventually nephrocalcinosis.

Although renal calculi occur in the majority of patients with primary hyperoxaluria, because this inherited disorder is rare, it is present in less than 1% of patients who form stones. Of all the various conditions that may cause nephrolithiasis, this has the worst prognosis.[13]

Intestinal disease Intestinal disease accounts for only a small number of renal calculi.[4] In a number of conditions, including small bowel resection, small bowel diverticula with bacterial overgrowth, small bowel disease with malabsorption, chronic pancreatitis and cirrhosis, there may be increased absorption of dietary oxalate and a raised incidence of oxalate stones. This happens because bile acids are not being reabsorbed; when they enter the colon they increase the permeability of its wall to oxalate.[20] Also, when steatorrhoea is present, the fatty acids make complexes with the calcium in the colon contents; this decreases the amount of calcium available for binding to oxalate and more oxalate is left free to be absorbed.[13,20]

Excessive ingestion of oxalate Cocoa, tea, rhubarb, spinach, strawberries, cranberries, grapes, chocolate, parsley, pepper, peanuts, beetroot and turnip leaves, and the juice of citrus fruits, contain particularly large amounts of oxalate. Dietary excess of these foods may, in a few people, lead to hyperoxaluria and increase their liability to stone formation. It has been suggested that they develop hyperoxaluria because they absorb a higher fraction of their dietary intake of oxalate than most people.[15,20]

Decrease in the volume of urine

Previously normal people from temperate climates who reside for long periods in tropical countries have a higher incidence of renal stones than do their counterparts who stay at home.[21] In patients being treated for recurrent calcium oxalate and phosphate stones, a urinary volume of less than 1400 ml/day carries an increased risk of recurrence of stone formation. From these observations it is inferred that a fluid intake inadequate to maintain normal hydration and a relatively dilute urine predisposes to crystal formation.

Aetiology

The cause of calcium oxalate and mixed calcium oxalate and phosphate stones is unknown in 75% of patients, because in addition to the 25% who have no known predisposing factors, there are the 50% with idiopathic hypercalciuria.

In the 25% of patients in whom the cause is reasonably clear, the detailed mechanisms involved are often uncertain. The best understood are the 5% of patients who have primary hyperparathyroidism, the 5% with hyperoxaluria, the 3% with renal tubular acidosis, and the roughly 2% with other causes of hypercalcaemia. The defect in the 10% of patients with medullary sponge kidneys is ill-defined and our understanding of what is happening is incomplete.

Pathogenesis

How calcium oxalate and mixed calcium oxalate and calcium phosphate stones are formed is still unclear. For stones to be made in the urine in the kidney crystal formation must be initiated and then the crystals must be retained, aggregate and grow.[2,13]

Crystal initiation

The initiation of crystal formation (*nucleation*) requires the urine to be supersaturated with stone-forming salts. This requirement is always satisfied because urine is normally supersaturated with these salts but is in such a physicochemical state that they do not crystallize spontaneously.[2,13]

If the degree of supersaturation is greatly increased then the physicochemical state is altered, the ions in solution can combine with one another into a solid phase, and spontaneous crystal formation (*homogeneous nucleation*) is likely to occur. This happens in those patients who develop hyperoxaluria and hypercalciuria. Causes of such oversecretion of stone-forming salts are discussed on pages 533 and 536.[2,13]

Nucleation is also more likely to occur if the ions can orient themselves on the surface of an existing different crystal, such as uric acid or calcium phosphate (*heterogeneous nucleation*). Patients who form calcium oxalate or mixed oxalate and phosphate stones often have hyperuricosuria; if at any time the hydrogen ion concentration of their urine becomes depressed crystals of uric acid appear which can act as heterogeneous nuclei and initiate calcium oxalate or calcium phosphate crystallization. Other heterogeneous nucleators may be urinary mucoproteins, including Tamm–Horsfall protein, and the surface of abnormal urothelial cells. All these nucleators are sometimes referred to as *promoters of crystal formation*.[2,13] However, the proteins and urothelial cells probably do not play any major role in the initiation of crystals composed of calcium oxalate or calcium phosphate.

In most patients who form stones the degree of supersaturation of the urine with calcium phosphate and oxalate is only marginally greater than in normal individuals. Nevertheless, in the presence of even slight hypercalciuria, precipitation of calcium phosphate is easily initiated by variations in the hydrogen ion concentration in the urine and precipitation of calcium oxalate by variations in the oxalate concentration. The two processes may alternate or coexist.[13] Whichever salt precipitates first, its crystallization will tend to cause precipitation of the other by heterogeneous nucleation.

There are postprandial and diurnal variations in the urinary excretion of calcium and oxalate; longer term cyclic and seasonal variations also occur.[4] The excretion of calcium, oxalate and octocalcium phosphate is increased in the summer months, with low values in the winter. These variations are often quite small in absolute terms, but they exert a marked effect on the degree of supersaturation of stone-forming salts in the urine.[4] These changes are thought to reflect increased vitamin D synthesis in the skin during summer, which promotes increased absorption of calcium from the gut leaving more oxalate available for absorption and excretion. This hypothesis is compatible with the 50% higher rate of stone formation by recurrent stone formers in the summer compared with the winter.[4] The diurnal variations in the degree of urine saturation with stone-forming salts, due to changes in the rate of flow of urine and its hydrogen ion concentration, increase the liability to crystallization at certain times of the day. These relatively minor seasonal and diurnal changes may allow the formation of microcrystals of calcium oxalate and calcium phosphate.

It is thought that microcrystals are most often first formed in the collecting ducts in the papillae, where the urine is concentrated: it is in this part of the nephron that concretions may be observed on histological examination.

Crystal retention

When first formed, crystals are minute and they are liable to be swept away with the urine that flows continuously down the collecting ducts and through the renal pelvis into the ureter.[2] The rate of crystal growth, even in the most supersaturated urine, is not fast enough to account for crystal retention. Attempts to explain this phenomenon usually involve some form of crystal fixation allowing subsequent growth and aggregation.[2] One suggestion is that Tamm–Horsfall protein, aggregated and precipitated as the urine becomes concentrated during its passage along the renal tubule, enmeshes any microcrystal and delays its expulsion from the terminal collecting ducts, giving it an opportunity to grow.[4,5] Another possibility is that the microcrystal adheres to the luminal surface of the uroepithelium; it is envisaged that this happens because the surface is in some way abnormal; it is known that microcrystals will not adhere to normal uroepithelium.[5] The original notion that stone formation begins intracellularly and leads first to localized areas of nephrocalcinosis in the renal papillae (Randall's plaques) is no longer widely favoured, although it still has some proponents.[22]

Crystal aggregation and growth

Once a microcrystal of any of the stone-forming salts has formed it will tend to cause precipitation of other salts by either heterogeneous nucleation or epitaxy, a phenomenon which involves the growth of one crystal on another when the dimensions of the atomic network in one or more commonly occurring faces of each type of crystal are similar.[5] As was mentioned earlier, calcium and oxalate ions can orient themselves on the surfaces of, for example, uric acid, to form a calcium oxalate stone.

Opposing the build-up of a single microcrystal into a renal stone are various *inhibitors of crystal formation*. These substances are found in normal urine and act at extremely low concentrations; they block crystal aggregation and growth probably by being adsorbed to the crystal surface.[2] The main naturally occurring inhibitors of calcium oxalate growth are citrate, pyrophosphate, glycosaminoglycan, fragments of RNA[2] and an acidic glycoprotein called nephrocalcin.[23] The principle inhibitors of calcium phosphate growth are magnesium, citrate, pyrophosphate and nephrocalcin.[2]

The propensity to stone formation in a particular urine depends, therefore, on a balance between the degree of saturation with stone-forming salts and the protective effect of these physiological inhibitors of crystallization.[4] Measurement of the degree of saturation and the inhibitory potency of a urine specimen and their expression as a saturation-inhibitor index, using a discriminant function analysis, show differences between patients with hyperparathyroidism who form stones and those who do not.[4,13]

The relative importance of the various inhibitors has yet to be determined. There is some evidence that nephrocalcin in patients who develop recurrent stones is abnormal in that it lacks gamma-carboxyglutamic acid and has altered surface properties.[23] Some forms of treatment increase the quantity of these inhibitors of crystal growth; this may help in the prevention of recurrent stone formation.[2] It is interesting that normal women excrete more citrate and less calcium than normal men; perhaps that is why calcium oxalate stones are more frequent in men.

MAGNESIUM AMMONIUM PHOSPHATE STONES

Magnesium ammonium phosphate calculi are composed of struvite ($MgNH_4[PO_4]\cdot 6H_2O$) and carbonate apatite ($Ca_{10}[PO_4]\cdot CO_3$). They are sometimes referred to as 'triple-phosphate', 'urease', 'struvite' or 'infection' stones.[24] They account for approximately 15% of renal calculi and are the result of alkalinization of the urine by recurrent urinary tract infections with urease-producing microorganisms.[24]

Clinical features

Magnesium ammonium phosphate stones are twice as common in females as in males, presumably because of the greatly increased susceptibility of females to urinary infection.[24] They particularly occur in patients who are unduly liable to develop chronic urinary infection. For example, they affect 8% of patients with a spinal cord injury and are more common in patients with complete and upper motor neurone lesions;[24] struvite stones also occur in 5–30% of patients with urinary diversion to ileal loops.

The patient may present with bacteriuria, or the signs and symptoms of cystitis or acute pyelonephritis. The organism in the urine is almost always a urease-producing bacterium; in about 70% of cases it is of the *Proteus* species. Less commonly it is a member of one of the more than 45 other species that are capable of producing urease; these include *Klebsiella, Pseudomonas, Providencia* and *Staphylococcus*. Occasionally a urease-producing mycoplasma, *Ureaplasma urealyticum*, is isolated.[25] Culture of the stone material is essential to identify the responsible pathogen and to determine appropriate antimicrobial treatment; urine cultures only identify 13% of the causative organisms.[25]

There may also be recurring manifestations of obstruction. Progressive loss of renal function occurs in many patients if the calculus is not removed. Ureteral colic is not common because struvite stones tend to stay in the renal pelvis. The stones may be initially radiolucent but ultimately they become radiopaque as their content of calcium phosphate rises.

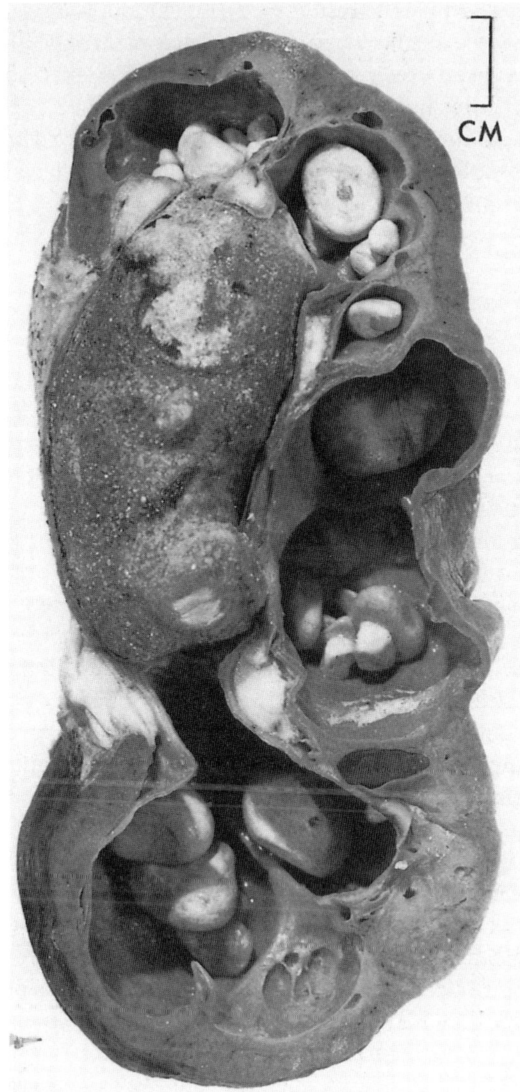

Fig. 14.1 Nephrolithiasis. There is a large magnesium ammonium phosphate stone in the renal pelvis (left of centre, and above); numerous smaller stones are seen in the dilated calyces.

Renal changes

Struvite stones are off-white or grey, and irregular in shape; they may be massive and branched, filling the entire pelvis and calyces, forming what is often known as a *stag-horn calculus* (Fig. 14.1). They vary in consistency; some are hard, but others are soft and crumble easily into fragments which may lodge in the ureter. The matrix is often soft and gelatinous and contains desquamated epithelial cells, leucocytes, red cells and bacteria.

Complications

Abscesses are common in the kidney; they also occasionally occur in the perinephric space as the result of erosion of a stone through the pelvic wall. *Hydronephrosis* and *pyonephrosis* are frequent and may ultimately result in a non-functioning kidney, especially when there is also obstruction of the distal ureter by stone fragments. Patients with infection-induced struvite stones may have coexistent metabolic stones and vesicoureteric reflux. Complications following treatment by shock wave lithotripsy are discussed on page 533.

Prognosis

Patients with untreated struvite renal calculi often follow a relentless downhill course. Failure to remove a unilateral stone results in death of 60% of the patients within 15 years; if bilateral branched stones are left in the kidneys 50% of the patients die within 5 years.[26] Cure can only be achieved by removal of all the calculi, eradication of the infection and correction of any renal anatomical abnormalities. Urease-producing bacteria are present in the interstices of the calculi and if stone fragments are left behind the condition recurs. To avoid this, large struvite calculi are usually removed by percutaneous lithotripsy followed by extracorporeal shock-wave lithotripsy to shatter any remaining stone fragments, followed by re-examination by the percutaneous method to verify that the kidney is free of stones. After successful elimination of all stone material, the mortality at 10 years is approximately 7%. However, because the removal of calculi is often incomplete and correction of any underlying abnormality is often not possible, infection persists in about 40% of patients and 27% have recurrent stones within 6 years.[24]

Urease inhibitors, such as acetohydroxamic acid, are effective in preventing stone growth. They are sometimes employed to potentiate antimicrobial treatment; but toxicity limits their usefulness.[21] Acidification of the urine with salts, such as ammonium sulphate, interferes with stone formation, but at present there is only one report on the prolonged use of this chemical in patients.[27]

Pathogenesis

Struvite calculi are the result of the action of the enzyme urease produced by the bacteria infecting the urinary tract. Urease splits the urea in the urine, producing ammonium and hydroxyl ions which make the urine alkaline; the hydrogen ion concentration (pH) commonly rises to 8.0–9.0. The change in pH increases the free ion activity of phosphate and carbonate, inducing a supersaturated state in the urine for several solutes, sufficient for crystallization of struvite, carbonate apatite and hydroxyapatite. The stone that results is usually a mixture of the crystals of these substances.[28] Approximately 50% of infection-induced stones form primarily in this way; the others develop upon pre-existing stones of other types.

The glycocalyx secreted by the urease-producing bacteria that are adhering to the uroepithelium binds the microcrystals of struvite and apatite as they are formed. This ensures retention of the crystals and permits them to aggregate and grow.[29] As the stone forms it is initially soft and radiolucent (*matrix stone*), but as the matrix of bacterial glycocalyx and trapped urinary mucoproteins is progressively replaced by struvite and carbonate apatite crystals, the stone hardens and becomes radiopaque.[30]

URIC ACID STONES

Uric acid stones occur most commonly in men: nine of every 10 patients are male. Both sexes are usually 40 years or more old when the stones are first detected. A family history of urolithiasis or gout or both is frequent but most cases are idiopathic and no underlying cause can be found. Uric acid stones account for approximately 7% of renal calculi.[2,13]

Clinical features

Uric acid stones may be clinically silent or present with renal colic, haematuria or a history of recurrent urinary infections. Small stones are sometimes passed with little or no discomfort. Very rarely patients with bilateral stones impacted in the ureters present with acute renal failure. In the cases where no predisposing cause can be found the serum uric acid and the urinary excretion of uric acid are often, but not always, normal. The pH of the urine is persistently low.[13] Analysis of any stone that is passed in the urine should be by an enzymic differential spectrophotometric method using uricase in order to distinguish uric acid from 2,8-dihydroxyadenine (see p. 543).[4]

Renal changes

Uric acid stones are yellowish-brown, hard and smooth. They are usually multiple and seldom exceed 2 cm in their largest dimension. When composed solely of uric acid they are radiolucent, but commonly they are faintly radiopaque because of impurities.

Complications

The complications of uric acid stones are *acute* and *chronic pyelonephritis* (see pp. 432 and 444), *hydronephrosis* (see p. 468) and *obstructive nephropathy* (see p. 467). Other complications may occur following treatment by shock-wave lithotripsy; these are discussed on page 533.

Predisposing conditions

Persistently low urinary hydrogen ion concentration (pH)

The most common disorder associated with uric acid nephrolithiasis is a persistently low urinary pH. The serum uric acid and the amount of uric acid excreted in the urine are normal, and there is no recognizable disorder of purine metabolism. What causes the low pH of the urine is not known. Patients with this disorder who develop stones are often included in a group said to have idiopathic uric acid nephrolithiasis.[13]

Gout

Approximately 25% of patients with uric acid stones have gout (see p. 339). Gouty patients who are treated with uricosuric agents, without ensuring that their fluid intake is increased and their urine made alkaline by citrate administration, are particularly likely to form stones soon after treatment starts.[13]

Myeloproliferative disorders

When these disorders are associated with increased purine metabolism, uric acid production may be raised producing excessive hyperuricosuria and the formation of uric acid stones. The chances of stone formation are greatly increased during treatment with chemotherapy and radiotherapy. The use of xanthine oxidase inhibitors in myeloproliferative disorders has reduced the frequency of complicating stones.[13]

Bowel disease

Uric acid stones may occur in patients with ileostomy and in those who have severe diarrhoea. In both these situations there is excessive loss of water and bicarbonate. The urine volume falls and the urinary pH is often about 5.0; the endogenously produced uric acid load is then too great for this urine volume and pH, and crystallization occurs. As these patients may be unable to absorb adequate fluid and base to rectify the situation, treatment with allopurinol is often needed.[13]

Obstructive uropathy

Elderly men with benign hyperplasia of the prostate often have difficulty and discomfort in urinating; sometimes they try to minimize the problem by severely reducing their fluid intake. The urine volume may decrease to less than 700 ml/day and the pH to less than 5.5. Uric acid crystallizes, producing small stones, and some of these are passed in the urine: this is sometimes termed 'bladder gravel'.[13]

Specific enzyme defects

Three rare specific enzyme defects make a patient liable to develop uric acid stones.

Deficiency of hypoxanthine-guanine phosphoribosyl-transferase (HGPRTase) Deficiency of the purine reutilization enzyme HGPRTase leads to an inability to salvage purine bases and a greatly increased degradation of these substances to uric acid.[13,31] The condition is present from birth (see p. 106); it is X-linked and the enzyme deficiency varies in degree, hemizygotes being greater overproducers of uric acid than heterozygotes. In its most severe form it is associated with the Lesch–Nyman syndrome (see p. 106). Uric acid calculi are frequent in these patients; they develop particularly at times when the urine is concentrated and acid. In the severe forms of this condition uric acid stones may block both ureters and cause renal failure.[13]

Hyperactivity of 5-phosphoribosyl pyrophosphate (5-PRPP) Hyperactivity of 5-PRPP leads to increased purine synthesis and overproduction of uric acid (see p. 340). Renal stone formation is not so common in this condition as it is in HGPRTase deficiency.[13]

Glucose-6-phosphate deficiency In von Gierke's glycogen storage disease hyperuricaemia is common and many patients develop gout in adolescence (see p. 103). This is associated with a liability to form uric acid stones in the kidneys.[13]

Prognosis

The prognosis is good because by utilizing the factors that affect supersaturation, most uric acid stones can be dissolved in 3 months or less. The important steps necessary to bring about this result are to increase the fluid intake, which lowers the concentration of uric acid in the urine; to make the urine alkaline with citrate, which greatly increases the solubility of uric acid; and to give the patient allopurinol, which reduces the absolute concentration of uric acid in the urine. Unless the patient has gout or a myeloproliferative disorder, the administration of allopurinol can be stopped once the stones have dissolved.[13]

Pathogenesis

When the pH is below 5.5, the urine volume must be nearly 2 litres to dissolve 600 mg of uric acid, the amount excreted in a day by a normal man. In patients who form uric acid stones the urinary pH is low and there may be hyperuricosuria; under these circumstances uric acid readily crystallizes. Sometimes these changes are secondary to one of the predisposing causes mentioned earlier (see p. 541) or they may be idiopathic with no obvious explanation. Hyperuricosuria on its own rarely causes stones unless it is massive; modest hyperuricosuria only produces stones when there is a concomitant reduction in the pH of the urine. In some patients who eat large quantities of meat there is lowering of the urinary pH and modest hyperuricosuria, sufficient to cause stone formation.[13]

CYSTINE STONES

Cystine stones account for approximately 3% of renal calculi.[2,13] Although an excess of cystine may be present in the urine in a number of conditions (e.g. cystinosis and hepatolenticular disease), cystine stones form only in cases of primary cystinuria. Primary cystinuria is an inherited impairment in the reabsorption of cystine, lysine, arginine and ornithine from the glomerular filtrate by the cells of the proximal segment of the tubules; there is a similar functional defect in the mucous membrane of the small intestine. The urine contains large amounts of the four basic amino acids and the massive amino aciduria continues with little or no change throughout life. Cystinuria is transmitted as an autosomal recessive characteristic. The homozygous abnormality is present in about one in 20 000 people. Stone formation occurs in about 65% of homozygotes and, rarely, in some heterozygotes. The only recognizable clinical disorder or pathological change in cystinuria is cystine urolithiasis (see p. 96).[13]

Clinical features

The tendency to form stones is typically manifested in children from the age of 10 years, but it can occur at any age; calculi are almost invariably present by the age of 30 years. In children cystine excretion may be lower than 400 mg/24 hours but it usually increases to more than this amount as they reach puberty. Individual adult homozygotes vary in the amount of cystine that they excrete; some produce as much as 1000 mg/day in their urine. Stone formation occurs particularly in those patients whose output is in the higher range. The patient may present with bacteriuria, or the signs and symptoms of cystitis or acute pyelonephritis. The microscopic demonstration of hexagonal flat cystine crystals in the urine, or identification of a stone as cystine by analysis, confirms the diagnosis. Radiographically, cystine stones are moderately radiopaque because of their high sulphur content, and very homogeneous.[13]

Renal changes

Cystine stones are yellowish and waxy; they become darker after removal from the kidney. They are multiple, smooth, rounded and usually small; occasionally they may fill the entire pelvis and calyces and become stag-horn shaped.

Complications

Hydronephrosis (see p. 468), *acute* and *chronic pyelonephritis* (see pp. 432, 444) and *obstructive nephropathy* (see p. 467) may occur. If shock-wave lithotripsy is used to dissipate the stones complications may occur related to this procedure (see p. 533).

Prognosis

Stone formation in many patients can be controlled by increasing the fluid intake to maintain the volume of urine excreted in 24 hours at or above 3 litres. Increasing the urinary pH to 7.5 will dissolve many of the stones but will cause secondary calcium phosphate crystallization. Reducing the patient's methionine intake requires a diet unacceptably restricted in protein. Penicillamine lowers the urinary excretion of cystine but has side-effects, including membranous glomerulonephritis (see p. 523); it is usually reserved for patients excreting more than 1000 mg of cystine per 24 hours in their urine. The stones are often resistant to shock-wave lithotripsy, but percutaneous ultrasound is extremely effective in removing them and is very safe. The prognosis is therefore very good if the stone formation is recognized before irreversible renal damage has occurred.[13]

Pathogenesis

Cystine is relatively insoluble and crystallizes readily in acid urine. Normal urine can hold in solution about 300 mg of cystine per litre; the cystine precipitates if its concentration in the urine exceeds this level. This may occur at night, for instance, when the urine is at its greatest concentration; similarly, the character of a person's diurnal rhythm of urine flow may play a part in making one homozygote more liable than another to form stones.[13]

OTHER STONES

Very rarely, renal stones are composed of almost pure xanthine, 2,8-dihydroxyadenine, silica or some chemical foreign to the body.

Xanthine stones

Xanthine stones are extremely rare. They are caused by an autosomal recessive hereditary deficiency of xanthine oxidase which normally degrades hypoxanthine and xanthine to uric acid.[13] Patients with the deficiency have low concentrations of plasma and urine urate and uric acid, and excrete excessive amounts of xanthine and hypoxanthine. Xanthine is less soluble in acid urine then uric acid and readily crystallizes. Patients are prone to recurrent xanthine stone formation in the urine and deposits of xanthine in the soft tissues.

The administration of xanthine oxidase inhibitors, such as allopurinol, only very rarely leads to xanthine stones; this is because the drugs decrease the overall production of oxypurines and only patients who have disorders associated with massive overproduction of uric acid are liable to develop xanthine stones.[32]

Pure xanthine stones are radiolucent but impurities often result in some degree of opaqueness to X-rays.

2,8-Dihydroxyadenine stones (2,8-DHA)

2,8-DHA stones are very rare. They occur in patients with an autosomal recessive hereditary deficiency in the enzyme adenine phosphoribosyltransferase which is responsible for the reutilization of adenine. In the absence of the enzyme, adenine is oxidized to 2,8-DHA which is relatively insoluble in urine and readily crystallizes to form radiolucent stones which are usually diagnosed in childhood. Identification of a stone passed in the urine as 2,8-DHA requires infrared spectroscopy. The disease can be effectively treated with allopurinol, which prevents the formation of 2,8-DHA.[13]

Silica

Silica stones are seldom reported. They occur in patients who ingest, over a period of many years, large quantities of magnesium trisilicate for indigestion. Macroscopically, the calculi resemble calcium oxalate stones; they are only recognized as silica stones if they are analyzed by infrared spectroscopy or X-ray energy spectroscopy.[33]

Foreign chemicals and compounds

Any foreign chemical or its metabolites that are removed from the body via the urinary tract may occasionally become involved in urinary calculi, but this is usually a passive process in pre-existing stones and of no clinical significance. Rarely, the process is an active one and the chemical initiates stone formation; this has occurred, for example, with sulphadiazine. Modern sulphonamides, correctly prescribed to adequately hydrated patients, are unlikely to crystallize out in renal tubules.

NEPHROCALCINOSIS

Calcium salts may be deposited in the kidneys in the course of many renal diseases. The term nephrocalcinosis is usually reserved, rather arbitrarily, for substantial calcification developing in the course of certain systemic diseases and states, particularly those accompanied by hypercalcaemia. Small scanty deposits of calcium are found in approximately 20% of kidneys examined routinely at autopsy;[34] they are also common in renal biopsies, particularly from children. Renal calcification of local origin, for example, in cases of renal infarction, cortical necrosis, tuberculosis and papillary necrosis, is not generally referred to as nephrocalcinosis; some authors, however, do include in this term the calcification that occurs in renal cortical necrosis with recovery.[4]

CAUSES OF NEPHROCALCINOSIS

Conditions accompanied by hypercalcaemia

Hypercalcaemia is an elevation of total serum calcium levels above 2.62 mmol/l (10.5 mg/dl) when serum protein values are normal. It is caused by increased calcium mobilization from bone, or an increase in calcium absorption from the gastrointestinal tract. There are also a few miscellaneous causes.

Increased calcium mobilization from bone

Calcium is mobilized from bone and may cause nephrocalcinosis in cases of cancer, hyperparathyroidism, prolonged immobilization and vitamin D intoxication.

Malignant disease Cancer is the commonest cause of hypercalcaemia. Usually this results from the osteolytic effects of metastatic deposits in bone; sometimes there is myelomatosis or lymphoma. In myelomatosis mild to moderate nephrocalcinosis has been reported in about 40% of cases at autopsy.[35] Occasionally hypercalcaemia occurs in some types of cancer without bony metastases: carcinoma of the bronchus and renal adenocarcinoma are the tumours usually involved. When nephrocalcinosis occurs in patients with cancer it is generally not extensive.[13]

Primary hyperparathyroidism Primary hyperparathyroidism is the cause of about 30% of cases of hypercalcaemia; it is commoner in women. It is frequently associated with nephrocalcinosis and renal calculi. Nephrocalcinosis was once found in 50–70% of patients with primary hyperparathyroidism, but with earlier diagnosis it is now detected in about 25%. Primary hyperparathyroidism is due to a single adenoma in a parathyroid gland in approximately 80% of cases. Double adenomas occur in 2–3% of patients and carcinomas in another 2–3%. In about 15% there is diffuse hyperplasia of all the parathyroid glands. The treatment of this condition is parathyroidectomy.[13]

Secondary hyperparathyroidism Most forms

of chronic renal disease can produce parathyroid hyperplasia mainly because of hypocalcaemia which stimulates the secretion of parathormone. Hypocalcaemia arises in chronic renal disease as a result of decreased reabsorption of calcium by the tubules. Secondary hyperparathyroidism may be complicated by nephrocalcinosis which can be very severe and detectable by radiography during life.[36]

Secondary hyperparathyroidism persists after successful renal transplantation in about 11% of patients; it may last for years and the hypercalcaemia may lead to nephrocalcinosis in the graft. The nephrocalcinosis is rarely severe.

Prolonged immobilization Hypercalcaemia is common in patients with multiple fractures who are immobilized. Nephrocalcinosis is infrequent and rarely severe.[13]

Vitamin D intoxication Vitamin D and its metabolites increase intestinal calcium absorption and bone reabsorption. When the vitamin is given in excess these effects lead to hypercalcaemia. Some patients develop nephrocalcinosis which may be marked.[13]

Increased calcium absorption from the gastrointestinal tract

Sarcoidosis (see p. 258) Approximately 20% of patients with sarcoidosis have mild hypercalcaemia secondary to an increase in calcium absorption. Of those with hypercalcaemia approximately 40% develop nephrocalcinosis.[37]

Vitamin D intoxication (see above) Vitamin D and its metabolites increase intestinal calcium absorption in addition to having a direct effect on bone reabsorption.

Milk-alkali syndrome (see p. 535) Patients with this syndrome may develop severe hypercalcaemia and extensive nephrocalcinosis.

Miscellaneous causes of hypercalcaemia

Berylliosis (see p. 508) Hypercalcaemia may follow occupational exposure to beryllium. This sometimes causes nephrocalcinosis. The altered calcium metabolism in chronic berylliosis is probably related to increased sensitivity to vitamin D associated with reduced circulating parathyroid hormone levels.

Other conditions

Renal tubular acidosis

Nephrocalcinosis is commonly found in type I renal tubular acidosis (see p. 534).

Primary hyperoxaluria

In primary hyperoxaluria (see p. 536) there is nephrocalcinosis in addition to recurrent formation of calcium oxalate stones.

Renal failure

Nephrocalcinosis is common in end-stage renal failure. It is often accompanied by deposition of oxalate crystals because oxalate is only excreted in the urine and when the kidneys fail plasma oxalate levels rise and crystals are deposited, particularly in the kidneys and heart (see page 34). The severity of the oxalosis is related to the duration of the renal failure.[38]

CLINICAL FEATURES

The clinical features of nephrocalcinosis vary with the underlying cause. In patients with hypercalcaemia there is often nausea, vomiting, polyuria, polydipsia, muscle weakness and lethargy. There may be evidence of renal failure. Hypertension is present in 20–30% of patients. Acute pain and haematuria may occur if stones are also present, as is often the case. In many patients the condition is silent. Sometimes the deposits of calcium salts in the kidneys are sufficiently large and extensive to be detectable on X-ray examination. The characteristic abnormality of hypercalcaemic nephropathy is an inability to concentrate the urine. The level of parathyroid hormone is elevated in hyperparathyroidism.

RENAL CHANGES

Gross appearance of the kidneys

The kidneys are usually normal in size, although the subcapsular surface may be scarred. When they are sliced, the knife grates on the calcific deposits, which can often be seen as whitish granules on the cut surface, particularly in the outer parts of the medulla.

Microscopic appearances

The calcium salts are deposited on the basement membranes of the tubules, in the cytoplasm of the tubular epithelial cells, in the lumens of the tubules, in the interstitium and in Bowman's capsule (Fig. 14.2). Sometimes the walls of arterioles and arteries are patchily calcified. The calcium stains deep purplish-blue with haematoxylin and usually dark brown with von Kossa's reagent; calcium oxalate deposits may not be stained by von Kossa's agent unless calcium carbonate or calcium phosphate is also present.[39]

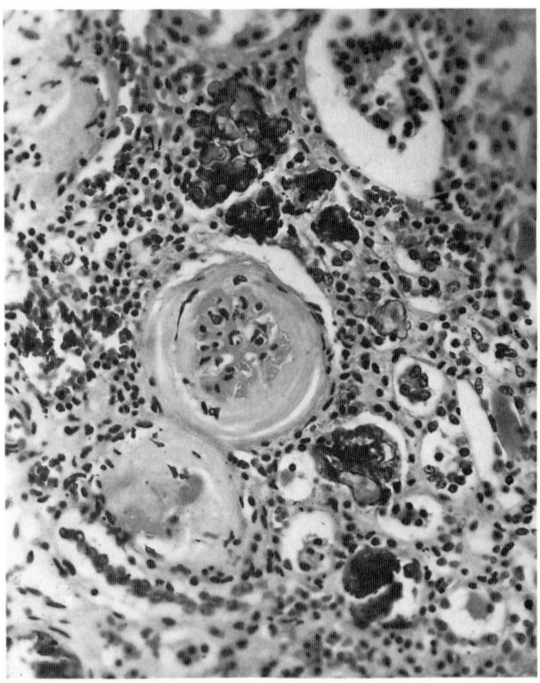

Fig. 14.2 Nephrocalcinosis. Deposits of calcium salts are present in the tubules and have extended into the interstitium. Much of the deposited material is strongly haematoxyphil and appears as rounded or amorphous black masses. There is extensive tubular atrophy and glomerular sclerosis in relation to the mineral deposits. Haematoxylin-eosin × 240

Although calcification is generalized in the kidneys, it tends to be mainly in the outer medulla; scarring is patchy and alternates with areas of normal parenchyma. In the scars there is atrophy and loss of tubules, periglomerular fibrosis, fibrosis internal to Bowman's capsule with collapse of glomerular tufts, interstitial fibrosis, and infiltration by lymphocytes. The scarring may be related to obstruction of collecting ducts by calcified concretions and possibly to chronic pyelonephritis in those cases that are associated with stones and obstruction.

PROGNOSIS

The prognosis will depend very largely upon the reversibility or otherwise of the underlying condition. Once calcium has been deposited in the kidneys it is usually not removed, even in those cases where, following treatment, the underlying cause ceases to operate. If the nephrocalcinosis that remains is marked then hypertension and renal insufficiency may occur. There are few reports dealing with the long-term follow-up of such patients: in one such study of 25 patients after parathyroidectomy, nine died 3–11 years after operation from hypertension with or without renal failure.[40]

PATHOGENESIS

In experimental animals made hyperglycaemic the earliest histological change in the kidneys is an increase in the number and size of vacuoles in the tubular epithelial cells; this is followed by calcium deposition in the vacuoles and in the mitochrondria.[41] Whether the vacuolation is caused by a direct toxic effect of calcium on the tubular cells, as some investigators claim, is not known.[42] Varying numbers of the epithelial cells are often shed and form casts in the tubular lumen; further deposition of calcium occurs in the casts. The intraluminal debris obstructs larger collecting ducts, causing their collapse; the proximal and distal tubules that join these ducts then atrophy.[43] Superimposed infection may produce an interstitial nephritis.

It has been suggested that tubular damage secondary to calcium deposition may initiate a progressive autoimmune response against antigens exposed by the damage; IgA has occasionally been reported on the tubular basement membranes in nephrocalcinosis but there is no evidence that this is harmful to the tubular cells.

REFERENCES

Nephrolithiasis (renal calculi)

1. Boyce WH. Organic matrix of human urinary concretions. Am J Med 1968; 45: 673–683.
2. Smith LH. The medical aspects of urolithiasis: an overview. J Urol 1989; 141: 707–710.
3. Andersen DA. The incidence of urinary calculi. Hosp Med 1968; 2: 1024–1033.
4. Watts RWE. Urinary stone disease (urolithiasis). In: Weatherall DJ, Ledingham JGG, Warrell DA, eds. Oxford textbook of medicine, 2nd edn. Oxford: Oxford University Press, 1987; 1: 18.87–18.95.
5. Gill WB. Urolithiasis update: biophysical and radiological advances enhance antistone therapy. Am J Kidney Dis 1981; 1: 66–90.
6. Guerin V, Rabian C, Noël LH et al. Anti-glomerular-basement-membrane disease after lithotripsy. Lancet 1990; 1: 856–857.
7. Rigatti P, Colombo R, Centemero A et al. Histological and ultrastructural evaluation of extracorporeal shock wave lithotripsy-induced renal lesions: preliminary report. Eur Urol 1989; 16: 207–211.
8. Lehmann J, Gray RW. Idiopathic hypercalciuria. J Urol 1989; 141: 715–718.
9. Broadus AE. Primary hyperparathyroidism. J Urol 1989; 141: 723–728.
10. Parks JH, Coe FL, Strauss AL. Calcium nephrolithiasis and medullary sponge kidney in women. N Engl J Med 1982; 306: 1088–1091.
11. Buckalew VM. Nephrolithiasis in renal tubular acidosis. J Urol 7 1989; 141: 731–737.
12. Caruana RJ, Buckalew VM. The syndrome of distal (type 1) renal tubular acidosis. Clinical and laboratory findings in 58 cases. Medicine (Baltimore) 1988; 67: 84–99.
13. Smith LH. Urolithiasis. In: Schrier RW, Gottschalk, CW, eds. Diseases of the kidney, 4th edn. Boston: Little, Brown, 1988; 1: 785–813.
14. Orwoll ES. The milk-alkali syndrome: current concepts. Ann Intern Med 1982; 97: 242–248.
15. Goldfarb S. Dietary factors in the pathogenesis and prophylaxis of calcium nephrolithiasis. Kidney Int 1988; 34: 544–555.
16. Schneider H-J. Epidemiology of urolithiasis. In: Schneider H-J, ed. Urolithiasis. Berlin: Springer, 1985: 143.
17. Lemann J, Piering WF, Lennon PJ. Possible role of carbohydrate-induced calciuria in calcium oxalate kidney-stone formation. N Engl J Med 1969; 280: 232–237.
18. Scott R, Cunningham C, McLelland A, Fell GS, Fitzgerald-Finch OP, McKellar N. The importance of cadmium as a factor in calcified upper urinary tract stone disease – a prospective 7 year study. Br J Urol 1982; 54: 584–589.
19. Stoeckle JD, Hardy HL, Weber AL. Chronic beryllium disease. Long-term follow-up of sixty cases and selective review of the literature. Am J Med 1969; 46: 545–561.
20. Williams HE, Wandzilak TR. Oxalate synthesis, transport and the hyperoxaluric syndromes. J Urol 1989; 141: 742–747.
21. Blacklock NJ. The pattern of urolithiasis in the Royal Navy. In: Nordian BEC, Hodgkinson A, eds. Proceedings of the Renal Stone Research Symposium. London: Churchill, 1969; 235.
22. Cifuentes Delatte L, Minon-Cifuentes JLR, Medina JA. Papillary stones: calcified renal tubules in Randall's plaques. J Urol 1985; 133: 490–494.
23. Kaiser ET, Bock SC. Protein inhibitors of crystal growth. J Urol 1989; 141: 750–752.
24. Lerner SP, Gleeson MJ, Griffith DP. Infection stones. J Urol 1989, 141: 753–758.
25. Fowler J. Bacteriology of branched renal calculi and accompanying urinary tract infection. J Urol 1984; 131: 213–215.
26. Priestley JT, Dunn JH. Branched renal calculi. J Urol 1949; 61: 194–203.
27. Pizarelli F, Peacock M. Effect of chronic administration of ammonium sulfate on phosphate stone recurrence. Nephron 1987; 46: 247–252.
28. Griffith DP. Struvite stones. Kidney Int 1978; 13: 372–382.
29. Nickel JC, Emtage J, Costerton JW. Ultrastructural microbial ecology of infection-induced urinary stones. J Urol 1985; 133: 622–627.
30. Griffith DP, Osborne CA. Infection (urease) stones. Miner Electrolyte Metab 1987; 13: 278–285.
31. Emmerson BT, Gordon RB, Johnson LA. Urate kinetics in hypoxanthine-guanine phosphoribosyltransferase deficiency: their significance for the understanding of gout. Q J Med 1976; 45: 49–61.
32. Brock WA, Golden J, Kaplan GW. Xanthine calculi in the Lesch-Nyhan syndrome. J Urol 1983; 130: 157–159.
33. Levison DA, Crocker PR, Banim S, Wallace DMA. Silica stones in the urinary bladder. Lancet 1982; 1: 704–705.

Nephrocalcinosis

34. Pyrah LN, Raper FP. Renal calcification and calculus formation. Br J Urol 1955; 27: 333–351.
35. Kapadia SB. Multiple myeloma: a clinicopathologic study of 62 consecutively autopsied cases. Medicine (Baltimore) 1980; 29: 380–392.

36. Vaughan JH, Sosman MC, Kinney TD. Nephrocalcinosis. Am J Roentgenol 1947; 58: 33–45.
37. Romer FK. Renal manifestations and abnormal calcium metabolism in sarcoidosis. Q J Med 1980; 49: 233–247.
38. Salyer WR, Keren D. Oxalosis as a complication of chronic renal failure. Kidney Int 1973; 4: 61–66.
39. Williams HE, Smith LH. Primary hyperoxaluria. In: Stanbury JB, Wyngaarden BB, Fredrickson DS, eds. The metabolic basis of inherited disease, 5th edn. New York: McGraw-Hill, 1983; 204–228.
40. Rienhoff WF. The surgical treatment of hyperparathyroidism with a report of 27 cases. Ann Surg 1950; 131: 917–944.
41. Caulfield JB, Schrag PE. Electron microscopic study of renal calcification. Am J Pathol 1964; 44: 365–381.
42. Scarpelli DG. Experimental nephrocalcinosis. A biochemical and morphological study. Lab Invest 1965; 14: 123–141.
43. Nguyen HT, Woodward JC. Intranephronic calculosis in rats. Am J Pathol 1980; 100: 39–47.

15

K. A. Porter

Renal disease in pregnancy

RENAL STRUCTURAL AND PHYSIOLOGICAL CHANGES IN NORMAL PREGNANCY

CHANGES IN STRUCTURE

The kidneys enlarge during pregnancy because of increases in the volume of the interstitium and of the blood vessels secondary to systemic vascular changes: compensatory hypertrophy plays no part in the enlargement and in fact does not occur.[1] The calyces, renal pelvis and ureters become dilated, the right side being more affected than the left: an erroneous impression of obstructive uropathy is often given. These changes are thought to be related to hormonal factors, particularly progesterone, and to mechanical compression of the ureters by the enlarged uterus.[2]

The structural alterations have important clinical implications. Dilatation of the urinary tract may lead to collection errors in tests based upon timed urine volume collections (e.g. 24-hour creatinine or protein excretion); in rare instances it may precipitate acute hydronephrosis or hydroureter (see p. 469). Urinary stasis within the ureters may also predispose to the development of pyelonephritis in women with asymptomatic bacteriuria (see p. 432).[3] The dilatation of the urinary tract may persist beyond delivery for as much as 12 weeks.

CHANGES IN PHYSIOLOGY

Extracellular fluid and plasma volume expand during pregnancy, producing so-called 'physiological hypervolaemia' and elevated cardiac output. Maternal volume receptors sense these changes as normal. Plasma osmolality decreases shortly after conception because of a fall in plasma sodium and associated anions; the osmioreceptor system resets to accept and preserve this new level of osmolality.[3]

The glomerular filtration rate and effective renal plasma flow increase 50–70% in the first two trimesters and fall in the third to a level 40% above that in the non-pregnant woman.[3] Since the glomerular filtration rate increases without substantial alterations in the production of creatinine and urea, the plasma levels of these solutes decrease in the third trimester to 47 µmol/l and 3.1 mmol/l, respectively. Corresponding levels in the non-pregnant woman are 73 µmol/l and 4.3 mmol/l. These physiological changes are important because values considered normal in non-pregnant women may reflect impaired renal function during pregnancy.[3] Urinary protein excretion is increased so that proteinuria in pregnancy should not be considered abnormal until it reaches 300 mg/24 hours. Glycosuria is usual; glucose excretion may be ten times greater than in the non-pregnant state.[3]

Blood pressure decreases early in pregnancy, then increases slowly, approaching pre-pregnancy values shortly before delivery. The cause of the initial hypotension is a marked decrease in peripheral vascular resistance, particularly in the kidneys, uterus and skin, mediated by increased prostaglandin levels; the later rise in the blood pressure is due to increasing vasoconstrictor tone.[3] Diastolic levels of blood pressure of 75 mmHg in the second trimester and 85 mmHg in the third trimester are often considered as the upper limits of normal.[4]

PREGNANCY IN RENAL TRANSPLANT RECIPIENTS

It has been estimated that of 50 women of childbearing age who have a functioning renal transplant one becomes pregnant, but this approximation is almost certainly too low because many pregnancies go unreported. The renal anatomical and physiological changes characteristic of pregnancy, including the increase in glomerular filtration rate, all occur in exactly the same way in renal allografts.[3]

In most cases pregnancy presents few problems to the mother if the renal allograft is functionally normal at the time of conception and continues to function satisfactorily during pregnancy. The risks to the fetus are increased.

URINARY TRACT CONDITIONS

INFECTION

Asymptomatic bacteriuria

Bacteriuria unaccompanied by any symptoms or signs of acute urinary tract infection occurs in 4–7% of pregnancies, an incidence similar to that in sexually active non-pregnant women.[4] In most instances, asymptomatic bacteriuria is discovered at the first examination during the pregnancy and is usually an expression of an abnormality acquired earlier in life. The most common organism is *Escherichia coli*. When present early in pregnancy asymptomatic bacteriuria progresses to symptomatic urinary tract infection in 20–40% of patients. More than half the infections are confined to the bladder. Treatment of asymptomatic bacteriuria lowers the incidence of subsequent symptomatic urinary tract infections by about 90%. An increased rate of premature delivery and fetal mortality has been reported in asymptomatic bacteriuric women with involvement of the upper urinary tract.[4]

Acute pyelonephritis and cystitis

Symptomatic urinary tract infections occur in 1–2% of pregnancies. *E. coli* is the most prevalent organism. Either cystitis or acute pyelonephritis may be produced; cystitis is the more common. The clinical manifestations and pathology of cystitis are discussed on page 705.

Acute pyelonephritis is the most common renal complication of pregnancy, occurring in about 1% of all pregnancies.[3] It appears, most commonly, after the 20th week of pregnancy. The symptoms and signs are the same as those of pyelonephritis occurring apart from pregnancy (see p. 434).

Acute pyelonephritis in pregnancy may result in septic shock, transient renal dysfunction, retardation of growth of the fetus, premature labour, fetal respiratory distress syndrome and fetal death.[4]

NEPHROLITHIASIS

The prevalence of renal calculi in pregnancy is between 0.03 and 0.35%, which is the same as in non-pregnant women. Stones are the most common cause of non-uterine abdominal pain requiring admission to hospital during pregnancy. The major adverse effect of urolithiasis is an increased frequency of urinary tract infections; urinary tract obstruction is very rare.[3,4]

ACUTE HYDRONEPHROSIS AND HYDROURETER

Very occasionally pregnancy may precipitate acute hydronephrosis or hydroureter. Obstruction may be at any level above the pelvic brim. The clinical manifestations are recurrent episodes of loin or low abdominal pain radiating to the groin. Typically, the pain is usually relieved by ureteric catheterization. The cause is unknown; one possibility is that due to the physiological changes of pregnancy an underlying compensated obstruction at the pelviureteric junction becomes decompensated and symptomatic.[4]

PRE-EXISTING RENAL DISEASE

Effect of pre-existing maternal renal disease on the fetus

Pre-existing renal disease may affect pregnancy adversely. As renal function declines, so does the ability to conceive and to sustain a viable pregnancy. Degrees of renal dysfunction that do not cause symptoms may still jeopardize pregnancy. In one series of cases with relatively mild pre-existing renal disease (plasma creatinine levels less than 150 μmol/l), perinatal mortality and the incidence of premature delivery and intrauterine growth retardation were higher than in healthy pregnancies.[5]

The same general principles apply to renal transplants. The risks to the fetus depend upon the level of renal function and blood pressure at the time of conception and during pregnancy. Additional risks are rejection of the transplant and transmission of the mother's original renal disease to the transplant during pregnancy (see p. 663).

Effect of pregnancy on mother's pre-existing renal disease

The majority of reports indicate that in most instances pregnancy does not affect the natural course of the pre-existing renal disease adversely, provided renal function is impaired only mildly and hypertension is absent at the time of conception.[3–5] In one collaborative study from three university medical centres in the USA significant hypertension (160/110 mmHg or higher) occurred in 23% of pregnancies in patients with relatively mild pre-existing renal disease, and a slight to moderate decrease in renal function occurred in 16%; in most of the patients, blood pressure and renal function reverted to pre-pregnancy levels after delivery. Increased proteinuria, often into the nephrotic range, was the most common effect of pregnancy on the diseased kidneys; this may reflect the tendency for increased protein excretion that occurs in normal pregnancy.[5] If, however, more severe renal insufficiency is present at the time of conception, pregnancy may accelerate the decline in renal function.[3] The same is true of renal allografts: whether the natural course of chronic rejection or any other disease in the renal transplant is affected by pregnancy will depend upon the level of renal function and blood pressure at the time of conception.

The statements given above are true when all forms of pre-existing disease are considered together. However, various underlying diseases have different outcomes. The effect of some particular diseases on the fetus and on the mother's pre-existing renal disease are considered below.

CHRONIC GLOMERULONEPHRITIS

Effect of pre-existing maternal glomerulonephritis on the fetus

Fetal loss in one large series of cases of primary maternal glomerulonephritis reported from Australia was 26%, comprising a perinatal mortality rate of 14% and an abortion rate of 12%.[6] This compares with an overall perinatal mortality rate of 0.7–1% in the Australian population during the same period. The worst fetal outcome was in the cases of focal segmental glomerulosclerosis, followed by IgA nephropathy, membranous glomerulonephritis and mesangiocapillary glomerulonephritis type I in that order. Cases of diffuse mesangial proliferative glomerulonephritis had the smallest fetal loss rate.[6] In another series membranous glomerulonephritis had the worst fetal loss rate and IgA nephropathy the smallest.[7] A transitory nephrotic syndrome, resolving spontaneously within 3 weeks, has been recorded in two newborn babies of patients with focal segmental glomerulosclerosis.[8] This observation is in keeping with the hypothesis that there is a circulating humoral factor in patients with focal segmental glomerulosclerosis that causes heavy proteinuria (see p. 209). The transient nephrotic syndrome in these babies may be comparable to the rapid reappearance of the nephrotic syndrome that occurs when some patients with focal segmental glomerulosclerosis receive a renal allograft (see p. 663).

Effect of pregnancy on mother's pre-existing glomerulonephritis

The maternal outcome in the Australian series cited above[6] was that impaired renal function occurred in 15% of the pregnancies, hypertension of 160/110 mmHg in 18% (but hypertension as defined by a diastolic blood pressure of 90 mmHg or higher on at least two successive readings occurred in 52%) and increased proteinuria in 59%.[6] After delivery, 5% of all the women were left with irreversible impairment of renal function, 18% who developed hypertension for the first time in pregnancy remained hypertensive, and 15% of all the women had a persistent increase in proteinuria.[6] The highest rate of persistent renal impairment was in patients with primary focal segmental glomerulosclerosis, and the greatest incidence of irreversible hypertension and proteinuria was in mesangiocapillary glomerulonephritis type I. The incidence of these persistent complications was lowest in diffuse mesangial proliferative glomerulonephritis.[6]

There is still a paucity of high quality data on this subject, but, in summary, it appears that in pregnant women with pre-existing primary glomerulonephritis the glomerular disease often worsens during pregnancy. This deterioration usually abates after delivery; occasionally it does not, in which case irreversible renal damage may hasten the progression of the disease. The question of progression, however, is particularly controversial because of the lack of adequate data.[9] Uncontrolled hypertension seems to be the main factor in bringing about the renal deterioration. The prognosis for the mother with primary glomerular disease is best in women who still have normal kidney function and who are not hypertensive at the onset of pregnancy.[9]

SYSTEMIC LUPUS ERYTHEMATOSUS

Effect of maternal systemic lupus erythematosus on the fetus

The overall rate of fetal loss in pregnant women with lupus nephritis is approximately 13%;[10] the fetal death rate is highest (45%) when manifestations of systemic lupus erythematosus first appear during pregnancy. When systemic lupus erythematosus has been present for some time before conception the prognosis for the fetus will depend upon whether the mother's disease has advanced to the stage of manifest impairment of renal function, hypertension or heavy proteinuria. The presence of these factors has an adverse affect on the survival of the fetus even when the systemic lupus erythematosus is immunologically inactive. The increased fetal mortality rate may be in part due to the formation of immune complexes in the decidual vessels with resulting placental ischaemia and infarction. The rate of fetal loss is not significantly greater in mothers who have systemic lupus erythematosus with circulating lupus anticoagulant than in those without the anticoagulant factor. A high anticardiolipin level in the blood of pregnant women with systemic lupus erythematosus is a sensitive predictor of fetal growth retardation and intrauterine fetal death.[11] Occasionally in patients with anti-Ro (SS-A) or anti-La (SS-B) antibodies or both in their blood, the newborn baby has the skin changes or atrioventricular block or both that the neonatal lupus syndrome comprises (see p. 240).

Effect of pregnancy on maternal lupus nephritis

The effect of pregnancy on the course of the mother's lupus nephritis is especially marked when systemic lupus erythematosus develops during pregnancy. About half the patients develop the nephrotic syndrome and a steep rise in serum creatinine; renal biopsy reveals a diffuse proliferative glomerulonephritis in almost all these cases. Treatment with high-dose corticosteroids brings some improvement to most patients but a few progress to end-stage renal failure within 3 years.[10]

When systemic lupus erythematosus precedes the pregnancy the prognosis for the mother depends upon whether she has been in stable clinical remission for some months before conception. If she has, then the chances of exacerbation of her systemic lupus erythematosus are small (about 7%); any exacerbations are usually mild and easily controlled by corticosteroid therapy. In contrast, if the woman has active disease at conception then the chances of exacerbation are high (about 60%) and in approximately a third of those with exacerbation the mother's renal disease suddenly worsens either during the pregnancy or in the first few weeks postpartum. The severe exacerbation of renal disease, often called a 'flare', usually consists of hypertension, decreasing renal function, thrombocytopenia and microangiopathic haemolytic anaemia;[12] corticosteroid therapy fails to reverse the renal failure in approximately 60% of flares and the patients rapidly progress to end-stage renal disease.[10]

OTHER PRE-EXISTING DISEASES

Diabetes mellitus

Effect of maternal diabetes mellitus on the fetus

Fetal loss associated with maternal diabetes mellitus is approximately 6%. Among the surviving babies there is a high rate of respiratory distress syndrome, hypoglycaemia, hypocalcaemia and jaundice; about 40% are large for gestational age and major congenital anomalies occur in about 9%.[13]

Effect of pregnancy on mother's pre-existing diabetes mellitus

During the course of gestation the serum creatinine rises by more than 35% in about a third of pregnancies in women with diabetic nephropathy. Most patients have significant increases in proteinuria and the nephrotic syndrome occurs in the third trimester in about 70%. The blood pressure rises in about 60% of the women. Renal function is usually stable except in those patients with severe hypertension. Following delivery, these changes are reversed and return to values observed in the first trimester; the long-term course of these patient's diabetic renal disease is almost always consistent with that expected in non-pregnant women.[13]

Reflux nephropathy

Pregnancy has no appreciable adverse effect on renal function in patients with reflux nephropathy when plasma creatinine does not exceed 200 μmol/l at conception. If conception occurs when the creatinine is above this value there is a risk that renal function will deteriorate, particularly if uncontrolled hypertension exists; at times the deterioration may be rapid, leading to end-stage renal failure within 2–3 years of delivery. In patients with hypertension and renal failure the outlook for the fetus is poor, with a mortality as high as 73%.[14]

PRE-EXISTING HYPERTENSION

Essential hypertension is present in about 3% of pregnant women when a diastolic pressure over 90 mmHg is used as the criterion. In another 0.5% there is secondary high blood pressure due to endocrine tumours, renal artery stenosis, a variety of renal diseases or coarctation of the aorta (see p. 316).

Essential hypertension

Essential hypertension is usually detectable from the time of conception; occasionally it is masked in the early stages of gestation and only becomes obvious in the last 3 months of pregnancy and is then categorized clinically as 'late hypertension' (see p. 564).

Pregnant women with essential hypertension may be more prone to develop pre-eclampsia, but otherwise gestation seems to have little influence on the course of the underlying disease. The pathological features of essential hypertension in pregnancy are no different from those in non-pregnant women (see p. 306). Fetal survival in these patients is related to the extent of renal damage prior to conception and to the occurrence of superimposed pre-eclampsia, its timing and severity.[15] The majority of patients have uncomplicated and successful pregnancies.

Secondary hypertension

Pregnancy may have a severely deleterious effect on patients who have hypertension secondary to phaeochromocytoma, systemic sclerosis or polyarteritis. *Phaeochromocytoma* may be associated with maternal mortality rates of 40% or more, in most instances because the diagnosis was missed and the condition thought to be pre-eclampsia. If the diagnosis is made quickly and the tumour resected or managed with alpha-adrenergic antagonists the prognosis for both mother and child is good. Plasma catecholamine levels and urinary catecholamine or vanillylmandelic acid secretion should be measured whenever hypertension is discovered early in pregnancy.

Fetal mortality is high in Cushing's disease.[15]

PRE-ECLAMPSIA AND ECLAMPSIA

Pre-eclampsia is a syndrome characterized by hypertension, proteinuria, oedema and, at times, coagulation abnormalities or hepatic abnormalities or both: it occurs during the latter part of pregnancy in women who are apparently healthy at the beginning of pregnancy.[15] In defining the syndrome oedema is often not included because it is a feature of normal pregnancy, can be assessed only subjectively and is not invariably present. Hypertension is taken as a diastolic blood pressure of 90 mmHg or more on two or more consecutive occasions 4 or more hours apart. Proteinuria is the presence of 300 mg or more of total protein in a 24-hour urine collection;[16] it may be heavy (more than 5 g/day) and it is moderately selective in terms of the molecular size of the filtered protein. The proteinuria is not preceded by a phase of microalbuminuria and it increases until delivery. Pre-eclampsia is the commonest cause of the nephrotic syndrome in pregnancy.

Pre-eclampsia is found most commonly in women having their first child (primigravidae), usually after the 20th week of gestation; in 50–70% it begins betweeen the 30th and 36th weeks. An onset earlier than the 20th week usually indicates that the disease is superimposed either upon pre-existing essential hypertension or upon some renal disease: in pure pre-eclampsia the blood pressure is normal in the first few weeks of gestation. Pre-eclampsia is also occasionally associated with hydatidiform mole or non-immune fetal hydrops.[17]

Pre-eclampsia can progress rapidly to a phase in which convulsions occur. This life-threatening condition is termed *eclampsia.* It is thought to result from intense vasoconstriction of small cerebral vessels with secondary thrombosis. Convulsions are often preceded by severe headache, visual disturbances, marked epigastric pain and heightened autonomic spinal reflexes, but they may occur unheralded in a seemingly stable patient with only slightly elevated blood pressure.[17] Delivery of the fetus terminates both pre-eclampsia and eclampsia and if carried out before irreversible damage has occurred, such as cerebral haemorrhage, recovery is complete and rapid.

Pre-eclampsia occurs six to eight times as frequently in primigravidae as in multiparous women; in first pregnancies the chances of developing it are five times as great if it is a twin pregnancy.[18] It also occurs more commonly in women with renal allografts.[19] Most primigravidae who develop pre-eclampsia have no recurrence in subsequent pregnancies, whereas pre-eclampsia in multiparous women is associated with a greater incidence of hypertension in later gestations.

The prevalence of pre-eclampsia varies considerably in different parts of the world, ranging from 0.05 to 27%. In Britain and the USA it develops in 5–10% of all pregnancies.[20]

There is a genetic predisposition to pre-eclampsia. It has been reported from Edinburgh that this inherited susceptibility is associated with HLA-DR4.[21] Susceptibility seems to depend upon a combination of fetal and maternal genotypes and the Edinburgh data are consistent with the involvement of a single recessive gene shared by mother and fetus. However, recent results show that it is unlikely that there is close linkage between HLA-DRβ and any maternal loci affecting pre-eclampsia.[22] Also a repetition of the study of HLA-DRβ alleles in the Edinburgh maternal population with polymerase chain reaction (PCR) amplification and allele-specific oligonucleotide probes in place of serological techniques has failed to confirm an association between HLA-DR4 and pre-eclampsia.[23] An association also exists between pre-eclampsia and trisomy 13.[24]

Hypertension in pre-eclampsia is characteristically labile and the normal circadian blood pressure rhythm is often reversed so that the highest levels occur at night. Dangerous blood pressure rises are sometimes missed when only day-time levels are recorded. The glomerular filtration rate and renal plasma flow decrease, but because their values are normally raised in pregnancy, measurements in pre-eclampsia may still be at or above levels that are normal in non-pregnant women.

There are disagreements concerning the incidence and importance of blood-clotting abnormalities in pre-eclampsia, but it is generally accepted that there is thrombocytopenia, and antithrombin III levels are often reduced compared to those in normotensive pregnant women.[20] Other reports indicate that the blood levels of prostacycline are lower and those of thromboxane higher than normal. There is usually haemoconcentration with elevation of haematocrit and haemoglobin levels. Hyperuricaemia and hypocalcaemia are common. The degree of hyperuricaemia corresponds with the extent of the renal lesions. Increased sodium retention occurs and the plasma aldosterone concentration is reduced.

Renal changes

The renal changes in pre-eclampsia and eclampsia are basically the same; they differ only in degree. The extent of the pathological alterations correlates with the severity of the clinical manifestations.

Gross appearance of the kidneys

The kidneys show no distinctive changes visible to the naked eye. They are usually normal in size. The cortex is pale and the glomeruli are prominent.[25]

Light microscopy

The important changes are in the glomeruli; the alterations in other structures are variable and non-specific.

Glomeruli The glomeruli are all enlarged and bloodless with tuft cellularity that is either normal or slightly increased (Fig. 15.1).[26] The enlargement is about 10% over normal glomerular size and is due to swelling of the endothelial and mesangial cells. The endothelial swelling is sometimes referred to as 'endotheliosis'. Fine lipid droplets are sometimes present in the endothelial cells, producing intracapillary foam cells. The capillary lumens, which may be dilated, are obliterated by the swollen cells and devoid of erythrocytes. There are no neutrophil granulocytes and the number of mesangial or endothelial cells is either normal or mildly increased. Some of the capillary loops become unfolded and develop an elongated cigar shape. Mesangial cell interposition is usually present and may result in a partial double contour appearance in the capillary walls.[26] Subendothelial deposits can usually be seen and are often large and slug-like, contributing substantially to the narrowing of the capillary lumens.[26,27] Herniation of the swollen capillary loops into the proximal convoluted tubules is common.[28] Thrombosis may occur rarely in the glomerular capillary loops; it is only found in se-

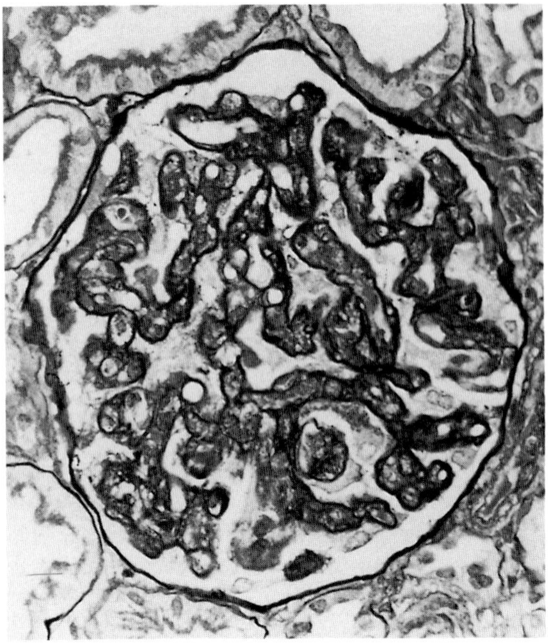

vere cases or when pre-eclampsia or eclampsia is superimposed upon, or complicated by, other obstetrical or renal diseases.[28] The amount of mesangial matrix is a little increased. The epithelial cells are swollen and their cytoplasm often contains numerous prominent protein transport droplets – a response to the increased protein load in the glomerular filtrate.[26,28] Crescents occasionally form in unusually severe cases.

Juxtaglomerular apparatus and peripolar cells Juxtaglomerular regions are not usually prominent and the cells are poorly granulated.[26,29]

Fig. 15.1 Pre-eclampsia: 24 weeks' gestation. The glomerulus is swollen and bloodless. A few of the capillaries have become unfolded and appear elongated. Some of the capillary walls have double contours.
Periodic acid-Schiff × 350

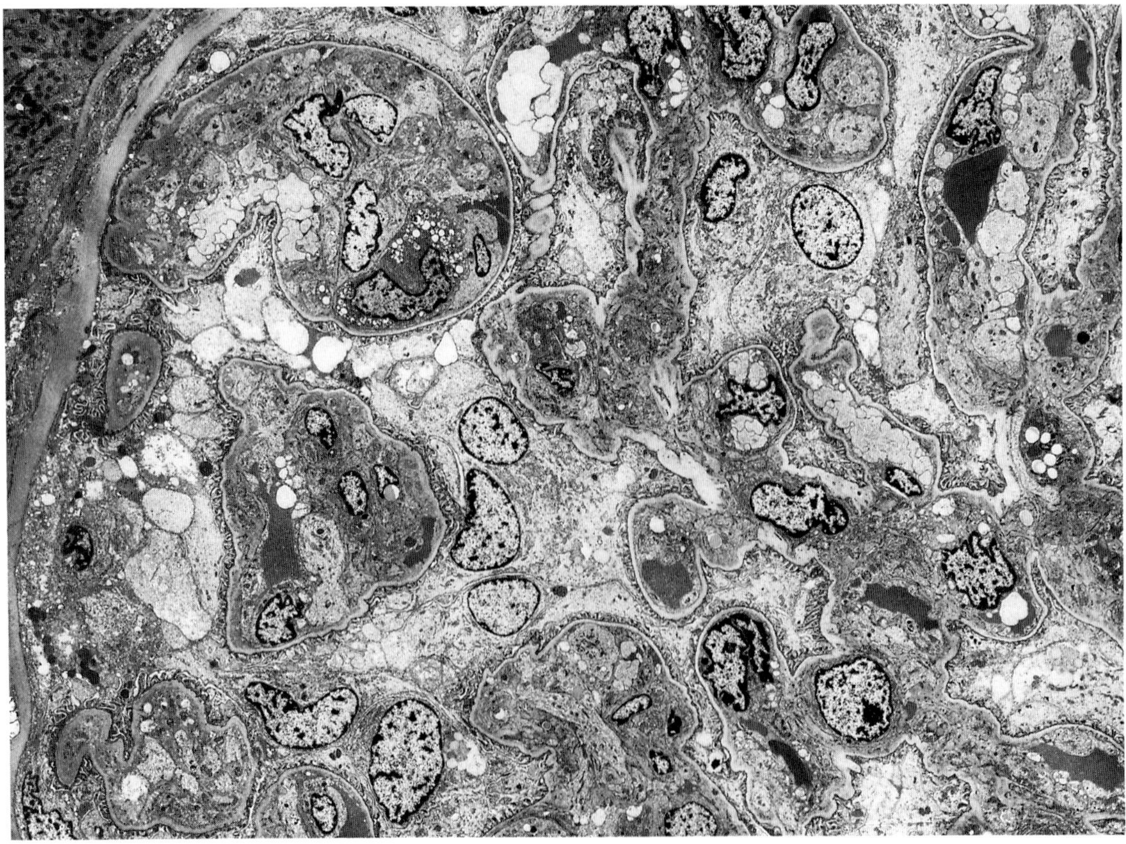

Fig. 15.2 Pre-eclampsia: 33 weeks' gestation. Electron micrograph of part of a glomerulus. The endothelial cells, which are swollen and have vacuolated cytoplasm, are obstructing most capillary lumens.
× 2025

The predominant cell is the type I or small cell which is believed to be functionally not very active. Glomerular peripolar cells with characteristic granules are occasionally seen but their numbers are not increased.[26,29] There have been a few descriptions of juxtaglomerular cell hyperplasia, with[30] or without[31] increased granularity of myoepithelioid cells.

Tubules and interstitium The tubules and interstitium show no specific changes. The proximal convoluted tubules often contain protein transport droplets (hyaline droplet change).

Blood vessels The arteries are normal in pure pre-eclampsia. In patients who have pre-eclampsia or eclampsia superimposed on essential or secondary hypertension there are hypertensive changes in the arterioles and arteries (see p. 306).

Electron microscopy

The glomerular capillary loops are partially or completely occluded by swollen endothelial and mesangial cells, and by electron-dense deposits on the subendothelial aspects of the capillary basement membranes (Figs. 15.2–15.4).[26,27] There are also various degrees of circumferential interposition of mesangial cell cytoplasm and mesangial matrix material along the inner aspect of the glomerular basement membrane, although this is rarely the dominant feature (Fig. 15.3).[26] The endothelial and mesangial cells contain vacuoles and electron-dense droplets. The subendothelial deposits vary in size and appearance: some are uniform and finely granular, others contain fibrillar material with the periodicity of fibrin (Fig. 15.5).[26] In some places the subendothelial space is widened by electron-lucent material. The

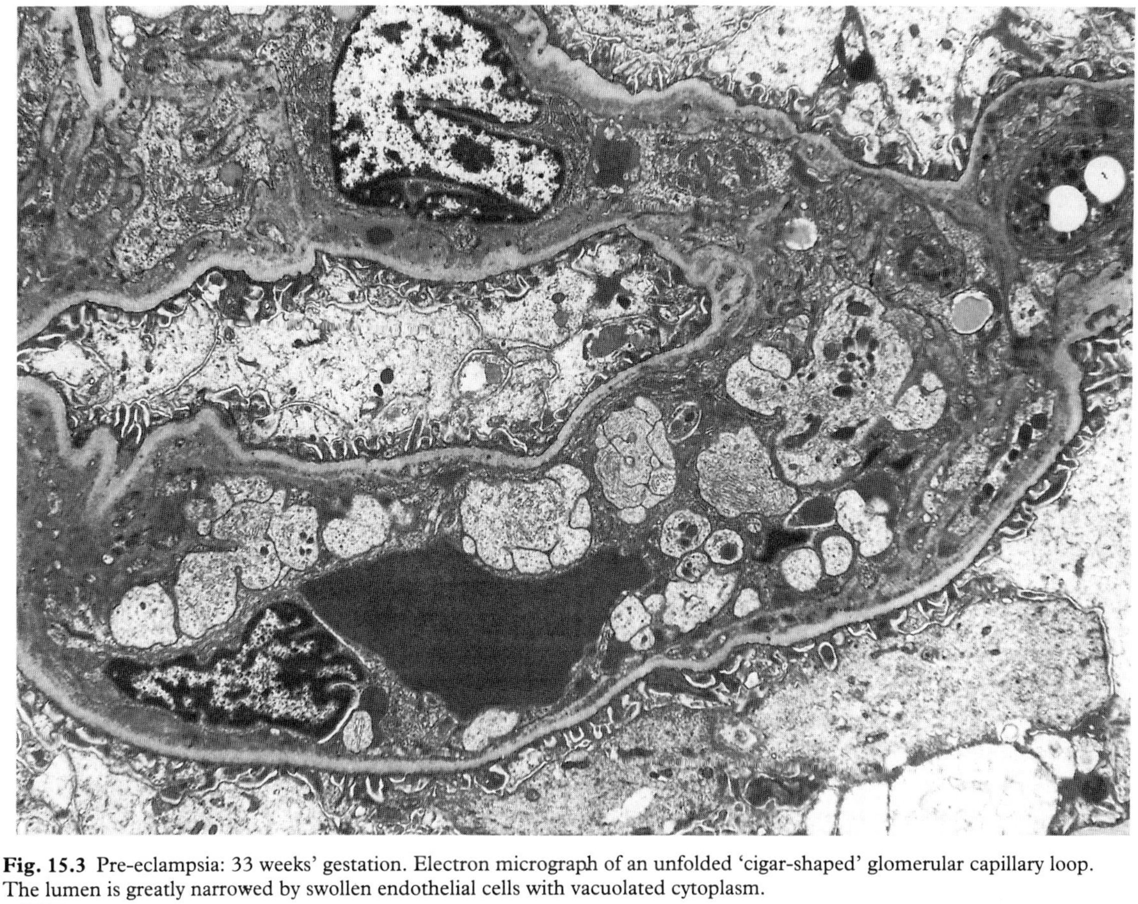

Fig. 15.3 Pre-eclampsia: 33 weeks' gestation. Electron micrograph of an unfolded 'cigar-shaped' glomerular capillary loop. The lumen is greatly narrowed by swollen endothelial cells with vacuolated cytoplasm. × 8000

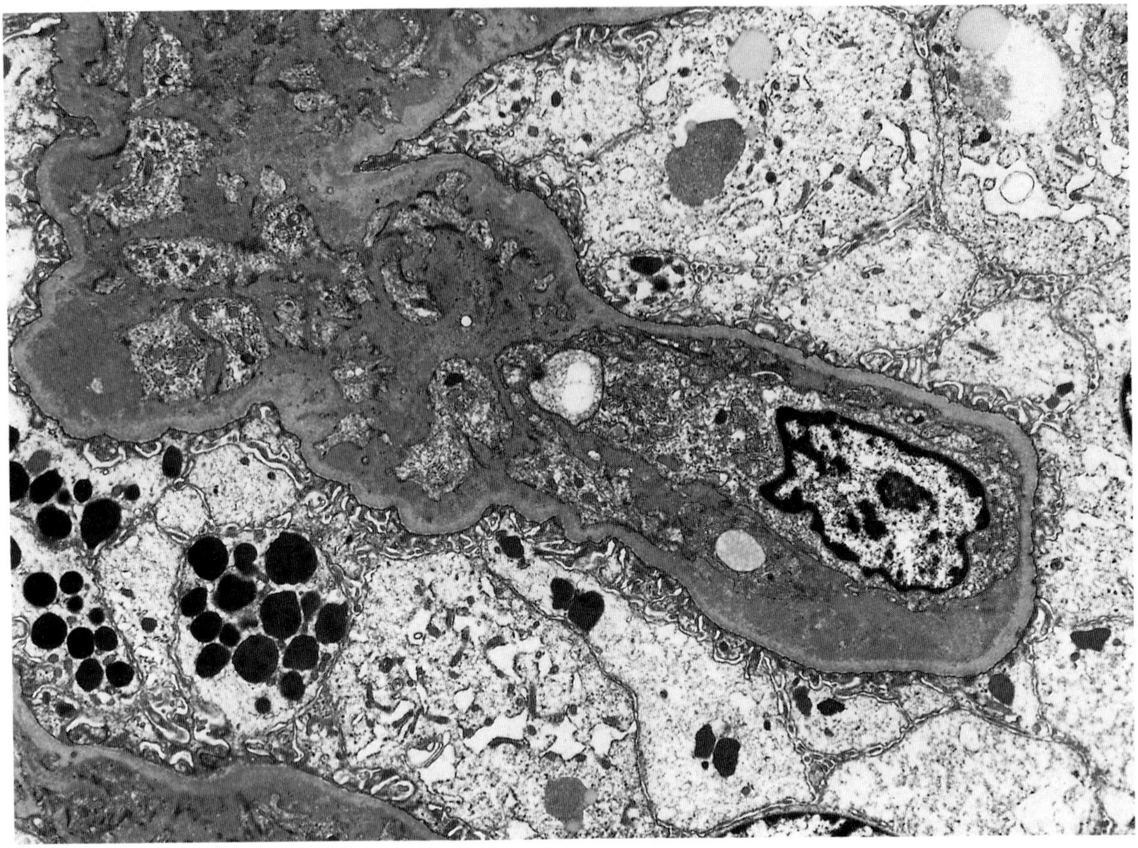

Fig. 15.4 Pre-eclampsia: 27 weeks' gestation. Electron micrograph of glomerular capillary. The lumen is obstructed by swollen endothelium. There is also some mesangial cell interposition and subendothelial and mesangial electron-dense deposits. The visceral epithelial cells are swollen and have vacuolated cytoplasm and some electron-dense granules. × 8000

mesangium is expanded and usually contains electron-dense deposits.[26] The visceral epithelial cells are often swollen and have vacuolated cytoplasm (Fig. 15.4). Most of the epithelial foot processes are normal; only focal areas of effacement are present.[26]

Immunofluorescence/immunoperoxidase microscopy

Focal or diffuse granular deposition of predominantly IgM and often fibrinogen, with smaller amounts of IgG, IgA, C3, C4 and C1q, in various combinations, is often present in the glomerular capillary walls, with some foci in the mesangium.[26,30] The thickened glomerular capillary walls contain, in addition to these plasma proteins, proteins derived from the glomerular matrix such as laminin, type IV collagen, fibronectin and proteoglycan.[32]

Immuno-electronmicroscopy

Immuno-electronmicroscopy has shown that the IgM is located in the subendothelial deposits.[33]

Changes in other organs

Liver

Moderate elevations in transaminase levels can often be detected in women with mild to moderate pre-eclampsia. Rarely, a patient may develop marked liver abnormalities accompanied by microangiopathic haemolytic anaemia and coagu-

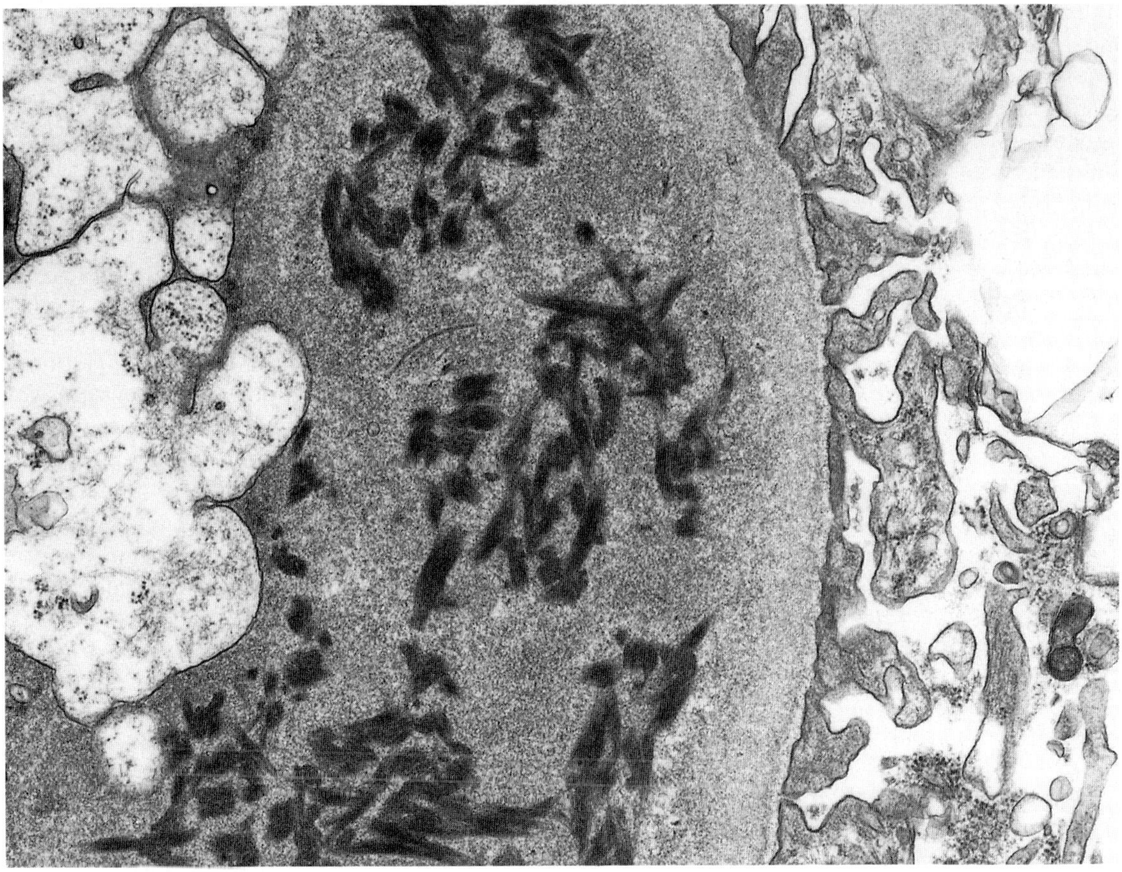

Fig. 15.5 Pre-eclampsia: 33 weeks' gestation. Electron micrograph of part of a glomerular capillary. The subendothelial deposit contains collections of fibrin.
× 40 000

lation abnormalities – the so-called HELLP syndrome (*h*aemolysis, *e*levated *l*iver enzymes, and *l*ow *p*latelet count).[34] This is a life-threatening condition necessitating emergency termination of pregnancy. In this syndrome, and in women who die of eclampsia, examination of the liver reveals a wide range of lesions that vary in severity from petechiae to infarcts and subcapsular haematomas. Periportal haemorrhagic necrosis is also commonly seen at autopsy.[25]

Brain

Haemorrhages, ranging from petechiae to large collections of blood, are found in the brains of women dying within 2 days after having eclamptic convulsions; cerebral haemorrhage causes 15–20% of deaths from eclampsia.[25] There may also be small vessel thromboses and cerebral oedema.

Heart and pituitary

Haemorrhagic changes similar to those seen in the brain are often found in the heart and anterior pituitary of patients dying from eclampsia.[25]

Uterus and placenta

In the first half of a normal pregnancy, the uterine spiral arteries of the placental bed become infiltrated by trophoblasts; this process causes these arteries to dilate, which enables the uteroplacental blood flow to increase normally in the second half of pregnancy.[35] In pre-eclampsia the process fails; one third to one half of the spiral arteries escapes invasion by trophoblasts and does not subsequently dilate.[36] The ensuing reduction in placental perfusion is exacerbated by the development of fibrinoid necrosis and subendothelial accumulation of lipid-laden foamy macrophages in the walls of the spiral arteries, a condition called acute atherosis. The placenta becomes ischaemic; infarcts, which occur in normal full-term placentas, are larger and more numerous in pre-eclampsia and eclampsia and there is increased evidence of villous ischaemia. Retroplacental haematomas are also more common than in a normal pregnancy.

Differential diagnosis

Although characteristic the renal changes in pre-eclampsia and eclampsia are not pathognomonic and a number of other possibilities have to be considered. These possibilities are not the same when a biopsy of a woman's own (native) kidneys is being examined as when the biopsy is of a renal transplant.

Differential diagnosis in native kidneys

Pre-existing or de novo mesangiocapillary glomerulonephritis type I The principal distinctions are that in mesangiocapillary glomerulonephritis type I, glomerular tuft cellularity and mesangial expansion are much greater than in pre-eclampsia, due mainly to mesangial cell proliferation; also endothelial swelling is absent, whereas it is the dominant feature in pre-eclampsia. Another difference is that the subendothelial and mesangial electron-dense deposits in mesangiocapillary glomerulonephritis type I contain predominantly IgG and/or C3, rather than IgM and/or fibrinogen as in pre-eclampsia.

Pre-existing or de novo lupus nephritis The distinction between lupus nephritis and pre-eclampsia can sometimes be very difficult if there is also a pregnancy-induced isolated hypertension, because the latter condition may superimpose circumferential mesangial cell interposition and expansion of the subendothelial space by electron-lucent material on the subendothelial electron-dense deposits of the lupus. Usually in lupus nephritis the dominant proteins in the subendothelial deposits will be IgG and/or C1q rather than IgM and/or fibrin. Differentiation is often possible on the serology by looking for DNA binding (see p. 227). On rare occasions, serial biopsies and/or serology postpartum may be necessary to establish the nature of the glomerular lesions.

Isolated hypertension late in pregnancy Isolated hypertension may be associated with glomerular changes that are indistinguishable from those of pre-eclampsia (see p. 564).[37] The distinction has to be a clinical one: in pre-eclampsia there is proteinuria of 300 mg or more per day; in isolated hypertension the urine contains less than 300 mg protein per day.

De novo haemolytic uraemic syndrome De novo haemolytic uraemic syndrome should not be a serious diagnostic problem because arterial lesions are a dominant feature in this condition, whereas in pre-eclampsia the arteries are normal. Real difficulty is only likely to be met if the pre-eclampsia is complicated by a superimposed malignant-phase hypertension due to some pre-existing renal or endocrine disease; severe hypertension can produce arterial lesions indistinguishable morphologically from haemolytic uraemic syndrome. The distinction in this very rare set of circumstances will depend upon the clinical findings.

De novo diffuse endocapillary proliferative glomerulonephritis In the very rare event of diffuse endocapillary glomerulonephritis complicating pregnancy the distinction from pre-eclampsia is usually easy on a biopsy. In endocapillary proliferative glomerulonephritis glomerular tuft cellularity is much greater than in pre-eclampsia and is largely due to infiltrating neutrophil granulocytes which are not found in pre-eclampsia; also, large scattered subepithelial electron-dense deposits ('humps'), common in endocapillary proliferative glomerulonephritis, do not occur in pre-eclampsia.

Differential diagnosis in renal transplants

Different conditions have to be considered when a biopsy of a renal transplant is being examined.

Acute transplant glomerulopathy Acute transplant glomerulopathy is discussed on page 649. The main point of distinction between this disease and pre-eclampsia is that in acute transplant glomerulopathy the glomerular capillary lumens are obstructed not only by swollen endothelial cells but also by large numbers of monocytes and macrophages which are not found in pre-eclampsia. There is usually also some evidence of acute tubulointerstitial rejection (see p. 636) and/or acute vascular rejection (see p. 645) in acute transplant glomerulopathy.

Chronic transplant glomerulopathy Chronic transplant glomerulopathy is discussed on page 656. Endothelial swelling with narrowing and obliteration of the glomerular capillaries does not occur in chronic transplant glomerulopathy, whereas it is the dominant feature in pre-eclampsia.

Recurrent mesangiocapillary glomerulonephritis type I The points of distinction between pre-eclampsia and mesangiocapillary glomerulonephritis type I are the same as in native kidneys (see above).

Recurrent or de novo haemolytic uraemic syndrome The differentiation of the renal changes in pre-eclampsia and the haemolytic uraemic syndrome are the same as in native kidneys (see above).

De novo diffuse endocapillary proliferative glomerulonephritis Features that enable diffuse endocapillary proliferative glomerulonephritis to be differentiated from pre-eclampsia are the same as in native kidneys (see above).

Complications involving the kidneys

Focal segmental glomerulosclerosis

In the early postpartum period, biopsies of kidneys of women who have had pre-eclampsia sometimes show focal segmental glomerulosclerosis (FSGS) in addition to the changes characteristic of pre-eclampsia.[38–41]

In one report of a series of women biopsied at this time because their pre-eclampsia had been either severe or atypical, FSGS affecting 4–10% of the glomeruli was found in 35% of the kidney specimens.[38] In the majority the FSGS was accompanied by arteriosclerosis and in about half by small numbers of cellular crescents. The authors suggest, on the basis of the arteriosclerosis, that the most probable explanation for the occurrence of FSGS in these kidneys is that the patients had undiagnosed chronic hypertension at the time of conception, and that the FSGS was secondary to the ischaemia induced by the hypertension. The clinical course of these patients was not given in the report.

Another four cases with FSGS and arteriosclerosis, in addition to the lesions of pre-eclampsia, reported from a different centre, could be interpreted in the same way.[40] However, these patients all lost completely their proteinuria and hypertension and regained a normal glomerular filtration rate within 5–15 months of delivery. To explain this recovery it would be necessary to postulate that the arteriosclerosis alone was insufficient to induce further FSGS and that the lesions present at the time of delivery regressed or in some other way ceased to induce proteinuria postpartum. The authors reject this explanation and suggest that the FSGS was induced during pregnancy by the same mechanism as caused the pre-eclampsia.

Several of the cases of FSGS described in the kidneys of a third series of patients who had had pre-eclampsia cannot readily be explained by the hypothesis of pre-existing hypertension. Only about a third of the kidneys had arteriosclerosis and 82% of the women lost their proteinuria and became normotensive within 3 months after delivery.[39] The authors suggest that the FSGS in these cases was induced by glomerular hyperfiltration brought about by the hypertension of pre-eclampsia compounded perhaps by the renal haemodynamic alterations of pregnancy.

In summary, FSGS is occasionally found in patients who have had pre-eclampsia but it seems not to be progressive and does not produce proteinuria, hypertension or renal dysfunction in the first 2 years postpartum. The lesions may be induced by glomerular hyperfiltration produced either by chronic hypertension present before conception or by the pre-eclampsia. In both instances the haemodynamic stimulus may be amplified by the alterations in the circulation that occur in pregnancy; when this extra stimulus is removed after delivery the FSGS lesions are insufficient to induce proteinuria.

Acute tubular necrosis

Acute tubular necrosis, which is discussed on page 492, may complicate pre-eclampsia. One of the precipitating causes is concealed accidental haemorrhage (abruptio placentae).

Haemolytic uraemic syndrome (Idiopathic postpartum acute renal failure)

Haemolytic uraemic syndrome, which is discussed on page 565, may complicate pre-eclampsia. It occurs within days or weeks after delivery.

Cortical necrosis

Cortical necrosis is a serious but rare complication of pre-eclampsia. There is a strong association between this disease and concealed accidental haemorrhage (premature placental separation), which is more frequent in pre-eclampsia. Cortical necrosis is discussed on page 303.

Evolution of lesions and prognosis

Pre-eclampsia progresses relentlessly but varies in the speed with which it evolves into eclampsia. In some patients it lasts 2–3 days only; in others it may extend to 3 weeks. With normal obstetric care pre-eclampsia and eclampsia are brief episodes because conservative management can only usually prolong the pregnancy by approximately 12 days before uncontrollable hypertension, deteriorating renal function, clotting or hepatic abnormalities, vomiting or impending fetal death, neccessitate delivery.[42] If this is carried out before a life-threatening, irreversible complication (such as cerebral haemorrhage or rupture of the liver capsule) has occurred, the primigravida or multigravida with no pre-existing renal disease or hypertension makes a complete and rapid clinical recovery. Residual proteinuria is rare, although excess protein excretion may occasionally take several months to disappear. The blood pressure usually quickly returns to pre-pregnancy levels, and the frequency distribution of systolic and diastolic pressures up to 34 years later is identical with that in age-matched women in the general population.[4,43]

Pre-eclampsia or eclampsia superimposed upon pre-existing chronic hypertension or renal disease has a poorer prognosis. In multigravidae, in whom this problem is most frequently encountered, there is a higher incidence of persistent hypertension and proteinuria, and the long-term age-specific death rate is about three times greater than expected, mainly because of hypertension.[15,43]

Although studies of sequential renal biopsies in pre-eclampsia are few, the evidence suggests that in most patients the morphological changes resolve with no permanent damage. The rapidity with which regression occurs seems to vary; occasionally all the lesions vanish within the first few hours after delivery,[44] but usually the mesangial and subendothelial deposits gradually become less prominent and may not completely resolve for weeks or even months.[45–48] The histological lesions seem to clear in sequence, with the subendothelial fibrinogen and IgM deposits disappearing more rapidly than the endothelial and mesangial swelling. Mesangial cell interposition and production of new basement membrane are often prominent 7–14 days post-partum when the endothelial swelling is waning or has gone; they may represent a healing phase in the resolution of pre-eclampsia.[27,49]

The placental ischaemia in pre-eclampsia leads to slowing of fetal growth and later to hypoxaemia, acidosis and asphyxiation of the fetus; intrauterine death is a likely outcome if delivery is delayed.

Prevention

Low dose aspirin therapy seems to protect against the appearance of pre-eclampsia in high-risk patients. This treatment probably exerts its effect by preventing intravascular coagulation, primarily by inhibiting the production of platelet thromboxane, while having little effect on endothelial prostacycline.[20] Prevention of pre-eclampsia by aspirin is currently being assessed in large multicentre trials.

Pathogenesis

The aetiology and pathogenesis of pre-eclampsia and eclampsia are unknown. Several factors, however, seem to be relevant.[4]

Hereditary and familial influences

Studies of the frequency of pre-eclampsia in blood relatives of women who have had the disease show that susceptibility to the condition is highly heritable.[22] Most of the pedigree data suggest a major role for the maternal genotype, while the association between susceptibility and HLA implicates the fetal genotype.[22] A recent hypothesis that pre-eclampsia occurs when both mother and fetus are homozygous for the same single HLA-linked recessive gene was based on the report that the disease is associated with sharing of HLA-DR4 between mother and fetus.[21] However, these data are being questioned[23] and it seems increasingly unlikely that there is such a close linkage between HLA and any maternal loci affecting pre-eclampsia.[22] Another suggested explanation for the association of HLA with susceptibility to pre-eclampsia is that there are fetally expressed HLA-linked genes which act as modifiers of the effect of maternally expressed susceptibility genes which lie elsewhere in the genome.[22]

The role of the placenta and uterus

An insufficient blood supply to the placenta appears to be an important factor in the aetiology and pathogenesis of pre-eclampsia and eclampsia;[42] this is supported by the finding that experimental placental ischaemia in the rabbit results in a syndrome resembling eclampsia.[50] In patients with pre-eclampsia and eclampsia placental ischaemia is associated with failure of trophoblasts to infiltrate as many of the uterine spiral arteries as in normal pregnancies (see p. 559). Why the trophoblastic replacement of muscle in the arterial walls is so incomplete in pre-eclampsia is not known. One suggestion is that a normal gene product is a placental growth factor necessary for adequate trophoblast invasion. It is supposed that this factor would be synthesized by either maternal or fetal (paternally derived) placental tissue. When a defective allele is present in both mother and father the normal gene product is absent and placental ischaemia results.[21] Hypertension may be caused by release of a humoral pressor factor from the ischaemic placenta.

The role of sodium and the renin-angiotensin-aldosterone system

Women destined to develop pre-eclampsia manifest increased pressor responsiveness to infused angiotensin II prior to the manifestation of clinical signs of the disease; this is in contrast to normal pregnant women who are resistant to the pressor effect of angiotensin II.[51]

The role of prostaglandins

A current hypothesis is that pre-eclampsia may occur under two circumstances: first, if the production of prostacycline or prostaglandin E_2 (PGE_2) decreases or that of thromboxane increases; second, if there is an imbalance between the production or release of vasodilator and vasoconstrictor eicosanoids. These suggestions are based on the assumption that increased PGE_2 and prostacycline are responsible for the vasodilatation and the resistance to vasoconstrictors (such as angiotensin II) that occur during normal pregnancy. It is an attractive idea because prostaglandins may not only influence uteroplacental blood flow but are known to induce platelet activation.[20]

Disturbances of coagulation

Coagulation abnormalities are common in pre-eclampsia and eclampsia; some of these may indicate chronic intravascular coagulation. The glomerular changes both in pre-eclampsia and eclampsia are compatible with a pathogenetic mechanism that involves intravascular coagulation. What triggers these changes in coagulation is unknown; they might result, at least in part, from the release of circulating thromboplastins from the ischaemic placental site.[4]

Immunological factors

The evidence that pre-eclampsia may be a disorder of the immunological mechanism involved in the normal response of the mother to the fetus includes an association with primigravidae, the protection afforded in subsequent pregnancies of the same paternity, the possibility of pre-eclampsia occurring in a subsequent pregnancy by a different father, and the protective effect of previous exposure to paternal antigens.[52] Much of this evidence, however, is weak and whether the immune system has a role in the aetiology and pathogenesis of pre-eclampsia remains very much an open question.[53]

ISOLATED HYPERTENSION LATE IN PREGNANCY

Some women develop isolated hypertension in the last 3 months of pregnancy, having been normotensive up to that time. The rise in blood pressure is mild to moderate in degree and is not associated with proteinuria, abnormal urinary sediment or urinary tract infection; the blood pressure returns to normal limits within 10 days after delivery. Most patients with isolated late hypertension are primigravidae.

Approximately half the primigravidae who manifest this condition have renal pathological changes that are indistinguishable from those of pre-eclampsia. In one series, the kidneys of 28 such patients were biopsied in the first 10 days after delivery. By light and electron microscopy and by immunofluorescence, lesions analogous to, but often less severe than, those of pre-eclampsia were observed in 13 (46%). Hyperuricaemia was found in all the patients with the lesions of pre-eclampsia, but not in the others.[37] Pathologically, these are cases of pre-eclampsia and in the older clinical classifications, such as that of Nelson,[54] they would have been accepted as 'mild grade' pre-eclampsia, along with the other 15 patients in this group whose disease on biopsy was essential hypertension, not pre-eclampsia. Most recent clinical classifications, in an attempt to exclude cases of essential hypertension, insist upon proteinuria as well as hypertension if a diagnosis of pre-eclampsia is to be made.

The other cases of isolated late hypertension either have normal-looking kidneys or show arteriolar hyalinization or arteriosclerosis or both.[37] In a few of those with vascular lesions there will be scattered small foci of glomerulosclerosis, tubular atrophy and interstitial fibrosis. Pathologically, these are cases of essential hypertension. It has been observed that the blood pressure of approximately 20% of patients with essential hypertension rises in the last trimester of pregnancy, the rise in many having been preceded by a fall earlier in pregnancy.[55] In recent clinical classifications of hypertension during pregnancy these cases are rightly not labelled as pre-eclamptic.

In summary, hypertension without proteinuria, appearing for the first time in the last 3 months of pregnancy, is caused either by pre-eclampsia or by essential hypertension which is masked in the early stages of pregnancy by the physiological fall in blood pressure that occurs at that time.

ACUTE RENAL FAILURE

Acute renal failure has become a rare complication of pregnancy in industrialized countries. This is largely because of liberalization of abortion laws and improvement in perinatal care, which have resulted in reductions in the frequency of complications such as sepsis, hypovolaemia, severe haemorrhage and eclampsia. In consequence, the current incidence of acute renal failure in pregnancy and the early postnatal period is probably less than 0.01% but it still has the classic bimodal distribution corresponding to septic abortion in early pregnancy and pre-eclampsia/eclampsia and haemorrhage in the third trimester.[3,56,57] Elsewhere in the world the incidence of acute renal failure in pregnancy remains high.

The great majority of obstetrical patients with acute renal failure have acute tubular necrosis, a substantial group have cortical necrosis, and a few have the haemolytic uraemic syndrome.

ACUTE TUBULAR NECROSIS

In pregnancy, acute tubular necrosis may occur in severe pre-eclampsia and eclampsia, concealed accidental haemorrhage (abruptio placentae), uterine haemorrhage from other causes, and miscellaneous conditions such as sepsis (including acute pyelonephritis and septic abortion), amniotic fluid embolism, incompatible blood transfusion and hyperemesis gravidarum. The morphological changes in the kidneys are the same as in acute tubular necrosis in non-pregnant patients (see p. 493).

In the rare condition of idiopathic acute fatty liver of pregnancy (see below), in which acute renal failure is common,[58] the underlying renal lesion may occasionally be acute tubular necrosis with the added features of bile-stained casts and leucine crystals in the tubules or interstitium as in other causes of the hepatorenal syndrome; more often the lesions are those of the haemolytic uraemic syndrome or of disseminated intravascular coagulation.

CORTICAL NECROSIS

Bilateral cortical necrosis occurs in approximately 20% of cases of acute renal failure in pregnancy.[56] Concealed accidental haemorrhage (abruptio placentae) is the most common precipitating event. Much less frequent causes are other forms of uterine haemorrhage, prolonged retention in the uterus of a dead fetus, sepsis (including septic abortion), amniotic fluid embolism and severe pre-eclampsia or eclampsia.[56,57] The pathological findings are discussed on page 303.

Bilateral renal cortical necrosis should be suspected when acute renal failure develops between the 26th and 30th weeks of pregnancy. It is characterized by anuria or severe oliguria lasting 15 days or more. The diagnosis is based on selective arteriography and/or renal biopsy.[56,57]

Many patients with bilateral cortical necrosis in pregnancy recover renal function over a period of 1 year. In one series, 10 of 13 patients recovered function permanently; in two function improved initially and then progressively declined to end-stage renal failure 5 and 9 years later respectively.[57]

It is unclear why pregnant women are more prone to develop cortical necrosis. Contributing factors may be the severe disturbances of coagulation, including enhanced capacity to produce fibrin and depressed fibrinolytic activity, that are found in cases of abruptio placentae and, to a lesser extent, in the other conditions associated with cortical necrosis in pregnancy.[56]

HAEMOLYTIC URAEMIC SYNDROME

The haemolytic uraemic syndrome occasionally causes acute renal failure in association with pregnancy. It most frequently does this in the post-partum period, producing what is often referred to as idiopathic post-partum acute renal failure.[59,60]

Idiopathic post-partum acute renal failure (post-partum haemolytic uraemic syndrome)

This form of acute renal failure is rare, accounting for approximately 2% of cases of acute renal failure;[61] it occurs 3 days to 10 weeks after an apparently normal pregnancy and delivery. Respiratory or gastrointestinal symptoms frequently precede the appearance of rapidly progressive oliguria and renal failure. The renal manifestations are accompanied by a microangiopathic haemolytic anaemia and thrombocytopenia. Although the blood pressure may be normal or only slightly raised at the outset, severe hypertension usually develops later.[62]

The pathological changes do not differ from those seen in the haemolytic uraemic syndrome occurring in other circumstances (see p. 283).

The prognosis is poor.[60] Death occurred in approximately 60% of the reported cases, and only 10% of the women regained normal renal function.[57] Recently the prognosis has improved, although renal sequelae are common. The reasons for the improvement are difficult to assess because plasma infusion, plasma exchange and agents that prevent platelet aggregation have all been used in uncontrolled studies.[60] Rapid delivery is indicated in most cases. Renal transplantation is often successful; in a few cases the disease is transmitted to the graft (see p. 669).

The aetiology and pathogenesis are unknown. The primary lesion seems to be damage to the vascular endothelium. In non-pregnant individuals the association between haemolytic uraemic syndrome and infection by verotoxin-producing *Escherichia coli* has been increasingly noted (see p. 281); such an organism may also play a role in women with post-partum haemolytic uraemic syndrome.[63] The raised levels of oestrogen in women post-partum may predispose them to the syndrome.

Idiopathic acute fatty liver of pregnancy

Acute fatty liver of pregnancy is rare, occurring approximately once in every 13 000 deliveries.[58] It presents in late pregnancy or the early post-partum period. The illness is fulminant and results in acute hepatic failure, a bleeding diathesis and coma;[58] there is often an accompanying acute renal failure.[57] Maternal mortality is 10–30%, with death resulting primarily from the hepatic damage. Various pathological changes have been described in the kidneys; often these have had the characteristics of the haemolytic uraemic syndrome.[64]

REFERENCES

Renal structural and physiological changes in normal pregnancy

1. Davison JM, Lindheimer MD. Changes in renal haemodynamics and kidney weight during pregnancy in the unanaesthetised rat. J Physiol 1980; 301: 129–136.
2. Fried AM, Woodring JH, Thompson DS. Hydronephrosis in pregnancy: a prospective sequential study of the course of dilatation. Ultrasound Med Biol 1982; 2: 255–259.
3. Davison JM. The kidney in pregnancy: a review. J R Soc Med 1983; 76: 485–501.

Urinary tract conditions

4. First MR, Pollak VE. Pregnancy and renal disease. In: Schrier RW, Gottschalk CW, eds. Diseases of the kidney, 4th edn. Boston: Little, Brown, 1988; 3: 2533–2559.

Pre-existing renal disease

5. Katz AI, Davison JM, Hayslett JP, Singson E, Lindheimer MD. Pregnancy in women with renal disease. Kidney Int 1980; 18: 192–206.
6. Packham DK, North RA, Fairley KF et al. Primary glomerulonephritis and pregnancy. Q J Med 1989; 71: 537–553.
7. Jungers P, Forget D, Henry-Amar M et al. Chronic kidney disease and pregnancy. Adv Nephrol 1986; 15: 103–141.
8. Lagrue G, Niaudet P, Guillot F, Lang P. Pregnancy and glomerulonephritis. Lancet 1989; 2: 1037 (letter).
9. Katz AI, Lindheimer MD. Does pregnancy aggravate primary glomerular disease? Am J Kidney Dis 1985; 6: 261–265.
10. Bobrie G, Liote F, Houillier P, Grünfeld JP, Jungers P. Pregnancy in lupus nephritis and related disorders. Am J Kidney Dis1987; 9: 339–343.
11. Lockshin MD, Druzin ML, Goei S et al. Antibody to cardiolipin as a predictor of fetal distress or death in pregnant patients with systemic lupus erythematosus. N Engl J Med 1985; 313: 152–156.
12. Imbasciati E, Surian M, Bottino S et al. Lupus nephropathy and pregnancy. A study of 26 pregnancies in patients with systemic lupus erythematosus and nephritis. Nephron 1984; 36: 46–51.
13. Hayslett JP, Reece EA. Effect of diabetic nephropathy on pregnancy. Am J Kidney Dis 1987; 9: 344–349.
14. Jungers P, Forget D, Houillier P, Henry-Amar M, Grunfeld JP. Pregnancy in IgA nephropathy, reflux nephropathy, and focal glomerulosclerosis. Am J Kidney Dis 1987; 9: 334–338.

Pre-existing hypertension

15. Davison JM, Lindheimer MD. Hypertension and pregnancy. In: Schrier RW, Gottschalk CW, eds. Diseases of the kidney, 4th edn. Boston: Little, Brown, 1988; 2: 1653–1686.

Pre-eclampsia and eclampsia

16. Davey DA, MacGillivray I. The classification and definition of the hypertensive disorders of pregnancy. Am J Obstet Gynecol 1988; 158: 892–898.
17. Lindheimer MD. Diagnosis and management of hypertension complicating pregnancy. Am J Kidney Dis 1989; 13: suppl 1, 17–27.
18. MacGillivray I. Some observations on the incidence of pre-eclampsia. J Obstet Gynaecol 1958; 65: 536–539.
19. Davison JM, Lindheimer MD. Pregnancy in women with renal allografts. Semin Nephrol 1984; 4: 240–247.
20. Lindheimer MD, Katz AI. Preeclampsia: pathophysiology, diagnosis and management. Ann Rev Med 1989; 40: 233–250.

21. Kilpatrick DC, Gibson F, Livingstone J, Liston WA. Pre-eclampsia is associated with HLA-DR4 sharing between mother and fetus. Tissue Antigens 1990; 35: 178–181.
22. Wilton AN, Cooper DW, Brennecke SP, Bishop SM, Marshall P. Absence of close linkage between maternal genes for susceptibility to pre-eclampsia/eclampsia and HLA DRβ. Lancet 1990; 336: 653–657.
23. Hayward C, Gilfillan A, Livingstone J et al. HLA-DR and pre-eclampsia in Edinburgh. Lancet 1990; 335: 1458–1459 (letter).
24. Boyd PA, Lindenbaum RH, Redman C. Pre-eclampsia and trisomy 13: a possible association. Lancet 1987; 2: 425–427.
25. Sheehan HL, Lynch JB. Pathology of toxaemia of pregnancy. Edinburgh: Churchill Livingstone, 1973.
26. Hill PA, Fairley KF, Kincaid-Smith P, Zimmerman M, Ryan GB. Morphologic changes in the renal glomerulus and the juxtaglomerular apparatus in human pre-eclampsia. J Pathol 1988; 156: 291–303.
27. Packham DK, Mathews DC, Fairley KF, Whitworth JA, Kincaid-Smith PS. Morphometric analysis of pre-eclampsia in women biopsied in pregnancy and post-partum. Kidney Int 1988; 34: 704–711.
28. Gaber LW, Spargo BH, Lindheimer MD. Renal pathology in pre-eclampsia. Clin Obstet Gynecol 1987; 1: 971–995.
29. Sheehan HL. Renal morphology in pre-eclampsia. Kidney Int 1980; 18: 241–252.
30. Fisher KA, Luger A, Spargo BH, Lindheimer MD. Hypertension in pregnancy: clinicopathological correlations and remote prognosis. Medicine (Baltimore) 1981; 60: 267–276.
31. Sommers S. Uterine, placental, renal biopsies and fibrin deposits in toxemia of pregnancy. Diagn Gynecol Obstet 1982; 3: 193–205.
32. Foidart JM, Nochy D, Nusgens B et al. Accumulation of several basement membrane proteins in glomeruli of patients with preeclampsia and other hypertensive syndromes of pregnancy. Possible role of renal prostaglandins and fibronectin. Lab Invest 1983; 49: 250–259.
33. Tribe CR, Smart GE, Davies DR, MacKenzie JC. A renal biopsy study in toxaemia of pregnancy. J Clin Pathol 1979; 32: 681–692.
34. Weinstein L. Syndrome of hemolysis, elevated liver enzymes, and low platelet count: a severe consequence of hypertension in pregnancy. Am J Obstet Gynecol 1982; 142: 159–167.
35. Brosens I, Robertson WB, Dixon HG. The physiological response of the vessels of the placental bed to normal pregnancy. J Pathol Bacteriol 1967; 93: 569–579.
36. Robertson WB, Khong TY. Pathology of the uteroplacental bed. In: Sharp F, Synonds EM, eds. Hypertension in pregnancy. Ithaca, New York: Perinatology Press, 1987: 101–113.
37. Nochy D, Biremaut P, Hinglais N et al. Renal lesions in the hypertensive syndromes of pregnancy: immunomorphological and ultrastructural studies in 114 cases. Clin Nephrol 1980; 13: 155 162.
38. Gaber LW, Spargo BH. Pregnancy-induced nephropathy. The significance of focal segmental glomerulosclerosis. Am J Kidney Dis 1987; 9: 317–323.
39. Nochy D, Hinglais N, Jacquot C, Gaudry C, Remy P, Bariety J. De novo focal glomerular sclerosis in pre-eclampsia. Clin Nephrol 1986; 25: 116–121.
40. Kida H, Takeda S, Yokoyama H, Tomosugi N, Abe T, Hattori N. Focal glomerular sclerosis in pre-eclampsia. Clin Nephrol 1985; 24: 221–227.
41. Heaton JM, Turner DR. Persistent renal damage following pre-eclampsia: a renal biopsy study of 13 patients. J Pathol 1985; 147: 121–126.
42. Redman CWG. Hypertension in pregnancy: a case discussion. Kidney Int 1987; 32: 151–160.
43. Chesley LC, Annitto JE, Cosgrove RA. The remote prognosis of eclamptic women: sixth periodic report. Am J Obstet Gynecol1976; 124: 446–459.
44. Pollak VE, Nettles JB. The kidney in toxemia of pregnancy: a clinical and pathological study based on renal biopsies. Medicine (Baltimore) 1960; 39: 469–526.
45. Furukawa T, Shigematsu H, Aizawa T, Oguchi H, Furuta S. Residual glomerular lesions in postpartal women with toxaemia of pregnancy. Acta Pathol Jpn 1983; 33: 1159–1169.
46. Fiaschi E, Nacoarato R. The histopathology of the kidney in toxaemia. Serial renal biopsies during pregnancy, puerperium and several years post-partum. Virchows Arch [Pathol Anat] 1968; 345: 299–309.
47. Hopper J, Farquhar MG, Yamauchi H, Moon HD, Page EW. Renal lesions in pregnancy. Obstet Gynecol 1961; 17: 271–293.
48. Mautner W, Churg J, Grishman E, Dachs S. Pre-eclamptic nephropathy. Lab Invest 1962; 11: 518–530.
49. Oe PL, Ooms ECM, Uttendorfsky OT, Stolte LAM, van Delden L, Graaff P. Post-partum resolution of glomerular changes in edema-proteinuria-hypertensive gestosis. Renal Physiol 1980; 3: 375–379.
50. Abitbol MM, Gallo GR, Pirani CL, et al. Production of experimental toxemia in the pregnant rabbit. Am J Obstet Gynecol 1976; 124: 460–470.
51. Gant NF, Worley RF, Everett RB et al. Control of vascular responsiveness during human pregnancy. Kidney Int 1980; 18: 253–258.
52. Serhal PF, Craft I. Immune basis for pre-eclampsia: evidence from oocyte recipients. Lancet 1987; 2: 744 (letter).
53. Kilpatrick DC. Immune mechanisms and pre-eclampsia. Lancet 1987; 2: 1460–1461 (letter).

Isolated hypertension late in pregnancy

54. Nelson TR. A clinical study of pre-eclampsia. Part I. J Obstet Gynaecol Br Emp 1955; 62: 48–57.
55. Morris WIC. The course of pregnancy complicated by essential hypertension. In: Morris NF, Browne JCM, eds. Symposium on non-toxemic hypertension in pregnancy. Boston: Little, Brown, 1958: 44.

Acute renal failure

56. Grünfeld J-P, Pertuiset N. Acute renal failure in pregnancy: 1987. Am J Kidney Dis 1987; 9: 359–362.
57. Grünfeld J-P, Ganeval D, Bournerias F. Acute renal failure in pregnancy. Kidney Int 1980; 18: 179–191.
58. Pockros PJ, Peters RL, Reynolds TB. Idiopathic fatty liver of pregnancy: findings in 10 cases. Medicine (Baltimore) 1984; 63: 1–11.
59. Robson JS, Martin AM, Rickley FA, MacDonald MK. Irreversible post-partum renal failure. Q J Med 1968; 37: 423–435.

60. Hayslett JP. Postpartum renal failure. N Engl J Med 1985; 312: 1556–1559.
61. Stratta P, Canavese C, Dogliani M, Todros T, Gagliardi L, Vercellone A. Pregnancy-related acute renal failure. Clin Nephrol 1989; 32: 14–20.
62. Morel-Maroger L, Kanfer A, Solez K, Srater J-D, Richet G. Prognostic importance of vascular lesions in acute renal failure with microangiopathic hemolytic anemia (hemolytic-uremic syndrome): clinicopathologic study in 20 patients. Kidney Int 1979; 15: 548–558.
63. Steele BT, Goldie J, Alexopoulou I et al. Postpartum haemolytic uraemic syndrome and verotoxin-producing *Escherichia coli*. Lancet 1984; 1: 511 (letter).
64. Morrin PAF, Handa SP, Valberg LS, Bencosme SA, Kipkie GF, Wyllie JC. Acute renal failure in association with fatty liver in pregnancy: recovery after fourteen days of complete anuria. Am J Med 1967; 42: 844–851.

16

K. A. Porter

Tumours of the kidneys and renal complications of extrarenal cancer

Many tumours of the kidney are small and unimportant, being for the most part incidental findings in nephrectomy specimens or at necropsy. 'Adenomas', renomedullary interstitial cell tumours, leiomyomas, lipomas and adrenal rests in the renal parenchyma account for the majority of these. Other tumours, which may be larger but usually behave in a benign fashion, are oncocytomas and angiomyolipomas. Very rarely a haemangioma, a lymphangioma or a juxtaglomerular cell tumour or a nodule of endometriosis may be encountered. Occasionally a haemangioma, transitional cell papilloma, inverted papilloma or fibroepithelial polyp may occur in the renal pelvis.

Primary clinically significant malignant tumours of the kidney are not common; they are found in approximately 0.4% of autopsies and constitute 2.5% of all malignant neoplasms.[1] The only frequent primary malignant tumours of the renal parenchyma are renal cell carcinoma (renal adenocarcinoma) and nephroblastoma (Wilms' tumour); rarities include sarcomas and carcinoid tumours. Primary malignant tumours of the renal pelvis are relatively unusual: the majority are transitional cell carcinomas; occasionally squamous cell carcinomas, adenocarcinomas and sarcomas occur.

The kidneys are frequently the site of metastatic tumours.

PRIMARY EPITHELIAL TUMOURS OF THE RENAL PARENCHYMA

RENAL CELL CARCINOMA

Commonly used synonyms for renal cell carcinoma are renal adenocarcinoma, clear cell carcinoma, hypernephroma and Grawitz tumour. The use of the term 'renal adenocarcinoma' has been challenged because the nephron is of mesodermal origin; clear cell carcinoma describes the commonest but not universal cellular pattern encountered in renal cell carcinoma; hypernephroma is a vestige from the days when renal cell carcinoma was thought to arise from adrenal rests; Grawitz was the man who described the tumour in 1883.

Renal cell carcinoma is a malignant epithelial tumour of the renal parenchyma; it is the commonest primary malignant tumour of the kidneys. It is rarely found in children and its incidence increases with advancing age; it is most frequently recognized in patients aged 50–60 years. It affects men nearly three times more often than women.

Incidence rates for renal cell carcinoma, adjusted for age, show a considerable variation over the world.[2] The highest rates are found in Scandinavia (e.g. 12.2 per 100 000 per annum for males in Iceland). Relatively high rates, in the range of five to seven per 100 000, are found in North America and continental Europe. The rates in England and Wales are lower, around 3.5 per 100 000. Very low rates, below three per 100 000 in males, occur in Africa, South America, Spain and Asia. In countries with relatively high rates the incidence of renal cell carcinoma appears to be increasing over time; in Connecticut, a two-fold increase was observed for males during the period 1935–1973.[3] The reason for the variation between countries is not known.

Clinical features

Haematuria (which may be painless or accompanied by a constant dull ache in the loin or abdomen), fatigue, weight loss, persistent fever and the discovery of a greatly enlarged kidney are the commonest presenting manifestations of renal cell carcinoma. Approximately 10% of patients present with signs or symptoms referable to metastases.[4] Sudden onset of a left scrotal varicocele occasionally occurs due to obstruction by tumour of the testicular vein at its entry point into the left renal vein. Anaemia and hypertension are common. Hepatic dysfunction is detected in about 15% of patients; in the absence of metastases liver function may return to normal when the tumour is removed.[5] Occasionally an arteriovenous anastomosis within the tumour causes high output cardiac failure.

Plain abdominal X-ray may show a mass, sometimes with calcification. Distortion of the calyces and renal pelvis may be revealed by intravenous pyelography and nephrotomography; ultrasonography will differentiate between a cyst and a solid tumour. Computed tomography is more accurate than arteriography in confirming the diagnosis of a tumour; it will also determine whether the regional lymph nodes are involved and whether there are distant metastases, thereby aiding staging of the tumour.

Biopsy and aspiration cytology in general are not very helpful; they are useful in only a few limited circumstances, e.g. to distinguish lymphoma from renal cell carcinoma, to check a diagnosis before treatment in inoperable cases, or to verify metastases. Urine cytology is a poor method for detecting renal cell carcinoma and is ineffective as a screening procedure.[6]

Endocrine activity

A few renal cell carcinomas produce endocrine secretions.[7]

Hypercalcaemia, with low or normal levels of phosphate in the serum, occurs in some patients in the absence of metastases in bone. In such cases the tumour may be found to be secreting a substance that is immunologically indistinguishable from parathyroid hormone. Removal of the tumour restores the serum calcium level to normal.[8] In some patients the tumour produces other bone-resorbing substances such as prostaglandins and the elevated levels of these substances in the blood may contribute to the production of hypercalcaemia.[9] Ectopic adrenocorticotrophic hormone is occasionally produced by a renal cell carcinoma, leading to Cushing's syndrome and marked hypercalcaemia.[10]

Approximately 4% of renal cell carcinomas are associated with an increase in erythropoietin activity of the blood and consequent erythrocytosis. The blood picture returns to normal after removal of the tumour. It is probable that the renal cell carcinoma in some of these cases secretes erythropoietin.[11]

Galactorrhoea, with high levels of circulating

prolactin, was observed in the case of a woman with a renal cell carcinoma producing this hormone.[7] Occasional renal cell carcinomas secrete renin producing hypertension,[12] or gonadotrophins leading to gynaecomastia. One tumour produced glucagon, leading to enteropathy and protein loss.[13]

Predisposing factors

There are few known predisposing factors. The most important are acquired cystic disease of the kidney (see p. 39) and von Hippel–Lindau's disease (see p. 69). Tobacco has been loosely incriminated[14] and there seems to be a higher risk in cadmium workers who smoke.[15] Rarely a dominantly inherited chromosomal aberration imposes a high risk of developing a renal cell carcinoma on members of a family.

Acquired cystic disease of the kidney

Cysts progressively appear in the kidneys of patients on dialysis, affecting males more than females (see p. 39). In one radiological study acquired cystic disease was found in 58% of patients who had been on dialysis for 2–4 years, 73% of those with 4–8 years of dialysis and 92% of those who had been on this treatment for more than 8 years.[16] Renal cell tumours arise in these cysts. Microscopic 'adenomas' are found in 10–20% of cases of acquired renal cystic disease after about 3 years on dialysis; another 3–6% will have renal cell carcinomas after about 5 years.[17] The tumours occur in patients of all ages; the mean is about 45 years. When acquired renal cystic disease is first detected metastases are present in 27% of patients.[17] The cystic disease appears to cause almost a 50-fold increase in the incidence of renal cell carcinoma and to lead to the appearance of this tumour 20 years earlier than in the general population.

Von Hippel–Lindau disease

Von Hippel–Lindau disease (VHLD; see p. 69) has a prevalence of about 1 in 40 000. Renal cell carcinoma occurs in approximately 28% of patients;[18] the tumours may be multiple or bilateral. The VHLD locus is close to that for the RAF-1 oncogene on chromosome 3p25 and in renal cell carcinomas arising in VHLD there is partial deletion of 3p. It is thought that the normal VHLD gene acts as a tumour suppressor.

Inherited predisposition to develop renal cell carcinoma

Familial renal cell carcinoma is rare. In two families with this condition the tumour has been found to be consistently associated with a heritable translocation between chromosomes 3 and 8 and 3 and 11 respectively.[19,20] The break took place in the proximal end of 3p in the region of 3p13.[19]

Each carrier of the genetic abnormality has a high risk of developing renal cell carcinoma at all ages, with an eventual cumulative risk in one of the families of 87% by the age of 59 years.[19] The median age of onset of the tumour is considerably lower than for renal cell carcinoma in the general population. Multifocal tumours are common and the probability that primary tumours will arise in both kidneys steadily increases with age.

Renal changes

Gross appearance of the kidneys[2]

Renal cell carcinomas are found in the renal cortex. They occur with equal frequency in either kidney and their intrarenal distribution is random. Typically they form an irregular, bosselated, soft mass which protrudes beneath the renal capsule. When the kidney is bisected the tumour is usually spheroidal with a sharply defined lobulated outline; it may appear to be encapsulated (Fig. 16.1). Most tumours at the time of nephrectomy are about 7.5 cm in diameter but they may be as large as 25 cm or as small as 0.5 cm in diameter. The cut surface bulges and is usually orange or yellow, mottled with deep red recent and old haemorrhages and traversed by grey bands. Necrotic areas are common, particularly in large tumours; they may be gelatinous or cystic. Occasionally the tumour is predominantly cystic. Infrequently there are foci of calcification. The tumour is usually unilateral and solitary; multiple tumurs occur in about 5% of patients and bilateral tumours in about 1%.

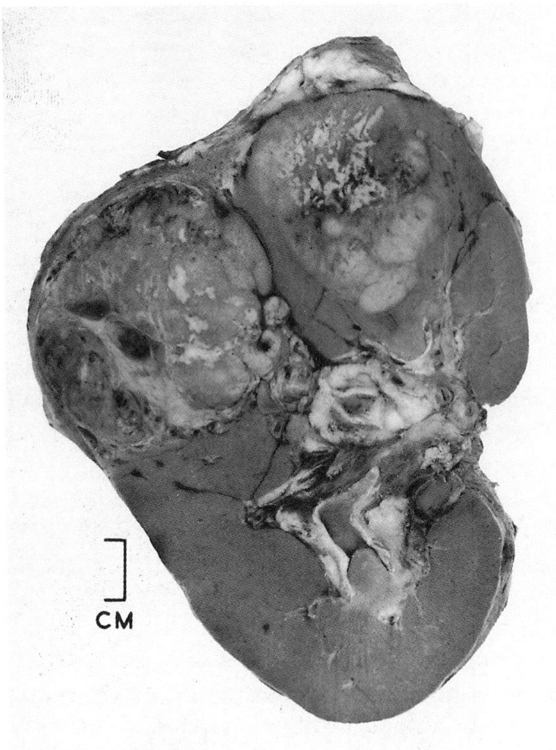

Fig. 16.1 Renal cell carcinoma. The tumour protrudes from the cortical surface of the kidney. The variegated pattern of the cut surface is due to haemorrhage, necrosis and some fibrosis.
Reproduced by permission of the Curator, Gordon Museum, Guy's Hospital, London, UK

Extension of the tumour through the renal capsule into the perirenal fat may be visible. In some cases processes of tumour tissue extend within the lumen of the main renal vein and even into and along the inferior vena cava, often resulting in thrombosis.

Light microscopy[2]

Most renal cell carcinomas are composed of a mixture of clear cells and granular cells; either type of cell may predominate.

The clear cells are so called because in paraffin wax-embedded material their cytoplasm is vacuolated and lacks granularity (Fig. 16.2) The reason for this appearance is that the cytoplasm is rich in lipid or glycogen or both but contains few cytoplasmic organelles. The fat is not visible in paraffin sections because it has been dissolved out in the processing; it can be seen only in frozen sections stained with fat-soluble dyes such as oil red O, Sudan IV or Sudan black. The glycogen is reduced in amount by formalin fixation, but some can still be demonstrated with the periodic acid-Schiff stain.

The granular cells lack fat and glycogen but have many mitochondria and other organelles which impart a granular eosinophilic appearance to their cytoplasm (Fig. 16.3).

Neither clear nor granular cells have intracytoplasmic mucin, although they may have abundant glycocalyx on their surfaces. Clear cells predominate in approximately 45% of renal cell carcinomas and granular cells in 25%; in the others the two types of cell are present in nearly equal numbers. The parts of the tumour that are composed of clear cells appear yellow to the naked eye.

In a few cases the tumour cell cytoplasm stains positively with Hale's acid iron colloid. These tumours have been referred to as *chromophobe renal cell carcinomas*; they are considered on page 580.

Both clear and granular cells are polygonal and are arranged in sheets, tubules, trabeculae and papillary formations. Cases in which vascularized connective tissue stalks invested by neoplastic cells make up 50% or more of the tumour are considered separately as a variant of renal cell carcinoma (*papillary renal cell carcinoma*: see p. 578). Typically there is little cellular or nuclear pleomorphism; mitotic figures are rare. The stroma is usually relatively inconspicuous and contains many fine capillaries. Sometimes there are small clusters of fat-laden macrophages and foci of calcification. Occasionally laminated calcified concretions (psammoma bodies) and foci of cartilaginous and osseous metaplasia occur in the stroma. Haemosiderin-laden macrophages are found in areas of old haemorrhage. Cholesterol clefts, groups of infiltrating mononuclear cells and variable amounts of fibrosis are common when necrosis is present.

Approximately 2% of renal cell carcinomas are either focally or completely composed of poorly differentiated cells that resemble a sarcoma. These so-called *sarcomatoid renal cell carcinomas* are discussed on page 581.

Very rarely a metastasis from another tumour

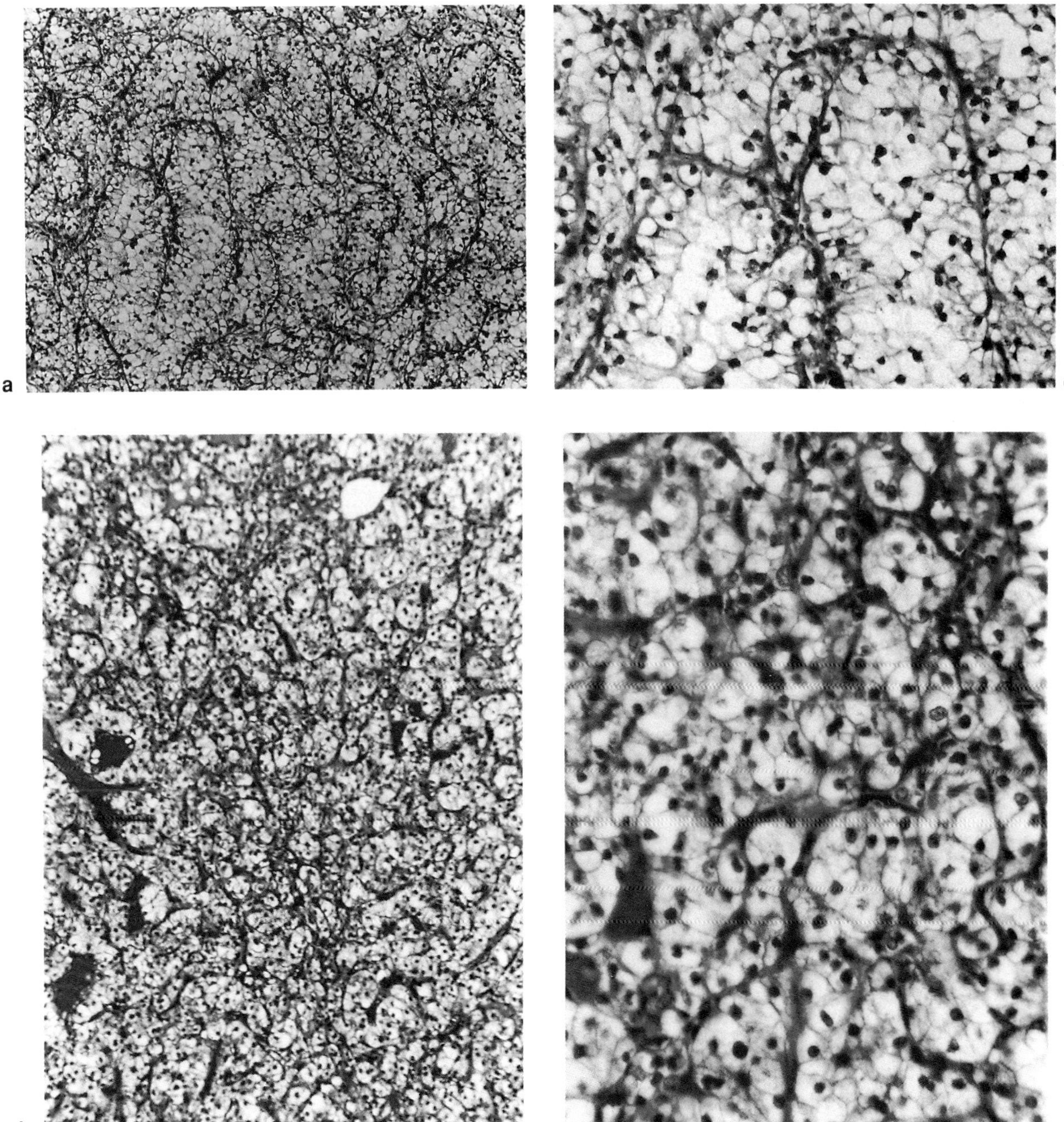

Fig. 16.2 a–d Renal cell carcinoma (predominantly clear celled). The tumour cells are polygonal and arranged in sheets, tubules and trabeculae. Clear cells predominate. Their cytoplasm appears to be empty as a result of loss of lipid and glycogen during histological processing.
Haematoxylin-eosin: (**a**),(**b**) × 110; (**c**),(**d**) × 350

elsewhere in the body may be found in a renal cell carcinoma. Secondaries from bronchial carcinoma, breast carcinoma and a malignant melanoma have all been recorded in renal cell carcinomas.[21]

Electron microscopy[3,22]

In many areas of a renal cell carcinoma the cells, whether clear or granular, have microvilli; these are quite variable, ranging from a brush border

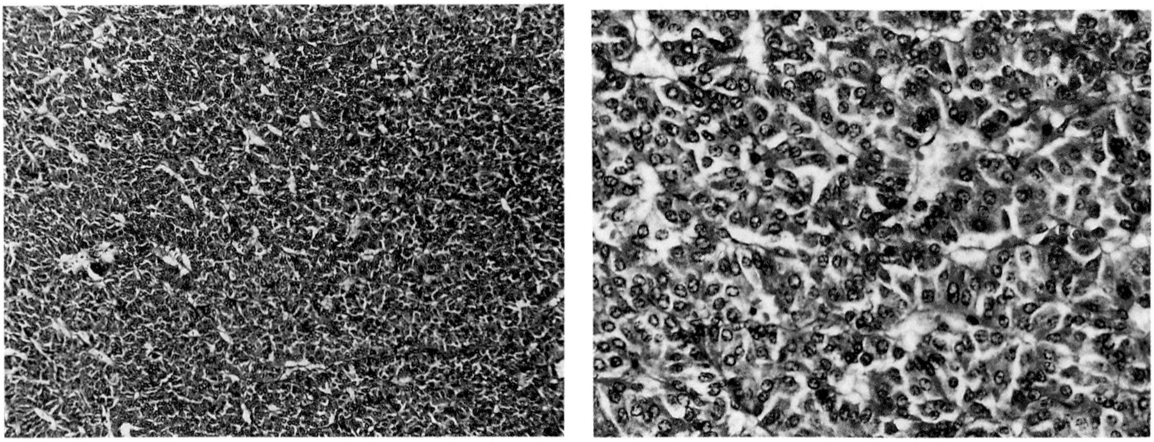

a b

Fig. 16.3 a, b Renal cell carcinoma (predominantly granular celled). The tumour cells are polygonal and arranged in sheets, tubules and acini. Most of the cells have granular cytoplasm.
Haematoxylin-eosin: (**a**) × 110; (**b**) × 350

of mainly straight or slightly curved protrusions into the lumen of a gland to a few short projections from a free cell surface. Microvilli are often lacking on carcinoma cells in solid areas. Abundant cytoplasmic glycogen and variable numbers of lipid droplets are features of clear cells. In contrast, glycogen and lipid are scanty in granular cells but organelles are more numerous.

The scattered renin-containing cells in a tumour that secreted this hormone had membrane-bound granules in their cytoplasm that were morphologically consistent with renin storage granules.[12]

Immunohistochemistry

Renal cell carcinomas usually express antigens characteristic for proximal tubules of the normal kidney. The use of monoclonal antibodies recognizing intermediate-sized filament proteins (components of the cytoskeleton) show that the tumour cells contain both vimentin and cytokeratin.[23,24] Several monoclonal antibodies to renal cell carcinoma-associated antigens have been described; the most specific (called G250) recognizes renal cell carcinoma and does not stain normal renal tissue or benign renal tumours.[25]

Cytogenetic analysis

Non-papillary renal cell carcinoma is characterized by recurrent deletion of the short arm (p) of one of the two homologous chromosomes 3. The breakpoint is localized in most cases at 3p 13–14. There are also non-random secondary chromosomal aberrations, such as trisomy of the 5q 22-qter segment.[26] This is in contrast to the papillary variant of renal cell carcinoma which fails to show any rearrangement of the chromosome 3p segment.[26]

In cases with familial occurrence of renal cell carcinoma inherited translocations involving the short arm (p) of chromosome 3 (3;8 and 3;11 translocations) have been observed; in families with these abnormalities the breakpoints on chromosome 3 are between the 3p 13 and 14 bands.[19]

Genotyping

Genotyping confirms the deletion of specific chromosome 3p segments and shows loss of heterozygosity for loci at 3p in non-papillary renal cell carcinomas.[27] Restriction analysis of the mitochondrial DNA fails to show the autoradiographic band that occurs in oncocytomas (see p. 585).

Spread

Renal cell carcinomas spread by direct invasion of adjacent tissues and by way of the lymphatics and blood stream. Local invasion is manifest in involvement of the renal pelvis, the perinephric tissue, the adjacent adrenal gland or the liver. Lymphatic spread results in involvement of lumbar lymph nodes, which occurs in about one-third of the cases.

Blood-borne metastasis is frequently a feature of the disease, but its occurrence is unpredictable. Tumours may become very large without metastasis taking place; in contrast, some small tumours produce numerous and widespread haematogenous secondary deposits: rarely, these are the presenting manifestation of the disease. Haematogenous deposits are found with particular frequency in the lungs (which are involved in about 55% of cases), liver (about 33%), bones (also about 33%), adrenal (about 20%), opposite kidney (about 10%) and brain (about 6%).[2] The deposits in bone are osteolytic and predispose to pathological fracture.

A renal cell carcinoma occasionally produces a solitary metastatic focus – for instance, in a lung or bone. It is often stated that excision of a solitary metastasis may result in 5-year survival rates equivalent to those of patients with Robson's stage I disease (see p. 576).[28] This is probably an uncommon outcome; in most cases the beneficial effects of excision of the metastasis are limited to improved short-term survival postoperatively.[29]

Renal cell carcinoma is unusual in that it may, though very rarely, metastasize to another tumour elsewhere in the body. For example, in one case a secondary deposit developed in a phaeochromocytoma.[30]

Invasion of the renal vein may lead to growth along the vena cava and into the right atrium. Spread into the left renal vein may result in involvement of the testicular or ovarian vein and retrograde tumour embolism of the pampiniform or ovarian plexus and consequent development of metastatic deposits in the spermatic cord, epididymis, broad ligament, ovary, vagina or vulva.

Spontaneous regression of metastases

Spontaneous regression of metastases has occasionally been described. Usually it is lung secondaries which are said to regress, but in many cases the presence of these metastases is based on radiological findings without any confirmatory histopathology. However, in one series 19 cases had histological confirmation of metastatic renal cell carcinoma and the reality of regression is difficult to dispute.[31]

The most popular, but as yet unsubstantiated, explanation for this phenomenon is that it is a manifestation of some undefined immunological process.

Differential diagnosis

Renal cell carcinoma in which clear cells predominate may on occasion be mimicked by *malakoplakia* and *xanthogranulomatous pyelonephritis*. The distinction from these conditions is discussed on pages 451 and 448.

Very rarely an *adrenal adenocarcinoma* arises in ectopic adrenal tissue in the kidney (see p. 607). These tumours usually lack glycogen, and by electron microscopy show endocrine rather than tubular features. The presence of epithelial markers should distinguish them from renal cell carcinomas.[32]

A poorly differentiated renal cell carcinoma involving both the kidney and the renal pelvis may be difficult to distinguish from a *pleomorphic transitional cell carcinoma of the renal pelvis*. Usually, a careful search through multiple sections will disclose areas where the tumour is sufficiently well differentiated for its origin to be identifiable. Occasionally, electron microscopy is helpful but microvilli and brush borders are often not present in poorly differentiated renal cell carcinomas. Immunohistochemical studies do not help because both tumours may express the same antigens including the renal cell carcinoma-associated antigen G250. The distinction between renal cell carcinoma and *oncocytoma* is discussed on page 585.

Infrequently the problem arises of distinguishing between a renal cell carcinoma and *metastatic carcinoma*. The tumours most commonly metastasizing to the kidneys are carcinomas of the lungs, breasts, stomach, ovaries and intestine. Usually the distinction can be made on light microscopy. In difficult cases variations in the expression of tumour-related antigens may be helpful. For example, bronchial carcinomas are usually strongly positive when stained with monoclonal antisera specific for carcinoembryonic antigen (CEA) whereas renal cell carcinomas are negative; breast carcinomas commonly express non-specific cross-reacting antigen (NCA) which is not expressed in renal cell carcinomas; colonic carcinomas consistently express both CEA and NCA.[33] Gastric carcinomas do not stain with monoclonal antibody G250, which recognizes the antigen expressed on cell membranes of renal cell carcinomas.[25] Eighty per cent of ovarian carcinomas do not express G250, but in 15% up to half of the tumour cells stain and in 5% more than half of the cells are positive.[25]

Complications

Amyloidosis

Systemic amyloidosis occurs in approximately 3% of patients with renal cell carcinoma[34] compared with 0.1–0.4% among all cancers. Deposits are nearly always present in the kidneys and may involve the stroma of the tumour.[35] This may lead to the nephrotic syndrome and renal failure. Gastrointestinal amyloid deposits are also relatively common in such patients and may give rise to diarrhoea. The patient may even present with slowly progressive muscle weakness or distal paraesthesia due to amyloid polyneuropathy.[36]

In many cases the amyloid associated with renal cell carcinoma seems to be AA in type (see p. 344);[35,37] in two cases associated with polyneuropathy[36] and in one case with a concomitant multiple myeloma[35] the amyloid was of lambda (AL) light chain immunoglobulin origin. There is some evidence to suggest that in the cases with AA amyloid chronic inflammation may be the contributing stimulus that leads to amyloid formation;[35] in the AL cases there seems to be a plasma cell dyscrasia that may be overt or occult.[36]

Glomerulonephritis

Examination of the uninvolved parenchyma in kidneys resected for renal cell carcinoma reveals in approximately 18% of cases a moderate to marked diffuse or focal, segmental or global increase in the amount of mesangial matrix and the number of mesangial cells.[38] In these, and in an additional 17% of kidneys that show only mild mesangial expansion, immunofluorescence microscopy reveals fine granular mesangial deposits of IgM which are often associated with C3.[38] Membranous glomerulonephritis (see p. 191) may occur but this is unusual.[39] Isolated cases with minimal change glomerulonephritis (see p. 135)[40] or mesangiocapillary glomerulonephritis type 1 (see p. 164)[41] have also been recorded.

The mesangial proliferative glomerulonephritic lesions are occasionally associated with mild proteinuria; usually they are clinically silent.[38] The patients with membranous or mesangiocapillary glomerulonephritis often develop a nephrotic syndrome which may resolve after the renal cell carcinoma is removed.[39]

The pathogenesis of these glomerular changes is not understood. Attempts to implicate tumour or renal tubular antigens have failed.[39]

Prognosis

Renal cell carcinoma is notoriously unpredictable in its behaviour. In attempting to determine the prognosis the extent to which the tumour has spread is the most important factor. The histological grade gives little guidance. Morphometry and cytometry are still at the development stage; their value, if any, in assessing expected survival in individual cases after nephrectomy for renal cell carcinoma is not yet known (see below).

Stage of tumour spread

The staging system that currently is in general use was proposed by Robson and his colleagues in 1969;[42] it remains popular because of its simplicity. The systems proposed by the American Joint Committee for Cancer (AJCC)[43] and the Union Internationale contre le Cancer (UICC)[44] are more complex and consequently less widely used.

Robson system There are four stages in the Robson system:

Stage I Tumour confined to the kidney.
Stage II Tumour extends through the renal capsule, invades the perinephric fat but is contained within the renal fascia (Gerota's fascia).

Stage III Tumour has invaded the renal vein or the regional lymph nodes or both, with or without involvement of the vena cava or perinephric fat.

Stage IV Tumour has metastasized to distant sites (including distant lymph nodes) or has extended through the renal fascia to involve contiguous structures.

When 5-year and 10-year survival rates after radical nephrectomy are assessed according to this staging system they are 65% and 56%, respectively, for stage I carcinoma; 47% and 20%, respectively, for stage II carcinoma; 51% and 37%, respectively, for stage III carcinoma; and 8% and 7%, respectively, for stage IV carcinoma.[4]

These survival rates immediately highlight the great shortcoming of Robson's staging system. Patients with renal vein involvement but without involvement of perinephric fat or lymph nodes often have survival rates that are similar to those in patients with stage I disease.[45] Inclusion of these patients in stage III accounts for the anomalous overall 5-year and 10 year survival rates for this stage that exceed those for stage II. It is now generally agreed that the single most important prognostic factor is extension into the perinephric tissues.

TNM (tumour, nodes, metastases) classification of UICC There are also four stages in the TNM classification:

Stage I Tumour 2.5 cm or less in greatest dimension, limited to the kidney (T1). No regional lymph nodes involved (NO). No distant metastases (MO).

Stage II Tumour more than 2.5 cm in greatest dimension, limited to the kidney (T2). Metastases in single lymph node 2 cm or less in greatest dimension (N1). No distant metastases (MO).

Stage III Tumour extends through the renal capsule but not beyond the renal fascia, or tumour extends into adrenal or renal vein (T3). Metastases in single lymph node more than 2 cm but not more than 5 cm in greatest dimension or involvement of multiple lymph nodes none more than 5 cm in greatest dimension (N2). No distant metastases (MO).

Stage IV Tumour extends beyond renal fascia (T4). Metastases in one or more lymph nodes 5 cm or more in greatest dimension (N3). Distant metastases (M1).

The worst prognostic features of a case decide the stage grouping, e.g. a T1 N2 tumour would be stage III. The TNM classification is used in Europe and in international trials of treatment. The universal acceptance of this system ensures that comparable groups of patients are treated, allowing a comparison between different methods. The main limitation of the classification is that the TNM stage assigned to a tumour will depend on the thoroughness of the clinical and radiological investigation, so this too has to be standardized in a therapeutic trial. The TNM classification has the same basic weakness as the Robson system in giving undue weight to renal vein involvement.

Histological grade

Histological grading is particularly difficult because the degree of cell differentiation often varies from one part of the tumour to the next. There is no uniformly accepted system for the histological grading of renal cell carcinoma. Various complex methods of analysis have been proposed but none has proved of great value in assessing prognosis. Statistical analysis has shown that the grade of nuclear pleomorphism has a significant bearing on survival.[46] Nevertheless, histological grading remains far less important than accurate staging in determining prognosis.

There may be a limited role for histological grading in determining which Robson's stage I tumours are likely to metastasize. Reliable forecasts have been claimed when the grading has been done by a single very experienced histopathologist working at a single institution.[47]

Morphometry and cytometry

Computed cell morphometry should reduce some of the problems of subjectivity and reproducibility in histological grading. Early attempts to use this technique to analyse Robson stage I tumours have been promising.[48]

Flow cytometry has been used to analyse the nuclear DNA patterns in renal cell carcinoma. Several studies have shown a correlation between nuclear DNA ploidy and tumour stage. It has also been reported that in Robson stage I tumours the existence of abnormal nuclear DNA histogram patterns correlates significantly with the subsequent development of metastases.[49]

Pathogenesis

Classic renal cell carcinoma (as distinct from some of the variants such as papillary renal cell carcinoma and collecting duct carcinoma of the kidney) is thought to arise from differentiated cells of the proximal renal tubules. This is based on electron microscopic features and on histochemical and immunohistochemical evidence.[22] The events that lead to malignant transformation of these cells are not known.

Inherited[19,20] and sporadic[27,50] renal cell carcinomas are both characterized by the loss of alleles at loci on the short arm (p) of chromosome 3. The variability of the breakpoint between 3p11.2 and 3p13 and the absence of a consistently translocated segment from another chromosome suggest deletion of a recessive tumour suppressor gene. This gene may be responsible for the regulation of normal growth of proximal tubular cells. The functional loss of both its alleles may permit neoplastic proliferation of these cells. A fuller understanding of the molecular biology of renal cell carcinoma and its phenotypic variants must await cloning of the putative renal cell tumour suppressor gene.

The role of environmental factors in initiating these events in sporadic renal cell carcinoma is not known. Regular consumption of phenacetin-containing analgesic mixtures appears to double the risk of developing a renal cell carcinoma.[51,52] The carcinogenic effect of phenacetin is thought to result from the potent alkylating action of the N-O sulphate and glucuronide conjugates of N-hydroxyphenacetin (see p. 462).[53]

Variants

The wide range of histological patterns encountered in renal cell carcinomas has tempted many authors to subclassify this neoplasm, mostly with little practical benefit. Variants that are currently recognized are papillary, chromophobe, sarcomatoid and collecting duct renal carcinoma. Only in the papillary variant is there evidence of a karyotypic difference from the more common forms of renal cell carcinoma. There is reliable evidence that the sarcomatoid variant is associated with a poor prognosis; anecdotal evidence indicates that the collecting duct variant may also have a poor outcome. It has been suggested that the papillary and chromophobe variants have a better survival rate but evidence for this is equivocal.

Papillary renal cell carcinoma

Papillary structures comprise at least 50% of the tumour in approximately 15% of renal cell carcinomas.[54] These cases differ from other forms of renal cell carcinoma not only in their morphological characteristics, but also in their karyotype and perhaps in their prognosis.

Clinical features The clinical features, sex and age distribution of papillary renal cell carcinomas do not differ significantly from those in non-papillary tumours. Angiographically they appear avascular or very hypovascular and radiologically about a third show calcification at the periphery of the tumour.

Gross appearance of the tumour[54,55] The most striking macroscopic feature of the tumour is the presence of massive necrosis which is seen in more than two-thirds of the cases; this is accompanied in many by marked cystic degeneration and complete or almost complete capsule formation. Hence the terms cystadenocarcinoma[56] and papillary cystic carcinoma which are sometimes applied to this variant.

Light microscopy[54,55] Microscopically the viable tumour is often composed entirely of papillary structures; in the others there are tubular areas. The papillae are usually covered by a single row of cells which in about half the cases have scanty cytoplasm (Fig. 16.4). In many of the tumours the vascularized connective tissue stalks of the papillae are infiltrated by numerous macro-

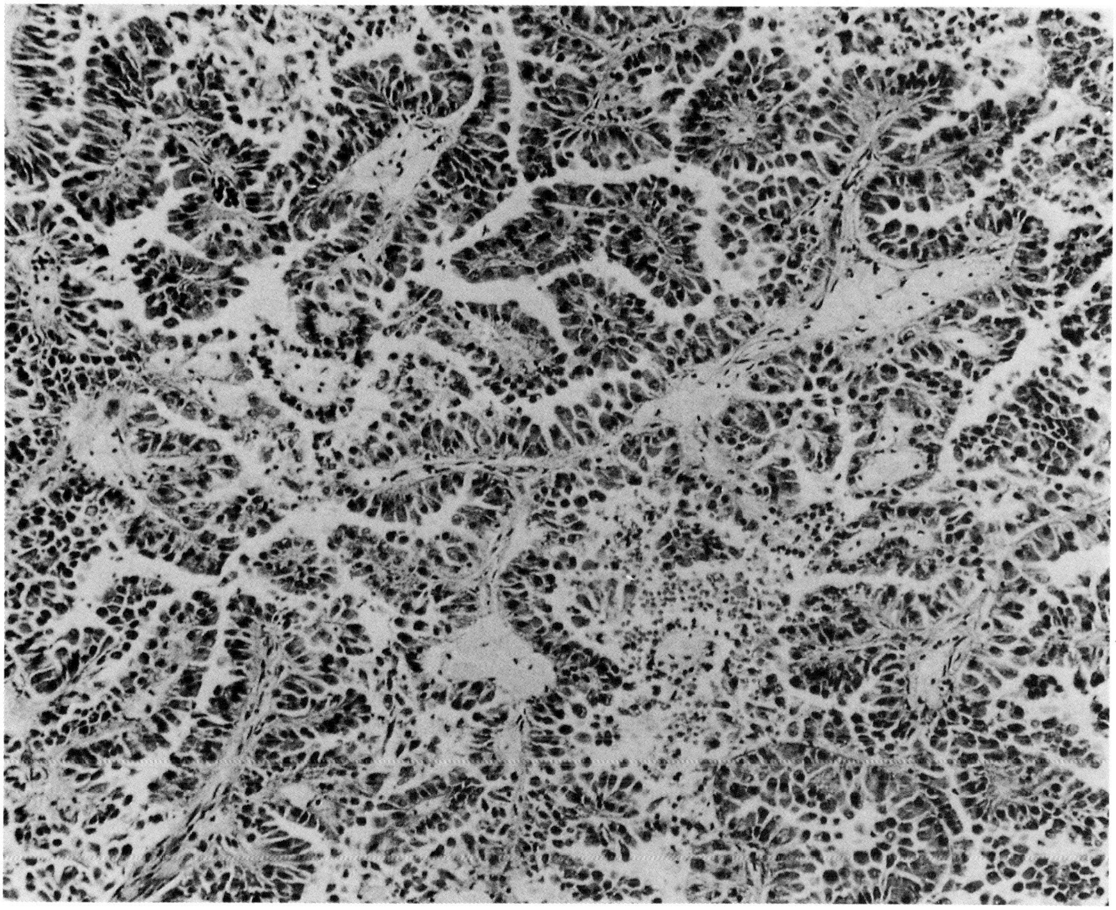

Fig. 16.4 Papillary renal cell carcinoma composed of papillae with delicate connective tissue cores covered by a single layer of epithelial cells.
Haematoxylin-eosin × 150
Reproduced by permission from: Mancilla-Jimenez R, Stanley RJ, Blath RA. Cancer 1976;38:2469 (Fig. 6)

phages with foamy cytoplasm (Fig. 16.5) and sometimes also with lymphocytes, granulocytes or both. Focal calcification and psammoma bodies are sometimes present. There is often extensive cellular infiltration around the fibrous capsule of the tumour.

Immunohistochemistry The few papillary renal cell carcinomas that have been studied have expressed antigens characteristic for distal and collecting tubules of the normal kidney. The tumour cells contain cytokeratin; most lack vimentin.[56,57] It is not yet known whether they stain for the renal cell carcinoma-associated antigen G250 (see p. 574).

Cytogenetics Cytogenetic studies show that papillary renal cell carcinomas differ from the non-papillary forms of this cancer in that they fail to show any rearrangement of the chromosome 3p segment or trisomy of the 5q 22-qter segment. Also they show trisomy of chromosome 17 which does not occur in non-papillary renal cell carcinoma.[55]

Prognosis Patients with papillary renal cell carcinoma have been reported as having a much better survival rate at 5 years than those with non-papillary tumours. This is mainly because at the time of diagnosis 85% of papillary renal cell carcinomas are still at Robson's stage I, but even

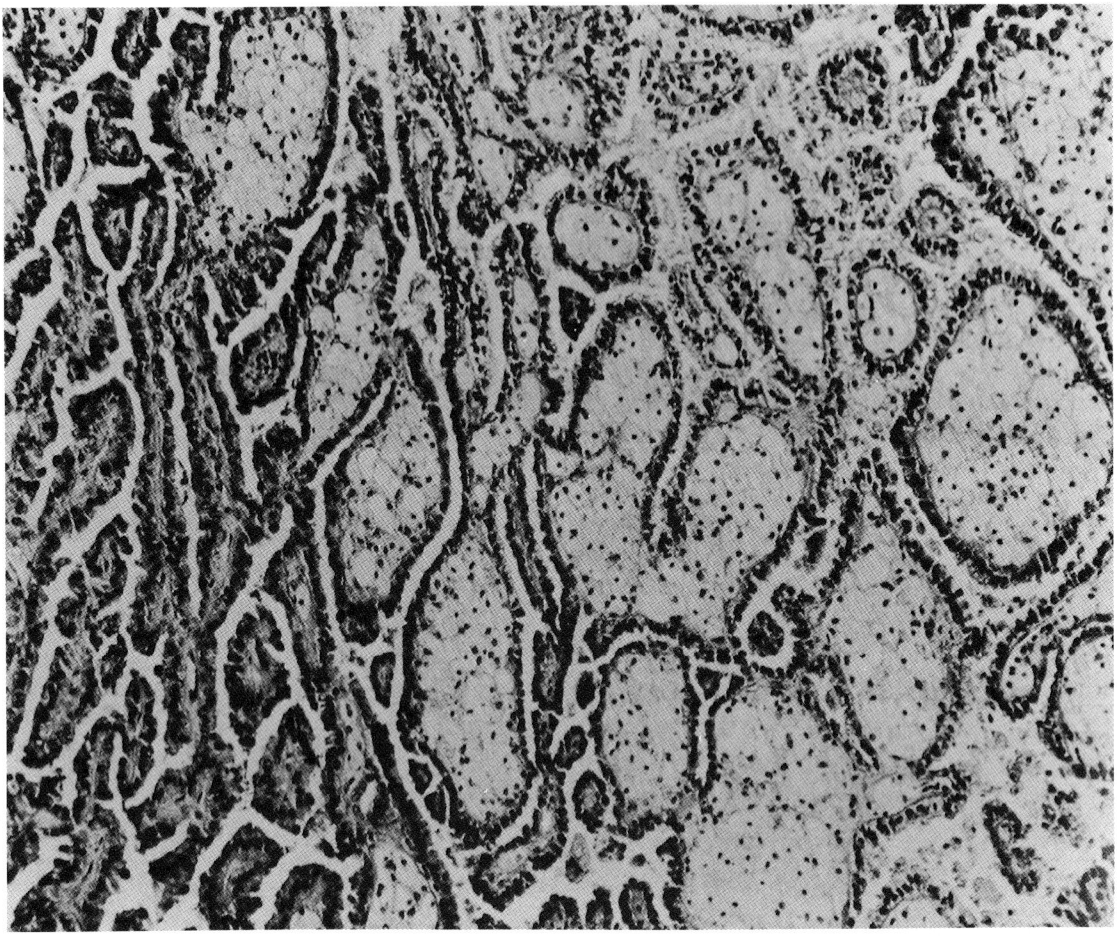

Fig. 16.5 Papillary renal cell carcinoma. The papillary structures are covered by small basophilic cells. The connective tissue stalks are expanded and infiltrated by numerous macrophages with foamy cytoplasm.
Haematoxylin-eosin × 150
Reproduced by permission from: Mancilla-Jimenez R, Stanley RJ, Blath RA. Cancer 1976;38:2469 (Fig. 8)

stage by stage the survival curve for papillary renal cell carcinoma is slightly better than that for the usual types of renal cell carcinoma.[54]

Chromophobe renal cell carcinoma[58]

In approximately 5% of renal cell carcinomas the cytoplasm of the tumour cells stains positively with Hale's acid iron colloid which detects polyanionic compounds. Both clear and granular cells may show this staining reaction. The term chromophobe renal cell carcinoma has been used to describe this group of tumours. It is claimed that they also differ from other renal cell carcinomas in having an abundance of microvesicles in their cytoplasm.

Like oncocytomas (see p. 583) and papillary renal carcinomas (see p. 578), they are said to contain cytokeratin but not vimentin; this is in contrast to other non-papillary renal cell carcinomas which stain for both intermediate filaments. It is not known whether chromophobe tumours stain for the renal cell carcinoma-associated antigen G250 (see p. 574). There are no reports of cytogenetic or genotyping studies on these cases.

Follow-up suggests that the prognosis may be better than for most renal cell carcinomas but the number of patients studied is very small and the period of observation short. Information about this variant has come entirely from one centre; so far there have been no reports, confirmatory or otherwise, from elsewhere.

Sarcomatoid renal cell carcinoma[2]

Approximately 2% of renal cell carcinomas either contain large foci of poorly differentiated cells that resemble sarcoma cells or are almost entirely composed of such cells (Fig. 16.6). These so-called sarcomatoid renal cell carcinomas most commonly contain spindle cells with many mitoses and the deposition of collagen; they may closely resemble a malignant fibrous histiocytoma or a fibrosarcoma. Sometimes they are composed of strap-like cells, giant cells and multinucleate giant cells intermixed with the spindle cells and they may mimic a rhabdomyosarcoma. Less frequently they look like liposarcomas or leiomyosarcomas.

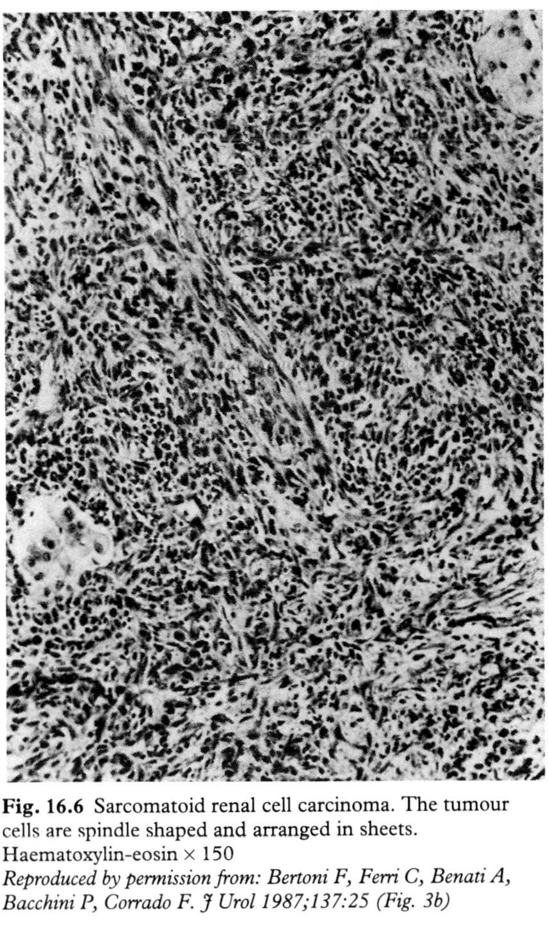

Fig. 16.6 Sarcomatoid renal cell carcinoma. The tumour cells are spindle shaped and arranged in sheets. Haematoxylin-eosin × 150
Reproduced by permission from: Bertoni F, Ferri C, Benati A, Bacchini P, Corrado F. J Urol 1987;137:25 (Fig. 3b)

Sarcomatoid renal cell carcinomas resemble typical renal cell carcinomas in that they express both cytokeratin and vimentin (see p. 574).[57,59] It is not known whether they contain the renal cell carcinoma-associated G250 antigen (see p. 574). There is no information about the karyotyping of these tumours and whether they show aberrations of chromosome 3.

The distinctive feature of sarcomatoid renal cell carcinoma is the presence of some ordinary clear or granular renal cell carcinoma. However, the quantity of such tissue may be very small, and difficult to find, and the differential diagnosis can be very demanding. They have to be distinguished from primary renal sarcomas (see p. 602), pleomorphic transitional cell carcinomas of the renal pelvis (see p. 609), nephroblastoma (see p. 590) and various secondary tumours. The adult nephroblastoma usually has a distinctive mixture of immature or embryonal renal structures (see p. 590). Sarcomatoid renal cell carcinomas can often be distinguished from a sarcoma by the presence of microvilli on the cell surfaces of the former. The expression of cytokeratin and anti-epithelial membrane antigen by sarcomatoid renal cell carcinomas and not by sarcomas is another distinguishing feature,[57] but the results of staining to demonstrate them can be equivocal.

The prognosis is poor. Sarcomatoid renal cell carcinomas are highly malignant. In about half the patients the tumour is at Robson's stage IV when the diagnosis is made. Nephrectomy appears to be ineffective – in one series 86% of the patients died within 1 year of operation;[60] in another series the median postoperative survival was 6.3 months.[61]

Collecting duct carcinoma of the kidney[62,63]

It is postulated that about 2% of renal cell carcinomas arise from the collecting ducts. The most common symptom is gross haematuria. Macroscopically the tumour mass is usually firm, grey, poorly circumscribed and lies in the renal medulla with irregular extensions into the adjacent cortex. Massive necrosis or haemorrhage is not a feature.

Microscopically the main tumour is a papillary adenocarcinoma with minimal nuclear pleomorphism and infrequent mitoses; the extensions into the adjacent renal parenchyma are tubular, with considerable nuclear pleomorphism and many mitoses and a marked fibroblastic interstitial reaction. Atypical hyperplastic changes are present in the epithelium lining the medullary collecting ducts; in a few cases these changes amount to carcinoma in situ.

The few tumours that have been studied have expressed antigens characteristic for distal and collecting tubules of the normal kidney. The tumour cells contain cytokeratin and vimentin.[63,64] Cytogenetic and genotyping studies have not been reported.

In a series of seven cases, four of the patients were at Robson's stage III or IV at presentation and three died of the disease within 3½ years.[63,64]

Evidence that these tumours arise from collecting ducts is indirect.

ONCOCYTOMA

An oncocytoma is a neoplasm composed predominantly of oncocytes, i.e. large cells with abundant eosinophilic finely granular cytoplasm that contains large numbers of mitochondria. Oncocytomas probably account for approximately 7% of all renal parenchymal neoplasms,[65] but with increasing use of computed tomography and awareness of the tumour more cases are being recognized each year. They usually behave as benign tumours. Most are found in patients aged 50–80 years but they may occur in people as young as 15 years; they are twice to three times as common in men as in women.

Clinical features

The majority of oncocytomas do not produce symptoms; they are diagnosed incidentally during radiological study or surgical exploration for an unrelated disease or they are discovered at autopsy. Occasionally they produce flank pain, haematuria and a renal mass. Rarely they have been associated with the nephrotic syndrome or hypertension. There are no pathognomonic angiographic patterns but about half have a radiating arterial arrangement.[66] On computed tomography scans they have almost homogeneous enhancement.[67]

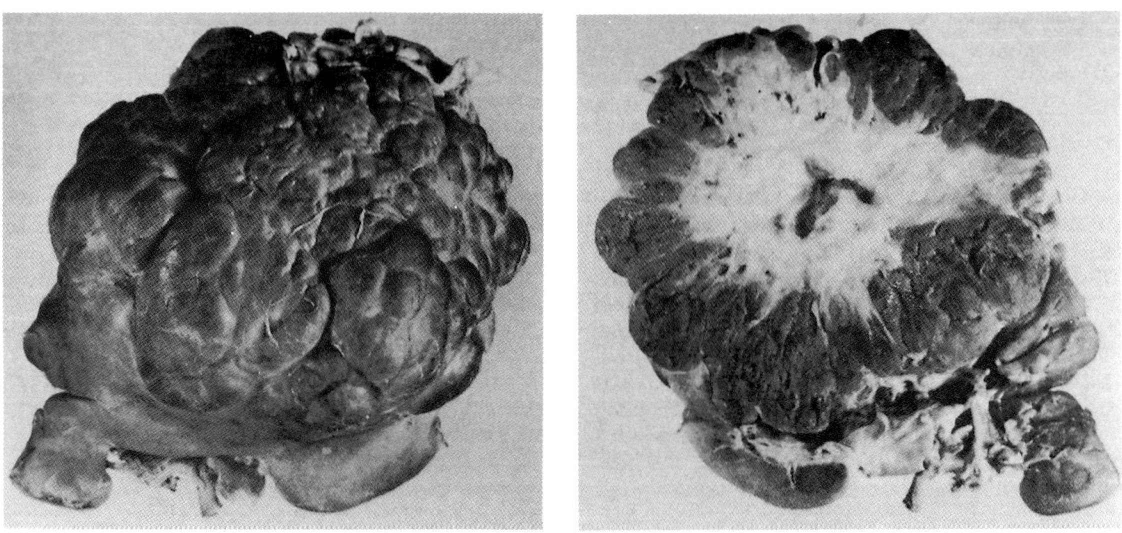

a b

Fig. 16.7 Oncocytoma. (**a**) External bosselated surface of tumour. (**b**) Cut surface showing central fibrous region and radiating bands of fibrous tissue.
Reproduced by permission from: Eble JN, Hull MT. Hum Pathol 1984;15:1054 (Fig. 1)

Renal changes

Gross appearance of the kidneys

Oncocytomas are usually well circumscribed, homogeneous and reddish-brown. Sometimes when the tumour is cut a central stellate region of fibrosis can be seen (Fig. 16.7); haemorrhage and necrosis are noticeably absent. When discovered most of the tumours are 5–10 cm in diameter. In approximately 10% of cases the tumours are multiple;[68] they are bilateral in about 3%.[69] In one patient innumerable small oncocytomas were scattered throughout both kidneys.[70]

Light microscopy

The tumour consists of sheets and groups of big cells each with large amounts of eosinophilic finely granular cytoplasm and a round to oval central vesicular nucleus (Fig. 16.8). Sometimes the cells are arranged in tubules and trabeculae; clusters of oncocytes embedded in oedematous stroma may be present. Nuclear pleomorphism is rare. Mitotic figures are not seen.[71]

Electron microscopy

The cytoplasm contains huge numbers of abnormally large, round, densely packed mitochondria rich in cristae (Fig. 16.9). Blunt microvilli are usually present on some cell surfaces; brush borders of parallel microvilli do not occur.[71,72]

Immunohistochemistry

Renal oncocytomas usually express antigens characteristic for distal and collecting tubules of the normal kidney; some express antigens associated with proximal tubular epithelium.[23] The tumour cells contain cytokeratin but lack vimentin.[24]

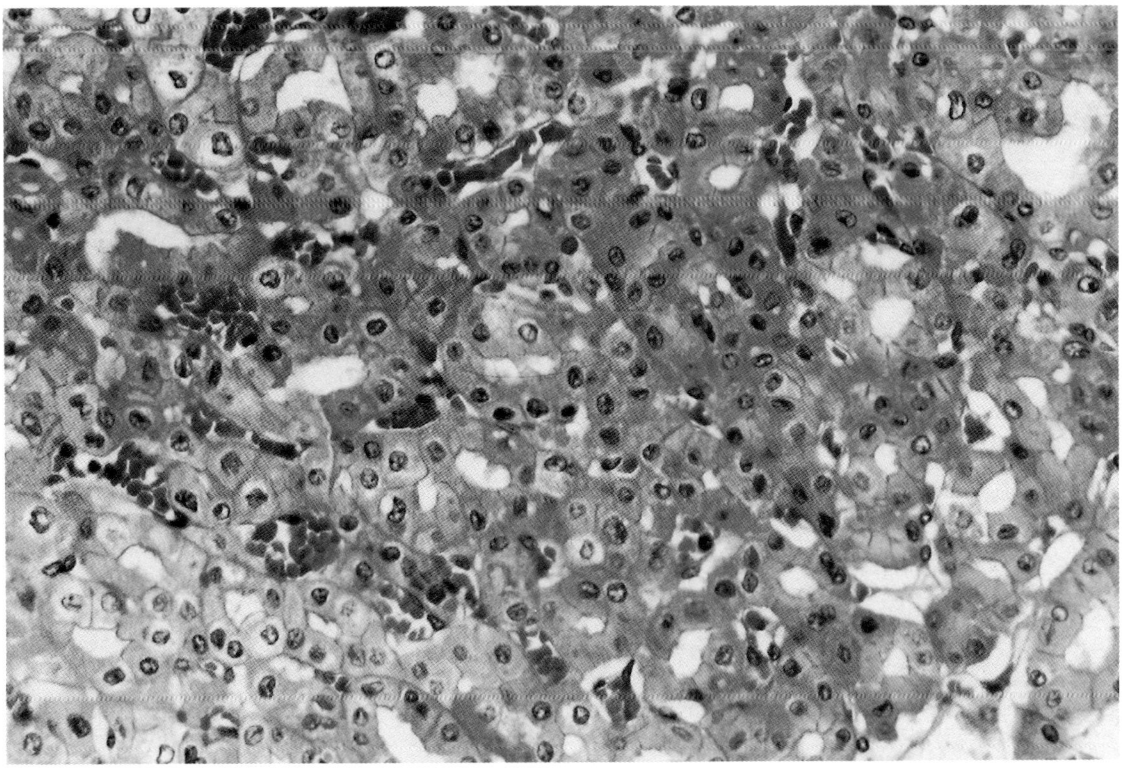

Fig. 16.8 Oncocytoma. Large cells with abundant eosinophilic cytoplasm and round nuclei are arranged in tubules, trabeculae and small nests.
Haematoxylin-eosin × 225

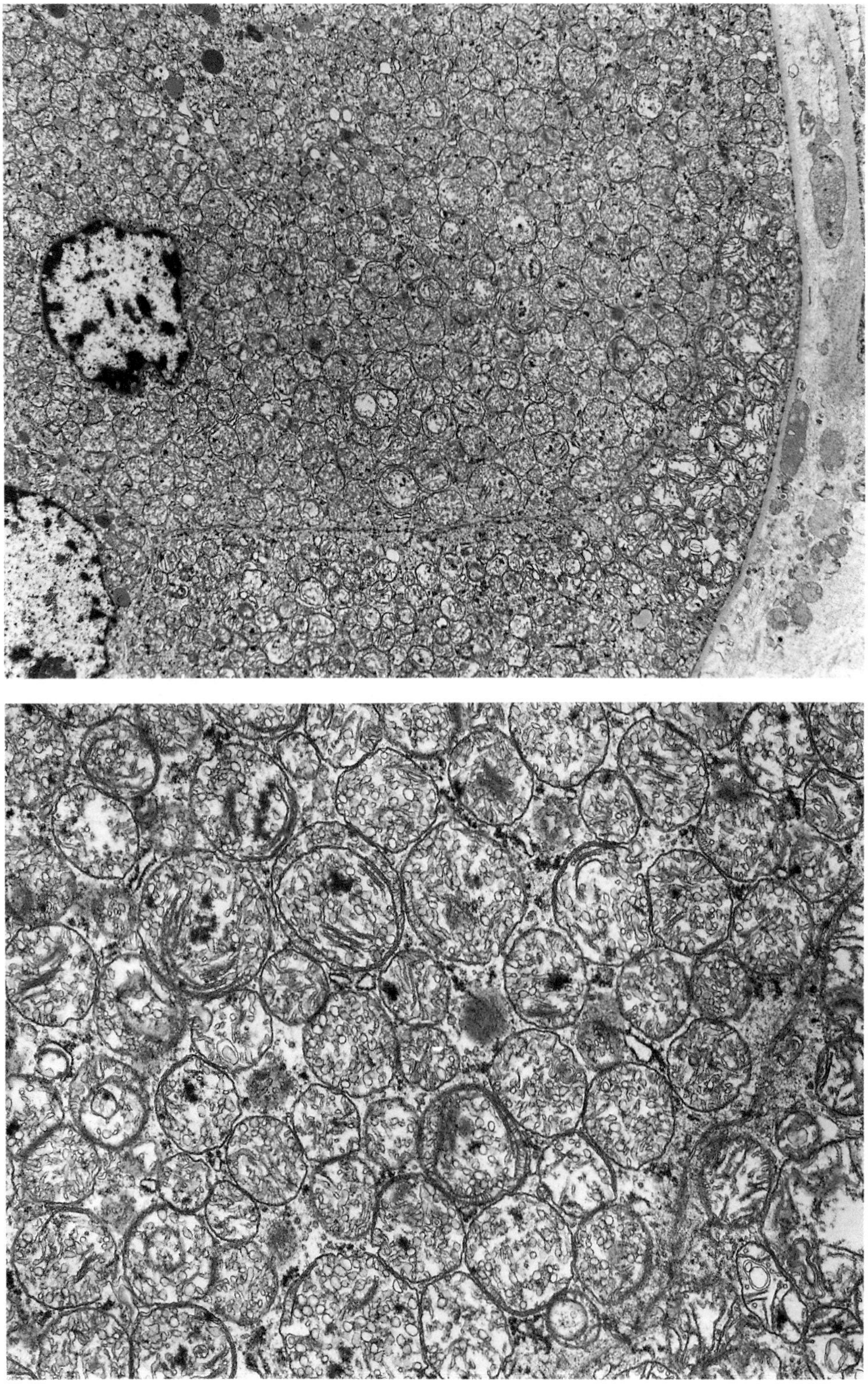

Fig. 16.9 a, b Oncocytoma. Electron micrograph of tumour cell. The cytoplasm is full of mitochondria. (**a**) × 5795; (**b**) 21 525

Cytogenetic analysis

Of the few oncocytomas that have been analysed cytogenetically most have shown a mosaic pattern of normal and aberrant karyotypes with no common abnormalities.[73] One tumour showed a structural chromosomal rearrangement t(9;11) (p23;q12) as the only change; this might be primary and just possibly specific for oncocytoma.[74]

Genotyping

No recurrent chromosome aberration and no rearrangement of the short arm (p) of chromosome 3 occur in renal oncocytoma; this is in contrast to non-papillary renal cell carcinoma where there is deletion of specific chromosome 3p segments and loss of heterozygosity for loci at 3p (see p. 574). Restriction analysis of the mitochondrial DNA has revealed a new autoradiographic band of about 50 basepairs in size occurring exclusively in oncocytomas.[73]

Spread

Renal oncocytoma is considered to be a benign tumour but there are a few reports of extension into perinephric tissue,[75,76] colon[77] and veins.[78] Metastases have been occasionally reported but usually in so-called grade II renal oncocytoma; these are cases showing foci in which there are atypical nuclei and variation in cell size and configuration.[75] In one case with spread to the cervical lymph nodes mitotic figures were present in the primary renal tumour;[79] most investigators would maintain that if this feature is present the tumour should have been classified as a renal cell carcinoma.

Differential diagnosis

Because the typical course of an oncocytoma differs markedly from that of a renal cell carcinoma (see below), separation of oncocytomas from other renal neoplasms is of great importance.

The diagnosis is usually not difficult when the clinical picture and the gross and microscopic features are considered. Tumours showing mitotic activity, foci of necrosis, or cells with clear cytoplasm and widespread atypical nuclei should not be called oncocytomas.

However, there are still times when a distinction between renal cell carcinoma, carcinoid and renal oncocytoma may be difficult because large cells with granular cytoplasm are also occasionally present in the first two of these conditions.[72] In these cases electron microscopy usually enables a differentiation to be made. If appropriately fixed material is not available this technique can still be undertaken using formalin-fixed paraffin-embedded tissue after reprocessing.

In the few cases in which electron microscopy is not conclusive,[72] monoclonal antibodies recognizing intermediate sized filaments should be used. Oncocytomas only express cytokeratin. No staining reaction occurs for vimentin, in contrast to its invariable expression in renal cell carcinoma (see p. 574).[23,24]

If for any reason the results of immunohistochemical studies are equivocal then the characteristic restriction pattern of mitochondrial DNA in renal oncocytoma should be sought.[73]

Definitive diagnosis of oncocytoma by frozen section is potentially hazardous because in a renal cell carcinoma there may be large areas which by light microscopy are compatible with oncocytoma. Similarly, needle biopsies and aspirates can also lead to the wrong diagnosis.

Complications

Instances of haemorrhage into an oncocytoma and the occurrence of an oncocytoma in one kidney and a renal cell carcinoma in the other kidney[76] have been reported. High erythropoietin levels and erythrocytosis were present in one case with multiple bilateral oncocytomas; both abnormalities were reversed after removal of the tumours.[80]

Prognosis

Renal oncocytoma usually follows a benign clinical course. A favourable prognosis may still be anticipated even if multiple tumours are present in the kidney so long as none of them are renal cell carcinomas.

The relatively small number of oncocytomas that show atypical nuclei and variation in cell size and configuration (so-called grade II tumours), however, are potentially malignant. In one series 14% of grade II renal oncocytomas eventually metastasized.[76] It may be that grade II oncocytomas are really renal cell carcinomas with oncocytic features; increasing application of cytogenetic analysis and genotyping should resolve this question.

Flow cytometry

Flow cytometry performed on 51 specimens from the archives showed that 39% of renal oncocytomas had an increase in the tetraploid DNA peak, while 11% showed a distinct aneuploid peak.[81]

Pathogenesis

Renal oncocytomas arise from differentiated renal tubular cells. Immunohistochemical studies show that these tumours predominantly stain for distal tubular antigens and it is therefore thought that the majority are derived from distal tubular epithelium.[23,82] In a few cases staining with lectins has suggested a proximal tubular origin.[83]

For the development of an oncocytoma all that may be needed is a small submicroscopic chromosomal deletion, a mutation, or a gene conversion. Another possibility is that a mitotic recombination occurs that is not detectable by cytogenetic methods or molecular genetic approaches using the DNA probes currently available.[73] What induces the initial change is not known.

Variant

A renal oncocytoma with the unusual gross appearance of a cystic tumour has been described.[84] The cysts were multiple and ranged from 0.1 to 1.6 cm in diameter. They were filled with either clear or blood-stained fluid.

Microscopically much of the tumour was composed of varying sized dilated tubuloalveolar structures lined by typical oncocytes, their cytoplasm packed with mitochondria. There was no evidence of prior necrosis to account for the cysts.

'ADENOMA'

Small, well-defined, rounded, yellowish nodules are common findings in the renal cortex. Approximately 7% of adults examined at autopsy have such nodules.[85] Microscopically they are mostly well differentiated glandular tumours; their ultrastructural and immunocytochemical features suggest a proximal tubular origin.[86] They often show papillary proliferation but cystic, tubular, acinar, trabecular and solid patterns are also found; clear cells and granular cells may occur alone or together in these nodules (Fig. 16.10).

Traditionally such tumours have been regarded as adenomas. However, there are no light microscopic, histochemical or electron microscopic features that distinguish these glandular tumours

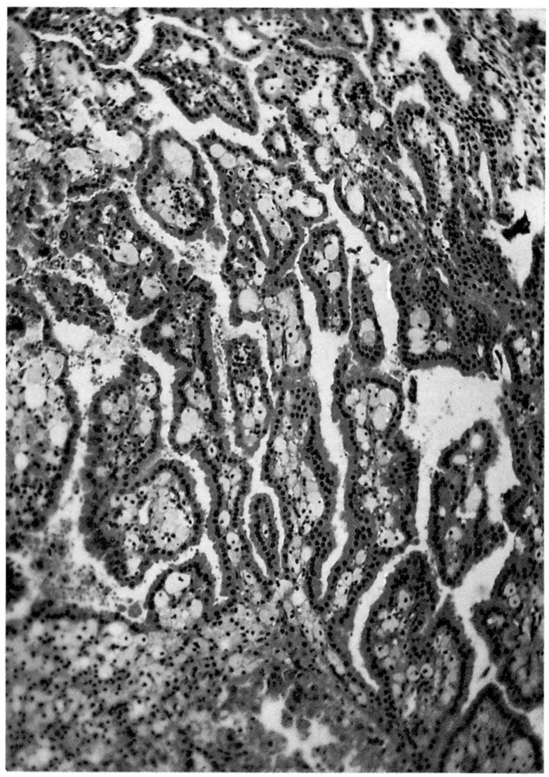

Fig. 16.10 Small papillary 'adenoma' of the renal cortex. For the most part the villous processes are covered by a single layer of epithelium. There are lipid-containing macrophages in the stroma of the processes. Haematoxylin-eosin × 105

from renal cell carcinoma. Like renal cell carcinomas they are much more common in males, they are only rarely found in people under 30 years old and they show an increasing incidence with age. The development of these small renal epithelial tumours is associated with renal scarring; adenomas are not independent age-related phenomena.[87]

This failure to be able to distinguish between renal adenoma and carcinoma means that in an individual case deciding whether a particular cortical tumour is likely to metastasize is impossible. When a small glandular tumour is found at autopsy whether one calls it an adenoma or a renal cell carcinoma that has not yet produced metastases is of little significance. However, if the tumour is found at surgery the terminology becomes all important. A diagnosis of renal adenoma in these cases does not warn the clinician that such tumours occasionally metastasize; the diagnosis of renal cell carcinoma brings foreboding to the patient, may have wide implications within the family and interferes with the patient's ability to obtain insurance.

On balance it is now widely accepted that all 'adenomas', regardless of size, should be considered Robson's stage I renal cell carcinomas (see p. 576).[88] If the tumour is tiny, and the cells are uniform and the acini regular, nephrectomy is not indicated. When the tumour is larger or more variable in structure nephrectomy may be indicated. An arbitrary separation on a basis of size (3 cm in diameter) is unsatisfactory – small growths may certainly metastasize. Because of the uncertainty of their behaviour, all cases of renal cell tumour should be carefully followed up.

Cytogenetic analysis

It is not yet known what proportion of small well-differentiated renal cortical glandular tumours have the recurrent deletion of the short arm of one of the two homologous chromosomes 3 that characterizes renal cell carcinomas (see p. 574). A recent study of large 'adenomas' in three men found that each tumour showed a consistent combination of recurrent chromosomal abnormalities: tetrasomy 7 (+7, +7), trisomy 17 (+17) and loss of the Y chromosome (–Y).[89] None of the tumours showed alterations of chromosomes 3p and 5q, the most common changes in renal cell carcinomas (see p. 574). If these findings are corroborated they may provide a means of defining a subgroup of 'adenomas' which have a benign course and differentiating them from renal cell carcinoma.

EMBRYONAL TUMOURS OF THE RENAL PARENCHYMA

NEPHROBLASTOMA (WILMS' TUMOUR)

Nephroblastomas are malignant tumours of primitive nephroblastic tissue which form structures resembling those of embryonic kidney.[90] They occur predominantly in children, constituting approximately 6% of all cancers (including leukaemia and lymphomas) in patients less than 15 years of age.[91] The tumour is seen in all parts of the world with a remarkably constant, stable incidence of 7.7 cases annually per million children under 15 years.[91] Males and females are affected equally. Most nephroblastomas are discovered before the age of 7 years; the maximum incidence occurs in the first 4 years with a peak at the age of 3 years – only 15% are recognized in the first year of life.[92] Very occasionally a nephroblastoma becomes evident in an adult.[93] The tumour may occur in families (see p. 589); such cases have an earlier mean age at diagnosis. It may sometimes be associated with congenital abnormalities, in particular aniridia and hemihypertrophy (see below – 'Predisposing factors').

The outlook for patients with this tumour is good, largely because of the efficacy of nephrectomy followed by combined treatment with actinomycin D, vincristin and radiotherapy. The 4-year survival rate for cases in which the tumour is confined to the kidney is 96%; even for those with metastases at the time of diagnosis it is 73%.[94]

Clinical features

An abdominal mass is often the only sign of the tumour, but there may be fever, abdominal pain, anorexia, nausea and vomiting. Hypertension has been observed in many cases; in some it has been shown to be associated with secretion of renin by the tumour.[95] Most patients have high levels of renin in their plasma, but most of this is biologically inactive prorenin. There is direct evidence that the renin is synthesized by the tumour.[96] Microscopic haematuria occurs in up to one-third of cases but gross haematuria is uncommon. Occasionally the tumour may press on the inferior vena cava and cause ascites and leg oedema. Venous obstruction can also lead to the sudden appearance of a varicocele. Metastases are present in about a quarter of the patients and may be the presenting manifestation.

Intravenous pyelography is the most helpful radiological procedure to differentiate nephroblastoma from other causes of an abdominal mass; there is usually distortion of the calyces with splaying of contrast medium around the tumour. Ultrasonography or computed tomography will determine whether the mass is solid or cystic and also indicate involvement of other organs. As the most common site of metastases from a nephroblastoma is the lungs, chest X-ray and lung tomography are indicated. Needle biopsy should be avoided; it increases the risk of tumour dissemination.

Predisposing factors

Several uncommon congenital malformations, inherited and non-inherited, are associated with an increased risk of nephroblastoma. The most frequent are sporadic aniridia, hemihypertrophy, pseudohermaphroditism with glomerulonephritis (Drash syndrome), Beckwith–Wiedemann syndrome and horseshoe kidney (see p. 57). Rarely a dominantly inherited chromosomal aberration confers a high risk of developing a nephroblastoma on members of the family.

Infants in whom foci of embryonic metanephric tissue persist after the end of nephrogenesis (approximately 36 weeks' gestation) probably have a higher risk of developing a nephroblastoma than those born without such foci in their kidneys. The various forms of persistent renal blastema are grouped under the general heading of nephroblastomatosis (see pp. 589, 595).

Sporadic aniridia[97]

Complete or partial absence of the iris appears in the general population with a frequency of approximately 1 : 82 000; the frequency among children with nephroblastoma is 1 : 50 and the frequency of nephroblastoma among children with aniridia is 1 : 3. The majority of children with both nephroblastoma and aniridia have hemizygous constitutional deletions on the short arm (p) of chromosome 11, with 11p13 the region most commonly involved.

Hemihypertrophy

Enlargement of a portion or an entire side of the body occurs in approximately 3% of patients with nephroblastoma.[98]

Pseudohermaphroditism and the Drash syndrome

The frequency of dysgenic male pseudohermaphroditism in children with nephroblastoma is approximately 1 : 180.[98] Although the association of these two conditions may occur without other abnormalities it is more common to find a nephropathy as well as the nephroblastoma and dysgenic male pseudohermaphroditism. The combination of the three anomalies is commonly known as the Drash syndrome after the first-named author of the paper in which it was first suggested that these anomalies were linked and constituted a syndrome.[99] The glomerulopathy is usually diffuse mesangial sclerosis (see p. 84);[100] it manifests itself very early, between the ages of 2 weeks and 18 months. Most patients present with the nephrotic syndrome, often with hypertension. Progression to end-stage renal failure occurs within a few months to 2 years from the onset.[100] It has been suggested that patients with the nephropathy and only one of the other two components may have an incompletely expressed form of Drash's syndrome. In one such case where preoperative investigation and postoperative gross examination of the kidney had failed to provide any evidence of a tumour, serial slicing of the resected kidney revealed a nephroblastoma 0.5 cm in diameter.[101]

Beckwith–Wiedemann syndrome

The main features of the Beckwith–Wiedemann syndrome are exomphalos, macroglossia and gigantism; hydramnios and prematurity are also common. Nephroblastoma occurs more frequently in patients with this congenital syndrome than in other infants. The syndrome is associated with trisomy 11p15.[102]

Horseshoe kidney

Nephroblastomas are approximately twice as common in patients with horseshoe kidneys (see p. 57) than in the general population.[103] The reason for this is not known.

Familial nephroblastoma

Occasionally nephroblastomas occur in more than one member of a family, with siblings or cousins most often affected. Pedigrees imply autosomal dominant transmission in these cases. Familial nephroblastomas usually present earlier than sporadic nephroblastomas and are more likely to be bilateral.[104] The incidence of nephroblastomas in the children of successfully treated nephroblastoma patients appears to be very low, but the numbers studied have been small.[105] Genetic analysis of two families with a history of nephroblastomas suggests that in these cases the locus conferring the inherited predisposition to the tumour lies somewhere other than in the 11p13 and 11p15 regions of the short arm of chromosome 11.[106]

Nephroblastomatosis

The term nephroblastomatosis is most commonly used to describe abnormal persistence and focal accumulation in a kidney of blastemal cells with neoplastic potential.[107]

Microscopic nodules of embryonic nephrogenic tissue may persist into the postnatal period and are found in the kidneys in approximately 1% of routine autopsies on infants under 3 months of age[108] and in 25–40% of kidneys with nephroblastomas.[109] They are also found in increased numbers in association with sporadic aniridia, pseudohermaphroditism, the Beckwith–Wiedemann syndrome and trisomy 18 (Edwards' syndrome).[107] The terms *persistent renal blastema*[90] and *nephrogenic rests*[110] are usually used to describe these lesions. The nodules are most frequently composed of predominantly blastemal cells, but varying degrees of tubular differentiation occur. Stromal sclerosis is common; when marked the descriptive term *sclerosing metanephric hamartoma* is sometimes used.[111]

The nodules of persistent renal blastema are characteristically found at the periphery of the renal lobes, just beneath the renal capsule (perilobar nephrogenic rests); they may also occur in the centres of the columns of Bertin and in the medulla (intralobar nephrogenic rests). The perilobar nodules are almost always sharply demarcated from the adjacent cortex and are usually multifocal (Fig. 16.11); the intralobar nodules are often poorly demarcated and solitary.[110]

Most nodules of renal blastema remain dormant and gradually regress by progressive involutional sclerosis during early infancy. A few nodules undergo diffuse overgrowth, producing a grossly visible lesion. The hyperplasia may affect several nodules simultaneously and the enlarged nodules sometimes then fuse, forming a diffuse rind on the surface of the renal lobe. Some authors restrict the term nephroblastomatosis to these diffuse hyperplastic lesions that produce renal enlargement but preserve the normal shape of the kidney. The lesions have also been referred to as *massive renal blastema*.[90]

Occasionally a rapidly expanding focus of proliferation arises within either a dormant or a hyperplastic lesion of nephroblastomatosis. This compresses the remainder of the nodule and may form a grossly visible small nephroblastoma. It has been estimated that less than 1% of infants born with foci of persistent nodular renal blastema develop a nephroblastoma.[109] The risk is increased once a tumour has developed; in about 5% of cases with perilobar nodules and 16% of those with intralobar nodules in the resected kidney, a nephroblastoma develops subsequently in the remaining kidney.[109]

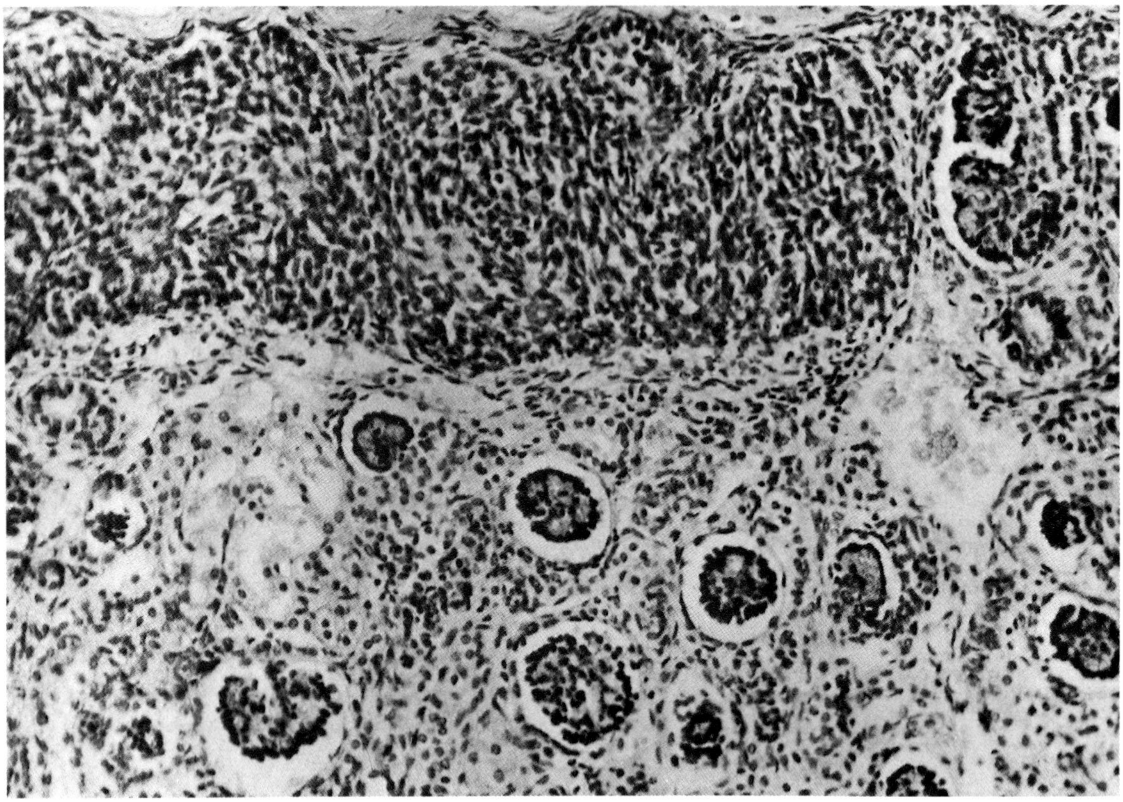

Fig. 16.11 Nephroblastomatosis. Persistent nodular renal blastema (perilobar nephrogenic rests). Several nodules of embryonic nephrogenic tissue are present beneath the renal capsule.
Haematoxylin-eosin × 100
Reproduced by permission from: Bennington JL, Beckwith JB. Atlas of tumor pathology, 2nd series, fascicle 12. Tumors of the kidney, renal pelvis, and ureter. Washington DC: Armed Forces Institute of Pathology, 1975 (Fig. 22)

Not all forms of nephroblastomatosis carry an increased risk of developing a nephroblastoma. For example, nodules of persistent renal blastema are very common in trisomy 18 but nephroblastomas are rare in this condition. Similarly, an exceedingly rare form of nephroblastomatosis, sometimes referred to as *pancortical diffuse nephroblastomatosis*,[90,111,112] does not appear to be linked with nephroblastoma.[107] The term nephroblastomatosis was first coined to describe this pancortical diffuse nephroblastosis,[112] which presents as a usually fatal symmetrical diffuse enlargement of the kidneys in a newborn infant. The entire renal parenchyma is composed of non-cystic abnormal nephrons interspersed with excess stroma and renal blastema. The renal changes are accompanied by congenital abnormalities in other organs. Pancortical diffuse nephroblastomatosis probably represents a genetically determined form of hyperplastic renal dysplasia or dysgenesis.[107]

Renal changes

Gross appearance of the kidneys[108]

Nephroblastomas are usually large (median diameter of tumour 12 cm) when first detected. The tumour is commonly soft; those with abundant stroma are firmer. The cut surface is white or grey and bulges; it is usually homogeneous but there may be cystic spaces (Fig. 16.12). Infrequently there are foci of haemorrhage or necrosis; calcification is rare. The tumour is often surrounded by a pseudocapsule. In some cases the growth can be seen to have spread into the perirenal tissue or into the renal vein or into both. Nephroblastomas

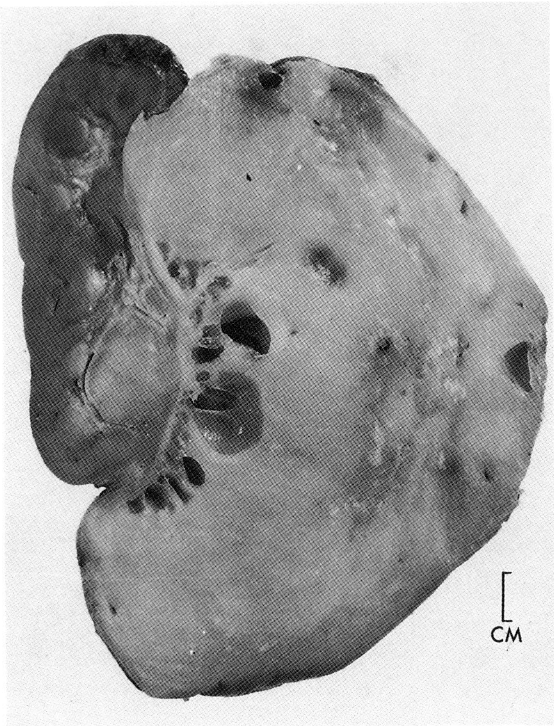

Fig. 16.12 Nephroblastoma. The tumour is large and pale, mostly homogeneous but in places cystic

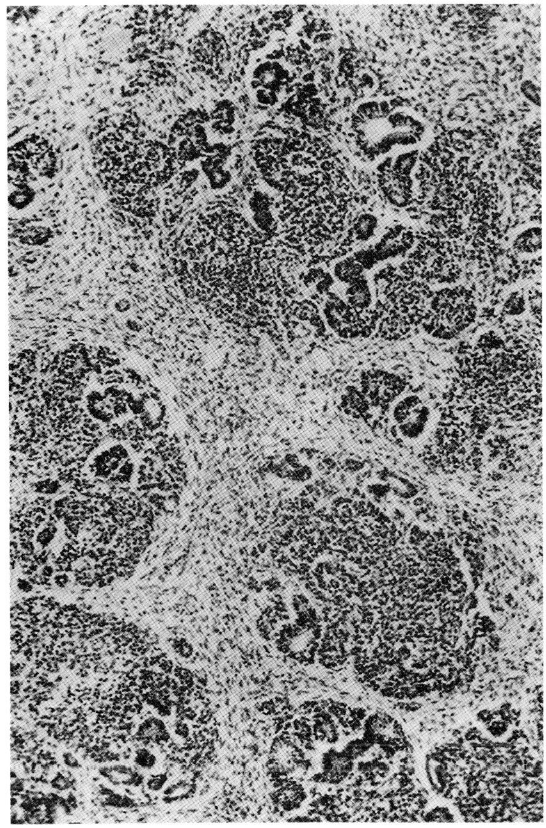

Fig. 16.13 Nephroblastoma. Islands of blastemal cells with scattered primitive tubules are surrounded by broad bands of stroma.
Haematoxylin-eosin × 60

are most commonly unilateral and solitary; they show no predilection for either kidney. The tumour is bilateral in about 5% of cases and multicentric in 7%.[91]

Light microscopy[108]

Nephroblastomas vary greatly in microscopical structure (Fig. 16.13). Typically there is a mixture of blastemal, stromal and epithelial elements; any one of these may predominate. Most tumours are of mixed histological pattern; approximately 22% are predominantly blastemal, 10% epithelial and 3% stromal. The blastemal cells are small, slightly oval, stain darkly with haematoxylin and eosin and have scanty cytoplasm. They are often closely packed together and arranged in nodules or trabeculae that are separated from one another by septa composed of stromal cells. The stromal cells are spindle shaped and embedded in varying amounts of matrix. The epithelium is primitive and often forms tubules; these are usually randomly distributed within and around trabeculae of blastemal cells. The tubules may mimic various stages in fetal development. Unvascularized glomeruloid structures are common.

Enclosed within tissue formed of these three main components there are commonly small clusters of tissue elements that are not normally seen in the kidneys at any stage of development. Of these skeletal muscle is the commonest (Fig. 16.14), but neural elements, cartilage, bone and other tissues occasionally occur.

Despite great differences in structure between individual nephroblastomas, most solitary tumours have a relatively uniform pattern. Multicentric tumours may have diverse microscopic appearances.

Approximately 7% of nephroblastomas show anaplasia as defined by cellular pleomorphism and

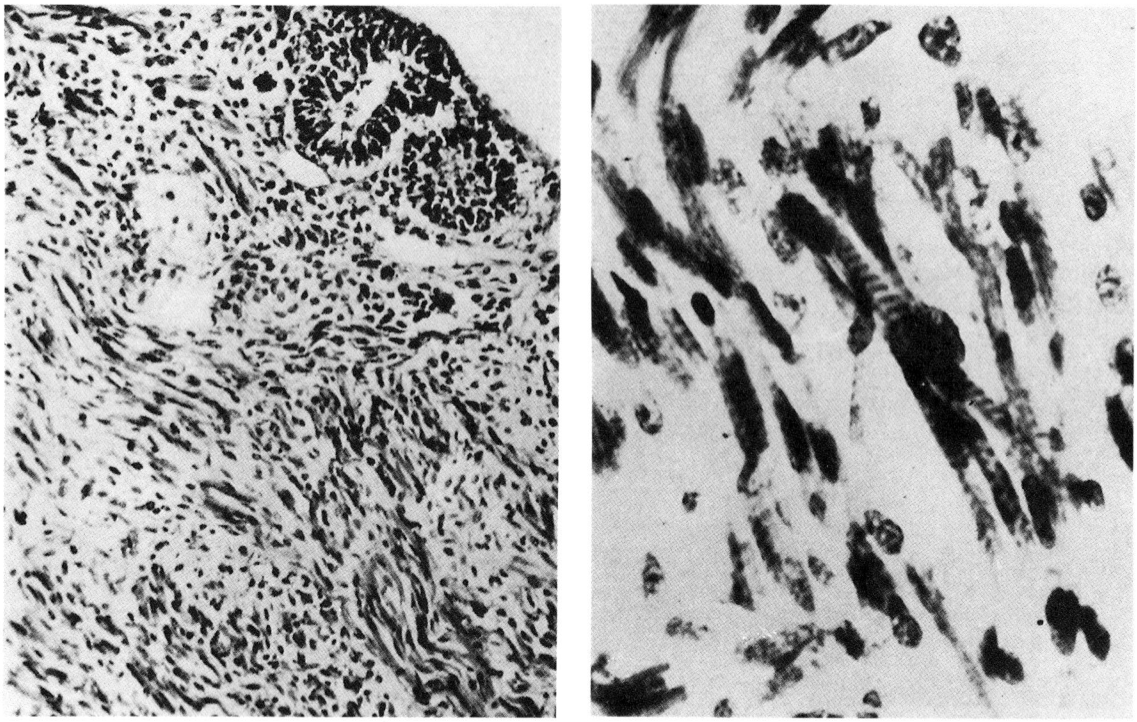

Fig. 16.14 a, b Nephroblastoma. A group of striated muscle cells lies in stroma. The cross-striations are visible (**b**). (**a**) Haematoxylin-eosin × 100; (**b**) Masson trichrome × 1500
Reproduced by permission from: Allen AC. The kidney. Medical and surgical diseases. London: Churchill, 1952 (Plate 305)

the presence of markedly enlarged, hyperchromatic, bizarre nuclei with multipolar mitoses, i.e. several metaphase plates in a single nucleus. Focal anaplasia is commoner than diffuse anaplasia.[113]

Electron microscopy[114]

The stromal cells appear remarkably primitive and closely resemble the non-aggregated nephrogenic mesenchyme before induction by branches from the ureteric bud. The blastemal cells usually have well-developed cell junctions and a coating of floccular material on their surface; cilia are occasionally present.

Immunohistochemistry

The epithelial component of the tumour stains for cytokeratin and epithelial membrane antigen; the blastemal component is negative for both antigens. Stains for vimentin react with the stromal cells and the endothelial cells of the tumour vessels. The blastemal cells stain equivocally for vimentin.[115] A polysialic acid oncodevelopmental antigen that is normally present during the differentiation of the metanephros (see p. 48), but absent in mature nephrons, occurs on both the blastemal and tubular components of nephroblastomas. The stroma is not stained.[116]

Cytogenetic analysis

Cytogenetic analysis of patients with nephroblastoma and aniridia has shown constitutional deletions on the short arm (p) of chromosome 11. The breakpoint is localized in most cases at 11p13.[97] In patients with Beckwith–Wiedemann's syndrome there is trisomy 11p15.[102] Analysis of sporadic and familial cases of nephroblastoma has generally failed to show any constitutional rearrangement of the chromosome 11p.[106] Tumour-specific 11p13 deletions, however, have been observed in several sporadic nephroblastomas,[117] the deletions being detectable in the tumour cells, but not in normal cells.

Genotyping

Molecular analysis confirms the deletion of specific segments on the short arm of chromosome 11 in cases of nephroblastoma associated with aniridia[97] and in some isolated cases of sporadic nephroblastoma.[118] Deleted sequences on chromosome 11 have also been detected that were not visible on cytogenetic analysis. The deletions have enabled investigators to pinpoint the site of the locus responsible for the tumour to band 11p13 on chromosome 11 and to clone a gene at that locus that may be the cause of nephroblastoma.[119,120] The candidate gene has tumour-suppressing properties and partial sequencing of the gene shows that it contains a region thought to be a hallmark of transcription factors: proteins that bind to DNA and either enhance or suppress gene expression. The normal function of the gene that has been isolated seems to be concerned with the formation of the kidneys in the developing fetus.[121]

This recent discovery, however, does not fully resolve the question of how nephroblastomas begin: there is evidence that changes in several other genes – some not even on chromosome 11 – may be involved in tumour initiation.[122,123] In some sporadic tumours the expression of the gene coding for insulin-like growth factor-2 (IGF-2), localized to the 11p15 region, has been shown to be markedly increased compared with the adjacent normal kidney.[124]

Spread

Nephroblastomas may spread by direct invasion of neighbouring structures, by lymphatics or by the blood stream. Local extension through the renal capsule is usually a late occurrence; it is often accompanied by infiltration of the tumour into the renal pelvis. Local extension into the renal vein is common. Lymphatic spread to the renal lymph nodes adjoining the renal hilum and other lateral aortic lymph nodes is found in approximately 25% of cases at the time the tumour is removed. About 12% of the patients present with haematogenous metastases.[125] The tumour deposits are particularly likely to be in the lungs: 85% of patients with metastases have pulmonary secondaries.[125] Involvement of the liver and mediastinal lymph nodes is much less frequent. Other sites, such as bone, are rarely involved. Cerebral and spinal cord involvement occurs occasionally. If metastases occur in patients who have been treated they usually do so within 2 years. Metastases often show marked differences in histological pattern from the primary tumour.

Differential diagnosis[126]

Two conditions in particular need to be considered in the differential diagnosis: teratoma and neuroblastoma.

Teratoma

It may at times be difficult to distinguish a nephroblastoma from a true teratoma. Renal teratomas are very rare. They usually contain germ cells and extraembryonic cell types, and they often show areas in which there are attempts at formation of non-renal somatic organs. These features do not occur in nephroblastomas.

Neuroblastoma

A neuroblastoma is sometimes mistaken for a nephroblastoma. In a neuroblastoma the rosettes differ from the tubules in a nephroblastoma by lacking lumens and basal laminae, and being multilayered. Also the stroma is fibrovascular rather than fibromyxoid and the tumour is monomorphous, lacking the variegated patterns usually present in nephroblastoma.

Prognosis

In determining the prognosis the extent to which the tumour has spread and the histopathological characteristics are both important. Morphometry and cytometry may refine the histopathological assessment; their value has not yet been adequately assessed.

Stage of tumour spread

The staging system currently used by the large multi-institutional National Wilms' Tumor Study in the USA is widely employed because of its relative simplicity.[125,127] The system adopted jointly by the Union Internationale contre le Cancer (UICC), the American Joint Committee for Cancer (AJCC) and the International Society of Pediatric Oncology (SIOP) is more complex and less widely used.[44] There are five stages in the National Wilms' Tumor Study system:

Stage I	Tumour confined to the kidney and completely excised.
Stage II	Tumour extends through the renal capsule, with or without invasion of the renal vein or involvement of periaortic lymph nodes. Resection complete with no apparent residual tumour.
Stage III	Residual non-haematogenous tumour confined to abdomen.
Stage IV	Haematogenous metastases, e.g. in lung, liver, bone and brain.
Stage V	Bilateral renal tumours.

Nephroblastomas respond very well to nephrectomy and combination chemotherapy. When 4-year survival rates after treatment are assessed according to the National Wilms' Tumor Study staging system they are 96.5% for stage I nephroblastoma, 92.2% for stage II nephroblastoma, 86.9% for stage III nephroblastoma, and 73% for stage IV nephroblastoma.[127] Few deaths occur after 4 years. The 3-year survival rate for stage V tumours is 76%. Patients with bilateral tumours are usually treated by chemotherapy followed by local excision or partial nephrectomy rather than nephrectomy.[128]

Lymph node involvement is an unfavourable prognostic sign: in stage II and III tumours combined survival rates at 2 years are 54% for those with lymph node involvement compared with 82% for those without.[127] Tumour in the lumen of the renal vein, even when extending into the inferior vena cava, does not confer an unfavourable prognosis.[125]

The prognosis in adults seems to be poorer than in children. In a series of 31 patients, the 3-year survival rate was 48% for stages I and II and 11% for stages III and IV.[129]

Histological grade

The National Wilms' Tumor Study recognizes two categories:[128]

Unfavourable histology	Anaplasia is the only criterion for assigning a true nephroblastoma to this category.
Favourable histology	All cases without anaplasia.

Only about 7% of true nephroblastomas have unfavourable histology.[113] Unfavourable histology has no apparent adverse significance in stage I nephroblastomas, but in patients with other stage tumours it is associated with a worse prognosis; survival rates at 2 years are 54% for patients with nephroblastomas showing unfavourable histology compared with 90% for those with tumours of favourable histology.[127]

Patients with unfavourable histology are more likely to relapse if they also have anaplasia in extrarenal tumour sites (either direct extensions or metastases) or if the nephroblastoma has a predominantly blastemal pattern. In a recent series patients manifesting either or both of these features experienced a relapse-free survival rate of 17% at 2 years, compared with 61% if both were absent.[130]

Morphometry and cytometry

Recent studies suggest that flow cytometry is a promising means of detecting anaplasia in nephroblastoma.[131,132] Computed cell morphometry has been little used so far in the analysis of this tumour.

Pathogenesis

Nephroblastomas most probably arise from foci of persistent metanephrogenic mesenchyme (renal blastema or nephrogenic rests; see p. 589). Data from morphological studies favour this origin[133] and immunohistochemical evidence, based on the presence of polysialic acid, indicates that the blastema of nephroblastomas represents the malignantly transformed equivalent of the nephrogenic caps, the first developmental stage of the induced metanephrogenic mesenchyme.[116]

What initiates tumour formation is not known. A widely accepted hypothesis is that two mutations occur which inactivate, in turn, each allele of a regulatory recessive gene on the short arm (p) of chromosome 11. Both copies of the gene are damaged or deleted, resulting in homozygocity or hemizygocity for the recessive allele.[104] Unimpaired expression of this gene is probably necessary for normal renal differentiation. It is assumed that the regulatory gene is an anti-oncogene (suppressor gene) which regulates other genes (oncogenes), allowing them to be expressed only during embryogenesis. The oncogenes are thought to code for substances involved in the regulation of differentiation and proliferation; several such genes are known to exist on chromosome 11. The insulin-like growth factor 2 (IGF-2) gene is located in the 11p14 band, the neural cell adhesion molecule (NCAM) gene is in the 11q23 band and the genes for Thy-1 and the delta chain of the T3–T cell receptor complex are also on 11q23.[116,124] It is suggested that inactivation of both copies of the anti-oncogene alleles results in uncontrolled continuous expression of these growth-regulating genes.

Supporting this concept is the known increased expression of the IGF-2 gene in nephroblastomas.[124] This may contribute to the malignant process by stimulating cell proliferation and inhibiting cell differentiation. Increased IGF-2 production may also be responsible for the gigantism that occurs in the Beckwith–Wiedemann syndrome (see p. 589) and the hemihypertrophy that is associated with some nephroblastomas. Direct evidence that genetic information capable of controlling the expression of the malignant phenotype of nephroblastoma is present on chromosome 11 has been obtained: the introduction of a normal chromosome 11 into nephroblastoma cells results in suppression of their malignant properties.[134]

In nephroblastomas associated with aniridia the first mutation is in the germ line; it is inherited from a parent and is already present in every cell of the body from the time of conception. Tumour development then simply requires a second mutation in any single cell of the metanephric blastema. Sporadic nephroblastomas arise in hitherto genetically normal individuals only when the two mutations occur de novo in a single blastemal cell.[104]

On the basis of the evidence obtained from cytogenetic and molecular studies it has been proposed that the germ cell mutations in nephroblastomas associated with aniridia[97] and the somatic mutations in some sporadic nephroblastomas[135] occur at a locus at chromosomal band 11p13. In Beckwith–Wiedemann syndrome the evidence suggests the existence of a locus at 11p15.[102] A putative nephroblastoma gene (Wg) has been isolated, cloned and characterized (see p. 593): there may, however, be changes in other genes.

Whether an environmental factor is involved in the induction of the mutations is not known. Epidemiological studies have shown weak associations with lead, and several chemical carcinogens and retroviral infections can cause nephroblastomas in various animals, but there is as yet no clearly identified causative factor.[136]

NEPHROBLASTOMATOSIS

Blastemal cells with metanephrogenic potential usually disappear from the fetus 4–6 weeks before term in a normal human gestation. Occasionally they persist and are present in the renal cortex after birth. The various morphological forms that these accumulations of blastemal cells may assume are often grouped together under the general term 'nephroblastomatosis'. Several lines of evidence suggest that some types of 'nephroblastomatosis' are important in the development of a nephroblastoma.

Nephroblastomatosis is discussed on page 589 under factors predisposing to nephroblastoma.

CONGENITAL MESOBLASTIC NEPHROMA

Congenital mesoblastic nephroma is a rare, usually benign, mesenchymal tumour of early infancy.[137,138] It is by far the commonest renal neoplasm in the first 3 months of life and accounts for approximately 3% of paediatric renal tumours.[139] Extremely rarely the tumour has been encountered in older children and in adult life. Boys are affected a little more often than girls.

Clinical features

The tumour usually presents as an abdominal mass that is obvious at birth. Polyhydramnios is a frequent associated condition. Hypertension with inappropriately high levels of plasma renin is sometimes reported and may be more common than is currently appreciated.[140]

Renal changes

Gross appearance of the kidneys

The tumour is usually large (mean diameter in one series 6.2 cm), spherical and always unilateral. The cut surface often resembles a uterine fibroid in colour and consistency (Fig. 16.15). It is homogeneously rubbery or firm and has a whorled pattern; less often it is softer and bulges. The tumour is not encapsulated and often extends beyond the renal capsule. There may be foci of haemorrhage, necrosis or cyst formation; these are most common in cellular congenital mesoblastic nephroma (see below).[141]

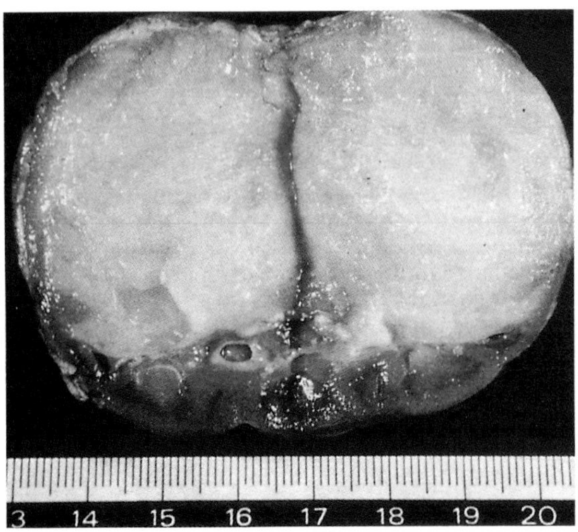

Fig. 16.15 Congenital mesoblastic nephroma – classical type. The large tumour replaces most of the kidney. Its cut surface has a whorled, coarsely trabeculated appearance.
Reproduced by permission from: Pettinato G, Manivel JC, Wick MR, Dehner LP. Hum Pathol 1989;20:682 (Fig. 1)

Light microscopy[137,138,141–143]

Classical congenital mesoblastic nephroma
Typically a congenital mesoblastic nephroma is composed predominantly of spindle-shaped cells resembling fibroblasts or smooth muscle cells; they are arranged in sheets or bundles with variable quantities of collagen between the cells (Fig. 16.16). The surrounding renal structures are not usually compressed and at the tumour's edge long narrow bundles of spindle cells extend into the adjacent kidney. Extrarenal infiltration of spindle cells is common, especially into the perihilar fat (Fig. 16.16); invasion of the psoas muscle, renal vein wall and renal vein lumen also occurs.[141] Well-differentiated dysplastic tubules and glomeruli are often scattered throughout the tumour; islands of cartilage and foci of erythropoiesis may also be present. Entrapped tubules and glomeruli are common at the margin of the tumour. Many tumours contain small areas in which the spindle cells are closely packed together, collagen is minimal and mitoses are frequent, giving a sarcomatous appearance.

Cellular congenital mesoblastic nephroma
In approximately two-thirds of examples of congenital mesoblastic nephroma the whole tumour is hypercellular and there is a high mitotic rate (Fig. 16.17).[143] The tumours may be either sharply demarcated or extend into the surrounding renal parenchyma.[141]

Electron microscopy

The spindle cells have the ultrastructural features of fibrocytes and fibroblasts. Myofibroblastic features have been described in some cases.[144] In classical congenital mesoblastic nephroma the intercellular space contains small numbers of collagen fibrils; in cellular congenital mesoblastic nephroma the spindle cells have an increased nuclear to cytoplasm ratio and prominent nuc-

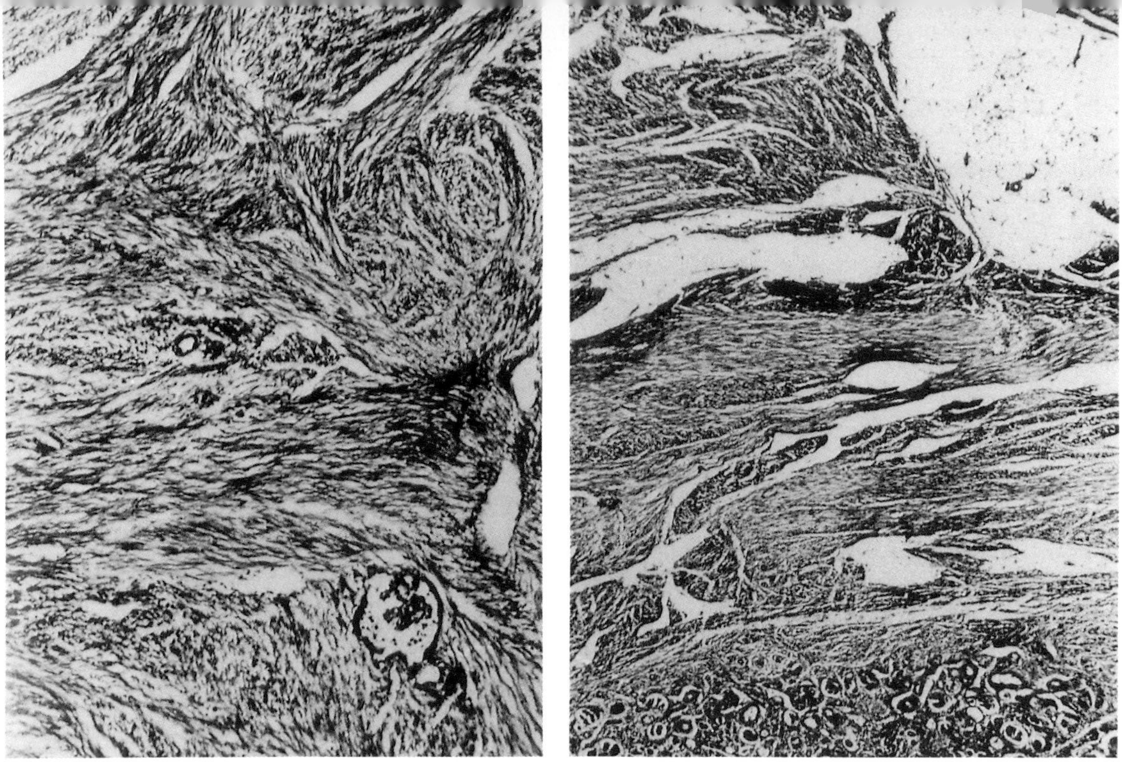

a b

Fig. 16.16 Congenital mesoblastic nephroma – classical type. (**a**) Intersecting bundles of uniform spindle cells entrap a glomerulus. (**b**) Spindle cells infiltrate through the renal capsule into the peritubular fat. Normal kidney is present at the bottom of the picture.
(**a**),(**b**) Haematoxylin-eosin × 30
Reproduced by permission from: Pettinato G, Manivel JC, Wick MR, Dehner LP. Hum Pathol 1989;20:682 (Fig. 2)

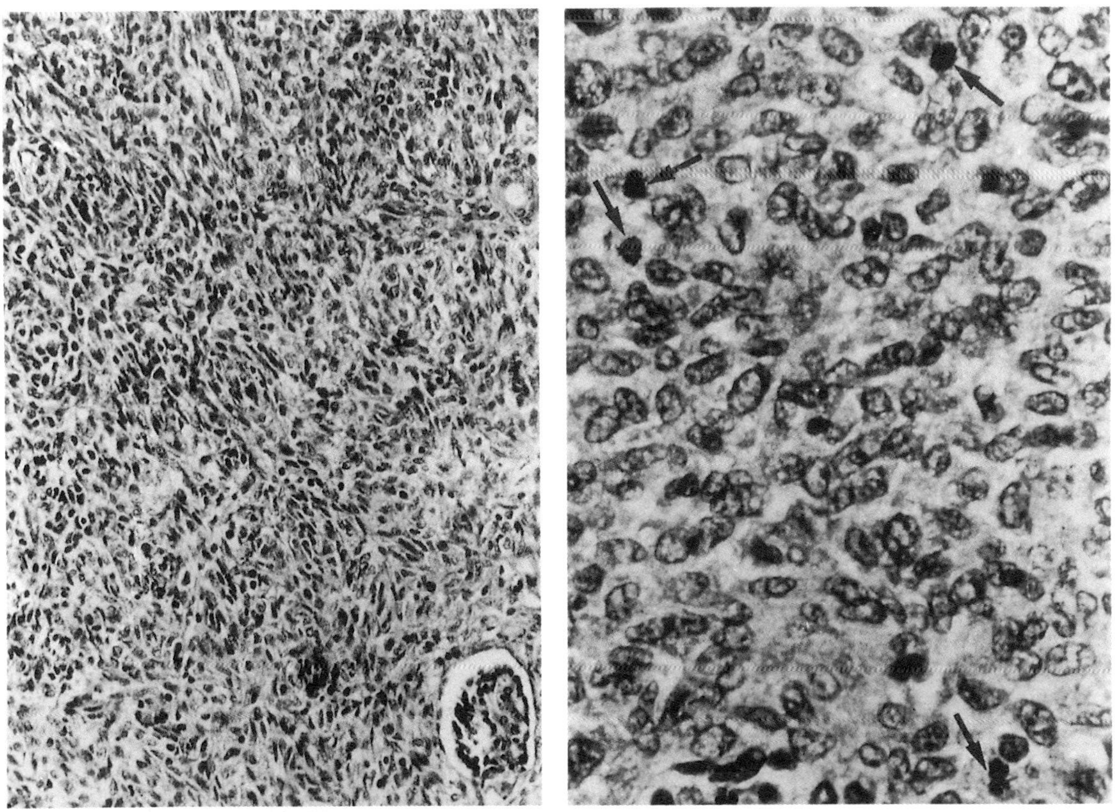

a b

Fig. 16.17 Congenital mesoblastic nephroma – cellular type. (**a**),(**b**) The irregularly arranged spindle cells are closely packed and mitotic figures (arrows) are frequent.
Haematoxylin-eosin: (**a**) × 80; (**b**) × 480
Reproduced by permission from: Pettinato G, Manivel JC, Wick MR, Dehner LP. Hum Pathol 1989;20:682 (Fig. 3)

leoli, and there are no collagen fibrils or basal laminae.[141]

Immunohistochemistry

Congenital mesoblastic nephromas contain fibronectin and vimentin but lack laminin.[141,145] Actin is present in all classical tumours, but in only a few of the cellular cases.[141] There is focal staining for the muscle-specific intermediate filament desmin in most of the tumours.[141] In infants with hyperreninism immunoreactive renin has been demonstrated particularly in the cells of afferent arterioles supplying glomeruli entrapped at the periphery of the tumour but also in the walls of vessels within the tumour itself.[140]

Differential diagnosis

The main distinction that has to be made is from a *nephroblastoma* in which stroma predominates (see p. 591), or from a nephroblastoma that has been subjected to chemotherapy or radiotherapy before resection. Large areas of spindle cells are infrequent in nephroblastomas and if present suggest the tumour is most probably a congenital mesoblastic nephroma. The finding of foci of blastemal cells or skeletal muscle almost always indicates that the tumour is a nephroblastoma. Cellular congenital mesoblastic nephromas must also be differentiated from variants of *clear cell sarcoma of the kidney* (see p. 601).

Prognosis

In the majority of cases the prognosis is good following nephrectomy, provided a wide margin is taken on all sides of the kidney to remove infiltrative growth which is not obvious macroscopically. The pathologist must ensure that adequate margins have been obtained.[109] Cases of completely removed classical congenital mesoblastic nephroma need no adjuvant therapy and do well. The same is true of cellular congenital mesoblastic nephroma in infants under 3 months of age. Inadequate excision of either type of the tumour may be followed by recurrence: chemotherapy is therefore usually given when removal is incomplete.[146]

Cellular congenital mesoblastic nephromas in infants 3 months old and over occasionally recur or metastasize even after complete resection. In such tumours, therefore, the presence of haemorrhage, necrosis, dense cellularity and high mitotic rates should lead to careful follow-up.[146,147]

Morphometry and cytometry

Despite morphological differences between classical and cellular congenital mesoblastic nephromas no correlation is apparent between DNA content and clinical behaviour. Flow cytometric studies have shown that although the classical tumours are invariably diploid, the cellular tumours may be either diploid or aneuploid.[141] In one case the aneuploid cells in a hypercellular part of the tumour had 54 chromosomes.[148] In another cellular tumour a series of monosomies and structural alterations were discovered on karyotypic analysis.[149]

Pathogenesis

Little is known about the aetiology and pathogenesis of this tumour. The demonstration of fibronectin in the absence of laminin in the neoplastic cells suggests that they arise from early primitive nephrogenic mesenchyme prior to or in the absence of the inductive influence of the ureteric bud.[133,145]

MULTILOCULAR CYSTS (CYSTIC NEPHROMA)[133,150,151]

Multilocular cysts of the kidney in children (see p. 68) are widely thought to represent mature variants of nephroblastoma; they are sometimes referred to as cystic nephromas. The septa in these tumours contain only mature elements, predominantly collagenous fibrous tissue. Cystic nephromas are benign. Nephrectomy is curative.

CYSTIC PARTIALLY DIFFERENTIATED NEPHROBLASTOMA[151,152]

Multilocular cysts in which some of the septa contain immature tissue elements resembling those of nephroblastoma are often described as cystic partially differentiated nephroblastomas. Usually they are benign. In one series of 18 cases only one recurred locally after resection; none metastasized. Nephrectomy should be followed by regular surveillance.

Cystic partially differentiated nephroblastomas in which the entire tumour is multicystic, should be distinguished from nephroblastomas with foci of cystic change.

MISCELLANEOUS TUMOURS OF THE RENAL PARENCHYMA

RHABDOID TUMOUR OF THE KIDNEY

Rhabdoid tumour of the kidney was first recognized in 1978.[153] It represents approximately 2% of primary renal tumours of childhood and is characterized by onset in infancy and by great malignancy. The median age at diagnosis is 11 months;[154,155] boys are affected more often than girls. The tumour is occasionally associated with marked hypercalcaemia and raised levels of parathormone.[156] Approximately 13% are associated with a medulloblastoma in the central nervous system.[155,157]

Renal changes

Gross appearance of the kidneys

The tumour is usually large (mean weight at resection 389 g), solitary and unilateral. Most have a soft, bulging, homogeneous cut surface and lack a pseudocapsule.[155]

Light microscopy

The neoplasm is composed of sheets or cords of cells with nuclei that contain a prominent single large central nucleolus, and abundant eosinophilic cytoplasm with hyaline inclusions (Fig. 16.18). The neoplastic cells often resemble skeletal muscle myoblasts but lack the cytoplasmic striations, ultrastructural features and immunohistochemical markers that characterize these cells.[126,153] Vascular invasion and mitotic figures are usually present. Entrapped residual tubules and glomeruli are often seen in the tumour.

Electron microscopy

The cytoplasmic inclusions are composed of tightly whorled masses of intermediate filaments.[158] These are not diagnostic; they occur in a number of other tumours. However, they are useful in distinguishing between rhabdoid tumours and congenital mesoblastic nephroma.

Immunohistochemistry

Vimentin and epithelial membrane antigen are demonstrable in the tumour cell cytoplasm; a low molecular weight cytokeratin is coexpressed in some.[133,159,160]

Differential diagnosis

Rhabdoid tumour of the kidney is distinguished from a *nephroblastoma* by the lack of blastemal, epithelial and stromal components. Tumours that stain positively for myoglobin should be classified as *rhabdomyosarcomas* (see p. 602).[161] *Congenital mesoblastic nephroma* can be differentiated from rhabdoid tumour because mesoblastic nephroma cells lack hyaline cytoplasmic inclusions.[133]

Prognosis

The tumour is very malignant. In the earlier trials of the National Wilms' Tumor Study 71% of patients with rhabdoid tumour of the kidney died within the first year following nephrectomy; more died subsequently.[154] In the latest trial of combination chemotherapy 75% of the patients were dead at the end of 2 years.[94] Even when the tumour is stage I at the time of diagnosis (using the system of staging described on p. 594), death from tumour progression usually occurs despite intensive antitumour therapy.

Pathogenesis

Very little is known about the aetiology and pathogenesis of this tumour. The immunohistochemical and ultrastructural data suggest a mesenchymal

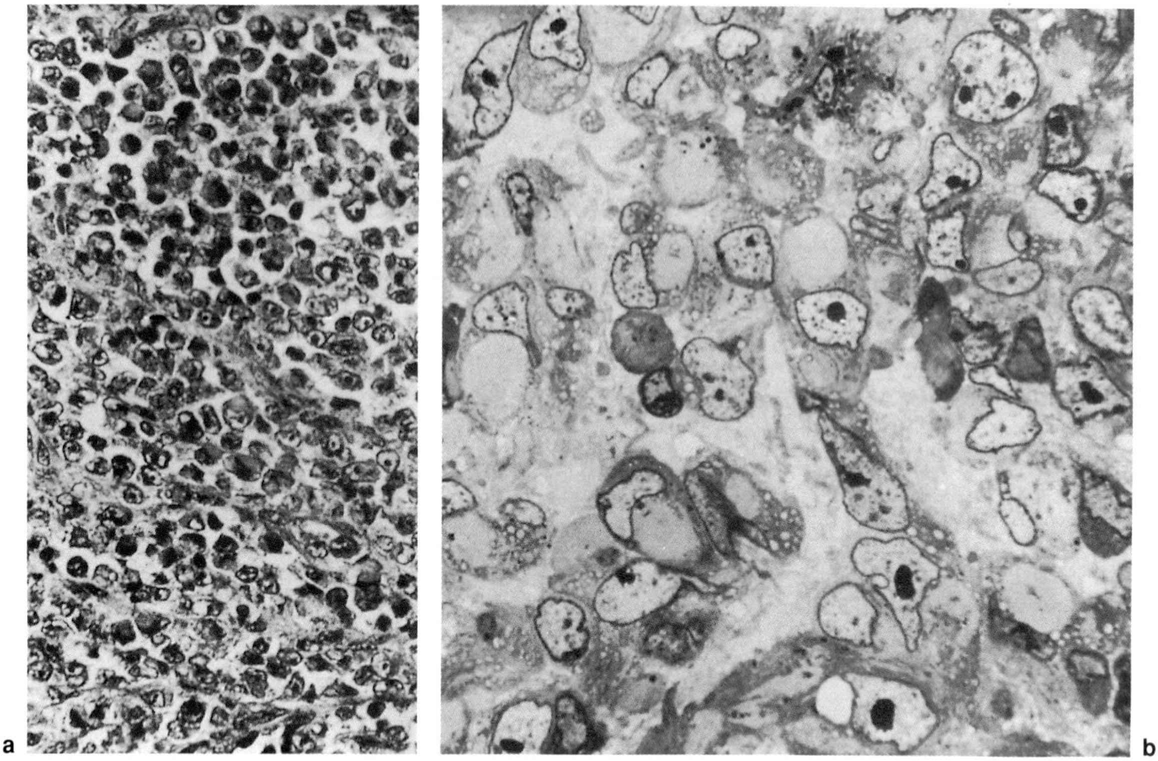

Fig. 16.18 a, b Rhabdoid tumour of the kidney. The tumour cells contain prominent central nucleoli and hyaline cytoplasmic inclusions.
(**a**) Haematoxylin-eosin × 400; (**b**) Toluidine blue × 600
Reproduced by permission from: Seo IS, Min KW, Brodhecker C, Mirkin LD. Histopathology 1988;13:657 (Fig. 3)

origin. One proposal is that it might arise from primitive cells involved in the formation of the renal medulla.[155]

CLEAR CELL SARCOMA OF THE KIDNEY ('BONE METASTASIZING RENAL TUMOUR OF CHILDHOOD')

Clear cell sarcoma of the kidney is a rare highly malignant tumour of early childhood.[153,162, 163] It constitutes about 4% of renal tumours encountered in that age group and is the commonest renal sarcoma of childhood.[126,163] The age distribution is the same as that of nephroblastoma (see p. 587), the mean age at diagnosis being approximately 3 years. Boys are affected slightly more often than girls. The clinical features do not differ from those seen in nephroblastoma; an abdominal mass and haematuria are the usual presenting signs.[163] The predisposing factors associated with nephroblastoma (see p. 588) are not found in clear cell sarcoma of the kidney.

Renal changes

Gross appearance of the kidneys

The tumour is solitary and large. The average tumour weight in one series of clear cell sarcomas in boys was 899 g.[163] The cut surface bulges and is usually a homogeneous grey or tan; there are often cysts near the periphery. The tumour often appears to arise in the medulla.

Light microscopy

Typically the tumour is composed of cords or

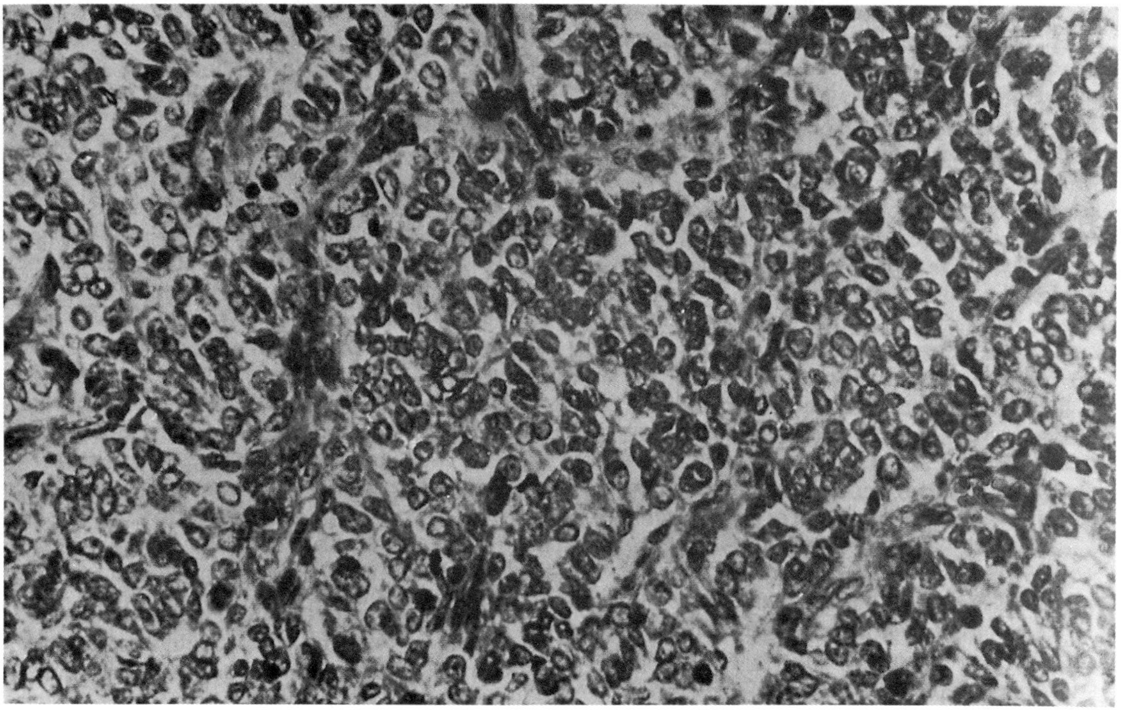

Fig. 16.19 Clear cell sarcoma of the kidney. The cords and clusters of cells with vacuolated cytoplasm are separated from one another by septa containing small blood vessels.
Haematoxylin-eosin × 350
Reproduced by permission from: Lawler W, Marsden HB. J Clin Pathol 1979;32:608 (Fig. 1)

nests of polygonal cells with small round nuclei. Cell boundaries are indistinct and cytoplasmic vacuolation is frequent (Fig. 16.19); the cells do not contain excess lipid or glycogen. Mitoses are often sparse and nucleoli inconspicuous. The groups of tumour cells are separated from one another by septa containing small blood vessels and spindle cell stroma. There are no metanephroblastic elements in the tumour. Peripherally the neoplastic cells infiltrate the surrounding parenchyma, isolating and entrapping tubules and rarely glomeruli; the entrapped tubules may become cystic.

Variations on this basic pattern occur. For example, there may be areas within the tumour in which expansion of the stromal component occurs, giving the appearance of a spindle cell sarcoma, and mucoid or hyaline ground substance may accumulate between the tumour cells. Palisading reminiscent of a neurilemmoma (schwannoma) has been described.[126]

Electron microscopy

The tumour cells have a high nuclear to cytoplasmic ratio and their cytoplasm is poor in organelles.[163]

Immunohistochemistry

Stains for laminin, fibronectin, cytokeratin and epithelial membrane antigen are negative. Vimentin has been demonstrated in approximately 50% of reported cases.[159]

Cytogenetic analysis and genotyping

No cytogenetic or genotyping studies of clear cell sarcoma of the kidney have been reported.

Spread

The tumour spreads widely by lymphatics and by

the blood stream. Metastases to bone are a distinctive feature of clear cell sarcoma of the kidney,[109,162] in contrast to nephroblastoma which only infrequently produces secondaries in bone, hence the synonym 'bone metastasizing renal tumour of childhood' for clear cell sarcoma. The skull is very commonly involved.[163]

Differential diagnosis

The variations that occur in the tumour can make diagnosis difficult. It is sometimes hard to distinguish from *congenital mesoblastic nephroma* (see p. 595), but electron microscopy will display the characteristic fibroblastic and myofibroblastic cells in the latter: these cells are quite unlike any that occur in clear cell sarcoma.

Prognosis

The prognosis after the standard treatment that is so successful in nephroblastoma is poor. Clear cell sarcomas of the kidney are highly malignant and systemic metastases occur early. In one series of 21 patients, 11 died from the tumour 5 months to 8 years 9 months after diagnosis.[163] However, the addition of adriamycin to the treatment appears to have markedly increased the survival rates. In the Third Wilms' Tumor Study 72.6% of children with clear cell sarcoma of the kidney were alive at 4 years.[94]

Pathogenesis

Little is known about the aetiology and pathogenesis of this tumour. Electron microscopy and immunohistochemistry give no clear indication of the cell of origin.

OTHER SARCOMAS

Other primary sarcomas of the kidney are rare, constituting about 3% of all malignant renal tumours.[164,165] They are highly malignant and the prognosis is poor. Leiomyosarcomas are the most common; liposarcomas are much less frequent. Only isolated examples of rhabdomyosarcoma, fibrosarcoma, osteosarcoma, malignant fibrous histiocytoma, angiosarcoma and chondrosarcoma have been reported. The morphology of these tumours is identical to those arising in other sites.

Leiomyosarcoma[164,165]

Leiomyosarcomas occur in adults; after the age of 20 years they increase in frequency with advancing age. They are not found in children. They are slightly more common in women. Leiomyosarcomas are rarely detected while still confined to the kidney. They usually present with haematuria, flank pain and an abdominal mass. Typically they form a firm lobulated mass 10–15 cm in diameter protruding from the cortical surface of the kidney and often adherent to perirenal structures. The cut surface is grey or pale brown and has a whorled pattern. There may be foci of haemorrhage and cysts.

Few patients survive for long after nephrectomy; in one series 14 of the 15 patients died of their tumour in 4 months to 5½ years.[164] In another series seven of the eight patients died from metastases within 18 months.[165]

Radiation and chemotherapy are of little avail.

Liposarcoma[165,166]

Liposarcomas arising in the kidneys are very rare. Their frequency in the past was exaggerated because of failure to distinguish them from angiomyolipomas and retroperitoneal sarcomas invading the kidney. The majority of liposarcomas occur between the ages of 40 and 60 years. They are typically very large, lobulated and localized to the capsular region of the kidney. The cut surface is frequently slimy.

The prognosis is not clear from the limited data that are available. In one series published in 1968, three of five patients died of their tumour 1 month, 1½ years and 13 years after nephrectomy.[164] However, in eight more recent cases followed up for 8 months to 14 years, all were alive. Recurrence was observed in only one of the seven cases in whom nephrectomy was performed.[166]

LYMPHOMA

Lymphomas very rarely arise primarily in the kidneys. This is in contrast to secondary renal involvement by lymphomas, which is common (see p. 607). They occur at all ages.

CARCINOID TUMOUR

Primary renal carcinoid tumours are very rare. Most patients are 60–70 years old. The tumours are solid, well demarcated and show foci of haemorrhage and necrosis. They do not differ morphologically from carcinoid tumours arising in the gut. The granules in the tumour cells are argyrophil, staining positively with the Grimelius stain and negatively with Fontana. There are reports of cases which have metastasized.[167]

TERATOMA

Primary teratomas have rarely been recorded in the kidney. They are distinguished from nephroblastomas by the presence of extraembryonic cell types and of germ cells; there are also often attempts at formation of non-renal somatic organs.

NEUROBLASTOMA AND GANGLIONEUROMA

Neuroblastomas and ganglioneuromas, apparently of intrarenal origin, occasionally occur in infants or small children. They must be distinguished from nephroblastomas (see p. 593).

NEURILEMMOMA (SCHWANNOMA)

Neurilemmomas very rarely occur in the kidney. Their natural history is not known because they have all been diagnosed after nephrectomy. Neurilemmomas usually are benign when they arise in peripheral nerves; some of those reported in the kidney have behaved in a malignant fasion.[168,169]

ANGIOMYOLIPOMA

Angiomyolipomas are composed of a mixture of mature adipose tissue, tortuous thick-walled blood vessels and sheets of smooth muscle. They are most probably hamartomas. Approximately 40% of patients with angiomyolipomas have one or more features of tuberous sclerosis (see p. 113). Angiomyolipomas account for about 1% of all surgically resected renal tumours.[170] In patients without tuberous sclerosis the mean age is 41 years, with a range of 26–72 years; females are more commonly affected than males.[171]

Angiomyolipomas have a benign clinical course.

Clinical features

Angiomyolipomas that are less than 4 cm in diameter are usually asymptomatic.[171] Common signs and symptoms of larger tumours are pain in the flank or abdomen, which may be sudden and severe, gross haematuria and hypertension. Diminishing renal function occasionally occurs in patients with bilateral and multiple lesions. Computerized tomography is useful in distinguishing the lesion from carcinoma; the fat in an angiomyolipoma is demonstrated by its low (negative) attenuation value, which differs from that of normal renal parenchyma or malignant tissue. The only other tumour giving such low values is a liposarcoma.

Renal changes

Angiomyolipomas in patients with tuberous sclerosis are usually multiple and often bilateral; many are less than 4 cm in diameter (see p. 113). Those tumours in patients with tuberous sclerosis that cause symptoms are almost always unilateral and solitary; they are larger, their mean diameter being 9.4 cm.[172]

The gross and microscopic appearances of the renal tumours are in general the same whether the patient has tuberous sclerosis or not. They are described on page 114. However, it has recently been suggested that angiomyolipomas in tuberous sclerosis are more likely to be associated with multiple small scattered foci composed of fat or smooth muscle in the kidneys in addition to the main tumour. They are also more likely to extend into the adjacent kidney and to contain tubular inclusions and calcification than are angiolipomas in patients without tuberous sclerosis.[173]

Changes in other organs

Rarely angiomyolipomas are also present in the regional lymph nodes[174] or spleen.[175] As the clinical course has remained benign in these cases it is generally thought that such tumours probably represent multicentric growth and not metastasis.

Differential diagnosis

Angiomyolipomas are most likely to be misdiagnosed as malignant tumours such as *fibrosarcomas, liposarcomas* and *leiomyosarcomas*, because of their propensity for extension through the renal capsule and the presence of mitoses and hyperchromatic and moderately pleomorphic nuclei (see p. 114). However, the absence of atypical mitoses and the presence of prominent, irregular, thick-walled blood vessels surrounded by collarettes of smooth muscle help distinguish the angiomyolipoma from a sarcoma.[173]

Complications

Life-threatening *bleeding* occasionally occurs from an angiomyolipoma. Patients with tuberous sclerosis and an angiomyolipoma may develop an incidental *renal cell carcinoma*. This occurred in 4.4% of such cases in one series.[176] The renal cell carcinoma may occur in the same kidney as the angiomyolipoma;[177] in one report malignant tumours involved both kidneys.[178] The limited data available suggest that renal cell carcinomas are commoner in patients with tuberous sclerosis than in the general population.

Prognosis

Angiomyolipomas behave as benign tumours. The tumour or tumours may be discovered during the deliberate screening of the kidneys of asymptomatric patients with tuberous sclerosis or during the investigation of any patient with symptoms and signs that might be related to a renal lesion. No treatment is needed in most asymptomatic patients; in those with symptoms tumour enucleation or other limited surgery may be necessary. Regular computerized tomography to detect renal cell carcinoma is advisable in older children and adults (see above).[176]

Pathogenesis

The majority view is that angiomyolipomas are hamartomas, i.e. congenital tumours composed of tissues that normally are present in a given organ but that are abnormal in quantity, arrangement or degree of maturation and that may grow and behave as benign neoplasms.[179]

RENOMEDULLARY INTERSTITIAL CELL TUMOUR (MEDULLARY FIBROMA)

Tiny pale grey nodules ranging in size from 0.1 to 0.7 cm are found in the renal medulla in approximately 30% of all patients autopsied in general hospitals.[180] They are particularly common in people aged over 50 years; they occur with equal frequency in men and women. The nodules are usually solitary but may be multiple and bilateral. There have usually been no signs and symptoms to suggest their presence.

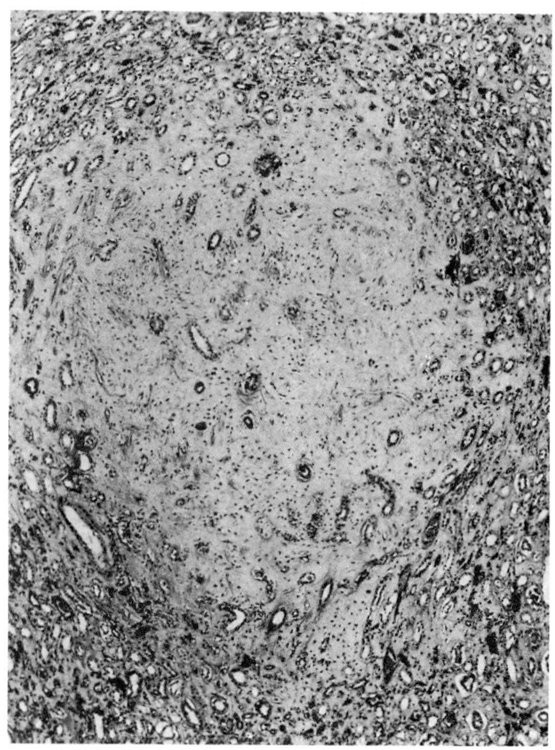

Fig. 16.20 Renomedullary interstitial cell tumour. The nodule is composed predominantly of collagen and is not encapsulated. There is entrapment of renal tubules. Haematoxylin-eosin × 50

Microscopically they are unencapsulated and composed of variable proportions of cells and stroma (Fig. 16.20). The cells are oval or irregularly shaped with vesicular nuclei; their cytoplasm contains neutral fat. Ultrastructurally they resemble medullary interstitial cells rather than fibroblasts.[180] The stroma contains abundant collagen but no reticulin or elastic tissue; amorphous material staining intensely for acid mucopolysaccharide is also present together with some lipid.

These nodules are considered to represent either hyperplasia or benign neoplasia of the interstitial cells that are normally present in the medulla (see p. 23). The lack of fibroblasts suggests that they are not fibromas; the absence of cells other than interstitial cells is incompatible with their being hamartomas.

Because medullary interstitial cells are thought to produce an antihypertensive factor, it has been suggested that renomedullary interstitial cell tumours arise as a response to hypertension. Current evidence does not support this idea.[181]

HAEMANGIOMA[182]

Haemangiomas are rare in the kidneys. The majority are detected between the ages of 20 and 40 years. Males and females are affected equally. The presenting symptom is haematuria, often accompanied by colicky pain due to passage of blood clots. Renal haemangiomas may be associated with haemangiomatosis involving other parts of the body, as, for example, in the Sturge–Kalischer–Weber syndrome.

Haemangiomas may be situated anywhere in the renal parenchyma; they are most common at the apex of a pyramid or in a calyx. The tumours are red and usually tiny (0.3–0.4 cm in diameter). Most of them are of the capillary type.

Simple excision is curative.

LYMPHANGIOMA[167]

Lymphangiomas are exceedingly rare. They are found particularly in women and often produce haematuria. The tumours are usually large, well demarcated, soft, honeycomb-like masses. Microscopically they are composed of widely dilated, thin-walled vessels lined by a single layer of flattened endothelial cells. They should be distinguished from multilocular cysts, which contain dilated tubules lined by epithelium (see p. 68). Lymphangiomas do not recur or metastasize after removal.

LEIOMYOMA AND LIPOMA

Small leiomyomas and lipomas are found in approximately 5% of all patients over 60 years of age who are autopsied at a general hospital.[183] They are six times as frequent in women as in men. Most leiomyomas and lipomas are found either in the superficial cortex or in the renal capsule; the two tumours sometimes coexist multifocally in the same kidney. They are almost always incidental findings but occasionally large pure leiomyomas or lipomas produce signs and symptoms. Those diagnosed in life have followed a benign course.

A leiomyoma may superficially resemble a mesoblastic nephroma (see p. 595), but is sharply circumscribed and does not contain entrapped tubular and glomeruloid structures. Also, mesoblastic nephroma is found almost exclusively in the first few weeks of life and is more frequent in boys than girls.

JUXTAGLOMERULAR CELL TUMOUR

Tumours of juxtaglomerular cells are very rare. They occur mainly in children and young adults of both sexes and are associated with high arterial blood pressure, persistently high levels of renin in the blood and secondary hyperaldosteronism.[184–186] In most cases removal of the tumour results in cure of the hypertension. The level of renin in the plasma is very low in the first few days after the operation; later it becomes normal. Neither recurrence nor metastasis has been reported. Persistent hypertension occurs in approximately a quarter of the patients, probably as a result of irreversible hypertensive arteriolar and arterial changes in the kidneys (see p. 307).[186]

The tumour is usually subcapsular, small (0.2–4.5 cm in diameter), solitary, well circumscribed and grey or brownish grey with areas of haemorrhage. Microscopically it consists of sheets of polygonal tumour cells arranged between large numbers of thin-walled blood vessels (Fig. 16.21). The nuclei are generally uniform in size and there are no mitoses. The cytoplasm of the tumour cells is basophilic when stained by haematoxylin and eosin. Immunoperoxidase staining of deparaffinized sections with a conjugated antibody to pure human renin reveals that the tumour cells contain renin. When assayed the tumour contains about a hundred times the renin activity of normal renal cortex.[187] Electron microscopy reveals abundant secretory granules (Fig. 16.22) of the various morphological types found in the granular cells of the normal juxtaglomerular apparatus (see p. 17).[188] The tumour also contains sympathetic nerve fibres.

When the tumour cells are grown in tissue culture, renin is released into the medium. It seems clear that the hypertension associated with these tumours is the result of secretion of active renin. The secretion is not entirely unregulated; it is

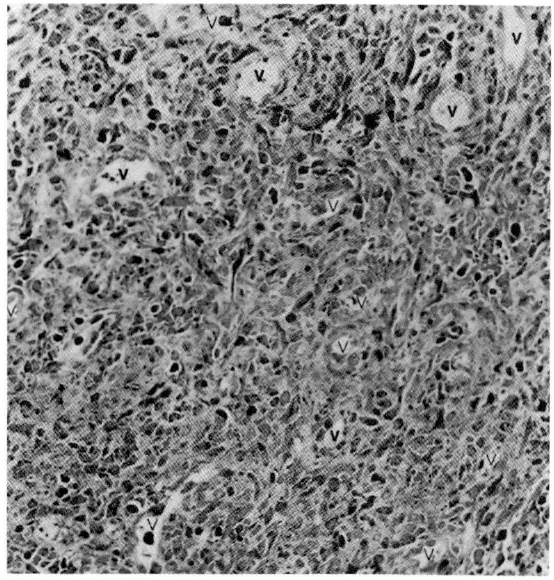

Fig. 16.21 Juxtaglomerular cell tumour. Sheets of tumour cells surround small blood spaces (v) lined by endothelium. Bowie stain × 140
Reproduced by permission from: Barajas L, Bennett CM, Connor G, Lindstrom RR. Lab Invest 1977;37:357 (Fig. 2)

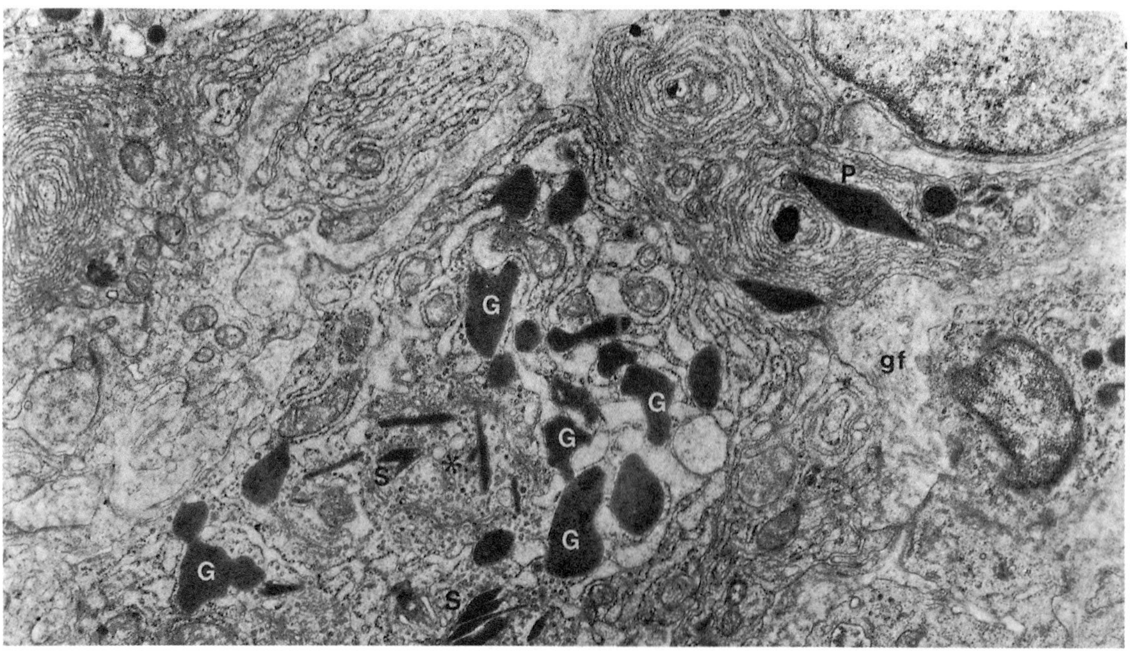

Fig. 16.22 Juxtaglomerular cell tumour. Electron micrograph of tumour cells showing granules in the cytoplasm that are structurally identical to those seen in the granular cells of the normal juxtaglomerular apparatus. G, mature granules; P, protogranule; S, sac containing protogranules; gf, granular fibrillar material.
× 12 000
Reproduced by permission from: Barajas L, Bennett CM, Connor G, Lindstrom RR. Lab Invest 1977;37:357 (Fig. 8)

responsive to posture, hypotension and the administration of spironolactone but not to alterations in sodium balance.

Although juxtaglomerular cells may be present in renal angiomyolipomas, and although nephroblastomas and renal cell carcinomas can secrete renin, the histopathological features of a juxtaglomerular cell tumour are characteristic and readily distinguished from those of other renal tumours. A retroperitoneal soft tissue haemangiopericytoma involving the kidney appears similar histopathologically but the tumour cells do not contain renin.

The presence of a tubular component in about half the cases and of sympathetic nerves in most supports the opinion that juxtaglomerular cell tumours are hamartomas.[188]

SECONDARY TUMOURS INVOLVING THE RENAL PARENCHYMA

The kidneys are frequently the site of macroscopically obvious metastatic tumours. Approximately 8% of all patients who die of malignant tumours have such renal metastases at autopsy.[189] Both kidneys are usually involved. The commonest source of metastases is a bronchial carcinoma. Secondary deposits of bronchial carcinoma are twice as commonly seen in the kidneys as primary renal tumours. Other common sources are carcinomas of the breast and large intestine; malignant melanoma of the skin and malignant thymomas also have a particular tendency to spread to kidneys.[189]

Tumour deposits that are visible only microscopically are often present, frequently in the glomerular tufts. Sometimes the malignant cells are confined to Bowman's space; very rarely such deposits affect the majority of the glomeruli, giving an overall appearance at low magnification reminiscent of crescentic glomerulonephritis.[190]

Secondary tumours in the kidneys do not usually cause clinical manifestations. In about 10% of cases there is haematuria, and in about 5% there is pain in the flank.

The kidneys are involved in approximately a third of patients dying from Hodgkin's disease and other lymphomas.[191] Infiltration by the tumour most commonly takes the form of multiple nodules.

In leukaemia the renal cortex may be massively infiltrated by neoplastic cells, usually with enlargement of the kidneys to two to three times their normal size. The kidneys are involved in approximately 42% of patients with lymphoid leukaemia and 24% with myeloid leukaemia.[192] The leukaemic infiltrates produce grey mottling, particularly of the outer cortex.

TUMOUR-LIKE CONDITIONS OF THE RENAL PARENCHYMA

ADRENAL RESTS

Adrenal rests are accessory nodules of adrenal tissue. When they occur in the kidneys they are usually situated immediately under the capsule at the lateral margin of the upper pole. Ectopic adrenal tissue in the kidney is an incidental finding in approximately 6% of autopsies.[193] Males and females are affected equally. In 10% of cases the adrenal rests are multiple.

The adrenal rest usually appears as a small yellow-orange rather flattened disc or plaque, up to 2 cm in diameter; less often it is nodular. Microscopically the ectopic tissue consists exclusively of adrenal cortex; some normal zoning into glomerulosa and fasciculata may be present. Adrenal rests usually lack a capsule and merge into the adjacent renal cortex.

Adrenocortical carcinoma has been reported arising in an adrenal rest and presenting with raised cortisol levels and a renal mass, but such an event is exceedingly rare.[194]

ENDOMETRIOSIS[195]

Involvement of the kidney by endometriosis is rare. The renal lesion is often the only demonstrable focus. If the lesion is symptomatic it usually produces flank pain and gross haematuria. The diagnosis depends upon finding typical endometrial glands with accompanying stroma. Unless the possibility of endometriosis is considered, the lesion is likely to be misdiagnosed as a primary or metastatic adenocarcinoma.

PRIMARY EPITHELIAL TUMOURS OF THE RENAL PELVIS

CARCINOMA OF THE RENAL PELVIS

Carcinoma of the renal pelvis is a rare tumour that arises in the pelvic epithelium; it accounts for approximately 5% of the clinically evident primary malignant neoplasms of the kidneys.[196] Data on its incidence are scanty because until recently carcinomas of the renal pelvis were included with those of the renal parenchyma in many large epidemiological studies. In Denmark approximately 26 new cases are diagnosed annually per million of the total population.[197]

Carcinomas of the renal pelvis are manifestations of a single, potentially multifocal, disease that may involve any part of the urothelium. Tumours elsewhere in the urinary tract may precede or coexist with a carcinoma of the renal pelvis or develop at a later stage (see pp. 689, 718). In one series of cases 20% had simultaneous carcinoma in the ureter;[198] in another series 40% of patients had a carcinoma in the bladder at some stage.[199]

Men are affected three to four times as commonly as women.[196,200] Most of the patients are aged from 60 to 80 years; the age range in one series was 29–88 years with an average of 62 years.[196] The tumour is very rare in children.

Clinical features

Haematuria is the most frequent clinical manifestation. It is usually intermittent, gross and painless; it may be profuse and sometimes accompanied by colic due to passage of a blood clot down the ureter. Less common signs and symptoms are loin pain and frequency or dysuria. Sometimes the tumour causes obstructive hydronephrosis and in a thin patient may present as a palpable mass. Occasionally there is malaise, weight loss and fever.

Cytological examination of the urine in patients with haematuria is useful in establishing the diagnosis (see p. 733); a positive result has been reported in 80% of patients with carcinoma of the renal pelvis.[201] The tumour appears as a radiolucent filling defect on intravenous pyelography; retrograde pyelography will distinguish between it and a radiolucent calculus or a blood clot.

Predisposing factors

Unlike renal cell carcinoma and nephroblastoma there is no indication of a relationship between carcinoma of the renal pelvis and any hereditary diseases. The most important of the few known predisposing factors are contact with an aromatic amine, excessive phenacetin consumption and inhalation of cigarette smoke (see p. 613).

Renal changes

The great majority of carcinomas of the renal pelvis are transitional cell in type. Very few are squamous cell carcinomas; in one large series only 1.4% were of this type.[196] Even rarer are adenocarcinomas or undifferentiated carcinomas.

Gross appearance of the kidneys[202]

The tumour occurs on either side with equal frequency. Most tumours are solitary; approximately 1–2% are bilateral.[196,198]

About 75% of the transitional cell tumours are papillary and consist of processes arising from the lining of the renal pelvis (Fig. 16.23). They are soft, bulky and pinkish-brown. The processes may be long and delicate, and attached to the mucosa by a slender pedicle; more often they are short and attached by a broad base. The tumour may fill the renal pelvis and calyces. Approximately 25% of transitional cell carcinomas are solid, non-papillary tumours which form flattened or nodular, firm masses that may infiltrate the renal pelvic wall to a variable depth and that are frequently ulcerated on their free surface. In situ tumours can sometimes be recognized as areas of mucosal thickening or granularity that may be accompanied by congestion.

Most squamous cell and undifferentiated carcinomas are solid, flat, non-papillary tumours. Adenocarcinomas are nodular and may have a mucoid or gelatinous appearance.

Tumours that partially block the outflow of urine will produce the changes that are associated with obstructive uropathy (see p. 467).

Light microscopy

Transitional cell carcinomas Microscopic-

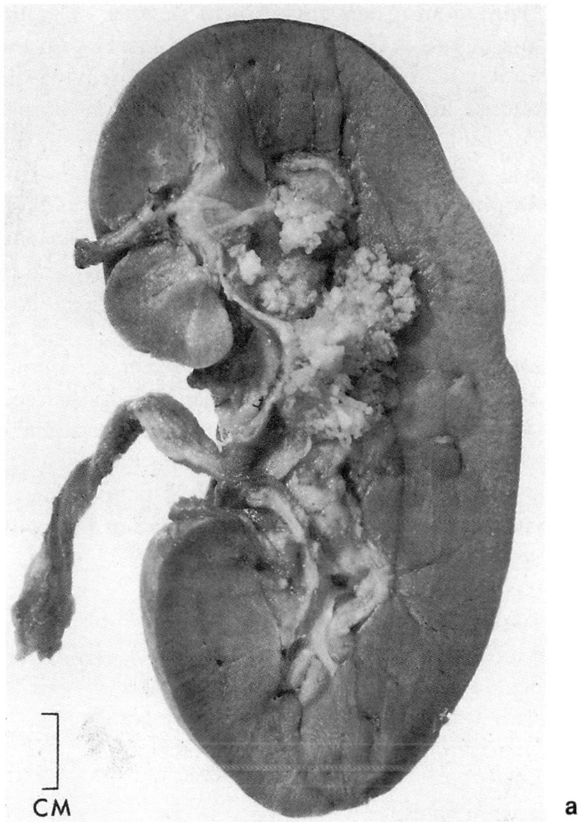

Fig. 16.23 Transitional cell carcinoma of the renal pelvis. The papillary tumour involves particularly the upper part of the renal pelvis and the adjacent calyces.

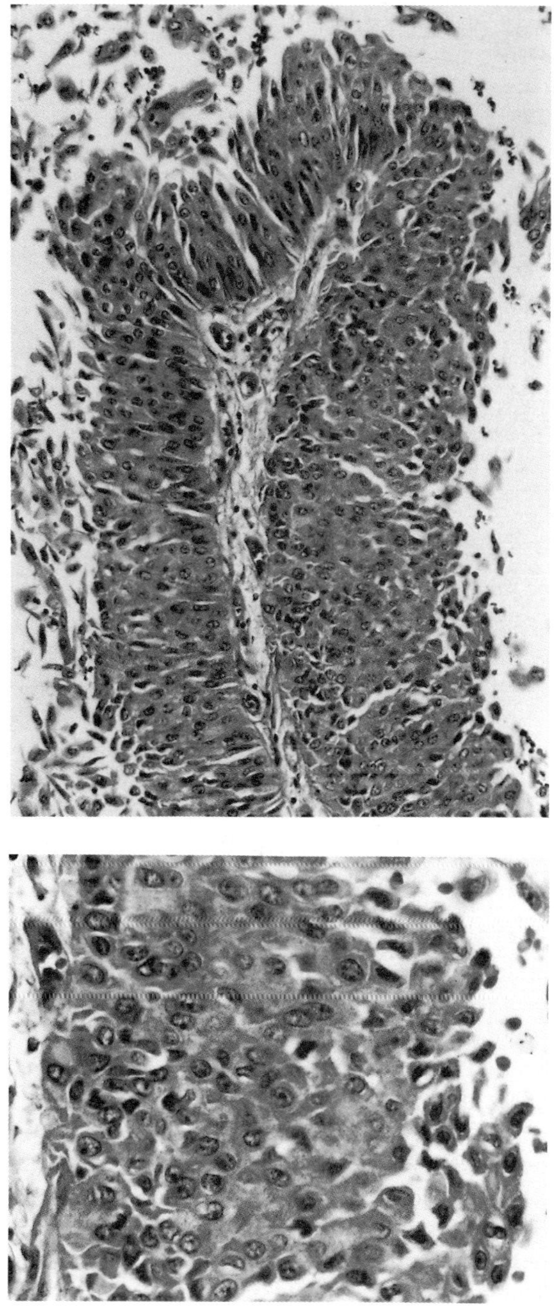

Fig. 16.24 a, b Transitional cell carcinoma of the renal pelvis. Grade I, stage pTa. Part of one of the papillary fronds. Haematoxylin-eosin: (a) × 150; (b) × 400

ally these tumours do not differ from their counterparts in the bladder (see p. 723) and ureter (see p. 689). They are divided into three grades according to the amount of epithelial dedifferentiation present.[203]

Grade I lesions are the most differentiated (Fig. 16.24). The epithelial cells covering the fronds of the papillary tumour are clearly of transitional type and have a low nucleus to cytoplasm ratio. However, the number of layers of these cells is increased to 10 or more. There is slight nuclear enlargement and hyperchromasia in a few cells. Occasional mitoses may be present (see p. 725).

Grade II lesions can still be recognized as being of transitional cell origin. The number of cell layers is markedly increased and there is loss of cell polarity. The nuclei are moderately enlarged and up to 50% show moderate hyperchromasia and variability in size. Mitoses are frequent.

Grade III lesions show such a degree of cellular pleomorphism and irregularity, loss of polarity and nuclear irregularity and hyperchromasia that it is often no longer immediately obvious that they have originated from transitional epithelium (see

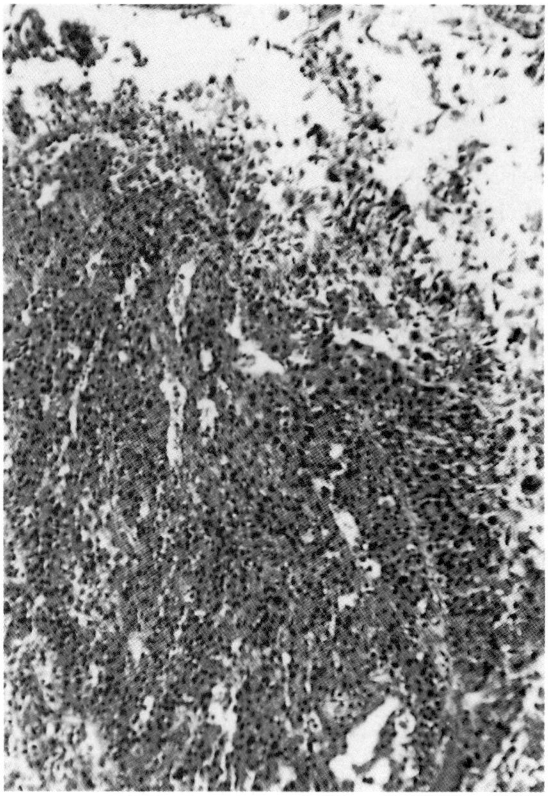

Fig. 16.25 Transitional cell carcinoma of the renal pelvis. Grade III.
Haematoxylin-eosin × 70

p. 725). The nucleus to cytoplasm ratio is high, and mitotic figures are common; giant cells and bizarre nuclear forms are not unusual. Single cell necrosis is common (Fig. 16.25).

Some authors separate out from this third grade those rare tumours with extreme nuclear pleomorphism, bizarre nuclear forms and atypical mitoses and denote them *grade IV*. Most pathologists consider this additional grade unwarranted.

Metaplastic foci of squamous or glandular change, occurring singly or in combination, may be found in any transitional cell tumour (see p. 725).

In many cases examination of the macroscopically normal pelvic epithelium adjacent to the tumour will reveal dysplasia or in-situ carcinoma. The severity of these changes generally corresponds to the grade of the transitional cell carcinoma.[199]

Transitional cell carcinoma in situ Carcinoma in situ is characterized by an increase in the number of cell layers in an area or areas of the mucosa lining the renal pelvis. This is accompanied by failure of differentiation of cells from the base to the surface of the epithelium, cellular pleomorphism and loss of polarity. There is also crowding and hyperchromasia of the nuclei and the presence of mitoses above the basal layer of cells (see p. 726).

Squamous cell carcinoma Pure squamous cell carcinomas (as distinct from transitional cell carcinomas showing foci of metaplastic squamous cell change) are rare.[204] There is usually keratin formation and tumour grading is possible, as with squamous carcinomas elsewhere in the body (see p. 728).

Adenocarcinoma Pure adenocarcinomas are extremely rare.[167] There is usually a clearly recognizable glandular pattern and the tumours can be graded using the criteria that are applicable to adenocarcinomas at other sites (see p. 729).

Electron microscopy[202]

The ultrastructural features of normal transitional epithelium persist in grade I transitional cell carcinomas. These features are: attachment of basal cells to the basement membrane by hemidesmosomes, connection of lateral cell surfaces by discrete attachments, and the presence of intracellular tonofilaments and lateral cisternae. In grade II tumours the characteristic lateral cisternae are lost. In grade III and IV tumours all distinguishing features have usually disappeared (see p. 732).

Immunohistochemistry

Immunostaining for ABH (ABO) blood-group-related antigens reveals that about 50% of tumours tested lack ABH antigen expression (even after excluding group O non-secretors which are a source of false-negative results). Absence of ABH expression correlates significantly with subsequent deep invasion and metastasis by the tumour.[205] Transitional cell carcinomas express cytokerakin polypeptides. As a tumour becomes more malignant the expression of the various polypeptides changes.[206] Although at present this is only of interest in research, it may be that in the future a selected panel of antibodies to different cytokeratin polypeptides could help in tumour grading and staging.

Cytogenetic analysis and genotyping

Cytogenetic analysis has been reported on only about four cases of renal transitional cell carcinomas, and no common chromosome changes have been found. Trisomy of chromosome 7 was present in one of the cases.[207] In transitional cell carcinoma of the bladder monosomy 9 has been found repeatedly, even as a sole abnormality, suggesting that it may represent a primary aberration.[208] Trisomy for chromosome 7 is also quite frequent in bladder cancer and has been reported as the only karyotypic abnormality in a primary transitional cell carcinoma of the ureter.[209]

Morphometry and cytometry

Analysis of DNA ploidy by flow cytometry is being used widely for research and clinical purposes in the study of bladder cancer (see p. 732). So far there is only one preliminary report of its use in renal pelvic carcinoma.[205] Flow cytometry ploidy results did not correlate with prognosis in this study on 42 cases of transitional cell carcinoma of the renal pelvis.[205]

There is little information about the usefulness of computed cell morphometry in the analysis of renal pelvic cancers.

Spread

Any of the tumours that arise in the renal pelvis may spread directly into the adjacent tissues and by lymphatics and blood stream to other parts of the body. Extension through the wall of the pelvis into the retroperitoneum or renal parenchyma is quite common once the tumour has become invasive. The abundant lymphatics in the renal pelvis are invaded early by infiltrating tumour. Blood-borne secondaries are present in at least a third of the fatal cases but they are not as common as in renal cell carcinoma. Metastases occur most frequently in the bones, lungs and liver; the bone deposits are osteolytic. The onset of metastatic spread may be long delayed.

Differential diagnosis

The differential diagnosis of renal pelvic carcinoma is similar to that of bladder cancer which is discussed on page 730.

Complications

The commonest and most important complication is obstruction to the urinary outflow tract giving rise to *hydronephrosis* (see pp. 444, 468). This may be accompanied or followed by *pyelonephritis*, either acute or chronic (see p. 432). *Calculi* are more frequent than in people without a carcinoma of the renal pelvis (see p. 531).

Prognosis

Removal of the primary transitional cell carcinoma is often followed by recurrence of the neoplasm or by the formation of fresh primary tumours. Even the ureteric stump left behind after nephrectomy develops a transitional cell carcinoma in approximately 10% of patients.[199]

In attempting to determine the prognosis the extent to which the tumour has spread and the histological grade are both important. The latter is more subjective; computed cell morphometry has been little used so far to improve the objectivity of histological grading. Useful additional prognostic information is provided by ABH status (see p. 610).[205] The role, if any, of establishing DNA ploidy of the tumour by flow cytometry is uncertain; the little evidence that is available is not encouraging.[205]

Tumour penetration of the muscle of the renal pelvic wall, poor differentiation of the tumour and multifocal tumour formation are the main features which adversely affect the prognosis.

Stage of tumour spread

In Europe the TNM (tumour, nodes and metastases) staging system proposed by the Union Internationale contre le Cancer in 1978[44] is often used:

pTa papillary non-invasive carcinoma
pT1 tumour not extending beyond lamina propria
pT2 invasion of superficial muscle
pT3 invasion of deep muscle
pT4 invasion of kidney or other structures outside the renal pelvis.

The problem with this system, which is widely used for the staging of bladder tumours (see p. 729), is that the thinness of the pelvic musculature makes it difficult to distinguish between pT2 and 3.

In the USA a number of staging systems are in use, most based upon Gittes' modification of a system first proposed by Grabstal or upon Marshall's adaption of the Jewett system. Most are very similar and the following is representative:[210]

Stage 0 non-invasive carcinoma
Stage A tumour not extending beyond lamina propria
Stage B invasion of muscle of wall of renal pelvis
Stage C invasion into peripelvic tissue or renal parenchyma
Stage D tumour accompanied by regional or distant metastases.

The staging system proposed by the Armed Forces Institute of Pathology, Washington, USA, is similar for the first three stages except that 0 is called stage I, A is stage II and B is stage III. The significant difference is that C and D are merged to give stage IV.[202]

Most transitional cell tumours of the renal pelvis are non-invasive or only superficially invasive when staged by one or other of these methods. In only about a third of cases is there evidence of spread into or beyond the muscle coat. In one series approximately 42% were non-invasive (pTa), 23% had breached the basement membrane to invade the stromal cores of the papillae but had not extended beyond the lamina propria (pT1), 7% had superficially invaded the muscle coat (pT2), 14% had invaded the deep muscle (pT3) and 12% had penetrated beyond the renal pelvis (pT4).[196]

The 5-year survival rate after nephrectomy for patients with tumours not penetrating beyond the midpoint of the muscle coat of the pelvis (pTa, pT1 and pT2) is approximately 70%; for patients with tumours invading deeply into or beyond the muscle (pT3 and 4) it is about 30%.[196] These data indicate that penetration of the muscle by the tumour predisposes to a poor prognosis.

Histological grade

Most centres use the system proposed by the Armed Forces Institute of Pathology for the histological grading of bladder tumours (see p. 609).[203] Graded in this way the majority of transitional cell carcinomas of the pelvis are well differentiated. In one series 64% fell into grade I, 22% into grade II and only 13% into grade III.[196]

The 5-year survival rate for patients with solitary, well-differentiated tumours (grade I) is approximately 73%, for those with tumours of intermediate grade (grade II) it is approximately 40% and for those with poorly differentiated tumours (grade III) it is approximately 33%. Therefore, the poorer the differentiation the worse the prognosis.

Multiplicity of tumours

Multifocal tumour formation is associated with a poor prognosis. The 5-year survival rate of patients with a grade I transitional cell carcinoma of the renal pelvis who have a similar carcinoma in the ureter is 50%, compared with 73% for those patients with only a renal pelvic tumour of the same grade and no ureteric tumour.[196]

Squamous cell carcinoma of the renal pelvis

The prognosis of squamous cell carcinomas is poor. Only about 33% are alive 1 year after operation; the 5-year survival rate is approximately 17%. Many cases are inoperable when discovered.[199]

Adenocarcinoma of the renal pelvis

The prognosis of adenocarcinomas is poor. The 5-year survival rate is approximately 10%.[167]

Pathogenesis

Renal pelvic carcinoma is thought to arise from

differentiated cells of the pelvic epithelium. The aetiology and pathogenesis of the malignant change in most of these tumours are unknown; in a few instances there is a clear link with an environmental factor such as contact with an aromatic amine, excessive phenacetin consumption or inhalation of cigarette smoke. An exceptionally high incidence of renal pelvic cancer in a tiny area of the Balkans suggests that an environmental agent is responsible but the agent has yet to be isolated.

Chemical agents

Carcinoma of the renal pelvis is sometimes seen as an occupational disease of workers in the rubber, aniline dye, cable, plastic and gas industries.[211] The carcinogens responsible are particular aromatic amines, principally β-naphthylamine, benzidine, *para*-aminodiphenyl and 2-acetylaminofluorene. Metabolites of these substances are excreted in the urine (see p. 719).

Excessive phenacetin consumption and renal papillary necrosis

There seems to be a causal link between excessive ingestion of phenacetin-containing analgesics and the occurrence of tumours of the renal pelvis (see p. 461). Transitional cell carcinomas are more common in analgesic abusers;[212,213] approximately 8% of patients with analgesic nephropathy in Sweden and Switzerland develop urothelial tumours.[213,214] It is estimated that in some areas in Switzerland transitional cell tumours of the renal pelvis occur 77 times more frequently in analgesic abusers than in non-abusers.[215] The tumours are more common in women, in contrast to the usual 3 : 1 ratio of males to females with renal pelvic cancers not associated with analgesic abuse. The mean induction time for analgesic-associated renal pelvic carcinomas is about 22 years.[216]

Morphologically the neoplasms do not differ from other transitional cell tumours of the renal pelvis. They are reputed to have a worse prognosis, the major contributing factor being the coexisting chronic nephropathy.[217] They are frequently multiple and there is often an accompanying extensive urothelial dysplasia, with focal carcinoma in situ.

Epidemiological surveys indicate that it is the regular consumption of analgesics containing phenacetin rather than of those containing no phenacetin that confers an increased risk of cancers of the renal pelvis.[218] The carcinogenic effect of phenacetin probably is due to the potent alkylating action of the N-O-sulphate and N-O-glucuronide conjugates of N-hydroxyphenacetin.[53]

Renal papillary necrosis (see p. 459) has been found in 75% of reported cases of analgesic-associated carcinoma of the renal pelvis. Evidence suggests that excessive phenacetin consumption and renal papillary necrosis are independent risk factors for renal pelvic carcinoma and that when they coexist they have sequential effects.[219]

Balkan endemic nephropathy

Carcinoma of the renal pelvis is unusually frequent among the inhabitants of a few villages in a small area in the vicinity of the Danube and its tributaries in adjacent parts of Romania, Yugoslavia and Bulgaria.[220] This is the same population that is affected by an obscure chronic tubulointerstitial nephritis called Balkan endemic nephropathy (see p. 481). Carcinoma of the renal pelvis is found in about a third of patients dying from Balkan endemic nephropathy.[221,222] In affected villages households occur in which two or even three members are affected by renal pelvic or ureteral tumours.[223] Although there is a high frequency of carcinoma of the renal pelvis and ureters, the incidence of bladder cancer in these regions is not particularly raised.[223]

The pathogenesis of Balkan endemic nephropathy is not known and the postulated environmental agent responsible for the tumours of the urothelium has not been identified (see p. 482).

Cigarette smoking

Cigarette smoking has been implicated as a factor in the causation of carcinoma of the renal pelvis. Population-based case control studies have shown that smokers are six to seven times more likely to develop a renal pelvic cancer than non-smokers. There is a dose–response relationship, heavy smokers being 11 times more likely than non-smokers to get the disease. It has been estimated that 82% of carcinomas of the renal pelvis among males and 61% of those among females in Minneapolis, USA, are due to cigarette smoking.[224]

TRANSITIONAL CELL PAPILLOMA

It is very difficult to make a sure distinction between a benign papilloma arising from the transitional epithelium of the renal pelvis and the corresponding grade I non-invasive transitional cell carcinoma. For this reason many authors, particularly in the USA, do not retain the transitional cell papilloma as a separate entity, but regard it as a very well-differentiated carcinoma. They often describe a range of transitional cell carcinomas from the most differentiated (grade 0) to the least differentiated (grade 4). British authors, however, still find it useful to retain the term 'papilloma', as defined by the Armed Forces Institute of Pathology in Washington,[203] to describe a papillary tumour covered by no more than seven layers of regular transitional cells that are indistinguishable from those that line the renal pelvis (Fig. 16.26). The individual cells are slender and lie parallel to each other at right angles to the basement membrane. The nuclei are regular in size and staining; mitoses are absent. Using these strict criteria only about 3% of all primary tumours of the renal pelvis fall into this category.

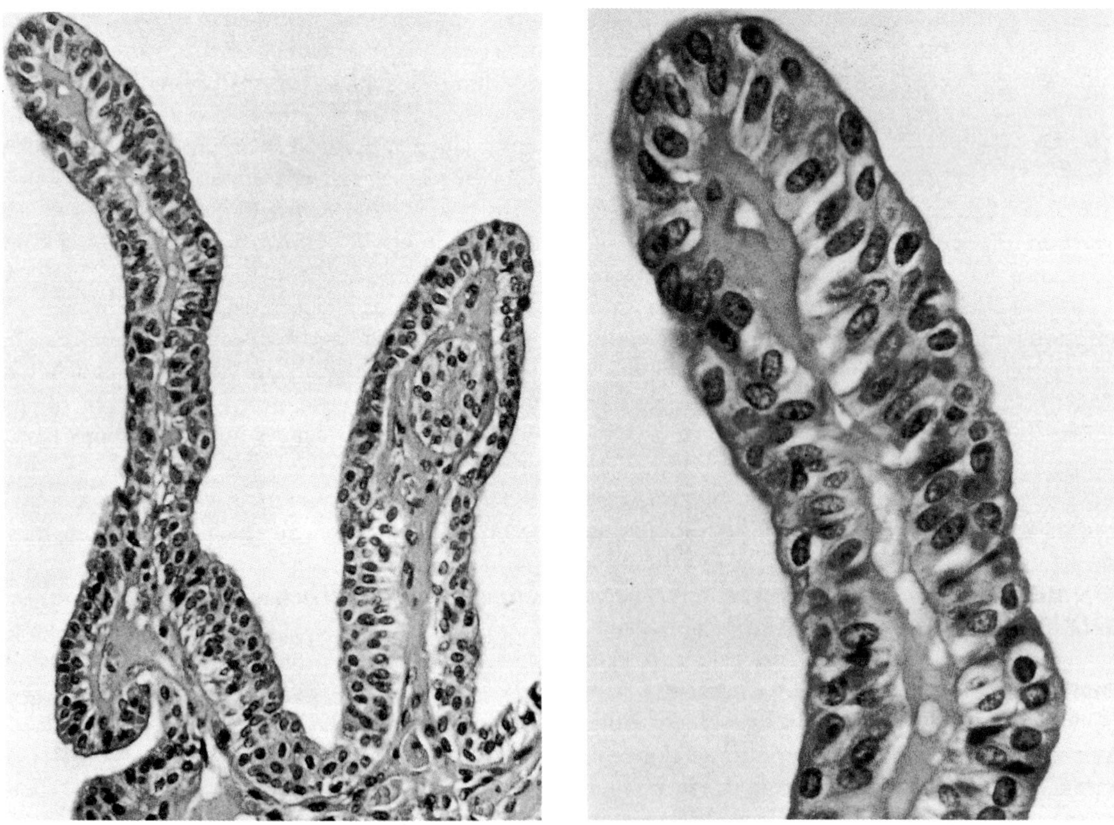

a b

Fig. 16.26 a, b Transitional cell papilloma. The finger-like processes are covered by normal transitional cell epithelium. Haematoxylin-eosin: (**a**) × 250; (**b**) 650
Reproduced by permission from: Koss LG. Tumors of the urinary bladder. Atlas of tumor pathology, 2nd series, fascicle 11. Washington DC: Armed Forces Institute of Pathology, 1975 (Figs. 16,17)

MISCELLANEOUS TUMOURS OF THE RENAL PELVIS

HAEMANGIOMA

Haemangiomas only very rarely arise in the mucosa of the renal pelvis.[225] So-called renal pelvic haemangiomas are usually renal parenchymal tumours that are situated at the tips of the papillae, producing nodular elevations of the calyceal mucosa; occasionally they protrude into the renal pelvis as a polypoid mass.

The most frequent clinical manifestations of renal pelvic haemangiomas are gross haematuria and renal colic secondary to the passage of blood clots.

OTHER RARITIES

Isolated cases of leiomyoma, neurilemmoma (schwannoma)[169] and leiomyosarcoma have been described.

SECONDARY TUMOURS INVOLVING THE RENAL PELVIS

Direct spread of a renal cell carcinoma into the renal pelvis is common, and invasion of the renal pelvis by a retroperitoneal sarcoma is occasionally seen. Metastasis to the renal pelvis from distant sites has only been recorded on a few occasions.

TUMOUR-LIKE CONDITIONS OF THE RENAL PELVIS

VON BRUNN'S NESTS, PYELITIS CYSTICA AND PYELITIS GLANDULARIS[202,203]

The urothelium lining the renal pelvis commonly responds to injury or irritation (e.g. infection, calculi and hydronephrosis) by forming buds of transitional epithelium which extend into the lamina propria. The buds may eventually lose their continuity with the surface epithelium, becoming discrete masses of cuboidal and fusiform epithelial cells – Von Brunn's nests (see p. 715). The nests are either solid or contain small cavities which dilate and eventually become cysts. The cystic changes are referred to as *pyelitis cystica*. As the cysts enlarge the lining epithelium undergoes metaplastic transformation to columnar mucus-secreting cells and the lumen fills with secretion. The term *pyelitis glandularis* is used to describe these metaplastic glandular changes. Occasionally, when the glandular metaplasia is florid and extensive, it may be difficult to distinguish pyelitis glandularis from an adenocarcinoma.

Von Brunn's nests are sometimes found in association with in-situ carcinoma in the overlying renal pelvic mucosa.

INVERTED PAPILLOMA[226]

The inverted papilloma is a rare tumour which is usually found in the bladder (see p. 730) but occasionally occurs in the renal pelvis. It appears as a small submucosal nodule composed of interconnected papillae and cords of transitional epithelial cells which extend into the underlying loose fibrous tissue.

FIBROEPITHELIAL POLYP[227]

Fibroepithelial polyps are uncommon and usually occur in the upper part of the ureter (see p. 688). Occasionally they occur in the renal pelvis and cause colicky flank pain in a child or young adult.

RENAL COMPLICATIONS OF EXTRARENAL CANCER

A wide range of renal complications may occur during the course of neoplastic disease (Table 16.1).

INVASION OF KIDNEYS BY THE NEOPLASM

Metastatic spread of an extrarenal tumour to the

Table 16.1 Renal complications of extrarenal cancer

1. Invasion of kidneys by the neoplasm
2. Glomerulonephritis
   (a) Diffuse membranous
   (b) Minimal change disease
3. Obstructive uropathy
   (a) Intrarenal
      (i) Uric acid nephropathy
      (ii) Myeloma cast nephropathy
      (iii) Renal calculi associated with hypercalcaemia
   (b) Extrarenal – obstruction of ureters, bladder or urethra
      (i) by tumour
      (ii) by urinary calculi
4. Fluid and electrolyte disturbances
   (a) Prerenal azotaemia and ischaemic ATN
   (b) Hypokalaemia and tubular vacuolation
   (c) Hypercalcaemia and nephrocalcinosis
5. Changes caused by treatment
   (a) Radiation nephritis
   (b) Drug-induced nephrotoxicity
      (i) cytotoxic drugs
      (ii) analgesics and antibiotics
6. Miscellaneous
   (a) Disseminated intravascular coagulation
   (b) Amyloidosis

kidneys is frequent (see page 607); direct invasion of the renal pelvis by a retroperitoneal sarcoma occurs occasionally (see p. 615). The invasive tumour rarely impairs renal function although proteinuria is almost always present and about 30% of patients have microscopic haematuria.[228]

GLOMERULONEPHRITIS

Several types of glomerulonephritis may arise in people with cancer. This has been increasingly recognized since the report in 1966 by Lee and his colleagues that of 101 patients with the nephrotic syndrome 11 had cancer.[229] The most frequent occurrence is diffuse membranous glomerulonephritis in patients with carcinomas and minimal change disease in those with Hodgkin's lymphoma.[230] Other forms of glomerulonephritis are only rarely associated with a cancer.

Membranous glomerulonephritis and carcinomas

Incidence

Cancer has been reported in 1.4% to 10.9% of patients with membranous glomerulonephritis; in a recent study of 128 biopsy proven cases of membranous glomerulonephritis, carcinomas were found in 4 (3.12%) of the patients.[231] This is a higher incidence than would occur by chance in an age-matched control group. It is sensible, therefore, to look carefully for cancer in any nephrotic patient of 40 years or over and to maintain close medical follow up, even if the initial examination is negative.[231] The cancers associated with membranous glomerulonephritis have included a variety of histological types from different primary sites, but the most common have been carcinomas of the lung and adenocarcinomas of the gastrointestinal tract.[231]

Autopsy studies of patients with a variety of neoplasms have failed to detect a raised incidence of membranous glomerulonephritis.[232] This failure is almost certainly because insufficiently large numbers of cancer patients were surveyed; glomerulonephritis is a very rare occurence in patients with neoplasms.

Clinical features

When diffuse membraneous glomerulonephritis occurs in a patient with a cancer, proteinuria is the first clinical manifestation; its severity soon becomes sufficient to induce the nephrotic syndrome.

Renal changes

The glomerular lesions in cancer-associated membranous glomerulonephritis do not differ histopathologically from those in the idiopathic form of of the disease (see page 192).

Pathogenesis

The search for specific immune complexes containing antigens of the associated cancer in the deposits on the glomerular capillary basement membranes has been only partly successful; the evidence obtained is suggestive but inconclusive.[230,232] It is still uncertain whether antigens from the cancer initiate the process which produces the glomerulonephritis. An alternative or additional possibility is that the cancer, by interfering with immune function or regulation, predisposes the patient to the development of an immune complex nephritis involving other exogenous or endogenous antigens; any tumour antigen present in the glomerular deposits might be there because of non-specific trapping.[232]

Prognosis

In some patients there has been remission of the nephrotic syndrome after resection of the carcinoma; in others the clinical manifestations have persisted even in cases in which subsequent biopsies have shown that the subepithelial glomerular deposits have disappeared.[232]

Minimal change disease and Hodgkin's lymphoma

There is a well-established but rare association between Hodgkin's lymphoma and minimal change disease. Surveys of large numbers of patients with Hodgkin's lymphoma have found minimal change disease in approximately 0.4%;[232] this is greater than the expected incidence based on chance. The nephrotic syndrome disappears when tumour regression occurs in response to antineoplastic therapy; it recurs with tumour relapse.[228]

Attempts to explain this association mostly involve linking the defect in T lymphocyte function that is present in Hodgkin's disease with the production by the patient of various lymphokines and other humoral agents that alter the permeability of the glomerular capillary basement membranes. At present there is little evidence to support any of the suggestions.[232]

Glomerular lesions are so rare in non-Hodgkin's lymphomas and leukaemia that it is difficult to be sure that the occurrence is anything other than incidental.

OBSTRUCTIVE UROPATHY

Intrarenal

Hyperuricaemic acute renal failure has become a major clinical problem since the development of effective chemotherapy for leukaemias and lymphoma. Uric acid excretion may be increased dramatically in patients with very responsive malignant neoplasms and uric acid crystals may precipitate in the nephrons leading to intrarenal obstruction and severe *uric acid nephropathy* (see page 341).

In multiple myeloma precipitation of Bence Jones protein in the lumen of the nephrons may occur leading to intrarenal obstruction (*myeloma cast nephropathy*) and acute renal failure (see page 358).

Patients with hypercalcaemia may develop *renal calculi* and these may give rise to obstructive nephropathy (see page 467).

Extrarenal

Neoplasms of the pelvic organs and genitourinary tract, retroperitoneal tumours and metastases from distant tumours may invade or press on some part of the urinary outflow tract and produce unilateral or bilateral obstructive uropathy.

FLUID AND ELECTROLYTE DISTURBANCES

It is not within the scope of this book to discuss the numerous electrolyte disturbances that may occur in patients with cancer. For further information on this subject the reader is referred to recent texts of nephrology. However, three disorders deserve brief mention because they are common and produce morphological renal lesions.

Prerenal azotaemia

Vomiting, diarrhoea and inadequate fluid intake are common in cancer patients and may lead to hypovolaemia which, if severe or prolonged, may give rise to ischaemic acute tubular necrosis (see page 492).

Hypokalaemia

Colorectal cancers lead to diarrhoea and potassium loss; hypokalaemia also occurs in cases of adrenal carcinoma and of neoplasms producing ectopic adrenocorticotrophic hormone (ACTH). Prolonged hypokalaemia causes tubular vacuolation (see page 97).

Hypercalcaemia

Hypercalcaemia occurs in the course of a variety of neoplasms. This may be due to the tumour destroying bone or producing parathormone-like substances. In bedridden patients it may simply be the immobilization that leads to the release of calcium from the bones. Both acute and chronic hypercalcaemia may produce renal injury (see page 544).

CHANGES CAUSED BY TREATMENT

Radiation nephritis

Radiation nephritis may still occur when irradiation of the kidneys cannot be avoided in treating, for example, neuroblastomas, seminomas and some retroperitoneal tumours. The damage that may be done to the kidneys is discussed on pages 477 to 480.

Drug-induced nephrotoxicity

Cytotoxic drugs

Several agents used in cancer chemotherapy are nephrotoxic. Examples are *cisplatin* which causes a nephrotoxic acute tubular necrosis (see page 516), *methotrexate* which may precipitate as crystals in the distal tubules causing intrarenal obstruction, and *mitomycin C* which, when combined with *5-fluorouracil*, can produce the haemolytic uraemic syndrome (see page 281).

Drugs used in supportive care

Cancer patients are frequently given *antibiotics* and some of these may damage the kidneys (see page 457). *Analgesics* are also commonly used and if given frequently for long periods may lead to analgesic nephropathy (seee page 458).

MISCELLANEOUS COMPLICATIONS

Disseminated intravascular coagulation

Disseminated intravascular coagulation may occur in cancer patients, possibly because certain tumour products act as procoagulants. It has particularly been associated with acute promyelocytic leukaemia (M3) and may involve the kidneys (see page 290).

Amyloidosis

Among extrarenal tumours amyloidosis is most likely to occur in multiple myeloma (see page 359); it only rarely complicates other tumours.

REFERENCES

1. Bennington JL, Beckwith JB. Tumors of the kidney, renal pelvis, and ureter. Atlas of tumor pathology: fascicle 12. Washington, DC Armed Forces Institute of Pathology, 1975; 26.

Primary epithelial tumours of the renal parenchyma

2. Bennington JL, Beckwith JB. Tumors of the kidney, renal pelvis, and ureter. Atlas of tumor pathology: fascicle 12. Washington, DC: Armed Forces Institute of Pathology, 1975; 93–199.
3. Muir CS, Nectoux J. Geographical distribution and aetiology of kidney cancer. In: Sufrin G, Beckley SA, eds. Renal adenocarcinoma. UICC technical report series: 49. Geneva: International Union against Cancer, 1980; 133–155.
4. Skinner DG, Colvin RB, Vermillion CD, Pfister RC, Leadbetter WF. Diagnosis and management of renal cell carcinoma. A clinical and pathologic study of 309 cases. Cancer 1971; 28: 1165–1177.
5. Utz DC, Warren MM, Gregg JA, Ludwig J, Kelalis P. Reversible hepatic dysfunction associated with hypernephroma. Mayo Clin Proc 1970; 45: 161–169.
6. Piscioli F, Pusiol T, Scappini P, Luciani L. Urine cytology in the detection of renal adenocarcinoma. Cancer 1985; 56: 2251–2255.
7. Altaffer LF, Chenault OW. Paraneoplastic

endocrinopathies associated with renal tumours. J Urol 1979; 122: 573–577.
8. Buckle RM, McMillan M, Mallinson C. Ectopic secretion of parathyroid hormone by a renal adenocarcinoma in a patient with hypercalcaemia. Br Med J 1970; 4: 724–726.
9. Cummings KB, Robertson RP. Prostaglandin: increased production by renal cell carcinoma. J Urol 1977; 118: 720–723.
10. Riggs BL, Sprague RG. Association of Cushing's syndrome and neoplastic disease. Arch Intern Med 1961; 108: 841–849.
11. Sytkowski AJ, Richie JP, Bickness KA. New human renal carcinoma line established from a patient with erythrocytosis. Cancer Res1983; 43: 1415–1419.
12. Lindop GBM, Leckie B, Winearls CG. Malignant hypertension due to a renin-secreting renal cell carcinoma – an ultrastructural and immunocytochemical study. Histopathology 1986; 10: 1077–1088.
13. Gleeson MH, Bloom SR, Polak JM, Henry K, Dowling RH. Endocrine tumour in kidney affecting small bowel structure, motility, and absorptive function. Gut 1971; 12: 773–782.
14. Bennington JL, Laubscher FA. Epidemiologic studies on carcinoma of the kidney. 1. Association with smoking. Cancer 1968; 21: 1069–1071.
15. Kolonel LN. Association of cadmium with renal cancer. Cancer 1976; 37: 1782–1787.
16. Mickisch O, Bommer J, Bachmann S, Waldherr R, Mann JFE, Ritz E. Multicystic transformation of kidneys in chronic renal failure. Nephron 1984; 38: 93–99.
17. Hughson MD, Buckwald D, Fox M. Renal neoplasia and acquired cystic kidney disease in patients receiving long-term dialysis. Arch Pathol Lab Med 1986; 110: 592–601.
18. Editorial. Von Hippel-Lindau disease. Lancet 1991; 337: 1065.
19. Cohen AJ, Li FP, Berg S et al. Hereditary renal-cell carcinoma associated with a chromosomal translocation. N Engl J Med 1979; 301: 592–595.
20. Pathak S, Strong LC, Ferrell RE, Trindade A. Familial renal cell carcinoma with a 3;11 chromosome translocation limited to tumor cells. Science 1982; 217: 939–941.
21. Singh EO, Benson RC, Wold LE. Cancer-to-cancer metastasis. JUrol 1984; 132: 340–342.
22. Mackay B, Ordóñez NG, Khoursand J, Bennington JL. The ultrastructure and immunocytochemistry of renal cell carcinoma. Ultrastruct Pathol 1987; 11: 483–502.
23. Van Keieken JHJM, Oosterwijk E, Lycklama À, Nijeholt AAB, Ruiter DJ. Renal oncocytoma: a report of two cases with immunohistochemical evaluation. Hum Pathol 1988; 19: 460–464.
24. Pitz S, Moll R, Störkel S, Thoenes W. Expression of intermediate filament proteins in subtypes of renal cell carcinomas and in renal oncocytomas: distinction of two classes of renal cell tumors. Lab Invest 1987; 56: 642–653.
25. Oosterwijk E, Ruiter DJ, Hoedemaeker PJ et al. Monoclonal antibody G250 recognizes a determinant present in renal-cell carcinoma and absent from normal kidney. Int J Cancer 1986; 38: 489–494.
26. Kovacs G, Frisch S. Clonal chromosome abnormalities in tumour cells from patients with sporadic renal cell carcinomas. Cancer Res 1989; 49: 651–659.
27. Kovacs G, Erlandsson R, Boldog F et al. Consistent chromosome 3p deletion and loss of heterozygosity in renal cell carcinoma. Proc Natl Acad Sci USA 1988; 85: 1571–1575.
28. O'Dea MJ, Zincke H, Utz DC, Bernatz PE. The treatment of renal cell carcinoma with solitary metastasis. J Urol 1978; 120: 540–542.
29. Dineen MK, Pastore RD, Emrich LJ, Huben RP. Results of surgical treatment of renal cell carcinoma with solitary metastasis. JUrol 1988; 140: 277–279.
30. Beatty PG, Oates JA, Oldham RK. Renal cell carcinoma metastatic to a pheochromocytoma. J Urol 1979; 122: 544–545.
31. Freed SZ, Halpern JP, Gordon M. Idiopathic regression of metastases from renal cell carcinomas. J Urol 1977; 118: 538–542.
32. Wick MR, Cherwitz DL, McGlennen RC, Dehner LP. Adrenocortical carcinoma. An immunohistochemical comparison with renal cell carcinoma. Am J Pathol 1986; 122: 343–352.
33. Ellis IO, Hitchcock A. Tumour marker immunoreactivity in adenocarcinoma. J Clin Pathol 1988; 41: 1064–1067.
34. Dictor M, Hasserius R. Systemic amyloidosis and nonhematologic malignancy in a large autopsy series. Acta Pathol Microbiol Scand [A] 1981; 89: 411–416.
35. Somer TP, Tornroth TS. Renal adenocarcinoma and systemic amyloidosis. Immunohistochemical and histochemical studies. Arch Pathol Lab Med 1985; 109: 571–574.
36. Dalakas MC, Fujihara S, Askanas V, Engel WK, Glenner GG. Nature of amyloid deposits in hypernephroma. Immunocytochemical studies in 2 cases associated with amyloid polyneuropathy. Am J Pathol 1984; 116: 447–454.
37. Pras M, Franklin EC, Shibolet S, Frangione B. Amyloidosis of the AA type associated with renal cell carcinoma. Am J Med1982; 73: 426–428.
38. Beaufils H, Patte R, Aubert P et al. Renal immunopathology in renal cell carcinoma. Virchows Arch [A] 1984; 404: 87–97.
39. Kerpen HO, Bhat JG, Feiner HD, Baldwin DS. Membranous nephropathy associated with renal cell carcinoma. Evidence against a role of renal tubular or tumor antibodies in pathogenesis. Am J Med 1978; 64: 863–867.
40. Dupond JL, Apffel L, Collas JM, Leconte des Floris R. Syndrome néphrotique à lésions glomérulaires minimes révélateur d'un cancer du rein. Nouv Presse Méd 1980; 9: 884–885.
41. Lee JC, Yamauchi H, Hopper J. The association of cancer and the nephrotic syndrome. Ann Intern Med 1966; 64: 41–51.
42. Robson CJ, Churchill BM, Anderson W. The results of radical nephrectomy for renal cell carcinoma. J Urol 1969; 101: 297–301.
43. Beahrs OH, Myers MH. Manual for staging of cancer, 2nd edn. Philadelphia: Lippincott, 1983.
44. Spiessel B, Beahrs OH, Hermanek P et al. TNM–atlas: illustrated guide to the TNM/pTNM classification of malignant tumours, 3rd edn. Berlin: Springer, 1989.
45. Libertino JA, Zinman L, Watkins E. Long term results of resection of renal cell cancer with extension into inferior vena cava. JUrol 1987; 137: 21–24.

46. Delahunt B, Nacey JN. Renal cell carcinoma II. Histological indicators of prognosis. Pathology 1987; 19: 258–263.
47. Fuhrman SA, Lasky LC, Limas C. Prognostic significance of morphologic parameters in renal cell carcinoma. Am J Surg Pathol1982; 6: 655–663.
48. Tosi P, Luzi P, Baak JPA et al. Nuclear morphometry as an important prognostic factor in stage I renal cell carcinoma. Cancer 1986; 58: 2512–2518.
49. Rainwater LM, Hosaka Y, Farrow GM, Lieber MM. Well differentiated clear cell renal carcinoma: significance of nuclear deoxyribonucleic acid patterns studied by flow cytometry. J Urol 1987; 137: 15–20.
50. Zbar B, Brauch H, Talmadge C, Linehan M. Loss of alleles of loci on the short arm of chromosome 3 in renal cell carcinoma. Nature 1987; 327: 721–724.
51. McLaughlin JK, Mandel JS, Blot WJ, Schuman LM, Mehl ES, Fraumeni JF. A population-based case-control study of renal cell carcinoma. J Natl Cancer Inst. 1984; 72: 275–284.
52. McCredie M, Ford JM, Stewart JH. Risk factors for cancer of the renal parenchyma. Int J Cancer 1988; 42: 13–16.
53. Mulder GJ, Hinson JA, Gillette JR. Generation of reactive metabolites of *N*-hydroxyphenacetin by glucuronidation and sulfation. Biochem Pharmacol 1977; 26: 189–196.
54. Mancilla-Jimenez R, Stanley RJ, Blath RA. Papillary renal cell carcinoma. A clinical, radiologic, and pathologic study of 34 cases. Cancer 1976; 38: 2469–2480.
55. Kovacs G. Papillary renal cell carcinoma. A morphologic and cytogenetic study of 11 cases. Am J Pathol 1989; 134: 27–34.
56. Reznicek SB, Narayana AS, Culp DA. Cystoadenocarcinoma of the kidney: a profile of 13 cases. J Urol 1985; 134: 256–259.
57. Medeiros LJ, Michie SA, Johnson DE, Warnke RA, Weiss LM. An immunoperoxidase study of renal cell carcinomas: correlation with nuclear grade, cell type, and histologic pattern. Hum Pathol 1988; 19: 980–987.
58. Thoenes W, Storkel ST, Rumpelt H-J, Moll R, Baum HP, Werner S. Chromophobe cell renal carcinoma and its variants – a report on 32 cases. J Pathol 1988; 155: 277–287.
59. Harris SC, Hird PM, Shortland JR. Immunohistochemistry and lectin histochemistry in sarcomatoid renal cell carcinoma: a comparison with classical renal cell carcinoma. Histopathology 1989; 15: 607–616.
60. Bertoni F, Ferri C, Benati A, Bacchini P, Corrado F. Sarcomatoid carcinoma of the kidney. J Urol 1987; 137: 25–28.
61. Tomera KM, Farrow GM, Lieber MM. Sarcomatoid renal carcinoma. J Urol 1983; 130: 657–659.
62. Fleming S, Lewi HJE. Collecting duct carcinoma of the kidney. Histopathology 1986; 10: 1131–1141.
63. Kennedy SM, Merino MJ, Lineham WM, Roberts JR, Robertson CN, Neumann RD. Collecting duct carcinoma of the kidney. Hum Pathol 1990; 21: 449–456.
64. Bane B, Grignon DJ, Friedman G, Verani R, Ro JY, Ayala AG. Collecting duct carcinoma (CDC) of the kidney: a distinct clinicopathologic entity. Lab Invest 1989; 60: 5A (abstr).
65. Choi H, Almagro UA, McManus JT, Norback DH, Jacobs SC. Renal oncocytoma. Cancer 1983; 51: 1887–1896.
66. Bonavita JA, Pollack HM, Banner MP. Renal oncocytoma: further observations and literature review. Urol Radiol 1981; 2: 229–234.
67. Levine E, Huntrakoon M. Computed tomography of renal oncocytoma. Am J Radiol 1983; 141: 741–746.
68. Raspa RW, Fernandes M, Ward JN. Bilateral renal oncocytoma: report of 2 cases and review of literature. J Urol 1985; 133: 458–461.
69. Zhang G, Monda L, Wasserman NF, Fraley EE. Bilateral renal oncocytoma. Report of 2 cases and literature review. J Urol 1985; 133: 84–86.
70. Warfel KA, Eble JN. Renal oncocytomatosis. J Urol 1982; 127: 1179–1180.
71. Eble JN, Hull MT. Morphologic features of renal oncocytoma: a light and electron microscopic study. Hum Pathol 1984; 15: 1054–1061.
72. Thoenes W, Störkel S, Rumpelt HJ. Histopathology and classification of renal cell tumors (adenomas, oncocytomas and carcinomas). Pathol Res Pract 1986; 181: 125–143.
73. Kovacs G, Welter C, Wilkens L, Blin N, Deriese W. Renal oncocytoma. A phenotypic and genotypic entity of renal parenchymal tumors. Am J Pathol 1989; 134: 967–971.
74. Walter TA, Pennington RD, Decker H-JH, Sandberg AA. Translocation t(9;11)(p23;q12): a primary chromosomal change in renal oncocytoma. J Urol 1989; 142: 117–119.
75. Akhtar M, Kott E. Oncocytoma of the kidney. Urology 1979; 14: 397–400.
76. Lieber MM, Tomera KM, Farrow GM. Renal oncocytoma. J Urol 1981; 125: 481–485.
77. Landier JF, Desligneres S, Boccon-Gibod L, Steg A. Les oncocytomes du rein. Semin Hôp Paris 1979; 55: 1275–1279.
78. Kay S, Armstrong KS. Oncocytic tubular adenoma of the kidney: report of three cases with 28 year follow up on one. Prog Surg Pathol 1980; 2: 259–268.
79. Engel U, Horn T, Nielsen OS, Olsen JH. Renal oncocytoma. Acta Pathol Microbiol Immunol Scand [A] 1987; 95: 107–111.
80. Stefenelli T, Silberbauer K, Ulrich W, Sommeregger K, Zechner O.Cardiac decompensation caused by hypertension and polyglobulia associated with multiple renal oncoctyomas. Clin Nephrol 1985; 23: 307–311.
81. Rainwater LM, Farrow GM, Lieber MM. Flow cytometry of renal oncocytoma: common occurrence of deoxyribonucleic acid polyploidy and aneuploidy. J Urol 1986; 135: 1167–1171.
82. Cohen C, McCue PA, Derose PB. Histogenesis of renal cell carcinoma and renal oncocytoma. An immunohistochemical study. Cancer 1988; 62:1946–1951.
83. Eble JN, Hull MT. Glycoconjugate expression in human renal oncocytomas. A lectin histochemical study. Arch Pathol Lab Med1988; 112: 805–808.
84. Ogden BW, Beckman EN, Rodriguez FH. Multicystic renal oncocytoma. Arch Pathol Lab Med 1987; 111: 485–486.
85. Newcomb WD. The search for truth, with special reference to the frequency of gastric ulcer cancer and the origin of Grawitz tumours of the kidney. Proc R Soc Med 1936; 30: 113–136.

86. Wallace AC, Nairn RC. Renal tubular antigens in kidney tumors. Cancer 1971; 29: 977–981.
87. Budin RE, McDonnell PJ. Renal cell neoplasms. Their relationship to arteriolonephrosclerosis. Arch Pathol Lab Med 1984; 108: 138– 140.
88. Bennington JL, Beckwith JB. Tumors of the kidney, renal pelvis, and ureter. Atlas of tumor pathology: fascicle 12. Washington, DC: Armed Forces Institute of Pathology, 1975; 94–99.
89. Dal Cin P, Gaeta J, Huben R, Li FP, Prout GR, Sandberg AA. Renal cortical tumors. Cytogenetic characterization. Am J Clin Pathol 1989; 92: 408–414.

Embryonal tumours of the renal parenchyma

90. Mostofi FK, Sesterhenn IA, Sobin LH. Histological typing of kidney tumours. Geneva: World Health Organization, 1981.
91. Young JL, Ries LG, Silverberg E, Horn JW, Miller RW. Cancer incidence, survival, and mortality for children younger than age 15 years. Cancer 1986; 58: 598–602.
92. Breslow NG, Beckwith JB. Epidemiological features of Wilms' tumor. Results of the National Wilms' Tumor Study. J Natl Cancer Inst 1982; 68: 429–436.
93. Babaian RJ, Skinner DG, Waisman J. Wilms' tumor in the adult patient. Diagnosis, management, and review of the world medical literature. Cancer 1980; 45: 1713–1719.
94. D'Angio GJ, Breslow N, Beckwith JB et al. Treatment of Wilms' tumor. Results of the Third National Wilms' Tumor Study. Cancer 1989; 64: 349–360.
95. Spahr J, Demers LM, Shochat SJ. Renin-producing Wilms' tumour. J Pediatr Surg 1981; 16: 32–34.
96. Lindop GBM, Duncan K, Millan DWM et al. Renin gene expression in nephroblastoma. J Pathol 1990; 161: 93–97.
97. Davis LM, Stallard R, Thomas GH et al. Two anonymous DNA segments distinguish the Wilms' tumor and aniridia loci. Science 1988; 241: 840–842.
98. Pendergrass TW. Congenital anomalies in children with Wilms' tumor. Cancer 1976; 37: 403–409.
99. Drash A, Sherman F, Hartmann WH, Blizzard RM. A syndrome of pseudohermaphroditism, Wilms' tumor, hypertension and degenerative renal disease. J Pediatr 1970; 76: 585–593.
100. Habib R, Loirat C, Gubler MC et al. The nephropathy associated with male pseudohermaphroditism and Wilms' tumor (Drash syndrome): a distinctive glomerular lesion – report of 10 cases. Clin Nephrol 1985; 24: 269–278.
101. Feiner HD, Camuto P, Wolman SR. Subclinical Wilms' tumor in incomplete Drash syndrome. Hum Pathol 1987; 18: 1077 (letter).
102. Turleau C, de Grouchy J, Chavin-Colin F, Martelli H, Voyer M,Charlas R. Trisomy 11p15 and Beckwith–Wiedemann syndrome. A report of two cases. Hum Genet 1984; 67: 219–221.
103. Mesrobian H-GJ, Kelalis PP, Hrabovsky E, Othersen H, de Lorimier A, Nesmith B. Wilms' tumor in horseshoe kidneys: a report from the National Wilms' Tumor Study. J Urol 1985; 133: 1002–1003.
104. Knudson AG, Strong LC. Mutation and cancer: a model for Wilms' tumor of the kidney. J Natl Cancer Inst 1972; 48: 313–324.
105. Li FP, Gimbrere K, Gelber RD et al. Outcome of pregnancy in survivors of Wilms' tumor. JAMA 1987; 257: 216–219.
106. Grundy P, Koufos A, Morgan K, Li FP, Meadows AT, Cavenee WK. Familial predisposition to Wilms' tumour does not map to the short arm of chromosome 11. Nature 1988; 336: 374–376.
107. Bove KE. Nephroblastomatosis. An overview. Arch Pathol Lab Med 1989; 113: 723–724.
108. Bennington JL, Beckwith JB. Tumors of the kidney, renal pelvis, and ureter. Atlas of tumor pathology: fascicle 12. Washington, DC: Armed Forces Institute of Pathology, 1975; 31–91.
109. Beckwith JB. Wilms' tumor and other renal tumors of childhood: an update. J Urol 1986; 136: 320–324.
110. Beckwith JB. Wilms' tumor and other renal tumors of childhood. Mod Probl Pathol 1986; 18: 313–332.
111. Bove KE, McAdams AJ. The nephroblastomatosis complex and its relationship to Wilms' tumor. A clinicopathologic treatise. Perspect Pediatr Pathol 1976; 3: 185–223.
112. Hou LT, Holman RL. Bilateral nephroblastomatosis in a premature infant. J Pathol 1961; 82: 249–255.
113. Bonadio JF, Storer B, Norkool P, Farewell VT, Beckwith JB, D'Angio GJ. Anaplastic Wilms' tumor: clinical and pathologic studies. J Clin Oncol 1985; 3: 513–520.
114. Mierau GW, Beckwith JB, Weeks DA. Ultrastructure and histogenesis of the renal tumors of childhood. An overview. Ultrastruct Pathol 1987; 11: 313–333.
115. Garvin AJ, Sullivan JL, Bennett DD, Stanley WS, Inabnett T, Sens DA. The in vitro growth, heterotransplantation, and immunohistochemical characterization of the blastemal component of Wilms' tumor. Am J Pathol 1987; 129: 353–363.
116. Roth J, Zuber C, Wagner P, Blaha I, Bitter-Suermann D, Heitz PU. Presence of the long chain form of polysialic acid of the neural cell adhesion molecule in Wilms' tumor. Identification of the cell adhesion molecule as an oncodevelopmental antigen and implications for tumor histogenesis. Am J Pathol 1988; 133: 227–240.
117. Slater RM, de Kraker J, Voute PA, Delemarre JFM. A cytogenetic study of Wilms' tumor. Cancer Genet Cytogenet 1985; 14: 95–109.
118. Schroeder WT, Chao L-Y, Dao DD et al. Nonrandom loss of maternal chromosome 11 alleles in Wilms' tumors. Am J Hum Genet 1987; 40: 413–420.
119. Gessler M, Poustka A, Cavenee W, Neve RL, Orkin SH, Bruns GAP. Homozygous deletion in Wilms' tumours of a zinc-finger gene identified by chromosome jumping. Nature 1990; 343: 774–778.
120. Call KM, Glaser T, Ito CY et al. Isolation and characterization of a zinc finger polypeptide gene at the human chromosome 11 Wilms' tumor locus. Cell 1990; 16: 509–520.
121. Pritchard-Jones K, Fleming S, Davidson D et al. The candidate Wilms' tumour gene is involved in genitourinary development.Nature 1990; 346: 194–197.
122. Hoffman M. One Wilms' tumor gene is cloned; are there more? Science 1989; 246: 1387.
123. Francke U. A gene for Wilms' tumour? Nature 1990; 343: 692–694.
124. Scott J, Cowell J, Robertson ME et al. Insulin-like

growth factor-11 gene expression in Wilms' tumor and embryonic tissues. Nature 1985; 317: 260–262.
125. Breslow NE, Churchill G, Nesmith B et al. Clinicopathologic features and prognosis for Wilms's tumor patients with metastases at diagnosis. Cancer 1986; 58: 2501–2511.
126. Beckwith JB. Wilms' tumor and other renal tumors of childhood: a selective review from the National Wilms' Tumor Study Pathology Center. Hum Pathol 1983; 14: 481–492.
127. D'Angio, GJ, Breslow N, Beckwith JB et al. Treatment of Wilms' tumor. Results of the Third National Wilms' Tumor Study. Cancer 1989; 64: 349–360.
128. Blute ML, Kelalis PP, Offord KP, Breslow N, Beckwith JB, D'Angio GJ. Bilateral Wilms' tumor. J Urol 1987; 138: 968–973.
129. Byrd RL, Evans AE, D'Angio GJ. Adult Wilms' tumor: effect of combined therapy on survival. J Urol 1982; 127: 648–651.
130. Zuppan CW, Beckwith JB, Luckey DW. Anaplasia in unilateral Wilms' tumor: a report from the National Wilms' Tumor Study Pathology Center. Hum Pathol 1988; 19: 1199–1209.
131. Douglass EC, Loo AT, Webber B et al. Hyperdiploidy and chromosomal rearrangements define the anaplastic variant of Wilms' tumor. J Clin Oncol 1986; 4: 975–981.
132. Schmidt D, Wiedemann B, Keil W, Sprenger E, Harms D. Flocytometric analysis of nephroblastomas and related neoplasms. Cancer 1986; 58: 2494–5000.
133. Mierau GW, Beckwith JB, Weeks DA. Ultrastructure and histogenesis of the renal tumors of childhood: an overview. Ultrastruct Pathol 1987; 11: 313–333.
134. Weissman BE, Saxon PJ, Pasquale SR, Jones GR, Geiser AG, Standbridge EJ. Introduction of a normal human chromosome 11 into a Wilms' tumor cell line controls its tumorigenic expression. Science 1987; 226: 175–180.
135. Fearon ER, Vogelstein B, Feinberg AP. Somatic deletion and duplication of genes on chromosome 11 in Wilms' tumours. Nature 1984; 309: 176–178.
136. Hard GC. Comparative oncology 1. Nephroblastoma in laboratory animals. In: Pochedly C, Baum ES, eds. Wilms' tumor. Clinical and biological manifestations. New York: Elsevier, 1984; 147–167.
137. Bolande RP, Brough AJ, Izant RJ. Congenital mesoblastic nephroma of infancy. A report of eight cases and the relationship to Wilms' tumor. Pediatrics 1967; 40: 272–278.
138. Bolande RP. Congenital mesoblastic nephroma of infancy. Perspect Pediatr Pathol 1973; 1: 227–250.
139. Gonzalez-Crussi F. Wilms' tumor (nephroblastoma) and related renal neoplasms of childhood. Florida: CRC Press, 1984; 92–100.
140. Cook HT, Taylor GM, Malone P, Risdon RA. Renin in mesoblastic nephroma: an immunohistochemical study. Hum Pathol 1988; 19: 1347–1351.
141. Pettinato G, Manivel JC, Wick MR, Dehner LP. Classical and cellular (atypical) congenital mesoblastic nephroma: a clinicopathologic, ultrastructural, immunohistochemical, and flow cytometric study. Hum Pathol 1989; 20: 682–690.
142. Marsden HB, Newton WA. New look at mesoblastic nephroma. J Clin Pathol 1986; 39: 508–513.
143. Sandstedt B, Delemarre JFM, Krul EJ, Tournade MF. Mesoblastic nephromas: a study of 29 tumours from the SIOP nephroblastoma file. Histopathology 1985; 9: 741–750.
144. Favara BF, Johnson W, Ito J. Renal tumors in the neonatal period.Cancer 1968; 22: 845–855.
145. Kumar S, Marsden HB, Carr T, Kodet R. Mesoblastic nephroma contains fibronectin but lacks laminin. J Clin Pathol 1985; 38: 507–511.
146. Beckwith JB, Weeks DA. Congenital mesoblastic nephroma. When should we worry? Arch Pathol Lab Med 1986; 110: 98–99.
147. Gormley TS, Skoog SJ, Jones RV, Maybee D. Cellular congenital mesoblastic nephroma: what are the options? J Urol 1989; 142: 479–483.
148. Kovacs G, Szucs S, Maschek H. Two chromosomally different cell populations in a partly cellular congenital mesoblastic nephroma. Arch Pathol Lab Med 1989; 111: 383–385.
149. Varsa EW, McConnell TS, Dressler LG, Duncan M. Atypical congenital mesoblastic nephroma. Report of a case with karyotypic and flow cytometric analysis. Arch Pathol Lab Med 1989; 113: 1078–1080.
150. Boggs K, Kimmelstiel P. Benign multilocular cystic nephroma: report of two cases of so-called multilocular cyst of the kidney. J Urol 1956; 76: 530–541.
151. Joshi VV, Beckwith JB. Multilocular cyst of the kidney (cystic nephroma) and cystic, partially differentiated nephroblastoma. Cancer 1989; 64: 466–479.
152. Joshi VV, Banerjee AK, Yador K, Pathak IC. Cystic, partially differentiated nephroblastoma. A clinicopathologic entity in the spectrum of infantile renal neoplasia. Cancer 1977; 40: 789–795.

Miscellaneous tumours of the renal parenchyma

153. Beckwith JB, Palmer NF. Histopathology and prognosis of Wilms' tumor: results of the National Wilms' Tumor Study. Cancer 1978; 41: 1937–1948.
154. Palmer NF, Sutow WW. Clinical aspects of the rhabdoid tumor of the kidney: a report of the National Wilms' Tumor Study Group. Med Pediatr Oncol 1983; 11: 242–245.
155. Weeks DA, Beckwith JB, Mierau GW, Luckey DW. Rhabdoid tumor of kidney. A report of 111 cases from the National Wilms' Tumor Study Pathology Center. Am J Surg Pathol 1989; 13: 439–458.
156. Mayes LC, Kasselberg AC, Roloff AJ, Lukens J. Hypercalcemia associated with immunoreactive parathormone in a malignant rhabdoid tumour of the kidney (rhabdoid Wilms' tumor). Cancer1984; 54: 882–884.
157. Bonnin JM, Rubinstein LJ, Palmer NF, Beckwith JB. The association of embryonal tumors originating in the kidney and in the brain. A report of seven cases. Cancer 1984; 54: 2137–2146.
158. Haas JE, Palmer NF, Weinberg AG, Beckwith JB. Ultrastructure of malignant rhabdoid tumor of the kidney. Hum Pathol 1981; 12: 646–657.
159. Kumar S, Carr T, Marsden HB, Clabuig-Crespo ML. Study of childhood renal tumours using antisera to fibronectin, laminin and epithelial membrane antigen. J Clin Pathol 1986; 39: 51–57.

160. Vogel AM, Gown AM, Caughlan J, Haas JE, Beckwith JB. Rhabdoid tumors of the kidney contain mesenchymal specific and epithelial specific intermediate filament proteins. Lab Invest 1984; 50: 232–238.
161. Weeks DA, Beckwith JB, Mierau GW. Rhabdoid tumor. An entity or a phenotype? Arch Pathol Lab Med 1989; 113: 113–114.
162. Marsden HB, Lawler W, Kumar PM. Bone metastasizing renal tumor of childhood. Morphological and clinical features and differences from Wilms' tumor. Cancer 1978; 42: 1922–1928
163. Sotelo-Avila C, Gonzalez-Crussi F, Sadowinski S, Gooch WM, Pena R. Clear cell sarcoma of the kidney: a clinicopathologic study of 21 patients with long-term follow-up evaluation. Hum Pathol 1985; 16: 1219–1230.
164. Farrow GM, Harrison EG, Utz DC, ReMine WH. Sarcomas and sarcomatoid and mixed malignant tumors of the kidney in adults – Part I. Cancer 1968; 22: 545–550.
165. Srinivas V, Sogani PC, Hajdu SI, Whitmore WF. Sarcomas of the kidney. J Urol 1984; 132: 13–16.
166. Mayes DC, Fechner RE, Gillenwater JY. Renal liposarcoma. Am J Surg Pathol 1990; 14: 268–273.
167. Peterson RO. Urologic pathology. Philadelphia: JB Lippincott; 1986.
168. Somers WJ, Terpenning B, Lowe FC, Romas NA. Renal parenchymal neurilemmoma: a rare and unusual kidney tumor. J Urol 1988; 139: 109–110.
169. Fein RL, Hamm FC. Malignant Schwannoma of the renal pelvis: a review of the literature and a case report. J Urol 1965; 94: 356–361.
170. Farrow GM, Harrison EG, Utz DC, Jones DR. Renal angiomyolipoma. A clinicopathologic study of 32 cases. Cancer 1968; 22: 564–570.
171. Oesterling JE, Fishman EK, Goldman SM, Marshall FF. The management of renal angiomyolipoma. J Urol 1986; 135: 1121–1124.
172. Price EB, Mostofi FK. Symptomatic angiomyolipoma of the kidney. Cancer 1965; 18: 761–774.
173. Van Baal JG, Becker AE, Fleury P, Brummelkamp WA. Renal angiomyolipomas: could the histology serve as a marker for tuberous sclerosis? Histopathology 1990; 17: 180–182.
174. Brecher ME, Gill WB, Strauss FH. Angiomyolipoma with regional lymph node involvement and long-term follow-up study. Hum Pathol 1986; 17: 962–963.
175. Hulbert JC, Graf R. Involvement of the spleen by renal angiomyolipoma: metastatic or multicentricity? J Urol 1983; 130: 328–329.
176. Stillwell TJ, Gomez MR, Kelalis PP. Renal lesions in tuberous sclerosis. J Urol 1987; 138: 477–481.
177. Graves N, Barnes WF. Angiomyolipoma in tuberous sclerosis. J Urol 1986; 135: 122–123.
178. Shapiro RA, Skinner DG, Stanley P, Edelbrock HH. Renal tumours associated with tuberous sclerosis: the case for aggressive surgical management. J Urol 1984; 132: 1170–1174.
179. Albrecht E. Ueber Hamartome. Verh Dtsch Pathol Ges 1904; 7: 153–157.
180. Lerman RJ, Pitcock JA, Stephenson P, Muirhead EE. Renomedullary interstitial cell tumour (formerly fibroma of renal medulla). Hum Pathol 1972; 3: 559–568.
181. Stuart R, Salyer WR, Salyer DC, Heptinstall RH. Renomedullary interstitial cell lesions and hypertension. Hum Pathol 1976; 7: 327–332.
182. Edward HG, De Weerd JH, Woolner LB. Renal haemangiomas. Mayo Clin Proc 1962; 37: 545–551.
183. Colvin SH. Certain capsular and subcapsular mixed tumours of the kidney herein called 'capsuloma'. J Urol 1942; 48: 585–600.
184. Robertson PW, Klidjian A, Harding LK, Walters G, Lee MR, Robb-Smith AHT. Hypertension due to a renin-secreting renal tumour. Am J Med 1967; 43: 963–976.
185. Baruch D, Corvol P, Alhenc-Gelas F et al. Diagnosis and treatment of renin-secreting tumours. Report of three cases. Hypertension 1984; 6: 760–767.
186. Squires JP, Ulbright TM, Deshryver-Kecskemeti K, Engelman W. Juxtaglomerular cell tumor of the kidney. Cancer 1984; 53: 516–523.
187. Tomita T, Poisner A, Inagami T. Immunohistochemical localization of renin in renal tumors. Am J Pathol 1987; 126: 73–80.
188 Camilleri J-P, Hinglais N, Bruneval P et al. Renin storage and cell differentiation in juxtaglomerular cell tumours: an immunohistochemical and ultrastructural study of three cases. Hum Pathol 1984; 15: 1069–1079.

Secondary tumours involving the renal parenchyma

189. Willis RA. Secondary tumours of the kidneys. In: The spread of tumours in the human body, 3rd edn. London: Butterworths, 1973; 193–213.
190. Perl SI, Yong JC, Higgins SG. Tumor crescents from intraglomerular metastases. Clin Nephrol 1987; 27: 260–262.
191. Richmond J, Sherman RS, Diamond HD, Craver LF. Renal lesions associated with malignant lymphomas. Am J Med 1962; 32: 184–207.
192. Sternby NH. Studies in enlargement of leukaemic kidneys. Acta Haematol 1955; 14: 354–362.

Tumour-like conditions of the renal parenchyma

193. Apitz K. Die Geschwülste und Gewebsmissbildungen der Nierenrinde. 1. Die intrarenalen Nebenniereninseln. Virchows Arch [A]1944; 311: 285–305.
194. Case records of the Massachusetts General Hospital (case 50 – 1986). N Engl J Med 1986; 315: 1595–1606.
195. Bazaz-Malik G, Saraf V, Rana BS. Endometrioma of the kidney: case report. J Urol 1980; 123: 422–423.

Primary epithelial tumours of the renal pelvis

196. Booth CM, Cameron KM, Pugh RCB. Urothelial carcinoma of the kidney and ureter. Br J Urol 1980; 52: 430–435.
197. Palvio DHB, Anderson JC, Falk E. Transitional cell tumors of the renal pelvis and ureter associated with capillarosclerosis indicating analgesic abuse. Cancer 1987; 59: 972–976.
198. Latham HS, Kay S. Malignant tumours of the renal pelvis. Surg Gynecol Obstet 1974; 138: 613–622.

199. Lauritzen AF, Kvist E, Bredesen J, Luke M. Primary carcinoma of the upper urinary tract. Acta Pathol Microbiol Immunol Scand [A]1987; 95: 7–10.
200. Olsen S. Tumours of the kidney and urinary tract. Copenhagen: Munksgaard, 1984; 140.
201. Cullen TH, Popham RR, Voss HJ. Urine cytology and primary carcinoma of the renal pelvis and ureter. Aust NZ J Surg 1972; 41: 230–236.
202. Bennington JL, Beckwith JB. Tumors of the kidney, renal pelvis, and ureter. Atlas of tumor pathology: fascicle 12. Washington, DC: Armed Forces Institute of Pathology, 1975; 243–310.
203. Koss LG. Tumors of the urinary bladder. Atlas of tumor pathology: fascicle 11. Washington, DC: Armed Forces Institute of Pathology, 1975; 13–38.
204. Gahagan HQ, Reed WK. Squamous cell carcinoma of the renal pelvis: three case reports and review of the literature. J Urol 1950; 63: 61–65.
205. Paulson J, Grignon D, Ro J, Ayala A, Brooks T, Ordonez N. Renal pelvis transitional cell carcinoma: prognostic significance of tumor ploidy and ABH status. Lab Invest 1989; 60: 71A (abstr).
206. Schaafsma HE, Ramaekers FCS, van Muijen GNP et al. Distribution of cytokeratin polypeptides in human transitional cell carcinomas, with special emphasis on changing expression patterns during tumor progression. Am J Pathol 1990; 136: 329–343.
207. Vanni R, Nieddu M, Scarpa RM, Migliari R, Usai E. Trisomy 7 in a case of transitional cell carcinoma of the kidney. Cancer Genet Cytogenet 1989; 41: 149–151.
208. Vanni R, Scarpa RM, Nieddu M, Usai E. Cytogenetic investigation on 30 bladder carcinomas. Cancer Genet Cytogenet 1988; 30: 35–42.
209. Sandberg AA, Berger CS, Haddad FS, Kerr D, Hecht F. Chromosome change in transitional cell carcinoma of ureter. Cancer Genet Cytogenet. 1986; 19: 335–340.
210. McCarron JP, Chasko SB, Gray GF. Systematic mapping of nephroureterectomy specimens removed for urothelial cancer: pathological findings and clinical correlations. J Urol 1982; 128: 243–246.
211. Poole-Wilson DS. Occupational tumours of the renal pelvis and ureter arising in the dye-making industry. Proc R Soc Med 1969; 62: 93–94.
212. Hultengren N, Lagergren C, Ljungqvist A. Carcinoma of the renal pelvis in renal papillary necrosis. Acta Chir Scand 1965; 130: 314–320.
213. Bengtsson U, Angervall L, Ekman H, Lehman L. Transitional cell tumours of the renal pelvis in analgesic abusers. Scand J Urol Nephrol 1968; 2: 145–150.
214. Gloor FJ. Changing concepts in pathogenesis and morphology of analgesic nephropathy as seen in Europe. Kidney Int 1978; 13: 27–33.
215. Mihatsch MJ, Manz T, Knüsli C et al. Phenacetinabusus. III. Schweiz Med Wochenschr 1980; 110: 255–264.
216. Johansson S, Wahlqvist L. Tumours of urinary bladder and ureter associated with abuse of phenacetin-containing analgesics. Acta Pathol Microbiol Scand [A] 1977; 85: 768–774.
217. Johansson S, Angervall L, Bengtsson U, Wahlqvist L. A clinicopathologic and prognostic study of epithelial tumors of the renal pelvis. Cancer 1976; 37: 1376–1383.
218. McCredie M, Stewart JH, Ford JM. Analgesics and tobacco as risk factors for cancer of the ureter and renal pelvis in man. J Urol 1983; 130: 28–30.
219. McCredie M, Stewart JH, Carter JJ, Turner J, Mahony JF. Phenacetin and papillary necrosis: independent risk factors for renal pelvic cancer. Kidney Int 1986; 30: 81–84.
220. Radovanović Z, Krajinović S, Petković S, Hall PW. Papillary transitional cell tumours, Balkan nephropathy, and β_2-microglobulin. Lancet 1981; 2: 689 (letter).
221. Petković S, Mutavdzic M, Petronic V, Markovic M. Comparative incidence pattern of urothelium tumours in and beyond endemic nephropathy regions. In: Puchlev A, Dincu IV, Milev B, Doichinov D, eds. Proceedings of the Second International Symposium on Endemic Nephropathy. Sofia: Bulgarian Academy of Sciences, 1974; 114–116.
222. Atanassov N, Donovski L, Kumanov H. Tumours of the urinary passages in endemic nephropathy. In: Puchlev A, Dincu IV, Milev B, Doichinov D, eds. Proceedings of the Second International Symposium on Endemic Nephropathy. Sofia: Bulgarian Academy of Sciences, 1974; 117–123.
223. Petkovic SD. Epidemiology and treatment of renal pelvic and ureteral tumors. J Urol 1975; 114: 858–865.
224. McLaughlin JK, Blot WJ, Mandel JS, Schuman LM, Mehl ES, Fraumeni JF. Etiology of cancer of the renal pelvis. J Natl Cancer Inst 1983; 71: 287–291.

Miscellaneous tumours of the renal pelvis

225. Bartone NF, Greco RV. Renal hemangioma. JAMA 1968; 205: 118–121.

Tumour-like conditions of the renal pelvis

226. Anderstrom C, Johansson P, Pettersson S. Inverted papilloma of the urinary tract. J Urol 1982; 127: 1132–1134.
227. Wolgel CD, Parris AC, Mitty, Schapira HE. Fibroepithelial polyp of renal pelvis. Urology 1982; 19: 436–439.

Renal complications of extrarenal cancer

228. Fer MF, McKinney TD, Richardson RL, Hande KR, Oldham RK, Greco FA. Cancer and the kidney: renal complications of neoplasms. Am J Med 1981; 71: 704–718.
229. Lee JC, Yamauchi H, Hopper J. The association of cancer and the nephrotic syndrome. Ann Intern Med. 1966; 64: 41–51.
230. Eagen JW, Lewis EJ. Glomerulopathies of neoplasia. Kidney Int 1977; 11: 297–306.
231. Brueggemeyer CD, Ramirez G. Membranous nephropathy: a concern for malignancy. Am J Kidney Dis 1987; 9: 23–26.
232. Alpers CE, Cotran RS. Neoplasia and glomerular injury. Kidney Int 1986; 30: 465–473.

17

K. A. Porter

Renal transplantation

INTRODUCTION

Renal transplantation has an established role, along with dialysis, in the treatment of chronic renal failure. The transplanted kidney, from a living or dead donor, is usually placed in the iliac fossa, with anastomosis of its vessels to the iliac vessels and implantation of the ureter into the bladder.

Almost all kidneys that are transplanted are grafts between individuals of different genetic constitution (allogeneic homografts, or *allografts*). Occasionally, a kidney is transplanted from one of a pair of identical twins to the other (syngeneic graft or *isograft*). Sometimes it is necessary to move a kidney from its natural position to another site in the same individual (*autograft*).

Autografts and isografts are accepted by the recipient; allografts induce an immune response which, if not circumvented or suppressed, will lead to destruction of the transplanted kidney (*rejection*). The ability of the patient to reject the kidney is impaired by various combinations of immunosuppressive drugs. Cyclosporin or azathioprine are commonly used; they are usually combined with steroids, and sometimes supplemented by polyclonal antilymphocyte serum or monoclonal antibodies directed against particular subsets of T lymphocytes. Usually the recipient is tissue typed and the best matched kidney available for transplantation is chosen.

The short-term prognosis after cadaveric renal transplantation is very good; most national registries report 1-year graft survival rates of 80% and 5-year survival rates of around 65%. Patient survival is at least 90% at 1-year and about 80% at 5-years. The results after transplantation of a kidney from a living related donor are even better. In the long term various limiting factors come into play, in particular the ever present risk of infection, a higher rate and earlier onset of cardiovascular disease and a continuing slow attrition of grafts from chronic rejection.

The histological appearances of a renal graft may be altered as a result of disease present in the donor kidney before transplantation, technical problems encountered during transplantation, rejection, immunosuppressive treatment, transmission of disease from the host (*recurrent disease*), or the development of a disease not present in the recipient (*'de novo' disease*). These changes are considered in sequence below.

DISEASE IN DONOR KIDNEY

Sometimes a kidney obtained from an asymptomatic donor is found, when biopsied at the time of transplantation, to be diseased. The incidence of significant lesions is not known because very few transplantation units routinely biopsy donor kidneys before transplantation.

It is very likely that *arteriolar hyalinization* is common in kidneys collected from individuals who have died from subarachnoid or intracerebral haemorrhage, because many of these donors have been hypertensive for some years before their death. Also, when older donors are used various degrees of *glomerular sclerosis, interstitial fibrosis* and *tubular atrophy* are bound to be present (for the effects of ageing on the kidney see p. 23). A knowledge of these changes becomes important when one is trying to decide whether or not arteriolar hyalinization or interstitial fibrosis in a transplant is due to cyclosporin toxicity (see p. 661).

Rarely, the donor kidney is found to be affected by unsuspected *glomerulonephritis*. By far the commonest form of glomerulonephritis to be encountered in this way is *IgA nephropathy* (see p. 157).[1,2] After transplantation the IgA deposits in the mesangium usually remain asymptomatic and gradually disappear; this resolution may take months or even years. Occasionally, the IgA deposits increase in amount and there is proteinuria, haematuria and a slow decline in renal function.[3,4] The majority of such progressive cases have been reported from Japan where there is a high incidence of IgA nephropathy, donor and recipient have usually been related, and the recipient's original disease in a significant proportion was IgA nephropathy. Some of the apparent progressions of donor disease might, therefore, represent recurrence of recipient IgA disease occurring in a transplant that already contains IgA in its mesangium at the time of transplantation.[5]

Other very rare diseases, such as *Fabry's disease*,[6] may be found in the donor kidney, and occasionally a *malignant neoplasm* may be present. Malignant tumours are important because approximately 60% of immunosuppressed patients receiving such a kidney develop distant metastases within 2 years.[7] In about a third of the patients the metastases regress, and often disappear, if the recipient's immunosuppressive treatment is discontinued.

Bacterial infections such as tuberculosis, fungal infections such as histoplasmosis, and parasites such as *Plasmodium vivax* may occasionally be detected in the graft. Viruses, such as *cytomegalovirus*, can sometimes be demonstrated in the graft by culture but their presence is rarely appreciated by conventional microscopy, although the viral nucleic acids may be detected by using *in situ* hybridization and labelled DNA probes.

Very rarely donor kidneys known to be diseased have been used in transplantation. This has occurred in countries where there is an acute shortage of suitable donors. In two such cases kidneys with diabetic glomerulosclerosis were transplanted;

subsequent biopsies and the course of the patients suggested that the lesions regressed during the first 7 months after transplantation.[8]

CHANGES CAUSED BY TECHNICAL DIFFICULTIES BEFORE OR DURING TRANSPLANTATION

GENERAL ISCHAEMIC INJURY

Some degree of ischaemic injury is almost inevitably present in a renal allograft. If the transplant is from a donor who died of acute circulatory arrest or following a prolonged period of hypotension the damage may be marked. Examination by light microscopy of a biopsy specimen taken from the transplant immediately after completion of the vascular anastomoses may underestimate the severity of the ischaemic injury because there has been insufficient time for the full morphological changes to become evident. In biopsies taken 1 or 2 days after transplantation, various degrees of tubular damage from acute tubular necrosis up to complete cortical necrosis may be seen. The changes in the tubules are usually accompanied by a moderate degree of cellular infiltration: this can be confused with the picture of acute tubulointerstitial rejection (see p. 637). The infiltrate usually consists of small lymphocytes, plasma cells, macrophages and some granulocytes. Lymphoblasts, which are a characteristic feature in acute tubulointerstitial rejection (see p. 638), usually constitute less than 3% of the cells that accumulate as a result of ischaemic changes.

When *acute tubular necrosis* occurs in a renal allograft, function may not commence for hours, days or weeks depending upon the severity of the damage. If rejection or other complications do not occur in the anuric period, acute tubular necrosis has little adverse effect on graft or patient survival. Recovery is usual and excellent function may eventually be attained.[9]

Compared with acute tubular necrosis in non-transplanted kidneys (see p. 493), acute tubular necrosis in renal allografts shows less flattening of the proximal tubular epithelium, less damage to the tubular brush border, more necrotic tubular cells, fewer casts, more birefringent oxalate crystals, and more mononuclear cells infiltrating the interstitium.[9]

Tubular necrosis is particularly prominent in patients being treated with cyclosporin because the damage inflicted by the drug augments the ischaemic injury.[10] To minimize this problem most treatment regimens aim at giving as little cyclosporin as possible during the critical period immediately after transplantation when the donor kidney is undergoing repair.

INJURY TO THE ARTERIAL SUPPLY

Failure to preserve the small arterial branches that contribute to the blood supply of those donor kidneys that have multiple arteries may result in localized infarction.

Overzealous removal of adipose tissue from the vicinity of the pelvis and ureter may impair the blood supply to the lower part of the ureter and lead to necrosis of its wall and the formation of a fistula, or the development of stenosis due to ischaemic fibrosis.[11]

INJURY TO THE VENOUS DRAINAGE

Difficulties in effecting the venous anastomosis, or positioning of the transplant in such a manner that the renal vein is kinked, may cause thrombosis of the veins and consequent venous infarction (see p. 302). Ligation of one of the major vessels draining a donor kidney that has multiple veins may lead to massive proteinuria and to interstitial fibrosis in the graft.[12]

PERFUSION INJURY

It is commonly the practice to flush the donor kidney with an appropriate cold electrolyte solution before storing the organ in an iced saline slush. Cooling depresses the metabolism of the kidney and minimizes damage while the donor is tissue typed, the organ is transported, a suitable recipient is selected, a cross-match between donor and recipient is performed, and the recipient is prepared for surgery. Such simple flushing and surface cooling allows ischaemia to be tolerated for up to 12 hours. After this procedure IgG is often deposited in a linear pattern on the walls of the glomerular capillaries of the graft. The IgG is not antiglomerular-basement-membrane (anti-GBM) antibody and is not accompanied by complement: it has no prognostic significance.[13]

Continuous machine perfusion of the kidney with a recirculating volume of oxygenated plasma-derived perfusate at 4°C extends the storage period to 72 hours. The perfusion pump may provide either a pulsatile or a non-pulsatile flow. Machine perfusion is only used frequently in the USA; it is rarely employed in European countries, including Britain. The procedure causes a 15% greater proportion of graft failure after transplantation than occurs after simple cold storage preservation. The increase in the rate of failure is due mainly to mechanical injury to the glomerular capillary endothelium and, much less frequently, to injury by cytotoxic alloantibodies in the plasma used for perfusion.[14] After mechanical damage the endothelium is lost from large areas of the glomerular capillary wall and intracapillary thrombosis follows.[15] After injury by antibodies the structural and immunofluorescent changes are the same as those that occur in hyperacute rejection due to anti-HLA antibodies in presensitized recipients (see p. 631). The incidence of thrombosis of the renal artery is also increased after mechanical perfusion because of damage to the intima.[16]

LYMPHOCELE

A pocket of lymph may develop round the graft and in the graft wound as the result of outpouring from lymphatics severed during dissection in the iliac fossa;[17] there is probably also some contribution from divided lymphatics at the hilum and surface of the graft. It occurs in about 3% of renal transplants.[18] The collection of fluid can obstruct the ureter and, through compression of the iliac veins, lead to oedema of the ipsilateral leg.

The clinical manifestations of a lymphocele may mimic rejection. Lymphocele can usually be prevented by meticulous ligation of divided lymphatics.

CHANGES ASSOCIATED WITH REJECTION

Allografts provoke an immune reaction in the host and are accepted only if this process of rejection can be either avoided or suppressed. Suppression of the immune response requires that most recipients of renal allografts be treated for an indefinite period with immunosuppressant drugs. Immunosuppressive treatment is accompanied by various hazards; some of these are discussed on page 661.

The antigens in the transplanted kidney responsible for evoking rejection are glycoproteins (*histocompatibility antigens*) on the surface of cells. The most important of these antigens are governed by a single genetic complex, the *major histocompatibility complex* (MHC). In humans the MHC is known as the *HLA system* (the human leucocyte antigen system) because transplantation antigens were first identified in peripheral blood leucocytes: it is composed of a series of many closely linked genes which are grouped in a very small segment of the short arm of chromosome 6.[19] The loci of the MHC and their cell surface protein products are divided into two classes according to their tissue distribution, the structure of the expressed antigens and their functions.

Class I antigens are present on most nucleated cells but their concentration on the cell surface varies widely. They are responsible for presenting foreign antigen, usually viral, on the surface of normal cells to cytotoxic T lymphocytes of the CD8 phenotype. Three class I loci have been identified in humans: HLA-A, -B, and -C.[19] In the kidney, class I antigens are normally expressed on the vascular endothelial cells, particularly those lining the arteries, and on the tubular, interstitial and mesangial cells.[20]

Class II antigens have a more limited tissue distribution. They are mainly responsible for presenting soluble foreign antigen, including transplantation antigen, to helper T lymphocytes of the CD4 phenotype. This process is facilitated by specialized antigen-presenting cells. The role of displaying transplantation antigens makes HLA class II antigens particularly important: in kidney grafting, matching class II antigens is more necessary than matching those of class I. The presently known class II loci are divided into three families – DR, DQ and DP.[19] In the kidney, class II antigens are normally expressed on glomerular and peritubular capillary endothelial cells, on mesangial cells and on those interstitial cells that have a dendritic shape. HLA-DR is also expressed on proximal, but not distal, tubular cells in approximately 70% of people.[20]

There are at least 18 alleles at the A locus, 41 at B, eight at C, 20 at DR, three at DQ and six at DP. Each allele is identified by a number preceded by the letter of the locus within which it is found, for example A17, B2 or DR7. Every person may have up to 12 different alleles, two from each of the six loci. These can create about 80 000 million different combinations, an extraordinarily high level of polymorphism.[21]

In the attempt to avoid rejection it is usual to try to select donors whose tissues are compatible with the recipient. The main difficulty with tissue typing is that because of the extreme polymorphism of the products of the HLA loci, complete matching is rarely possible; usually it can only be partial. To obtain good matches between donor and recipient, cadaveric kidneys for transplantation have to be shared and made available to a very large pool of recipients. When this is done the percentage of grafts with very long cold ischaemia times increases (because of the distances the donor kidneys have to be transported): this leads to more transplants developing delayed function. Despite this, recent data suggest that the long-term benefits of histocompatibility outweigh any disadvantages from sharing.[22]

The basic physiological function of the MHC molecules is to bind peptide fragments of selected antigens in a special groove on the HLA molecule to produce a new antigenic determinant that is recognized by T lymphocytes. Antigen-specific T lymphocytes can recognize these foreign peptides only if the lymphocytes share MHC molecules with the cells presenting the peptides (*self MHC restriction*). However, the much more frequent allospecific T lymphocytes, whose response leads to the rejection of a renal transplant, do not appear to have their powers of recognition of the foreign peptides restricted by self MHC: the graft's own cells can present graft peptides to the recipient's alloreactive T lymphocytes.[23]

In addition to the MHC, the *ABO red cell antigen system* acts as a histocompatibility system, and a non-HLA *endothelial cell antigen system* has been demonstrated (see p. 630). There must also be many *minor histocompatibility systems*; our ignorance of these is largely due to our inability to raise antisera against them; in the mouse, in which breeding experiments can be used to aid their detection, over 30 minor histocompatibility loci have been identified.[24]

Matching of donor and recipient HLA antigens, and ensuring ABO compatibility, improve the survival of renal allografts and lead to better function in those that survive.[25] But even if complete HLA identity between donor and recipient is achieved, approximately 10% of grafts are still rejected in the first year after transplantation, largely because of incompatibilities in the endothelial cell antigen system and the minor histocompatibility systems.

The magnitude of the beneficial effect of tissue typing in any individual transplantation unit will depend upon the baseline rate of graft loss in that centre (*the centre effect*)[26] and upon whether the recipient has been given *pretransplantation blood transfusions*. In transplantation units where the baseline rate of graft loss is high, the effect of matching will be large and easily seen; where the rate of loss is low the effect in the short term may be difficult to detect. However, even in the very best centres the benefits of tissue matching become obvious when 10-year graft survival rates are considered.

A graft is likelier to survive if the patient has previously been given numerous random blood transfusions.[27] Before the advent of the powerful immunosuppressive drug cyclosporin, the benefits of prior blood transfusions were so marked that it was considered mandatory to ensure that recipients of cadaveric grafts had received several blood transfusions before transplantation; the recipient of a renal transplant from a living related donor, when donor and recipient shared only one haplotype, was usually transfused with blood from the donor before transplantation. Since cyclosporin came into general use the improvement in graft survival in untransfused recipients has been such that the overall differences between transfused and non-transfused recipients is now small.[28] At present the benefits of blood transfusions may sometimes be considered to be outweighed by the hazards of the procedure, in particular the chance of transmission of hepatitis virus or human immunodeficiency virus to the recipient, and the risk of sensitizing the patient to histocompatibility antigens in the proposed or subsequent grafts.

How blood transfusions improve graft survival is still not known. They probably induce a state of immunological unresponsiveness in the recipient; this hypothesis is supported by evidence that the activity of suppressor T lymphocytes is increased, anti-idiotypic antibodies are produced against the T lymphocyte antigen receptor, blocking antibodies against the Fc receptor may appear, and clonal deletion sometimes occurs.[29]

Rejection

In spite of attempted matching of donor and recipient by tissue typing, of pretransplant blood transfusions, and of continuous immunosuppressive treatment, most patients with renal allografts undergo at least one clinical episode of *acute rejection*. Some also develop *chronic rejection*.

Mismatched kidneys, transplanted into hypersensitized recipients who have circulating cytotoxic antibodies aimed at some of the donor antigens, are often rejected within a few minutes or hours. Such an immediate failure is commonly described as *hyperacute rejection*. Mismatched kidneys, transplanted into recipients who are sensitized to donor antigens but do not have detectable circulating antidonor cytotoxic antibodies, may undergo severe rejection within the first week after transplantation. This is sometimes described as *accelerated rejection*.

HYPERACUTE REJECTION

Any individual who receives into his or her body any of the cells of other people may thereby be sensitized to a wide spectrum of histocompatibility antigens. The most potent cause of hypersensitization, with the production of circulating lymphocytotoxic antibodies which react with many of the lymphocytes from a panel of randomly selected people, is the previous loss of one or more renal allografts by rejection. A significant number of parous women who are given a blood transfusion also become highly sensitized. Multiple pregnancies alone may result in women developing antibodies against any incompatible paternally inherited HLA antigens in the fetus, but few of the women become hypersensitized. Blood transfusions alone only occasionally lead to severe hypersensitivity.

If the presensitized individual later requires a renal transplant, he or she may be found to have circulating cytotoxic antibodies against either some of the donor's HLA class I antigens or non-HLA endothelial histocompatibility antigens or against both. Where this is the case, the circulating antibody immediately binds to the histocompatibility antigen molecules that are expressed on the vascular endothelium of the graft. The bound antibody stimulates fixation of complement, platelet activation, damage to the endothelium and activation of the coagulation system with obstruction of the capillaries and arterioles. As a result irreversible graft failure rapidly occurs.

Inadvertent perfusion of a kidney before transplantation with plasma that contains cytotoxic antibodies directed against the donor's histocompatibility antigens, may also cause hyperacute rejection by an identical mechanism.[14] A closely related state of affairs is present in some cases of major ABO blood group incompatibility between donor and recipient. Recipients lacking the A_1 or B antigen almost always have natural circulating antibodies against the missing antigen; in the sera of blood group O patients titres of agglutinating antibody in excess of 1 : 8 are present to A_1 antigen in 80% and to B antigen in 55%.[30] Red cell ABO group incompatibility between donor and recipient may result in the allogeneic kidney encountering high titres of circulating isohaemagglutinins which bind to the A_1 or B antigens that are present on the vascular walls of the ABO-incompatible graft. Blood group A_2 is the exception since antibody titres to this determinant may be low; only 25% of type O patients have titres of agglutinating antibody of 1 : 8 or higher against A_2 antigen and 17% have no detectable antibody.[30]

A slightly different situation is where the recipient has circulating IgM cold agglutinins. Primarily these are directed against the host's erythrocytes and cause hyperacute rejection by agglutinating these cells as they enter a kidney that has been cooled for preservation and not warmed just before it is transplanted: less frequently cold agglutinins also react with donor antigens.

Incidence

Classic hyperacute rejection is now rarely reported because it can be avoided. Kidneys are not usually transplanted in the presence of either an ABO blood group incompatibility or incompatibility between the donor's lymphocytes and the recipient's sera. When all categories of hyperacute rejection are grouped together, the incidence is approximately 0.5%.[31] However, the percentage of grafts that are recorded as having never functioned is significantly higher in patients who have previously received one or more renal allografts than in those receiving their first graft. There is a 5% difference between first and second grafts and an 11% difference between first and third grafts. These percentage differences probably represent the incidence of undetected hyperacute rejection.[31] Hyperacute rejection may be missed because either some of the cross-matching methods in common use are insufficiently sensitive, or the circulating cytotoxic antibody is directed against antigens on endothelial cells[32] or granulocytes and is not being discovered by the standard cross-match which uses lymphocytes as the target cells.

Clinical features

When the blood flow is re-established the transplanted kidney becomes pink and firm. Within 10–20 minutes the organ softens, and mottled blue areas appear on its surface despite good pulses at the renal hilum. The flow of blood through the organ quickly falls, urine flow ceases and the kidney becomes deep purple and flabby. Over the next 24–48 hours arteriography reveals progressive cortical necrosis.

If the characteristic gross changes in the kidney and the cessation of function do not occur until after the wound is closed the diagnosis may be missed; if the changes in tone and colour happen extremely quickly and function is fleeting, the graft may be thought not to have functioned.[31]

Laboratory findings

In the first few minutes after revascularization, platelets, neutrophil granulocytes, complement, fibrinogen and coagulation factors II, V and VIII accumulate in the graft and the level of the cytotoxic antibodies in the serum drops abruptly. Once the graft has been saturated with antibodies, or when the graft is removed, the circulating antibodies return to pretransplant levels.[33]

Renal changes

Gross appearance of the graft

Shortly after the onset of anuria the kidney is soft, flabby and blotchily or uniformly deep bluish-purple. If the graft is left *in situ* for some days there is cortical necrosis.

Light microscopy

Biopsy specimens taken within a few minutes of transplantation show focal and segmental obstruction of glomerular capillaries by amorphous masses of platelets and some sludged red cells (Figs 17.1,17.2).[34] Similar focal changes are present in the peritubular capillaries. The aggregated platelets usually appear pale pink and slightly granular in sections stained with haematoxylin and eosin; they are barely stained by periodic acid-Schiff.

Soon afterwards, neutrophil granulocytes[35] and fibrin[36] appear in the lumens of the capillaries (Fig. 17.3); within a few hours most of the capillaries and arterioles of the kidney are blocked by microthrombi. The interstitium becomes oedematous and contains focal haemorrhages; infiltrating mononuclear cells are rare.

A few days later there is complete cortical necrosis; masses of fibrin fill the capillaries and more or less completely obstruct the arterioles and small arteries.[37]

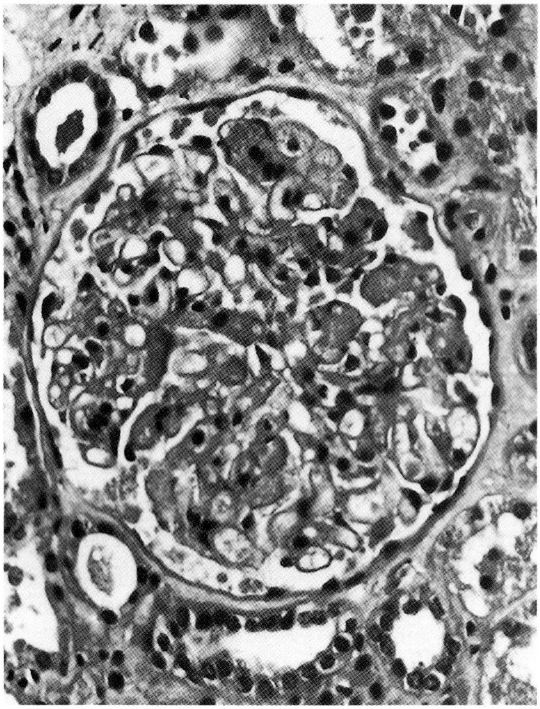

Fig. 17.1 Hyperacute rejection. Biopsy of a renal allograft 20 minutes after transplantation. Many of the glomerular capillaries contain aggregated platelets and sludged red blood cells. See also Figure 17.2.
Periodic acid-Schiff × 280

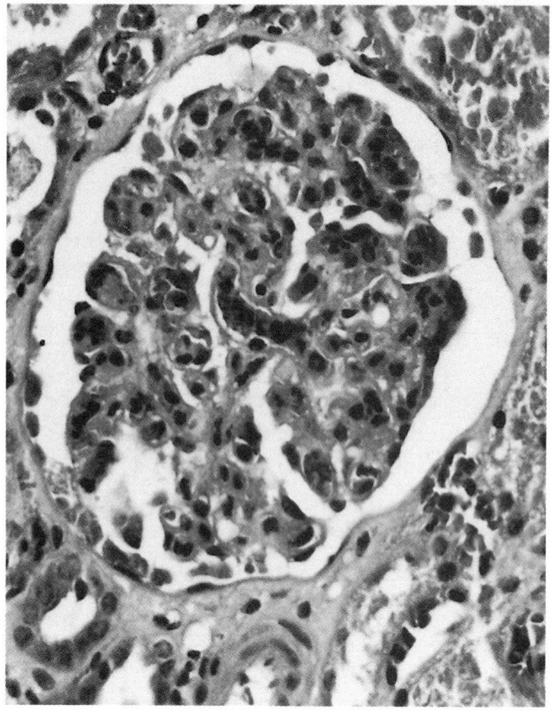

Fig. 17.3 Hyperacute rejection. Biopsy of a renal allograft 30 minutes after transplantation. The glomerular capillaries contain neutrophil granulocytes and fibrin in addition to platelets and sludged red cells. See also Figure17.4.
Haematoxylin-eosin × 320

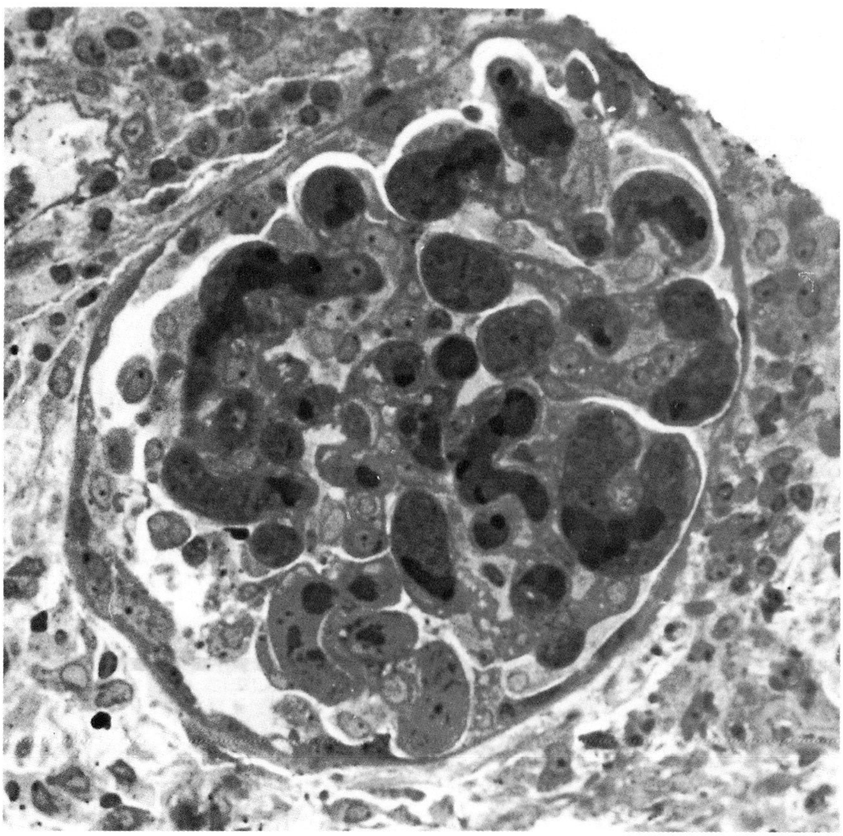

Fig. 17.2 Hyperacute rejection. Same case as illustrated in Figure17.1. In this thin section of the tissue embedded in resin, the aggregated platelets and sludged red blood cells can be seen more easily.
Epon-embedded tissue, section 0.5 μm thick; azure II × 300

Electron microscopy

In the very early stages the lumens of the glomerular and peritubular capillaries contain aggregated platelets with intact granules. Soon afterwards, neutrophil granulocytes appear in increasing numbers, lining the capillary walls (Fig. 17.4); the platelets degranulate, fibrin is deposited and is accompanied by groups of sludged red cells. The capillary endothelial cells show acute damage and areas of capillary basement membrane are exposed.[34]

Immunofluorescence/immunoperoxidase microscopy

Biopsies taken within minutes of the kidney becoming cyanotic show segmental linear and granular localization of IgG and C3 on the walls of the glomerular and peritubular capillaries (Fig. 17.5). Later, there is marked staining for fibrinogen along the capillary walls and in the capillary lumens, but often no specific localization of immunoglobulin or complement. If there is staining for immunoglobulin or complement it is often focal and granular.[34]

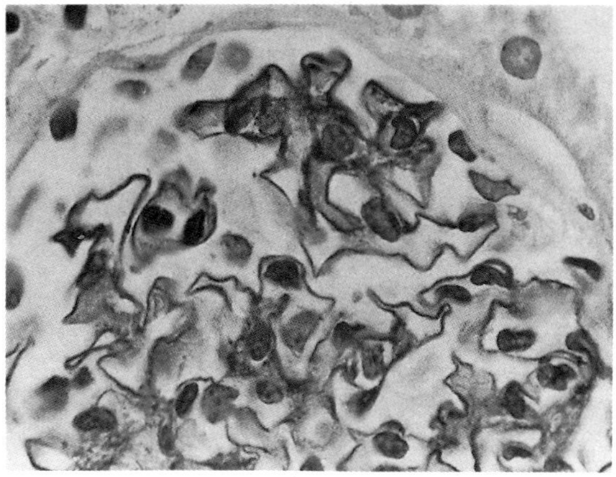

Fig. 17.5 Hyperacute rejection. Part of a glomerulus from a renal allograft 10 minutes after transplantation. There is linear deposition of IgG in the walls of the capillaries. Immunoperoxidase × 600

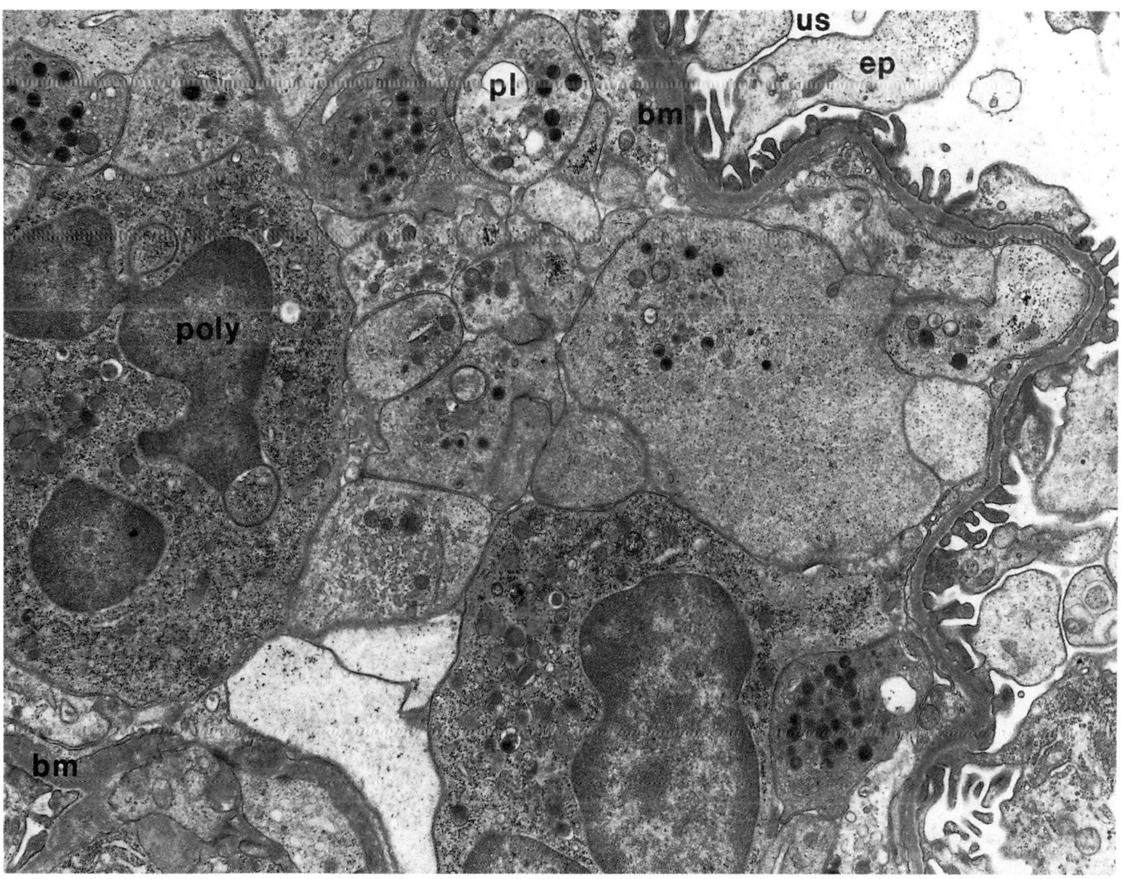

Fig. 17.4 Hyperacute rejection. Same case as illustrated in Figure 17.3. Electron micrograph of a glomerular capillary loop. The lumen is distended with neutrophil granulocytes (poly) and aggregated, partly degranulated, platelets (pl). bm, capillary basement membrane; ep, epithelial cell; us, urinary space.
× 4200

Elution studies

Donor specific anti-HLA[38,39] and anti-endothelial antigens[32] have been eluted from kidneys that have undergone hyperacute rejection in patients hypersensitized to these antigens.

Differential diagnosis

When a kidney is found to be blue and flaccid after transplantation inadequate arterial blood flow and faulty preservation of the kidney before transplantation should be considered. *Inadequate blood flow* is best checked by the surgeon; if the renal artery pulsation is weak, the anastomoses should be re-examined and torsion of the vessels at the hilum of the kidney excluded. If, in a biopsy taken within the first few hours after the graft has become blue, the endothelium has disappeared from large areas of the glomerular wall, causing thrombosis, then *preservation injury* is more likely than hyperacute rejection. The presence of many neutrophil granulocytes in the capillaries favours hyperacute rejection. However, the differentiation between these two causes by morphology is sometimes impossible. Under these circumstances attempts should be made to elute immunoglobulin from the graft.

Complications

A *microangiopathic haemolytic anaemia* sometimes occurs.[40] This is not unexpected since fibrin deposits in the lumen of small vessels in the kidney are thought to fragment red cells. The blood changes revert to normal following removal of the graft.

Prevention

Hyperacute rejection can be prevented by ensuring that the donor and recipient are ABO-compatible, screening the recipient for antibodies against the donor's tissues, looking for cold agglutinins, and undertaking a final cross-matching before transplantation, using a sensitive technique such as flow cytometry. The screen most often omitted is that for anti-endothelial antibodies.

Recently, there have been successful attempts to exploit the frequently low or absent titres of antibody to blood group A_2 antigen in the circulation of many people by deliberately transplanting A_2 kidneys into O or B recipients. Of the 56 cases reported 4% underwent hyperacute rejection, 13% were lost to either accelerated or acute rejection and 54% were functioning normally 5 months to 7½ years after transplantation.[41,42] Two factors seem to be important in determining the survival of A_2 grafts in O or B recipients: one is the quantity of isohaemagglutination in the recipient's circulation at the time of transplantation, although patients with low titres of anti-A_2 antibody do not always do well; the second is the quantitative and qualitative differences in the expression of A determinants that exist in the kidneys of A_2 donors.[43]

The more difficult problem of preventing hyperacute rejection occurring in known major ABO blood group incompatible recipients, other than by A_2 grafts to O recipients, has been tackled by attempting to eliminate the circulating antibodies. Before renal transplantation the antibodies were removed by extracorporeal immunoabsorption or plasmapheresis and the patient's ability to reform antibodies was hindered by splenectomy and treatment with immunosuppressive drugs. With this regimen only 3% of the grafts were lost to hyperacute rejection and 7% to accelerated or acute rejection.[44] Sixty-eight per cent were functioning normally 2 months to 4 years 10 months after transplantation even though high titres of IgG and IgM antibodies often eventually returned in the circulation. The reason for the lack of damage to the graft by these antibodies may be that the graft ceases after a time to express blood group antigens. These results are impressive but such treatment can be justified only exceptionally because of the long-term increased mortality from infection following splenectomy.

Pathogenesis

Experiments on animals have shown that perfusion of an allogeneic renal transplant with cell-free plasma obtained from an animal previously hyperimmunized by tissue grafts from the donor produces rapid destruction of the graft.[45] As soon as the plasma flows into the kidney, IgG becomes bound to the walls of the arterioles, glomerular capillaries, peritubular capillaries and venules; platelets and neutrophil granulocytes accumulate in the affected vessels and microthrombi form. Passive transfer of the IgG fraction of the hyperimmune plasma produces the same effects. These results, taken in conjunction with the absence of lymphoid cell infiltration in hyperacutely rejecting grafts, suggest that this form of rejection is mediated solely by antibody.

The anti-donor cytotoxic antibody binds to the vasculature of the kidney because the HLA or non-HLA endothelial antigen molecules against which it is directed are expressed on the endothelium. The binding of antibody stimulates platelet aggregation and degranulation; it also causes activation of the complement system which results in the assembly of the membrane-attack complex that disrupts the endothelial cells. The stimulated endothelial cells release platelet activating factor,[46] which causes further recruitment, aggregation and degranulation of platelets, and later the accumulation of neutrophil granulocytes. Release of adenosine diphosphate and thromboxane A_2 from the platelets leads to yet more platelet aggregation; the thromboxane A_2 also probably causes the afferent arterioles and interlobular arteries to constrict. The release of tissue factors from the damaged endothelium, in combination with platelet factors, activates the coagulation sequence. The platelet mass and trapped red cells become enmeshed in fibrin and form microthrombi. Eventually obstruction of arteries leads to acute ischaemic necrosis, manifested as infarctions and finally widespread cortical necrosis.

In cases of ABO blood group incompatibility similar changes are induced by binding of the recipient's natural isohaemagglutinins to the A_1 and B antigens which, in secretors, are present in the walls of the blood vessels of the graft. In non-secretors hyperacute rejection may not occur.

Cold agglutinins act by causing aggregation of red cells and obstruction of the vessels when the blood flows through a kidney that has been cooled to 10°C prior to transplantation, rewarming having been omitted.

Prognosis

Hyperacute rejection is an irreversible condition. At best, treatment can only postpone its inevitable outcome by a few hours.

ACCELERATED REJECTION (ACCELERATED ACUTE REJECTION)

Accelerated rejection is a clinical term sometimes used to describe severe rejection occurring within the first week after transplantation. Most episodes are recognized on the second or third day post-transplantation. Clinical manifestations such as fever, hypertension, graft swelling and tenderness are severe and response to standard anti-rejection therapy is poor.[47]

Microscopically there is severe acute vascular rejection (see p. 645). The amount of mononuclear cell infiltration is variable. Often it is moderate to severe in density; in about 30% it is minimal.

This response is very similar to that which occurs in many sensitized (but not massively hypersensitized) dogs. It differs from hyperacute rejection in its delayed onset and the invariable presence of at least a few infiltrating mononuclear cells. The antibodies responsible for the humoral component of the response may be directed against either HLA class I antigens[48] or endothelial antigens.[49]

Accelerated rejection occasionally occurs in kidneys from living related donors where the recipients have been deliberately pretreated with donor-specific blood transfusions.[50]

Recently seven presensitized patients have been reported who had antibody against donor HLA class I antigens. Unlike most cases of accelerated rejection the main histological features were the presence of neutrophil granulocytes and scattered fibrin thrombi and platelet aggregates in the glomerular and peritubular capillaries. Evidence of acute vascular rejection and acute tubulo-interstitial rejection was minimal or absent.[48]

Pathogenesis

Prior exposure of the recipient to graft alloantigens leads to immunization to those antigens. Memory cells are generated and these are activated when a renal transplant is inserted that carries some of the previously encountered transplantation antigens. The requirements for lymphocyte activation in these circumstances are less stringent and specific than for a primary response (see p. 643).

The host's T lymphocytes are stimulated by alloantigen on any of the graft's cells; the antigen does not have to be presented by macrophages or dendritic cells. Activation of the host's T lymphocytes does not need the release of interleukin-1 (IL-1) by the antigen-presenting cell as a second signal. The host's CD8-positive T lymphocytes can also become effective cytotoxic cells without help from CD4-positive T lymphocytes.

The recipient's B lymphocyte memory cells are stimulated by the renewed encounter with the graft's alloantigens to rapidly generate plasma cells. These B cells produce specific antibody which is released into the circulation and binds to the vasculature of the graft.

By these two mechanisms various blends of the pathological changes associated with acute tubulointerstitial rejection and hyperacute rejection are produced.

ACUTE REJECTION

Most patients with renal allografts undergo at least one clinical episode of acute rejection, particularly during the first few weeks after transplantation. These episodes are not so frequent and are clinically less severe in patients treated with cyclosporin than in those treated with azathioprine. Acute rejection is uncommon after a year.

A renal allograft that is undergoing acute rejection may show varying degrees and combinations of interstitial, tubular, vascular and glomerular damage. The exact pattern produced will depend on many factors, the most important being the genetic differences between donor and recipient, the degree and type of immune impairment achieved by the immunosuppressive agents being used, and the number of pretransplant blood transfusions.

Because of the prognostic implications, it is useful to distinguish those cases in which there is acute tubulointerstitial nephritis without vascular or glomerular lesions (so-called *acute tubulointerstitial rejection* or *acute cellular rejection*) from those in which there is an acute vasculitis (*acute vascular rejection, acute humoral rejection*) or an acute endocapillary proliferative glomerulonephritis (*acute transplant glomerulopathy, acute allograft glomerulopathy*). Acute tubulointerstitial rejection is usually reversed by prompt treatment with a short high-dose course of prednisolone or an anti-T-lymphocyte antibody preparation. Acute vascular rejection and acute transplant glomerulopathy respond less readily and completely, and may progress to chronic rejection.

Acute tubulointerstitial rejection (acute cellular rejection)

Clinical features

Acute tubulointerstitial rejection is rare before the fifth day after transplantation; earlier episodes are usually the result of presensitization and are often referred to as accelerated rejection (see p. 635). There is sudden deterioration in renal function with a rise in serum creatinine. This is often accompanied by fever, a rise in blood pressure, some swelling and tenderness of the kidney, and oliguria; these signs are usually fewer and less obvious in patients treated with cyclosporin than in those treated with azathioprine.[11] Ultrasonographic examination demonstrates that the graft is enlarged with no dilatation of the renal pelvis or ureter. The total blood flow to the kidney falls, and the percentage supplying the cortex decreases as rejection proceeds. Proteinuria increases or recurs, and the urine contains interleukin-2 (IL-2) and large numbers of lymphocytes and tubular cells (particularly those from the collecting ducts).[51] This is in contrast to cyclosporin nephrotoxicity in which abnormal tubular cells are accompanied by granulocytes, not lymphocytes, and IL-2 is absent. Increased ratios of CD4-positive T lymphocytes to CD8-positive T lymphocytes occur in the blood of approximately 60% of patients during acute rejection; as a similar change is found in about a quarter of patients with acute tubular necrosis or with infections, and in some who have cyclosporin toxicity or no clinical evidence of rejection, measurement of this ratio has little value in the clinical management of patients.[52]

If a renal allograft fails to function adequately in the first few weeks because of acute tubular necrosis, recognition of the onset of rejection can be difficult. In some centres transplants that are not functioning are routinely biopsied at 5 or 7 days to detect hidden acute rejection and perhaps exclude cyclosporin nephrotoxicity.

Patients who develop acute rejection often present evidence of infection by cytomegalovirus or other members of the herpesvirus group. The role, if any, of the viruses in provoking or accelerating graft rejection is still not clear.

Gross appearance of the graft

The graft is swollen and may be up to three times heavier than normal.[53] The cortex is pale or mottled and bulges when cut; the medulla is usually congested. The ureteric wall is oedematous and pale.

Light microscopy

Interstitium There is generalized oedema and a dense infiltration of the cortex by mononuclear cells (Fig. 17.6). The infiltrate appears diffuse in about 75% of cases, although usually with focal accentuation; in about 25% it is purely focal.[54] It affects predominantly the cortex; a similar, but less pronounced, cellular infiltration is often present in the outer medulla.[55]

The area of interstitium infiltrated by mononuclear cells is considerably greater in acute rejection than in well-functioning grafts. Morphometric analysis of grafts routinely biopsied at 7 and 21 days after transplantation, irrespective of their function, showed that the mean percentage area occupied by infiltrating mononuclear cells was 21% in biopsies obtained during a clinical episode of acute rejection, compared with 12% in biopsies from clinically stable grafts.[56] There is often more cellular infiltration in patients treated with azathioprine than in those treated with cyclosporin, but the difference is not significant.[54,56]

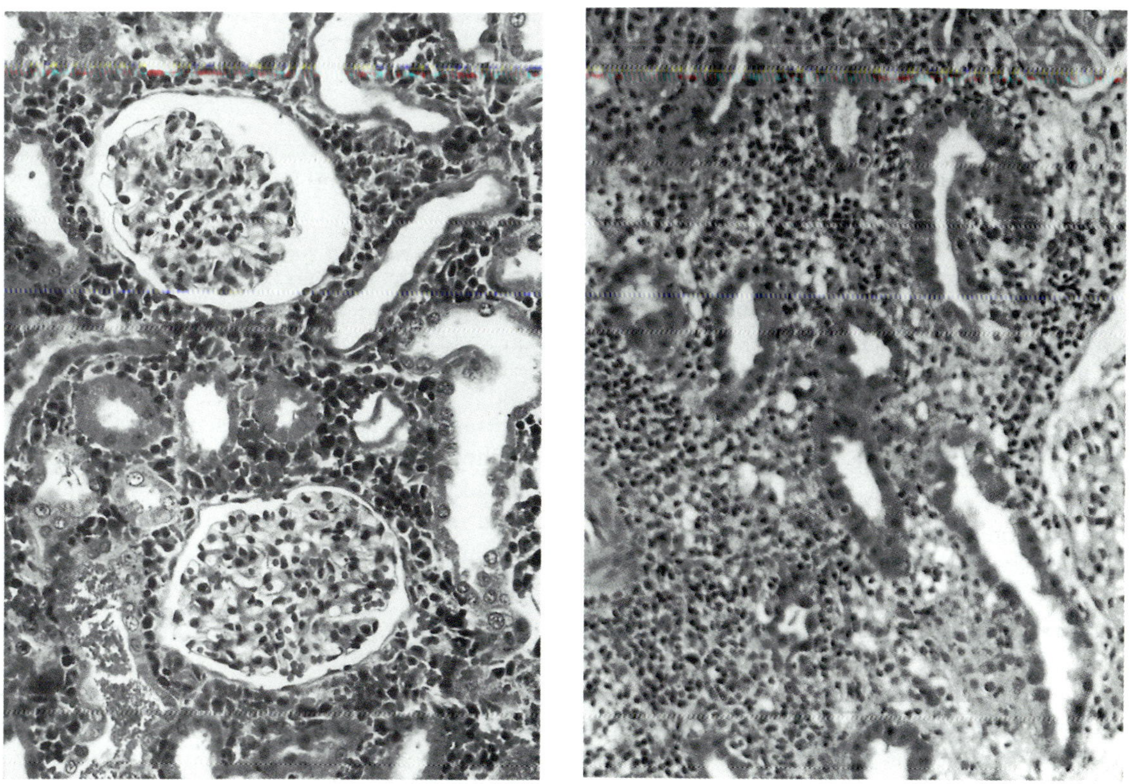

a b

Fig. 17.6 a, b Acute tubulointerstitial rejection. Mononuclear cells fill the peritubular capillaries and lymphatics and diffusely infiltrate the oedematous interstitium. The glomeruli appear normal. See also Figures 17.7 and 17.8.
(**a**),(**b**) Haematoxylin-eosin × 120

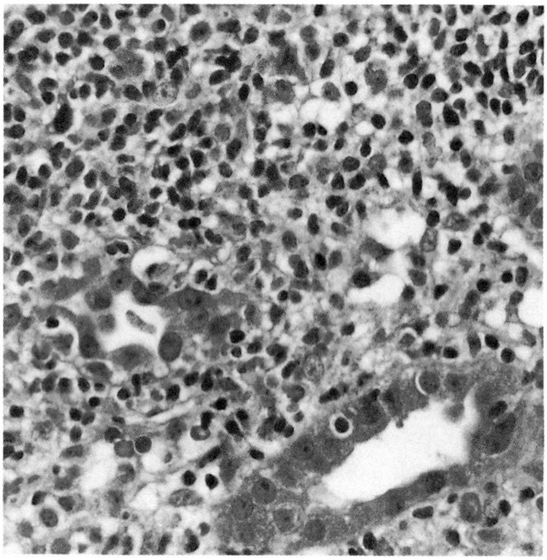

Fig. 17.7 Acute tubulointerstitial rejection. Mixture of lymphoid cells and macrophages in oedematous interstitium of rejecting renal allograft. See also Figures 17.6 and 17.8. Haematoxylin-eosin × 360

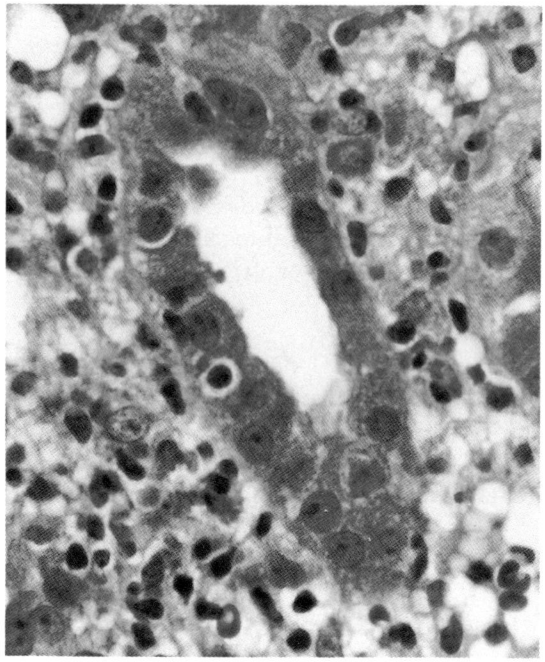

Fig. 17.8 Acute tubulointerstitial rejection. Tubulitis. Two lymphocytes are present between the tubular epithelial cells. See also Figures 17.6 and 17.7. Haematoxylin-eosin × 425

In haematoxylin and eosin stained sections the mononuclear cells appear to be a mixture of lymphocytes and macrophages, the former usually predominating (Fig. 17.7). Lymphoblasts are always present and in severe acute rejection up to a third of the lymphoid cells may be of this form. The cytoplasm of the lymphoblasts and often of many of the other lymphoid cells stains red with methyl green pyronin because it is full of ribosomes containing ribonucleic acid (RNA). Usually a few of the lymphoblasts are in mitosis. Small numbers of plasma cells and eosinophils are also present. The number of plasma cells is greater in second or subsequent episodes of acute tubulointerstitial rejection. Collections of Tamm–Horsfall protein are common, particularly at the corticomedullary junction.[57]

Tubules In about 75% of grafts undergoing acute rejection lymphoid cells and macrophages are present between the tubular epithelial cells and in the tubular lumens – a process often referred to as '*tubulitis*' (Fig. 17.8).[58,59] It only occurs where the interstitium is infiltrated by mononuclear cells, it affects particularly the distal tubules, and it is commonly accompanied by tubular dilatation and by tubular necrosis.[58]

Blood vessels and lymphatics The peritubular capillaries, venules and lymphatics contain increased numbers of lymphoid cells and monocytes.

Glomeruli Slightly increased numbers of T lymphocytes and monocytes or macrophages are commonly found in the glomerular capillaries. There may also be swelling of endothelial cells, mild expansion of the mesangium and a small segmental increase in the number of mesangial cells. These minor changes are sometimes referred to as '*glomerulitis*'.[58]

Ureter There is widespread marked oedema and diffuse interstitial infiltration by mononuclear cells, predominantly in the lamina propria. The infiltration may be focally accentuated. Lymphoid cells and macrophages are also present between the transitional epithelial cells.[60]

Electron microscopy

A little over half the infiltrating mononuclear cells have the ultrastructure of lymphocytes; about a quarter are macrophages, some could be natural killer cells and small numbers are plasma cells. Of the lymphocytes about 30% are lymphoblasts.[61] Lymphocytes and macrophages can be seen traversing the walls of the peritubular capillaries through endothelial cell junctions[34] and moving across the tubular walls between the epithelial cells.[59] There is evidence of focal injury to peritubular capillaries[34] and tubules.[59]

Immunofluorescence/immunoperoxidase microscopy

Immunoglobulin and complement deposits are not usually present in the blood vessels and glomeruli.

Phenotyping of mononuclear cells infiltrating interstitium

Phenotyping of the cells infiltrating the interstitium, using monoclonal antibodies and frozen sections, has demonstrated that most of the cells are T lymphocytes and macrophages, and that of the lymphocytes both CD4-positive and CD8-positive subsets are present; but there is no consensus on the relative frequency of these cell types.[56,62,63] This failure to achieve agreement, despite large numbers of studies, is probably because of variations in the potency and specificity of the monoclonal antibodies used by the different investigators, the form of basic immunosuppression given to the patients, and the time when the biopsy was taken in relation to the onset of clinical rejection. Other differences between series were whether high-dose steroid treatment had started before the biopsy was taken, whether areas of focal or diffuse cellular infiltration were biopsied, and the failure to use morphometric methods in most of the studies. There is some evidence that CD8-positive T lymphocytes predominate when the interstitial infiltrate is diffuse, while CD4-positive T lymphocytes tend to be more numerous in focal perivascular aggregates and in biopsies taken earlier in the course of acute rejection.[62]

Expression of activation markers by mononuclear cells infiltrating the interstitium

The activation of T lymphocytes by antigen is characterized by the synthesis of IL-2 and the appearance of IL-2 (CD25) and transferrin receptors, CD38 (T10) and MHC class II antigens, and proliferation antigens. These antigens are not expressed by resting cells. Because the number of activated cells in a graft undergoing rejection tends to be small and the expression of the markers transient, they are difficult to demonstrate. In one study, which claimed to have overcome these difficulties, it was found that activated and proliferating cells were almost always present in rejection, but were usually absent in other circumstances.[63]

HLA expression on the tubular epithelium

During clinical episodes of rejection there is a generalized increase in HLA class II expression in approximately 60% of renal allografts.[64] The distal tubular epithelium becomes intensely positive for HLA-DR, -DP and -DQ antigens and their expression on glomerular cells, vascular endothelium and proximal tubules is increased. In about 10% of grafts the increase is focal; in 30% it remains normal.[65] The intensity of HLA class II antigen induction is closely correlated with the number of T lymphocytes infiltrating the interstitium; it is probably a local response to gamma interferon produced by these cells when activated. Once induced, enhanced HLA class II antigen expression often persists for some weeks.[64]

Adhesion molecule expression

In acute rejection host lymphocytes and macrophages adhere to endothelial and other cells of the graft by the interaction of adhesion receptors on the leucocytes with appropriate ligands on the target cells. As might therefore be expected the expression of adhesion ligands, such as intercellular adhesion molecule-1 (CAM-1, CD54), increases in the graft in acute rejection.[66,67] The increased expression, like that of HLA class II antigens, is probably induced by inflammatory mediators released by the infiltrating mononuclear cells.

Flow cytometric analysis of graft cells

If part of a graft biopsy is cut into 1-mm pieces and digested with collagenase, the freed cells can be stained with combinations of fluorescein- and phycoerythrin-labelled antibodies. A single cell suspension can then be analysed in a two-colour flow cytometer and sorter. Using this technique and five different mononuclear antibodies (defining CD3, CD8, CD16, CD45 and HLA-DR) it has been claimed that during acute rejection the numbers of lymphocytes and HLA-DR-positive renal tubular cells increase, and the proportions of CD8-positive lymphocytes and CD16-positive NK-like cells are raised. The number of suppressor-induced (CD45R- and CD4-positive) T lymphocytes and suppressor effector (CD11b- and CD8-positive) T lymphocytes are reduced. Multivariate analysis then allowed a precise and rapid diagnosis of acute tubulointerstitial rejection.[68]

Fine needle aspiration cytology

Because the needle used in this technique is very fine, repeated aspiration biopsies can be obtained from a graft with far less risk than after most conventional needle biopsies. Application of immunocytochemical techniques to the cells obtained enables the onset of acute tubulointerstitial rejection to be detected and allows monitoring of the effects of immunosuppressive treatment.[69] Relatively minor problems are that the method requires considerable cytological skills for accurate interpretation, and it can be difficult to avoid contamination of the aspirate with peripheral blood cells.

The great disadvantage of fine needle aspiration cytology is that vascular damage cannot be detected in the material obtained so that the coexistence or development of acute vascular rejection will be missed. In most circumstances this is too great a penalty because a knowledge of whether acute vascular rejection is present or not is crucial in estimating the prognosis and deciding the best form of treatment.

Fine needle aspiration cytology must therefore be backed up by conventional needle biopsy to obtain a core of tissue. When this has to be done it removes the safety advantage that initially makes fine needle aspiration cytology seem so attractive. Moreover, the aspirate provides no more information than can be obtained from flow cytometric analysis of single cell suspensions.

Changes in other organs

Changes in rejection are not confined to the transplant. Large lymphoid cells with pyroninophilic cytoplasm accumulate around the postcapillary venules in the paracortical area of the draining lymph nodes and in the periarteriolar lymphoid sheaths of the splenic white pulp.[70]

Differential diagnosis

The histological and immunohistochemical features of acute tubulointerstitial rejection are not pathognomonic. Just because a graft contains a mononuclear cell infiltrate it cannot be assumed that the kidney is undergoing clinical rejection. All renal allografts contain considerable numbers of such cells in the first weeks after transplantation and lesser numbers for much longer periods, even when the transplanted kidneys are functioning normally.[56,71] Well-functioning grafts, when routinely biopsied 7 days after transplantation, have on average 12% of the area of the biopsy sections occupied by infiltrating mononuclear cells; the area infiltrated is still much the same at 21 days.[56] However, the extent of the cellular infiltrate in a clinical episode of acute tubulointerstitial rejection can be excluded (with a 95% probability) if the infiltrating mononuclear cells occupy less than 8% of the area of the sections in a graft biopsy from a patient treated with cyclosporin.[72] Experienced histopathologists will make this assessment without morphometry, but in equivocal cases point counting[73] or image analysis (which is faster)[74] can be helpful.

In cases where the area of biopsy occupied by mononuclear cells exceeds 8%, five conditions need to be considered in the differential diagnosis.

They are acute tubular necrosis, cyclosporin toxicity, cytomegalovirus infection, pyelonephritis, and lymphoproliferative disorders.

Acute tubular necrosis Acute tubular necrosis is usually associated with an interstitial mononuclear cell infiltrate and this sometimes occupies more than 8% of the area of the sections. However, the composition of the infiltrate differs from that in acute rejection. In acute tubular necrosis lymphoblasts, lymphocytes with pyronin-positive cytoplasm and mononuclear cells in mitosis are rare; in acute tubulointerstitial rejection there are usually a few infiltrating cells in mitosis, and pyronin-positive cells and lymphoblasts are frequent. Increased HLA-class II expression on tubules is not a useful discriminant in individual cases because up to 26% of grafts undergoing rejection do not show enhanced HLA expression.[65] Interstitial oedema is usually greater in acute tubulointerstitial rejection than in acute tubular necrosis, but, because of overlap, estimations of the quantity do not help in individual cases. Tubulitis, although more marked in rejection, also occurs in both conditions. The amount of tubular damage is unhelpful because it may be extensive in acute tubulointerstitial rejection. Ultimately the distinction between acute tubular necrosis and acute tubulointerstitial rejection on a particular biopsy has to be made on the nature of the cellular infiltrate; this may be aided by the immunocytochemical demonstration of activated cells (as shown by anti-Tac and anti-transferrin monoclonal antibodies) and proliferating cells (as indicated by anti-Ki-67) which are common in acute tubulointerstitial rejection and rare in acute tubular necrosis.[63] The value of two-colour flow cytometry and multivariate analysis of cell suspensions from the graft using multiple monoclonal antibodies has yet to be proved.

Cyclosporin nephrotoxicity Cyclosporin nephrotoxicity is not associated with any pathognomonic histological changes.[54] However, there is evidence that after a period of continuous treatment with cyclosporin, arteriolar hyalinization and isometric vacuolation of tubular cells occur, and the expression of HLA class II antigens is inhibited (see p. 661).

The vascular change affects the afferent arterioles and is characterized by subintimal and medial hyaline deposits with focal replacement of pericytes;[75,76] the deposits contain IgM, C3 and Clq.[75] This lesion cannot be clearly differentiated from the arteriolar hyalinization that occurs in benign phase hypertension and in diabetes mellitus (see p. 307). In cyclosporin nephrotoxicity the arteriolar hyaline change is probably preceded by vasoconstriction which is reversible. Arteriolar hyalinization may cause focal ischaemic tubular atrophy and interstitial fibrosis which may have a striped form.

The isometric vacuolation affects the straight segment of the proximal tubules and is due to dilatation of the smooth and rough endoplasmic reticulum which produces vacuoles that are free of lipid; it is indistinguishable from osmotic nephrosis (see p. 495).[75]

The failure to induce the expression of HLA class II antigens on the distal tubules is in contrast to acute rejection;[77] however, as up to a quarter of patients undergoing an acute clinical rejection episode do not show enhanced expression of HLA class II antigens, this feature cannot be used in individual cases to distinguish between rejection and cyclosporin nephrotoxicity.

Histologically, therefore, cyclosporin nephrotoxicity is a diagnosis of exclusion made when evidence of acute rejection and other possible causes of graft dysfunction are not present.[78] In certain circumstances the diagnosis of cyclosporin nephrotoxicity may be strongly suspected. For example, if a biopsy of a graft at the time of transplantation shows no arteriolar lesions, and the patient remains normotensive following transplantation and does not develop diabetes mellitus, then the discovery of arteriolar hyaline lesions in a subsequent biopsy, taken at a time of graft dysfunction, is strongly suggestive of cyclosporin nephrotoxicity because arteriolar hyalinization is not produced by acute rejection.[78]

Cytomegalovirus infection Cytomegalovirus infection (see p. 403) is a common complication of renal transplantation.[79] It is associated with focal mononuclear cell infiltration of the interstitium. The diagnosis depends upon either finding viral inclusions, which are rare and usually within the tubular cells, or demonstrating the presence of the viral nucleic acids using in situ hybridization and labelled DNA probes.[80] Viral nucleic acids may be present in the infiltrating mononuclear cells of many grafts that do not show inclusions by light microscopy. It should be remembered, however, that identification of cytomegalovirus in the graft does not exclude an associated acute tubulointerstitial rejection; the two conditions frequently coexist.

Pyelonephritis Pyelonephritis is uncommon in renal allografts, but when it occurs it must be distinguished from rejection. The distinction is made largely on the nature of the interstitial cellular infiltrate. In acute pyelonephritis there are many more neutrophil granulocytes than in acute tubulointerstitial rejection. In chronic pyelonephritis activated and proliferating lymphocytes and macrophages are very infrequent or absent, in contrast to acute tubulointerstitial rejection in which they are a major component of the mononuclear infiltrate.

Lymphoproliferative disorders When graft dysfunction occurs some weeks after transplantation and a biopsy of the transplant contains a dense mononuclear cell infiltrate, it is important to exclude a lymphoproliferative disorder.[81,82] Although rare, lymphoproliferative disorders are almost 60 times more frequent than would be expected in an age-matched population;[83] they involve the graft in about 2.5% of renal transplant patients who are treated with cyclosporin and steroids.[84] In many the diagnosis is obvious but in several the appearances on the initial biopsy have been confused with severe acute tubulointerstitial rejection. There is a focal or diffuse, dense proliferation of lymphoid cells of B lymphocyte origin. Staining of frozen sections with appropriate monoclonal antibodies should therefore differentiate lymphoproliferative disorders from acute tubulointerstitial rejection in which the infiltrate is composed of a mixture of T lymphocytes and macrophages. In B-cell lymphoproliferative disease there is a strong association with Epstein-Barr virus and the viral DNA can often be demonstrated in the proliferating cells by DNA hybridization.

The extremely rare T-cell lymphoproliferative lesions can be more difficult to differentiate from acute tubulointerstitial rejection. However, they tend to be composed almost entirely of uniform sheets of predominantly large atypical lymphoid cells with nuclear aberrations.[85] The lesions lack macrophages and small lymphocytes, which are a feature of acute tubulointerstitial rejection.

Complications

Occasionally the greatly swollen and tense graft ruptures (see p. 660).

Prognosis

Acute tubulointerstitial rejection is usually promptly reversed either by treatment with high doses of steroids for 3 days, or by a short course of antilymphocyte globulin or a monoclonal anti-T-lymphocyte antibody. Improvement in the clinical condition is generally apparent within 24 hours and renal function quickly returns to normal. In a few patients one or more further episodes of acute tubulointerstitial rejection occur after an interval of days or weeks; most of these later episodes are also usually reversible.

Occasional episodes of acute tubulointerstitial rejection are resistant to treatment; this is more likely to occur in patients who have already had one or more previous episodes of reversible acute tubulointerstitial rejection[11] and they are usually associated with the appearance of acute vascular rejection (see p. 645). Such episodes often progress to chronic rejection (see p. 653).

There is some evidence that the number of reversible acute rejection episodes that the patient undergoes is directly related to the long-term survival of the graft. Those who have no rejection episodes are much more likely to have a functioning graft 5 and 10 years after transplantation than those who undergo two or more episodes of rejection in the first 2 months after the transplantation.[86]

After acute tubulointerstitial rejection has been clinically reversed the initial mononuclear cell infiltrate is usually reduced in amount to about 7% of the area of biopsy sections in cyclosporin-treated patients.[65] The phenotypic composition of the cellular infiltrate remains unaltered,[56] but the lymphoblasts and lymphoid cells with pyroninophilic cytoplasm and mitoses disappear, and the infiltrating cells no longer stain with monoclonal antibodies that act as markers for the presence of activation and proliferation (such as anti-Tac, anti-transferrin and Ki-67).[63] The increased expression of HLA class II antigens on the tubular cells persists, often for some weeks.

The density of the interstitial cellular infiltrate and the area it occupies do not correlate with graft survival. There is some evidence, however, that a diffuse infiltrate of predominantly CD8-positive T lymphocytes is associated with increased resistance to treatment and a poorer prognosis.[87] Infiltrates that contain more than 4% of eosinophils also seem to be more difficult to reverse.[88]

Pathogenesis

For rejection to occur there must usually be incompatability between donor and host for antigens of the HLA or the endothelial cell antigen system. Mismatching for either class I or class II HLA antigens can initiate rejection; some evidence suggests that class II incompatibility causes a more marked reaction. Where there is compatibility for these antigen systems multiple differences in the minor histocompatibility antigens can probably sometimes lead to rejection.

When the graft is introduced the foreign HLA class II antigens are recognized by some of the host's T-helper lymphocytes. The lymphocytes of this group are referred to as *alloreactive T lymphocytes,* in contrast to the rest of the T lymphocytes which respond to other antigens and are usually called *antigen-specific T lymphocytes.* About 1% of T-helper lymphocytes are strongly alloreactive without prior sensitization, which is a far greater percentage than responds to any other antigen. The alloreactive and the antigen-specific T lymphocytes probably belong to the same lineage and use the same antigen receptors.

The antigen determinant recognized by alloreactive T lymphocytes is composed of allogeneic peptide fragments which have been bound in a special groove on the HLA molecule[23] (see p. 629). Recognition is facilitated by presentation of the antigenic determinant on an appropriate donor cell.[89] The essential characteristics of these cells are their capacity to take up, process and display the transplant's antigen in the grooves of the HLA molecules on their cell surface. They also have a high natural ability to express both class I and class II HLA molecules and the capacity to release interleukin-I (IL-1). In the transplanted kidney the two most important types of antigen-presenting cells are the *dendritic cells in the interstitium* and the *vascular endothelial cells.* In rodents the dendritic cells migrate out of an allograft via the blood stream and settle in the white pulp of the recipient's spleen where they associate predominantly with CD4-positive T lymphocytes.[90] This provides a direct route for central sensitization of the host, i.e. recognition by the host's alloreactive helper T lymphocytes in the spleen of the foreign HLA antigens carried by the donor's dendritic cells. When the alloantigen is presented to the host's lymphocytes by the graft's endothelial cells, recognition occurs peripherally, i.e. in the transplant.

Both central and peripheral modes of sensitization are probably important in humans who receive a renal allograft. In rodents the interstitial dendritic cells are crucial because the endothelial cells within the graft do not initially express MHC class II antigens. In patients the role of the dendritic cells is unlikely to be so critical because the vascular endothelial cells in the renal graft naturally express HLA class II antigen molecules. The endothelial cells, therefore, probably play a significant role in sensitizing patients.

T lymphocytes also recognize the allograft antigen when they are processed and presented by the host's dendritic cells and macrophages (as distinct from comparable donor cells from the transplant). The foreign histocompatibility antigens are partly degraded, then released on the cell surface and presented by the host cells to the host's alloreactive T lymphocytes as peptides in the grooves of host class II HLA antigens. This response may cause rejection by the activation of lymphokines, but not by direct cytotoxicity because the target cells in the graft do not express host HLA antigen molecules (see self MHC restriction on p. 629).

The alloreactive T lymphocytes that recognize the graft as foreign are usually CD4-positive helper cells that respond to those HLA class II molecules that are present in the transplant but not in the recipient. Occasionally the HLA class II antigens of donor and recipient will be compatible. In these circumstances incompatibilities in the HLA class I antigens will be recognized by CD8-positive T lymphocytes. Both phenotypes therefore play an essential role in the triggering and effecting of rejection in a previously unsensitized host.

Recognition of alloantigen occurs during a complicated interaction involving not only the T-cell receptor and HLA–peptide complexes, but also the CD3 complex on the surface of the T lymphocytes and numerous other cell surface molecules on the donor antigen-presenting cells and the recipient's lymphocytes.[23]

Activation of the host's CD4-positive helper T lymphocytes involves two signals: the first is provided in some way through the cross linking of the receptors on the lymphocyte and the antigen-presenting cells; the second is the release of IL-1 by the antigen-presenting cell. The results include a rapid increase in cytoplasmic calcium concentration, expression of the IL-2 receptor, and secretion of IL-2. The helper T lymphocyte begins to synthesize RNA and protein, enlarges to form a lymphoblast with pyroninophilic cytoplasm, and then divides and releases other lymphokines, including IL-3, IL-4, IL-5 and gamma interferon. IL-2 is an essential growth factor for clonal expansion and massive cell division follows leading to the proliferation of large numbers of non-specific, as well as specific, effector and memory cells.[23]

Some of the T lymphocytes generated are cytotoxic. Division of cytotoxic T lymphocytes is dependent on IL-2 which the cytotoxic cells do not make; the IL-2 is largely provided by T-helper lymphocytes which are therefore very important in facilitating a cytotoxic T lymphocyte response. The CD8-positive cytotoxic T lymphocytes damage the cells of the graft. They bind to a target cell after recognizing the foreign HLA antigen plus HLA class I antigens on its surface. The process is assisted by accessory molecules such as the lymphocyte-function-associated molecules LFA-1 and LFA-3. The lymphocyte then produces a pore-forming protein (perforin) which inserts itself into the membrane of the graft cell, polymerizes and forms a hole in the membrane which causes osmotic death of the cell.[91]

B lymphocytes are also activated by direct interaction with transplantation antigens through their surface immunoglobulin receptors. Contact with T-helper lymphocytes or with lymphokines, such as IL-4, is then necessary for the B lymphocytes to be stimulated to proliferate and differentiate into antibody-secreting plasma cells.

The release of lymphokines also leads to an assortment of non-specific effects. Some of the soluble factors, such as macrophage-chemotactic factor, and macrophage-activating factor, attract macrophages into the graft and activate them. The macrophages cause non-specific tissue destruction by the release of proteases and reactive oxygen species. They also secrete a host of mediators that promote inflammation. The production of gamma interferon increases the concentration of class I and II HLA antigens on cells already expressing the antigen, and also induces the transcription of class II genes in cells which are normally negative.[92] Enhanced expression of class II HLA antigens on the vascular endothelial cells and new expression of the same antigens on the tubular cells augment the process of recognition of the graft and create targets for the cytotoxic T lymphocytes.

An additional consequence of lymphokine release is that vascular endothelial cells are induced to express molecules, such as HLA-1, that facilitate migration of lymphocytes into the adjacent tissue. The lymphocytes recruited into the graft in this way are non-specific, but they become activated and proliferate when exposed to the lymphokines, such as IL-2 and IL-3, that are being released by the specifically activated T lymphocytes. This results in a massive accumulation of activated cells in the graft, the majority of which have no specificity for antigens in the graft. The lymphokines also directly kill cells; for example, tumour necrosis factor beta is cytotoxic and gamma interferon is cytostatic.

The primary target of the host's immune attack is the vascular endothelium, much of which in humans expresses both class I and class II HLA antigens and intercellular adhesion molecules such as ICAM-1, LFA-1 and LFA-3.

Marked cortical ischaemia occurs during the process of rejection. The cause is still not resolved. The widespread obstruction and destruction of peritubular capillaries by cytotoxic T lymphocytes and perhaps other cells, or by lymphokines, undoubtedly lead to profound changes in the haemodynamics of the graft. Vasoconstriction also plays a role; it is caused by thromboxane A_2 and other arachidonic acid metabolites such as leukotriene B_4 and leukotriene C_3 which are produced by the cellular infiltrate, in particular by the macrophages.

Acute vascular rejection (acute humoral rejection)

Clinical features

Acute vascular rejection presents as an acute rejection episode which differs only in its severity from that which accompanies acute tubulointerstitial rejection (see p. 636).

Laboratory findings

The laboratory findings are mostly the same as those associated with acute tubulointerstitial rejection (see p. 636). Platelet sequestration in the graft is, however, sometimes a feature. The blood platelet count is often low at the onset of clinical evidence of rejection and labelling the platelets with ^{51}Cr or ^{111}In has shown that many collect in the graft. Platelet sequestration in the graft is rare in acute tubulointerstitial rejection but does occur in those cases of cyclosporin nephrotoxicity in which arteriolar lesions are found (see p. 641). Some studies suggest that cytotoxic alloantibodies to B lymphocytes, especially those directed against donor HLA-DR, are particularly associated with acute vascular rejection.

Gross appearance of the graft

The graft is initially swollen and oedematous. The subcapsular surface is speckled with petechial haemorrhages; similar haemorrhages are present on the cut surface of the cortex. Later, there are often scattered small infarcts, particularly in the cortex.

Light microscopy

Arterioles and arteries Mononuclear cells, neutrophil granulocytes or both, may be seen adhering to the endothelium of arteries, a process usually called *'margination'*. There is also often focal infiltration of mononuclear cells beneath the endothelium which is lifted from its basement membrane; this may be associated with swelling, patchy necrosis and loss of endothelial cells. These changes are sometimes referred to as *'endothelialitis'* (Fig. 17.9).[93] Margination or endothelialitis or both occur in 37–46% of patients treated with azathioprine and prednisolone who are clinically in acute rejection;[93,94] the incidence is lower in patients treated with cyclosporin. Vascular leucocyte margination and endothelialitis are sometimes grouped together and referred to as *acute cellular arteritis*.[95]

In severe cases foci of *fibrinoid necrosis* are present in the walls of arterioles and small arteries (Fig. 17.10). The media is particularly affected; sometimes the damaged wall is infiltrated by mononuclear cells. The lesions are often accompanied by rupture of the internal elastic lamina. Fibrin, platelets and neutrophil granulocytes adhere to the damaged areas of the vessel wall; the lumen of some vessels becomes obliterated by these thrombi. Fibrinoid necrosis of arterioles

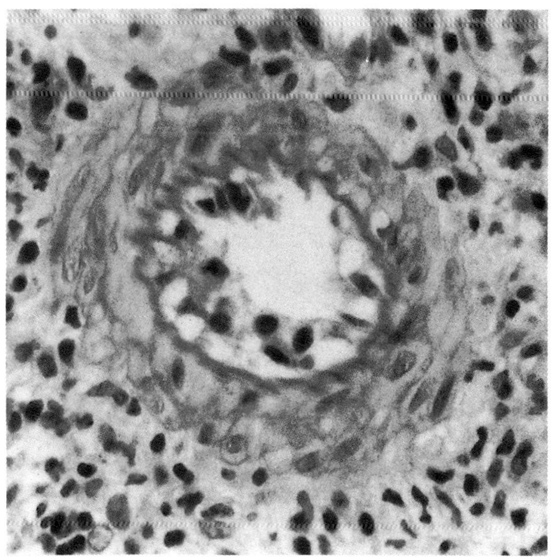

Fig. 17.9 Acute vascular rejection. 'Endothelialitis'. A small interlobular artery shows a subintimal mononuclear cell infiltrate.
Periodic acid-Schiff × 500

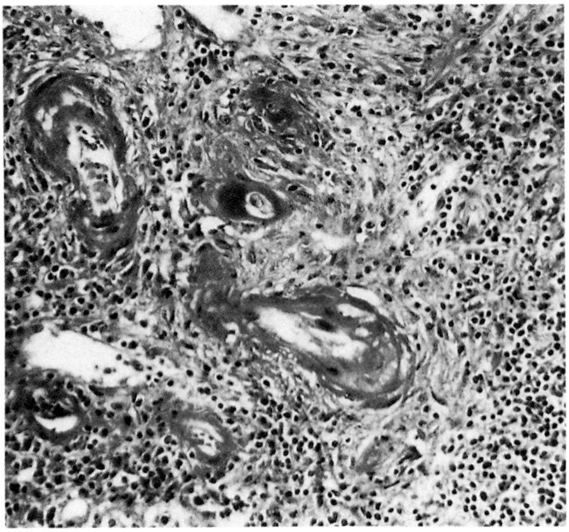

Fig. 17.10 Acute vascular rejection. Fibrinoid necrosis. The walls of several arterioles are necrotic with replacement of smooth muscle by material staining for fibrin. There is focal mononuclear cell infiltration in the adjacent interstitium. Haematoxylin-eosin × 170

and arteries or both is present in 16–23% of azathioprine- and prednisolone-treated patients in acute rejection.[93,94] The arteriolar and arterial fibrinoid necrotic lesions are sometimes classified as *necrotizing arteritis*.[95]

Glomeruli Thrombosis of capillaries or segmental necrosis may occur in variable numbers of glomeruli. These lesions were present in 31% of one series of grafts undergoing acute rejection in patients treated with azathioprine and prednisolone.[94]

Interstitium Focal haemorrhages and collections of fibrin are frequent. They were present in 29% of one series of grafts biopsied during acute rejection.[94] In severe cases foci of necrosis and small infarcts occur. Mononuclear cell infiltration is slight to moderate in amount.

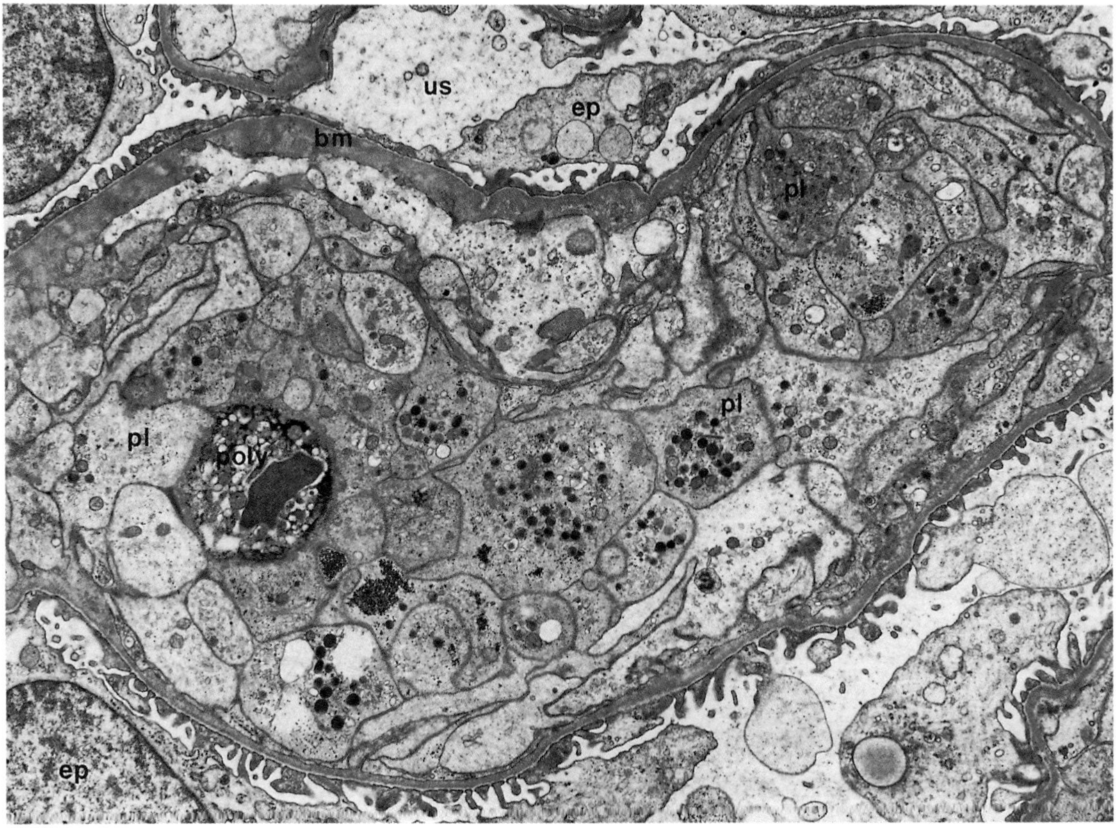

Fig. 17.11 Acute vascular rejection. Electron micrograph of a glomerular capillary loop. The lumen is obstructed by aggregated platelets (pl) and a dead neutrophil granulocyte (poly). bm, capillary basement membrane; ep, visceral epithelial cell; us, urinary space.
× 6450

Ureter Endothelialitis and leucocyte margination are common in the periadventitial arteries and arterioles. Fibrinoid necrosis of these vessels also occurs.[60] Thrombosis of the small veins is frequent.

Electron microscopy

Platelet aggregates are common in variable numbers of glomerular and peritubular capillaries (Fig. 17.11). Serial biopsies have shown that fibrin and neutrophil granulocytes soon appear and the resulting microthrombi are indistinguishable from those found in hyperacute rejection.[96]

In the arterioles and small arteries the smooth muscle cells of the media are focally necrotic. Where there is loss of endothelial cells, microthrombi are present on the exposed basement membrane (Fig. 17.12).[96]

Immunofluorescence/immunoperoxidase microscopy

IgG, IgM and particularly Clq and C3 and fibrinogen are common in the walls of arterioles, arteries and glomerular and peritubular capillaries.[97] The glomerular deposits tend to be segmental and linear rather than granular. The mononuclear cells involved in vascular leucocyte margination and endothelialitis include CD8-positive and CD4-positive T lymphocytes and lymphoblasts, and monocytes. When the lesions are severe CD8-positive T lymphocytes predominate, suggesting that that HLA class I antigens are the primary target.[98]

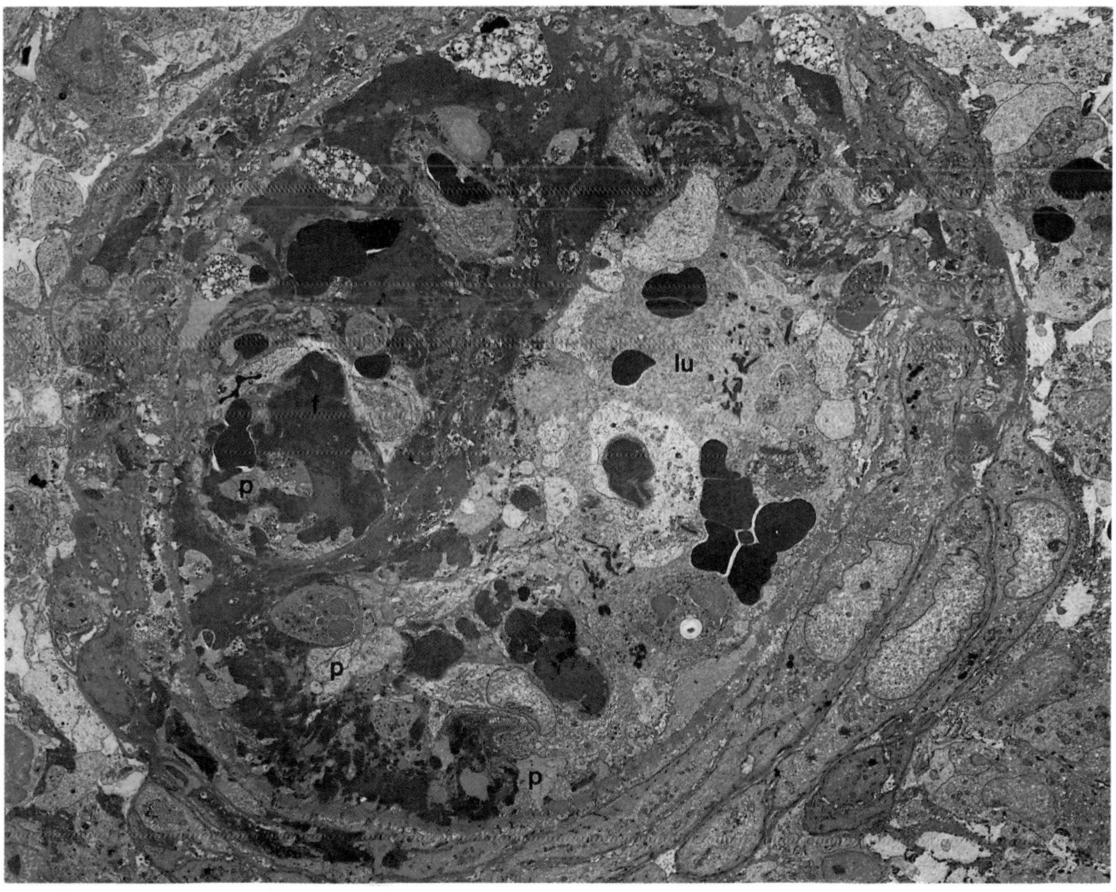

Fig. 17.12 Acute vascular rejection. Electron micrograph showing mural thrombus in a small artery. There is necrosis of smooth muscle and loss of endothelial cells in part of the vessel wall. Fibrin (f), platelets (p) and neutrophil granulocytes form a thrombus over the damaged area. lu, arterial lumen.
× 1000
Reproduced by permission from: Porter, KA. Int Rev Exp Pathol 1972;11;73 (Fig. 6)

Changes in other organs

As in acute tubulointerstitial rejection, changes occur in the spleen and lymph nodes (see p. 640).

Differential diagnosis

The histological and immunohistochemical features of acute vascular rejection are not pathognomonic. Six conditions need to be considered in the differential diagnosis. They are cyclosporin nephrotoxicity, severe hypertension, recurrent haemolytic uraemic syndrome, recurrent Henoch–Schönlein purpura, recurrent thrombotic thrombocytopenic purpura and accelerated rejection.

Cyclosporin nephrotoxicity When margination, endothelialitis or fibrinoid necrosis of arterioles and small arteries is present in an allograft biopsy cyclosporin nephrotoxicity is unlikely because vascular lesions in this latter condition take the form of arteriolar hyalinization. If in the biopsy there is arteriolar hyalinization and a focus of interstitial haemorrhage or necrosis, serial sections should be searched for focal arterial fibrinoid necrosis because interstitial haemorrhage and necrosis are rare in cyclosporin nephrotoxicity and frequent in acute vascular rejection. Glomerular capillary thrombosis in a biopsy taken during a period of acute graft dysfunction is more commonly an indication of acute vascular rejection than cyclosporin nephrotoxicity. Despite claims that such thrombi are one of the features of cyclosporin nephrotoxicity,[99] a comparison of biopsies taken routinely from patients at 7 and 21 days after transplantation showed that glomerular capillary thrombosis occurred less frequently in patients on cyclosporin than in those being treated with azathioprine and steroids.[100]

Severe hypertension The vascular effects of severe hypertension are histologically indistinguishable from those produced by acute vascular rejection. The distinction must be made on clinical evidence.

Recurrent haemolytic uraemic syndrome Haemolytic uraemic syndrome frequently recurs (see p. 669) and histologically may be indistinguishable from acute vascular rejection. The patient's original disease must be known before diagnosing acute vascular rejection.

Recurrent Henoch–Schönlein purpura Henoch–Schönlein purpura (see p. 669) frequently recurs but it can be easily distinguished from acute vascular rejection by immunofluorescence. In Henoch–Schönlein purpura mesangial accumulations of IgA are a characteristic feature; they are not found in acute vascular rejection.

Recurrent thrombotic thrombocytopenic purpura Thrombotic thrombocytopenic purpura occasionally recurs (see p. 290). The lesions in the graft can be indistinguishable from acute vascular rejection. Diagnosis depends upon knowing the patient's original disease.

Accelerated rejection The histological lesions in accelerated rejection and acute vascular rejection may be identical. The distinction is fairly arbitrary and depends upon the time of onset of the rejection episode; accelerated rejection becomes clinically apparent in the first 1–4 days after transplantation; acute vascular rejection is apparent only from the fifth day onwards. Some do not think this distinction worth making (see p. 649).

Prognosis

Severe acute vascular rejection is difficult to reverse and the outlook is poor. In one study 82% of the grafts with acute vascular rejection ceased functioning within 4½ years; most of the losses occurred within 2 months of the failure to respond to the first high-dose course of steroids.[101]

The presence of medial necrosis of arteries and arterioles, glomerular thrombosis or necrosis or both, and interstitial haemorrhage, either singly or together, in a graft biopsy taken during the first 3 months after transplantation, is a very sensitive and accurate indicator of early failure of the transplant. In Herbertson's important study[94] less than 10% of 65 grafts with one or more of these features of acute vascular rejection, regardless of severity, were capable of supporting life 1 year after transplantation. Endothelialitis, if severe, was also associated with less than 10% graft survival at 1 year after transplantation. There was also a significant association between poor subsequent graft function and lesser grades of endothelialitis and cellular margination. Other investigators have reported similar findings. These studies were all performed before the advent of cyclosporin; since then, although the accumulative incidence of acute rejection in the first year has been approximately halved, acute vascular rejection continues to occur and seems as difficult to reverse.

It is mainly because of their better prognosis that vascular cellular margination and the lesser grades of endothelialitis are sometimes grouped together and referred to as *acute cellular arteritis*. This clearly separates them from the arteriolar and arterial medial fibrinoid necrotic lesions with their associated glomerular thrombosis or necrosis, interstitial haemorrhage and poor prognosis, which are classified as *necrotizing arteritis* (see p. 646).[95]

Pathogenesis

In the severe necrotizing arteritis form of acute vascular rejection the histology of the affected blood vessels resembles in many ways that seen in hyperacute rejection, antibodies of donor specificity are often present in the circulation, and antibody and complement can be shown to be present in the lesions. Some renal allografts irreversibly damaged by necrotizing arteritis have been found to contain anti-HLA antibodies bound to them;[102] in others anti-endothelial non-HLA antibodies have been detected.[103] For these reasons it is usually considered that necrotizing arteritis is antibody mediated. However, it has not been unequivocally shown that the appearance of antibody is essential before acute necrotizing arteritis can occur, and the lesions are often preceded or accompanied by endothelialitis with its infiltrating CD8-positive T lymphocytes and macrophages; similar cells are sometimes present in the media. It is therefore equally possible that cell-mediated mechanisms are reponsible.

Acute cellular arteritis is often thought to be mediated by T cells rather than antibodies,[95] but very similar lesions are encountered in presensitized patients with rejection associated with antibodies against donor class I HLA antigens and these are thought to be mediated by the antibody.[48]

Whatever the basic underlying effector mechanism, it is likely that the end result is endothelial injury which triggers platelet aggregation, activation of the coagulation cascade and an inflammatory response as in hyperacute rejection (see p. 634).

It is often difficult to know whether the immune response that causes acute vascular rejection is primary or secondary. If there is evidence that the patient has been presensitized to some of the donor's antigens then the changes should be considered as accelerated rejection (see p. 635). Because of this difficulty Colvin[95] does not differentiate between accelerated rejection and necrotizing arteritis but groups them together under the latter term.

Acute transplant glomerulopathy (acute allograft glomerulopathy)

From 4 to 10% of renal allografts develop a distinctive glomerular lesion characterized by occlusion of the capillary lumens by swollen endothelial cells and mononuclear cells. The lesion usually occurs in the first 2 months after transplantation but it is occasionally found much later. It is resistant to treatment and associated with poor graft survival.

Clinical features

Acute transplant glomerulopathy presents as an acute rejection episode (see p. 636); usually there is nothing particularly distinctive about the signs and symptoms.

Light microscopy

In more than 50% of glomeruli the capillaries are distended and occluded by a combination of swelling of the endothelium and accumulation of mononuclear cells in the lumen (Fig. 17.13).[98,104] The changes usually involve the whole of each affected glomerulus, but they may be segmental. The number of mesangial cells is slightly increased and the mesangium is a little expanded. A few segments of the capillary basement membrane show double contours. Sometimes fine webs of

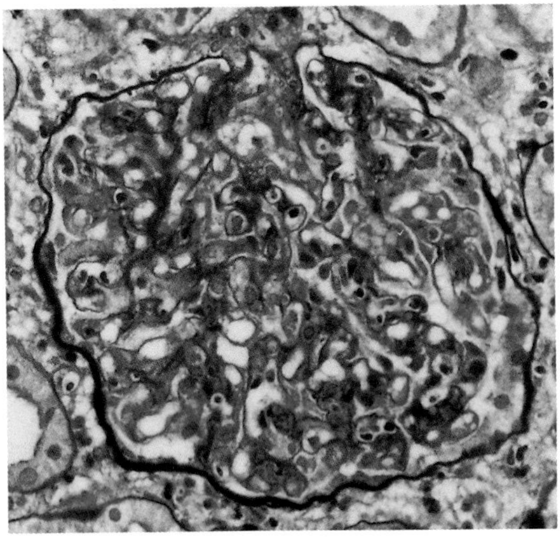

PAS-positive material extend across the capillary lumen.

Most patients have an accompanying tubulo-interstitial rejection of at least moderate intensity; acute vascular rejection is present in about 18% of cases.

Electron microscopy

The enlarged endothelial cells contain increased numbers of ribosomes and prominent nucleoli;

Fig. 17.13 Acute transplant glomerulopathy. The capillaries in the glomerulus are distended and occluded by a combination of swelling of the endothelium and accumulation of mononuclear cells in the lumen. See also Figure 17.14.
Periodic acid-Schiff × 280

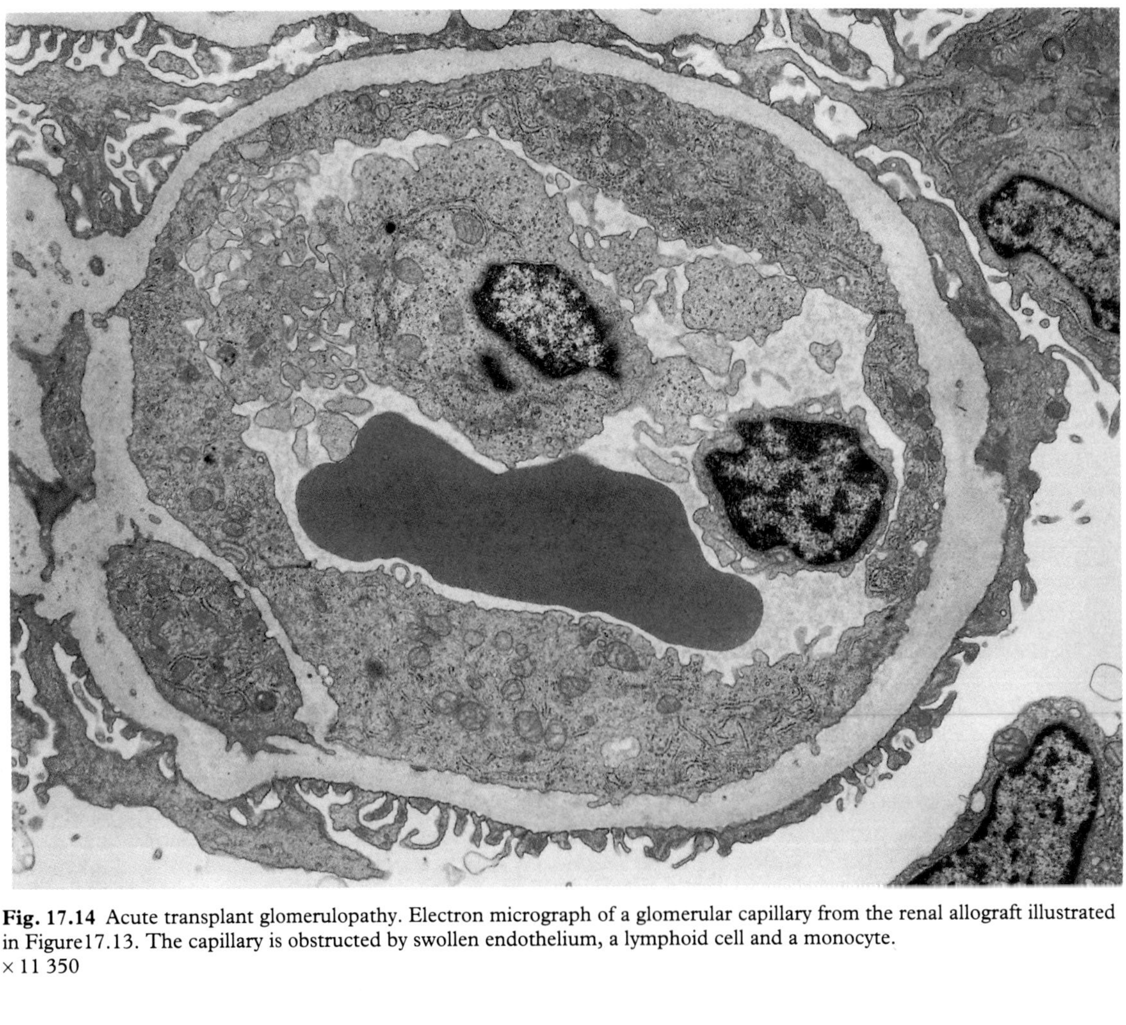

Fig. 17.14 Acute transplant glomerulopathy. Electron micrograph of a glomerular capillary from the renal allograft illustrated in Figure17.13. The capillary is obstructed by swollen endothelium, a lymphoid cell and a monocyte.
× 11 350

the cytoplasm covering the capillary walls is thick and lacks fenestrations. The mononuclear cells in the capillary lumens are lymphocytes and monocytes (Figs 17.14,17.15). There are no electron-dense deposits.[98,104]

Immunofluorescence/immunoperoxidase microscopy

In about 50% of the cases there is focal and segmental staining of glomerular capillary walls for C3 and IgM. There is often C3 in the arteriolar walls; sometimes this is accompanied by IgM.[104]

Immunohistochemistry

Approximately 50% of the glomerular intracapillary cells are T lymphocytes, mostly of the CD8 phenotype.[98] The other cells are monocytes, macrophages and cells of the CD57 phenotype which may be natural killer cells. Vascular and tubular expression of HLA class I antigens, but not class II, tends to be more diffuse and intense than in transplants with acute tubulointerstitial rejection without glomerulopathy.

Differential diagnosis

The diagnosis can only be made unequivocally on a graft biopsy. Acute transplant glomerulopathy is a distinctive lesion and it is only likely to be confused with *diffuse endocapillary proliferative glomerulonephritis*; this may arise either de novo or in response to the horse protein in polyclonal antilympho-

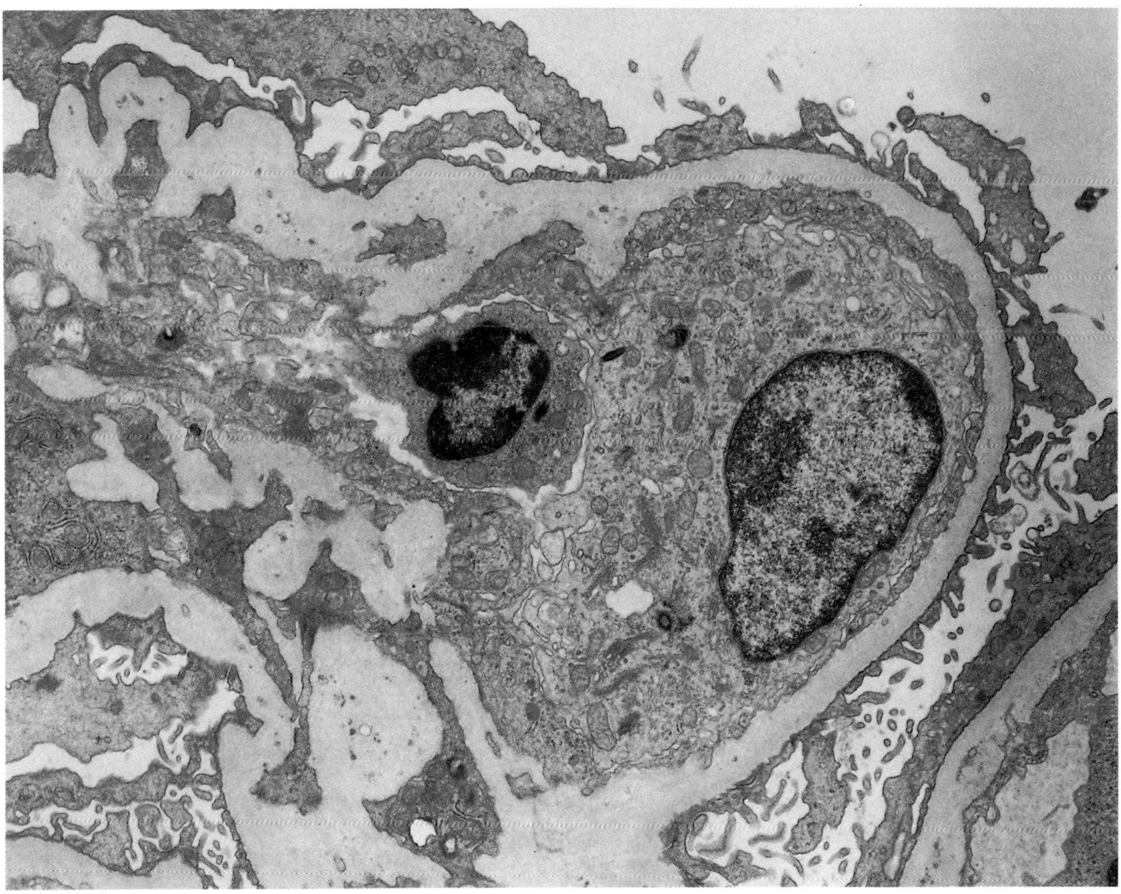

Fig. 17.15 Acute transplant glomerulopathy. Electron micrograph of a glomerular capillary which is obstructed by a large monocyte and a lymphocyte.
× 11 350

cyte globulin (ALG) or antithymocyte globulin (ATG). De novo and ALG-related endocapillary proliferative glomerulonephritis are both rare, particularly during the first few weeks after transplantation. The distinction between acute transplant glomerulopathy and endocapillary proliferative glomerulonephritis is not difficult. In diffuse endocapillary proliferative glomerulonephritis there are subepithelial, and often subendothelial and intramembranous, electron-dense deposits and numerous intracapillary and often intramesangial neutrophil granulocytes. These lesions do not occur in acute transplant glomerulopathy. Diffuse endocapillary glomerulonephritis secondary to antilymphocyte globulin has the added unique feature that glomerular deposits of horse protein can be demonstrated by immunofluorescence in the glomerular capillary walls.[105]

Prognosis

Acute transplant glomerulopathy does not usually respond to treatment with short courses of high doses of steroids given intravenously (high pulse doses) and the prognosis is poor; in one series 67% of the grafts survived for less than 6 months.[106] Sequential biopsies usually show the development of mesangial cell interposition (Fig. 17.16) and progression of the glomerular lesions to chronic transplant glomerulopathy.[104,107] There is also often accompanying evidence of acute vascular rejection.

Pathogenesis

The pathogenesis is obscure. Acute transplant glomerulopathy is frequently associated with

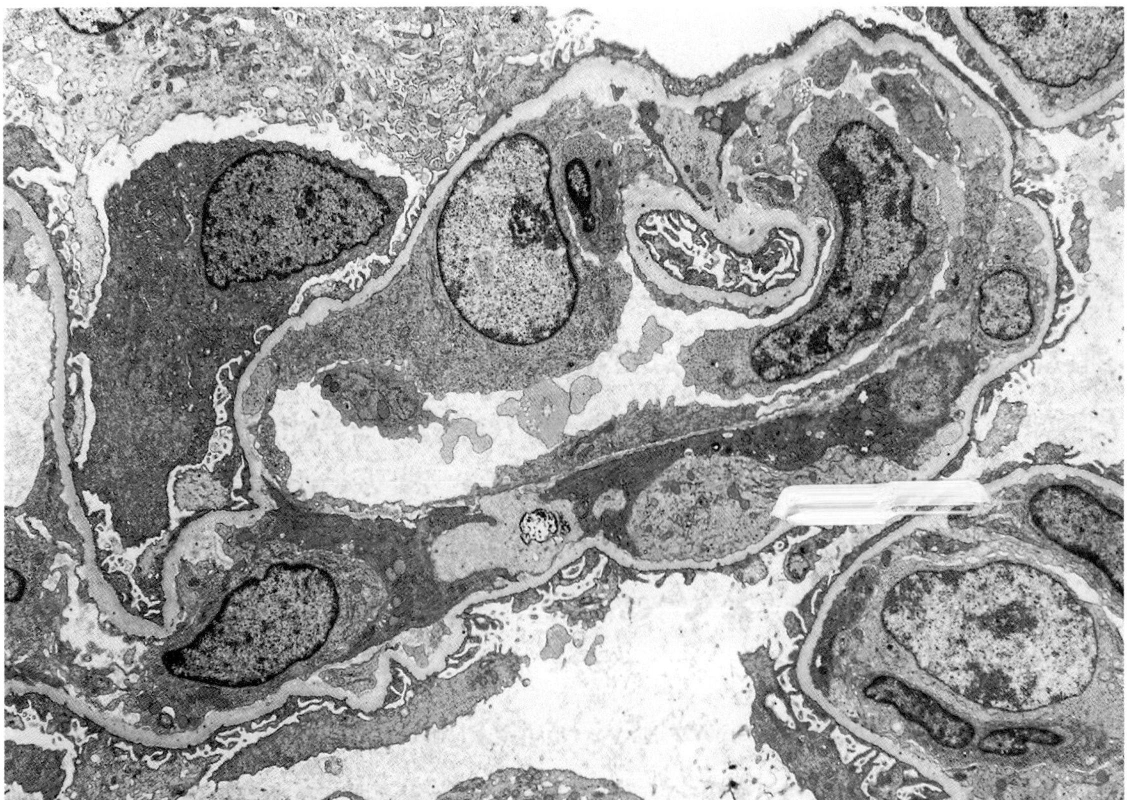

Fig. 17.16 Acute transplant glomerulopathy. Electron micrograph of part of a glomerulus showing development of mesangial cell interposition.
× 8000

cytomegalovirus infection, but the incidence of infection is no higher than in patients with acute rejection but no glomerular lesions,[107] and there is no evidence that the virus is directly responsible for the glomerulopathy. A possibility that has not been entirely excluded is that the cytomegalovirus infection may sometimes indirectly promote the glomerular injury by increasing the density of HLA antigens on the surface of the glomerular capillary endothelium through mediators such as the interferons.[98] Some of the patients have been presensitized to the donor's HLA-DR antigens and have had a positive B lymphocyte cross-match. In these cases the glomerular cells, which express HLA-DR antigens particularly densely, may be special targets for the recipient's alloreactive T lymphocytes. Reaction between lymphocytes and endothelium would bring about the release of lymphokines, inducing an influx of monocytes into the glomerular capillaries.[98]

CHRONIC REJECTION

Chronic rejection may occur as a sequel to one or more episodes of acute rejection that are only partially responsive to high-dose steroid treatment, or it may appear insidiously without any obvious preceding acute rejection. The term chronic refers to the relatively slow deterioration in renal function that commonly occurs.

Kidneys undergoing chronic rejection show obliterative arterial intimal thickening (chronic vascular rejection) or thickening of the glomerular capillary walls (chronic transplant glomerulopathy), or both. Very rarely the predominant change is tubular atrophy with interstitial fibrosis (chronic tubulointerstitial rejection).

Chronic vascular rejection (chronic allograft arteriopathy; transplant atherosclerosis)

Clinical features

The first indication of chronic vascular rejection is usually a gradual deterioration in renal function which generally commences some months or years after transplantation; occasionally it occurs much earlier. The renal dysfunction is almost always accompanied by a slow rise in blood pressure; sometimes hypertension is the first indication of chronic vascular rejection. Commonly there is a history of two or more clinical episodes of acute rejection during the first 2 months after transplantation.

Laboratory findings

Fibrin degradation products usually reappear in the urine. Circulating antibodies against renal endothelial antigens are present in approximately 50% of the patients; donor-specific lymphocytotoxic antibodies can sometimes be demonstrated. Lymphocytes and tubular cells are rare in the urine; IL-2 levels in urine and plasma are often within the normal range.

Gross appearance of graft

The graft is often normal in size or enlarged; compensatory hypertrophy ensures that even after considerable ischaemic damage the kidney will weigh 150–200 g. The subcapsular surface is usually pale and smooth and often, after bisection, a variable number of the arcuate arteries are seen to have thickened walls and narrowed lumens. The larger arteries, including the main renal artery, also may appear narrowed.[108]

Light microscopy

Blood vessels Arterial narrowing is commonest in the interlobular and arcuate arteries, but vessels of any calibre may be involved. Sometimes the narrowing starts at the anastomosis.[108] The intima is thickened, usually concentrically, by an accumulation of elongated cells and a few mononuclears lying in a matrix that takes up little stain in haematoxylin and eosin preparations, but may stain positively for acid mucopolysaccharide (Fig. 17.17). Variable numbers of cells with foamy cytoplasm that contains fat are also present. As the lesion ages collagen is laid down in the thickened intima. The internal elastic lamina is often ruptured; rarely it is reduplicated. The media may be atrophic. The endothelium is usually intact.

Sometimes there is prominent hyalinization of the afferent and efferent arterioles. This change

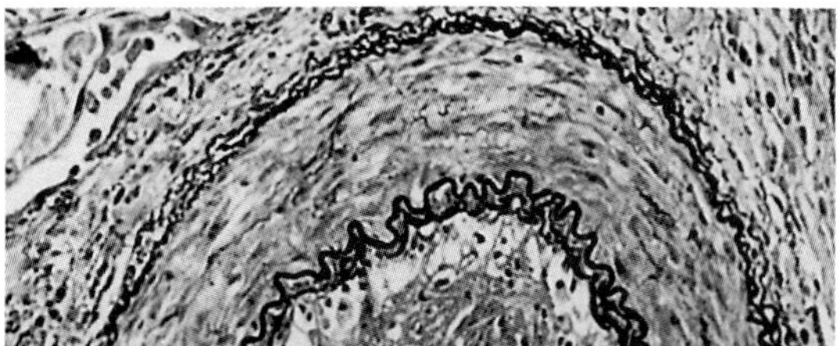

Fig. 17.17 Chronic vascular rejection. An arcuate artery is narrowed by intimal thickening. There is rupture of the internal elastic lamina.
Hart-Sheridan elastic fibre stain; neutral red × 45

is most common when there is also chronic transplant glomerulopathy.[109]

The arterial narrowing is usually accompanied by ischaemic atrophy of tubules and interstitial fibrosis, most marked in the superficial part of the cortex. There may be some interstitial oedema in the early stages, and there is almost always some patchy infiltration of the interstitium by mononuclear cells; this is usually particularly marked adjacent to arteries. Nephrectomy specimens may contain a dense diffuse mononuclear cell infiltrate as in acute tubulointerstitial rejection because immunosuppressive therapy is frequently stopped before the graft is removed.

As the disease progresses variable numbers of glomeruli develop ischaemic wrinkling and collapse of capillary walls, and focal segmental glomerulosclerosis appears and gradually becomes more widespread. The juxtaglomerular apparatus is frequently hyperplastic.[109]

Chronic vascular rejection often affects the periadventitial arteries in the ureter.[60]

Electron microscopy

The thickened intima is composed of myointimal and smooth muscle cells lying in an amorphous electron-lucent ground substance that contains deposits of finely granular, electron-dense material. Fine collagen fibrils are also present and their number increases with time.[109] Fat is normally confined to the cytoplasm of the myointimal cells.

Immunofluorescence/immunoperoxidase microscopy

The thickened intima frequently contains IgM, complement and fibrinogen; IgG is found less frequently.[110]

Immunohistochemistry

Phenotypic analysis reveals that the thickened intima contains actin-positive proliferating smooth muscle cells, activated T lymphocytes and macrophages. A few S100-protein-positive dendritic cells of host origin are also present, particularly during the period when the intima is rapidly thickening.[111,112]

Differential diagnosis

The characteristic obliterative arterial changes are not pathognomonic. Four conditions should be considered in the differential diagnosis: hypertension, atherosclerosis (arteriosclerosis), recurrent haemolytic uraemic syndrome and recurrent systemic sclerosis. Cyclosporin nephrotoxicity is not associated with changes in vessels larger than arterioles.[78]

Hypertension The intimal thickening of interlobular arteries (endarteritis fibrosa or productive endarteritis; see p. 312) that occurs in *severe hypertension* can, in biopsies, be indistinguishable histologically from chronic vascular rejection. If the whole kidney can be examined the distinction can usually be made because in chronic vascular rejection the intimal thickening extends throughout the renal arterial tree up to the anastomosis with the recipient's internal iliac artery; in severe hypertension the arcuate and larger arteries are usually normal.

In *benign phase hypertension* the intimal thickening of interlobular arteries is characterized by multiple concentric layers of elastic tissue (*elastosis*; see p. 307) and the media is usually normal. In contrast, the thickened intima in chronic vascular rejection lacks the multiple layers of elastic and the media is usually thinner than normal.

Atherosclerosis (arteriosclerosis) The thickening of the intima of the interlobular arteries that occurs in atherosclerosis is fibroelastic and, even in the absence of hypertension, the amount of elastic tissue is much greater than is ever seen in chronic vascular rejection. The fibrous intimal thickening that occurs in the arcuate and larger arteries can be histologically indistinguishable from chronic vascular rejection; it is, however, not characterized by ruptures in the internal elastic lamina, which commonly occur in chronic vascular rejection.

Recurrent haemolytic uraemic syndrome Haemolytic uraemic syndrome frequently recurs in grafts (see p. 669). Histologically the lesions can be very like those of chronic vascular rejection. If the patient's original disease was haemolytic uraemic syndrome then evidence of recurrence must be sought clinically and from laboratory data before any arterial lesions in the graft are attributed to chronic rejection.

Recurrent systemic sclerosis Systemic sclerosis possibly recurs in grafts (see p. 671). It cannot be differentiated histologically from chronic vascular rejection. If the patient's original disease was systemic sclerosis then the clinical and laboratory findings should be reviewed for evidence of recurrence.

Prognosis

Chronic vascular rejection is the principal cause of the approximately 8% loss of kidneys that occurs per year after the first year following transplantation; it remains the major limitation to the long-term success rate of renal transplantation.[113] There is generally no sustained response to high-dose steroids, anti-T-lymphocyte antibodies or plasma exchange. Even when there is evidence that the vascular lesions are no longer progressing, renal function may go on declining because of superimposed focal segmental glomerulosclerosis (see p. 205).

It has been claimed that the relentless fall in renal function, independent of immune mechanisms, can be slowed by reducing the patient's dietary protein, which decreases glomerular hyperfiltration (see p. 28).

At present the only known reliable way to lower the toll of chronic vascular rejection is by prevention: tissue matching reduces the rate of graft loss to about 3% per year.[113]

Pathogenesis

There is no direct evidence that chronic vascular rejection is initiated by immune mechanisms. It has been suggested that the intimal endothelial damage may be caused by cold storage; the injury may be potentiated by factors like leukotrienes, platelet-activating factor, thromboxane A_2 and free radicals that are released (during reperfusion of the organ) from leucocytes and platelets adhering to the vessel wall.[114] Against this hypothesis is the fact that renal autografts, which are often stored in the cold for long periods, do not develop arterial intimal thickening. Favouring an initial immune insult is the fact that the rate of long-term graft loss from this lesion in recipients who are well matched by tissue biopsy is less than in poorly matched recipients, and the fact that the number of early acute rejection episodes is a risk factor in relation to chronic vascular rejection.

Even if the likelihood of an initiating immune mechanism is accepted the pathogenesis is unclear. One hypothesis is that chronic vascular rejection is the end stage of unimpeded acute vascular rejection. Serial biopsies of kidneys undergoing rejection have shown that the morphological changes of chronic vascular rejection seem to arise as a result of continued or intermittent formation of platelet and fibrin aggregates on the vessel wall.

The mural deposits become covered by endothelium and are incorporated into the interstitium. The platelets break down, smooth muscle enters the thickened intima, and collagen fibres are deposited.[96] The hyperlipidaemic state of the recipient may in some cases contribute to the number of foam cells.

Repeated endothelial injury may take place during episodes of rejection by cytotoxic T cells, complement and antibody. The injury will initiate platelet adhesion with release of growth factors, such as platelet-derived growth factor; these factors induce smooth muscle proliferation and migration into the interstitium.

The resemblance of the arterial lesions of chronic vascular rejection to atheroma is to be expected because, although the initial insult in the two conditions is different, the subsequent changes in the vessel wall are probably very similar.[115]

Chronic transplant glomerulopathy

Clinical features

Chronic transplant glomerulopathy occurs in approximately 4% of renal allografts.[107,116,117] It is associated with proteinuria of more than 1 g/day which is persistent and progressive; some patients develop a nephrotic syndrome.[118] The onset may be at any time but it is generally a few months after transplantation. There are no characteristic laboratory findings.

Gross appearance of graft

The graft is usually pale and normal in size or enlarged. The subcapsular surface is smooth.

Light microscopy

The walls of the glomerular capillaries are thickened and the mesangium is expanded (Fig. 17.18).[107,116,117,119,120] These changes rarely affect all the glomeruli; they are focal rather than diffuse, and some segments of the glomeruli are involved more than others. The capillary wall thickening is caused by a combination of widening of the subendothelial zone and extensive mesangial cell interposition which gives a double

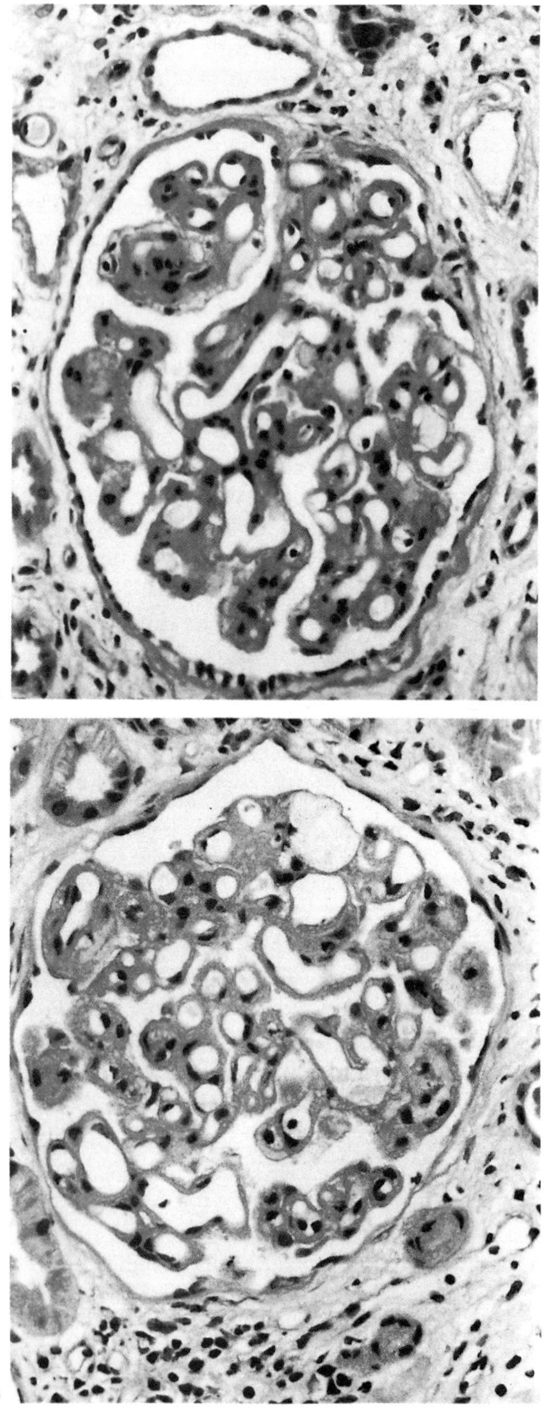

Fig. 17.18 a, b Chronic transplant glomerulopathy. The glomerular capillary walls are segmentally and variably thickened; some have a double contour. The amount of mesangial matrix is segmentally increased. Tuft cellularity is slightly increased in a few segments.
(**a**), (**b**) Periodic acid-Schiff × 300

contour pattern. There is usually some slight focal and segmental increase in the amount of mesangial matrix and in the number of mesangial cells. The mesangial cells are often enlarged. Rarely there are occasional crescents.

The afferent and efferent arterioles sometimes contain large hyaline deposits in their walls. Hyaline deposits are also occasionally seen in the basement membranes of the peritubular capillaries.

Electron microscopy

The subendothelial zone of the glomerular capillary basement membranes is markedly widened by material which resembles the plasma precipitate in the capillary lumen. Within this electron-lucent substance there are collections of finely granular amorphous electron-dense material, fine filaments and microfibrils (Figs 17.19,17.20).[107,117,119–121] Strands of new basement membrane are often present immediately beneath the endothelium (Fig. 17.21). Circumferential mesangial cell interposition is common (Figs 17.20,17.21). Small foci of mesangiolysis have been described in some grafts.[121] Obliteration of epithelial foot processes and loss of endothelial fenestrations are also often present. Occasionally there are scanty subendothelial, subepithelial or mesangial dense deposits.[96]

Immunofluorescence/immunoperoxidase microscopy

Global or segmental finely granular deposits of IgM, sometimes accompanied by Clq and C3, are often found in the affected glomeruli. Occasionally IgG, with or without complement, is deposited in a linear pattern in the glomerular capillary walls.[110,116,117]

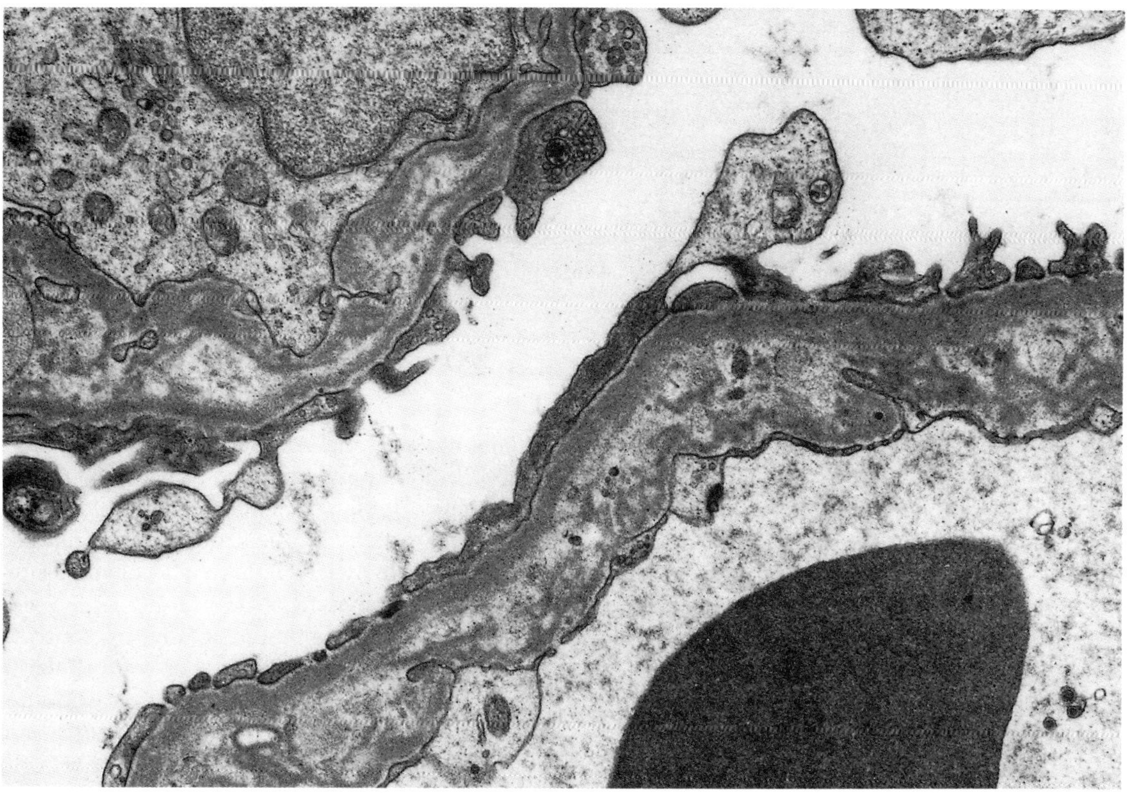

Fig. 17.19 Chronic transplant glomerulopathy. Electron micrograph of parts of two glomerular capillary loops, showing widening of the subendothelial zone.
× 9200

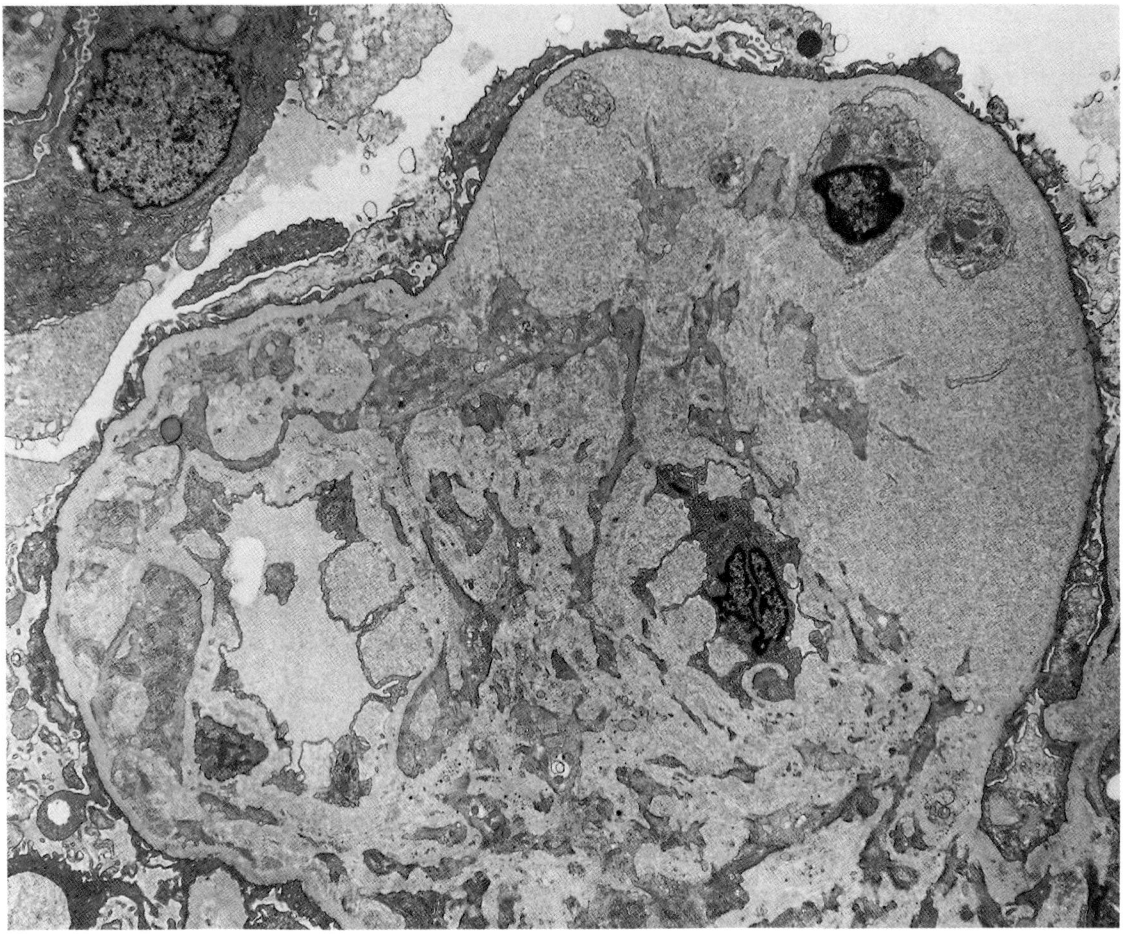

Fig. 17.20 Chronic transplant glomerulopathy. Electron micrograph of part of a glomerulus. The subendothelial zone of the capillary on the right is greatly widened by material which resembles precipitated plasma. On the left a capillary wall is thickened by mesangial cell interposition.
× 8000

Differential diagnosis

The lesions of chronic transplant glomerulopathy are distinctive but not pathognomonic. Four conditions should be considered in the differential diagnosis: de novo or recurrent mesangiocapillary glomerulonephritis type I, recurrent haemolytic uraemic syndrome, pre-eclamptic toxaemia and ischaemic glomerular injury.

De novo or recurrent mesangiocapillary glomerulonephritis type I The distinction between chronic transplant glomerulopathy and mesangiocapillary glomerulonephritis type I is usually not difficult. Although both show double contouring of the glomerular capillary basement membranes, mesangiocapillary glomerulonephritis type I is usually a diffuse disease with marked glomerular tuft hypercellularity and obvious subendothelial and mesangial electron-dense deposits. Chronic transplant glomerulopathy, by contrast, is focal and segmental, glomerular tuft cellularity is only slightly increased, and typical subendothelial and mesangial electron-dense deposits are either absent or present in only tiny numbers. In about 10% of cases of chronic transplant glomerulopathy the degree of tuft cellularity is confusingly high, but even in these grafts the disease remains

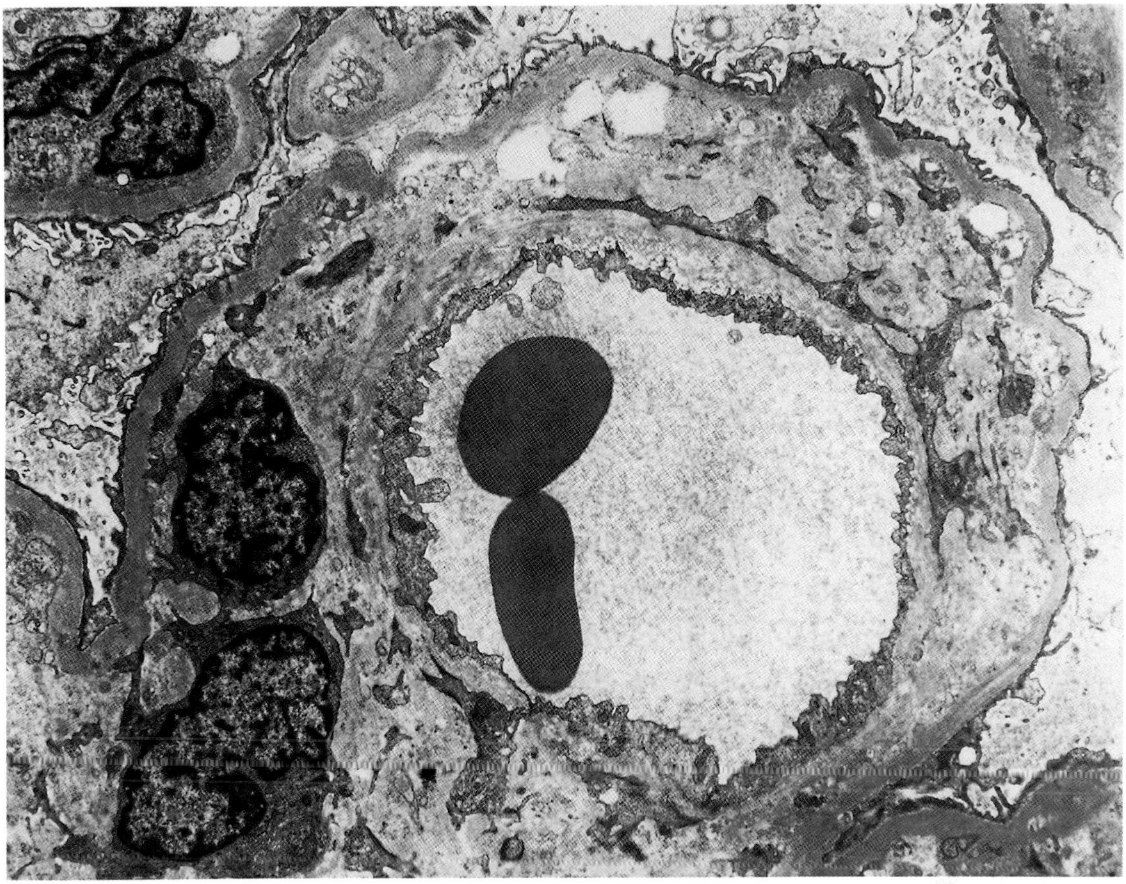

Fig. 17.21 Chronic transplant glomerulopathy. Electron micrograph of a glomerular capillary. The capillary wall is greatly thickened by mesangial cell interposition. A new layer of basement membrane has formed beneath the endothelium. × 8000

essentially patchy, and subendothelial electron-dense deposits are very scarce or absent.[116,122]

Recurrent haemolytic uraemic syndrome The morphological lesions in haemolytic uraemic syndrome may be indistinguishable from those in chronic transplant glomerulopathy. If the patient's original disease was haemolytic uraemic syndrome, evidence of recurrence must be sought clinically and from laboratory data.

Pre-eclamptic toxaemia This diagnosis must be thought about in renal transplant patients who are pregnant. The morphological lesions may be remarkably like those in chronic transplant glomerulopathy.[107]

Ischaemic glomerular injury It is not difficult to differentiate chronic transplant glomerulopathy from ischaemic glomerular injury due to chronic vascular rejection. By light microscopy, in ischaemia the glomeruli show wrinkling and thickening of capillary basement membranes and accumulation of collagen on the inner aspect of Bowman's capsule; ultrastructurally, there is no expansion of the subendothelial layer of the capillary wall by electron-lucent plasma-like material, and mesangial cell interposition is not found (see p. 306).

Prognosis

The proteinuria usually becomes gradually more severe and a nephrotic syndrome often develops.

Insidious loss of renal function may also occur. In one group of 30 reported cases, 23 (77%) of the grafts failed at periods up to 10 years 8 months after transplantation.[107] The decline in renal function is sometimes associated with the development of a superimposed focal and segmental glomerulosclerosis.

Pathogenesis

It seems most probable that chronic transplant glomerulopathy arises from the host's immune response to the graft because glomerulopathy is found more frequently in patients mismatched for HLA.[119] In some instances it has been shown by sequential biopsies to have been preceded by acute transplant glomerulopathy (see p. 649).[107,116]

Repeated endothelial damage, produced either by cytotoxic antibodies to HLA or endothelial antigens, or by mononuclear cells and the cytokines they produce and induce, may be followed by penetration by plasma constituents into the subendothelial space. Mesangial cell interposition will be provoked by the plasma and the cytokines.

Chronic tubulointerstitial rejection

Tubular atrophy, interstitial fibrosis and focal, sparse infiltration of the interstitium by mononuclear cells are common in chronic vascular rejection and chronic transplant glomerulopathy. Occasionally the tubulointerstitial changes are particularly severe, out of proportion to the degree of vascular or glomerular damage, and accompanied by circulating anti-tubular-basement-membrane antibodies; these severe cases are sometimes referred to as chronic tubulointerstitial rejection. In some of these patients anti-tubular-basement-membrane antibodies have been eluted from the renal allograft.[123,124]

However, although evidence from animal experiments has shown that anti-tubular-basement-membrane antibodies can produce tubulointerstitial nephritis with deposits of immunoglobulin and complement along the tubular basement membrane, there is little to indicate that anti-tubular-basement-membrane antibodies are responsible for chronic tubulointerstitial rejection in patients. Circulating IgG antibodies of various subclasses directed against the tubular basement membranes of the graft develop in about 3% of renal transplant recipients.[125] Neither tubular nor interstitial injury has been shown to be significantly associated with these antibodies and graft survival is no different in patients with antibodies than in those without.[125]

Differential diagnosis

Chronic tubulointerstitial rejection has no distinctive features. In the differential diagnosis *cyclosporin toxicity* must be considered. Band-like zones of fibrosis (striped fibrosis) occur with cyclosporin[78] but the pattern of scarring is insufficiently unique to enable a distinction to be made from chronic rejection in an individual biopsy. Tubulointerstitial nephritis induced by *analgesics* (see p. 459) and *aminoglycosides* (see p. 519) should be excluded. *Renal artery stenosis*, due to causes other than chronic rejection (see p. 298), and *reflux nephropathy* (see p. 440) may produce very similar tubulointerstitial changes, as may the rare occurrence of late *ureteric obstruction* due to stricture, stone, ball of fungus or other causes. Appropriate investigations should enable these simulants to be identified.

RUPTURE OF THE TRANSPLANTED KIDNEY

Two to six per cent of renal allografts rupture. Rupture occurs predominantly in grafts from cadavers, as an accompaniment of acute rejection during the first 2 weeks after transplantation.[126]

The patient suffers sudden pain over the graft, local swelling is seen, the blood pressure falls, the pulse rate rises, and secretion of urine stops. The graft is swollen and in cases treated with azathioprine usually shows the other changes of acute rejection (see p. 637). Since the introduction of cyclosporin treatment rupture has been particularly associated with renal vein thrombosis,[127] probably because of the thrombotic tendency and reduced renal blood flow caused by cyclosporin.

The tear is usually along the convexity and is ragged and confined to the cortex.[126] Occasionally there are second tears. Microscopically, most cases treated with azathioprine show the changes of acute tubulointerstitial rejection with marked interstitial oedema. Occasionally there is no evidence of rejection.[126] Cases treated with cyclosporin and having renal vein thrombosis only show interstitial oedema and haemorrhage.[127]

The cause of rupture of the transplant is not known. It is probably a direct complication of the acute swelling brought about by the interstitial oedema, the cortex of the acutely swollen organ tearing spontaneously along the line of greatest tension.

CHANGES INDUCED BY IMMUNOSUPPRESSIVE TREATMENT

CYCLOSPORIN NEPHROTOXICITY

Treatment with cyclosporin increases the survival of renal allografts but its use is complicated by acute and chronic nephrotoxicity. *Acute/subacute toxicity* is not always associated with any renal lesions discernible by light microscopy. Sometimes, however, isometric vacuolation of the cells of the straight part of the proximal tubule (Fig. 13.11)[75] or arteriolar hyalinization (Figs. 13.12,13.13), or both, are present (see p. 521).[78] The expression of HLA class II antigens is inhibited.[77] The tubular damage is not associated with any appreciable loss of function; the arteriolar damage is preceded by a period of vasoconstriction and is associated with acute renal insufficiency which initially is reversible.[75] It is also claimed that cyclosporin nephrotoxicity causes glomerular capillary thrombosis but this is controversial.[99,100]

The *chronic cyclosporin-induced lesion* is interstitial fibrosis, which often shows a striped form. It is associated with tubular atrophy, glomerular sclerosis and progressive impairment of renal function.[76]

Acute/subacute cyclosporin nephrotoxicity is related to trough cyclosporin blood levels; chronic nephrotoxicity to cumulative cyclosporin dose. Patients who experience acute cyclosporin nephrotoxicity do not appear to have a great risk of developing chronic nephrotoxicity.

Because cyclosporin nephrotoxicity causes renal allograft dysfunction it has to be continually thought about when diagnosing rejection in a transplant biopsy. The practical difficulty is that cyclosporin nephrotoxicity may produce no discernible morphological lesions and even when there are lesions they are non-specific. The diagnosis of cyclosporin nephrotoxicity in an allograft biopsy is, therefore, almost always one of exclusion.[78]

GLOMERULONEPHRITIS CAUSED BY ANTILYMPHOCYTE OR ANTITHYMOCYTE GLOBULIN

Antilymphocyte globulin (ALG) and antithymocyte globulin (ATG) are gamma globulin preparations raised in various animal species by immunization with human splenic or thymic lymphocytes. Occasionally their use is complicated by *serum sickness* and the production of a *diffuse endocapillary proliferative glomerulonephritis* in the graft. Although the clinical presentation is usually characteristic, there have been occasions when the serum sickness reaction has been misinterpreted as acute rejection.[105] On biopsy the differentiation from rejection is straightforward (see p. 651).

INFECTIONS

Immunosuppressive treatment increases the likelihood and danger of general infection by bacteria, viruses, fungi, protozoa and helminths. Sometimes the transplant is involved in the course of such infections, with development of extensive or localized lesions.

Viral inclusions are occasionally found in transplants. Cytomegalovirus is most frequently responsible for such infections; the changes characteristic of its presence are seen particularly in the epithelial cells of the tubules and much less frequently in the endothelial cells of the glomeruli.

Swelling and proliferation of the epithelial cells of the lining of the ureter of the transplant may result from infection by a papovavirus (BK virus) and lead to obstruction. Indeed, this is how the virus was first identified in a patient, B- K-, at St Mary's Hospital, London.[128]

Fungal infections may cause papillary necrosis. In some cases a ball colony of a fungus may form in the pelvis of the transplant and obstruct it. Both these conditions are most frequently caused by species of candida.

HYPERTENSION

Approximately half the patients who have received a renal graft develop persistent hypertension. Currently used maintenance doses of cyclosporin are responsible for some of this hypertension. The incidence is difficult to determine because of the problems of differentiating cyclosporin from the other causes of post-transplant hypertension such as chronic vascular rejection, stenosis of the renal artery of the graft, the presence of the patient's own diseased kidneys, recurrent glomerulonephritis and steroid excess. Cyclosporin-induced hypertension differs from most of the other forms of post-transplantation hypertension in being more responsive to sodium restriction and being associated with vasoconstriction that is not mediated by the renin-angiotensin system.[129]

Large doses of prednisolone in the first 6 months after transplantation may contribute to the development of early hypertension; it is unlikely that the small maintenance dose is responsible for late persistent hypertension.

In the graft the lesions of benign hypertensive nephrosclerosis (see p. 306) are often present, frequently superimposed on those of chronic rejection.

LIPID ABNORMALITIES

Hyperlipidaemia is one important consequence of chronic renal failure (see p. 35); it continues to affect approximately 60% of patients after renal transplantation.[130] Corticosteroid administration is probably a major factor in causing persistence of the hyperlipidaemia. Hypercholesterolaemia is the dominant lipid abnormality, although the triglyceride levels, particularly in cyclosporin-treated patients, are also raised. There is some evidence that cyclosporin also produces an elevation in the low density (LDL) cholesterol fraction.[131]

Hypertension and hyperlipidaemia are probably the most important conditions contributing to the high cardiovascular morbidity and mortality that occur after renal transplantation. Approximately a third of all deaths in patients with renal grafts are from cardiovascular causes.[132]

Hyperlipidaemia is probably responsible for the excessive amounts of fat that are found in the thickened intima of the arteries in the graft in cases of chronic vascular rejection (see p. 306).

MALIGNANT NEOPLASIA

Immunosuppressive treatment is accompanied by an increased incidence of cancer.[133] The most common malignancies encountered in allograft recipients, particularly in countries where there is a lot of sunshine, are those of the skin. The second most common are neoplasms of B lymphocytes. Carcinoma of the cervix and Kaposi's sarcoma are also particularly increased in frequency. Many of these cancers are associated with viral infections: human papillomavirus in squamous neoplasms of the skin and cervix[134] and Epstein–Barr virus in lymphomas.[135]

Most of the tumours originate in the tissues of the host and the transplant is only rarely involved. The exception is the lymphomas which frequently invade the graft. In two reported series of lymphomas in patients with renal transplants, 17%[82] and 41%[136] of the tumours first presented in the graft.

When the graft is affected the infiltrating B-cell lymphoma must be distinguished in a biopsy from the predominantly T lymphocyte and macrophage infiltrate of acute tubulointerstitial rejection (see p. 637). T-cell lymphomas are extremely rare and only three have been reported that involved the graft.[137] The differential diagnosis in a biopsy between a T-cell lymphoma infiltrating a renal transplant and acute tubulointerstitial rejection is considered on page 642.

Occasionally a tumour arising in the transplant can be shown to have originated from donor cells. Most such tumours have been present at the time of transplantation, but overlooked: they grow quickly in the recipient and metastases occur at an early stage (see p. 626).

TRANSMISSION OF DISEASE FROM HOST TO GRAFT

TRANSMISSION OF PRIMARY GLOMERULONEPHRITIS (RECURRENT GLOMERULONEPHRITIS)

Published figures for the incidence of transmission of glomerulonephritis from the host to the graft (recurrence) vary considerably. One of the reasons for this is that a diagnosis of recurrent disease requires precise histological confirmation of the patient's original glomerulonephritis and this is commonly lacking. Many patients first come to the clinic in advanced renal failure, and renal biopsy may not be performed. If tissue is obtained, the glomerular changes may be at too late a stage to allow them to be classified. Another reason is that there must be certainty that the donor kidney was free of glomerulonephritis at the time of transplantation: this is frequently not possible because few grafts are biopsied before completion of the vascular anastomoses. Thirdly, an accurate and detailed assessment of the glomerular lesions and the cause of graft failure in a transplant thought to be showing recurrence of disease are essential. It is particularly important to differentiate allograft glomerulopathy from recurrence of glomerulonephritis. To make this assessment, data from immunofluorescence, immunoperoxidase and ultrastructural studies need to be available: often they are not.[138] A fourth reason is that only certain forms of glomerulonephritis recur frequently and the occurrence of these in different series will be very different depending upon the age and the country of residence of the population being studied.

In one series in which most of these conditions were met, glomerulonephritis recurred in 31% of patients whose original disease was glomerulonephritis.[139] Even this figure may be an underestimate of the true incidence because recurrent glomerulonephritis is often clinically silent for long periods and in most transplant units the policy is to biopsy the graft only when there is proteinuria, haematuria or graft dysfunction. In one paediatric transplant centre where all grafts were in addition routinely biopsied 18 months after transplantation, even if the patients were symptomless and had normal renal function, recurrent glomerulonephritis was detected in 49% of renal allografts.[116]

Several categories of recurrent glomerulonephritis, even when they produce clinical disease, progress slowly and only occasionally cause renal failure and loss of the graft in the first 5 years after transplantation. There are a few notable exceptions to this generalization, but even so the risk of recurrence of glomerulonephritis is rarely a contraindication to transplantation.

All types of glomerulonephritis have been reported to recur after transplantation, but some are much more likely to do so than others.[138] The approximate transmission rates for the various categories of glomerulonephritis are: dense deposit disease 90%; IgA nephropathy 50%; membranoproliferative glomerulonephritis type I 40%; focal segmental glomerulosclerosis 30%; and membranous glomerulonephritis 10%. Transmission rates in the other forms of glomerulonephritis are less than 5%. Recurrence is most serious in focal segmental glomerulosclerosis because clinical manifestations are usually immediate and major, and over half the affected grafts fail in the first 5 years after transplantation.

Focal segmental glomerulosclerosis

Focal segmental glomerulosclerosis (FSGS) is transmitted in 25–33% of cases to kidneys that are transplanted into patients who have FSGS that has produced a steroid-resistant nephrotic syndrome and end-stage renal failure.[139] The three most important risk factors for recurrence are age, mesangial cellularity and time taken to progress to renal failure. Approximately 50% of grafts placed in children under 15 years of age develop recurrent disease, while recurrence is rare over the age of 30 years. Recurrence occurs in about 50% of patients who have focal or diffuse mesangial hypercellularity in the original biopsy of their own diseased kidneys, but in only about 10% of those with normal glomerular cellularity at the time of diagnosis. Patients whose original disease progressed to renal failure in less than 3 years have a higher incidence of recurrent disease than do patients with a more slowly evolving disease.[140,141] Once transmission of disease has occurred in the first graft, there is an increased chance of recurrence in the second and third grafts.[142]

Clinical features

In the majority of patients massive persistent proteinuria commences immediately after transplantation; in the others heavy proteinuria occurs within 2 months after transplantation. The protein loss is usually associated with the nephrotic syndrome.[139] Microscopic haematuria is common and hypertension frequent.

Changes in the renal allograft

At first the only change is diffuse obliteration of the foot processes of the glomerular epithelial cells.[142] At about 1 month after recurrence focal and segmental epithelial cell swelling and degeneration appear; the adjacent glomerular capillaries partially collapse and may become occluded by leucocytes or swollen endothelial cells.[142] Over the next few weeks or months the segmental lesions gradually alter so that they become indistinguishable from the lesions seen in FSGS when it affects untransplanted kidneys (see p. 205). Mesangial cell proliferation often also occurs.[141,143,144]

Differential diagnosis

The main problem is to exclude *de novo focal segmental glomerulosclerosis* which occurs in approximately 10% of grafts, usually in association with ischaemia secondary to chronic rejection, and occasionally in association with reflux nephropathy. This exclusion often cannot be done because the individual glomerular lesions in de novo and recurrent focal and segmental glomerulosclerosis are indistinguishable morphologically, and the lesions of chronic rejection are not confined to grafts with de novo disease. It is therefore only possible to be certain of the diagnosis of recurrent disease in transplants in the absence of significant evidence of chronic rejection or reflux nephropathy.

Prognosis

Recurrent FSGS leads to renal dysfunction and loss of the graft in many recipients. Approximately 60% fail within the first 4 years after transplantation[116] and by 10 years about 85% have ceased to function.[140,142] In a few patients the loss of protein in the urine is so great that the graft has to be removed in the first few days or weeks after transplantation.[140] The proteinuria is resistant to high doses of steroids and to cyclophosphamide. Early plasmapheresis, before the FSGS lesions appear, has been reported to have been beneficial in some cases.[144]

Pathogenesis

It would appear that there is some circulating factor in the recipient that immediately enhances glomerular permeability in the graft. No such humoral factor has yet been discovered.

Mesangiocapillary glomerulonephritis type I

Transmission of mesangiocapillary glomerulonephritis type I to one or more grafts has been reported in approximately 40% of patients with this disease.[139,145,146] This may be an underestimate of the frequency because clinically silent microscopic recurrence is only detected in those centres where grafts are routinely biopsied: in one such centre the incidence of recurrence was found to be 70% in patients whose original disease was mesangiocapillary glomerulonephritis type I.[116] Once transmission of disease has occurred, the chances of recurrence are increased in subsequent grafts.

Clinical features

The major clinical manifestation is proteinuria which often becomes sufficient to produce the nephrotic syndrome. There is usually also microscopic haematuria. Later, some patients develop progressive renal dysfunction; this may be accompanied by gross haematuria.[147] The urine changes are first detected at about 1 year 9 months but they may occur as early as 2 months or as late as 7½ years after transplantation.[139] Complement levels are often within the normal range and bear little relationship to the activity of the recurrent disease. Recurrence seems to be more common in allografts from living related donors, but this is not statistically significant.

Microscopy

Sequential biopsies show that the first evidence of recurrence is the appearance of electron-dense deposits in the mesangium. By light microscopy the glomeruli appear mildly hypercellular, and the mesangium is expanded; there are mesangial deposits of C3.[116] Later, subendothelial electron-dense deposits appear in the glomerular capillary walls accompanied by mesangial cell interposition; the mesangial hypercellularity increases and tuft lobularity becomes accentuated. Immunofluorescence usually shows strongly positive staining for C3 and IgG in a granular distribution along the capillary walls and often in the mesangium.[148] Sometimes there is a peripheral lobular type of staining[149] and there may be staining for C3 but not immunoglobulin.[147] The condition in the graft may be complicated by the appearance of abundant crescents.[149]

Differential diagnosis

Five conditions need to be considered in the differential diagnosis; chronic transplant glomerulopathy, acute transplant glomerulopathy, recurrent antiglomerular-basement-membrane-antibody disease (anti-GBM antibody disease) or crescentic glomerulonephritis, de novo mesangiocapillary glomerulonephritis type I and diabetic glomerulosclerosis. The most important of these is chronic transplant glomerulopathy.

Chronic transplant glomerulopathy Usually there is no difficulty in differentiating chronic transplant glomerulopathy from mesangiocapillary glomerulonephritis type I. Although both show double contouring of the glomerular capillary basement membranes and mesangial expansion, chronic transplant glomerulopathy is typically a focal and segmental disease; the number of mesangial cells is only slightly increased and there are no classic subendothelial or mesangial electron-dense deposits. If there are immune deposits they are finely granular and composed of IgM and sometimes C3. Recurrent mesangiocapillary glomerulonephritis type I, by contrast, is typically a diffuse and global disease with marked increase in the number of mesangial cells, and obvious subendothelial and mesangial electron-dense deposits. Immune deposits are invariably present, coarsely granular, and composed of IgG and C3 or of C3 alone. In about 10% of cases of chronic transplant glomerulopathy, mesangial cell hypercellularity is considerably increased, but it remains essentially focal with great variation in the amount of mesangial cell proliferation between glomeruli.[116,123]

For a diagnosis of recurrent mesangiocapillary glomerulonephritis type I, all or most glomeruli should contain obvious subendothelial electron-dense deposits, the predominant immune deposits should be IgG in the capillary walls and C3 in the mesangium, and double contours should be present in several capillary loops in the great majority of glomeruli.

Acute transplant glomerulopathy Although the lesions may be diffuse, this condition is usually easily differentiated from recurrent mesangiocapillary glomerulonephritis type I because the increased tuft cellularity is due to large numbers of monocytes within the glomerular capillary lumens and to swelling and proliferation of endothelial cells. Such endocapillary proliferation is not a feature of recurrent mesangiocapillary glomerulonephritis type I. Occasionally recurrent mesangiocapillary glomerulonephritis type I has an endocapillary component in its acute phase but the cellular increase remains predominantly mesangial. In acute transplant glomerulopathy it is always predominantly endocapillary.

Recurrent anti-GMB antibody disease and crescentic glomerulonephritis Some cases of recurrent mesangiocapillary glomerulonephritis type I develop large numbers of crescents. In these cases it is important to check the patient's original kidneys and the graft lesions for linear staining for IgG on the glomerular capillary walls. If it is present anti-GBM antibodies should be sought in the recipient's blood. If there is granular staining for IgG or C3 the recipient's original kidneys should be reviewed to make sure that the disease underlying the crescents was mesangiocapillary glomerulonephritis type I.

De novo mesangiocapillary glomerulonephritis type I This possibility can be excluded by checking the biopsy material originally obtained from the patient's own kidneys.

Recurrent or de novo diabetic glomerulosclerosis Although on light microscopy diabetic glomerulosclerosis may resemble recurrent mesangiocapillary glomerulonephritis type I, the distinction is easily made on electron microscopy and immunofluorescence: diabetic lesions do not display subendothelial electron-dense deposits, double contouring of the glomerular capillary walls or granular deposits of IgG or C3, all of which are present in recurrent mesangiocapillary glomerulonephritis type I.

Prognosis

Patients who are asymptomatic when diagnosed by routine biopsy as having recurrence, may remain symptomless and with normal urine for long periods, sometimes for more than 8 years.[116] The patients with proteinuria usually become nephrotic and then slowly develop renal impairment. In approximately 40% renal dysfunction occurs more rapidly, leading to loss of the graft about 2½ years after transplantation.

Pathogenesis

Although the frequent recurrence of mesangiocapillary glomerulonephritis type I in transplanted kidneys suggests that humoral factors mediate the disease, the pathogenesis remains obscure.

Dense deposit disease

Dense deposit disease is transmitted to over 90% of kidneys transplanted into patients with the disease.[116,150,151] This high rate of recurrence is only evident if the grafts are routinely biopsied, because approximately one-third of the patients with recurrence lack clinical manifestations. When transmission of disease has occurred, the chances of recurrence in subsequent renal allografts is increased.

Clinical features

Approximately 70% of the patients with recurrent dense deposit disease develop mild to moderate proteinuria and microscopic haematuria. These urinary changes usually commence about 7 months after transplantation, but there is great variation and they may commence as early as 2 months or as late as 7 years after transplantation. In about 40% of the patients the proteinuria becomes progressively greater, the nephrotic syndrome develops and renal function slowly declines.

Microscopy

Ribbon-like bands of very electron-dense material start to replace the lamina densa of the glomerular capillary basement membrane of the graft as early as 3 weeks following transplantation.[116,151] At first the recurrence only affects the hilum of a few glomeruli;[151] in most patients this is followed by slow progressive involvement of the peripheral capillary walls and the capsular and tubular basement membranes. Mesangial nodules are slow to appear. Double contouring of the capillary walls and mesangial cell proliferation only occur in some patients. Crescents and segments of necrosis appear in the glomeruli of grafts that are failing.[116,150]

Differential diagnosis

The collections of electron-dense material are pathognomonic. They do not occur in rejection or any other renal disease. So long as electron microscopy is used it is easy to make the diagnosis of recurrence. The difficult part is to decide, in a case with coexisting rejection changes, the relative importance of the two lesions in bringing about graft loss.

Prognosis

Approximately 40% of grafts with recurrent dense deposit disease eventually progress to end-stage renal failure. This process may take many years; occasionally it occurs within months of transplantation.[150] In about 60% of grafts that fail the recurrent disease is responsible; in the other 40% acute or chronic rejection plays an important, sometimes a dominant, role in destroying the graft.[116] Graft failure occurs more frequently in males, in those whose original disease ran a rapidly progressive course, and in those who develop the nephrotic syndrome following transplantation. The presence or degree of hypocomplementaemia does not correlate with graft loss.[150]

Pathogenesis

The appearance of the very electron-dense material within the basement membranes throughout the transplant would seem to depend upon some factor in the recipient's circulation that persists following transplantation. No evidence has been provided that might lead to the identification of such a factor.

IgA nephropathy

Renal transplantation in IgA nephropathy is often followed by the reappearance of IgA within the glomerular mesangium, but this histological recurrence is only occasionally accompanied by anything more than minimal clinical manifestations. Recurrence, therefore, is particularly likely to go undetected unless the transplant unit has a policy of routine biopsy after treatment or some other indication for biopsy arises. The incidence of recurrence is probably at least 50%. In two centres where routine biopsy is practised, IgA deposits in the graft have been detected in 53%[152] and 75%[116] of kidneys transplanted into patients whose original disease was IgA nephropathy. Recurrence is commoner in kidneys from living related donors; this probably reflects the known HLA linkages of the disease (see p. 158). There is an increased chance of recurrence in second and third grafts after transmission has occurred in a first graft.

Clinical features

Approximately 30% of patients with recurrence remain asymptomatic and have normal urine.[152] The remainder develop minimal proteinuria or microscopic haematuria or both. These clinical manifestations usually remain mild and often intermittent,[152] but about 10% of the patients with symptoms develop progressively heavier proteinuria and haematuria, and then declining renal function.[138,146,153–155]

Microscopy

The first indication of recurrence, which may occur as early as 1 month after transplantation, is the appearance of diffuse and global staining of the glomerular mesangium for IgA and C3, with focal and segmental electron-dense deposits in the paramesangium. The glomeruli appear normal by light microscopy with no increase in the number of mesangial cells.[152] The deposits increase in amount for a few years and then become stable. Occasionally a small amount of focal and segmental mesangial cell proliferation occurs. The few patients who pursue a rapidly progressive course to end-stage renal failure usually develop diffuse global mesangial hypercellularity, endothelial swelling and proliferation, and many circumferential cellular crescents.[5,153,154]

Differential diagnosis

Recurrent IgA nephropathy cannot be distinguished from *IgA nephropathy that is present in the donor kidney* at the time of transplantation (see p. 626). Only a biopsy of the transplant taken just before the vascular anastomoses are completed will make this distinction. Donor IgA nephropathy is a particular problem in countries, such as Japan, where there is a high incidence of IgA nephropathy and transplantation from a live related donor is common.[3–5] Similarly, morphology cannot distinguish between recurrent and *de novo IgA nephropathy*; examination of a biopsy of the patient's own kidneys is necessary to exclude this possibility. There should not be any confusion between recurrent IgA nephropathy and acute or chronic transplant glomerulopathy – IgA deposits do not occur in rejection.

Prognosis

Most cases do not progress to the nephrotic syndrome or renal dysfunction. In the few patients who do develop renal failure the final phase of deterioration may be rapid as the lesions of crescentic glomerulonephritis are superimposed on the IgA nephropathy.[153,154]

Pathogenesis

Why mesangial deposits of IgA recur in some patients and not others, and induce progressive disease in very few grafts, is not known.

Membranous glomerulonephritis

The frequency of recurrence of membranous glomerulonephritis is difficult to assess because most of the reports give no indication of the number of patients with biopsy-proven membranous glomerulonephritis and a renal transplant who were at risk.[138] In the largest series there was one recurrence in 10 graft recipients with known membranous glomerulonephritis.[146]

Clinical features

Patients with recurrent membranous glomerulonephritis develop persistent heavy proteinuria and usually the nephrotic syndrome. In most cases the onset is 1 year or more after transplantation. Renal function remains normal for long periods, but in approximately a third of the patients it gradually declines, leading to loss of the graft.

Microscopy

When first discovered the subepithelial deposits are generally at stage I or stage II (see p. 194), irregular in size and shape, and segmental rather than global. Later they become diffuse and more uniform. In one patient who went into rapid renal failure there was a superimposed crescentic glomerulonephritis.[156]

Differential diagnosis

De novo membranous glomerulonephritis must be distinguished; this can only be done by examination of the recipient's own kidneys. In the early stages of recurrent membranous glomerulonephritis, before the subepithelial deposits have become diffuse, there may be difficulty in differentiating these lesions from *chronic transplant glomerulopathy*, which is occasionally accompanied by a few small focal and segmental subepithelial deposits. Resolution of this problem has sometimes to await the findings on later biopsies.

Prognosis

Approximately 25% of the patients lose their graft as a direct result of the recurrent disease. In almost all cases graft failure has not occurred until at least 2 years after transplantation.

TRANSMISSION OF OTHER DISEASES

Antiglomerular-basement-membrane (anti-GBM) antibody disease

Renal transplantation in patients with anti-GBM antibody disease who have circulating antibodies results in immediate fixation of the antibodies to the glomerular capillary basement membranes of the graft in approximately 60% of the patients. In most cases antibody fixation induces little histological or functional damage and is compatible with excellent long-term graft function. However, about 40% of the grafts with bound antibody develop a crescentic glomerulonephritis accompanied by rapidly progressive renal failure and loss of the graft.[157]

The production of circulating antibody in patients with anti-GBM antibody disease generally only lasts weeks or months; if renal transplantation is postponed until anti-GBM antibody has not been detected in the recipient for 6 months, then there is little chance of recurrence. Delay before transplantation in cases of anti-GBM antibody disease is now the accepted policy in all transplant units. The exact risk of transmission of disease in these circumstances is not known; rare instances of recurrence are still reported.

Clinical features

Fixation of anti-GBM antibodies to the glomerular capillary basement membranes of the graft is often accompanied by transient proteinuria and haematuria.[158] In those cases that progress to crescentic glomerulonephritis, proteinuria persists, becomes heavy, and is often accompanied by haematuria; renal function deteriorates and the graft is lost in 6–12 weeks.

Microscopy

Clinically silent recurrence is associated with linear deposits of IgG and complement on the glomerular capillary basement membranes, but few other changes. In clinically overt disease there is, in addition, a segmental glomerulonephritis with tuft necroses and crescents; those patients with the most rapidly progressive course have the most crescents.

Differential diagnosis

Linear staining of the glomerular capillary basement membranes for IgG may occur in *chronic transplant glomerulopathy*, but this is focal and segmental, never diffuse and global. There may also be a few crescents, but the numbers rarely exceed 5%. Glomerular segmental necroses are rare in chronic transplant glomerulopathy; when they occur few glomeruli are affected. *De-novo anti-GBM antibody disease* should only be considered if there is clear biopsy and serological evidence that the patient's own disease was not anti-GBM antibody disease. If *diabetes mellitus* develops following transplantation this may cause diffuse linear staining of the glomerular basement membranes for IgG.

Prognosis

In the presence of circulating anti-GBM antibodies about 25% of renal allografts develop a rapidly progressive recurrent disease leading to graft loss within a year.[157] If the recipient with anti-GBM antibody disease has no circulating antibodies at the time of transplantation and antibodies have been absent for the previous 6 months, then recurrent disease occurs only very rarely.

Henoch–Schönlein purpura

Patients with Henoch–Schönlein purpura commonly develop mesangial IgA deposits in their renal transplants. Routine biopsy revealed an incidence of histological recurrence of 89% in one series of cases[116] and of 53% in another.[159] About 60% of these histological recurrences are accompanied by mild proteinuria and microscopic haematuria. Of the clinically overt cases of recurrence 30% eventually develop renal dysfunction which leads to loss of the graft.

Microscopy

Deposits of IgA appear in the paramesangial areas of variable numbers of glomeruli. Sometimes this happens as early as 1 month after transplantation.[159] In most cases the IgA deposits are accompanied by a mild increase in the number of mesangial cells. Focal and segmental proliferation and necrotic lesions with variable numbers of crescents occur in patients with clinically progressive disease.

Differential diagnosis

The lesions of clinically silent recurrent Henoch Schönlein purpura are indistinguishable morphologically from *IgA deposits that are present in the donor kidney* and persist after transplantation.[159] The distinction can only be made on a biopsy of the graft taken before the circulation is re-established. Recognition of *recurrent IgA nephropathy* depends upon reviewing the biopsies of the patient's own kidneys.

Prognosis

About 18% of renal allografts transplanted into patients with Henoch–Schönlein purpura fail after several years, primarily because of recurrent disease.[116,159]

Haemolytic uraemic syndrome

Patients whose original disease was haemolytic uraemic syndrome may develop the same syndrome after renal transplantation. The incidence seems to vary widely, being 50%,[160] 25%,[161] and 10%[162] in three recent series. The time of onset is mostly within 2 months of transplantation. Second and subsequent grafts may also be affected.

Differential diagnosis

Lesions morphologically identical to those of recurrence may be induced by *severe acute rejection, malignant hypertension* and the administration of *cyclosporin*. To diagnose recurrence of haemolytic uraemic syndrome with any confidence both the clinical and the pathological features of the syndrome must be present, there must be no evidence of rejection, the patient should not have been on cyclosporin and severe hypertension should not have occurred following transplantation.

Prognosis

The outlook is poor for those renal allografts that develop, for whatever reason, the morphological lesions of haemolytic uraemic syndrome (see p. 283). In approximately 70% of cases the graft ceases to function within a few weeks.

Pathogenesis

The haemolytic uraemic syndrome is brought about by a group of disorders of mixed aetiology, all of which act initially through the common mechanism of inducing endothelial cell damage (see p. 288). In some recipients the tendency to develop the syndrome in response to infections or other stimuli is inherited and lifelong, whereas in others it is acquired and brief.

Primary hyperoxaluria type I

If no safeguards are taken there is almost universal and rapid recurrence of disease in the transplanted kidney.[163] The prognosis is must better if intensive pretransplant haemodialysis is used to remove as much oxalate as possible, if the donor kidney is well matched to decrease rejection damage in which oxalate may deposit, and if long-term diuresis is induced after transplantation to inhibit crystallization of calcium oxalate in the urine.[164]

Diabetes mellitus type I

Recurrence of the renal lesions of diabetes mellitus is common, but the changes appear slowly and they have no adverse effect on renal function for a long period.

After the graft has been in the patient for at least 2 years the glomerular capillary basement membranes begin to thicken and then the mesangium starts to expand.[165,166] To detect these early changes electron microscopy with morphometric analysis is needed. Linear localization of IgG and albumin on the glomerular capillary basement membranes is also common.[165] The mesangial expansion is slowly progressive and in about 18% of grafts, by 13 years following transplantation, it has become severe and nodular producing Kimmelstiel–Wilson lesions.[167] Hyaline arteriosclerosis, affecting both afferent and efferent arterioles, occurs in approximately 50% of the grafts but this also occurs in grafts in which neither the donor nor the recipient is diabetic[109] and it is, therefore, not a useful indication of diabetic nephrosclerosis.

The early basement membrane thickening and mesangial expansion are associated with microalbuminuria; the severe nodular lesions are associated with marked proteinuria, sometimes with the nephrotic syndrome.

Recurrent disease accounts for only about 8% of graft failures in diabetics and it usually takes 12 years or more to destroy the graft.[168]

Amyloidosis

Amyloid develops in the graft in about 20–30% of cases in the first 2 years after transplantation into a patient with this disease.[169] The deposits are associated with proteinuria, but this does not usually commence until at least 11 months after transplantation. Graft failure occurs only occasionally. Patients are more likely to die from infection following immunosuppressive treatment of rejection, or from cardiovascular or other complications related to widespread amyloidosis.

Fabry's disease

Ceramide deposits in the graft are infrequent and

confined to the endothelial cells. They do not influence graft survival.[170]

Cystinosis

The interstitium of the transplant often becomes infiltrated by host macrophages that contain cystine:[171] they have little or no effect on renal function.

Systemic lupus erythematosus

Lupus nephritis very rarely recurs in a transplanted kidney. Up to 1989 only five well-documented cases had been reported.[172]

Systemic sclerosis

There are reports on 12 patients with end-stage renal failure caused by systemic sclerosis who were treated by renal transplantation. Two grafts rapidly failed: their arterioles and interlobular arteries showed a thickened mucoid intima containing IgM and complement.[173,174] Although these cases were interpreted as transmission of systemic sclerosis, the close resemblance between the morphological features of this condition and vascular rejection makes the diagnosis of recurrent disease very difficult to establish.

Sickle cell nephropathy

A kidney transplanted into a patient with sickle cell anaemia will be subject to the same influences that originally lead to the destruction of the patient's own kidneys (see p. 106). Surprisingly, therefore, only three grafts have been reported in which the disease was thought to have recurred.[175,176]

Hypercalcaemia

In one carefully studied group of renal graft recipients, hypercalcaemia (defined as a total plasma calcium greater than 2.70 mmol/l on three successive estimations, with correction for plasma albumin), was present in 11% of cases after transplantation.[177] The major cause was pre-existing secondary hyperparathyroidism which persisted after successful grafting and sometimes lasted for years.

The hypercalcaemia may lead to microscopic calcification in the graft. The amount is usually minor; the distribution is the same as in untransplanted kidneys (see p. 546).

DE NOVO DISEASE

The development of a disease (other than rejection) in the transplant that was not present in the donor, and that is not present in the recipient, is usually referred to as de novo disease. The most important de novo disease is glomerulonephritis.

DE NOVO GLOMERULONEPHRITIS

De novo glomerulonephritis is not as common as recurrent glomerulonephritis and much less frequent than transplant glomerulopathy (see p. 656). Morphologically it may assume a number of different patterns, including membranous glomerulonephritis, focal segmental glomerulonephritis and crescentic glomerulonephritis. The most common type of de novo glomerulonephritis is membranous glomerulonephritis.

Membranous glomerulonephritis

Membranous glomerulonephritis may develop in a renal allograft in a patient whose original disease was not membranous glomerulonephritis.[178–181] The incidence is reported to be approximately 2% in transplantation units in which grafts are not routinely biopsied;[180] in units practising routine biopsy the recognized incidence is about 9%.[178] De novo membranous glomerulonephritis occurs in any age group. There has been no reported association with any of the infections, systemic diseases or medications that are known to be linked to the development of membranous glomerulonephritis in non-transplanted kidneys. De novo membranous glomerulonephritis may occasionally affect more than one graft in a particular patient.[180]

Clinical features

The interval from transplantation to diagnosis is usually 1–2 years. Most patients develop persistent proteinuria, with or without the nephrotic syndrome; less frequently there is renal dysfunction.[178,180] Approximately a third have no clinical manifestations when they are diagnosed on routine biopsy; they may remain asymptomatic for many years before developing proteinuria.[178]

Microscopy

At diagnosis the morphological lesions in most cases are diffuse and global, and in stage I or II (see p. 194); in about a quarter they are focal and segmental. The subepithelial deposits are sometimes ill-defined and atypical compared with those in membranous glomerulonephritis in the non-transplanted kidney. Almost all the grafts with de novo disease show more interstitial mononuclear cell infiltration than would be expected at their particular period after transplantation, just over a half have evidence of vascular rejection, and approximately a third have chronic transplant glomerulopathy.[180] In a few patients the lesions progress to stages III or IV; reversal of the changes has not been recorded.

Differential diagnosis

Recurrent membranous glomerulonephritis is indistinguishable morphologically from the de novo disease; only clear biopsy evidence that the patient's original disease was not membranous glomerulonephritis enables a distinction to be made. *Chronic transplant glomerulopathy* is easily excluded if there are diffuse subepithelial deposits in the graft because these do not occur in rejection. A few focal and segmental subepithelial deposits in a transplant undergoing chronic rejection, in a patient whose disease was not membranous glomerulonephritis, should not be diagnosed as de novo disease; they should be regarded as suspicious: only if they can be shown in subsequent biopsies to progress to diffuse and global lesions can the diagnosis of de novo membranous glomerulonephritis be justified.

Prognosis

Grafts with proteinuria over 3 g/24 hours or with a serum creatinine greater than 115 μmol/l almost always fail.[180] When graft destruction occurs it is rarely due solely to the de novo membranous glomerulonephritis; a major factor is usually chronic rejection.

Pathogenesis

Unmasking or release of tubular antigens due to rejection could be responsible, acting through a mechanism rather like that which operates in Heymann's nephritis in the rat (see p. 202). The frequent association of the changes of chronic rejection with de novo membranous glomerulonephritis is in keeping with this explanation. Antibodies to tubular epithelial antigens have been demonstrated in several cases.[181] Another possibility is that antibodies directed against HLA antigens form immune complexes on the glomerular endothelial cells; the complexes are then shed and redistributed to a subepithelial position.[180]

Focal segmental glomerulosclerosis

De novo focal segmental glomerulosclerosis (FSGS) occurs in 1–9% of renal allografts that have survived for more than 6 months.[116,182] The main clinical manifestation is proteinuria; sometimes there is also haematuria and hypertension.[182] In contrast to recurrent FSGS (see p. 664), the proteinuria rarely commences before 4 months following transplantation and in only about a third of the patients is it severe enough to produce the nephrotic syndrome.

The lesions do not differ morphologically from those seen in idiopathic or recurrent FSGS. They are often associated with ischaemia secondary to chronic rejection and are commonest in the glomeruli of the outer cortex. The distinction between de novo and recurrent FSGS is discussed on page 664.

Most patients eventually develop a progressive decline in renal function leading to graft loss.

Anti-GBM antibody disease and crescentic glomerulonephritis

De novo anti-GBM antibody disease, with or without crescents, is rare. Among the cases reported there is an interesting subgroup which occurs in patients whose original disease was hereditary nephritis (Alport's syndrome; see p. 73). About 15% of these patients develop anti-GBM antibodies against the graft's Goodpasture antigen (see p. 11), which is absent from their own glomerular basement membranes and has therefore not been met previously by the host and is regarded as foreign. The antibodies bind to the glomerular capillary basement membranes of the transplant. In most cases this event produces no clinical manifestations but in some patients it results in urinary changes 1 month to 2 years after transplantation; occasionally it causes a progressive crescentic glomerulonephritis with rapid destruction of the graft.[183–185]

The patients with Alport's syndrome who do not produce anti-GBM antibodies may have a lesser reduction in the amount of Goodpasture antigen in the glomerular capillary basement membranes of their original kidneys.

REFERENCES

Disease in donor kidney

1. Jones B, Nanra RS, Hibberd AD, White K. Resolution of IgA nephropathy after renal allograft transplantation. Clin Nephrol 1990; 33: 53.
2. Silva FG, Chander P, Pirani CL. Disappearance of glomerular mesangial IgA deposits after renal allograft transplantation.Transplantation 1982; 33: 214–216.
3. Suganuma T, Morozumi K, Satoh K et al. Studies of IgA nephropathy in renal transplantation. Transplant Proc 1989; 21: 2123–2127.
4. Sugiyama S, Yamamoto T, Tsuyuki M, Ohshima S. Study of IgA nephropathy in the transplanted kidney – sequential changes in mesangial IgA deposits found in one hour post-transplantation kidney biopsies. Jpn J Nephrol 1986; 28: 729–737.
5. Brensilver JM, Mallat S, Scholes J, McCabe R. Recurrent IgA nephropathy in living-related donor transplantation: recurrence or transmission of familial disease? Am J Kidney Dis 1988; 12: 147–151.
6. Popli S, Molnar ZV, Leehey DL et al. Involvement of renal allograft by Fabry's disease. Am J Nephrol 1987; 7: 316–318.
7. Penn I. Transmission of cancer with donor organs. Transplant Proc 1988; 20: 739–740.
8. Abouna GM, Adnani MS, Kumar MSA, Samhan SA. Fate of transplanted kidneys with diabetic nephropathy. Lancet 1986; 1: 622–623.

Changes caused by technical difficulties before or during transplantation

9. Olsen S, Burdick JF, Keown PA, Wallace AC, Racusen LC, Solez K. Primary acute renal failure ('acute tubular necrosis') in the transplanted kidney: morphology and pathogenesis. Medicine (Baltimore) 1989; 68: 173–187.
10. Solez K, Racusen LC, Burdick JF, Keown PA, Olsen S. Transplant 'acute tubular necrosis' (ATN) in cyclosporine (CsA)-treated patients (pts). Kidney Int.1990; 37: 495
11. Tilney NL. The early course of a patient with a kidney transplant. In: PJ Morris, ed. Kidney transplantation. Principles and practice, 3rd edn. Philadelphia: Saunders, 1989; 263–283.
12. Abouna GM, Kogure H, Porter KA, Andres GA, Lutcher CL, Sobel RE. Massive early proteinuria following renal homotransplantation. JAMA 1973; 226: 631–635.
13. Dupont E, Dupuis F, Richard C. One-hour biopsy and kidney transplantation. Lancet 1974; 1: 64–65 (letter).
14. Light JA, Annable C, Perloff LJ et al. Immune injury from organ preservation. A potential cause of hyperacute rejection in human cadaver kidney transplantation. Transplantation 1975; 19: 511–516.
15. Evan AP, Gattone VH, Filo RS, Leapman SE, Smith EJ, Luft FC. Glomerular endothelial injury related to renal perfusion. Transplantation 1983; 35: 436–441.
16. Sheil AGR, Drummond JM, Boulas J. Vascular thrombosis in machine-perfused renal allografts. Transplantation 1975; 20: 178–179.
17. Ward K, Klingensmith WC, Sterioff S, Wagner HN. The origin of lymphoceles following renal transplantation. Transplantation 1978; 25: 346–347.
18. Zincke H, Woods JE, Aguilo JJ et al. Experience with lymphoceles after renal transplantation. Surgery 1975; 77: 444–450.

Changes associated with rejection

19. Bach FH, Sachs DH. Current concepts: immunology. Transplant Immunol. N Engl J Med 1987; 317: 489–492.
20. Fuggle SV, Errasti P, Daar AS, Fabre JW, Ting A, Morris PJ. Localization of major histocompatibility complex (HLA-ABC and DR) antigens in 46 kidneys: differences in HLA-DR staining of tubules among kidneys. Transplantation 1983; 35: 385–390.
21. Bodmer WF. The HLA system: structure and function. J Clin Pathol 1987; 40: 948–958.
22. Takiff H, Iwaki I, Cecka M, Terasaki PI. The benefit and underutilization of sharing kidneys for better histocompatibility. Transplantation 1989; 47: 102–105.
23. Krensky AM, Weiss A, Crabtree G, Davis MM, Parham P. T-lymphocyte-antigen interactions in transplant rejection. N Engl J Med 1990; 322: 510–517.
24. Simpson E, Tomonari K. Mapping minor H genes. Immunology Suppl 1989; 2: 42–48.
25. Opelz G. The role of HLA matching and blood transfusions in the cyclosporine era. Transplant Proc 1989; 21: 609–612.
26. Taylor RMR, Ting A, Briggs JD. Renal transplantation in the United Kingdom and Ireland: the centre effect. Lancet 1985; 1: 798–802.
27. Opelz G, Sengar DPS, Mickey MR, Terasaki PI. Effect of blood transfusion on subsequent kidney transplants. Transplant Proc 1973; 5: 253–259.

28. Opelz G. Comparison of the transfusion effect in North America and Europe. Transplant Proc 1988; 20: 1069–1070.
29. Wood ML, Okazaki H, Monaco AP. The effect of blood transfusions on the immune response. Transplant Proc 1988; 20: 1200–1203.
30. Cecka JM, Breidenthal SE, Terasaki PI. Low anti-A and anti-B titers in some type O patients may permit renal transplantation across the ABO barrier. Transplant Proc 1987; 19: 4507–4510.
31. Iwaki Y, Terasaki PI. Primary nonfunction in human cadaver kidney transplant: evidence for hidden hyperacute rejection. Clin Transplant 1987; 1: 125–131.
32. Brasile L, Rodman E, Shield C, Clarke J, Cerelli J. The association of antivascular endothelial cell antibodies with hyperacute rejection: a case report. Surgery 1986; 99: 637–640.
33. Starzl TE, Boehmig HJ, Amemiya H et al. Clotting changes, including disseminated intravascular coagulation, during rapid renal-homograft rejection. N Engl J Med 1970; 283: 383–390.
34. Porter KA. Clinical renal transplantation. Int Rev Exp Pathol 1972; 11: 73–176.
35. Myburgh JA, Cohen I, Gecelter L et al. Hyperacute rejection in human-kidney allografts – Schwartzman or Arthus reaction? N Engl J Med 1969; 281: 131–135.
36. Williams GM, Hume DM, Hudson RP, Morris PJ, Kano K, Milgrom F. 'Hyperacute' renal-homograft rejection in man. N Engl J Med 1968; 279: 611–618.
37. Kissmeyer-Nielson F, Olsen S, Petersen VP, Fjeldborg O. Hyperacute rejection of kidney allografts, associated with preexisting humoral antibodies against donor cells. Lancet 1966; 2: 662–665.
38. Lucas ZJ, Coplon N, Kempson R, Cohn RB. Early renal transplant failure associated with subliminal sensitization. Transplantation 1970; 10: 522–529.
39. Metzgar RS, Seigler HF, Ward FE, Rowland DT. Immunological studies on eluates from human renal allografts. Transplantation 1972; 13: 131–137.
40. Katz J, Lurie A, Kaplan BS, Krawitz S, Metz J. Coagulation findings in the hemolytic-uremic syndrome of infancy: similarity to hyperacute allograft rejection. J Pediatr 1971; 78: 426–434.
41. Nelson PW, Helling TS, Pierce GE et al. Successful transplantation of blood group A_2 kidneys into non-A recipients. Transplantation 1988; 45: 316–319.
42. Rydberg L, Breimer ME, Samuelsson BE, Brynger H. Blood group ABO-incompatible (A_2 to O) kidney transplantation in human subjects: a clinical, serologic, and biochemical approach. Transplant Proc 1987; 19: 4528–4537.
43. Welsh KI, Van Dam M, Koffman CG et al. Transplantation of blood group A_2 kidneys into O or B recipients: the effect of pretransplant anti-A titers on graft survival. Transplant Proc 1987; 19: 4565–4567.
44. Alexandre GPJ, Squifflet JP, De Bruyère M et al. Present experience in a series of 26 ABO-incompatible living donor renal allografts. Transplant Proc 1987; 19: 4539–4542.
45. Altman B. Tissue transplantation: circulating antibody in the homotransplantation of kidney and skin. Ann R Coll Surg Engl 1963; 33: 79–104.
46. Ito S, Camussi G, Tetta C, Milgrom F, Andres G. Hyperacute renal allograft rejection in the rabbit. The role of platelet-activating factor and of cationic proteins derived from polymorphonuclear leukocytes and from platelets. Lab Invest 1984; 51: 148–161.
47. Jordan SC, Malekzadeh MH, Pennisi AJ, Ettenger RB, Uittenborgaart SC, Fine RN. Accelerated acute rejection of primary renal allografts in pediatric patients. Transplantation 1980; 30: 5–8.
48. Halloran PF, Wadgymar A, Ritchie S, Falk J, Solez K, Srinivasa NS. The significance of the anti-class I antibody response. I. Clinical and pathologic features of anti-class I-mediated rejection. Transplantation 1990; 49: 85–91.
49. Paul LC, Class FHJ, van Es LA, Kalff MW, de Graeff J. Accelerated rejection of a renal allograft associated with pretransplantation antibodies directed against donor antigens on endothelium and monocytes. N Engl J Med 1979; 300: 1258–1260.
50. Salvatierra O. Advantages of continued use of kidney transplantation from living donors. Transplant Proc 1985; 17: suppl, 18–22.
51. Simpson MA, Madras PN, Cornaby AJ et al. Sequential determinations of urinary cytology and plasma and urinary lymphokines in the management of renal allograft recipients.Transplantation 1989; 47: 218–223.
52. Kahan BD. Immunologic monitoring: utility and limitations. Transplant Proc 1985; 17: 1537–1545.
53. Porter KA, Marchioro TL, Starzl TE. Pathological changes in 37 human renal homotransplants treated with immunosuppressive drugs.Br J Urol 1965; 37: 250–273
54. D'Ardenne AJ, Dunnill MS, Thompson JF. Cyclosporin and renal graft histology. J Clin Pathol 1986; 39: 145–151.
55. Bonsib SM, Reznicek MJ, Wright FH. Renal medulla in the diagnosis of acute cellular rejection. Transplantation 1989; 48: 690–691.
56. McWhinnie DL, Thompson JF, Taylor HM. Morphometric analysis of cellular infiltration assessed by monoclonal antibody labelling in sequential human renal allograft biopsies. Transplantation 1986; 42: 352–358.
57. Cohen AH, Border WA, Rajfer J, Dumke A, Glassock RJ. Interstitial Tamm-Horsfall protein in rejecting renal allografts. Identification and morphologic pattern of injury. Lab Invest 1984; 50: 519–525.
58. Sibley RK, Rynasiewicz J, Ferguson RM et al. Morphology of cyclosporine nephrotoxicity and acute rejection in patients immunosuppressed with cyclosporine and prednisolone. Surgery 1983; 94: 225–234.
59. Nadasdy T, Ormos J, Stiller D, Csajbak E, Szenohradszky P. Tubular ultrastructure in rejected human renal allografts. Ultrastruct Pathol 1988; 12: 195–207.
60. Katz JP, Hakki A, Katz SM, Simonian S. Rejection of the ureter: a new component of renal allograft rejection. Transplant Proc 1987; 19: 2200–2202.
61. Nabarra B, Descamps B. Ultrastructure of cells infiltrating human kidney allografts. Clin Exp Immunol 1976; 24: 300–309.
62. Sako H, Nakane Y, Okino K et al. Immunohistochemical study of the cells infiltrating human renal allografts by the ABC and the IGSS method using monoclonal antibodies. Transplantation 1987; 44: 43–50.
63. Séron D, Alezopoulos E, Raftery MJ, Hartley RB, Cameron JS. Diagnosis of rejection in renal allograft

biopsies using the presence of activated and proliferating cells. Transplantation 1989; 47: 811–816.
64. Fuggle SV, McWhinnie DL, Chapman JR, Taylor HM, Morris PJ. Sequential analysis of HLA-Class II antigen expression in human renal allografts. Induction of tubular class II antigens and correlation with clinical parameters. Transplantation 1986; 42: 144–150.
65. McWhinnie DL, Fuggle SV, Azevedo LS, Jones RM, Morris PJ. HLA class II induction and cellular infiltration are effectively suppressed by triple therapy in renal allografts. Transplant Proc 1987; 19: 3628–3629.
66. Bishop GA, Hall BM. Expression of leucocyte and lymphocyte adhesion molecules in the human kidney. Kidney Int 1989; 36: 1078–1085.
67. Randall JF, Starr RJ, Russ GR. Vascular endothelial cell expression of adhesion molecules and HLA antigens in renal allografts. Transplant Proc 1989–21: 316–317.
68. Tötterman TH, Hanås E, Bergstrom R, Larsson E, Tufveson G. Immunologic diagnosis of kidney rejection using FACS analysis of graft-infiltrating functional and activated T and NK cell subsets. Transplantation 1989; 47: 817–823.
69. Von Willebrand E, Häyry P. Fine needle aspiration cytology of the transplanted kidney. In: PJ Morris, ed. Kidney transplantation. Principles and practice, 3rd edn. Philadelphia: Saunders, 1989; 491–510.
70. Porter KA, Joseph NH, Rendall JM, Stolinski C, Hoehn RJ, Calne RY. The role of lymphocytes in the rejection of canine renal homotransplants. Lab Invest 1964; 13: 1080–1098.
71. Burdick JF, Beschorner WE, Smith WJ et al. Characteristics of early routine renal allograft biopsies. Transplantation 1984; 38: 679–684.
72. McWhinnie DL, Carter NP, Chapman JR, Taylor HM, Wood RFM, Morris PJ. Prediction of rejection by morphometric analysis of renal allograft biopsies. Transplant Proc 1986; 18: 1040.
73. Aherne WA, Dunnill MS. Morphometry. London: Arnold, 1982; 33–45.
74. Foot RA, Fuggle DL, McWhinnie DL, Carter NP, Morris PJ. The diagnosis of renal allograft rejection: an improved assessment of graft infiltration using image analysis. Transplant Proc 1989; 21: 1905–1906.
75. Versluis DJ, Ten Kate FJW, Wenting GJ, Jeekel J, Weimar W. Histological lesions associated with cyclosporin: incidence and reversibility in one year old kidney transplants. J Clin Pathol 1988; 41: 498–503.
76. Myers BD, Newton L, Boshkos C et al. Chronic injury of human renal microvessels with low-dose cyclosporine therapy. Transplantation 1988; 46: 694–702.
77. Barrett M, Milton AD, Barrett J et al. Needle biopsy evaluation of class II major histocompatibility complex antigen expression for the differential diagnosis of cyclosporine nephrotoxicity from kidney graft rejection. Transplantation 1987; 44: 223–227.
78. Racusen LC, Solez K. Cyclosporine nephrotoxicity. Int Rev Exp Pathol 1988; 30: 107–157.
79. Kurtz JB, Thompson JF, Ting A, Pinto A, Morris PJ. The problem of cytomegalovirus infection in renal allograft recipients. Q J Med 1984; 53: 341–349.
80. Gnann JW, Ahlmen J, Svalander C, Olding L, Oldstone MBA, Nelson JA. Inflammatory cells in transplanted kidneys are infected by human cytomegalovirus. Am J Pathol 1988; 132: 239–248.
81. Denning DW, Weiss LM, Martinez K, Flechner SM. Transmission of Epstein–Barr virus by a transplanted kidney, with activation by OKT3 antibody. Transplantation 1989; 48: 141–144.
82. Nalesnik MA, Jaffe R, Starzl TE et al. The pathology of posttransplant lymphoproliferative disorders occurring in the setting of cyclosporine A – prednisolone immunosuppression. Am J Pathol 1988; 133: 173–192.
83. Kinlen LJ, Sheil AGR, Peto J, Doll R. Collaborative United Kingdom–Australasian study of cancer in patients treated with immunosuppressive drugs. Br Med J 1979; 2: 1461–1466.
84. Starzl TE, Nalesnik MA, Porter KA et al. Reversibility of lymphomas and lymphoproliferative lesions developing under cyclosporin-steroid therapy. Lancet 1984; 1: 583–587.
85. Ulrich W, Chott A, Watschinger B, Reiter C, Kovarik J, Radaszkiewicz T. Primary peripheral T cell lymphoma in a kidney transplant under immunosuppression with cyclosporine A. Hum Pathol 1989; 20: 1027–1030.
86. Amend WJC, Vincenti F, Duca R et al. Prognostic features of early renal transplant rejections. Am J Kidney Dis 1982; 1: 281–287.
87. Sanfilippo F, Kolbeck PC, Vaughn WK, Bollinger RR. Renal allograft cell infiltrates associated with irreversible rejection. Transplantation 1985; 40: 679–685.
88. Kormendi F, Amend WJC. The importance of eosinophil cells in kidney allograft rejection. Transplantation 1988; 45: 537–539.
89. Mason DW, Morris PJ. Effector mechanisms in allograft rejection. Annu Rev Immunol 1986; 4: 119–145.
90. Larson CP, Morris PJ, Austyn JM. Migration of dendritic leukocytes from cardiac allografts into host spleens. A novel pathway for initiation of rejection. J Exp Med 1990; 171: 307–314.
91. Liu C-C, Rafii S, Granelli-Piperno A, Trapani JA, Young JD-E. Perforin and serine esterase gene expression in stimulated human T cells. Kinetics, mitogen requirements, and effects of cyclosporin A. J Exp Med 1989; 170: 2105–2118.
92. Collins T, Korman AJ, Wake CCT et al. Immune interferon activates multiple class II major histocompatibility complex genes and the associated invariant chain gene in human endothelial cells and dermal fibroblasts. Proc Natl Acad Sci USA 1984; 81: 4917–4921.
93. Matas AJ, Sibley R, Mauer M, Sutherland DER, Simmons RL, Najarian JS. The value of needle renal allograft biopsy. I. A retrospective study of biopsies performed during putative rejection episodes. Ann Surg 1983; 197: 226–237.
94. Herbertson BM, Evans DB, Calne RY, Banerjee AK. Percutaneous needle biopsies of renal allografts: the relationship between morphological changes present in biopsies and subsequent allograft function. Histopathology 1977; 1: 161–178.
95. Colvin RB. Renal allografts. In: Colvin RB, Bhan AK, McCluskey RT, eds. Diagnostic immunopathology. New York: Raven Press, 1988; 151–197.
96. Porter KA, Peart WS, Kenyon JR, Joseph NH, Hoehn RJ, Calne RY. Rejection of kidney homotransplants. Ann NY Acad Sci 1964; 120: 472–495.
97. Porter KA, Andres GA, Calder MW et al. Human renal transplants. II. Immunofluorescent and immunoferritin studies. Lab Invest 1968; 18: 159–171.
98. Tuazon TV, Schneeberger EE, Bhan AK et al. Mononuclear cells in acute allograft glomerulopathy. Am J Pathol 1987; 129: 119–132.

99. Neild GH, Reuben R, Hartley RB, Cameron JS. Glomerular thrombi in renal allografts associated with cyclosporin treatment. J Clin Pathol 1985; 38: 253–258.
100. Dunnill MS, Gatter KC, Mason DY, Morris PJ. Immunosuppression and thrombosis in renal transplantation: an immunohistological study. Histopathology 1990; 16: 79–82.
101. Banfi G, Imbasciati E, Tarantino A, Ponticelli C. Prognostic value of renal biopsy in acute rejection of kidney transplantation. Nephron 1981; 28: 222–226.
102. Vogeler U, Doxiadis I, Buchholz B et al. Cytotoxicity of antibodies eluted from rejected kidney allografts. Transplant Proc 1985; 17: 2630–2634.
103. Baldwin WM, Soulillou J-P, Claas FHJ, Peyrat M-A, van Es LA, van Rood JJ. Antibodies to endothelial antigens in eluates of 88 human kidneys: correlation with graft survival and presence of T-and B-cell antibodies. Transplant Proc 1981; 13: 1547–1550.
104. Axelsen RA, Seymour AE, Mathew TH, Canny A, Pascoe V. Glomerular transplant rejection: a distinctive pattern of early graft damage. Clin Nephrol 1985; 23: 1–11.
105. Cunningham E, Chi Y, Brentjens J, Venuto R. Acute serum sickness with glomerulonephritis induced by antithymocyte globulin. Transplantation 1987; 43: 309–312.
106. Boyce NW, Hayes K, Gee D et al. Cytomegalovirus infection complicating renal transplantation and its relationship to acute transplant glomerulopathy. Transplantation 1988; 45: 706–709.
107. Maryniak RK, First MR, Weiss MA. Transplant glomerulopathy: evolution of morphologically distinct changes. Kidney Int 1985; 27: 799–806.
108. Porter KA, Thomson WB, Owen K, Kenyon JR, Mowbray JF, Peart WS. Obliterative vascular changes in 4 human kidney homotransplants. Br Med J 1963; 2: 639–645.
109. Porter KA, Rendall JM, Stolinski C, Terasaki PI, Marchioro TL, Starzl TE. Light and electron microscopic study of biopsies from 33 human renal allografts and an isograft 1¾–2½ years after transplantation. Ann NY Acad Sci 1966; 129: 615–636.
110. Andres GA, Accinni L, Hsu KC et al. Human renal transplants: III. Immunopathologic studies. Lab Invest 1970; 22: 588–604.
111. Oguma S, Banner B, Zerbe T, Starzl T, Demetris AJ. Participation of dendritic cells in vascular lesions of chronic rejection of human allografts. Lancet 1988; 2: 933–936.
112. Demetris AJ, Zerbe T, Banner B. Morphology of solid organ allograft arteriopathy: identification of proliferating intimal cell populations. Transplant Proc 1989; 21: 3667–3669.
113. Terasaki PI, Mickey MR, Iwaki Y et al. Long-term survival of kidney grafts. Transplant Proc 1989; 21: 615–617.
114. Foegh ML. Chronic rejection – graft arteriosclerosis. Transplant Proc 1990; 22: 119–122.
115. Libby P, Salomon RN, Payne DD, Schoen FJ, Pober JS. Functions of vascular wall cells related to development of transplantation-associated coronary arteriosclerosis. Transplant Proc 1988; 21: 3677–3684.
116. Habib R, Antignac C, Hinglais N, Gagnadoux M-F, Broyer M. Glomerular lesions in the transplanted kidney in children. Am J Kidney Dis 1987; 10: 198–207.
117. Manaligod JR, Jao W, Mozes MF, Jonasson O. Glomerular changes in renal allografts. Am J Kidney Dis 1986; 7: 29–34.
118. Cheigh JS, Mouradian J, Susin M et al. Kidney transplant nephrotic syndrome: relationship between allograft histopathology and natural course. Kidney Int 1980; 18: 358–365.
119. Porter KA, Dossetor JB, Marchioro TL et al. Human renal transplants I. Glomerular changes. Lab Invest 1967; 16: 153–181.
120. Zollinger HU, Moppert J, Thiel G, Rohr H-P. Morphology and pathogenesis of glomerulopathy in cadaver kidney allografts treated with antilymphocyte globulin (clinical, light, electron and immunofluorescent optic examinations). Curr Top Pathol 1973; 57: 1–48.
121. Hsu H-C, Suzuki Y, Churg J, Grishman E. Ultrastructure of transplant glomerulopathy. Histopathology 1980; 4: 351–367.
122. Peng-fei Z, Rao KV, Anderson WR. An ultrastructural study of the membranoproliferative variant of transplant glomerulopathy. Ultrastruct Pathol 1988; 12: 185–194
123. Klassen J, Kano K, Milgrom F et al. Tubular lesions produced by autoantibodies to tubular basement membrane in human renal allografts. Int Arch Allergy Appl Immunol 1973; 45: 675–689.
124. Wilson CB, Lehman DH, McCoy RC, Gunnells JC, Stickel DL. Antitubular basement membrane antibodies after renal transplantation. Transplantation 1974; 18: 447–452.
125. Rotellar C, Noël L-H, Droz D, Kreis H, Berger J. Role of antibodies directed against tubular basement membranes in human renal transplantation. Am J Kidney Dis 1986; 7: 157–161.
126. Dryburgh P, Porter KA, Krom RAF et al. Should the ruptured renal allograft be removed? Arch Surg 1979; 114: 850–852.
127. Richardson AJ, Higgins RM, Jaskowski AJ, Murie J, Dunnill MS, Morris PJ. Renal allograft rupture and renal vein thrombosis. Transplant Proc 1990; 22: 1419.

Changes induced by immunosuppressive treatment

128. Gardner SD, Field AM, Coleman DV, Hulme B. New human papovavirus (B.K.) isolated from urine after renal transplantation. Lancet 1971; 2: 1253–1257.
129. Curtis JJ. Hypertension after renal transplantation: cyclosporine increases the diagnostic and therapeutic considerations. Am J Kidney Dis 1989; 13: suppl 1, 28–32.
130. Chan MK, Varghese Z, Moorhead JF. Lipid abnormalities in uremia, dialysis and transplantation. Kidney Int 1981; 19: 625–637.
131. Vathsala A, Weinberg RB, Schoenberg L et al. Lipid abnormalities in renal transplant recipients treated with cyclosporine. Transplant Proc 1989; 21: 3670–3673.
132. Raine AEG. Cardiovascular complications after renal transplantation. In: PJ Morris, ed. Kidney transplantation. Principles and practice. 3rd edn. Philadelphia: Saunders, 1989; 575–601.
133. Sheil AGR, Flavel S, Disney APS, Mathew TH, Hall BM. Cancer incidence in renal transplant patients treated with azathioprine or cyclosporine. Transplant Proc 1987; 19: 2214–2216.
134. Blessing K, McLaren KM, Morris R et al. Detection of human papillomavirus in skin and genital lesions of

renal allograft recipients by *in situ* hybridization. Histopathology 1990; 16: 181–185.
135. Ho M, Miller G, Atchinson W et al. Epstein–Barr virus infections and DNA hybridization studies in posttransplantation lymphomas and lymphoproliferative lesions: the role of primary infection. J Infect Dis 1985; 152: 876–886.
136. Hanto DW, Frizzera G, Gajl–Peczalska KJ et al. Epstein–Barr virus-induced B-cell lymphoma after renal transplantation. Acyclovir therapy and transition from polyclonal to monoclonal B-cell proliferation. N Engl J Med 1982; 306: 913–918.
137. Griffith RC, Saha BK, Janney CM et al. Immunoblastic lymphoma of T-cell type in a chronically immuno-suppressed renal transplant recipient. Am J Clin Pathol 1990; 93: 280–285.

Transmission of disease from host to graft

138. Mathew TH. Recurrence of disease following renal transplantation. Am J Kidney Dis 1988; 12: 85–96.
139. Morzycka M, Croker BP, Seigler HF, Tisher CC. Evaluation of recurrent glomerulonephritis in kidney allografts. Am J Med 1982; 72: 588–598.
140. Cameron JS, Senguttuvan P, Hartley B et al. Focal segmental glomerulosclerosis in fifty-nine renal allografts from a single centre: analysis of risk factors for recurrence. Transplant Proc 1989; 21: 2117–2118.
141. Axelsen RA, Seymour AE, Mathew TH, Fisher G, Canny A, Pascoe V. Recurrent focal glomerulosclerosis in renal transplants. Clin Nephrol 1984; 21: 110–114.
142. Striegel JE, Sibley RK, Fryd DS, Mauer SM. Recurrence of focal segmental sclerosis in children following renal transplantation. Kidney Int 1986; 30: S44–S50.
143. Korbet SM, Schwartz MM, Lewis EJ. Recurrent nephrotic syndrome in renal allografts. Am J Kidney Dis 1988; 11: 270–276.
144. Laufer J, Ettenger RB, Ho WG, Cohen AH, Marik JL, Fine RN. Plasma exchange for recurrent nephrotic syndrome following renal transplantation. Transplantation 1988; 46: 540–542.
145. Moritz MJ, Burke JF, Jarrell BE, Carabasi RA. The incidence of membranoproliferative glomerulonephritis in renal allografts.Transplant Proc 1987; 18: 2206–2207.
146. O'Meara Y, Green A, Carmody M. Recurrent glomerulonephritis in renal transplants: fourteen years' experience. Nephrol Dial Transplant 1989; 4: 730–734.
147. Zimmerman SW, Hyman LR, Uehling DT, Burkholder PM. Recurrent membranoproliferative glomerulo-nephritis with glomerular properdin deposition in allografts. Ann Intern Med 1974; 80: 169–175.
148. Glicklich D, Matas AJ, Sablay L et al. Recurrent membranoproliferative glomerulonephritis type I in successive renal transplants. Am J Nephrol 1987; 7: 143–149.
149. McCoy RC, Clapp J, Seigler HF. Membrano-proliferative glomerulonephritis. Progression from the pure form to the crescentic form with recurrence after transplantation. Am J Med 1975; 59: 288–292.
150. Eddy A, Sibley R, Mauer SM, Kim Y. Renal allograft failure due to recurrent dense intramembranous deposit disease. Clin Nephrol 1984; 21: 305–313.
151. Droz D, Nabarra B, Noël L-H, Leibowitch J, Crosnier J. Recurrence of dense deposits in transplanted kidneys: I. Sequential survey of the lesions. Kidney Int 1979; 15: 386–395.
152. Berger J. Recurrence of IgA nephropathy in renal allografts. Am J Kidney Dis 1988; 12: 371–372.
153. Bachman U, Biava C, Amend W et al. The clinical course of IgA-nephropathy and Henoch–Schönlein purpura following renal transplantation. Transplantation 1986; 42: 511–515.
154. Díaz-Tejeiro R, Maduell F, Diez J et al. Loss of renal graft due to recurrent IgA nephropathy with rapidly progressive course: an unusual clinical evolution. Nephron 1990; 54: 341–343.
155. Yussim A, Ben-Bassat M, Shapira Z et al. Post-transplant glomerulonephritis under conventional and cyclosporin A immunosuppression. Transplant Proc 1989; 21: 2119–2120.
156. Hill GS, Robertson J, Grossman R, Perloff L, Barker CF. An unusual variant of membranous nephropathy with abundant crescent formation and recurrence in the transplanted kidney. Clin Nephrol 1978; 10: 114–120.
157. Wilson CB, Dixon FJ. Anti-glomerular basement membrane induced glomerulonephritis. Kidney Int 1973; 3: 74–89.
158. Lerner RA, Glassock RJ, Dixon FJ. The role of antiglomerular basement membrane antibody in the pathogenesis of human glomerulonephritis. J Exp Med 1967; 126: 989–1004.
159. Hasegawa A, Kawamura T, Ito H et al. Fate of renal grafts with recurrent Henoch–Schönlein purpura nephritis in children. Transplant Proc 1989; 21: 2130–2133.
160. Hebert D, Sibley RK, Mauer SM. Recurrence of hemolytic uremic syndrome in renal transplant recipients. Kidney Int 1986; 30: S51–58.
161. Van den Berg-Wolf MG, Kootte AMM, Weening JF, Paul LC. Recurrent hemolytic uremic syndrome in a renal transplant recipient and review of the Leiden experience. Transplantation 1988; 45: 248–251.
162. Eijgenraam FJ, Conckerwolcke RA, Monnens LAH, Proesmans W, Wolff ED, van Damme B. Renal transplantation in 20 children with hemolytic-uremic syndrome. Transplantation 1990; 33: 87–93.
163. Barnes BA, Bergan JJ, Braun WE et al. Renal transplantation in congenital and metabolic diseases. A report from the ASC/NIH Renal Transplant Registry. JAMA 1975; 232: 148–153.
164. Scheinman JI, Najarian JS, Mauer SM. Successful strategies for renal transplantation in primary oxalosis. Kidney Int 1984; 25: 804–811.
165. Bohman S-O, Wilczek H, Tyden G, Jaremko G, Lundgren G, Groth CG. Recurrent diabetic nephropathy in renal allografts placed in diabetic patients and protective effect of simultaneous pancreatic transplantation. Transplant Proc 1988; 19: 2290–2293.
166. Mauer SM, Steffes MW, Connett J, Najarian JS, Sutherland DER, Barbosa J. The development of lesions in the glomerular basement membrane and mesangium after transplantation of normal kidneys to diabetic patients. Diabetes 1983; 32: 948–952.
167. Mauer SM, Goetz FC, McHugh LE et al. Long-term study of normal kidneys transplanted into patients with type I diabetes. Diabetes 1989; 38: 516–523.
168. Najarian JS, Kaufman DB, Fryd DS, McHugh L, Mauer SM, Sutherland DER. Survival into the second decade following kidney transplantation in type I

diabetic patients. Transplant Proc 1989; 21: 2012–2015.
169. Pasternack A, Ahonen J, Kuhlbäck B. Renal transplantation in 45 patients with amyloidosis. Transplantation 1986; 42: 598–601.
170. Friedlaedner MM, Kopolovic J, Rubinger D et al. Renal biopsy in Fabry's disease eight years after successful renal transplantation. Clin Nephrol 1987; 27: 206–211.
171. Spear GS, Gubler MC, Habib R, Broyer M. Renal allografts in cystinosis and mesangial demography. Clin Nephrol 1989; 32: 256–261.
172. Kumano K, Sakai T, Mashimo S et al. A case of recurrent lupus nephritis after renal transplantation. Clin Nephrol 1987; 27: 94–98.
173. Cannon PJ, Hassar M, Case DB, Casarella WJ, Sommers SC, LeRoy EC. The relationship of hypertension and renal failure in scleroderma (progressive systemic sclerosis) to structural and functional abnormalities of the renal cortical circulation. Medicine (Baltimore) 1974; 53: 1–46.
174. Merino GE, Sutherland DER, Kjellstrand CM, Simmons RL, Najarian JS. Renal transplantation for progressive systemic sclerosis with renal failure. Case report and review of previous experience. Am J Surg 1977; 133: 745–749.
175. Miner DJ, Jorkasky DK, Perloff LJ, Grossman RA, Tomaszewski JE. Recurrent sickle cell nephropathy in a transplanted kidney. Am J Kidney Dis 1987; 10: 306–313.
176. Barber WH, Deierhoi MH, Julian BA. Renal transplantation in sickle cell anemia and sickle disease. Clin Transplant 1987; 1: 169–175.
177. Cundy T, Kanis JA, Heynen G, Morris PJ, Oliver DO. Calcium metabolism and hyperparathyroidism after renal transplantation. Q J Med 1983; 52: 67–78.

De novo disease

178. Antignac C, Hinglais N, Gubler M-C, Gagnadoux M-F, Broyer M, Habib R. De novo membranous glomerulonephritis in renal allografts in children. Clin Nephrol 1988; 30: 1–7.
179. Gomez-Campdera FJ, Niembro E. 'De novo' membranous glomerulonephritis in renal allografts in children. Clin Nephrol 1989; 31: 279.
180. Truong L, Gelfand J, D'Agati V et al. De novo membranous glomerulonephropathy in renal allografts: a report of 10 cases and review of the literature. Am J Kidney Dis 1989; 14: 131–144.
181. Ward HJ, Koyle MA. Immunopathologic features of de novo membranous nephropathy in renal allografts. Transplantation 1988; 45: 524–529.
182. Cheigh JS, Mouradian J, Solman M et al. Focal segmental glomerulosclerosis in renal transplants. Am J Kidney Dis 1983; 2: 449–455.
183. McCoy RC, Johnson HK, Stone WJ, Wilson CB. Absence of nephritogenic GBM antigen(s) in some patients with hereditary nephritis. Kidney Int 1982; 21: 642–652.
184. Milliner DS, Pierides AM, Holley KE. Renal transplantation in Alport's syndrome. Anti-glomerular basement membrane glomerulonephritis in the allograft. Mayo Clin Proc 1982; 57: 35–43.
185. Savige JA, Mavrova L, Kincaid-Smith P. Inheritable anti-GBM antibody activity after renal transplantation in Alport's syndrome. Transplantation 1989; 48: 704–705.

PART 2

The Urinary Tract

R. C. B. Pugh, revised by I. D. Ansell

18

R. C. B. Pugh, revised by I. D. Ansell

The ureters

Although the renal pelvis has been referred to in the chapters of this volume that deal with the diseases of the kidneys, its pathology could equally well have been considered in these three final chapters on the ureter, bladder and urethra since all are concerned with the passage of urine from the nephron to the exterior. The continuous transitional epithelial lining of these structures – the urothelium – is subject to similar pathological influences (predominantly those within the urine) in all three sites and thus many conditions of the bladder have their counterpart in ureter and urethra such that the subdivision of the urinary tract into these named anatomical segments (and their separation from the renal pelvis) is to a significant degree artificial. Accordingly, the majority of conditions common to all parts of the urinary tract will be dealt with in the chapter devoted to the bladder: the chapters on the ureter and urethra will discuss mainly those conditions peculiar to the respective structure.

DEVELOPMENT[1,2]

The normal ureter develops as a solid bud which grows from the dorsal aspect of the lower part of the mesonephric (Wolffian) duct into the surrounding mesenchyme, which condenses to form the nephrogenic cap, the precursor of the kidney. The lower end of this ureter soon becomes incorporated into the trigone of the bladder and the upper part of the urethra, both of which are also derived from the Wolffian duct. The embryonic ureter is initially quite short but as it lengthens it becomes canalized; when fully developed constrictions can normally be seen at three levels – in the region of the pelviureteric junction, at the point where the ureter crosses the pelvic brim and just outside the bladder.

ABNORMALITIES OF DEVELOPMENT[2,3]

AGENESIS AND ATRESIA

Agenesis is failure of development of the ureteric bud and when bilateral it is, of course, incompatible with life. When agenesis is unilateral the corresponding half of the trigone of the bladder is absent and the opposite kidney usually hypertrophies. Should the developing ureteric bud fail to canalize *atresia* will result: in place of a normal kidney and ureter there is then a fibrous cord, which usually terminates with a nubbin of dense fibrous tissue (a dysplastic kidney) at its upper end. However, atresia is sometimes incomplete and only the upper part of the ureter fails to canalize; again there is usually a dysplastic kidney at its end.

ECTOPIA AND DUPLICATION[4]

If a ureter originates away from the usual site in the Wolffian duct its lower end will not be incorporated into the bladder in the normal way during the later stages of development; when development is completed the ureteric orifice will be either in the bladder below and medial to its normal position on the trigone or in an ectopic position elsewhere. In the male such ectopic ureteric orifices may be anywhere in the Wolffian duct territory (the ejaculatory duct, the seminal vesicle or the prostate) and in the female either in Wolffian remnants – such as Gartner's duct, which opens at the vestibule – or, if there is any communication between the Wolffian and Müllerian systems, in the vagina or uterus.

Ureteric duplication is one of the commonest malformations of the urinary tract and has been recorded in about 0.7% of autopsy material. Females are affected more frequently than males. The condition is often bilateral and there may be a definite familial tendency to its occurrence. Duplication is *incomplete* when the two ureters join before they enter the bladder and *complete* if there are two separate orifices. When the ureter is bifid (an example of the incomplete form of duplication) there are two renal pelves and two ureteric limbs that join to form a single channel, usually at about the level of the sacroiliac joint. Complete duplication is less common; each ureter then drains a separate renal pelvis, the normal or 'orthotopic' one from the lower part of the renal pelvis opening into the bladder in the usual position and the accessory ureter from the upper part of the pelvis entering either the area of the bladder neck or in an ectopic position. Although on occasions a single ureter is ectopic, it is much commoner for there to be ureteric duplication, with one normally situated ureteric orifice and a second accessory ectopic opening. Usually there is also an associated duplex kidney, the upper part of this being almost invariably dysplastic and draining into the ectopic ureter. Dribbling urinary incontinence occurs in the female if the ectopic ureteric orifice is in the lower part of the urethra or in the vestibule or vagina, and therefore below the level of the sphincters. Dribbling is not a feature if the opening is in the region of the bladder neck because, as in the male, continence is then preserved since entry is above the external sphincter; however, reflux and urinary tract infection are common.

URETEROCELE[4]

A ureterocele is a cystic dilatation of the lower (intravesical submucosal) portion of the ureter with an inner lining of ureteric epithelium and an external covering of bladder epithelium. Occasionally a ureter with a normally sited orifice is affected: the ureteric orifice itself is then usually stenosed. About four times as common is dilatation of an ectopic ureter (ectopic ureterocele) which occurs seven times as frequently in the female as in the male and is occasionally bilateral. It is an important anomaly which usually presents clinically in infancy or childhood but may not become evident until complications develop in adult life. The ectopic orifice is usually not stenosed and indeed is sometimes large enough to permit vesicoureteric reflux.

RARER ANOMALIES[5]

These include triplication of the ureter (which is almost always associated with a malrotated or dysplastic kidney), juxtavesicular diverticulum, blind-ending duplication and valves or kinks in the ureter. Sometimes abnormalities of the ureter result from anomalous development of other organs or tissues. For example, the ureter will be unduly long or short when there is renal ectopia with, respectively, a high thoracic kidney or a low pelvic one. In crossed ectopia, which affects males more than females, the two kidneys are found to be on the same side of the body; the ectopic one is lower than its fellow and its ureter crosses the mid-line to reach the bladder. Bilateral crossed ectopia is an extremely rare abnormality.

An anomalous course of the ureter can result from maldevelopment of the inferior vena cava and persistence of the right posterior cardinal or right subcardinal veins. There are several variants of the anomaly (such as postcaval or circumcaval ureter) which are of clinical importance because the ureter may be obstructed where it is in close relation to the inferior vena cava. There may also be abnormal development of the contralateral kidney.

'PRUNE BELLY' SYNDROME[3,6]

The very rare 'prune belly' syndrome (deficient abdominal musculature syndrome) is a diffuse disorder of mesenchymal development that affects males almost exclusively. The lack of underlying muscle produces redundant, loose, wrinkled skin of the anterior abdominal wall which has a striking resemblance to the skin of a dried prune. The many associated anomalies of the genitourinary system include a large bladder, patent urachus, tortuous ureters (in which fibrosis and scarcity of muscle bundles are found on microscopical examination), dysplastic kidneys, urethral abnormalities and undescended testes. There may or may not be vesicoureteric reflux. Other body systems may be affected and partial forms of the syndrome are recorded.

FUNCTIONAL ANATOMY

The ureters are thick-walled muscular tubes, the obvious function of which is to transmit the urine, continuously produced by the kidney, to the bladder for storage prior to being voided intermittently. The mechanisms thought to be involved have been studied for many years but it is only within the last two decades or so – thanks to the use of the electron microscope, histochemical methods, urodynamic techniques and conventional and more elaborate imaging methods – that a clearer understanding is emerging. It is well established that urine is passed down the ureter by a peristaltic wave and that the excised ureter is capable of contraction under experimental conditions. Much of the earlier work sought to relate these facts directly to the structure of the ureter and in particular to the arrangement of the muscle fibres in its wall. A 'braided' appearance of these fibres in the upper part of the ureter, interlacing spirals with inner longitudinal and outer circular fibres[7] and a helical arrangement[8] have been described by different authors and related to normal and disordered ureteric function.

Recent studies[9] of the normal ureter have shown that the muscle is of uniform thickness throughout. Morphologically distinct longitudinal and circular layers cannot be identified, but the inner fibres tend to be longitudinally disposed and the outer ones are circular or oblique in direction in the upper part of the ureter, whereas near the ureterovesical junction they are almost entirely oblique or longitudinal in orientation. Nerve fibres can be seen in the muscle coat and adventitia, but are not directly responsible for the peristaltic activity of the ureter. This is essentially a function of the muscle itself and intercellular connections, seen with the electron microscope,[10] form an anatomical pathway which allows the spread of electrical impulses from one muscle cell to the next.

The peristaltic waves start in the renal pelvis and it is postulated that they are initiated there either because of its passive stretching by the urine being secreted or because of activation of pacemakers in the minor calyces. When the volume of urine in the pelvis becomes sufficiently large the pelvic contractions pass through the pelviureteric junction as coordinated ureteric contractions. There is no definite evidence that pacemakers exist in the ureter, and the two elements essential for normal ureteric peristalsis are a distending 'bolus' of urine and electrical impulses transmitted along the ureteric muscle. Where the ureter enters the bladder the predominantly longitudinal muscle fibres, together with Waldeyer's sheath (made up of non-striated fibres of the detrusor muscle), are continued into the base of the bladder to form the superficial and deep muscles of the trigone.[11] These are anchored in the region of the verumontanum and the internal and external sphincter. The integrity of the ureterovesical junction depends on the oblique course of the intramural part of the ureter and the length of its submucosal segment, as well as on the resting tone of the muscles of the trigone and intravesical ureter and the state of the detrusor muscle. In a normal bladder this provides a firm muscular backing to the other components of the junction. Muscle tone suffices to keep the ureteric orifice closed except when a ureteric contraction wave forces a 'bolus' of urine through. When voiding occurs simultaneous contraction of the trigonal and detrusor muscles seals the orifice and prevents both efflux and reflux of urine.

ABNORMALITIES OF FUNCTION

Dilatation of the urinary tract may be due to mechanical obstruction, seen for instance when there is hydronephrosis or hydroureter secondary to an enlarged prostate or a ureteric calculus (see p. 686), or, in the absence of any such obvious cause, is indicative of disordered function and regarded as idiopathic. Two idiopathic forms are recognized, idiopathic hydronephrosis and primary megaureter; both are characterized by zones of abnormal function in the ureter (sometimes with obvious local narrowing) respectively at the pelviureteric junction and at the lower end of the ureter, with proximal dilatation.

IDIOPATHIC HYDRONEPHROSIS

In this condition there is dilatation of the renal pelvis and calyces, the ureter being of normal calibre or slightly narrowed (see pp. 467–473). Abnormal blood vessels crossing the external aspect of the pelviureteric junction,[12] sail-like adhesions in the same region, origin of the ureter from the upper part of the renal pelvis,[13] and a preponderance of longitudinal muscle bundles[7] (preventing normal peristalsis) have been suggested as possible causative factors.

It has been shown, however, that the disposition of the muscle fibres is normal, and failure of transmission of the peristaltic wave across the pelviureteric junction has been thought to be due to an increase of collagen which forms an inelastic collar in the upper part of the ureter that prevents distension of the pelviureteric junction.[14] Recently this view has been questioned by the finding of an increased amount of collagen more proximally in the wall of the renal pelvis, without any morphological or histochemical changes in the region of the pelviureteric junction and upper ureter.[15] Since obstruction of the pelviureteric junction is probably multifactorial in pathogenesis it is not surprising that a variety of pathological findings has been described.[16]

PRIMARY MEGAURETER (OBSTRUCTED MEGAURETER, NON-REFLUXING MEGAURETER, IDIOPATHIC MEGAURETER)

In this disorder the ureter is dilated and hypertrophied, and actively peristaltic throughout its length except at the distal end where there is an apparently narrowed segment. Although the ureteric lumen is slightly reduced in this area a probe can be passed through it and there is no reflux. The condition is more often unilateral than bilateral and may be accompanied by other abnormalities in the genitourinary system. Most cases are seen in childhood but clinical manifestations sometimes do not appear until adult life. The urodynamic findings are often difficult to interpret (as is also often the case in patients with idiopathic hydronephrosis)[17] and many theories have been put forward in an attempt to explain them and the clinical features. A preponderance of circular muscle[18] or a total muscular defect[14] at the lower end of the ureter had been suggested but recent work has shown that the changes seen with both the light microscope and the electron microscope have many similarities to those seen in the region of the pelviureteric junction in idiopathic hydronephrosis. There is an increase of collagen not only in the functionally inert segment of ureter but also in the dilated and hypertrophied ureter proximal to it.

It would appear, then, that in neither idiopathic hydronephrosis nor primary megaureter is the presence of areas of inelastic collagen in the ureteric wall the primary anomaly;[15] rather, there may be some primary developmental defect of the pelvic and ureteric smooth muscle with a secondary overproduction of collagen. It can, therefore, be fairly said that the true cause of both these disorders has yet to be determined, and it is interesting to note that both these functional obstructions occur at sites which are known to be constricted during fetal life.

MEGAURETER–MEGACYSTIS SYNDROME[19]

This uncommon condition is a disorder of childhood in which there is a very large thin-walled untrabeculated bladder with a large trigone and laterally placed, usually widely open, ureteric orifices. The bladder is capable of emptying without residue but there is frequently reflux of urine into grossly dilated ureters.

VESICOURETERIC REFLUX[20]

Any structural alteration of or interference with the action of the various components of the ureterovesical junction may permit reflux of urine into the ureter when the intravesical pressure rises, for whatever reason. Reflux may be regarded as primary when there is failure of development of the ureterovesical junction mechanism – for instance, when the intramural segment of the ureter is unduly short or there is lack of the firm muscular backing of the detrusor muscle in the region of the ureteric hiatus in the bladder wall. Reflux is classed as secondary when there is an obvious outflow obstruction due, for example, to urethral valves or a neuropathic bladder. Primary reflux in children may be recoverable and there is evidence of racial differences in incidence and possibly also of a familial prediposition. Reflux often occurs in urinary tract infection due, it is thought, to oedema or impaired muscular activity at the orifice. It may also be present in the rare 'prune belly' syndrome (see p. 683).

Reflux may be graded as mild (Grade 1) when urine enters the ureters only, as moderate (Grade 2) when there is also filling of the pelvicalyceal system without dilatation and as severe (Grade 3) when calyceal dilatation occurs. In itself reflux is not necessarily harmful but if the structure of the renal papillae permits intrarenal reflux, so that urine enters the kidney itself, parenchymal scarring (reflux nephropathy) is likely to supervene if the urine is infected (see pp. 436, 439–444, 472–473).

TRAUMA

Damage to the ureters by external violence is not at all common and in civilian practice is usually the result of a road traffic accident. The victim is almost always a pedestrian and more often a child than an adult. The most frequent type of injury is rupture or avulsion of the ureter at or within a short distance of the pelviureteric junction and clinically the lesion may be masked by the extent and severity of other injuries sustained in the accident.[21]

Ureteric injury due to penetrating wounds of the abdomen has been recorded in between 2 and 4% of battle casualties in World Wars I and II, and in Vietnam.[22] It was also noted in 2.25% of patients admitted to hospital during civil hostilities in Northern Ireland[23] after wounding by a variety of low and high velocity missiles, rubber bullets and other weapons. Low velocity missiles cause damage to structures directly in their path whereas with high velocity missiles there is, in addition, widespread and often very severe injury due to cavitation of the tissues by the blast waves generated by the projectile. The ureter may be completely or partially ruptured or if seen at laparotomy soon after wounding by a high velocity missile may appear only to be bruised. However, the blast wave is liable to cause vascular damage and this can result in necrosis in the bruised area followed by fistula formation. This may be evident within 2–4 days or it may be delayed.[24] Ureteric injury almost never occurs as an isolated event and it is usually accompanied by damage to other parts of the urinary tract, the bowel and other intra-abdominal organs and, as in road accident victims, these other injuries often mask the damage to the ureter.

The ureters are at risk in virtually all major abdominal operations and, for instance, may be crushed or inadvertently divided during the course of gynaecological operations, in excision of the rectum or during vascular reconstruction operations in the region of the pelvic brim. Damage may follow the passage of a stone or the use of the expanding Dormia basket for the endoscopic removal of stones[25] or after overvigorous attempts at retrograde ureteric catheterization. Residual local scarring is likely to cause a degree of outflow obstruction with, possibly, some renal damage as well. If urine escapes into the surrounding tissues a 'urinoma'[26] develops, with much fibroblastic proliferation and fibrosis, and sometimes fistula formation. So-called 'spontaneous' rupture is a rare complication of a ureteric stone.[27]

CALCULOUS DISEASE[28–32]

The vast majority of calculi found in the ureter have migrated there from the renal pelvis. Several types of stones occur; these have been described in Chapter 14 (see pp. 531–544).

Stones associated with infection of the urinary tract are composed of magnesium ammonium phosphate or calcium phosphate; they occur particularly as a consequence of infection by species of proteus and are predisposed to by anatomical or functional abnormalities such as an ectopic ureter or primary megaureter, or obstruction due to a ureteric tumour. Metabolic and idiopathic stones may acquire a coating of phosphate if the urine is infected. Stones occasionally form round foreign bodies in the ureter.[32]

Ureteric stones are commoner in men than in women and most are seen in patients between the ages of 20 and 50 years. In this age group men tend to have calcium oxalate stones, whereas in women phosphate stones associated with infection are more usual. In later life the reverse is often the case. Most stones that enter the ureter are small and are likely to traverse its full length, entering the bladder without any apparent difficulty and often without producing any symptoms. However, if a calculus is of any appreciable size it is likely to become impacted and this is liable to occur at one of the normally narrower parts of the ureter (at its origin from the renal pelvis, where it crosses the brim of the bony pelvis and where it enters the bladder – see p. 682) or where there is any pre-existing obstruction, for example, due to a tumour or a fibrous stricture. An impacted stone which does not completely occlude the lumen may gradually increase in size. Impaction will exacerbate any colic and may lead to proximal dilatation of the tract; pyonephrosis may follow if infection is present. At the site of impaction there is likely to be local inflammation, sometimes leading to ulceration and periureteritis or to a 'urinoma' and, later, to stricture formation.

INFLAMMATORY CONDITIONS

NON-SPECIFIC URETERITIS

Non-specific inflammation of the ureter is most commonly seen as part of a more widespread inflammatory process in the urinary tract, but occasionally complicates local pelvic disease in the female, for example salpingo-oophoritis, or bowel lesions such as diverticulitis. In the majority of cases of pyelonephritis and pyelitis the ureter is also involved in varying degree, and in many patients with lower urinary tract inflammation either or both of the ureteric orifices may become incompetent, permitting vesicoureteric reflux and the passage of infected urine into the ureter. Renal infection may follow; the most likely mechanism is an intraluminal mechanical transfer of organisms when there is a reflux of urine, although the blood stream and lymphatic channels cannot altogether be ruled out as possible alternative routes. Trauma to the mucosal surface by the passage of a stone or by instrumentation or the presence of any existing functional or organic obstruction is likely to aggravate or perpetuate infection.

The organisms most often concerned are those generally found in urinary tract infections, *Escherichia coli* and *Proteus* species being the commonest.[33] The tissue changes in acute and chronic ureteritis are non-specific, although in the acute stage local oedema may interfere with peristalsis. If the inflammation is more severe ulceration will occur and when this heals, or the infection becomes chronic, there will almost certainly be fibrosis and thickening of the ureteric wall. Permanent obstruction can result. Sometimes the mucosal surface of an inflamed ureter has a granular appearance because of subepithelial collections of lymphoid cells (ureteritis follicularis). Gangrenous ureteritis is a rare form of the disease which occasionally results from bacterial infection but, more commonly, complicates extensive pelvic operations and is then thought to be of ischaemic nature following damage to the blood supply.[34] The lower part of the ureter is most often affected and a ureterovaginal fistula is likely to develop.

TUBERCULOUS URETERITIS

Tuberculous ureteritis is always secondary to renal tuberculosis and results from spread from one or more foci of active disease in the kidney and renal pelvis, usually by extension along mucosal surfaces but occasionally by the lymphatics. In the earlier stages typical tubercles are seen in the lamina propria, often with much local oedema which is likely to narrow the lumen. As the disease progresses the tubercles coalesce, granulation tissue forms and fibrosis develops: the ureter becomes transformed into a rigid fibrous tube, and the lumen contains tuberculous material. Later, the ureter becomes increasingly narrow, periureteritis develops and the ureter becomes fixed to the surrounding tissues. Strictures are particularly liable to develop in the untreated case and are most often to be found in the lower part of the ureter, specially in the region of the ureterovesical junction; they sometimes occur in the region of the pelviureteric junction but are rare in the middle third.[35] So long as some vestige of lumen remains tuberculous material will continue to be discharged into the bladder, but if there is complete occlusion the renal pelvis and the ureter above the obstruction will slowly fill up with caseous debris. Modern chemotherapy combined with radical and reconstructive surgery has greatly improved the prognosis.[36]

Proliferative and reactive changes (von Brunn's nests and the cystic lesion traditionally referred to as ureteritis cystica) are often seen in the mucosa adjacent to or surrounding areas of inflammation or tumour formation. Similar changes occur elsewhere in the urinary tract and are described in detail later (see p. 712). Ureteritis cystica (Figs 18.1,18.2) is of interest as the cysts are occasionally of such a size as to produce a characteristic radiological appearance; they may even cause some degree of ureteric obstruction. Areas of adenomatous metaplasia ('nephrogenic adenoma') (see p. 718) may be seen also, as filling defects in a urogram.[37]

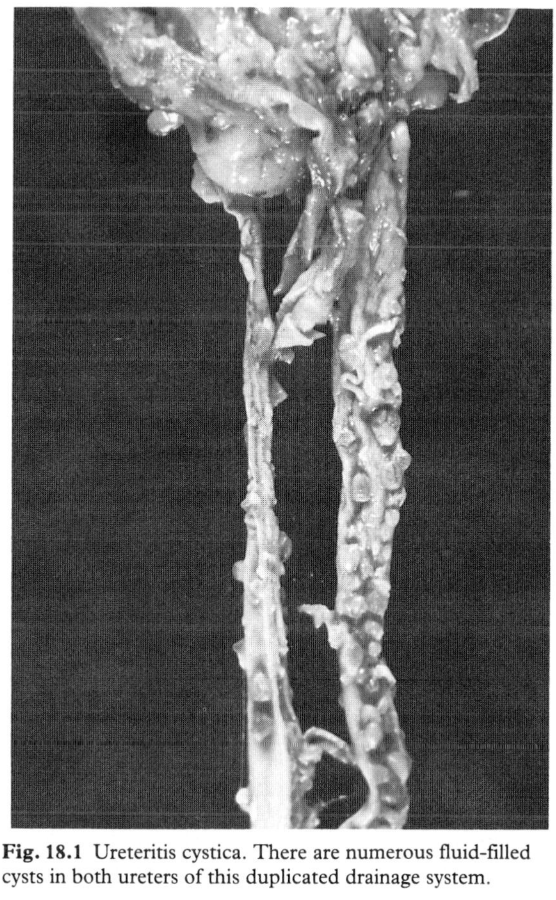

Fig. 18.1 Ureteritis cystica. There are numerous fluid-filled cysts in both ureters of this duplicated drainage system.

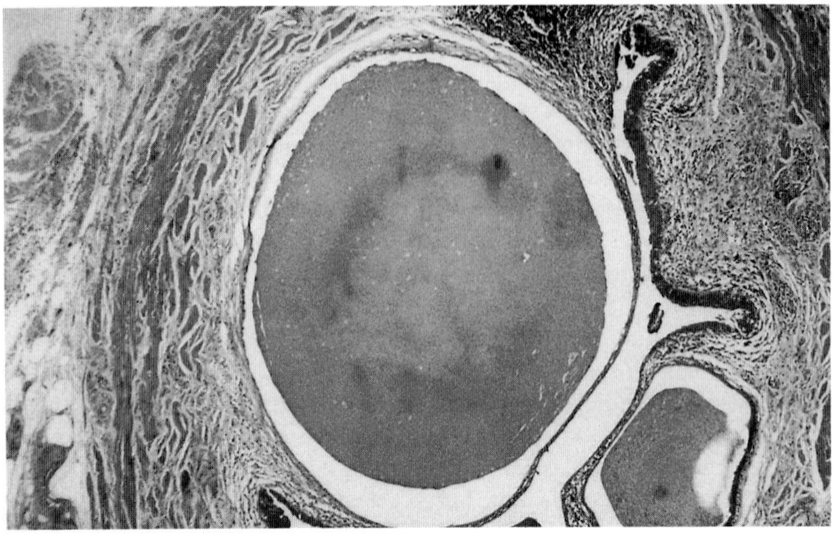

Fig. 18.2 Ureteritis cystica. Cysts are seen to be filled with coagulated fluid and to have a simple epithelial lining.
Haematoxylin and eosin × 34

PARASITIC INFESTATION

SCHISTOSOMIASIS (BILHARZIASIS)

Ureteric involvement with stricture formation is one of the most common and potentially serious manifestations of infestation with *Schistosoma haematobium*, which causes schistosomiasis in Egypt and in parts of Central and Southern Africa and the Middle East. The lesions are often bilateral but may be unilateral. In the acute stages of the disease lesions similar to those found in the bladder (see p. 713) occur in the lower part of the ureter with maximal involvement of the juxtavesical segment: they comprise sandy patches, polypi, ureteritis cystica and glandular change (ureteritis glandularis) as well as areas of ulceration. The upper part of the ureter is usually spared. The late stages are characterized by dense fibrosis and obstruction particularly affecting the juxtavesical and intramural segments.[38] The ureter above the obstruction usually dilates and becomes tortuous and, unless a free flow of urine is restored, urinary tract infection, stone formation and progressive impairment of renal function will follow. Ova, often heavily calcified, are commonly found in the fibrosed area. Schistosomal infestation in Natal (South Africa) has a much more favourable prognosis because of the lower incidence of mechanical obstruction of the ureter in the chronic stages of the disease.[39]

TUMOURS

BENIGN TUMOURS

The benign lesions most often seen in the ureter are *fibroepithelial polyps*; these occur particularly in children and young adults. The lesions are lobulated and have a slender stalk. They are usually single but may be multiple, and they are most frequently found in the upper third of the ureter (Fig. 18.3) where they produce an irregular filling defect in the intravenous urogram and cause some degree of ureteric obstruction.[40] Some polyps occur in the lower part of the ureter and may even protrude through the ureteric orifice. The free surface is covered by a layer of transitional epithelium continuous with the lining of the ureter and there is a central fibrovascular core which often includes some wisps of smooth muscle and is sometimes infiltrated by a few chronic inflammatory cells. The so-called 'inverted' papilloma has been recorded in the ureter[41] but most examples are seen in the bladder (see p. 730).

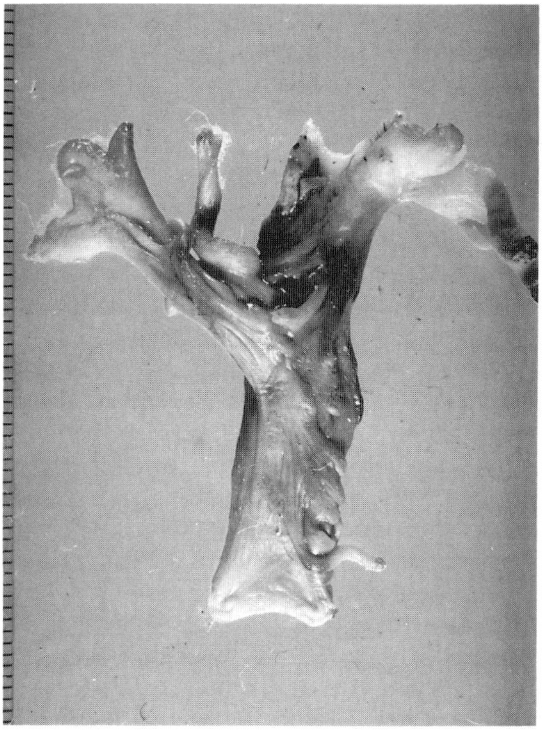

Fig. 18.3 Fibroepithelial polyp. Typical ureteric fibroepithelial polyp with branching 'antler-like' appearance which gives it its characteristic appearance in the intravenous pyelogram

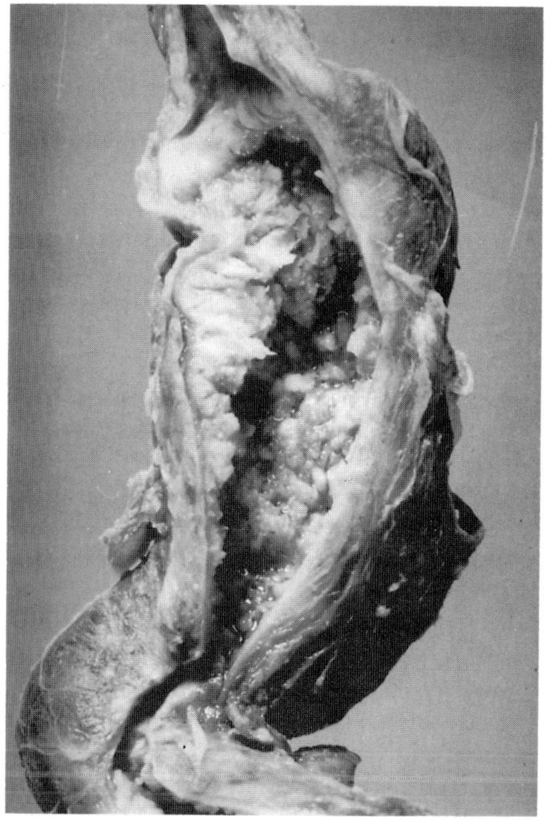

Fig. 18.4 Carcinoma of ureter. Non-invasive transitional cell carcinoma with typical fronded appearance and dilatation of the ureter above the growth.

On rare occasions a *fibroma, leiomyoma or angioma* is found in the ureter.

MALIGNANT TUMOURS

Primary malignant tumours are very much commoner in the ureter than benign ones. The majority are of epithelial origin, usually as part of a generalized urothelial neoplasia. Tumours elsewhere in the tract may precede or coexist with a ureteric carcinoma or develop at a later stage, and it is probable that in less than 5% of cases the ureter is the only part of the urinary tract to be involved. In generalized urothelial disease the tumours occur more commonly in the bladder and urethra than in the upper reaches of the tract.[42] Of the proximal tumours about 40% are found in the renal pelvis and calyces and about 45% in the ureter; in the remaining cases there are tumours both in the calyces and in the ureter. The right and left ureters are affected equally; most of the tumours are situated in the lower part of the ureter; they tend to assume a cylindrical shape and cause a variable amount of ureteric obstruction (Fig. 18.4). The ureter proximal to the obstruction becomes hypertrophic and later dilates. The majority of tumours are transitional cell carcinomas; when neoplasia is a complication of calculous disease the tumour is usually of squamous type and squamous carcinoma of the ureter is particularly infrequent in the absence of stone. In rare instances a ureteric tumour is a glandular carcinoma.

In general, ureteric tumours tend to be well differentiated and non-invasive or only superficially invasive (stages pTa to pT1; see p. 729) and in only about one-third of cases is there evidence of spread into or beyond the muscle coat. In many cases microscopy reveals dysplasia or in situ carcinoma in the urothelium adjacent to the ureteric tumour.[43] Widespread multifocal tumour formation, poor differentiation and penetration of the muscle are among the factors which determine a poor prognosis. The aetiology, age, sex incidence and general characteristics of ureteric tumours are similar to those of bladder cancer and are considered in detail on pages 719–730.

An uncommon lesion is the so-called 'stump tumour' which arises in the residual ureter months or even years after simple nephrectomy for malignant disease or for a benign condition such as nephrolithiasis.[44]

Tumours occasionally arise at the site of a ureterocolic anastomosis,[45] either within a short time (usually measured in months rather than years) after diversion necessitated by malignant disease or after a period of up to 20 or more years in patients with benign disease such as vesical exstrophy. It has been suggested that nitrosamines may have a role in carcinogenesis at this site.[46] Tumours are also on record at the ureteroileal anastomosis in an ileal conduit.[47]

Secondary tumours of the ureter are uncommon and are usually a result of direct extension from a primary growth in an adjacent organ (see p. 690). Haematogenous metastasis to the ureter is extremely rare.

URETERIC OBSTRUCTION AND DILATATION

Obstruction of the upper part of the urinary tract due to a disorder of function (megaureter) (see 'Idiopathic hydronephrosis' and 'Primary megaureter', page 684) has to be distinguished from obstruction due to mechanical or physiological causes. An obstruction can be caused by stricture formation or by kinking of the ureter and, depending upon how complete it is and the length of time it has been present, there will be a variable amount of proximal myohypertrophy and dilatation of the lumen.

Temporary obstruction often occurs during an episode of acute cystitis due to oedema of the ureteric orifice. Bilateral dilatation is also seen when there is bladder outflow obstruction, as occurs in patients with prostatic enlargement. In pregnancy, too, some ureteric dilatation is common; in the early stages this is attributed to hormonal influence on the ureteric musculature and in the later stages to pressure of the enlarging uterus on the structures at the pelvic brim.

Mechanical obstruction may be produced by lesions outside the ureter, for example, congenital anomalies (see retrocaval ureter, p. 683) or inflammatory conditions such as psoas abscess, diverticulitis and Crohn's disease, as well as by pelvic lipomatosis, retroperitoneal fibrosis and retroperitoneal tumours. It may also be caused by conditions affecting the wall of the ureter such as amyloidosis, endometriosis, schistosomiasis, ureteritis and neoplasms; and it may result when the lumen is occupied by calculi (probably the commonest of mechanical causes), tumour tissue, blood clot, fungus balls or inflammatory debris. Some of these conditions call for further comment.

NEOPLASTIC OBSTRUCTION

The ureter may be involved by direct extension of primary neoplasms of the cervix, bowel or ovary, or by malignant lymphoma in the retroperitoneal tissues[48] or in lymph nodes at the pelvic brim. Probably the tumours which most frequently cause obstruction are those arising in the bladder or prostate. The urothelial carcinomas are frequently multifocal and widespread, and ureteric obstruction occurs not only when there is an occluding intraluminal tumour, but also if tumour tissue overlies the ureteric orifice in the bladder. Ureteric obstruction is often bilateral in cases of prostatic carcinoma. It must not be forgotten that radiotherapy may result in fibrotic obstruction of one or both of the ureters.[49]

RETROPERITONEAL FIBROSIS [50,51]

The essential feature of this condition is the formation of excessive amounts of fibrous tissue in the retroperitoneal space. In the earlier stages of the disease this tissue is of fairly loose texture and is often diffusely or focally infiltrated with inflammatory cells. In the later stages a firm dense plaque forms and surrounds all the retroperitoneal structures. The process usually starts in the region of the pelvic brim and extends up on one or both sides, often reaching the level of the renal vessels or very occasionally the crura of the diaphragm. Many occluded vessels are seen in the typical plaque and although the ureters are surrounded by fibrous tissue they can often be dissected surprisingly easily during the operation of ureterolysis. Despite the evidence of functional obstruction and back pressure, the lumen of the ureter is usually patent on retrograde catheterization. The cause of the condition is as yet unknown. The cellular infiltration suggests an inflammatory origin and the presence of occlusive lesions in many of the vessels has prompted the idea of a primary vascular basis, while an association with certain drugs such as methysergide has also been noted.[51] Retroperitoneal fibrosis is also recorded as a complication of intravesical formalin therapy for a bladder carcinoma[52] and there is a well-known association with other forms of the fibromatoses such as primary mediastinal fibrosis.[51]

AMYLOIDOSIS[53]

Localized primary amyloidosis of the ureter is a very rare lesion which may be a cause of ureteral stricture and mural calcification.

ENDOMETRIOSIS[54]

Endometriosis of the ureter is rare and typically affects the distal third of the ureter in the third and fourth decades. Two forms of the disease are described – extrinsic, in which there is no invasion beyond the adventitia although the ureter may become compressed, and intrinsic, in which there is infiltration of the ureteric wall by the ectopic tissue, often with much local fibrosis (Fig. 18.5). The intrinsic form is particularly liable to be mistaken for carcinoma.

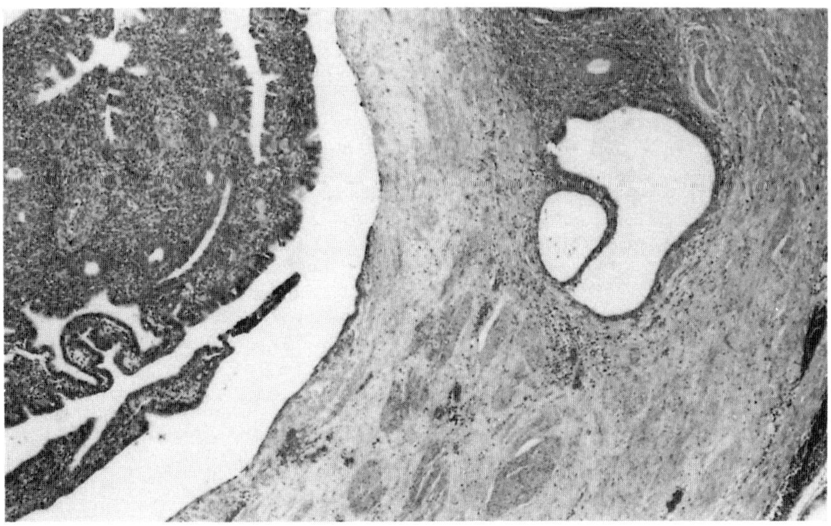

Fig. 18.5 Endometriosis of ureter. Intrinsic endometriosis with glands and stroma in the muscular wall of the ureter and also in the lamina propria.
Haematoxylin and eosin: × 100

REFERENCES

Development

1. Moffat DB. Development of the urogenital system in the male. In: Chisholm GD, Fair WR eds. Scientific foundations of urology, 3rd edn. London: Heinemann, 1990; 231–242.
2. Hill GS. Renal and ureteral abnormalities. In: Hill GS ed. Uropathology. Edinburgh: Churchill Livingstone, 1989; 1–13.

Abnormalities of development

3. Moffat DB. Developmental abnormalities of the urogenital system. In: Chisholm GD, Fair WR, eds. Scientific foundations of urology, 3rd edn. London: Heinemann, 1990; 242–256.
4. Williams DI. Ureteric duplications and ectopia. In: Williams DI, Johnston JH, eds. Paediatric urology, 2nd edn. London: Butterworth, 1982; 167–187.
5. Johnston JH. Upper urinary tract obstructions. In: Williams DI, Johnston JH, eds. Paediatric urology, 2nd edn. London: Butterworth, 1982; 189–213.
6. Hill GS. Prune-belly syndrome. In: Hill GS, ed. Uropathology. Edinburgh: Churchill Livingstone, 1989; 121–126.

Functional anatomy

7. Murnaghan CF. Mechanism of congenital hydronephrosis with reference to factors influencing surgical treatment. Ann R Coll Surg Engl 1958; 23: 25–46.
8. Tanagho EA. Ureteral embryology, developmental anatomy and myology. In: Boyarsky S, Tanagho EA, Zimskind P, Gottschalk D, eds. Urodynamics: hydrodynamics of the ureter and renal pelvis. New York: Academic Press, 1971; 3–74
9. Gosling JA, Dixon JS, Humpherson JR. Functional anatomy of the urinary tract. Edinburgh: Churchill Livingstone, 1983.
10. Whitaker RH. Pathophysiology of the ureter. In: Chisholm GD, Fair WR, eds. Scientific foundations of urology, 3rd edn. London: Heinemann, 1990; 260–266.
11. Tanagho EA, Pugh RCB. The anatomy and function of the ureterovesical junction. Br J Urol 1963; 35: 151–165.

Abnormalities of function

12. Quinby WC. Hydronephrosis. J Urol 1923; 10: 45
13. Ostling K. The genesis of hydronephrosis. Acta Chir Scand [Suppl] 1942; 72.
14. Hanna MK, Jeffs RD, Sturgis JM, Barkin M. Ureteral structure and ultrastructure. II. Congenital uretero-pelvic junction obstruction and primary obstructive megaureter. J Urol 1976; 116: 725–730.
15. Gosling JA, Dixon JS. Functional obstruction of the ureter and renal pelvis. A histological and electron microscopic study. Br J Urol 1978; 50: 145–152.
16. Hill GS. Ureteropelvic junction obstruction. In: Hill GS, ed. Uropathology. Edinburgh: Churchill Livingstone, 1989; 575–598.
17. Whitaker RH. Upper urinary tract obstruction: the use of dynamic studies. Rec Advanc Urol Androl 1981; 3: 45–50.
18. Hutch JA, Tanagho EA. Aetiology of non-occlusive ureteral dilatation. J Urol 1965; 93: 177–184.
19. Johnston JH. Bladder disorders. In: Williams DI, Johnston JH, eds. Paediatric urology, 2nd edn. London: Butterworth, 1982; 225–237.
20. Ransley PG. Pathogenesis and classification of vesico-ureteric reflux. Rec Advanc Urol Androl 1981; 3: 63–72.

Trauma

21. Palmer JM, Drago JR. Ureteral avulsion from non-penetrating trauma. J Urol 1981; 125: 108–111.
22. Selikowitz SM. Penetrating high velocity genito-urinary injuries. J Urol 1977; 118: 947–949.
23. Archbold JAA, Barros d'Sa AAB, Morrison E. Genitourinary injuries of civil hostilities. Br J Surg 1981; 68: 625–631.
24. Cetti NE. Delayed urinary fistula from high velocity missile injury to the ureter. Ann R Coll Surg Engl 1983; 65: 286–288.
25. Hodge J. Avulsion of a long segment of ureter with a Dormia basket. Br J Urol 1973; 45: 328.
26. Trapnell JE. Spontaneous rapture of the renal pelvis and ureter. Br J Surg 1969; 56: 33–39.
27. El-Boghdadly SA. Spontaneous rupture of the ureter proximal to ureteric stone. J R Soc Med 1985; 78: 255–257.

Calculous disease

28. Anderson DA. Historical and geographic differences in the pattern of incidence of urinary stones considered in relation to possible aetiological factors. In: Hodgkinson A, Nordin BEC, eds. Renal stone research symposium. London: Churchill, 1969.
29. Blacklock NJ. Urolithiasis: epidemiology. In: Chisholm GD, Fair WR, eds. Scientific foundations of urology, 3rd edn. London: Heinemann, 1990; 170–175.
30. Sutor DJ. Crystallographic analysis of urinary calculi. In: Chisholm GD, Williams DI, eds. Scientific foundations of urology, 2nd edn. London: Heinemann, 1982; 259–267.
31. Drach GW. Urinary lithiasis. In: Walsh PC, Gittes RF, Perlmutter AD, Stamey TA, eds. Campbells's Urology. Philadelphia: Saunders. 1986; 1094–1190.
32. Androulakakis P, Deliveliotis A. Ureteric stone formed on a polyester suture: case report. Int Surg 1982; 67: 83.

Inflammatory conditions

33. Crump J, Peal L, Maskell R. Urinary infections in general practice. Lancet 1976; 1: 1184–1185.
34. Michaels JP. Study of ureteral blood supply and its bearing on necrosis of the ureter following the Wertheim operation. Surg Gynecol Obstet 1948; 86: 36–44.
35. Gow JG. Genitourinary tuberculosis. In: Blandy JP, ed. Urology. Oxford: Blackwell Scientific, 1976; 222–260.
36. Gow JG, Barbosa S. Genitourinary tuberculosis. A study of 1117 cases over a period of 34 years. Br J Urol 1984; 56: 449–455.
37. Ford TF, Watson GM, Cameron KM. Adenomatous metaplasia (nephrogenic adenoma) of urothelium. An analysis of 70 cases. Br J Urol 1985; 57 427–433.

Parasitic infestation

38. Al-Shukri S, Alwan MH. Bilharzial strictures of the lower third of the ureter: a critical review of 560 strictures. Br J Urol 1983; 55: 477–482.
39. Naude JH. The natural history of ureteric bilharzia. Br J Urol 1984; 56: 599–601.

Tumours

40. Chang HH, Ray P, Ockuly E, Guinan P. Benign fibrous ureteral polyps. Urology 1987; 30 114–118.
41. Perrin P, Dutrieux N, Durand L. Inverted papilloma of the ureter. Br J Urol 1984; 56: 223.
42. Booth CM, Cameron KM, Pugh RCB. Urothelial carcinoma of the kidney and ureter. Br J Urol 1980; 52: 430–435.
43. Auld CD, Grigor KM, Fowler JW. Histopathological review of transitional cell carcinoma. Br J Urol 1984; 56: 485–489.
44. Wisheart JD. Primary tumours of the ureteric stump following nephrectomy. Br J Urol 1968; 40: 344–349.
45. Whitaker RH, Pugh RCB, Dow D. Colonic tumours following uretero-sigmoidostomy. Br J Urol 1971; 43: 562–575.
46. Stewart M, Hill MJ, Pugh RCB, Williams JP. The role of N-nitrosamine in carcinogenesis at the uretero-colic anastomosis. Br J Urol 1981; 53: 115–118.
47. Shousha S, Scott J, Polak J. Ileal loop carcinoma after cystectomy for bladder extrophy. Br Med J 1978; 2: 397–398.

Ureteric obstruction and dilatation

48. Ligthelm RJ, Lister TA. Malignant lymphoma of the ureter. Br J Urol 1985; 57: 587.
49. Sklaroff DM, Gnaneswaran P, Sklaroff RB. Post-irradiation ureteric stricture. Gynecol Oncol 1978; 6: 538.
50. Baker LRI, Mallinson WJW, Gregory MC et al. Idiopathic retroperitoneal fibrosis. A retrospective analysis of 60 cases. Br J Urol 1988; 60: 497–503.
51. Bullock N. Idiopathic retroperitoneal fibrosis. Br Med J 1988; 297: 240.
52. Ferrie BG, Smith PJB. Retroperitoneal fibrosis complicating intravesical formalin therapy. J R Soc Med 1983; 76: 831.
53. Farrands PA, Tribe CR, Slade N. Localised amyloid of the ureter – a case report and review of the literature. Histopathology 1983; 7: 613–622.
54. Klein RS, Cattolica EV. Ureteral endometriosis. Urology 1979; 13: 477–482.

19

R. C. B. Pugh, revised by I. D. Ansell

The bladder

DEVELOPMENT[1]

The greater part of the urinary bladder, the upper portion of the male urethra and the whole of the female urethra are of endodermal origin and develop from the vesicourethral canal. This is the upper part of the primitive urogenital sinus which forms when the primitive cloaca is divided into two by the urorectal septum as it grows down to reach the cloacal membrane. Later, mesoderm grows forwards from each side of the upper or cranial part of the primitive streak and passes between the ectodermal and endodermal layers of the cloacal membrane, fusing in the midline to form the genital tubercle. Initially the vesicourethral canal is continuous at its cranial end with the allantois but the lumen of this channel (the urachus) is obliterated gradually and the urachus becomes transformed into the median umbilical ligament. The trigone of the bladder and posterior wall of the urethra are also of mesodermal origin: they are derived from the lower ends of the mesonephric ducts as these are absorbed into the vesicourethral canal. The lower part of the abdominal wall, between the umbilicus and the symphysis pubis, is quite thin in its early development and consists of ectoderm and endoderm separated by a layer of mesoderm. Sheets of muscle later grow into the mesoderm from the somites and form the definitive abdominal musculature.

The *epithelium* lining the bladder is specialized to allow for continual distension and relaxation following urine storage and micturition. It is composed of three to six layers of basal and intermediate cells of similar appearance and a covering of large flatter more impervious 'umbrella' cells. This is traditionally called *transitional epithelium*, denoting that it is intermediate between squamous and glandular; more recently the term *urothelium* has been introduced to underline the fact that the epithelium lining renal pelves, ureters, bladder and urethra has an identical histological appearance and is subject to the same neoplastic and non-neoplastic lesions which follow exposure to urine and its contents.

ABNORMALITIES OF DEVELOPMENT[2]

Congenital abnormalities of the bladder are of several types and of varying complexity and severity, the rarest being agenesis (which is usually associated with other serious abnormalities), duplication and hourglass deformity. Diverticula, which may occur either at the ureteric hiatus in the bladder wall or in the region of the urachus, usually become evident only if there is lower urinary tract obstruction. The two most important groups of anomalies are lesions of the urachus and vesical exstrophy.

LESIONS OF THE URACHUS[3]

In the adult all that usually remains of the urachus outside the bladder is a midline fibrous band which runs between the apex of the bladder and the umbilicus (the median umbilical ligament) and sometimes contains a central column of epithelial cells. In the bladder wall itself cystic urachal remnants are found quite commonly in the region of the fundus: there is a small central lumen and the cyst wall consists of a layer of cuboidal, low columnar or transitional epithelium, a narrow connective tissue lamina propria and a smooth muscle sheath that is circumferentially arranged and distinct from the surrounding bladder muscle (Fig. 19.1).

Part or all of the urachus may remain patent after birth. If the entire canal is open (patent urachus or urachal fistula), urine will leak from the umbilicus. This is usually an isolated anomaly but is sometimes seen in infants with spina bifida or a neuropathic bladder, or in boys with the 'prune belly' syndrome (see p. 683) and obstruction of the membranous urethra due to stenosis or atresia. Patency at the vesical end leads to the formation of no more than a urachal diverticulum; if the other end is patent there is a urachal sinus at the umbilicus. A urachal cyst forms if both ends are closed and part of the intervening portion distends; such cysts may be solitary or multiple and occur most frequently in the lower part of the urachus. All these lesions are liable to episodes of infection and inflammation; the lining then often undergoes metaplasia to squamous or mucus-secreting columnar epithelium.

The majority of tumours arising in the urachus are derived from the epithelial lining and less commonly from the surrounding connective tissue and smooth muscle. The most frequent types are adenomas or adenocarcinomas (see p. 729), though squamous carcinomas and, more rarely, transitional cell carcinomas may occur. Adenomas are usually quite small and often are symptomless. Urachal adenocarcinomas arise from remnants within the bladder wall or outside it in the supravesical area where they form a mass that is often of considerable size. Involvement of the mucosal surface of the bladder is sometimes, but by no means invariably, seen. The prognosis is not

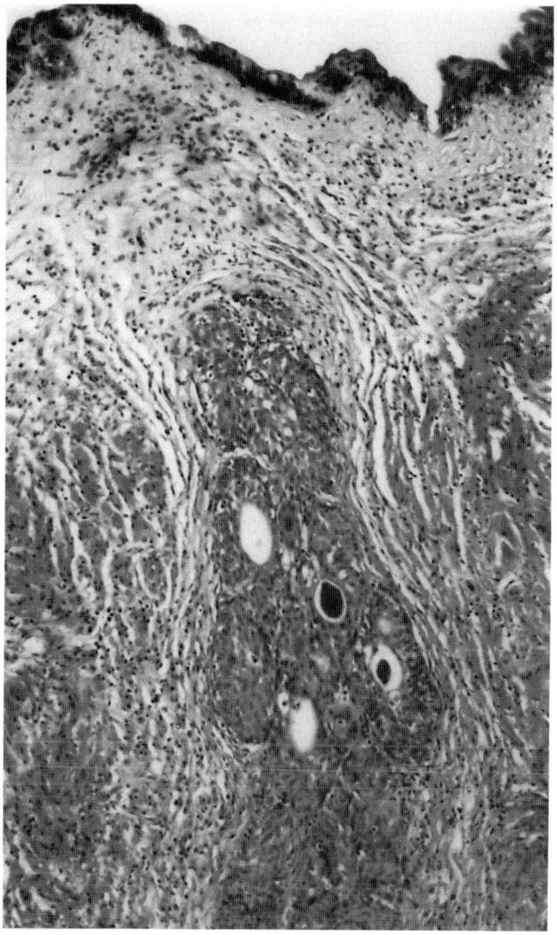

Fig. 19.1 Urachal remnant. Aggregate of urothelial cells with early cyst formation between muscle bundles of the detrusor. Haematoxylin–eosin × 90

good and wide excision of the affected part of the bladder wall and also of the tissues up to the umbilicus is necessary if local recurrence is to be avoided.

VESICAL EXSTROPHY[4,5]

In this condition the mesoderm that migrates forwards into the cloacal membrane from the primitive streak fails to reach the midline, possibly because the membrane is unduly large. The anterior bladder wall and the infraumbilical part of the anterior abdominal wall will therefore not develop normally; the genital tubercle will be displaced caudally and its two paired primitive components may be incompletely fused in the midline. The thin infraumbilical layers of ectoderm and endoderm break down, the exact type of the defect that results depending on the stage in intrauterine development at which this occurs.

The least severe anomalies are epispadias without exstrophy (see p. 743) and the rare condition of incomplete exstrophy or superior or inferior vesical fissure in which, because only part of the membrane fails to be invaded by mesoderm, the exstrophy is confined to the apical or basal part of the bladder respectively. The commonest lesion is complete vesical exstrophy; the most severe, and fortunately the least common, is cloacal exstrophy (vesical fissure).

In *complete exstrophy* the bladder, instead of being a closed sac, is everted and forms a moist protuberant reddened mass on the anterior abdominal wall, with the trigone and ureteric orifices occupying the lower part of the area. In the male the penis is rudimentary, epispadiac and flattened from side to side (see p. 743); its underside is normal with a midline raphe continuous with the scrotal raphe. The scrotum is sometimes bifid and the testes may be undescended. The abdominal muscles extend medially only as far as the lateral margins of the defect in the anterior abdominal wall and a sheet of fibrous tissue lies between the upper border of the everted bladder and the umbilicus, which is usually situated at a lower level than is normal. The appearances are very similar in the female and the clitoris is usually cleft. There is also failure of normal development of the symphysis pubis, with wide separation of the pubic bones so that the patient has a characteristic waddling gait.

The developmental abnormality in cases of *cloacal exstrophy* occurs before the urorectal septum forms, and both the hind gut and the urinary system are involved in the defect.[6] The anatomical details vary from patient to patient but the basic deformity consists of a central zone of intestinal mucosa with, on either side, bladder tissue and a ureteric orifice. The anus is usually imperforate and commonly there are also other congenital abnormalities, such as cystic, aplastic or dysplastic kidneys, undescended testes or spina bifida.

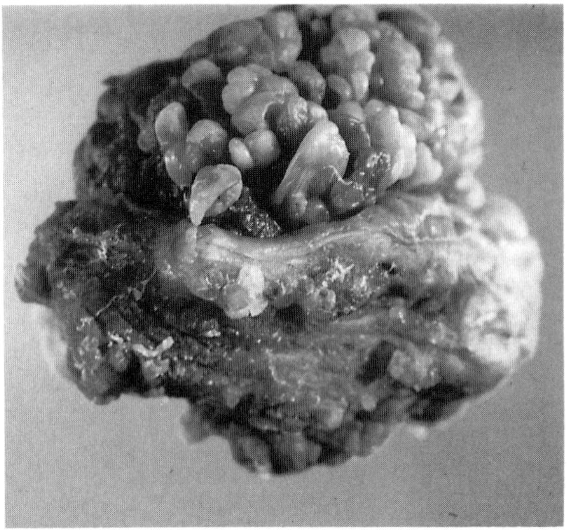

Fig. 19.2 Exstrophy. Resected portion of exstrophic bladder, with marked polypoid cystitis which microscopically showed widespread squamous metaplasia.

Exstrophy is present in about one in every 40 000 births and is more common in the male than in the female (the reported ratios varying from 2 : 1 to 7 : 1). At birth the exstrophied bladder is red and velvety, but within a very short time, because of repeated trauma and inflammation, the surface becomes covered with mucoid exudate, encrusted debris and granulations. The surface transitional cells present at birth very soon undergo metaplasia to squamous or glandular epithelium (Fig. 19.2). Repeated episodes of infection and surface ulceration and subsequent epithelial regeneration and growth often result in sequestration of islands of epithelium beneath the surface. This heterotopic epithelium is frequently of glandular type and should not be mistaken for adenocarcinoma, which may arise in this condition. The prognosis in untreated cases is poor and many patients die of upper urinary tract infection. Tumours may develop in those who survive into adult life, but are rare and tend to occur at a younger age than do the tumours in patients with normally developed bladders. Adenocarcinomas, which very rarely metastasize, are the commonest type.[7] Even after the exstrophy has been corrected surgically the risk of malignancy persists,[8] although these tumours should be distinguished from the tumours developing after diversion of the urine into the ileum or colon (see p. 690).

TRAUMA[9–12]

The bladder may be damaged by penetrating wounds caused by stabbing or by low or high velocity missiles, when frequently there is also injury to the bowel and other viscera or to the bony structures of the pelvis. It is sometimes opened inadvertently during the course of operations on other structures, such as a large sliding hernia, or from within during transurethral resection of bladder or prostatic lesions. It may also be damaged in attempts to procure an abortion.

Rupture can result from direct violence, such as a kick to the lower abdomen, and is seen quite commonly in the victims of road accidents, especially if the pelvis has been fractured. If the bladder is full at the time rupture into the peritoneal cavity is most likely, with a risk of general peritonitis. Extraperitoneal rupture, either by tearing or by penetration of the bladder wall by a bone spicule, is much more common and likely to cause pelvic cellulitis. Spontaneous rupture without any history of preceding trauma occasionally occurs in heavily inflamed (see p. 709) or neoplastic bladders.

MECHANISM OF MICTURITION[13, 14]

Micturition, which is normally under the full control of higher centres, is brought about by a modified sacral reflex that consists of a sustained detrusor contraction coupled with relaxation of both the internal sphincter (mediated by action of parasympathetic nerves originating in the second, third and fourth sacral cord segments) and the striated muscle of the pelvic floor. Afferent impulses that indicate the degree of distension of the bladder pass along autonomic nerves to the sacral region of the cord and also travel up the cord to centres in the pons, mid-brain, posterior hypothalamus and cerebral hemispheres. Inhibitory impulses that can be interrupted voluntarily will then be sent down the cord to suppress the motor side of the arc and prevent reflex emptying until such time as it is convenient for micturition to proceed. Micturition, once it commences, is usually assisted by the action of voluntary muscles of the abdominal wall and the pelvic floor. Detrusor function is normal (or 'stable') when contractions are initiated, continue under volitional control and are maintained until the bladder is completely empty. Detrusor function is described as 'unstable' when one or more of these stages is absent. Detrusor contraction can have one of two effects on the bladder neck depending on the arrangement of its fibres at that site: either the neck will be pulled further open and urine will flow, or it will be prevented from opening and there will be an effective barrier at the bladder neck. The term dyssynergia is used to indicate this incoordination of detrusor contraction and sphincter relaxation.

BLADDER OUTFLOW OBSTRUCTION

Obstruction to the outflow of urine during the act of micturition has many causes, some organic and others functional, located either in the bladder or in the lower urinary tract. Organic obstruction occurs, for instance, in children with congenital urethral valves or in older patients with a urethral stricture or an enlarged prostate. Functional obstruction may occur with spina bifida, with a neurological disease such as tabes dorsalis or multiple sclerosis, and when the spinal cord has been damaged by trauma or by a tumour (see p. 700).

Simple outflow obstruction of short duration will cause the bladder to dilate. The condition is reversible when the obstruction is removed, but with longer standing obstruction the bladder muscle hypertrophies and there is an increase in collagen due to the persistent and sustained rise in intravesical pressure. The bladder often becomes trabeculated (Fig. 19.3) and diverticula may form.[15] Later, decompensation will occur, the bladder wall becomes thin and the lumen dilates. Dilatation of the upper urinary tract with or without reflux is then likely and there is an ever present risk of infection, which may lead to serious and permanent renal damage. Cystoscopy in children with enuresis shows trabeculation, and there is an increase of collagen in their bladder wall.[16]

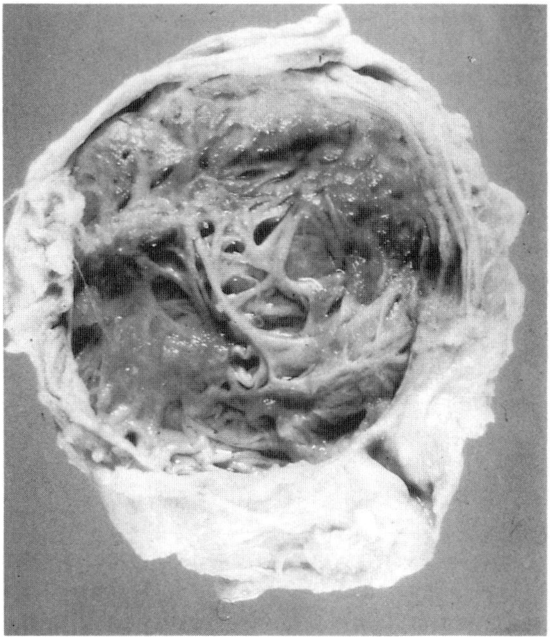

Fig. 19.3 Bladder outflow obstruction. Trabeculated bladder wall in patient with outflow obstruction due to a urethral stricture (not illustrated).

BLADDER NECK OBSTRUCTION

Obstruction at the bladder neck in the adult male without any evidence that it is due to prostatic enlargement is a condition of obscure aetiology formerly known as Marion's disease. It has been attributed to the mechanical effects of local fibrosis and myohypertrophy,[17] both of which have been demonstrated in biopsy specimens. Recent work has confirmed that there is an increased amount of local collagen but the present concept is that the primary defect may be in the innervation of the preprostatic muscle sphincter.[18] It is currently held that outflow obstruction in the male may be due either to detrusor failure or to incoordination of sphincter and detrusor action (dyssynergia), whereas in the female it results from weak detrusor action rather than dyssynergia.[19, 20]

There has been controversy, too, with regard to children with so-called 'idiopathic' bladder neck obstruction. Fibrotic and hypertrophic changes similar to those seen in the adult male have been described and fibroelastosis of the prostatic urethra has been suggested as the basic lesion in boys. Bladder neck obstruction as a primary lesion in childhood is now believed to be extremely rare and it is widely accepted that the diagnosis should only be considered when all possible neurogenic and sphincter disorders of organic or emotional cause have been excluded.[21]

NEUROGENIC BLADDER

Interruption of or damage to the various parts of the reflex arc and its connections in the cord with the higher centres lead to a number of lesions which collectively are referred to as the neuropathic bladder. If there is interruption of the sensory limb of the reflex arc, as occurs in tabes dorsalis, the bladder will become overdistended and overflow will occur because of the total lack of sensation and the patient's consequent unawareness of what is going on in the bladder. The bladder wall becomes thinned and its muscle atrophies. Loss of higher cerebral control in patients with a cerebral tumour or after a cerebrovascular accident will result in inability to inhibit emptying of the bladder and the patient will be incontinent. In all these patients, as in those with organic obstruction, urinary tract infection is a serious complication.

Damage to the spinal cord by trauma, inflammation or neoplastic disease is likely to have serious sequelae and produce the so-called 'cord bladder'.[14] The effects that follow trauma depend on the level of the lesion in the spinal cord and whether or not it is complete, and also on the amount of damage to the cord above and below the area of greatest injury. In the early stages there will be necrosis and haemorrhage into the cord, to be followed later by varying amounts of gliosis.

In lesions above the sacral region there is an initial period of spinal shock, with retention of urine and overflow. After an interval ranging from a few hours to several weeks there will be a gradual return of reflex activity and detrusor contraction in response to afferent stimuli from the bladder. However, it will be some time before the detrusor contractions are powerful enough or sustained enough to open the bladder neck: detrusor-sphincter dyssynergia often occurs. In many patients the reflex contractions are never adequate enough to empty the bladder completely and there will then always be a large volume of residual urine.

The effects produced by lesions of the cauda equina or conus depend on whether the damage to the sacral roots and sacral cord segments is complete or incomplete. If complete, there is permanent paralysis of the detrusor and of the striated muscle of the pelvic floor, which are supplied by the pudendal nerves that originate in the ventral horns of the second, third and fourth sacral segments. The bladder becomes a dilated, and occasionally trabeculated, sac that is incapable of contraction and can be emptied only by manual compression or abdominal straining. Incomplete cord damage will produce a mixed clinical picture with weak or absent reflex detrusor contractions, though reflex activity of the muscles of the pelvic floor and of the intrinsic urethral striated muscle will be retained. Detrusor-sphincter dyssynergia may be pronounced. In children interruption of the nervous pathways is more commonly partial than complete,[22] and the clinical picture is often a very complex one with varying degrees of detrusor and sphincter inactivity or hyperactivity. Most often there is a large flaccid bladder with overflow incontinence and vesicoureteric reflux. The commonest cause is a myelomeningocele[23] but sometimes the child has spinal dysraphism, diastematomyelia or transverse myelitis.

All patients who suffer neurological damage after injury to the spinal column and cord need to be thoroughly investigated by modern combined urodynamic and radiological studies and, on account of the urological complications that may develop, the urologist needs to be involved in clinical management from the outset. Upper tract dilatation during voiding is liable to occur with dyssynergia, and vesicoureteric reflux is recorded in between 17 and 25% of patients. Incomplete emptying of the bladder may be followed by infection which may affect both the upper and the lower parts of the urinary tract. Stone formation due to stasis and infection is not uncommon. Amyloidosis is a serious complication and together with chronic pyelonephritis and stone formation may cause fatal renal failure.[24] In a follow-up study of a series of World War II paraplegics[25] the prognosis was found to depend on the amount of residual bladder function: 50% of patients with good bladder function – that is, no reflux, residual urine less than one-third of the bladder volume, and no indwelling catheter – were alive after 25 years, compared with only 20% survival among patients with poor bladder function. Renal disease accounted for 40% of these fatalities. In a recent series of patients treated by a specialist spinal injuries team completeness of the cord lesion was one of the most important factors contributing to morbidity and death in renal failure.[26]

DIVERTICULA

Diverticula are most often seen in elderly men with hypertrophy and trabeculation of the bladder as a result of acquired outflow obstruction due to enlargement of the prostate. The diverticula may be single or multiple and usually develop in the posterolateral parts of the lower half of the bladder. The majority are from 3 to 4 cm in diameter but some grow to a considerable size and in rare instances become as large as the bladder itself. In children diverticula are sometimes found in the vicinity of the ureteric hiatus in the detrusor, which is the weakest part of the bladder wall. The protrusions form on either the medial or the lateral side of the ureter and occasionally develop with normal detrusor action in the absence of any significant outflow obstruction; more often, though, there is definite obstructive or neurological disease[21].

Diverticulum formation in the trabeculated bladder commences when, during micturition, small saccules lined by transitional epithelium are pushed out between the trabeculae and into the outer layers of the bladder muscle. The fully formed diverticulum protrudes through the muscular coat into the surrounding loose connective tissue. The lining epithelium may still be of transitional type but very commonly it is replaced in part or in whole by inflamed fibrogranulation tissue or squamous epithelium. The wall consists mostly of fibrous tissue; the muscle gradually thins and in many instances finally disappears altogether, and inflammatory changes may extend into the surrounding connective tissue. The stoma is often quite large but occasionally is so small that the cystoscopist has the greatest difficulty in lo-

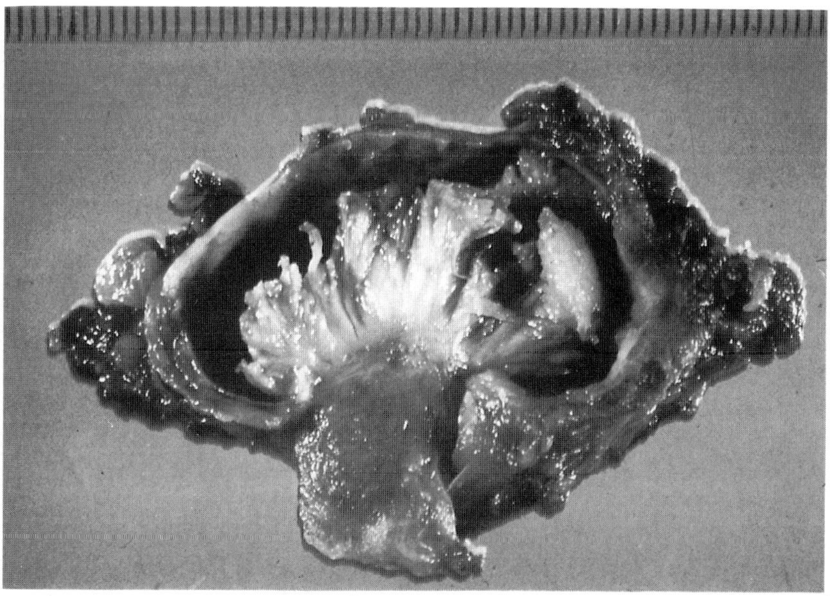

Fig. 19.4 Carcinoma in bladder diverticulum. This diverticulum is almost completely filled by a papillary carcinoma, the neck of the diverticulum can be seen to the right of the base of the tumour.

cating it amongst the trabeculae. The epithelium around the margins of the opening may be heaped up and resemble tumour and indeed it may become neoplastic.

Failure of a diverticulum to empty completely during micturition leads to urinary stasis, and repeated episodes of infection are common. Stones are sometimes formed within the sac and on very rare occasions a diverticulum perforates. Tumours may develop within the lumen (Fig. 19.4) but their frequency cannot be established at all accurately as in most hospitals it is not a regular practice to submit all excised diverticula for histological examination. The quoted figure of a 3.6% incidence of tumour formation[27] is without doubt a gross overestimate. What is certain, though, is that while transitional cell carcinoma is the tumour most often found, there is a higher incidence of squamous carcinoma within diverticula than in the bladder itself. The frequent association of stasis and epithelial metaplasia of the lining epithelium has suggested that they may play a part in tumour development, but there is evidence that stasis per se is not a risk factor.[28] Diagnostic problems sometimes arise when a patient with no overt tumour in the bladder or upper urinary tract has demonstrable tumour cells on cytological examination of the urine as a manifestation of an occult tumour within a diverticulum. Sometimes, too, a tumour arising within a diverticulum protrudes through the stoma into the lumen of the bladder and is mistaken on cytoscopy for a primary neoplasm of the bladder itself.

HERNIATION AND DISPLACEMENT

In elderly patients part of the bladder wall may become incorporated in an inguinal or femoral hernia and be at risk during operative repair of the hernia. A cystocele is a protrusion of the bladder into the vagina, most commonly seen in multiparae. In the condition of pelvic lipomatosis the bladder is pushed up out of the true pelvis by an accumulation of adipose tissue in the region of the bladder base and has a very characteristic inverted pear-shaped outline on cystography.

FISTULAE

A fistulous track can develop between the bladder and the female genital tract or the bowel, or open directly on to the skin surface. Some, such as those associated with the urachus or with exstrophy of the bladder, are of congenital origin, but the majority are due to trauma or to a variety of inflammatory diseases or neoplasms.

The commonest fistulae in relation to the female genital organs are the vesicovaginal type.[29] Some are of traumatic origin and result from pressure on the tissues during a prolonged or difficult labour, and others follow local damage during the course of a gynaecological operation or irradiation. Carcinoma of the cervix is a common cause, especially if the tumour has been irradiated, though occasionally a primary bladder tumour penetrates into the vagina. Much less common types are vesicosalpingeal fistulae, which may complicate salpingitis, and vesicouterine fistulae, which sometimes follow obstetrical damage or gynaecological operations, or occur when there is malignant disease in either the bladder or the uterus.

Vesicointestinal fistulae are very occasionally of congenital origin. Usually they are due to inflammatory or neoplastic disease; the primary disease is in the bowel more often than in the bladder.[30] Though any part of the bowel from the terminal ileum to the rectum may be involved, the fistulous opening is usually in either the sigmoid colon or the ileum. Sigmoid diverticulitis is the most frequent cause but carcinoma of the colon and Crohn's disease each account for a significant number of cases. Males are affected more often than females. The bladder and bowel may come into contact with each other (direct type of fistula) or may be separated by an intervening mass of fibrous tissue surrounding an abscess cavity (indirect type). In the earliest or incipient stages of fistula formation in cases of diverticulitis or Crohn's disease fibrinous adhesions bind the bladder and bowel together. These organize later into fibrous tissue and there is usually local thickening of adherent bladder and bowel. The inner surface of the bladder is inflamed and the epithelium is frequently heaped up or actually polypoid (see p. 717). The patient will complain of frequency, sometimes with haematuria, and on cystoscopy the changes in the bladder wall may resemble those of a primary bladder tumour. The local inflammatory thickening of the bladder wall may cause further confusion when a bimanual examination is performed, and a bladder biopsy is an essential part of the clinical investigation. Once a fistula is fully established, bowel contents will be detectable in the urine and there will be clinical evidence of cystitis; pneumaturia is a common symptom. Most fistulae develop in the posterolateral part of the bladder, usually about halfway between the fundus and trigone.

Carcinoma of the large bowel, and on very rare occasions carcinoma of the bladder, may be complicated by the development of a vesicointestinal fistula. The incipient stages, with local inflammation and polypoid changes in the bladder epithelium, are similar to those in cases of diverticulitis; bladder biopsy is likely to reveal an often rather confusing appearance with thickened, hyperplastic and polypoid transitional epithelium mixed with glandular tumour tissue. Whenever adenocarcinomatous tissue is found in a biopsy specimen from the bladder steps should be taken to exclude a primary growth in the bowel or in the female genital tract before the possibility of a primary adenocarcinoma of the bladder is considered. In the late stages of neoplastic disease of the bladder or female genitalia multiple fistulae may develop between adjacent viscera.

Extensive fistula formation with involvement of many viscera or openings on to the skin surface may follow gunshot wounds and other penetrating injuries of the abdomen.

CALCULOUS DISEASE[31]

Most of the caluli seen in the bladder originate in the upper urinary tract (see p. 531) in patients with 'idiopathic' stone disease; others form on a nucleus of dead tissue or a foreign body in the bladder and some are so-called 'endemic' stones. Small stones are likely to pass quite rapidly down the urethra and those that remain in the bladder for any length of time are liable to acquire an additional surface coating, especially if there is urinary stasis and an infection with urea-splitting organisms. Stasis is also an important factor in the formation of the so-called 'recumbency' calculi in patients confined to bed for a long time. Stone formation is much more common in males than females, largely due to the higher incidence of urinary stasis in men.

'Endemic' stone formation was seen frequently in former times in Europe and in certain parts of England – notably East Anglia in the eighteenth and nineteenth centuries. Children were more often affected than adults, and boys more often than girls, and the disease was ascribed to the poor socioeconomic conditions that prevailed and in particular to the high intake of cereals in the diet. As social conditions improved and the diet changed to contain less cereal so the incidence of the disease declined and it is now virtually non-existent in Britain. However, it does still exist today in certain areas of the world, such as parts of the Far and Middle East and in some Mediterranean countries where the cereal content of the diet is often high. The prevalence of the disease varies from country to country.[32] The composition of the diet is obviously not the only responsible factor, because feeding practices are not the same within different ethnic groups in any one country, and there is not always the same incidence in rural and urban dwellers. Endemic calculi are still seen much more often in children than in adults and in boys than in girls, and are usually composed of calcium oxalate, uric acid, and ammonium acid urate. In contrast, bladder stones in children in affluent societies are usually 'infection' stones composed of calcium phosphate or magnesium ammonium phosphate.

In adults with idiopathic stone disease the calculi are composed of pure calcium oxalate or of calcium oxalate and calcium phosphate; if the urine is infected, especially with urea-splitting organisms, the calculi are magnesium ammonium phosphate or calcium phosphate 'infection' stones.

Metabolic stones of aetiology similar to those seen in the ureter (see p. 686) also occur in the bladder and are likely to have a surface coating of phosphate if the urine is infected.

Phosphatic 'infection' calculi are grey or grey-white and may be hard or soft or of a friable consistency. Oxalate stones are usually hard and may be smooth and rounded, or nodular resembling a mulberry, or irregularly spiculated; if there has been much bleeding they may be black or very dark brown. Uric acid and urate stones are usually smooth, yellowish or brown, and round or oval. Cystine stones are hard, smooth and yellow and sometimes have a peculiar waxy look. Naked-eye appearances should never by relied on for identification and if possible every stone should be submitted to chemical analysis. Bisection will usually reveal a laminated structure and unless the central parts of the stone as well as the surface areas are analysed an underlying metabolic defect may be entirely overlooked. Whatever their eventual crystalline composition stones have a central core of mucoprotein matrix substance around which more mucoprotein is deposited in both lamellar and radial fashion. Crystals are deposited on and between the mucoprotein laminae and a calculus increases in size by further deposition of mucoprotein which in turn becomes mineralized.

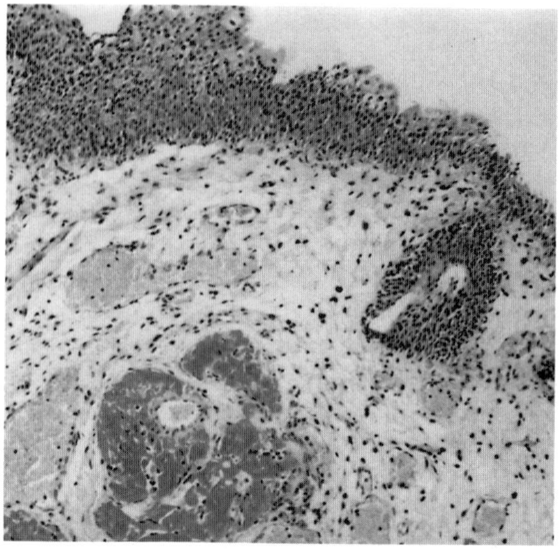

Fig. 19.5 Bladder amyloid. Deposit of densely eosinophilic material in oedematous lamina propria. Haematoxylin–eosin × 85

AMYLOIDOSIS[33]

Amyloidosis may be considered to occur in two forms – a *primary* (or localized) type that develops without any obvious or predisposing factor and a *secondary* (or systemic) type that occurs in patients with chronic infections (especially tuberculosis or osteomyelitis) and a variety of other conditions such as rheumatoid arthritis, Hodgkin's disease or myeloma. The secondary type is always generalized and affects many different organs and parts of the body – sometimes including the bladder – whereas in the primary type the lesions, though very occasionally generalized, are much more often localized to a single organ such as the bladder, a lung, the skin, the larynx or a ureter. Since the introduction of antibiotics secondary amyloidosis is seen less often than it was, though it still constitutes a serious hazard to paraplegics,[24] especially if there is extensive involvement of the urinary tract, when it may be a cause of profuse haematuria, with or without clot retention.[34] Vesical amyloidosis is an uncommon condition and in most cases is of the primary type; surprisingly, analysis of the amyloid material has shown it to be frequently of the AL variety more commonly associated with secondary amyloid.[35] Haematuria is a characteristic and common symptom. On cystoscopy the lesions, which may be single or multiple and which occur anywhere in the bladder (though usually sparing the trigone), are seen as ragged, haemorrhagic, and sometimes ulcerated, areas that may be mistaken for neoplasm.

In both forms of the disease amyloid is deposited mainly between the collagen bundles in the lamina propria, commonly forming a distinct layer immediately below the surface epithelium. The walls of blood vessels are often infiltrated as well and there may also be involvement of the detrusor muscle. There is frequently a local foreign body giant cell reaction, sometimes with calcification or, very rarely, bone formation.[36] The lamina propria is usually congested and oedematous and, because of the changes in the blood vessel walls, often contains areas of haemorrhage; sometimes the bleeding is extensive. The overlying epithelium is often irregularly thickened and hyperplastic, and is sometimes ulcerated and occasionally polypoid. A significant degree of epithelial dysplasia is commonly found; care has to be taken not to confuse this with malignant change.

ENDOMETRIOSIS[37]

Endometriosis of the bladder is a very rare condition that occurs most often in premenopausal women, usually between the ages of 25 and 50. The deposits of endometrial tissue are usually seen on the serosal surface but, in rare instances, they are found within the bladder wall, producing localized cystic swellings deep to the epithelium, usually in the region of the trigone or low down on the posterior wall. Clinically, there is often frequency and dysuria, and there may be cyclical haematuria. A filling defect that can resemble a neoplasm may be seen on cystography. In rare cases retention of urine has occurred when the lesions were in the region of the bladder neck. Vesical endometriosis has also been reported in male patients under treatment with oestrogens for carcinoma of the prostate.[38]

INFLAMMATORY CONDITIONS

Inflammatory changes in the bladder may be due to a wide variety of causes, acting singly or in combination. Bacterial infection is by far the commonest. Fungi, actinomycetes, metazoal parasites, viruses, chemical irritants (including some drugs used therapeutically), foreign bodies, irradiation and trauma may be responsible in some cases. Any congenital or acquired lesion that causes obstruction and stasis, even of quite short duration, is likely to increase the liability to infection or to exacerbate an infection that is already established. There are a number of metaplastic conditions of the urothelium which are not necessarily infective or inflammatory in origin but which are confusingly called cystitis; these are considered in the next section (see p. 715) although there is some degree of overlap or artificiality in distinguishing between the two groups.

BACTERIAL INFECTIONS

The bladder is very resistant to bacterial infection and under normal conditions is sterile. When an infection occurs the organisms usually reach the bladder either from the urethra after it has become contaminated with faecal organisms or, less commonly, from the upper tract when there is haematogeneous infection with staphylococci or Gram-negative organisms.[39]

Bacterial urinary tract infection is much more common in females than in males; the close proximity of the urethra and perineum in the female, which can facilitate the direct transfer of faecal organisms to the urethra, is obviously an important aetiological factor. It is also known that introital colonization with faecal organisms sometimes occurs and it has been shown that it is these organisms that cause urinary infections. Others factors likely to increase the risk of urethral contamination are any surgical procedures on the prostate or lower urinary tract and, in particular, the use of an indwelling catheter. Vaginal prolapse and local trauma during sexual intercourse may also be precipitating factors. Organisms that have become established in the urethra can ascend into the bladder by migration against the current of urine or by being transferred there mechanically by a catheter or other instrument; on reaching the bladder they either remain in the bladder urine or attach themselves to the surface of the epithelium, some adhering more readily than others. Organisms in the bladder will multiply there, but are exposed to the effects of a number of host defences. The most important of these defences is the bladder washout mechanism: this is the constant flow of urine down the ureters which, although it may be sufficient to prevent altogether any increase in the bacterial count in the bladder urine, will not have any significant effect on organisms attached to the mucosa. The washout effect will be vitiated in variable degree if there is any obstruction at the bladder neck or lower down in the urinary tract, or if there is vesicoureteric reflux, or if the organisms colonizing the urethra continue to ascend into the bladder. Incomplete bladder emptying, as may occur in the presence of a vesical diverticulum or in patients with a neuropathic bladder, will also reduce its efficiency.

Epithelial damage, due possibly to the action of bacterial endotoxins or to alterations in the surface mucin layer brought about by bacterial enzymes, and demonstrated with the scanning electron microscope, is usually more severe in chronic than in acute infections.[40] As the epithelial cells desquamate during the course of an infection any organism attached to them will be carried into the lumen of the bladder and pass out in the urine. Then, because of the loss of the surface cells, bacteria in the urine will be exposed to the action of the phagocytes in the bladder wall. The main inhibitors of bacterial growth in the urine itself are its urea content and its pH. The precise role of humoral factors is not clear, though there may be rises of IgA, IgG and IgM levels in the urine during the course of an infection. Secretory IgA is produced locally in the bladder wall but it originates in larger amounts in the urethra, where it may prevent bacterial attachment and colonization and thus protect the bladder from ascending infection. This may possibly explain the relative infrequency of cystitis as a complication of clinical urethritis. Circulating antibodies are unlikely to have any effect in reducing the incidence of ascending urinary tract infection.

The severity of an infection and whether or not it is likely to recur depend on several factors. Some organisms are very much more virulent than others and some, for example *Escherichia coli*, may produce an endotoxin. The ability of coliforms to adhere to the epithelium and therefore to colonize the urinary tract also varies from strain to strain and is related both to the surface structure of the bacteria and to the presence of K antigen. Strains with much K antigen are more invasive than those in which the antigen is absent. The importance, and indeed the danger, of infection with *Proteus* species is their ability to produce a urease which splits urinary urea to form ammonia. This will alkalinize the urine and this in turn will have two important effects: phosphate will be precipitated, which may lead to stone formation, and the activity of many therapeutic antimicrobial agents will be reduced.

The organisms responsible for bladder infection vary with the sex and age of the patient and depend also on whether the infection is contracted in the home environment or in hospital.[41] Most of the responsible organisms are Gram-negative aerobic bacteria, either Gram-negative rods (predominantly *E. coli* and *Proteus* species) or aerobic micrococci. Faecal streptococci are found less frequently and infection with *Staphylococcus saprophyticus* biotype 3 occurs only in infections acquired at home and is not seen in patients infected in hospital. With any invasive procedure on the urinary tract, particularly the use of catheters or other instruments, there is a liability to infection with *Klebsiella* species, *Pseudomonas* and *Serratia*. Cross-infection is also a hazard and each hospital is likely to have its own specific pattern of infecting bacteria.

In neonates of both sexes *E.coli* is the commonest organism to cause an infection. The same is true of young girls in whom about 90% of infections are due to coliforms; in the remainder *Proteus mirabilis*, *Streptococcus faecalis* and other organisms can be cultured. Contrasting figures are found in young boys in whom about one-third of infections are due to *E.coli* and nearly a half are due to *Proteus* species. In adults of both sexes *E. coli* can be cultured in between two-thirds and three-quarters of infections. Proteus infections are less common in the female than in the male; they are seen more often in older than in younger men.

It is often difficult to correlate the clinical and microbiological findings in patients with, or suspected of having, a bacterial urinary infection. Symptomatic cystitis may or may not be accompanied by bacteriuria and there is an important group of patients with 'asymptomatic bacteriuria' in whom there is no clinical suspicion of infection but who yet have bacteria in their urine.[42] For many years counts of bacteria in the urine have been one of the yardsticks for the diagnosis of infection and it is now widely accepted that, with certain provisos, a concentration of organisms of less then 100 000 per millilitre of urine almost certainly indicates contamination of the specimen and is not likely to be of clinical significance. It is nevertheless true that patients with symptoms of urinary infection may sometimes be found to have fewer than 100 000 organisms per millilitre in their urine. A count of more than 100 000 in a single specimen can be taken to mean, with 90% degree of certainty, that organisms are present and multiplying in the bladder urine. A similar concentration of bacteria in a second consecutive specimen indicates 95% certainty. The methods of collecting the urine specimens, the ways in which they are handled subsequently and the laboratory techniques used are of crucial importance in the interpretation of the results and their clinical significance; the details are beyond the scope of the present discussion and are to be found in the appropriate texts. It must be appreciated, though, that results expressed merely in terms of bacterial numbers may be of little or no significance if the bladder empties so frequently that there is insufficient time for bacteria to multiply there or if the urine is very highly concentrated or contains antibacterial agents. Some microbiologists emphasize that the purity of the bacterial culture rather than the density of organisms is the crucial diagnostic criterion. This observation is, however, of limited value in hospital practice as pure cultures are unlikely ever to be obtained from patients with indwelling catheters, neurogenic bladder or any structural abnormality in the urinary tract.

Symptomless bacteriuria occurs at all ages but with quite marked differences in prevalence in the two sexes. There are no very accurate figures for neonates but male infants are affected more often than females, probably because they have a higher incidence of congenital anomalies of the urinary tract. Schoolgirls, with a prevalence of about 1 – 2%, are affected up to 40 times more often than boys of comparable ages; the incidence in girls rises steadily with age. In adult life the female to male ratio drops to about 8 to 1. It has been estimated that from 10 to 20% of women have bacteria in their urine at some time during their lives. There is an increasing prevalence with increasing age; asymptomatic bacteriuria in early pregnancy may be followed by symptomatic urinary tract infection and, as term approaches, so the risk of upper urinary tract infection increases. Urinary tract infection is a common cause of morbidity and one of its particular dangers is the frequency with which it complicates or is complicated by vesicoureteric reflux and the presence of residual urine, thus predisposing to upper tract disease. Ultimately there may be chronic renal disease, hypertension and renal failure. Urinary infection in children is unlikely to cause permanent structural damage unless there is reflux.

For treatment to be effective it is important to recognize the site of an infection and in particular to distinguish between upper and lower urinary tract disease. This is often extremely difficult. There needs to be very close collaboration between the clinician and the laboratory and many techniques may have to be used, such as the collection of midstream or 'clean catch' urine specimens, ureteric catheterization, suprapubic aspiration, bladder washouts, detection of antibody-coated bacteria and the determination of serum antibodies to O antigens of *E. coli* as well as many other highly specialized investigations. Histological examination of biopsy specimens is of little or no value in the diagnosis of bacterial infection, though it may confirm that an infective process is present or reveal structural changes resulting from it. It may also confirm or exclude the presence of some underlying condition, such as a neoplasm. None the less, as will be described below, certain histological patterns of acute and chronic infection as well as some special forms of cystitis can be recognized in tissue specimens. But, with certain exceptions, notably tuberculosis, there is no clear correlation between the type or strain of organism isolated from the urine and the gross and microscopical features that will be found in the bladder.

Acute cystitis

In acute cystitis or in an exacerbation of a more chronic infection the pathological changes in the bladder wall are of varying severity and extent. In mild cases the mucosal surface is red and velvety and microscopically there is vascular congestion, local oedema and infiltration by polymorphonuclear leucocytes. When the infection is more severe the mucosal surface may have a somewhat ragged appearance; congestion and oedema are now more pronounced and the epithelium is either thickened and hyperplastic or ulcerated. There will be widespread inflammatory cell infiltration, predominantly with polymorphonuclear leucocytes, affecting the lamina propria and sometimes spreading down into the muscle coat as well. Small abscesses occasionally occur. The blood vessels are thick walled and their lining endothelial cells are frequently swollen, and there may be small perivascular haemorrhages.

Chronic non-specific cystitis

Chronic non-specific cystitis is seen in persistent infections or after repeated attacks of acute cystitis. The inner surface of the bladder is usually patchily congested and the epithelium may be deficient altogether or irregularly hyperplastic, or even polypoid. In longstanding cases there is often squamous metaplasia: this may be recognizable as pale areas on gross examination. The lamina propria is often much widened, contains more fibrous tissue than is usual and is congested and diffusely or focally infiltrated with inflammatory cells of all types. Lymphocytes and plasma cells predominate and sometimes the lymphoid cells are collected into follicles. The inflammatory process extends into the bladder wall to a variable depth and sometimes there is a considerable increase in fibrous tissue within the muscle coat. Blood vessels throughout the bladder wall are usually thick walled and many of them show hyaline or obliterative changes. In the late stages of the disease the fibrous tissue contracts and the bladder capacity will be correspondingly reduced, sometimes to an extreme degree. Ultrastructural studies of biopsy specimens[40] show that in acute bacterial cystitis the urothelium differs but little from normal, whereas in chronic cystitis there are pronounced changes, with absent cell junctions, alterations in microvilli, loss of surface cells and, in places, complete disruption of the epithelial layer. Bacteria may be seen on the surface in acute infections and in larger numbers and also deep to the surface in chronic cases.

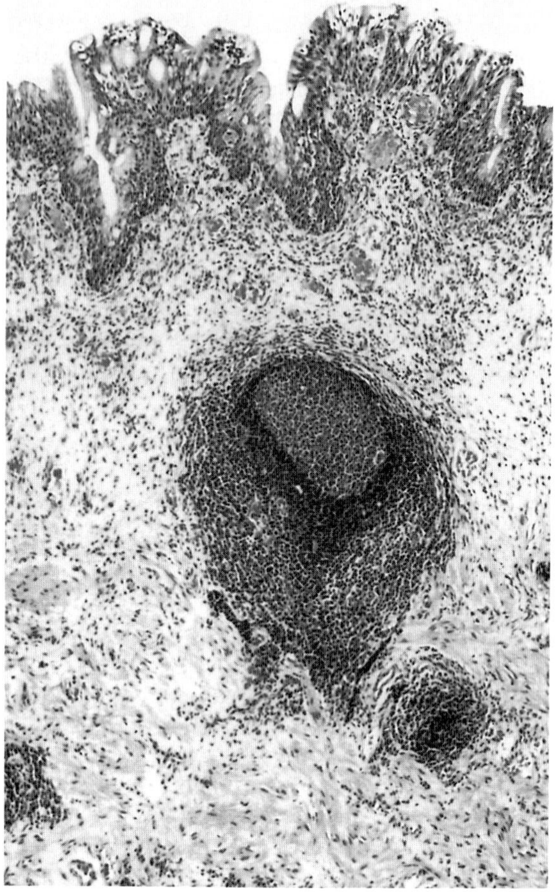

Fig. 19.6 Follicular cystitis. Oedematous somewhat polypoid bladder containing lymphoid aggregates with prominent germinal centres.
Haematoxylin–eosin × 90

The gross appearances in both acute and chronic cystitis vary from case to case and sometimes the predominant change is indicated by describing the lesions[43] as, for example, *haemorrhagic cystitis* (as may occur in patients treated with cyclophosphamide [see p. 711], or penicillin[44]) and *ulcerative cystitis*. *Follicular cystitis* (Fig. 19.6) is the term used to describe the accumulation of lymphoid cells seen in some patients with chronic disease and recognized as pale granular areas when seen through the cystoscope or in specimens of fixed tissue. *Bullous cystitis* is a rare condition in which localized oedema of the lamina propria produces a polypoid condition of the mucosa. There may be local haemorrhages and microscopically the cystic lesions may resemble the grape-like masses of embryonal sarcozma (see p. 735): however, the distribution is different as the apex of the bladder is affected more often than the base, which is the site of predilection of the embryonal tumour. *Emphysematous cystitis* is an uncommon condition in which there are gas-filled cysts in the lamina propria. Many of the patients are diabetic[45] and though in the majority of cases the infection is due to gas-forming aerobes, such as *E. coli*, on very rare occasions anaerobes are responsible.[46]

ABACTERIAL CYSTITIS

In a significant number of women with symptoms of cystitis organisms cannot be cultured from the urine using standard laboratory procedures. The condition (also known as the urethral syndrome, frequency/dysuria syndrome, symptomatic abacteriuria) is often recurrent and difficult to treat successfully. Many causes have been suggested, including infection with chlamydiae, viruses or slow-growing bacteria as well as infection of the urethra[47] or periurethral glands, stenosis of the urethral meatus and a variety of gynaecological conditions,[48] including cervical erosion and cervicitis. It is generally accepted that gynaecological disorders can be excluded from the aetiological causes. There is good evidence to suggest that an occult coliform infection might be responsible for the symptoms in many of these patients. This is supported by the knowledge that some patients with abacterial cystitis later develop bacteriuria and that some women known to have bacterial cystitis become abacteriuric on occasions. Sometimes there is squamous metaplasia[49] of the bladder epithelium in the region of the trigone, but this is not a change that is specific to this condition (see p. 716).

Some male patients with severe symptoms of cystitis may also be found to be abacteriuric on routine urine culture and infection with unusual organisms such as chlamydiae or mycoplasmas should be suspected. The inflammatory changes seen in the bladder are often severe and there may be mucosal ulceration.

VIRAL CYSTITIS

An acute haemorrhagic cystitis in children and in patients with bone marrow transplants has been attributed to adenovirus type II[50] when the virus can be isolated from the urine. Cystitis has also been reported as a result of infection with herpes simplex, herpes zoster, papovavirus and cytomegalovirus[43] – in these conditions the appropriate inclusions may be seen in voided urothelial cells.

GANGRENOUS CYSTITIS

Gangrenous cystitis (croupous, diphtheritic, membranous or pseudomembranous cystitis, vesical necrosis) is due to many causes including chemical irritation, physical damage by irradiation, infections, overdistension, pressure of a gravid uterus or injury to, or disease of, blood vessels. These causes either interfere with the blood supply of the bladder or produce severe local inflammatory changes.[51] Gangrenous cystitis has also been recorded as a complication of prostatectomy. The condition is an uncommon one and its incidence has declined in recent years because of the wider use of antibiotics, advances in obstetric care and the better management of bladder outflow obstruction. In the *pseudomembranous type* the mucosal surface of the bladder is covered with a layer of fibrinous material (the pseudomembrane) containing pus cells, degenerate epithelial cells and organisms; the mucosa and lamina propria form a slough which may be exfoliated in fragments or as a cast of the bladder.[52] Aerobic or anaerobic organisms may be cultured. Some of the more recent accounts describe full-thickness necrosis of the bladder wall (*vesical necrosis*)[53, 54] and stress that true necrosis must be distinguished from the pseudomembranous variety though its causes may be the same.

ENCRUSTED CYSTITIS

When the urine is infected with urea-splitting organisms, and especially when the bladder wall has been damaged by local irradiation, the passage of a stone or repeated diathermy, deposition of calcium magnesium phosphate may occur on the traumatized area. On gross examination grey or white gritty crusts or plaques are seen on the mucosal surface and around the margins and on the base of any ulcerated areas.[55] Microscopically, the epithelium is frequently hyperplastic and calculous material is found embedded in it or in the lamina propria where it sometime elicits a local foreign body giant cell reaction. There is usually a heavy local inflammatory cell infiltration.

IRRADIATION CYSTITIS

The bladder may be damaged by local or external irradiation applied either to the bladder wall itself or to adjacent organs. Initially there is vascular congestion and some oedema of the lamina propria which may progress to the formation of bullae. Epithelial desquamation usually follows and shallow ulcers form. Later there is often hyperplasia of the epithelium that remains, frequently with many bizarre and irregularly hyperchromatic cells that may be difficult to distinguish from malignant urothelial cells. Areas of squamous metaplasia are sometimes seen. Vascular changes are common and widespread: in acute cases necrotizing arteriolitis is present throughout the affected lamina propria, and in longstanding cases obliterative lesions are seen. A frequent finding is telangiectasia of the superficial vessels in the lamina propria which, because of persistent oozing, may be a source of heavy blood loss.[56] The lamina propria may contain radiation fibroblasts of stellate configuration and atypical nuclei which must be distinguished from the multinucleate cells of giant cell cystitis.[57] In *chronic irradiation cystitis* there is usually extensive fibrosis in all coats of the bladder wall, causing progressive reduction in bladder capacity. Bacterial infection is almost invariable and the bladder wall is usually heavily infiltrated with inflammatory cells. Encrustation may follow if urea-splitting organisms are present in the urine. If there has been severe tissue damage fistulae sometimes develop (see p. 702).

INTERSTITIAL CYSTITIS

This form of cystitis, often referred to as *Hunner's ulcer*,[58] is a severe disease of long duration which occurs characteristically in middle-aged or elderly women. It is usually resistant to therapy though temporary relief is sometimes obtained by distension of the bladder. The condition is characterized by distressing and disabling frequency of micturition, urgency, dysuria and suprapubic pain, although usually no evidence of urinary tract infection can be demonstrated. There is often haematuria and the symptoms are frequently intermittent rather than continuous. It is possible that this symptom complex encompasses a number of conditions and the term *painful bladder disease* has been suggested as an alternative.[59]

The bladder capacity is reduced and cystoscopy reveals erythematous patches which tend to fade or split when the bladder is filled. Linear scars, areas of ulceration and petechial haemorrhages also occur. Most of the changes are seen on the posterior wall or at the vault. Histologically, the epithelium may or may not be ulcerated; the most striking changes are found in the lamina propria, which is thicker and more fibrous than is usual, and diffusely infiltrated with inflammatory cells of all types: lymphocytes and plasma cells predominate but mast cells occur in significant numbers and are also present throughout the detrusor muscle[60] and remote from areas of mucosal ulceration. Whilst an increase of mast cells is suggestive of this diagnosis the histological appearances are by no means pathognomic; a significant increase in mast cells is only demonstrable in the muscle (not always present in bladder biopsies) and a proportion of patients with the clinical criteria for the diagnosis do not have a significant increase in mast cells.[61] The interfascicular septa in the muscle coat are widened and infiltrated with inflammatory cells, and the inflammatory process spreads through the full thickness of the bladder wall, justifying the term '*pancystitis*' sometimes given to this condition. Capillaries and small arterioles are usually very prominent and frequently have thickened walls.

The cause is not known but there is evidence to support the theory of an autoimmune basis as many of the patients also have allergic disorders or suffer from or have a family history of thyroiditis, rheumatoid arthritis or psoriasis.[62] Deposition of IgM, Clq and C3 on vessel walls has also been reported in some patients. It is suggested that mast cells, activated by C3, release histamine and that this may have an important role in the pathogenesis of the condition.[63]

Middle-aged or elderly men sometimes complain of the symptoms which in a woman would immediately suggest the diagnosis of interstitial cystitis. In a very few male patients this diagnosis might eventually prove to be correct, but it is much more likely that the symptoms result from malignant disease in the bladder. Very careful investigation is therefore essential: bladder biopsy should be repeated at frequent intervals and cytological examination of the urine is particularly useful as a follow-up procedure.

CYCLOPHOSPHAMIDE CYSTITIS

Cystitis may be due to the toxic effect of a number of chemicals of which cyclophosphamide is by far the most commonly responsible. The haemorrhagic cystitis that sometimes complicates this form of cytotoxic therapy is caused by the breakdown products of cyclophosphamide rather than by the drug itself and its occurrence is not dose dependent. The inflammation is often severe, and typically there is extensive bleeding into the more superficial layers of the lamina propria. In long-standing cases fibrosis of the bladder wall is likely. There is a case report of gas gangrene of the bladder complicating cyclophosphamide therapy.[64] Tumour formation is another unusual complication but one that is being reported with increasing frequency in patients being treated for lymphoproliferative or myeloproliferative disorders or being immunosuppressed after organ transplantation.[65] Most of the tumours are transitional cell carcinomas[66] but squamous or glandular lesions are also recorded. Whether neoplasia occurs because of alterations in the body's immune defence mechanisms or as a result of a direct carcinogenic or co-carcinogenic action of the drug has yet to be established.

Chemical cystitis has also been caused by ether (used to dissolve retained Foley catheters), by accidental or suicidal ingestion of turpentine and by formalin instilled into the bladder to control haemorrhage due to cyclophosphamide cystitis.

EOSINOPHILIC CYSTITIS[67]

This is a rare condition affecting children more often than adults and usually due to a food or drug allergy,[68] or to an infection or parasitic disease. There may be an accompanying blood eosinophilia. Cystoscopically the bladder mucosa is frequently polypoid and the appearances may resemble a tumour. Microscopically, the lamina propria is heavily and diffusely infiltrated with eosinophils and there is no sign of neoplasia. It is important to distinguish between true eosinophilic cystitis, which usually affects the bladder diffusely, and the local infiltration with eosinophils that is seen very commonly where the bladder wall has been recently biopsied or where the tip of an indwelling catheter has caused ulceration. Local eosinophilia is also a constant feature of the acute stages of bilharzial infestation (see p. 713).

MALAKOPLAKIA[69]

Malakoplakia is a chronic granulomatous disease first described by Michaelis and Gutmann,[69a] in 1902; though it is relatively uncommon, it occurs much more often than reports in the world literature would suggest. For many years it was thought that the lesions were confined to the urinary system but within the past 25 or so years the disease has been found to affect many other parts of the body and particularly the genitalia, gastrointestinal tract and retroperitoneum. Amongst the cases on record, the majority of lesions occur in the urinary tract; the bladder is most often affected, followed in order by the renal parenchyma, ureter and renal pelvis, with very infrequent involvement of the pelviureteric junction or of the urethra. The disease affects females about four times as often as males and occurs at any age, though most of the patients are more than 50 years old. In the bladder soft yellowish brown, round or oval plaques or, occasionally, polypoid lesions are scattered over the mucosal surface. The overlying epithelium is intact in early lesions but may break down and ulcerate later. Microscopically, the lamina propria is infiltrated by dense collections of large histiocytes (von Hansemann cells) whose cytoplasm contains many eosinophilic, periodic-acid-Schiff-positive granules. Small rounded, haematoxyphile, often concentrically laminated, target-like bodies (Michaelis–Gutmann bodies) that stain positively

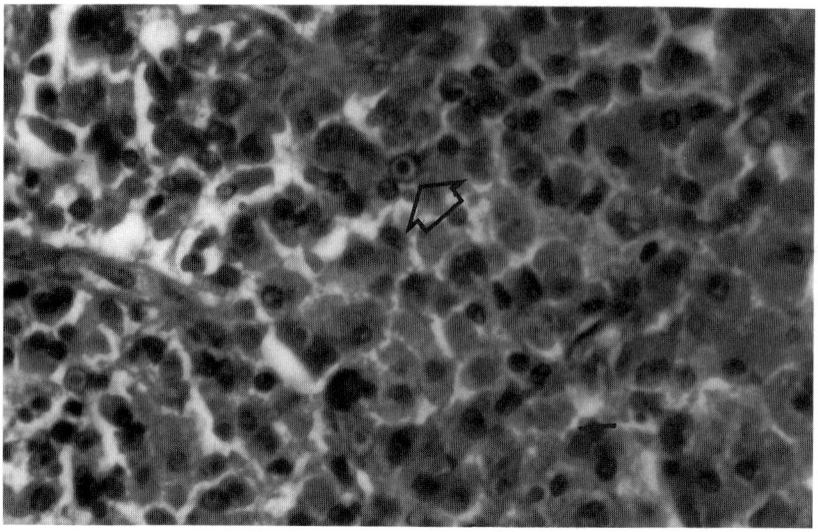

Fig. 19.7 Malakoplakia. Histiocytes containing target-like Michaelis–Gutmann bodies (arrowed).
Haematoxylin–eosin × 570

for iron and with the von Kossa and periodic-acid Schiff techniques are found extracellularly as well as within the histiocytes (Fig. 19.7). The origin of the Michaelis–Gutmann bodies and the nature of the disease process have been much debated. The condition is invariably associated with chronic urinary infection with coliform organisms and the bodies are thought to be altered bacteria or bacterial breakdown products within lysozomes that have become mineralized. The relatively high incidence in the general population of urinary tract infection with coliform organisms might be thought to favour the suggestion that these organisms could in some way be responsible agents, but the comparative rarity of malakoplakia indicates that some other factor must be involved in the pathogenesis. Whether this might be intercurrent systemic disease, an unusual strain of organism, abnormal lysozomes or an alteration in the immune responses remains uncertain. The disease is not always easy to eradicate and lesions near the ureteric orifice or in the ureter itself may cause obstruction.[70] Polypoid lesions in the bladder should not be mistaken for neoplasms. In a number of cases reported in the literature malakoplakic changes have been seen in the stroma of a tumour but this should not be taken as an indication that there is a direct relationship between malakoplakia and neoplasia.

GRANULOMATOUS CYSTITIS

A number of specific infections (tuberculosis, schistosomiasis) produce a granulomatous cystitis but are better considered individually (see below). Necrotizing palisaded granulomas are also seen in the bladder, following previous resection of a bladder tumour.[71] Cystitis has been recorded in the very rare chronic granulomatous disease of childhood in which the bactericidal activity of the leucocytes is depressed due to a genetic enzyme defect.[72]

TUBERCULOUS CYSTITIS[73]

Tuberculous involvement of the bladder is secondary to renal tuberculosis (see pp. 383–386). The early lesions are seen around one or other ureteric orifice as haemorrhagic or granular areas, usually with bullous oedema of the mucosa. Shal-

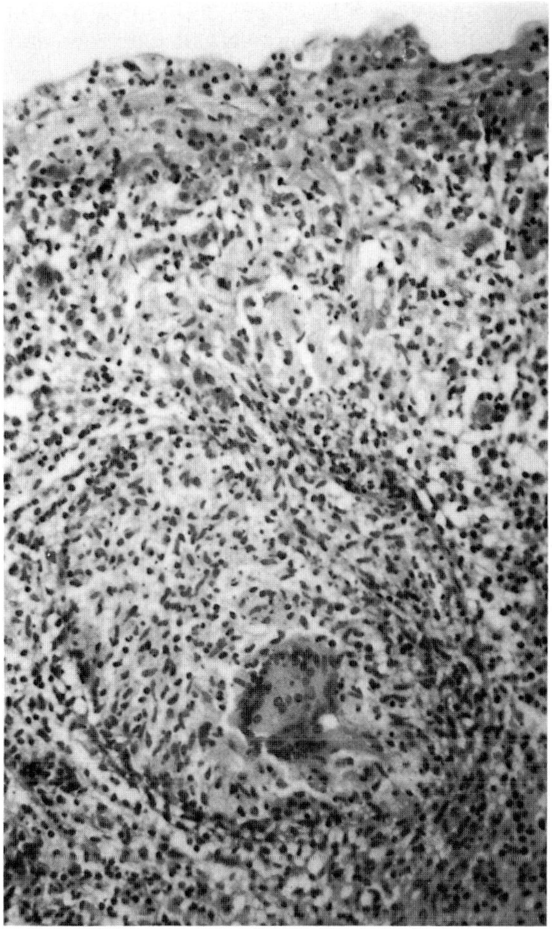

Fig. 19.8 Tuberculous cystitis. Giant cell granuloma of tuberculosis. Caseation and giant cells are not always obvious and a Ziehl–Neelsen stain should always be performed when granulomatous inflammation is seen. A similar appearance is produced after treatment of bladder cancer with Bacillus Calmette–Guérin (BCG). Haematoxylin–eosin × 230

low ulcers soon develop and subsequent fibrosis produces the characteristic 'golf hole' ureteric orifice and allows vesicoureteric reflux. Severe contracture of the bladder often develops in the late stages of the untreated disease. The histological appearances are similar to those seen in tuberculous lesions elsewhere in the body (Fig. 19.8). Sterile pyuria and an acid urine are common but in some patients the only urinary abnormalities may be proteinuria with or without a few red blood cells. Superimposed coliform urinary tract infection is quite common.

ACTINOMYCOTIC CYSTITIS

Actinomycosis of the urinary bladder, as of the other parts of the urinary tract, is an extremely uncommon condition; it has been reported as a complication of the use of intrauterine contraceptive devices.[74] A tendency to form fistulae or a palpable mass may suggest malignant disease on clinical examination.

FUNGAL CYSTITIS

Cystitis caused by fungi is almost always an opportunistic infection. It is seen in diabetics and in patients with indwelling catheters and, increasingly in recent years, after prolonged antibiotic therapy or treatment with steroids and immunosuppressive and antineoplastic agents. Females are more often affected than males. *Candida albicans* and other species of candida, which are normal inhabitants of the gut and vagina, reach the bladder by direct transfer, producing severe diffuse inflammatory changes, sometimes with a membranous type of exudate.[75] Vesical aspergillosis,[76] cryptococcosis and zygomycosis have also been recognized. Non-opportunistic mycotic infections of the bladder are rarely observed and are generally an incidental occurrence in the course of generalized haematogenous dissemination of the organisms in cases of histoplasmosis, blastomycosis and other primary mycoses.

SCHISTOSOMIASIS

Schistosomiasis due to infestation with *Schistosoma haematobium* is very common in Egypt and indeed it was there that Theodor Bilharz in 1851 first demonstrated this type of blood fluke as the cause of haematuria in a young boy. The disease is widespread in other parts of North Africa and in some countries in the Middle East as well as in parts of Central, East, West and Southern Africa. It is rife in those areas where the standards of sanitation are low and people come into contact with contaminated water.

The helminth has a sexual cycle of reproduction in man and an asexual cycle in an intermediate host, the fresh-water snail *Bulinus contortus*. The mature adult worms reside in the portal venous system of man and after fertilization the gravid females migrate to the venous plexuses in the bladder, ureter and prostate where ova are laid. Some of the ova die and become calcified and are eventually surrounded by fibrous tissue, but others pass through the lamina propria of the bladder wall and are voided in the urine. If the urine contaminates fresh water, free swimming miracidia are released from the ova by the process of osmosis and are able to enter the intermediate host where they mature into cercariae within sporocysts in the snail's liver. Rupture of the sporocysts allows the cercariae to leave the snail and swim around in the water, and to penetrate the skin of any human swimming or washing there, causing a transient skin weal – the so-called 'swimmer's itch'. The cercariae lose their tails in the blood stream of the human host and, as metacercariae, eventually reach the portal system and mature there into adult worms. When the ova are deposited in the bladder wall there is much local irritation and, usually, frequency of micturition and some haematuria. Microscopically the ova with their characteristic and diagnostic terminal spines will be seen in the lamina propria surrounded by a heavy accumulation of eosinophils. The lamina propria is also congested and there is a variable amount of local oedema; on rare occasions adult worms will be found there. Later, the reaction becomes granulomatous and the ova are surrounded by epithelioid cells and foreign body giant cells. Eosinophils are still a prominent feature at this stage but other types of inflammatory cell are also seen. The ova may remain viable or die and ultimately calcify. The follicular granulomatous lesions need to be distinguished from tuberculous foci but the large number of eosinophils should suggest the correct diagnosis. In the later stages of the disease there is dense fibrosis, often enclosing dead calcified ova, in the lamina propria and in the detrusor muscle. The bladder epithelium overlying or adjacent to the lesions in the lamina propria is almost always hyperplastic and thickened and frequently polypoid. Proliferative and metaplastic mucosal lesions are common and cystitis cystica (see p. 715), cystitis glandularis (see p. 715) and squamous metaplasia (see p. 716) occur frequently. The proliferative changes are often extreme and sometimes are difficult to distinguish from true neoplasia.

The microscopical changes are reflected in the appearances seen with the cystoscope or in resected tissue specimens. In the earlier stages there are raised reddened areas on the mucosal surface, often with petechial haemorrhages. The granulomas produce the characteristic bilharzial tubercles, which are pin-head-sized yellow specks, often surrounded by a hyperaemic zone, and situated on the trigone and posterior wall – a distribution that serves to distinguish them from tuberculous follicles which are usually most numerous around the ureteric orifices. 'Sandy patches' develop when the ova within the granuloma die and calcify. Ulcers develop when tubercles coalesce and the overlying mucosa sloughs away. Epithelial thickening and hyperplasia produce bilharzial nodules and 'papillomas' or polyps. Secondary bacterial infection is very common and in the late stages of the disease the bladder is contracted and fibrotic, often with a significant amount of chronic pericystitis and fibrosis.

In the areas where the disease is endemic almost continuous reinfestation is common and lesions in all stages of evolution may be found at any one time: in the majority of patients the pathological appearances in the bladder are by no means uniform.

Ova deposited in the urethra (see p. 744) or the lower part of a ureter (see p. 688) produce local lesions essentially the same as those seen in the bladder. Stricture formation is liable to occur at either site when the disease is untreated or in a late stage.

Patients with vesical schistosomiasis are particularly liable to develop carcinoma of the bladder. The tumours differ in several important respects from those that occur in patients not exposed to this helminth as they present at a very much earlier age and most are squamous carcinomas. It had been thought there was a direct association between schistosomiasis and carcinoma but it is now known that the extent and amount of infestation are not directly related to the incidence of tumours, which varies in the different countries in which schistosomiasis is endemic. There is evidence that this different incidence may be related to dietetic factors, and especially to the amount of nitrate in the diet, and also to the levels of nitrosamine in the urine.[78] Nitrosamine formation is related both to nitrate intake and to the presence of specific bacteria in the urine, and the incidence of urinary tract infection in the different populations at risk is clearly an important aetiological factor (see 'Mechanisms of carcinogenesis', p. 721).

NON-NEOPLASTIC PROLIFERATIVE AND METAPLASTIC MUCOSAL LESIONS

The many proliferative, reactive and metaplastic changes that are commonly seen, either singly or in combination, in the urothelium of the renal pelvis (see p. 615), ureter (see p. 687), bladder (see below) and urethra (see p. 745) in many different types of inflammatory, neoplastic or preneoplastic diseases are of variable importance and clinical significance.[79] Some may be confused on gross or microscopical examination with tumours.

VON BRUNN'S NESTS, CYSTITIS CYSTICA AND CYSTITIS GLANDULARIS

These three closely related lesions are commonly seen in the bladder in the human[80] as well as in the experimental animal. Opinion is divided as to their significance though there is broad agreement that to use the word 'cystitis' is not strictly accurate as cystic and glandular changes are found frequently in bladders that show no evidence whatever of inflammation. To describe them as cystic metaplasia and glandular metaplasia would certainly be more accurate but 'cystitis' has become so entrenched in the literature that its use will be continued here. Some writers have considered all these lesions to be preneoplastic and others judge them to indicate an instability of the mucosa which, though capable of returning sometimes to an entirely normal appearance, nevertheless has a malignant potential without necessarily being overtly preneoplastic. These somewhat contradictory opinions have been based very largely on the interpretation of biopsy specimens taken from patients with, or suspected of having, a vesical tumour. The report that these same metaplastic changes (as well as squamous metaplasia) were found in bladders that were normal on gross inspection and contained no obvious infection or inflammation has suggested that they are probably not preneoplastic and should be considered as normal variants of urothelium,[80] despite the undisputed fact that they are often found in the neoplastic bladder.

Von Brunn's nests

The structures known as Von Brunn's nests are formed when rounded buds of cells grow down from the deep aspect of the bladder transitional epithelium into the underlying lamina propria. Later the buds become surrounded by a layer of condensed connective tissue which eventually separates them altogether from the overlying epithelium. Sometimes the cells within the nests have a whorled appearance indicating early squamous change. The buds are by definition solid but very occasionally there is commencing central cavitation: this is not of sufficient degree to warrant describing the condition by the term cystitis cystica.

Cystitis cystica

Central cavitation of Von Brunn's nests or the infolding of the surface epithelium with the formation of crypts whose surface openings become obstructed leads to the production of the characteristic lesions of cystitis cystica. These vary considerably in size and when large can cause the epithelial surface to be irregular and granular. The small cysts are lined by cuboidal or low columnar cells with basal nuclei and eosinophilic cytoplasm, or by stratified epithelium. In the larger ones the lining cells are usually flattened and the lumen contains structureless eosinophilic material.

Cystitis glandularis

There has been confusion over the definition of this term. We should prefer to reserve it for those

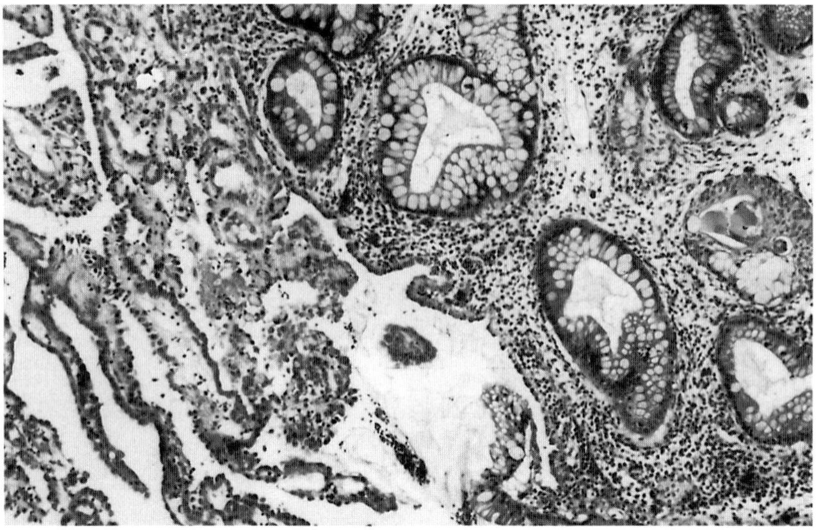

Fig. 19.9 Cystitis glandularis and adenomatous metaplasia. This bladder with florid metaplastic changes shows intestinal-type epithelium of cystitis glandularis on the right and the attenuated 'hob-nail' epithelium of adenomatous metaplasia (nephrogenic adenoma) on the left.
Haematoxylin–eosin × 85

cystic lesions which are lined by epithelium of intestinal type (Fig. 19.9). However, some authorities[81] apply the term cystitis glandularis to lesions of cystitis cystica type that are recognized only under the microscope and reserve the term cystitis cystica for lesions seen macroscopically: they suggest the lesions of both these types may be known together by the name cystitis glandularis et cystica. Others[79] use cystitis cystica only when there is an actual cyst containing eosinophilic secretion: they describe two types of cystitis glandularis, a common typical form composed of cuboidal and columnar urothelial cells and a rare lesion in which the cells are of intestinal type. Intestinal epithelium in the bladder has to be distinguished from adenocarcinoma, primary or metastatic. Extensive intestinal metaplasia of the bladder which is not a component of cystitis glandularis should be separately categorized as there is some evidence that it is a premalignant condition.[82]

SQUAMOUS METAPLASIA

Squamous metaplasia of urothelium should be subdivided into non-keratinizing and keratinizing varieties since they have completely different significance and natural history. Non-keratinized stratified squamous epithelium is seen as white patches on the lining of the bladder in the region of the bladder neck and in the trigone and is a common finding in women; occasionally it occurs in normal males.[79] The cells have a high glycogen content and because of the similarity to normal vaginal epithelium the condition, which is not in any way preneoplastic, is often referred to as vaginal metaplasia (Fig. 19.10). It has been described as a feature specific to and diagnostic of the 'urethral syndrome' (see p. 709) but it is now considered to be a normal variant.[80] A number of studies have suggested that it is a response to female hormones: oestrogen receptors have certainly been demonstrated in these cells.[83] Squamous metaplasia elsewhere in the bladder in patients of both sexes is often associated with chronic irritation caused, for instance, by stones or the tip of an indwelling catheter. It often occurs, too, in vesical diverticula: this accords with the higher incidence of squamous carcinoma in diverticula than in the bladder itself.

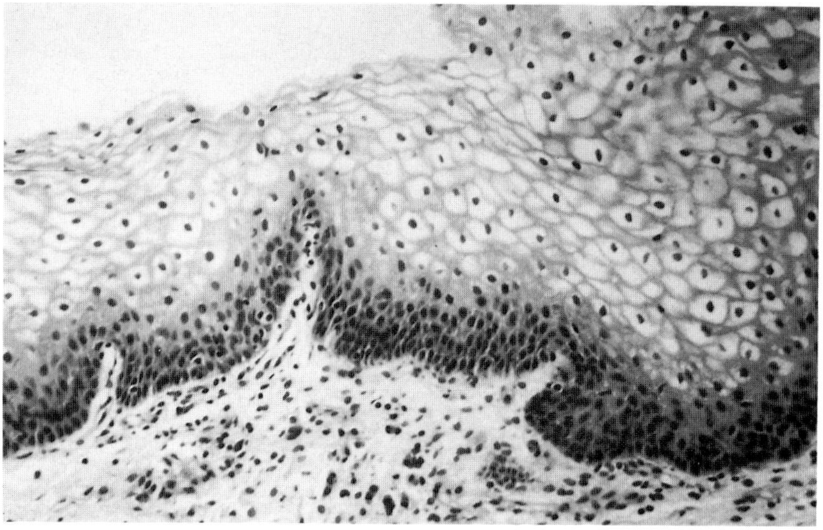

Fig. 19.10 Squamous metaplasia. This non-keratinized type of squamous metaplasia is often termed vaginal metaplasia.
Haematoxylin–eosin × 335

LEUKOPLAKIA

Although there is reluctance to continue to use this term in relation to other organs, it is convenient to retain it when considering the urinary bladder in order to differentiate the condition from non-keratinizing squamous metaplasia. Leukoplakia is a rare condition, commoner in men than in women, that is distinguished from squamous metaplasia by surface keratinization and the presence of intercellular bridges. It produces white or shaggy patches on the mucosal surface and is frequently associated with chronic or recurrent urinary tract infection and bladder stones. Atrophic and hypertrophic types have been described and each has an equal liability to become neoplastic.[84] Malignant change occurs in about one-third of cases[85] and is usually insidious, without any alteration to the surface detectable on cystoscopy. The resulting tumour, which is almost invariably a squamous carcinoma, is often in an advanced state by the time it is detected clinically.

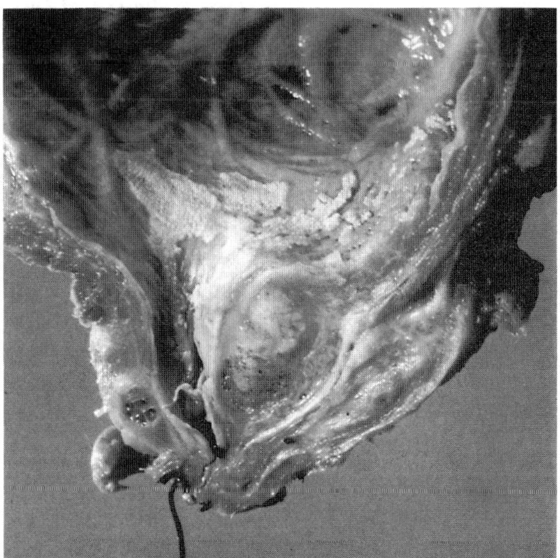

Fig. 19.11 Leukoplakia. Shaggy white plaques of keratinized squamous metaplasia at the bladder base.

POLYPOID CYSTITIS

In response to many different types of local stimulation the urothelium may be thrown into polypoid folds that project into the bladder lumen and simulate a fronded neoplasm on cystoscopic examination. If these folds are especially finger-like the term papillary cystitis may be used.[86] The change is commonly seen, for example, where the

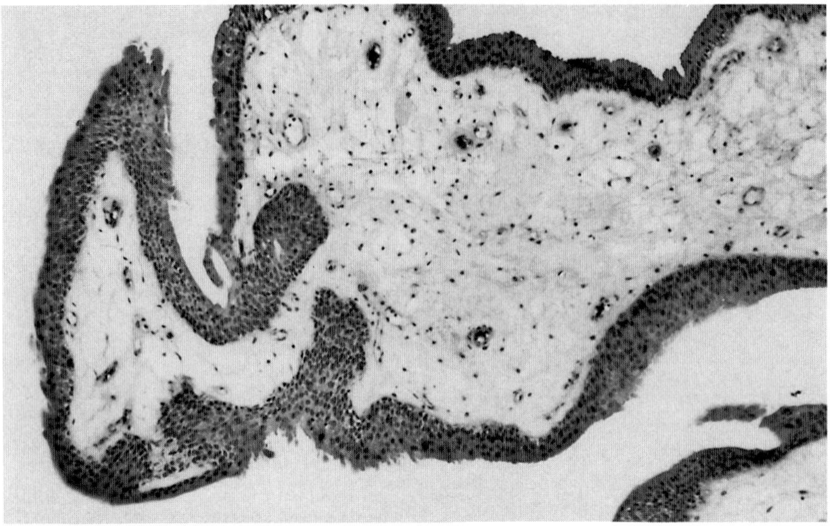

Fig. 19.12 Polypoid cystitis. Outgrowth of bladder epithelium of normal thickness and abundant oedematous stroma distinguishes this lesion from a papillary carcinoma. Haematoxylin–eosin × 85

tip of an indwelling catheter is in contact with the bladder mucosa and in such cases it has been fancifully called a catheter tumour.[87] It is also seen in at least two other circumstance – when an extravesical tumour is infiltrating the bladder wall (but has not yet erupted into the lumen) and around the edges of an established neoplastic fistula; it is not itself regarded as a preneoplastic change. Characteristically, the polyps are broad-based and taper towards their tip, contrasting with the fronds of a papillary tumour which are finger-like with parallel sides. The stroma is often coarser and more abundant than in a fronded tumour and there is usually a moderately heavy inflammatory cell infiltrate (Fig. 19.12). The covering epithelium is sometimes nearly normal but more often is hyperplastic, sometimes with a degree of reactive dysplasia which must be distinguished from true in-situ malignancy.

ADENOMATOUS METAPLASIA

This lesion, first described under the name 'nephrogenic adenoma'[88] because of a supposed likeness to renal tubules, occurs as a response to epithelial damage. Any part of the urinary tract may be involved but the majority of lesions are found in the bladder.[89] Many of the patients have a past history of calculous disease, tuberculosis, interstitial cystitis, or repeated urinary tract trauma by, for instance, a catheter. The individual lesions are flat or, more commonly, polypoid and have a surface covering of a single layer of regular cuboidal cells. In the underlying lamina propria and in continuity with the surface there are many small closely packed clusters of cells or small gland-like spaces lined by cuboidal cells some of which contain mucoid material (Fig. 19.9). Cellular pleomorphism is not a noticeable feature but mitotic figures are sometimes found. The lesion is not usually considered to be either neoplastic or preneoplastic, but it has been reported adjacent to a poorly differentiated mucus-secreting adenocarcinoma of the bladder.[90]

NEOPLASMS OF THE BLADDER

EPITHELIAL TUMOURS

The majority of bladder tumours arise from the lining urothelium and while for descriptive purposes it is often convenient to consider them

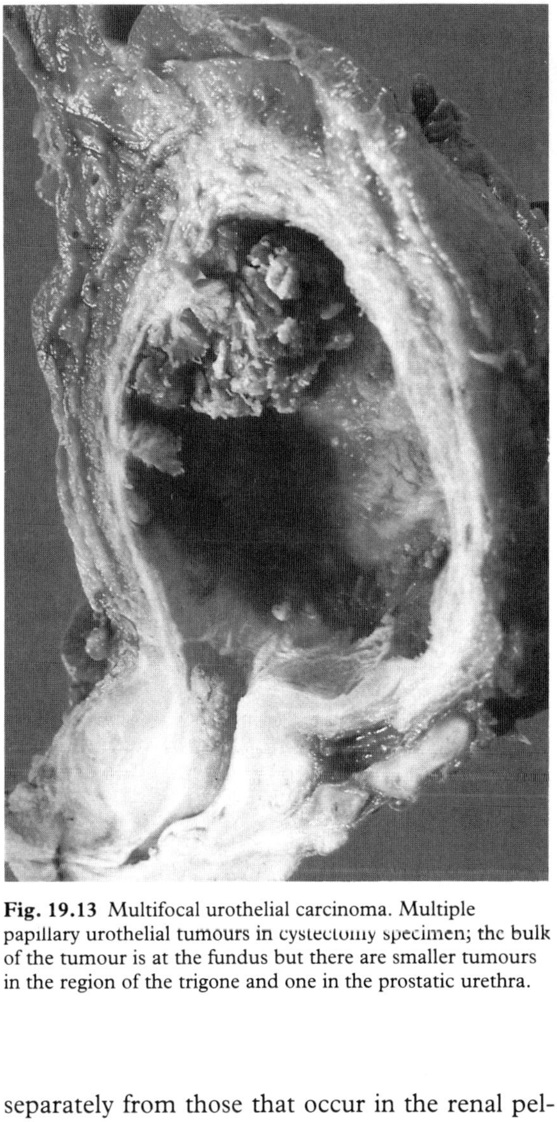

Fig. 19.13 Multifocal urothelial carcinoma. Multiple papillary urothelial tumours in cystectomy specimen; the bulk of the tumour is at the fundus but there are smaller tumours in the region of the trigone and one in the prostatic urethra.

separately from those that occur in the renal pelvis, ureter or urethra it is important to recognize that all urothelial tumours are manifestations of a single, potentially multifocal disease that may involve any part of the urinary tract. In a few patients the multifocal propensity is evident from the start as they present clinically with tumours simultaneously affecting all parts of the urinary tract, suggesting that there might be a single cause for the neoplasia (Fig. 19.13). In other cases the connection is much less obvious because the tumours are apparently confined to one area and the complete spectrum of the disease evolves over a relatively long period of time, often measured in years. For example, a renal pelvic tumour on one side with or without an accompany tumour in the ipsilateral ureter may be followed some months or years later by a bladder tumour, sometimes with urethral involvement later still. In such a case there may indeed be a common cause for the multiple tumours: obviously, other factors may also be significant, such as the possibility of implantation into the lower tract from a lesion higher up, or lymphatic spread, or direct spread of tumour cells by continuity along the surface of the urothelium. Local conditions, such as schistosomiasis (see p. 713) and exstrophy (see p. 697), often determine in which part of the urinary tract a tumour develops.

Incidence and frequency

Bladder cancer is not a particularly common disease and in England and Wales it accounts for about 7% of all cancers in males and about 3% of all cancers in females. The incidence is rising. It is commoner in males than females, in ratios of from 2 to 4 males to 1 female; it is rare in the first five decades of life with, thereafter, a sharp rise in incidence with increasing age.[91] The mortality rate rises with a decrease in social status. Very similar trends are seen in many other countries though the information is sometimes difficult to interpret because some registries include papillomas with the carcinomas in their statistics whereas others do not. In the USA, the incidence is higher in whites than in blacks. In Egypt bladder cancer accounts for 11% of all malignant disease.

Aetiology

An association between bladder cancer and industrial occupation was first recognized in aniline dye workers in Germany in 1895. Since then the list of occupations in which there is a definite (or 'recognized') risk has increased considerably and now includes the chemical, rubber and cable industries, gas retort-house workers, some rat catchers, and laboratory technicians.[92] There is a possible, though not yet fully established, risk to workers in the printing, leather and footwear trades. The distinction between a recognized occupational risk and a possible one is important in the UK as with the former, but not with the latter, a patient who has a bladder cancer is entitled to compensation and financial benefit if it can be proved that the tumour developed after exposure at work.[93] All forms of transitional cell carcinoma of the urothelium, including carcinoma in situ, are covered by the most recent British legislation.[94] In the dye-stuff industry it was first thought that the finished dyes themselves caused the tumours, but it was shown later that certain intermediate products were responsible. It is now known that the metabolic products of α- and β-naphthylamine, benzidine and 4-aminodiphenyl and orthotolidine, absorbed into the body by inhalation, ingestion or through the skin, are carcinogenic. Methylene-*bis*-orthochloraniline has recently been added to the list. Occupational tumours usually occur at an earlier age than spontaneous ones and one of their very characteristic features is that there is an induction period, sometimes as long as 20 or more years, between exposure to the chemical and clinical detection of the tumour. In some patients, though, the exposure time is very short indeed. In general, the longer the exposure the greater the risk of a tumour developing. It has been suggested that in certain heavily industrialized areas in the USA and UK about 20–30% of all bladder tumours may be associated with occupation.[95,96] Measures taken within recent years to control the use and manufacture of toxic substances are likely to reduce the risks. Grossly and microscopically, industrial tumours are no different from neoplasms that arise apparently spontaneously.

Endogenous carcinogens are sometimes considered to be wholly or partly responsible for tumour formation and it has been reported that 3-hydroxykynurenine, 3-hydroxyanthranilic acid and 2-amino-3-hydroxyacetophenone (all of which are orthoaminophenolic metabolites of tryptophan) may be excreted in the urine in larger amounts in patients with a bladder tumour than in normal individuals. These substances are known to be carcinogenic in mice.[97]

Increased consumption of phenacetin-containing analgesics is well established as a cause of serious renal damage, and in particular of renal papillary necrosis, and there is good evidence that it is also responsible for urothelial tumour formation. There is usually a long history of analgesic abuse and a relatively long interval between the onset of such abuse and the clinical appearance of tumours – a situation very reminiscent of the long induction period that characterizes occupational cancer. Most of the tumours occur in the upper urinary tract (see p. 613) but in a significant number of patients the ureter or bladder is also involved, either concurrently or sequentially.[98,99] Phenacetin itself, rather than other constituents of the analgesic mixtures, is believed to be the active carcinogen as it is an aniline derivative and produces orthoaminophenolic metabolites (see above). It has been suggested that analgesic abuse may be a much more important aetiological factor in urothelial malignancy than has hitherto been believed.[100]

There have been many epidemiological studies seeking to identify other extrinsic factors, such as smoking, coffee drinking and the use of artificial sweeteners, that might cause or contribute to tumour development. The data are commonly confusing and often contradictory but it is now evident that cigarette smoking is hazardous, though the carcinogen or carcinogens have yet to be identified fully; coffee drinking is not harmful, while the two sweeteners, saccharin and sodium cyclamate, may have a contributory rather than a primary causal role.[93]

The suggestion that there might be some significant environmental factor in the development of urothelial tumours first came from veterinary workers who reported an association in cows between the ingestion of bracken fern (*Pteris aquilina*) and the incidence of bladder cancer in some parts of Turkey and the Balkans.[101] But probably of greater significance to the human problem is the increased incidence of renal pelvic carcinoma recorded in certain geographical areas in Yugoslavia, where again some environmental agent may be operative (see p. 613).[102]

Local factors are often important and sometimes determine which part of the urinary system is first involved in tumour formation. Neoplasia in the exstrophied bladder is referred to on page 729; it is important to appreciate that a tumour may develop after surgical correction of the initial deformity. Similarly, after surgical diversion of the urinary flow the defunctioned bladder is at risk: pyocystis (empyema vesicae) is not at all uncommon and tumours occasionally occur.[103] Tumours occur in a variety of other conditions, as already discussed – in diverticula (see p. 701), after cyclophosphamide therapy (see p. 711), complicating leukoplakia (see p. 717), after ureterocolic anastomosis (see p. 690) and in schistosomiasis (see p. 713). The significance of the various types of proliferative and metaplastic mucosal lesions is considered on pages 715–718. Epithelial or connective tissue tumours have been recorded as complications of radiotherapy to pelvic organs. Calculous disease is sometimes cited as a cause of urothelial carcinoma, though it is more likely that the stones have a secondary role as mucosal irritants rather than an action as direct carcinogens. Urinary tract obstruction is a common finding in patients with vesical cancer.[104]

Mechanisms of carcinogenesis

Since the demonstration in 1938 that bladder tumours could be produced by feeding dogs with β-naphthylamine there has been a great deal of experimental work aimed at identifying the agents which could be responsible for tumour formation in the bladder and the ways in which they might act.[105] There is now good evidence that carcinogenesis in the bladder of the experimental animal is a multistage process,[106] comprising a stage of initiation in which cells are converted irreversibly into latent tumour cells followed by a stage of promotion in which the same cells are stimulated to divide and grow into actual tumours. Initiation may be produced by exposure to a large dose of a single carcinogen (possibly for only a very short time) or to lower doses of a single substance or to multiple agents – these may act synergistically with each other or even in a mutually antagonistic fashion. By contrast, promotion is always a much more protracted process which, at least in its early stages, is reversible.

Certain substances, such as N-methyl-N-nitrosourea (MNU) and N-butyl-4-(4-hydroxybutyl) nitrosamine (BBN), given to rats in a single dose, or in smaller doses over a long period of time, can act both as initiators and promoters. Tumour incidence is dose-related when the small dose regimen is used. With a single subthreshold non-carcinogenic dose of MNU the sweeteners saccharine and sodium cyclamate can act as promoters though neither is capable of acting as an initiator on its own. Similarly, tryptophan has been shown to promote tumours initiated by N-4-(5-nitro-2-furyl)-2-thiazolyl) (FANFT).[107] In all these experiments, and others, tumour incidence is related to the dose of the initiator but not to the amount of the promoter. Stones in the bladder acted as irritants causing epithelial hyperplasia and were an additional stimulus to tumour growth but not active on their own as tumour promoters.

Much of this experimental work has particular relevance to human bladder cancer. The clinical findings in man can best be explained by the action of a urine-borne carcinogen[108] that transforms urothelial cells at many different sites, thus producing the multifocal tumours that are so characteristic of the disease though, as stated earlier (see p. 719), multifocality may have other explanations. In cases of occupational bladder cancer, tumour initiation will occur when the individual is exposed to the toxic substance. If the dose of the latter is sufficiently large the same chemical substance probably acts as promoter as well. But if the dose is low other factors, such as tobacco smoke or excretion of tryptophan metabolites, may promote: in either event the process will be long drawn out so that typically there is a long induction period between exposure to the carcinogen and the clinical manifestation of the tumour. The high incidence of bladder cancer in some parts of the world where schistosomiasis (see p. 713) is endemic can be explained very readily by the hypothesis of two-stage carcinogenesis: nitrosamines produced in the bladder during episodes of urinary tract infection with nitrate-reducing bacteria are capable of initiating and promoting tumours while the ova, by their irritant effect on the bladder wall, add further stimulus to epithelial proliferation.

Gross appearances

Epithelial tumours in the bladder occur in papillary (non-invasive) or solid (invasive) or flat in-situ (non-papillary non-invasive) forms or in combinations of these three basic types. The *papillary tumours* (Fig. 19.14) range from finely fronded lesions, usually with slender stalks attach-

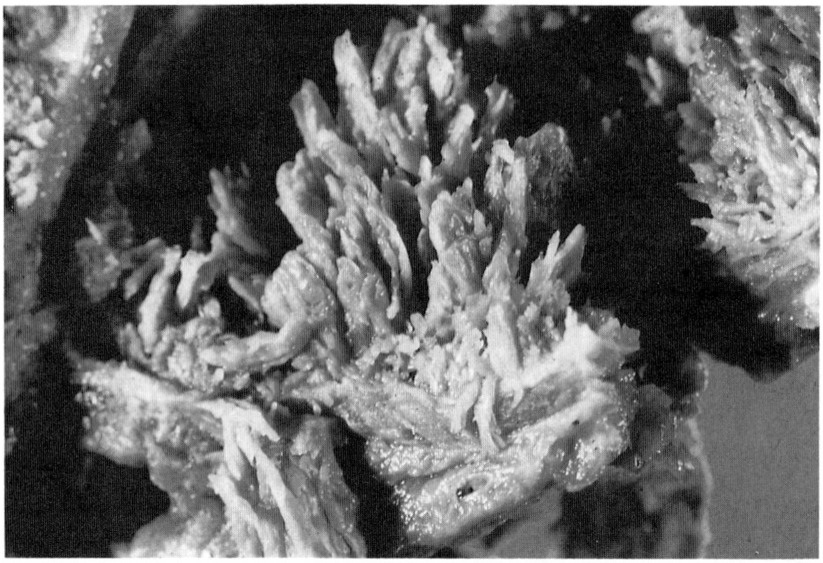

Fig. 19.14 Papillary carcinoma. Delicate fronds of a non-invasive papillary urothelial carcinoma.

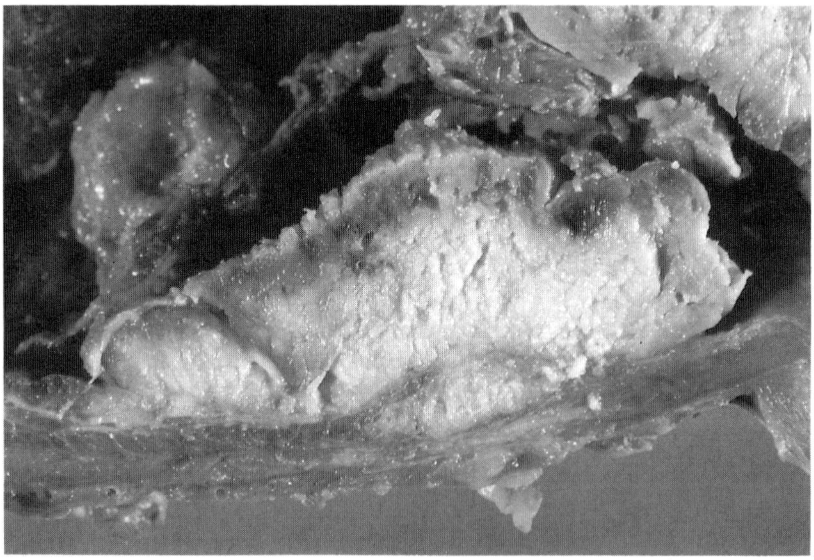

Fig. 19.15 Solid carcinoma. Compact nodule of tumour with partially ulcerated surface which can be seen to be infiltrating muscle in the centre of the photograph.

ing them to quite small areas of the mucosal surface of the bladder, to bulkier masses of larger and plumper papillae that often have a fairly broad basal attachment to the bladder wall. The *solid tumours* (Fig. 19.15) are sessile and form firm nodules that infiltrate the bladder wall to a variable depth and are frequently ulcerated on their free surfaces. In a papillary lesion that has a solid invasive element there will usually be thickening and infiltration of the bladder wall in the region of the tumour stalk. *In-situ tumours* may be recognizable as areas of mucosal reddening when seen through the cystoscope and there is often underlying capillary dilatation when the fixed tissue specimen is examined. Sometimes, however, in-situ disease may be found only on microscopic examination of bladder mucosa that appears to be normal on gross examination.

Tumours of the bladder may be single or multiple and occur in any site though most often on the trigone and near the ureteric orifices or on the posterolateral walls.

Microscopic appearances

Transitional cell carcinoma

A convenient way to describe any bladder tumour is to assess four specific features – the growth pattern, the cell type, the degree of differentiation (tumour grade) and the depth of invasion, if any, into the bladder wall (pathological stage).[109]

Growth pattern The pattern of growth, determined by examining histological sections with a hand lens or the low power of the microscope, corresponds to the gross forms already described and may therefore be papillary, solid, papillary and solid, or non-papillary and non-invasive (in-situ). The early stages of solid or invasive growth are likely to be detected only when the higher power of the microscope is used.

Cell type As regards the cell type, more than 90% of the bladder tumours seen in the UK are composed of transitional cells, often with varying amounts of squamous or glandular change in many of the less well differentiated ones. It is important to recognize these *focal areas of metaplasia* and to distinguish them from true squamous carcinomas or adenocarcinomas which are composed entirely of a single cell type and often have a rather different prognosis. In some countries, such as Egypt, where schistosomiasis is endemic and vesical carcinoma common, there is a very high incidence of squamous tumours and pure transitional cell carcinomas are in the minority. Aside from these endemic areas there is wide variation in the reported incidence of squamous tumours; figures from several registries in Britain range from 1 to 6%; even higher figures have been reported in some series from the USA and Scandinavia.[110] This almost certainly reflects confusion between tumours of a pure cell type and those in which there is metaplasia and it is probable that the true incidence of both squamous carcinoma and glandular carcinoma in the UK is from 1 to 1.5% of all bladder tumours.

Differentiation (tumour grade) Estimation of the degree of tumour differentiation (grade), based on the amount of dedifferentiation of the constituent cells of the tumour, is a contentious subject. Many of the problems stem from the lack of agreement about the histological structure of the bladder papilloma and the criteria which serve to distinguish it from a carcinoma. Indeed, several tumour registries make no distinction in their statistics between the two types of tumour. Also some authors dispense with the words papilloma and carcinoma altogether, and describe a range from the best differentiated (G0) through to the least differentiated (G4) tumours.[111] All of this causes confusion, especially when attempts are made to establish the incidence of bladder cancer in the area covered by a particular tumour registry or to compare the results obtained in different treatment centres. A practical solution to at least part of the problem is to use a very rigid definition of *papilloma* and to apply the term only to a papillary tumour of cylindrical shape with parallel sides, covered by up to four or five cell layers of regular transitional cells which are indistinguishable from those that line the bladder (Fig. 19.16). The individual cells are slender and lie parallel to each other at right angles to the basement membrane. The nuclei are regular in size and staining and mitoses are absent. There is a central core of loose delicate connective tissue. Using these criteria the papilloma will be diagnosed on only very rare occasions. All other papillary lesions should be regarded as carcinomas, provided that polypoid (papillary) cystitis has been excluded (see p. 717). The shape of the two lesions is an important distinguishing feature, the cylindrical papilloma contrasting with a broad-based tapering polypoid lesion whose covering epithelium often shows a significant amount of hyperplastic thick-

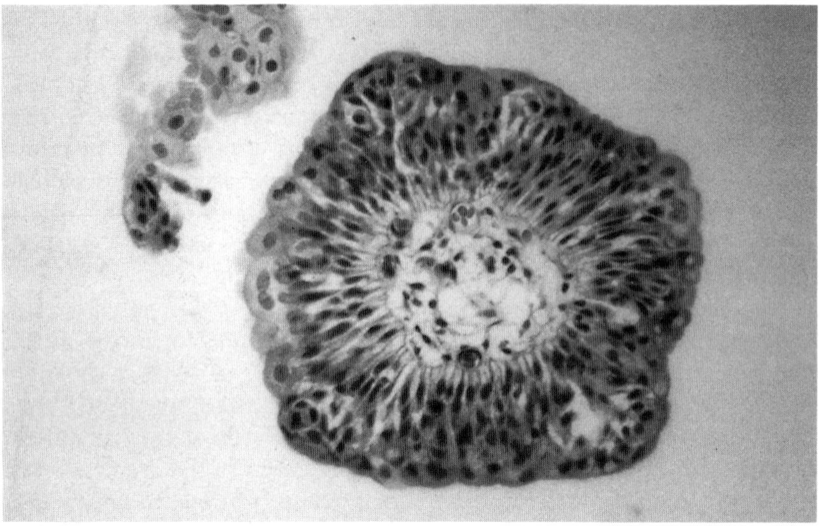

Fig. 19.16 Papilloma. Papillary bladder tumour composed of urothelium only four or five cells thick and with obvious superficial umbrella cells.
Haematoxylin–eosin × 335

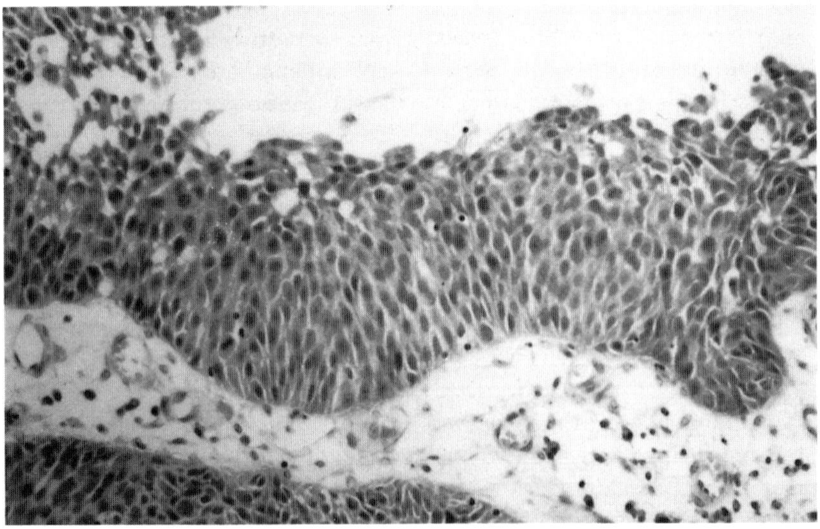

Fig. 19.17 Grade 1 carcinoma. Urothelium thicker than normal with minor degree of loss of polarity and increased nuclear hyperchromicity.
Haematoxylin–eosin × 335

ening and, quite frequently, a degree of dysplasia. This apparent contradiction in designating a non-invasive tumour as a carcinoma is retained because this is established common usage and because of the propensity of the tumours to recur. In a number of instances there is no doubt as to the histological diagnosis of carcinoma because there is penetration of the basement membrane and invasion of the bladder wall but the diagnosis of carcinoma can and should be made in the absence of such infiltration if the changes in the epithelium justify it (see 'Carcinoma in situ', p. 726).

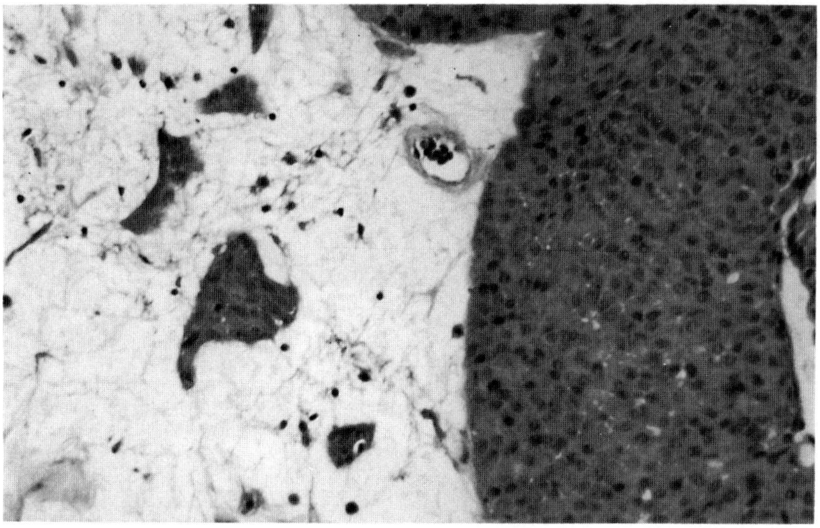

Fig. 19.18 Grade 2 carcinoma. This tumour shows invasion of underlying stroma. Assessment of invasion in tumour resections can be difficult due to tangential cuts; the stellate arrangement of this invasive tumour could not be produced by mere obliquity of section of a non-invasive tumour.
Haematoxylin–eosin × 250

Carcinomas can be separated into three *grades* according to the amount of epithelial dedifferentiation present[112]. In the most differentiated (*Grade 1*) papillary tumours the cells are obviously of transitional type but the criteria for the diagnosis of a papilloma are not met as there is an increase in the number of layers of cells in the surface epithelium in addition to some loss of the regular cell polarity and a minor degree of nuclear hyperchromicity (Fig. 19.17). There may be a few mitotic figures. Many authors would say that Grade 1 tumours never have invasive foci and it is certainly true that on follow-up the majority merely recur and do not evolve into invasive tumours. The intermediate (*Grade 2*) tumour can still be recognized as being of transitional cell origin (Fig. 19.18); there are more cell layers than in a papilloma or differentiated carcinoma and there is a more obvious loss of cell polarity, more pronounced nuclear irregularity and hyperchromicity and more mitotic activity than in a Grade 1 tumour. There may also be some irregularity and loss of continuity of the luminal aspect of the epithelium. All these abnormal features are very much more marked in the high grade and anaplastic or undifferentiated (*Grade 3*) tumours. These sometimes show such a degree of cellular pleomorphism and irregularity, loss of polarity, nuclear hyperchromicity and mitotic activity that it may no longer be immediately obvious that they have originated from transitional epithelium and many classifications assign such tumours to a fourth category – undifferentiated carcinoma (Fig. 19.19). Giant cells or bizarre nuclear forms are not unusual and an important diagnostic feature is the loosening and irregularity of the superficial cell layers, which are shed into the lumen of the bladder and provide the material that enables the cytologist to make an accurate diagnosis of a high grade lesion.

Metaplastic foci of squamous or glandular change, occurring singly or in combination, may be found in any transitional cell tumour and are especially common in the less differentiated types.

Solid transitional cell tumours can be graded using the same general principles although rarely, if ever, being of Grade 1.

It is inevitable that any grading system that depends entirely on a subjective analysis of a series of histological features will have its limitations. Differences and discrepancies between observers and in the interpretation of any individual observer on different occasions cannot be avoided, but practical experience, familiarity with the urothelium and

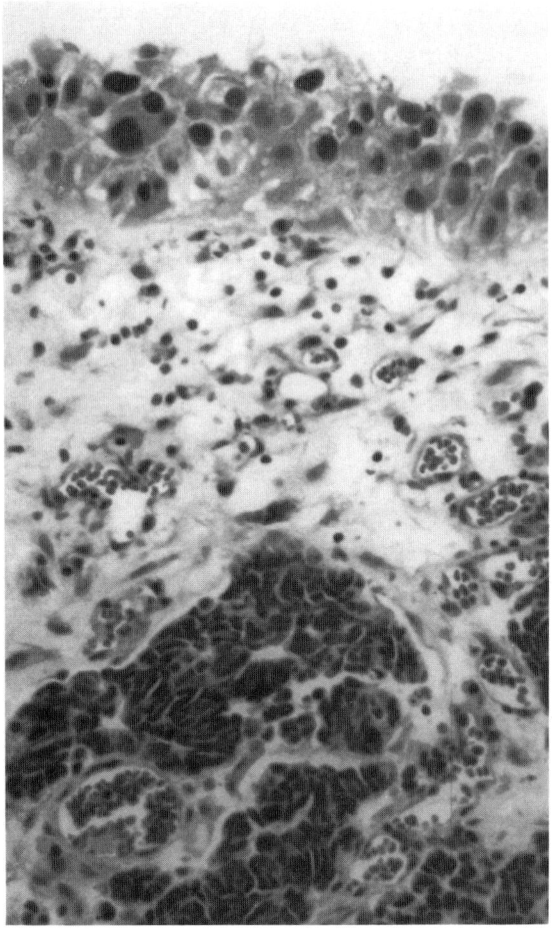

Fig. 19.19 Undifferentiated carcinoma. The invasive tumour at the base of this photomicrograph could be designated as oat cell carcinoma. Note flat in-situ carcinoma of overlying urothelium.
Haematoxylin–eosin × 370

the natural history of its many diseases, and close collaboration between histopathologist and clinician certainly reduce many of the problems to an acceptable level. There is no doubt though that cellular morphometry (at present a research tool rather than a technique in general use) will introduce a much needed measure of objectivity.[113] As will be discussed later (see p. 732), electron microscopy has a place in the assessment of urothelial disease and is providing useful objective information concerning the early stages of tumour development and the means of distinguishing between cystitis, preneoplasia and neoplasia.

Depth of invasion (pathological staging) The extent to which the bladder wall has been infiltrated by a tumour is the basis of *pathological staging* (which is distinct from clinical staging which takes account of factors other than the histological analysis). The larger the specimen the greater the accuracy of pathological staging, but even in small biopsy fragments it is often possible to see the very earliest evidence of bladder wall invasion as shown by breaching of the basement membrane. The pathological stage as defined by the World Health Organization (WHO) is the deepest point in the bladder wall to which the tumour has spread in continuity.[114] Permeation of lymphatics or blood vessels at a deeper level does not warrant increasing the stage though it should of course be noted and included in the histological assessment of the tumour.

Pathological staging is considered in more detail in a later section (see 'Grading and staging of bladder tumours' pp. 729–730) and at this point it suffices to note that bladder tumours can be divided conveniently into non-invasive (in-situ) types and those that invade the lamina propria (stage 1) or superficial muscle (stage 2) or deep muscle (stage 3) or extravesical structures (stage 4).

Carcinoma in situ[115]

Non-invasive, non-papillary, flat in-situ transitional cell carcinoma is an important type of tumour whose natural history has not yet been fully established. In unequivocal examples the histological diagnosis is not very difficult and most, if not all, of the following features will be seen – an increase in the number of cell layers, crowding of the nuclei, cellular pleomorphism, loss of cell polarity, hyperchromicity of the nuclei, failure of differentiation of cells from the base to the surface of the epithelium, increased mitotic activity (and, in particular, the presence of mitotic figures above the basal layers of cells), and, frequently, lack of mutual cohesion of the most superficial layers of cells, which desquamate into the lumen of the bladder (Fig. 19.20). There may also be an increased number of small capillary blood vessels in the underlying lamina propria. Sometimes it is

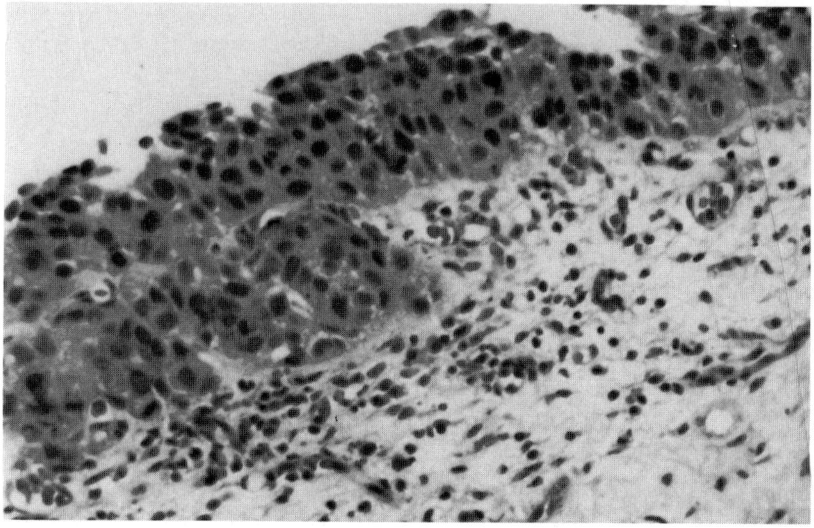

Fig. 19.20 Flat in-situ carcinoma. Complete disorganization of urothelium with obviously malignant cells and telangiectatic capillaries of underlying lamina propria. Early invasion is seen on the left of the picture.
Haematoxylin–eosin × 250

not at all easy to distinguish carcinoma in situ from reactive hyperplasia and most observers recognize a spectrum of change ranging from normal epithelium through the stages of hyperplasia, and of hyperplasia with atypia (dysplasia), to carcinoma,[116] though inevitably there is likely to be some disagreement about the exact point at which the diagnosis of carcinoma is felt to be justified. Unfortunately, there is not the uniformity of nomenclature for hyperplastic and atypical hyperplastic abnormalities of the urothelium as has been formulated for the uterine cervix and for the colonic mucosa in cases of longstanding ulcerative colitis, although there have been attempts to obtain a consensus view[117]. Some workers use a numerical grading scheme to classify the series of changes and correlate their grading with the clinical behaviour of the lesions. Epithelial hyperplasia and dysplasia often occur in inflammatory disease of the bladder, in bladders containing calculi,[118] following systemic administration of drugs,[118a] and as a result of local radiotherapy and topical drug administration.[116] These changes may mimic carcinoma in situ but are reversible and the epithelium returns to normal when the stimulus is withdrawn. It is widely believed that the epithelial changes in established in-situ disease are not reversible and that sooner or later papillary or invasive, or papillary and invasive, tumours will inevitably develop. It is important to note however, that in several early series significant numbers of patients have remained alive and apparently well for 10 or more years after in-situ disease has been diagnosed.[119] There are usually no specific histological features to distinguish the in-situ lesions that are likely to progress from those that will remain unaltered, though there is evidence to suggest that the loss of ABO isoantigen, detected by methods using blood-typing sera,[120] is a useful predictor of progression to invasion.

Variants of transitional cell carcinoma

Spindle cell tumour (sarcomatoid carcinoma[121]) Sometimes a poorly differentiated transitional cell carcinoma is composed in part or almost entirely of spindle cells and may very easily be mistaken for a sarcoma (Fig. 19.21). The recognition of this type of tumour depends on finding transitions between spindle and transitional cells but the search for this evidence is often very tedious. Reticulin impregnation is not always

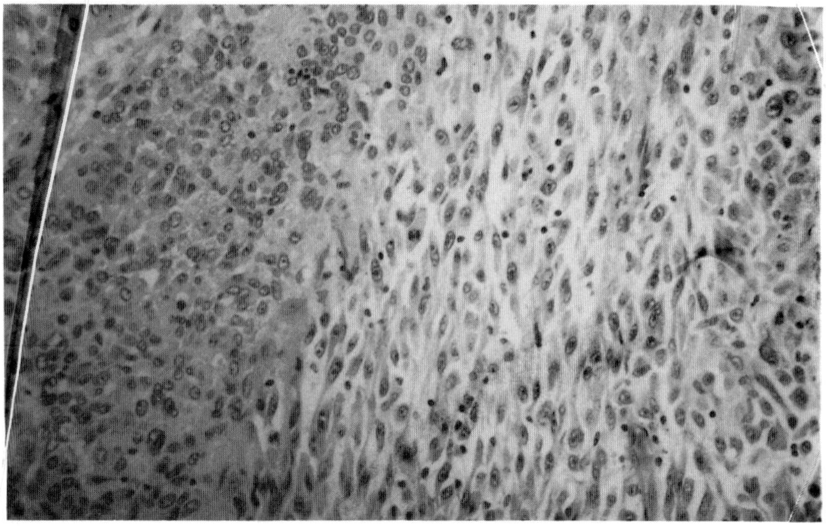

Fig. 19.21 Spindle cell tumour. Anaplastic carcinoma on the left with spindle cell element on right. Differentiation between sarcomatoid carcinoma and carcinosarcoma requires immunocytochemical techniques.
Haematoxylin–eosin × 250

very useful. The monoclonal antibody techniques against cytokeratins and epithelial membrane antigen will demonstrate the epithelial nature of the spindle cells. The prognosis of these tumours is not good.

Stromal metaplasia in transitional cell carcinosarcomas[122] On rare occasions metaplastic foci of cartilage or bone are seen in the stroma of an epithelial tumour and have to be distinguished from the even less common primary chondrosarcomas[123] (in which the overlying epithelium shows reactive changes only) or carcinosarcomas (see below). Another variant is of a pseudosarcomatous spindle cell change in the stroma of urothelial carcinoma;[124] these tumours can be differentiated by immunocytochemistry, which confirms the mesenchymal nature of the spindle-shaped cells.

Carcinosarcoma[122, 125]

The diagnosis of carcinosarcoma can be justified only when there is convincing evidence of malignant change in tissues that are clearly identifiable as having separate origin in both epithelium and mesenchyme. It is not always easy to distinguish them from the sarcomatoid carcinoma (see above) and the diagnosis is difficult, too, when there is any significant amount of pleomorphism in an area of stromal metaplasia. Most of these very uncommon tumours form bulky masses in the region of the trigone and bladder base and the prognosis is poor as the patient is usually elderly and often in poor condition. The epithelial element is usually a papillary or solid transitional cell carcinoma, with or without squamous and/or glandular metaplasia, though pure squamous or glandular tumours are found occasionally. The mesenchymal element is most commonly a chondrosarcoma or fibrosarcoma but leiomyosarcoma and osteogenic sarcoma also occur.

Squamous cell carcinoma

This term should be reserved for tumours that are entirely squamous and should not be employed for transitional cell carcinomas with areas of squamous carcinoma. Squamous carcinoma is a rare tumour[110] except where schistosomiasis is endemic (see p. 713), though it is not uncommonly seen in non-endemic areas in situations of chronic infection such as vesical diverticula, in ureteric stumps, in the surgically defunctioned bladder or in association with calculi. Papillary forms are unusual and most tumours are bulky, nodular, infiltrative masses, often with an ulcerated surface.[126] Microscopically there is usually evidence of keratin formation. Tumour grading is possible as with squamous carcinomas elsewhere in the body. The infiltrating trabeculae of malignant cells are frequently surrounded by an abundant fibroblastic stroma, and often there is squamous metaplasia of the adjacent bladder epithelium, usually of the keratinizing variety. In some patients there is a history of preceding leukoplakia (see p. 717).

Adenocarcinoma[126]

Primary adenocarcinoma of the bladder is a rare tumour[110] and may arise at the fundus from the urachus (see p. 696) and less frequently from areas of glandular metaplasia at the bladder base and from the columnar epithelium of an exstrophic bladder. A tumour should not be labelled adenocarcinoma unless totally of this appearance. There is usually a clearly recognizable glandular pattern and the tumours can be graded using the criteria that are applicable to glandular tumours at other sites. Histological variants described are signet-ring-cell carcinoma,[127] which has a very poor prognosis, and clear-cell carcinoma. It must be appreciated, though, that by far the greatest numbers of glandular tumours found in the bladder originate in extravesical structures, most commonly in the bowel or, in female patients, in an ovary or other pelvic viscera. Glandular tumours at the bladder base must be differentiated from primary prostatic carcinoma and here immunocytochemical staining for prostate-specific antigen and prostate-specific acid phosphatase are invaluable. Polypoid cystitis (see p. 717) may precede the eruption of an extravesical tumour through the urothelium into the bladder lumen or may be found around the margins of an area where the bladder epithelium has already been breached by the invading neoplasm. The finding of neoplastic glandular elements in a bladder biopsy always demands the exclusion of an extravesical tumour before the possibility of a primary adenocarcinoma can be considered.

Grading and staging of bladder tumours

There have been many attempts to classify the various pathological features of bladder tumours with the intention of establishing criteria that would enable the clinician to monitor the progression or regression of the disease in an individual, at the same time providing statistical material which would allow comparisons between different therapeutic regimens and the results obtained in different treatment centres. In some instances tumour grading[127] has provided the basis for categorization but in others the emphasis is on staging,[128] which, it should be stressed, has the great advantage of being a much less subjective undertaking than grading. Classifications that have received wide acceptance are that proposed by the World Health Organization (WHO),[114] which is concerned mainly with histological features, with particular emphasis on tumour grading, and that proposed by the International Union against Cancer (UICC), whose current TNM scheme provides a framework for the pretreatment clinical classification (TNM) and a postsurgical histopathological subdivision (pTNM) with greater weight given to staging than to grading (Table 19.1).[129] Several modifications of the earlier TNM schemes[130–132] are in use or have been proposed as experience has shown various practical difficulties or deficiencies in applying the latter. A common problem is the virtual impossibility of establishing the exact midpoint in the bladder muscle, which is the line of demarcation between the pT2 and pT3 tumours whose prognosis is so very different; this difficulty is especially

Table 19.1 pTNM post-surgical histopathological classification of urothelial carcinomas (Union internationale contre le cancer 1978)[129]

pTis	Pre-invasive (in-situ) carcinoma
pTa	Papillary non-invasive carcinoma
pT1	Tumour not extending beyond lamina propria
pT2	Invasion of superficial muscle
pT3	Invasion of deep muscle or perivesical tissue
pT4	Invasion of prostate or other extravesical structures
pT0	No tumour found
pTX	Extent of invasion cannot be assessed

Table 19.2 Institute of Urology (London) pathological staging (1981) of urothelial carcinoma

Pis	Flat pre-invasive carcinoma: carcinoma in situ
Pa	Papillary non-invasive carcinoma
Pla	Invasion limited to the core of a papilla
Plb	Invasion of true lamina propria
P2	Superficial muscle invasion
P3a	Deep muscle invasion
P3b	Invasion of perivesical tissues
P4a*	Invasion of prostate, uterus or vagina
P4b	Invasion of pelvic or abdominal wall

*P4a – tumours invading the prostate are further subdivided into:
P4aa invasion limited to prostatic ducts or acini only
P4ab invasion of fibromuscular interstitial tissues of the prostate

troublesome when dealing with transurethral resection specimens. A valid criticism of the present TNM scheme is that some of the stages lack refinement; there is good evidence, for instance, that the prognosis worsens with every increase in the stage of a tumour[133] and that it is therefore worthwhile to subdivide them further (Table 19.2)[134] When there is invasion of the prostate it is particularly important to indicate the earliest signs of infiltration and, because of their very different prognosis, to distinguish between the tumours that invade the interstitial tissues of the gland and those in which the malignant tissue is confined by the basement membrane within the lumen of the ducts and acini. Continuous reassessment of the tumour stage in serial bladder biopsies is also much preferred to the single initial assessment advocated by the UICC because it gives the clinician vital information about the current state of his patient's bladder and the way it is, or is not, responding to a particular treatment regimen.

Differential diagnosis

Many of the inflammatory and reactive lesions that sometimes need to be considered in the differential diagnosis of carcinoma have been considered already – von Brunn's nests (see p. 715), adenomatous metaplasia (see p. 718), polypoid cystitis (see p. 717), various forms of metaplasia (see p. 715), amyloidosis (see p. 704) and endometriosis (see p. 705). Malakoplakic lesions sometimes resemble neoplasms on cystoscopic or gross examination (see p. 711). The gross appearances in an irradiated bladder are often equally difficult to interpret (see p. 710).

The 'inverted papilloma'[135] is a localized proliferation of urothelial cells that forms a rounded

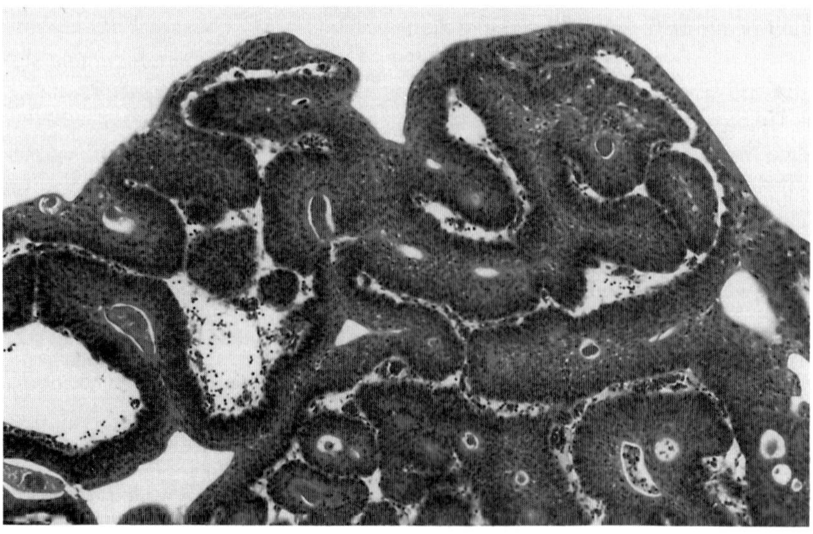

Fig. 19.22 Inverted papilloma. Circumscribed lesion composed of histologically benign urothelium and covered by a layer of similar but attenuated cells. Haematoylin–eosin × 40

or oval polypoid nodule in the superficial lamina propria and combines many of the histological features of von Brunn's nests and cystitis cystica (Fig. 19.22). Trabecular and glandular forms have been described.[136] The lesions are very much commoner in men than in women. They are usually situated at the base of the bladder. Though benign they may be mistaken for carcinoma; cytological examination of the urine will reveal normal or degenerate cells and help to exclude malignancy.[137] Occasionally an inverted papilloma and carcinoma coexist and sometimes transitional cell carcinomas have an inverted pattern of growth. The diagnosis of inverted papilloma can be made only when all its histological criteria are met.

Fragments of an epithelial tumour biopsied transurethrally from the base of the bladder are often a problem in histological diagnosis and it is important to appreciate that a bladder tumour not infrequently invades the prostate (stage P4a/pT4 – see Tables 19.1 and 19.2, pp. 729 and 730) and that occasionally a prostatic carcinoma spreads up into the bladder and masquerades as a primary bladder tumour. Less commonly a carcinoma of the bladder and a carcinoma of the prostate coexist.

Some of the histological features that may assist in the differential diagnosis are shown in Table 19.3 on this page, but beyond all doubt techniques such as the localization of prostate-specific antigen,[138] prostate-specific acid phosphatase, epithelial membrane antigen and carcinoembryonic antigen[139] provide valuable and reliable means of identification. The use of other monoclonal antibodies is now widespread and is invaluable in diagnosis, not only of this group of tumours but also of the spindle cell tumours, carcinosarcomas and connective tissue tumours and also when intestinal or genital tumours invade the bladder and are encountered in biopsy material.

Invasion of the bladder by intestinal tumours, with incipient or established vesicointestinal fistula, and preceded or accompanied by polypoid cystitis, is described on page 702. Tumours of the uterine cervix may spread into the base of the bladder. Metastatic spread to the bladder of tumours in more remote parts of the body include transcoelomic spread from upper abdominal cancers, haematogenous spread of malignant melanoma and, rarely, of carcinoma of the

Table 19.3 Differential diagnosis of tumours at the bladder base

	Carcinoma of bladder	Carcinoma of prostate
Pattern of growth	Large alveoli and trabeculae of cells	Slender trabeculae ('Indian file') more usual
Fibrous or fibroblastic tumour stroma	Common	Unusual
Alveoli and trabeculae of tumour cells with		
Squamous areas	Common in poorly differentiated tumours	Very rare or absent (except after oestrogen therapy)
Glandular areas	Common in poorly differentiated tumours	Usual, except in high-grade tumours
Cellular pleomorphism	Common	In high-grade tumours only
Cell nuclei	Pleomorphism and hyperchromicity common	Nucleoli often very prominent
Mitotic figures	Common	Unusual except in high-grade tumours
Overlying or adjacent transitional epithelium	Often continuous with tumour All varieties of hyperplasia, metaplasia or neoplasia often seen	No continuity: epithelium normal, or mild to moderate hyperplasia only

breast,[140] and implantation of renal parenchymal carcinomas that have invaded the pelvicalyceal system.

Spread of urothelial tumours

One of the most important methods of spread, and the one that is the basis of the staging classifications already described, is direct extension into the bladder wall with invasion of adjacent structures and eventual tethering of the bladder to the wall of the pelvis. Involvement of a ureteric orifice or of the intramural segment of a ureter may occur relatively early and often has a serious effect on prognosis.

The frequent association of vesical tumours with tumours in other parts of the urinary tract as a manifestation of multifocal urothelial disease has been noted on pages 719 and 721. Within the bladder itself tumours are often multiple, both in space and in time; new tumours found after local intravesical therapy may be true recurrences (if they grow at the original site) or further manifestations of multicentricity if they develop elsewhere in the bladder wall.

Lymphatic spread is common. When the superficial lymphatics in the lamina propria are invaded there will often be centrifugal spread deep to the surface producing a subepithelial plaque of tumour tissue. Invasion of the deep lymphatics is a particular feature of the less well differentiated tumours and leads to involvement of the regional lymph nodes along the iliac vessels and in the para-aortic region. Blood-borne metastasis often occurs in the later stages of the disease, with deposits in the liver, lungs, bone and adrenals; other sites include the heart, brain and kidneys.

Electron microscopy and ultrastructure of bladder tumours

Transmission and scanning electron microscopical studies have been used in an attempt to establish firm diagnostic criteria for identifying normal, premalignant and malignant urothelium.[141] The free surface of normal superficial cells is formed by an asymmetrical luminal membrane which prevents seepage of bladder urine into the bladder wall; by reason of its convolutions this membrane permits the bladder to expand and contract without loss of this unique property.[142] The superficial cells are joined by desmosomes and tight junctions. The basement membrane, seen as a PAS-positive band with the light microscope, consists of an electron-dense basal lamina superimposed on collagen fibrils.

With the transmission electron microscope alterations can be seen in the asymmetrical luminal membrane when a tumour develops;[143] pleomorphic microvilli occur on the surface of the cells and there is a loss of mutual cell attachment in higher grade tumours. Discontinuities of the basal lamina with microinvasion of the lamina propria are seen very much more frequently than would be expected from the light microscopical appearances.

A 'cobblestone' appearance on scanning electron microscopy, due to the presence of many microvilli on the surface of the cells, is recorded as characteristic of established carcinoma and preneoplastic epithelium; this appearance is not a feature of normal epithelium. The suggestion has been made that the presence of microvilli might be an indication of an increased tendency of a tumour to recur. It should be noted that microvilli are not pathognomonic of malignancy: this is evident from the fact that they have been seen in inflammatory lesions[40] and in polypoid cystitis.

Chromosomes in bladder tumours and flow cytometry

Non-invasive and superficially invasive transitional cell carcinomas have been found to have chromosome numbers within the diploid range: the presence of abnormal numbers of chromosomes indicates a liability to tumour recurrence, increasing ploidy being correlated with a fall in the 5-year survival rate in patients with bladder tumours.[144] Modern technology has identified markers for bladder cancer on chromosomes 1,5,7,9 and 11, but their significance is not yet known. Flow cytometry has been used extensively in the study of bladder carcinoma and the findings in large part mirror the earlier studies on chromosome content. Perhaps the most useful clinical application is in their use in non-invasive tumours in attempts to identify the small percentage which will progress to invasive cancer.[145]

Exfoliative cytology[116]

Urine cytology has an important place in the clinical management of patients known to have, or suspected of having, urothelial cancer. It is a particularly valuable and reliable means of screening those at risk from exposure to industrial hazards and an essential part of the laboratory investigation in any patient in whom there is a suspicion of in-situ carcinoma. Repeated cytological examination of the urine is also a useful and convenient way of assessing the course of established neoplastic disease following surgery, radiotherapy or chemotherapy and of detecting persistence of residual tumour or recrudescence of a previously treated one.

Voided bladder urine provides the cytologist with the most satisfactory specimens but bladder washouts[147] or mucosal brushing with soluble swabs[148] may be required in some cases. The reliability of the results depends on standardization of the methods of collecting and processing specimens but above all on the experience of the cytologist. False positives may occur with urinary tract infection but about three-quarters of urothelial tumours can be detected by the cytologist before they can be identified by the combined efforts of the cystoscopist, radiologist and histopathologist. Poorly differentiated tumours are much more easily diagnosed than well differentiated because of their tendency to desquamate the superficial cell layers and of the greater degree of atypicality of the nuclei. Many Grade 1 tumours will have negative cytology and reliable diagnosis of these tumours usually requires the presence of a fragment of the papillary tumour in the specimen of urine. Significant changes may be found in the exfoliated cells in patients with urinary calculi[118] or inverted papillomas.[137] Cytological interpretation of conduit urine after urinary diversion is difficult because of the large amounts of debris inevitably present in the specimens.

PHAEOCHROMOCYTOMA[149]

These rare tumours, first recognized in the bladder as recently as 1953,[150] arise from embryonic rests of chromaffin cells in the sympathetic plexuses in the bladder wall. Most are solitary lesions within the muscle or lamina propria: they occur anywhere in the bladder but most commonly at the dome or on the trigone. There is usually an overlying layer of intact urothelium. The tumour cells, which are polyhedral with granular cytoplasm and regular circular nuclei, are arranged in rounded nests or cords supported on a very well vascularized connective tissue stroma. The tumours occur at all ages, with the highest incidence in the first two decades, and are a little more common in males than in females.

In a few patients there are only non-specific symptoms, such as haematuria, but in the majority there is some evidence of hormonal activity due to the release of catecholamines into the circulation. Characteristically this causes paroxysmal hypertension with palpitation and sweating, with or without headaches or blurred vision, either when the bladder fully distends just prior to micturition or, more often, when the detrusor contracts during voiding. Removal of the tumour relieves these symptoms.[151] Persistent hypertension supervenes in some patients. Metastasis occurs in a very few. The diagnosis of malignancy is often very difficult, as in other endocrine tumours: the usual histological criteria are of little value as cellular pleomorphism and considerable mitotic activity often occur in phaeochromocytomas that behave quite benignly, and the finding of tumour cells deep in the muscle coat is a reflection of the site of their origin rather than evidence of invasiveness and malignancy. The only unequivocal evidence of malignancy is the finding of tumour deposits in those parts of the body normally devoid of chromaffin tissue and not in direct continuity with the primary growth. Chromaffin tissue has a wide distribution in the human fetus and this is reflected in the fact that phaeochromocytomas are multifocal in about 10% of patients.

CONNECTIVE TISSUE TUMOURS[123]

Connective tissue tumours are uncommon and account for less than 5% of all bladder neoplasms. Most are benign and there is probably no single non-urothelial component of the bladder wall which is not on record as having given rise to a benign or malignant tumour. Many of the references in the literature are to single case reports only and it is therefore difficult to estimate the true frequency of many of the individual types of tumour.

Benign connective tissue tumours

Fibromas and *leiomyomas* are the most common benign connective tissue tumours of the urinary bladder. They occur at any age and are usually found at the base and in the region of the trigone. Most of the leiomyomas are seen in young or middle-aged females and project into the bladder lumen as a polypoidal mass that may produce symptoms of bladder irritation or cause haematuria or retention. The surface may be ulcerated and covered with granulations which may make the histological diagnosis difficult in biopsy material.

Neurofibromas are uncommon. They are found in children as well as adults. The bladder may be the site of a solitary lesion but in many cases there is evidence of generalized neurofibromatosis. In the patients with generalized disease the bladder wall is either diffusely involved or contains localized, sometimes pedunculated, masses, usually in the region of the trigone or at the bladder neck. The lesion originates in the pelvic autonomic plexuses and is often extensive and apparently infiltrative, producing considerable thickening of the bladder wall. Sarcomatous change occurs in rare cases. Obstructive uropathy is one of the greatest dangers.

Angiomas occur in two forms. Tiny capillary lesions are sometimes seen in the lamina propria and occasionally cause haematuria. They are usually single and microscopically resemble the so-called senile haemangiomas of the skin (Campbell de Morgan spots). They have to be distinguished from the reparative granulomas which follow a previous biopsy. Much commoner, but still rare, are cavernous haemangiomas: they occur at any age but are seen more frequently in children than in adults. They may cause severe haemorrhage and occur more often as single lesions than multiple ones. They are found anywhere in the bladder though the trigone is usually spared. In about 20% of cases haemangiomas are also present on the external genitalia or elsewhere in the skin.

Malignant non-epithelial tumours

Lymphoma[152]

Though the bladder is a rare site of extranodal lymphoma, this is the second most common type of non-epithelial malignant neoplasm to occur in it, being outnumbered there only by tumours of muscle. Vesical lymphoma occurs at all ages, though middle-aged or elderly women are most commonly affected. An important clinical feature which may distinguish the lesion from invasive carcinoma is that back-pressure changes in the upper urinary tract are uncommon when a lymphomatous mass is situated near the ureteric orifice; a carcinoma in the same situation almost invariably causes upper tract obstruction.

Grossly the lesions may be single or multiple and characteristically they form smooth, solid, sometimes hemispherical, masses projecting into the bladder lumen and covered by a smooth layer of epithelium which sometimes shows areas of superficial ulceration.

Microscopically, the earliest changes, in contrast to those in an inflammatory lesion, are seen in the deeper layers of the lamina propria with later spread superficially towards the urothelial surface and deeply into the muscle coat. Perivesical spread is unusual. Circumferential infiltration of the walls of blood vessels is often seen and may assist in the differential diagnosis from carcinoma. Precise categorization, using one or other of the several classifications of malignant lymphoma, is not easy as the tumours are often of mixed type; many are of the centroblastic-centrocytic variety. A few cases of plasmacytoma have been recorded.

The prognosis is variable. In many patients who present with urological symptoms there is already evidence of widespread lymphomatous disease, but in a number of cases the lesion is confined to the bladder and responds to local irradiation or chemotherapy. It is sometimes argued that some at least of the latter group are examples of pseudolymphomas rather than true lymphomas – the use of immunocytochemistry should differentiate these two conditions. The two conditions most likely to be confused with lymphoma are severe chronic inflammation and anaplastic carcinoma.

Embryonic sarcoma[153]

This tumour has a potential field of origin from the mesenchyme at the bladder base, in the prostate and seminal vesicles, at the lower end of the ureters and the origin of the urethra and, in girls, in the vaginal vault. It is the commonest bladder tumour in children and occurs in boys more often than in girls, usually within the first 4 years of life.

The characteristic gross appearance is a pearly white rather translucent polypoid tumour (the 'grape-like sarcoma' or sarcoma botryoides) arising from a wide area of the base of the bladder. Subepithelial plaques of solid-looking tumour tissue often extend upwards towards the dome. Ureteric extension is not common but there is often involvement of the membranous urethra in boys and of the whole length of the urethra in girls. The epithelium overlying the tumour is either normal or thinned out, sometimes ulcerated or occasionally slightly thickened and hyperplastic.

Microscopically, the tumour usually occupies the full thickness of the lamina propria without any extension into the underlying bladder muscle. The neoplastic mesenchyme consists of small fusiform or stellate cells surrounded by an abundant, loose, mucinous type of stroma. Differentiation into striated muscle is found in many, but by no means all, tumours and all stages of rhabdomyoblast formation[154] may be seen, ranging from bulky round cells to more elongated or strap-like forms with abundant eosinophilic cytoplasm in which cross striations are present. The demonstration of cross-striations is not essential for the diagnosis of this highly malignant tumour, which should always be suspected when the typical stellate or fusiform cells are seen. The cells may have a single nucleus but many are multinucleated. Mitotic figures can usually be found. The use of histological markers will assist in distinguishing the tumour from the other small-cell tumours of childhood.[155]

Early diagnosis is imperative. The prognosis is not good though it has recently been improved by advances in radiotherapy and chemotherapy. Local spread to the regional lymph nodes usually occurs before distant metastases develop.

Other sarcomas

These include leiomyosarcomas, fibrosarcomas, fibroleiomyosarcomas and, very rarely, osteogenic sarcomas and chondrosarcomas. They occur at all ages and are most commonly seen in patients in the seventh decade; 80% of patients are over 50 years of age. Grossly the tumours are subepithelial in situation and form bulky, solid, pedunculated or sessile masses, often partly necrotic and usually with a variable amount of surface ulceration. In elderly patients the tumours are usually seen at the bladder base but in younger ones they are found more frequently in the region of the vault. Leiomyosarcomas, which are the commonest variety, sometimes have a rather gelatinous appearance on the cut surface. The better differentiated of them are distinguished from leiomyomas by the amount of nuclear pleomorphism and the finding of mitotic figures, though the dividing line is by no means always clear cut. The anaplastic forms cannot always be readily distinguished from the other types of sarcoma and are sometimes mimicked by poorly differentiated spindle cell carcinomas (see p. 727).

In the elderly patient in poor general condition it is often only an academic exercise to attempt to decide whether a tumour has originated in smooth muscle or is some other type of sarcoma. Because of their predominantly basal situation in the bladder and the almost inevitable urinary tract infection and obstructive uropathy the prognosis is uniformly bad. In younger patients the tumours are more often of a lower grade of malignancy and arise away from the bladder base and are therefore more amenable to wide local resection.

There have been a number of reports of spindle-celled pseudosarcomatous lesions, sometimes following surgery, that closely mimic sarcomas and that may be very difficult to differentiate from malignant tumours. Immunocytochemistry and electron microscopy will usually enable the correct diagnosis to be made.[156]

OTHER TUMOURS

Malignant melanoma

Both primary[157] and secondary[115] forms of malignant melanoma are among the rarest of bladder tumours.

REFERENCES

Development

1. Moffat DB. Development of the urogenital system in the male. In: Chisholm GD, Fair WR, eds. Scientific foundations of urology, 3rd edn. London: Heinemann, 1990; 231–242.

Abnormalities of development

2. Moffat DB. Developmental abnormalities of the urogenital system. In: Chisholm GD, Fair WR, eds. Scientific foundations of urology, 3rd edn. London: Heinemann, 1990; 242–256
3. Eble JN. Abnormalities of the urachus. In: Young RH, ed. Pathology of the urinary bladder. Edinburgh: Churchill Livingstone, 1989; 213–243.
4. Johnston JH. The exstrophic anomalies. In: Williams DI, Johnston JH, eds. Paediatric urology. London: Butterworth, 1982: 299–316.
5. Marshall VF, Muecke EC. Variations in exstrophy of the bladder. J Urol 1962; 88: 766–796.
6. Johnston JH, Poenn IA. Exstrophy of the cloaca. Br J Urol 1966; 38: 302–307.
7. O'Kane HOJ, Megaw J McI. Carcinoma of the exstrophic bladder. Br J Surg 1968; 55: 631–635.
8. Rudin L, Tannerbaum M, Lattimer JK. Histologic analysis of the exstrophied bladder after anatomical closure. J Urol 1972; 108: 802–807.

Trauma

9. Archbold JAA, Barros d'Sa AAB, Morrison E. Genitourinary tract injuries of civil hostilities. Br J Surg 1981; 68: 625–631.
10. Roberts M. Injuries of the lower urinary tract. In: Blandy JP, et al. Urology. Oxford: Blackwell Scientific, 1976; 954–962.
11. McConnell JD, Wilkerson MD, Peters PC. Rupture of the bladder. Urol Clin North Am 1982; 9: 292–296.
12. Carswel JW. Intraperitoneal rupture of the bladder. Br J Urol 1974; 46: 425–429.

Mechanism of micturition

13. Blaivas JG. Mechanism of micturition. In: Chisholm GD, Fair WR, eds. Scientific foundations of urology, 3rd edn. London: Heinemann, 1990; 273–286.
14. Thomas DG, Lucas MG. The urinary tract following spinal cord injury. In: Chisholm GD, Fair WR, eds. Scientific foundations of urology, 3rd edn. London: Heinemann, 1990; 286–299.

Bladder outflow obstruction

15. Gosling JA. The structure of the bladder and urethra in relation to function. Urol Clin North Am 1979; 6: 31–38.
16. Booth CM, Gosling JA. Histological and urodynamic study of the bladder in enuretic children. Br J Urol 1983; 55: 367–370.
17. Bodian M. Some observations on the pathology of congenital "idiopathic bladder neck obstruction" (Marion's disease). Br J Urol 1957; 29: 393–398.
18. Booth CM, Shah PJR, Milroy EJG, Thompson SA, Gosling JA. The structure of the bladder neck in male bladder neck obstruction. Br J Urol 1983; 55: 279–282.
19. Kirby RS, Fowler C, Gilpin SA, et al. Non-obstructive detrusor failure. A urodynamic, electromyographic, neurohistochemical and autonomic study. Br J Urol 1983; 55: 652–659.
20. Bates CP, Arnold EP, Griffiths DJ. The nature of the abnormality in bladder neck obstruction. Br J Urol 1975; 47: 651–656.
21. Johnston JH. Bladder disorders. In: Williams DI, Johnston JH, eds. Paediatric urology, 2nd edn. London: Butterworth, 1982; 227–237.
22. Eckstein HB, Williams DI. Neuropathic bladder. In: Williams DI, Johnston JH, eds. Paediatric urology, 2nd edn. London: Butterworth, 1982: 325–336.
23. Mundy AR, Shah PJR, Borzyskowski M, Saxton HM. Sphincter behaviour in myelomeningocele. Br J Urol 1985; 57: 647–651.
24. Tribe CR, Silver JR. Renal failure in paraplegia. London: Pitman, 1969.
25. Donelly J, Hackler RH, Bunts RC. Present urologic status of World War II paraplegics: 25 year follow-up. Comparison with status of the 20 year Korean war paraplegics and 5 year Vietnam paraplegics. J Urol 1972; 108: 558–562.
26. Webb DR, Fitzpatrick JM, O'Flynn JD. A 15 year follow-up of 406 consecutive spinal cord injuries. Br J Urol 1984; 56: 614–617.

Diverticula

27. Peterson LJ, Paulson DF, Glenn JF. The histopathology of vesical diverticula. J Urol 1973; 110: 62–64.
28. Fellows GJ. The association between vesical carcinoma and diverticulum of the bladder. Eur Urol 1978; 4: 185–18.

Fistulae

29. Slade N, Gaches C. Vesico-intestinal fistulae. Br J Surg 1972; 59: 593–597.

30. Pugh JI. On the pathology and behaviour of acquired non-traumatic vesico-intestinal fistula. Br J Surg 1964; 51: 644–657.

Calculous disease

31. Blacklock NJ. Urolithiasis: epidemiology. In: Chisholm GD, Fair WR, eds. Scientific foundations of urology, 3rd edn. London: Heinemann, 1990; 170–175.
32. Scott R. Epidemiology of stone disease. Br J Urol 1985; 57: 491–497.

Amyloidosis

33. Cohen AS, Connors LH. The pathogenesis and biochemistry of amyloidosis. J Pathol 1987; 151: 1–10.
34. Nurmi M J, Ekfors TO, Puntala PV. Secondary amyloidosis of the bladder: a cause of massive haematuria. J Urol 1987; 138: 44–45.
35. Fujihara S, Glenner GG. Primary localized amyloidosis of the genitourinary tract. Immunohistochemical study of eleven cases. Lab Invest 1981; 44: 45–60.
36. Thomas SD, Saunders PW, Pollack H. Primary amyloidosis of urinary bladder and ureter. Cause of mural calcification. Urology 1977; 9: 586–589.

Endometriosis

37. Shook TE, Nyberg LN. Endometriosis of the urinary tract. A review article. Urology 1988; 31: 1–6.
38. Pinkert TC, Catlow CE, Straus R. Endometriosis of the urinary bladder in a man with prostatic cancer. Cancer 1979; 43: 1562–1567.

Inflammatory conditions

39. O'Grady FO. Urinary tract infection. Initiation and ascent. In: Chisholm GD and Williams DI. eds. Scientific foundations of urology, 2nd edn. London. Heinemann. 1982; 199–204.
40. Elliott TSJ, Slack RCB, Bishop MC. Scanning electron microscopy of human bladder mucosa in acute and chronic urinary tract infection. Br J Urol 1984; 56: 38–43.
41. Maskell R. Urinary tract infection. London: Edward Arnold, 1982.
42. Asscher AW. Symptomless bacteriuria. In: Chisholm GD, Williams DI, eds. Scientific foundations of urology, 2nd edn. London: Heinemann, 1982; 184–191.
43. McClure J, Young RH. Infectious disease of the urinary bladder, including malacoplakia. In: Young RH, ed. Pathology of the urinary bladder. Edinburgh: Churchill Livingstone, 1989: 351–375.
44. Cook FV, Farrar E, Kreutner A. Hemorrhagic cystitis and ureteritis and interstitial nephritis associated with administration of penicillin G. J Urol 1979; 122: 110–111.
45. Rocca JM, McClure J. Cystitis emphysematosa. Br J Urol 1985; 57: 585.
46. West TE, Holley HP, Lauer AD. Emphysematous cystitis due to *Clostridium perfringens*. JAMA 1981; 246: 363–364.
47. Walpita P, Marsh FP. Do urethral *Escherichia coli* cause abacterial cystitis? J Clin Pathol 1983; 36: 224–227.
48. Stamey TA. Pathogenesis and treatment of urinary tract infection. Baltimore: Williams & Wilkins, 1980.
49. Packham DA. The epithelial lining of the female trigone and urethra. Br J Urol 1971; 43: 201–205.
50. Mufson MA, Belshe RB. A review of adenoviruses in the etiology of acute haemorrhagic cystitis. J Urol 1976; 115: 191–194.
51. Barrett JC. Gangrenous cystitis. Br J Urol 1962; 34: 312–317.
52. Walter S, Mogensen P, Jacobsen GK. Gangrenous cystitis: a case report. Scand J Urol Nephrol 1981; 15: 73–74.
53. Maggio AJ, Lupu A. Gangrene of the bladder. Urology 1981; 18: 390–391.
54. Khan AU, Stern JM, Posalaky Z. Vesical necrosis associated with acute bladder overdistension. Urology 1982; 19: 197–199.
55. Letcher HG, Matheson NM. Encrustation of the bladder as a result of alkaline cystitis. Br J Surg 1935; 23: 716–720.
56. Goldstein AG, d'Escrivan JC, Allen SD. Haemorrhagic radiation cystitis. Br J Urol 1968; 40: 475–478.
57. Wells HG. Giant cells in cystitis. Arch Pathol 1938; 26: 32.
58. Hunner CL. A rare type of bladder ulcer in women. Report of cases. Boston Med Surg J 1915; 72: 600.
59. Anonymous. Painful bladder diseases: interstitial or abacterial cystitis. Lancet 1988; 1: 337–338.
60. Larsen S, Thompson SA, Hald T, et al. Mast cells in interstitial cystitis. Br J Urol 1982; 54: 283–286.
61. Lynes WL, Flynn SD, Shortliffe LD, Stamey TA. The histology of interstitial cystitis. Am J Surg Pathol 1990; 14: 969–976.
62. Rosin RD, Griffiths T, Sofras F, James DCO, Edwards L. Interstitial cystitis. Br J Urol 1979; 51: 524–527.
63. Mattila J. Vascular immunopathology in interstitial cystitis. Clin Immunol Immunopathol 1982; 23: 648–658.
64. Galloway NTM. Gas gangrene of the bladder complicating cyclophosphamide cystitis. Br J Urol 1984; 56: 100–101.
65. Pearson RM, Soloway MS. Does cyclophosphamide induce bladder cancer? Urology 1978; XI: 437–447.
66. Ansel ID, Castro JE. Carcinoma of the bladder complicating cyclophosphamide therapy. Br J Urol 1975; 47: 413–418.
67. Hellstrom HR, Davis BK, Shonnard JW. Eosinophilic cystitis: a study of 16 cases. Am J Clin Pathol 1979; 72: 777–784.
68. Rubin L, Pincus MB. Eosinophilic cystitis: the relationship of allergy in the urinary tract to eosinophilic cystitis and the pathophysiology of eosinophilia. J Urol 1974; 112: 457–460.
69. Stanton MJ, Maxted W. Malacoplakia: a study of the literature and current concepts of pathogenesis, diagnosis and treatment. J Urol 1981; 125: 139–146.
69a. Michaelis L, Gutmann C. Ueber Einschlüsse in Blasentumoren. Z Klin Med 1902; 47: 208–215.
70. Feldman S, Levy LB, Prinz LM. Malakoplakia of the bladder causing bilateral ureteral obstruction. J Urol 1980; 123: 588–589.
71. Ansell ID. Granulomata in bladder and prostate after previous operations. J Clin Pathol 1984; 37: 104.
72. Cyr WL, Johnson H, Balfour J. Granulomatous cystitis as a manifestation of chronic granulomatous disease of childhood. J Urol 1973; 110: 357–359.
73. Laidlaw M. Renal tuberculosis. In: Chisholm GD, Fair WR, eds. Scientific foundations of urology, 3rd edn.

London: Heinemann. 1990; 148–152.
74. King DT, Lam M. Actinomycosis of the urinary bladder: association with an intra-uterine contraceptive device. JAMA 1978; 240: 1512–1513.
75. Zincke H, Furlow WL, Farrow GM. *Candida albicans* cystitis: report of a case with special emphasis on diagnosis and treatment. J Urol 1973; 109: 612–614.
76. Sakamota S, Ogata J, Sakazaki Y, Ikegami K. Fungus ball formation of aspergillus in the bladder. Eur Urol 1978; 4: 388–389.
77. Smith JH, Christie JD. Urinary schistosomiasis. In: Young RH, ed. Pathology of the urinary bladder. Edinburgh: Churchill Livingstone, 1989; 377–399.
78. Hicks RM, Walters Cl, Elsebai I, El-Asasser AB, El-Merzabani M, Gough PA. Demonstration of nitrosamines in human urine: preliminary observations on a possible aetiology for bladder cancer in association with chronic urinary tract infections. Proc R Soc Med 1977; 70: 713: 413–417.

Non-neoplastic proliferative and metaplastic mucosal lesions

79. Young RH. Non-neoplastic epithelial abnormalities and tumourlike lesions. In: Young RH, ed. Pathology of the urinary bladder. Edinburgh: Churchill Livingstone, 1989; 1–63.
80. Wiener DP, Koss LG, Sabla B, Freed SZ. The prevalence and significance of Brunn's nests, cystitis cystica and squamous metaplasia in normal bladders. J Urol 1979; 122: 317–321.
81. Murphy WM. Diseases of the urinary bladder, urethra, ureters and renal pelvis. In: Murphy WM, ed. Urological pathology. Philadelphia: WB Saunders, 1989; 34–146.
82. Bullock PS, Thori DE, Murphy WM. The significance of colonic mucosa (intestinal metaplasia) involving the urinary tract. Cancer 1987; 59: 2086–2090.
83. Stephenson TJ, Henry L, Harris Sc, Gini DD, Fox M, Underwood JCE. Pseudomembranous trigonitis of the bladder: hormonal aetiology. J Clin Pathol 1989; 42: 922–926.
84. Morgan RJ, Cameron KM. Vesical leukoplakia. Br J Urol 1980; 52: 96–100.
85. O'Flynn JD, Mullaney J. Vesical leukoplakia progressing to carcinoma. Br J Urol 1974; 46: 31–37.
86. Young RH. Papillary and polypoid cystitis. Am J Surg Pathol 1988; 12: 542–546.
87. Noble NM, Clarke T, Hammonds JC. Histological changes in the urinary bladder secondary to urethral catheterisation. Br J Urol 1989; 63: 354–357.
88. Friedmann NB, Kuhlenbeck H. Adenomatoid tumors of the bladder reproducing renal structures (nephrogenic adenomas). J Urol 1950; 64: 657–670.
89. Ford TF, Watson GM, Cameron KM. Adenomatous metaplasia (nephrogenic adenoma) of urothelium: an analysis of 70 cases. Br J Urol 1985; 57: 427–433.
90. Molland EA, Trott PA, Paris AMI, Blandy JP. Nephrogenic adenoma: a form of adenomatous metaplasia of the bladder. A clinical and electron microscopical study. Br J Urol 1976; 48: 453–462.

Neoplasms of the bladder

91. Skeet RG. Epidemiology of urogenital tumours. In: Chisholm GD, Fair WR, eds. Scientific foundations of urology, 3rd edn. London: Heinemann, 1990; 427–429.
92. Wallace DM. Occupational urothelial cancer. Br J Urol 1988; 61: 175–182.
93. Thompson IM, Fair WR. Occupational and environmental factors in bladder cancer. In: Chisholm GD, Fair WR, eds. Scientific foundations of urology, 3rd edn. London: Heinemann, 1990; 576–581.
94. The BAUS subcommittee on industrial bladder cancer. Occupational bladder cancer: a guide for clinicians. Br J Urol 1988; 61: 183–191.
95. Cole MP, Hoover R, Friedell GH. Occupation and cancer of the lower urinary tract. Cancer 1972; 29: 1250–1260.
96. Anthony H. Thomas GM. Tumors of the urinary bladder: an analysis of the occupation of 1300 patients in Leeds, England. J Natl Cancer Inst 1971; 45: 879–895.
97. Boyland E, Williams DC. Metabolism of tryptophan: metabolism of tryptophan in patients suffering from cancer of the bladder. Biochem J 1956; 64: 578–582.
98. Johansson S, Angervall L, Bengtsson U, Wahlqvist L. Uroepithelial tumors of the renal pelvis associated with the abuse of phenacetin-containing analgesics. Cancer 1974; 33: 743–753.
99. Johansson S, Wahlqvist L. Tumours of the urinary bladder and ureter associated with abuse of phenacetin-containing analgesics. Acta Pathol Microbiol Scand [A] 1977; 85: 768–774.
100. Lomax-Smith J, Symour AE. Unsuspected analgesic nephropathy in transitional cell carcinoma of the upper tract: a morphological study. Histopathology 1980; 4: 255–269.
101. Pamukcu AM, Govisoysus K, Price JM. Urinary bladder neoplasms induced by feeding bracken fern (*Pteris aquilina*) to cows. Cancer Res 1967; 27: 917.
102. Petkovic S, Mutavdzič, Petronic Vi, Markovič V. Les tumeurs du bassinet et de l'uretere. Recherches cliniques et étiologiques. J Urol Nephrol (Paris) 1971; 77: 429.
103. Silber SJ. Carcinoma in the bladder left behind. J Urol 1973; 110: 675–677.
104. Fellows GJ. The association between vesical carcinoma and urinary obstruction. Eur Urol 1978; 4: 187–188.
105. Hueper WC, Wiley FH, Wolfe HD. Experimental production of bladder tumors in dogs by administration of beta-naphthylamine. J Ind Hyg Toxicol 1938; 20: 46.
106. Hicks RM. Multistage carcinogenesis in the urinary bladder. Br Med Bull 1980: 36: 39–46.
107. Cohen SM, Arae M, Jacobs JB, Friedell GH. Promoting effect of saccharin and DL-tryptophan in urinary bladder carcinogenesis. Cancer Res 1979; 39: 1207–1215.
108. Wallace DMA. Development of bladder cancer. In: Chisholm GD, Fair WR, eds. Scientific foundations of urology, 3rd edn. London: Heinemann, 1990; 561–567.
109. Pugh RCB. The pathology of cancer of the bladder: an editorial overview. Cancer 1973; 32: 1267–1274.
110. Union Internationale contre le Cancer (UICC). Cancer incidence in five contients, vol. 2. Geneva: Springer, 1970.
111. Bergkvist A, Ljungqvist A, Moberger G. Classification

of bladder tumours based on the cellular pattern. Acta Chir Scand 1965; 130: 371.
112. Webb JN. Histopathology of bladder cancer. In: Chisholm GD, Fair WR, eds. Scientific foundations of urology, 3rd edn. London: Heinemann, 1990; 549–561.
113. Ooms ECM, Anderson WAD, Alons CL, Boon ME, Veldhuizen RW. Analysis of the performance of pathologists in the grading of bladder tumors. Hum Pathol 1983; 14: 140–143.
114. Mostofi FK, Sobin LH, Torloni H. WHO international histological classification of tumours – No. 10. Geneva: World Health Organization, 1973.
115. Koss LG. Tumors of the urinary bladder. Atlas of tumor pathology, 2nd series, fascicle 11. Washington, DC: Armed Forces Institute of Pathology, 1975.
116. Murphy WM. Atlas of bladder carcinoma. Chicago: American Society of Clinical Pathologists Press, 1986.
117. Friedell GH, Soloway MS, Milgar AG, Farrow GM. Summary of workshop on carcinoma in situ of bladder. J Urol 1986; 136: 1047–1048.
118. Highman WJ, Wilson E. Urinary cytology in patients with calculi. J Clin Pathol 1982; 35: 350–356.
118a. Pearson RM, Soloway MS. Does cyclophosphamide induce bladder cancer? Urology 1978; 11: 437–447.
119. Riddle PR, Chisholm GD, Trott PA, Pugh RCB. Flat carcinoma in situ of the bladder. Br J Urol 1975; 47: 829–833.
120. Gunter PA, de Abela-Borg J, Pugh RCB. Urothelium and the specific red cell adherence test. Br J Urol 1983, 55: 10–16.
121. Young RH, Wick MR, Wills SE. Sarcomatoid carcinoma of the urinary bladder. Am J Clin Pathol 1988; 90: 653–661.
122. Pang LSC. Bony and cartilaginous tumours of the urinary bladder. J Pathol Bacteriol 1958; 76: 357.
123. Walker AN, Mills SE, Young RH. Mesenchymal and miscellaneous other primary tumours of the bladder. In: Young RH, ed. Pathology of the urinary bladder. Edinburgh: Churchil Livingstone, 1985; 196–227.
124. Young RH, Wick MR. Transitional cell carcinoma of the urinary bladder with pseudosarcomatous stroma. Am J Clin Pathol 1988; 89: 216–219.
125. Young RH. Carcinosarcoma of the urinary bladder. Cancer 1987; 59: 1333–1339.
126. Young RH. Unusual variants of primary bladder carcinoma and secondary tumours of the bladder. In: Young RH, ed. Pathology of the urinary bladder. Edinburgh: Churchill Livingstone, 1989; 103–138.
127. Miller A, Mitchell JP. Brown NJ. The Bristol bladder tumour registry. Br J Urol 1969; 41: Suppl, 1–64.
128. Jewett HJ, Strong GH. Infiltrating carcinoma of the bladder. J Urol 1946; 55: 366–372.
129. UICC (Union Internationale contre le Cancer). In: Harmer MH, ed. TNM classification of malignant tumours, 3rd edn. Geneva: WHO, 1978.
130. Prout GR. Bladder carcinoma and a TNM system of classification. J Urol 1977; 117: 583–590.
131. Skinner DG. Current state of classification and staging of bladder cancer. Cancer Res 1977; 37: 2838–2842.
132. Chisholm GD, Hindmarsh JR, Howatson AG, Webb JN, Busuttil A, Hargreave TB, Newsam JE. TNM (1978) in bladder cancer: use and abuse. Br J Urol 1980; 52: 500–505.
133. Pryor JP. Factors influencing the survival of patients with transitional cell tumours of the urinary bladder. Br J Urol 1973; 45: 586–592.
134. Pugh RCB. Histological staging and grading of bladder tumours. In: Oliver RTD, Hendry WF, Bloom HJG, eds. Bladder cancer: principles of combination therapy. London: Butterworth, 1981.
135. Cameron KM, Lupton CH. Inverted papilloma of the lower urinary tract. Br J Urol 1976; 48: 567–577.
136. Kunze E, Schauer A, Schmitt M. Histology and histogenesis of two different types of inverted urothelial papillomas. Cancer 1983; 51: 348–358.
137. Highman WJ. Urinary cytology in inverted papilloma of the lower urinary tract. Acta Cytol 1978; 22: 335.
138. Nadji M, Tabel SZ, Castro A, et al. Prostatic specific antigen. An immunohistologic marker for prostatic neoplasms. Cancer 1981; 48: 1229–1232.
139. Heyderman E, Brown BME, Richardson TC. Epithelial markers in prostatic, bladder and colorectal cancer: an immunoperoxidase study of epithelial membrane antigen, carcinoembryonic antigen, and prostatic acid phosphatase. J Clin Pathol 1984; 37: 1363–1369.
140. Haid M, Ignatoff J, Khandekar JD, Graham J, Holland J. Urinary bladder metastases from breast carcinoma. Cancer 1980; 46: 229–232.
141. Herd ME, Williams G. Scanning electron microscopy of normal, neoplastic and inflamed human bladder. Histopathology 1984; 8: 601–610.
142. Newman J, Hicks RM. Detection of neoplastic and pre-neoplastic urothelia by combined scanning and transmission electron microscopy of the urinary surface of human and rat bladders. Histopathology 1977; 1: 125–136.
143. Tannenbaum M, Tannenbaum S, Romas NA. Conformational membrane changes in early bladder cancer. In: Connolly JG, ed. Carcinoma of the bladder. New York: Raven Press, 1981.
144. Raghaven D, Shipley WU, Garrick MB, Russel PJ, Richie JP. Biology and management of bladder cancer. N Engl J Med 1990; 322: 1129–1138.
145. Wick MR, Zarbo RJ, Hitchcock Cl. Special techniques for the pathological analysis of lesions of the urinary bladder. In: Young RH, ed. Pathology of the urinary bladder. Edinburgh: Churchill Livingstone, 1989; 285–350.
146. Weiss MA. Urinary cytology of transitional cell neoplasms of the urinary tract. In: Young RH, ed. Pathology of the urinary bladder. Edinburgh: Churchill Livingstone, 1989; 245–284.
147. Trott PA, Edwards LE. Comparison of bladder washings and urine cytology in the diagnosis of bladder cancer. J Urol 1973; 110: 664–66.
148. Trott PA. Detection of urethral carcinoma using a soluble swab. Br J Surg 1971; 58: 66–69.
149. Das S, Bulusu NV, Lowe P. Primary vesical pheochromocytoma. Urology 1983; 21: 20–25.
150. Zimmerman IJ, Biron RE, MacMahon HE. Pheochromocytoma of the urinary bladder. N Engl J Med 1953; 249: 25–26.
151. Higgins PM, Tresidder GC. Malignant pheochromocytoma of the urinary bladder. Br J Urol 1980; 52: 230.
152. Simpson RHW, Bridger JE, Anthony PP, James KA, Jury I. Malignant lymphoma of the lower urinary tract. A clinicopathological study with review of the literature. Br J Urol 1990; 62: 254–260.

153. Williams DI, Martin J. Tumours of the lower genito-urinary tract. In: Williams DI, Johnston HH, eds. Paediatric urology, 2nd edn. London: Butterworth, 1982; 411–422.
154. Horn RC, Enterline HT. Rhabdomyosarcoma: a clinicopathological study and classification of 39 cases. Cancer 1958; 11: 181.
155. Royds JA, Variend S, Timperley WRE, Taylor CB. Comparison of β-enolase and myoglobin as histological markers of rhabdomyosarcoma. J Clin Pathol 1985; 38: 1258–1260.
156. Hughes DF, Biggart JD, Hayes D. Pseudosarcomatous lesions of the urinary bladder. Histopathology: 1991: 18; 67–71.
157. Ironside WJ, Timperley WR, Madden JW, Royds JA, Taylor CB. Primary melanoma of the urinary bladder presenting with intracerebral metastases. Br J Urol 1985; 57: 593–594.

20

R. C. B. Pugh, revised by I. D. Ansell

The urethra

DEVELOPMENT

The male urethra is derived from the primitive urogenital sinus,[1] which is an endodermal structure that has become divided into an upper part, the vesicourethral canal (which develops into the bladder, see p. 695) and a more caudal portion, the definitive urogenital sinus, comprising a short pelvic part and a larger phallic portion which is flattened from side to side. Mesoderm from the primitive streak forms the genital tubercle and, more caudally, a pair of genital swellings, and medial to these, lying on either side of the urogenital sinus, is a pair of thin urethral folds. The phallic part of the sinus grows forwards on to the underside of the genital tubercle, which has now enlarged and forms the phallus, which has a ventral groove. This later becomes invaginated into the mesodermal core of the phallus by medial growth of the urethral folds which fuse to form the midline raphe. Urethral closure commences posteriorly and continues forward as far as the proximal part of the developing glans. The terminal portion of the urethra is formed in part by ectoderm and its development is linked with that of the preputial sac and the prepuce and the forward migration of the urinary meatus from just behind the glans to its tip.

The whole of the female urethra is developed from the vesicourethral canal.

ABNORMALITIES OF DEVELOPMENT

The congenital anomalies found in the lower urinary tract are often accompanied by abnormalities of the upper tract. That there may also sometimes be associated disorders of development of the gonads and alimentary system is hardly surprising in view of their common origin and close anatomical relationships.

ABNORMALITIES IN THE MALE[2,3]

Complete *atresia* is a rare anomaly usually affecting the membranous portion of the urethra and occurring in some cases of the 'prune belly' syndrome (see p. 683). *Ectopic urethral openings* may be seen at or below the level of the verumontanum (see p. 682) and *diverticula* occur in the posterior urethra just below the verumontanum or further forward in the region of the bulb or penoscrotal junction. *Utricular cysts* in the posterior urethra are thought to be persistent Müllerian duct structures. *Megalourethra* is an enormous dilatation of the penile urethra resulting from a defect of the cavernous tissues.

Urethral duplication occurs in two forms. In the commoner (sagittal) type the two channels lie one above the other; in the epispadiac variety the accessory urethra lies on the dorsum of the penis, which is curved upwards, whereas in the hypospadiac form one urethra opens in the normal position and the other is located on the underside of the phallus. The other main type (collateral duplication) is less common and usually associated with diphallus. Duplication is an error that occurs at a relatively early stage of development and is not uncommonly associated with other abnormalities such as absence of one kidney, tracheo-oesophageal fistula and imperforate anus.

Posterior urethral valves[4]

Posterior urethral valves, consisting of folds of mucosa on a fibrous tissue core, are the commonest abnormalities to cause obstruction of the lower urinary tract in the male infant. Three types are described: in the commonest type (type I)[5] a pair of mucosal folds runs downwards and outwards from the lower end of the verumontanum to meet in the midline anteriorly with a narrow slit-like urethra between them. The upward passage of an instrument is not obstructed in any way but during micturition the cusps come together and obstruct the outflow of urine. The posterior urethra dilates and the bladder hypertrophies, vesicoureteric reflux and hydronephrosis are common and the kidneys are frequently dysplastic. A type III valve[6] is an incomplete diaphragm in the region of the membranous urethra that causes some degree of obstruction to the passage both of instruments from below and of urine from above. Type II valves, comprising two folds that pass upwards from the upper end of the verumontanum, are now considered to be normal variants incapable of causing urinary obstruction.

Other causes of obstruction

Obstruction is occasionally caused by pedunculated *polyps* in the vicinity of the verumontanum or by *strictures,* sometimes of congenital origin, in the anterior or posterior parts of the urethra. Urinary tract anomalies are commonly found when there is agenesis of the terminal part of the bowel and an imperforate anus;[7] one or both kidneys may be absent or ectopic, and ureteric anomalies include duplication, megaureter, ureterocele and ectopia. The bladder may be exstrophic and the urethra sometimes contains valves or is hypospadiac. When the bowel lesion affects the rectum (rectal agenesis) there is almost always a rectourethral fistula which opens just below the verumontanum; with lower lesions (anal agenesis) there may be an anobulbar fistula.

Hypospadias

Hypospadias is a relatively common anomaly in which there is incomplete closure of the urethral groove, with the result that the urethra terminates at some point between the bulb and its normal position on the glans. The penis is bowed ventrally and the prepuce always has a characteristic 'hooded' appearance as it is deficient ventrally and overdeveloped dorsally and laterally. The site of the meatus may be glandular, coronal, penile, penoscrotal or in the perineum. In the glandular form the glans tends to be flattened and broadened; the meatus is often narrowed and stenotic, and a groove leads forwards on the underside of the glans from the urethral opening to its tip where there is a pit at the normal site of the meatus. Associated anomalies include undescended testis, testicular hypoplasia and abnormalities of the prostatic utricle.[8]

Epispadias

Epispadias (which is much less common than hypospadias) is an anomaly that rarely occurs alone and in its most severe form is frequently associated with vesical exstrophy (see p. 697). The penis is small, flattened from side to side and curved upwards; its underside is normal, with a midline raphe; the prepuce is usually incomplete. In a less severe form of defect (penopubic epispadias) a groove on the upper surface of the stunted penis leads into the bladder through a defect in the anterior abdominal wall. The least severe defects are the balanic and penile types of epispadias in which the urethral opening lies, respectively, on the glans (away from the usual site) or on the penile shaft.

ABNORMALITIES IN THE FEMALE[9]

Major abnormalities of the urethra are not at all common in the female and are usually seen only in association with defects in other systems. *Persistence of the urogenital sinus or cloaca* results in a common opening for the urinary, genital and alimentary tracts. Associated anomalies of the upper urinary tract, genitalia and bowel are often present and the urethra may either be absent altogether or unusually short and widened. In the condition of *female hypospadias* there is incomplete development of the posterior wall of the urethra which opens into the anterior vaginal wall at or within the introitus. The meatus is often stenosed. *Duplication* is a very rare anomaly, most often seen when there is duplication of the bladder. *Distal urethral obstruction*, which is said to cause difficulty in micturition and recurrent urinary tract infection, is a very controversial condition that has been ascribed to either sphincter spasm or the presence of a collagenous ring around the lower part of the urethra and the meatus.[10] There are, however, serious doubts as to both the existence of an organic obstruction and the concept of this as a pathological entity. *Ectopic ureteric openings* may be found in the lower urethra, vestibule or vagina (see p. 682).

TRAUMA[11]

Most of the urethral injuries seen in civilian practice occur as a result of major accidents or as a complication of open or transurethral surgical procedures, though self-instrumentation or the introduction of foreign bodies or of an abortifacient is occasionally responsible. Damage can also occur as a complication of prolonged labour, when compression of the urethra against the symphysis pubis by the fetal head produces ischaemic changes in its wall.

Rupture, more often partial than complete, is very much more common in males than in females and may occur when a fall astride a firm object or a kick in the perineum compresses the urethra against the symphysis pubis and crushes and lacerates the bulbar portion. If there is extensive pelvic trauma, for instance in a road accident, the anterior and posterior parts of the urethra may be torn away from each other by a shearing force with the triangular ligament acting as a fixed point. There is often a fracture-dislocation of the pelvis and damage to the bladder as well.

Extravasation is a serious complication of rupture and its extent will depend on whether the lesion is in the anterior urethra in front of the triangular ligament or affects the posterior urethra (the membranous or prostatic portions). When the anterior urethra is ruptured the external sphincter at first remains closed and the bladder distends. Extravasation follows later and urine will collect in the superficial tissues of the anterior abdominal wall, scrotum and penis and the anterior part of the perineum, but fascial attachments will prevent extension into the thigh. With rupture of the membranous or prostatic urethra extravasation occurs early as the bladder is usually displaced backwards because the puboprostatic ligaments have been torn through, allowing urine to escape into the extraperitoneal tissues in the pelvis and abdominal wall. Later complications include stricture formation, which may not develop for several years after the traumatic incident, and, in the male, sterility (in up to 30–60% of patients) or impotence.

Penetrating wounds, especially those caused by high velocity missiles,[12] are liable to cause severe, and often multiple, injuries. The anterior part of the urethra is more commonly involved than the posterior parts and injuries to the bladder, penis, scrotum and bowel are to be expected in most cases.

URETHRAL STRICTURE[13]

Although strictures of the urethra are sometimes the result of congenital maldevelopment most are the outcome of local trauma or are a complication of acute or chronic inflammatory disease or of a urethral tumour. Two types or stages of stricture formation are usually recognized, the 'soft' type and the 'hard' type. In the 'soft' type the mucosal surfaces, abraded by an instrument or foreign body, or involved in an inflammatory process, adhere to each other because of a local fibrinous exudate. In the 'hard' variety there is involvement of the underlying corpus spongiosum, leading to fibrosis there, probably as a result of local urinary extravasation: the urethra becomes shortened, rigid, inelastic and white, and its lumen becomes narrowed.[14]

Stricture formation is an uncommon complication of acute urethritis treated by modern methods[15] and occurs in only about 4% of patients with non-specific urethritis. However, it is by no means rare in neglected cases or after inadequate or injudicious treatment, and many such cases are seen in the less well developed parts of the world. Chronic inflammatory disease, such as tuberculosis, syphilis, lymphogranuloma inguinale and the late fibrotic phase of schistosomiasis, is sometimes responsible. Balanitis xerotica obliterans[16] is present in some cases of stricture but it is uncertain whether this is cause or effect. Strictures sometimes develop as a late complication of urethral catheterization (see p. 745).

After closed injury to the bulb a short stricture is likely whereas after injury to the membranous urethra, such as might occur when there is a fractured pelvis, there may be either a short sinuous channel between the prostatic urethra and the sphincters or a long gap filled by a mass of scar tissue. Strictures sometimes complicate prostatectomy and occur either in the penile urethra after perurethral resection or at the site of division of the urethra after open operations. Strictures may be complicated by extravasation of urine into the scrotum or around the urethra itself, or by a periurethral abscess which in turn may be followed by the development of a fistula. The classic 'watering-can perineum' results from the formation of multiple fistulae. Some patients with a urethral stricture develop urethral carcinoma (see p. 748). Any significant amount of stricturing, particularly if allowed to go untreated, is liable to be complicated by urinary tract infection.

DIVERTICULA AND CYSTS

In the male, diverticula may complicate surgical repair of a rectourethral fistula in cases of high imperforate anus or develop proximal to a stricture at the site of urethral trauma. Calculi sometimes develop within the diverticular lumen and infection is not uncommon. Cystic dilatation of the paraurethral glands as a result of blockage of their ducts by inflammatory exudate is a not uncommon complication of gonoccocal urethritis. Congenital cysts may arise in the utricle.

Diverticula of the female urethra are found in the posterior wall, usually in parous women, and it is uncertain whether they are congenital in origin (possibly representing the lower end of the Wolffian duct) or arise because of inflammation of the paraurethral glands. Large stones sometimes develop in the lumen, and occasionally a tumour is found within a diverticulum.

URETHRAL FISTULAE

Congenital rectourethral fistulae are seen in patients with imperforate anus (see above), and fistulae may complicate calculous disease and virtually any traumatic, inflammatory, cystic or neoplastic lesion of the urethra. Fistula formation is very much commoner in the male than in the female: the tracks are commonly tortuous and the openings, sometimes single but often multiple, are found on the skin of the penis, scrotum or perineum or in the vagina.

URETHRAL CALCULI

Most of the calculi entering the urethra from the bladder are small enough to be passed in the urine though their passage along the urethra is usually far from painless. Impaction of larger calculi, seen more often in males than females, is likely to occur at the site of a stricture or, in the male, in those areas (the prostatic urethra, bulb or fossa navicularis) where there is a natural relative narrowing of the calibre of the urethra. Partial or complete obstruction will occur and urethritis and periurethritis, sometimes with abscess formation, are likely. Fibrous scarring can follow. Fistulae sometimes develop as an even later complication. Continued surface deposition of phosphates sometimes causes a stone to enlarge so that eventually a cast of the urethral lumen forms. Foreign bodies introduced into the urethra can form the nucleus of a calculus and these, too, may eventually enlarge to form a luminal cast. Primary stone formation, due to stagnation of infected urine, is liable to occur in the lumen of any cyst or diverticulum and very large stones are sometimes found within urethral diverticula in women.

AMYLOIDOSIS

Primary localized amyloidosis of the urethra is a rare disorder which to date has been reported only in the male. The patients are usually middle-aged or elderly and complain of haematuria or retention of urine, and sometimes have a previous history of gonorrhoea. The anterior part of the urethra is involved more often than the posterior parts; clinically the lesions may be mistaken for carcinoma.[17]

URETHRAL CARUNCLE

The caruncle is a fleshy nodule up to about 1 cm in maximum size situated in the distal part of the urethra of women. The patients usually are over 40 years of age. The nodule protrudes from the urethra and is often exquisitely painful and may bleed; there is often a degree of urethral prolapse. Essentially the lesion consists of a core of connective tissue covered on its surface by transitional or squamous epithelium; glands are sometimes present. A number of histological 'types' are described but the subdivisions are not particularly important and lack specific diagnostic criteria. The *papillomatous* from is characterized by marked proliferation of the surface epithelium which, if glandular, has been designated *adenomatous*; the *granulomatous* variety has an inflamed central core of granulation tissue. In the *angiomatous* type there are many, sometimes quite large, vascular spaces within the core. The cause of caruncle formation is not known but the lesions are not thought to be either neoplastic or preneoplastic and probably result from local trauma and inflammation. Excision and careful histological examination is recommended as occasionally a neoplasm of the urethra may present at the meatus as a nodule which clinically resembles a caruncle.[18]

INFLAMMATORY CONDITIONS

The crucial role of the urethra in the initiation of infection in the bladder and upper urinary tract is considered on pages 705–707 and at this point it is necessary only to indicate again some of the factors that predispose to these infections. By far the most important is any operative procedure on the lower tract, especially when performed to relieve obstruction and accompanied or preceded by stasis and stagnation of urine necessitating the passage of catheters or other instruments. Other forms of urethral trauma, for example caused by foreign bodies or chemicals, are no less important. Recent studies of catheter-induced urethritis have shown that the material of which the catheter is made is often a critical factor, and that latex is very much more harmful to the tissues than materials such as silicone.[19] Stricture formation is a well-recognized complication of urethral catheterization (see opposite).

Urethritis occuring after sexual intercourse can be caused by a wide variety of bacteria, mycoplasmas, viruses, protozoa and fungi but for practical purposes the infections fall readily into two groups – the *gonococcal* and the *non-gonococcal*, the latter encompassing all the other infections.[20] It must be appreciated, though, that mixed infections are very common indeed. There has been a steady rise in the number of patients with sexually transmitted diseases attending departments of genitourinary medicine in England and Wales within the last 30 or so years and significantly many more of these patients are in the younger age groups than heretofore.

The reasons for these trends are complex and probably relate to the appearance of drug-resistant strains of some of the responsible organisms, notably the gonococcus, and to the changes in the social and sexual mores in the population.

GONOCOCCAL URETHRITIS

Between 2 and 5 days after infection by *Neisseria gonorrhoeae* the patient notices a urethral discharge which, initially mucoid, soon becomes purulent. The organisms attach themselves to the epithelial surface of the urethra and multiply there, as well as in the ducts and crypts of the paraurethral glands, causing inflammatory changes with heavy local accumulations of neutrophil granulocytes. The urethral mucosa may ulcerate and abscesses sometimes form in the glands or their ducts. In an uncomplicated case in the *male* the infection is confined to the structures distal to the triangular ligament, but if the posterior urethra becomes involved prostatitis, seminal vesiculitis and unilateral or bilateral epididymitis are likely to ensue. In most patients direct microscopy of a specimen of urethral discharge will reveal the characteristic Gram-negative intracellular diplococci but in about 10% of cases microbiological confirmation of the diagnosis is possible only after culture on selective media. Special laboratory procedures such as sugar fermentation and immunofluorescence are sometimes required to distinguish *N. gonorrhoeae* from other neisseriae.

In the *female* the infection involves the endocervix as well as the urethra. Direct microscopy of any vaginal discharge or of smears from the urethra and cervix is never a reliable means of diagnosis and culture of urethral and cervical swabs is essential and often has to be repeated before the organisms can be isolated. Bartholinitis or a Bartholin's abscess sometimes occurs as a local complication. The acute inflammation will usually resolve entirely without complication when treatment is prompt and adequate. Failure to respond may be because the organism is of a drug-resistant strain or, as happens fairly frequently, because the patient is reinfected.

Chronic gonococcal infection in men, or acute infection complicated by severe inflammation or abscess formation in the paraurethral glands, is sometimes followed by a urethral stricture (see p. 744). Pelvic inflammatory disease is the most serious sequela in women and occurs in about 10% of female patients: this condition is difficult to diagnose and treat satisfactorily and is often responsible for long-term morbidity, especially in patients living in poor communities.

Dissemination of gonococcal infection is rare and occurs more often in women than in men, causing tenosynovitis, joint pains (in the wrists, knees, elbows, ankles and hands), skin lesions and occasionally endocarditis or myocarditis. These complications may also be a manifestation of an immune response to the gonococcus.

NON-GONOCOCCAL URETHRITIS

Non-gonococcal urethritis encompasses all the infections of the urethra other than infection by *Neisseria gonorrhoeae*. By definition, the term includes not only cases infected during sexual intercourse but also those in which the changes in the urethra are part of a more generalized urinary tract infection, such as cystitis or pyelonephritis, produced by coliforms or proteus organisms. The infections may either be '*specific*', when the causal agent can be identified or, less commonly, '*non-specific*', when no such cause is recognized and the aetiology remains uncertain or unknown. In the specific group, which accounts for 75% of the cases attending some genitourinary clinics, *Chlamydia trachomatis* is the organism most often transmitted during sexual intercourse, though venereal infection with *Ureaplasma urealyticum, Trichomonas vaginalis, Candida albicans* or herpes simplex virus type 2 is not uncommon. The cases are usually divided into chlamydia-positive and chlamydia-negative types as the two groups respond differently to treatment. Non-specific urethritis is always sexually transmitted.

Chlamydial urethritis has an incubation period of 7–14 days. A purulent urethral discharge develops but the diagnosis is difficult and depends on serological investigations and culture of the organism (and not on its demonstration in the discharge, as in gonococcal urethritis in the male). In the female the organisms cause urethritis and endocervicitis. Male patients often present with epididymitis or prostatitis and their consorts may be found to have an asymptomatic infection.[21] The immediate complications are not unlike those seen in gonococcal infections: prostatitis, seminal vesiculitis and epididymitis in men and pelvic inflammatory disease in women; disseminated metastatic lesions, such as are seen occasionally in gonorrhoea, are not encountered. Chlamydial infections may be very persistent and difficult to eradicate.

Reiter's disease occurs in rare cases of non-gonococcal urethritis, more often in men than in women, and is characterized by urethritis, seronegative arthropathy (affecting the knees, ankles and feet), conjunctivitis and occasionally lesions of the mucous membranes, skin and nails.

The protozoon *Trichomonas vaginalis* is a common cause of sexually transmitted vaginitis, urethritis and cervicitis and usually produces a copious vaginal discharge. In males there may be a subacute or chronic urethritis. Infection with the fungus *Candida albicans* causes vulvovaginitis in women and balanitis and occasionally urethritis in their sexual partners.

Herpes genitalis, due to infection with herpes simplex virus type 2, is a disease very much on the increase; it has assumed almost epidemic proportions in some parts of the world. The lesions are initially vesicular but soon ulcerate. They are usually multiple and often very painful and they occur in the urethra and on the skin of the thighs in both sexes, sometimes with enlargement of the regional lymph nodes. In men the skin of the penis and scrotum may be involved and in women lesions occur on the cervix and external genitalia. The condition does not respond well to treatment and recurrent infections are common. Other sexually transmitted diseases are often present at the same time and it is particularly important to exclude syphilis by dark ground microscopy and appropriate serological tests.

Syphilitic urethritis is not common and is seen either in the primary stage of the disease, when a chancre develops in the terminal part of the urethra, or in the secondary stage when mucous patches are found. *Tuberculous urethritis* is also uncommon and occurs more often in males than females. The lesions develop either when tubercle bacilli are being passed in the urine from a focus in the bladder, ureters or kidneys, or by direct extension of the disease from the bladder or prostate. With modern therapy the urethral lesions usually heal completely though in very rare instances there is a residual stricture.[22]

Malakoplakia affects the urethra in very rare instances (see p. 711) and may cause obstructive symptoms.[23] Involvement of the lower genitourinary tract in *Wegener's granulomatosis* is very unusual, though a necrotizing type of urethritis with protrusion of a tumour-like mass into the urethral lumen has been recorded.[24]

The ova of *Schistosoma haematobium* are sometimes deposited in the wall of the urethra and in the male there is a particular liability to involvement of the prostatic urethra.[25] Granulomas similar to those seen in the bladder (see p. 713) develop; fibrous scarring in the later stages of healing may result in stricture formation, sometimes involving a considerable length of the urethra.

TUMOURS OF THE URETHRA

Malignant tumours, the majority occurring as part of a widespread multifocal urothelial neoplasia, far outnumber benign neoplasms. The latter will be considered first.

BENIGN TUMOURS AND TUMOUR-LIKE CONDITIONS

Condylomata acuminata (venereal warts) are the commonest benign tumour-like lesions of the urethra. They are caused by a papilloma virus belonging to the papovavirus group. They are nearly always transmitted by sexual contact and often coexist with other sexually transmitted diseases.

Lesions occur on the external genitalia in both sexes and sometimes also involve the perineum, anus and rectum. In males the external meatus is often involved and in rare cases typical lesions occur along the length of the urethra, occasionally extending to involve the bladder.[26] After an incubation period of about 3 months the characteristic painless, sharply demarcated, soft, friable, cauliflower-like papillae appear, sometimes singly but often at multiple sites. Microscopically, the appearances are those of a squamous papilloma with enlargement and elongation of the rete pegs, which typically extend evenly into the underlying tissue, to the same level and often to a considerable depth. They must be distinguished from the condyloma latum of secondary syphilis which has the typical endothelial hyperplasia and numerous plasma cells typical of this infection.

Fibroepithelial polyps similar in structure to those seen in the ureter (see p. 688) are rare lesions, occurring in young boys either in the region of the verumontanum[27] or in the anterior urethra.[28] They are probably not true neoplasms and are possibly of congenital origin. Polyps of prostatic origin are more frequent than generally thought;[29] they may be covered by prostatic columnar epithelium,[30] on occasions giving the appearance of a papillary adenoma[31] – these lesions must be distinguished from true clear cell carcinomas (see p. 729).

Non-epithelial benign tumours are extremely rare and include haemangiomas[32] and fibromas, both of which are more often seen in males, and leiomyomas, which are commoner in females.

MALIGNANT TUMOURS

Primary carcinoma

Primary carcinoma of the urethra unaccompanied by neoplasm in the upper urinary tract or bladder and with no history of such a tumour is rare in the UK. It is seen more often in women than in men.[33] A past history of gonorrhoea, urethral stricture or trauma (for instance, by repeated instrumentation) is common in male patients. The tumour sometimes develops after urethroplasty.[34] Most of the patients, both men and women, are in the sixth or seventh decades and complain of obstruction, haematuria, urinary tract infection, frequency or dysuria. There may be a palpable mass or even a fistula and the disease is often in an advanced state and inoperable when the patient is first seen. The tumours are polypoid, sessile or infiltrative or become ulcerated. The majority are squamous carcinomas[35] but approximately 15% are transitional cell carcinomas, and a few are adenocarcinomas. Some are so poorly differentiated that they cannot be categorized.

In men the tumour usually occurs in the bulb or bulbomembranous region. The anterior part of the urethra is less often the site.[36] This has an important bearing on prognosis: anterior urethral tumours tend to spread to the inguinal lymph nodes and therefore are likely to be recognized earlier and to be more amenable to surgery than the posterior ones. Carcinomas of the posterior part of the urethra present later and frequently metastasize to the external iliac and other intra-abdominal lymph nodes. Local spread of the tumour with extension into the corpora and periurethral tissues is common and tumours in the region of the bulb may invade the deep structures of the perineum, sometimes forming a fistula. It may be difficult to decide whether a papillary adenocarcinoma in the prostatic urethra arises from the periurethral glands or the prostatic ducts or from Wolffian or Müllerian remnants.[37]

In women[38] the tumour frequently involves the entire length of the urethra; in some reported series there are equal numbers in the anterior urethra (the distal third) and posterior urethra (the proximal two-thirds). The prognosis, especially of posterior urethral tumours, is not good as the lymphatic drainage is into the intraperitoneal nodes, as in cases of posterior urethral carcinoma in men. There may also be quite extensive local spread to involve the vaginal wall. The location of a tumour and its stage (the extent of its local spread) are more important as prognostic guides than the histological appearances.

Adenocarcinomas account for some 10% of primary urethral tumours in women; they may arise from periurethral glands or in rare instances within a diverticulum.[39] There are records of a few cases of a clear-cell adenocarcinoma with a tubulocystic pattern which it is suggested may be of mesonephric origin; well-differentiated examples must be distinguished form nephrogenic adenoma[40] (see p. 718).

Urethral involvement in multifocal urothelial carcinoma.

Most of the malignant tumours seen in the urethra occur in patients who concurrently have a urothelial tumour higher up in the urinary tract or who have a past history of such a tumour (Fig. 20.1). The possible causes of multiplicity of urothelial tumours have been considered on page 719. The finding of a tumour in the isolated urethra following simple cystectomy (see p. 719) has been reported in from 4 to 18%[41] of patients; in-situ carcinoma of the urethral mucosa has been found in 19% of cystectomy patients, occurring twice as often in cases of multiple papillary bladder tumours as in those with a single tumour or with a solid (non-papillary) tumour.[42] In some patients the neoplastic changes develop in the periurethral glands rather than in the urethral mucosa itself and this may make diagnosis by biopsy or cytological examination difficult. The frequency of urethral involvement in cases of bladder tumour and the length of time that may elapse before the urethral tumours develop, the problems of accurate histological and cytological diagnosis after simple cystectomy, and the practical difficulties of dealing adequately at a second operation with any tumour at the proximal end of the urethra in the region of the prostate or of the apex of the bladder have prompted many surgeons[43] to abandon simple cystectomy in favour of a one-stage en-bloc removal of the bladder, prostate and urethra in the male, and the bladder, urethra, uterus, tubes and ovaries in the female. This radical approach has been challenged by other surgeons[44] who suggest that careful monitoring of the cytology of the anterior part of the urethra may obviate the need for such extensive procedures.

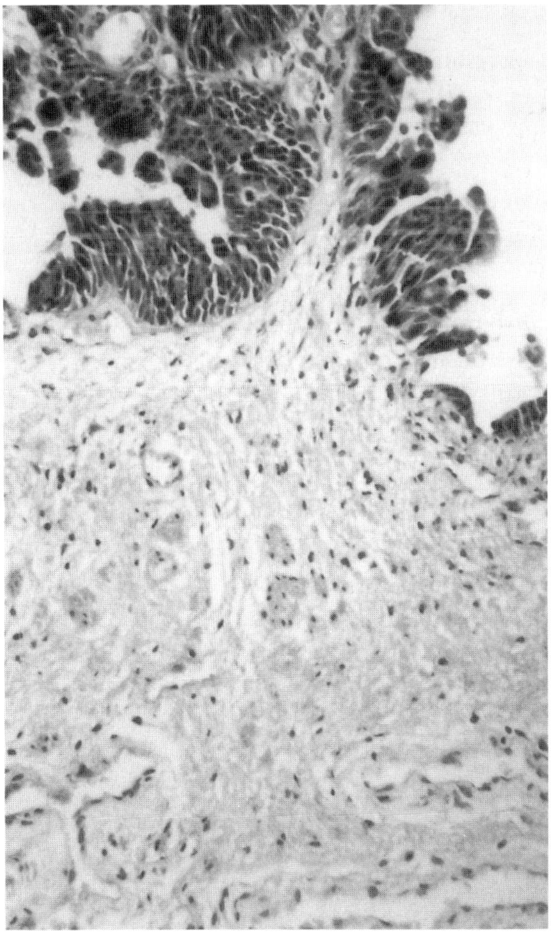

Fig. 20.1 Urothelial carcinoma of penile urethra. Papillary carcinoma in urethrectomy specimen removed at time of total cystectomy. Note vascular spaces of erectile tissue at base of photomicrograph. Haematoxylin–eosin × 185.

Melanoma

Primary melanoma of the urethra is a very rare tumour; it is seen most often in men in their late fifties and in women in their mid-sixties. The prognosis in both sexes is uniformly bad, with early recurrence and widespread metastasis. Many of the patients die within months and few survive more than 2 years. In men the tumour is more often single than multiple: three-quarters occur in the anterior part of the urethra and about half are found at the meatus (sometimes also with a lesion on the glans) or in the fossa navicularis.[45] In women most of the tumours occur near the meatus or in the anterior part of the urethra.[46] The urethra is occasionally the site of secondary deposits in patients with melanomatosis originating elsewhere in the body.

Primary connective tissue tumours

These are extremely rare. The embryonic sarcoma (rhabdomyosarcoma) of childhood may extend from the bladder into the proximal part of the urethra as a part of the 'field of origin' of this tumour (see p. 735).

Secondary tumours

Secondary tumours, other than those associated with urothelial carcinoma (see p. 749) or due to direct spread from adjacent organs such as the prostate, cervix or uterus, are very uncommon. They have included plasmacytoma,[47] and a leiomyosarcoma from a vesical primary.[48]

REFERENCES

Development

1. Moffat DB. Development of the urogenital system in the male. In: Chisholm GD, Fair WR, eds. Scientific foundations of urology, 3rd edn. London: Heinemann, 1990; 231–242.

Abnormalities of development

2. Moffat DB. Developmental abnormalities of the urogenital system. In: Chisholm GD, Fair WR, eds. Scientific foundations of urology, 3rd edn. London: Heinemann, 1990; 242–256.
3. Williams DI. Male urethral anomalies. In:Williams DI, Johnston JH, eds. Paediatric urology, 2nd edn. London: Butterworth, 1982; 239–250.
4. Williams DI. Male urethral obstruction. In:Williams DI, Johnston JH, eds. Paediatric urology, 2nd edn. London: Butterworth, 1982; 251–270.
5. Young HH, Frontz WA, Baldwin JC. Congenital obstruction of the posterior urethra. J Urol 1919; 3: 289.
6. Robertson WB, Hayes JA. Congenital diaphragmatic obstruction of the male posterior urethra. Br J Urol 1969; 41: 592–598.
7. Williams DI. Urinary tract complications of imperforate anus. In: Williams DI, Johnston JH, eds. Paediatric urology, 2nd edn. London: Butterworth, 1982; 271–278.
8. Shima H, Ikoma, F, Terakawa T, et al. Developmental anomalies associated with hypospadias. J Urol 1979; 122: 619–621.
9. Williams DI. Female urethral anomalies and obstructions. In: Williams DI, Johnston JH, eds. Paediatric urology, 2nd edn. London: Butterworth, 1982; 279–288.
10. Lyon NP, Smith DR. Distal urethral stenosis. J Urol 1963; 89: 414–421.

Trauma

11. Roberts M. Injuries of the lower urinary tract. In: Blandy JP, ed. Urology. Oxford:Blackwell Scientific, 1976; 954–962.
12. Archbold JAA, Barros d'SA AAB, Morrison E. Genitourinary tract injuries of civil hostilities. Br J Surg 1981; 68: 625–631.

Urethral stricture

13. Blandy JP. Urethral stricture and carcinoma. In: Blandy JP, ed. Urology. Oxford: Blackwell Scientific, 1976; 1014–1048.
14. Beard DE, Goodyear WE. Urethral stricture: a pathological study. J Urol 1948; 59: 619.
15. Dunlop EMC. Incidence in the male of stricture after urethritis. Br J Vener Dis 1961; 37: 64.
16. Bainbridge DR, Whitaker, RH, Shepheard BGF. Balanitis xerotica obliterans and urinary obstruction. Br J Urol 1971; 43: 487–491.

Amyloidosis

17. Vaudevan P, Stein AM, Pinn VW, Rao C. Primary amyloidosis of the urethra. Urology 1981; 17: 181.

Urethral caruncle

18. Marshall FC, Uson AC, Melicow MM. Neoplasms and caruncles of the female urethra. Surg Gynecol Obstet 1960; 110 723–733.

Inflammatory conditions

19. Nacey JN, Tulloch AGS, Ferguson AF. Catheter-induced urethritis: a comparison between latex and silicone catheters in a prospective clinical trial. Br J Urol 1985; 57: 325–328.
20. Hooton TM, Kreiger JN. Sexually transmitted disease. In Chisholm GD, Fair WR, eds. Scientific foundations of urology. London: Heinemann, 1990; 157–169.
21. Grant JBF, Brooman PJC, Chowdhure SD, Seueira P, Blacklock NJ. The clinical presentation of *Chlamydia trachomatis* in a urological practice. Br J Urol 1985; 57: 218–221.
22. Gow JG. Genito-urinary tuberculosis. In: Blandy JP, ed. Urology. Oxford: Blackwell Scientific 1976; 226–260.
23. Sharm TC, Kagan HN, Sheils JP. Malacoplakia of the male urethra. J Urol 1981; 125: 885–886.
24. Jensen KM-E, Neilsen KK, Kock K. Necrotising urethritis in Wegener's granulomatosis. Br J Urol 1982; 54: 434.
25. Zaher MF, El Deeb AA. Bilharzial urethritis cystica. J Urol 1969; 101: 870–873.

Tumours of the urethra

26. Bissada NK, Cole AT, Fried FA. Extensive condyloma acuminata of entire male urethra and bladder. J Urol 1974; 112: 201–203.
27. Williams DI, Abbasian A. Solitary pedunculated polyp of the posterior urethra in children. J Urol 1966; 96: 483.

28. Foster RS, Weigel JW, Mantz FA. Anterior urethral polyps. J Urol 1980; 124: 145–146.
29. Goldstein AMB, Bragin SD, Terry R, Yoell JH. Prostatic urethral polyps in adults: histopathologic variations and clinical manifestations. J Urol 1981; 129–131.
30. Chan JKC, Chow TC, Tsue MS. Prostatic-type polyps of the lower urinary tract: three histogenic types. Histopathology 1987; 11: 789–801.
31. Murad TM, Robinson LH, Beuschen AJ. Villous polyps of the urethra: a report of two cases. Hum Pathol 1979; 10: 478–481.
32. Sharm SK, Reddy MJ, Joshi VV, Bapha BC. Capillary haemangioma of male urethra. Br J Urol 1981;53:277.
33. Grabstald H. Tumors of the urethra in men and women. Cancer 1973; 32: 1236–1255.
34. Kirkman NF. Urethral carcinoma following urethroplasty. Br J Surg 1961; 48: 508.
35. Levine RL. Urethral cancer. Cancer 1980; 45: 1965–1972.
36. Hopkins SC, Nag SK, Soloway MS. Primary carcinoma of male urethra. Urology 1984; 23: 128.
37. Cantrell BB, Leifer G, de Klerk DP, Eggleston JC. Papillary adenocarcinoma of the prostatic urethra with clear-cell appearance. Cancer 1981; 48: 2661–2667.
38. Johnson DE, O'Connel JR. Primary carcinoma of female urethra. Urology 1983; 21: 42.
39. Reheis JP. Goldstein IS, Mogil RA. Papillary adenocarcinoma arising in a urethral diverticulum accompanied by adenocarcinoma of the bladder: case report and review of the literature. J Urol 1981; 126: 695–697.
40. Young RH, Scully RE. Clear cell adenocarcinoma of the bladder and urethra. Am J Surg Pathol 1985; 9: 816–826.
41. Schellhamer PF, Whitmore WF. Transitional cell carcinoma of the urethra in men having cystectomy for bladder cancer. J Urol 1976; 115: 56–60.
42. Hendry WF, Gowing NFC, Wallace DM. Surgical treatment of urethral tumours associated with bladder cancer. Proc R Soc Med 1974; 67: 304–306.
43. Wallace DM. Carcinoma of the urothelium. In:Blandy JP, ed. Urology. Oxford. Blackwell Scientific, 1976; 774–806.
44. Skinner DG, Crawford ED, Kaufmann JJ. Complications of radical cystectomy for carcinoma of the bladder. J Urol 1980; 123: 640–643.
45. Weiss J, Elder D, Hamilton R. Melanoma of the male urethra: surgical approach and pathological analysis. J Urol 1982; 128: 382–385.
46. Katz JI, Grabstald H. Primary malignant melanoma of the female urethra. J Urol 1976; 116: 454–457.
47. Campbell CM, Smith JA, Middleton RG. Plasmacytoma of the urethra. J Urol 1982; 127: 986.
48. Alabaster AM, Jordan WP, Soloway MS, Shippel RM, Young RM. Leiomyosarcoma of the bladder and subsequent urethral recurrence. J Urol 1981; 125: 583–585.

Index